# Revision Spine Surgery

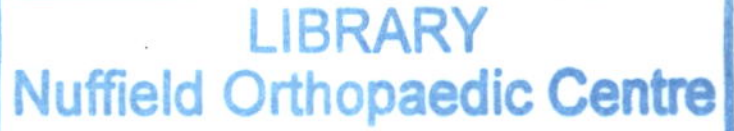
LIBRARY
Nuffield Orthopaedic Centre

WITHDRAWN



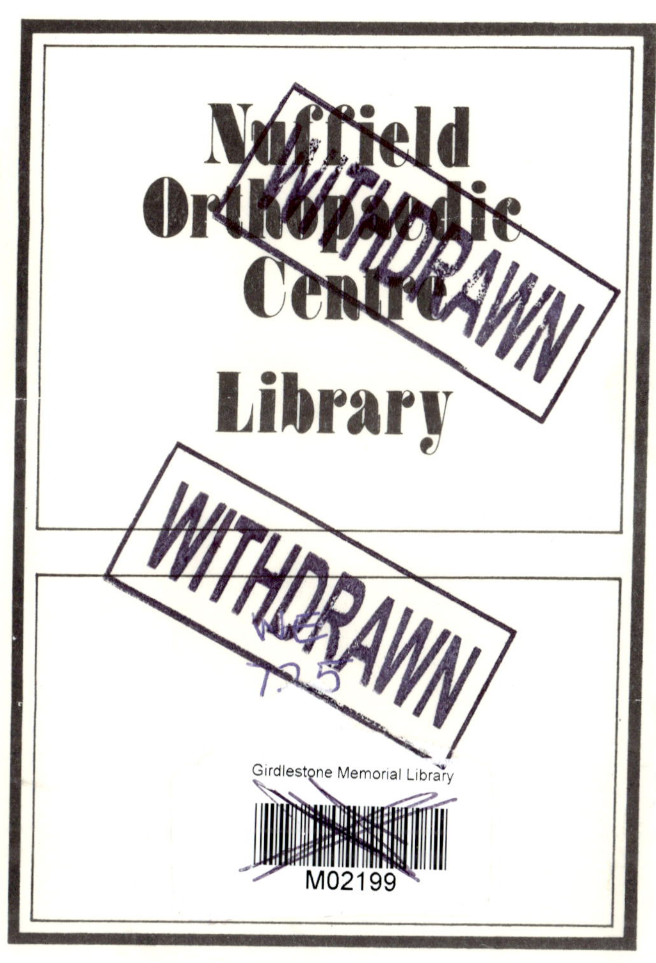
Nuffield
Orthopaedic
Centre
Library
WITHDRAWN
WITHDRAWN
Girdlestone Memorial Library
M02199

# Revision Spine Surgery

JOSEPH Y. MARGULIES, M.D., PH.D.
Associate Professor of Orthopaedic Surgery
Montefiore Medical Center
Albert Einstein College of Medicine
New York

MAX AEBI, M.D.
Professor and Chairman
Division of Orthopaedic Surgery
McGill University
Surgeon-in-Charge
Division of Orthopaedic Surgery
Royal Victoria Hospital
Montreal

JEAN-PIERRE C. FARCY, M.D.
Clinical Associate Professor of Orthopaedic Surgery
New York University Medical Center
Chief of Spine Service
Maimonides Medical Center
New York

*with* 116 *Contributors*

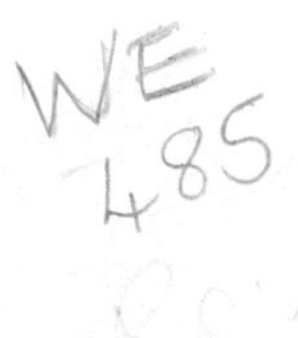


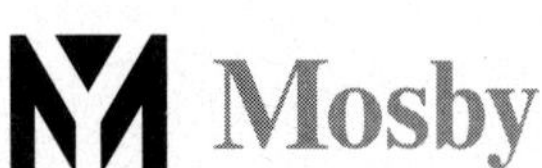

Mosby

St. Louis Baltimore Boston Carlsbad Chicago Minneapolis New York Philadelphia Portland
London Milan Sydney Tokyo Toronto

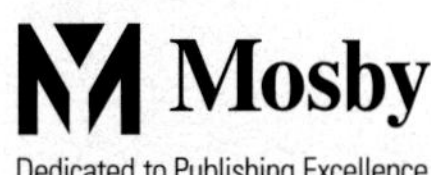

Dedicated to Publishing Excellence

A Times Mirror
Company

*Senior Editor:* Robert Hurley
*Developmental Editor:* Andrew C. Hall
*Project Manager:* David Orzechowski
*Production Editor:* Marian S. Hall
*Designer:* Carolyn O'Brien
*Cover Design:* Maria Bellano
*Manager of Production and Manufacturing—Philadelphia:* William A. Winneberger, Jr.
*Publisher:* Geoff Greenwood

1st Edition


Composition by ATLIS Graphics
Illustration work by Trinity Graphics
Printing/binding by Maple-Vail Press, Inc.

Mosby, Inc.
11830 Westline Industrial Drive
St. Louis, Missouri 63146

**Library of Congress Cataloging-in-Publication Data**
Revision spine surgery / [edited by] Joseph Y. Margulies, Max Aebi, Jean-Pierre C. Farcy ; with 116 contributors. — 1st ed.
p. cm.
Includes bibliographical references and index.
ISBN 0-8151-4591-8
1. Spine—Surgery. 2. Spine—Reoperation. I. Margulies, Joseph Y. II. Aebi, M. (Max) III. Farcy, Jean-Pierre C.
[DNLM: 1. Spinal Diseases—surgery. 2. Reoperation—methods. WE 725R454 1999]
RD768.R484 1999
617.5′6059—dc21
DNLM/DLC
for Library of Congress 98-36265
CIP

99 00 01 02 03 / 9 8 7 6 5 4 3 2 1

# CONTRIBUTORS

**Jean-Jacques Abitbol, M.D.**
Clinical Instructor, Department of Orthopaedic Surgery, State University of New York Health Science Center, Syracuse; Associate Clinical Professor, State University of New York, Stony Brook; Long Island Spine Specialists, New York

**Emre R. Acaroglu, M.D.**
Associate Professor of Orthopaedics, Hacettepe University, Ankara, Turkey

**Wayne H. Akeson, M.D.**
Professor of Orthopaedics, University of California, San Diego; University of California, San Diego Medical Center; Thornton Hospital; San Diego Veterans Administration Hospital, California

**David W. Amory, Jr., M.D.**
M.P.H., Fellow in Spine Surgery, Rush Medical College, Chicago, Illinois

**Paul A. Anderson, M.D.**
Clinical Associate Professor, Department of Orthopaedic Surgery, University of Washington, Seattle; Orthopaedic Spine Surgeon, Othopaedics International, Seattle

**Vincent Arlet, M.D.**
Assistant Professor of Surgery, Montreal Children's Hospital, Montreal, Canada

**Edouard F. Armour, M.D.**
Department of Orthopaedic surgery, Montefiore Medical Center, New York

**Marc A. Asher, M.D.**
Professor of Orthopaedic Surgery, University of Kansas Medical Center, Kansas City, Kansas

**Atul L. Bhat, M.D.**
Lenox Hill Hospital, New York

**Fabian D. Bitan, M.D.**
Spine and Pediatric Orthopaedic Surgeon, New York Spine Institute, Beth Israel Medical Center, New York

**Ohenebe Boachie-Adjei, M.D.**
Associate Clinical Professor, Cornell University Medical College; and Chief, Scoliosis Service, Hospital for Special Surgery, New York

**Scott D. Boden, M.D.**
Associate Professor of Orthopaedics, Emory Universtiy School of Medicine, Director, The Emory Spine Center, Atlanta, Georgia

**Ciaran Bolger, Ph.D., F.R.C.S.I. (SN)**
Senior Lecturer, Bristol University and Consultant Neurosurgeon, Frenchay NHS Trust, Frenchay Hospital, Bristol, United Kingdom

**Marco Brayda-Bruno, M.D.**
Vice-Chairman, Spine Surgery Department, Hospital Maria Adelaide, Turin, Italy

**Keith H. Bridwell, M.D.**
Professor, Department of Orthopaedic Surgery, Washington University School of Medicine; Chief, Spinal Surgery, Washington University Medical Center; Barnes-Jewish Hospital; St. Louis Children's Hospital; Shriners Hospitals for Children, St. Louis, Missouri

**Allen L. Carl, M.D.**
Professor of Surgery, Orthopaedic Surgery, Albany Medical College, New York

**Steven A. Caruso, M.Eng.**
Director, Orthopaedic Biomechanical Engineering, St. Vincent's Hospital and Medical Center of New York and Instructor of Orthopaedic Surgery, New York Medical College, New York

**Mark K. Chang, M.D.**
Keystone Orthopaedic Specialists, Hazel Crest, Illinois

**Jens R. Chapman, M.D.**
Associate Professor, University of Washington and Chief of Spine Service, Harborview Medical Center, Seattle

**William P. H. Charlton, M.D.**
Department of Orthopaedic Surgery, Thomas Jefferson University, Philadelphia, Pennsylvania

**Patrick J. Connolly, M.D.**
Associate Professor, Orthopaedic Surgery, State University of New York at Syracuse Health Science Center, Syracuse, New York

**Jerome M. Cotler, M.D.**
The Everett J. and Marion Gordon Professor of Orthopaedic Surgery, Thomas Jefferson University and Attending Orthopaedic Surgeon Jefferson Medical Center of Thomas Jefferson University, Philadelphia, Pennsylvania

**H.V. Crock, M.D., M.S., F.R.C.S., F.R.A.C.S., F.R.C.S. Ed. (Hon)**
Director, Spinal Disorders Unit, Cromwell Hospital, London; Consultant Spinal Surgeon (Formerly, Honorary Consultant), Royal Postgraduate Medical School, Hammersmith Hospital, London, United Kingdom

**Vincent J. Devlin, M.D.**
Department of Orthopaedic Surgery, Kaiser Permanente Fontana Medical Center, Fontana, California

**Ronald L. Dewald, M.D.**
Professor, Orthopaedic Surgery, Rush Medical College; Director, Spine Surgery, Rush Presbyterian-St. Luke's Medical Center, Chicago, Illinois

**John Dove, F.R.C.S.**
Senior Lecturer, Keele University; Director of Stoke-on-Trent Spinal Service, New Hartshill Orthopaedic and Surgical Unit, Hartshill, Stoke-on-Trent, United Kingdom

**Jean Dubousset, M.D.**
Professeur des Universités, Université René Descartes, Paris; Pratician Hospitalier, Hospital St. Vincent de Paul, Paris, France

**Marcel F. Dvorak, M.D., F.R.C.S.(C)**
Clinical Assistant Professor, Departemnt of Orthopaedics, University of British Columbia; Associate Director Acute Spinal Cord Injury Unit, Vancouver Hospital, Vancouver, British Columbia, Canada

**Thomas J. Errico, M.D.**
Associate Professor of Clinical Orthopaedics and Neurosurgery, New York University Medical Center, New York

**Stephen I. Esses, M.D.**
Professor of Orthopaedic Surgery and Director, Residency Program, Baylor College of Medicine, Houston, Texas

**Daniele A. Fabris, M.D., Ph.D.**
Department of Clinical Orthopaedics, Spinal Surgery Unit, University of Padova School of Medicine, Italy

**Charles G. Fisher, B.Sc., M.D., F.R.C.S.(C)**
Clinical Assistant Professor, Department of Orthopaedics, University of British Columbia; Spinal Surgeon, Vancouver General Hospital, Vancouver, British Columbia, Canada

**Yizhar Floman, M.D.**
Professor of Orthopaedic Surgery, Hadassah-Hebrew University Medical School; Chief, Spine Surgery, Hadassah University Hospital, Jerusalem, Israel

**Robert D. Fraser, M.D., M.B., B.S., F.R.A.C.S.**
Clinical Professor, The University of Adelaide and Head of The Spinal Unit, Royal Adelaide Hospital, Adelaide, Australia

**Stephen R. Freidberg, M.D.**
Chair Division of Surgery and Chair Department of Neurosurgery, Lahey Clinic, Burlington, Massachusetts

**Steven R. Garfin, M.D.**
Professor and Chair, University of California, San Diego; USCD Medical Center, Hillcrest and LaJolla, California

**Charles A. Gatto, M.D.**
Spine Surgeon, Mt. Sinai Hospital, New York

**Robert W. Gaines, Jr., M.D.**
Professor, University of Missouri and Spine and Pediatric Specialist, University of Missouri Hospital and Clinics, Columbia, Missouri

**Stanley D. Gertzbein, M.D., F.R.C.S.(C)**
Medical Director, The Spine Institute; Baylor College of Medicine, Houston, Texas

**Alexander J. Ghanayem, M.D.**
Assistant Professor of Orthopaedic Surgery and Rehabilitation and Neurosurgery, Chief Division of Spine Surgery, Loyola University Medical Center, Maywood, Illinois

**Federico P. Girardi, M.D.**
Orthopaedic Surgeon, Spine and Scoliosis Service, The Hospital for Special Services, New York; Orthopaedic Surgeon, New York Cornell Medical Center, New York

**Robert Goodkin, M.D.**
Associate Professor, University of Washington Medical School and Medical Center; Chief of Neurosurgery Section, Veterans Association Puget Sound Health Care System, Seattle

**Dieter Grob, Dr. Med., M.D., P.D.**
Chefarzt Spine Unit, Privatdozent Universital, Zurich; Shulthess Klinik, Zurich

**Robert Gunzburg, M.D., Ph.D.**
Eeuwfeestkliniek, Antwerp, Belgium

**Richard D. Guyer, M.D.**
Associate Clinical Professor of Orthopaedics, Southwestern School of Medicine, Fellowship Director; Chairman of the Board, Texas Back Institute Research Department, Plano, Texas

**Alexander G. Hadjipavlou, M.D.**
Professor of Orthopaedic Surgery and Neurosurgery, Radiology Chief, Division of Spine Surgery, Department of Orthopaedics and Rehabilitation, University of Texas Medical Branch, Galveston

**Thomas R. Haher, M.D.**
Professor of Orthopaedic Surgery, New York Medical College; Chairman, Orthopaedic Surgery, St. Vincent's Hospital and Medical Center, New York

**Jerome Hall, M.D.**
Adult and Pediatric Surgery, St. Joseph's Medical Center, Tacoma, Washington

**James W. Harkess, M.D., Ch.B.**
Former Kosair Professor of Orthopaedic Surgery, Jewish Hospital, Louisville, Kentucky

**Michael H. Heggeness, M.D., Ph.D.**
Associate Professor, Baylor College of Medicine; The Methodist Hospital; St. Luke's Episcopal Hospital, Houston, Texas

**Richard T. Holt, M.D.**
Clinical Associate Professor, Department of Orthopaedic Surgery, Tulane University, New Orleans; Volunteer Faculty, Division of Orthopaedic Surgery, University of Kentucky, Louisville, Kentucky

**Ken Y. Hsu, M.D.**
Director of Orthopaedic Surgery, St. Mary's Spine Center, San Francisco, California

**Cameron B. Huckell, M.D., F.R.C.S.**
State University of New York at Buffalo, New York

**Roger P. Jackson, M.D., F.A.C.S.**
Clinical Assistant Professor, Orthopaedic Surgery, University of Kansas School of Medicine; North Kansas City Hospital, North Kansas City, Missouri

**Parviz Kambin, M.D.**
Professor of Orthopaedic Surgery, Allegheny University of the Health Sciences and Director, Spine Diagnostic and Treatment Center, Allegheny University Hospitals MCP, Philadelphia, Pennsylvania

**Eldin E. Karaikovic, M.D.**
Orthopaedic Surgery Resident, University of Missouri and University of Missouri Hospital and Clinics, Columbia, Missouri

**Harpal S. Khanuja, M.D.**
Division of Orthopaedic Surgery, Albany Medical College, New York

**Won-Joong Kim, M.D.**
Assistant Professor, Inje University Sanggye Paik Hospital, Seoul, Korea

**Joshua A. King, M.D.**
Clinical Assistant Professor of Surgery, Albany Medical College; Attending in Plastic Surgery, Albany Medical Center Hospital, New York

**John R. Klein, M.D.**
Research Fellow, Division of Orthopaedic Surgery, Maimonides Medical Center, Brooklyn, New York

**Christine Kohler-Ekstrand, M.D.**
Department of Orthopaedic Surgery, Montefiore Medical Center, New York

**David Lamb, M.D.**
Department of Orthopaedics, Emory University School of Medicine, Atlanta, Georgia

**Lawrence G. Lenke, M.D.**
Assistant Professor, Department of Orthopaedic Surgery and Chief of Spine Surgery, St. Louis Shiners Hospital, St. Louis, Missouri

**Isador H. Lieberman, B.Sc., M.D., F.R.C.S.(C)**
Orthopaedics and Spinal Surgeon, The Cleveland Clinic Foundation, Cleveland, Ohio

**Douglas A. Linville, M.D.**
Assistant Professor Orthopaedic Surgery, Wake Forest School of Medicine; Attending Spinal Surgeon, Wake Forest University Baptist Medical Center, Winston-Salem, North Carolina

**Paul Lombardi, M.D.**
Chief Resident in Orthopaedic Surgery, Albany Medical Center, Albany, New York

**William Lorensen, M.S.**
General Electric Corporation Research and Development Center, Schenectady, New York

**Thomas G. Lowe, M.D.**
Associate Clinical Professor, University of Colorado; Denver Orthopaedic Specialists, Wheat Ridge, Colorado

**Gary L. Lowery, M.D., Ph.D.**
Medical Director, Research Institute International; Orthopaedic Spinal Surgeon, President, Florida Neck and Back Institute; Columbia North Florida Regional Medical Center, Gainesville, Florida

**John P. Lubicky, M.D.**
Professor of Orthopaedic Surgery, Rush Medical College; Chief of Staff, Shriners Hospital for Children, Chicago, Illinois

**Kurt Madsen, D.O.**
Associate Staff, Audrain County Hospital; Madison Orthopaedics, Madison Orthopaedics, Mexico, Missouri

**Mohammad E. Majd, M.D.**
Spine Surgery, PSC, Louisville, Kentucky

**John Mahan, M.D.**
Graduate of Tulane-Louisville Spine Fellowship; Perose-St. Francis and Memorial Hospitals, Colorado Springs, Colorado

**Dante G. Marchesi, M.D.**
Assistant Professor of Surgery, McGill University; M.D. Head Spinal Unit, Jewish General Hospital, Montreal, Canada

**Steven M. Mardjetko, M.D.**
Assistant Professor, Orthopaedics; Rush Presbyterian Hospital; St. Lukes Hospital; Rush Presbyterian Hospital; Shriners Hospital for Children; Lutheran General Hospital, University of Illinois, Cook County Hospital; Children's Memorial Hospital, Chicago

**Paul C. McAfee, M.D.**
Associate Professor of Orthopaedic Surgery, Johns Hopkins Hospital; Chief of Spine Surgery, St. Joseph's Hospital, Baltimore, Maryland

**Richard F. McDonough, B.S.**
Clinical Research Assistant, Research Institute International, Inc., Gainesville, Florida; Florida Neck and Back Institute, Miami, Florida

**Laurence E. Mermelstein, M.D.**
Attending Physician, Long Island Spine Specialists, Commack, New York

**Andrew A. Merola, M.D.**
Assistant Professor of Orthopaedic Surgery, SUNY HSC at Brooklyn; St. Vincent's Hospital and Medical Center of New York, New York

**Sohail K. Mirza, M.D.**
Assistant Professor, University of Washington, Harborview Medical Center, Seattle

**Russell T. Nevins, M.D.**
Department of Orthopaedic Surgery, Montefiore Medical Center, New York

**Jürgen Nothwang, M.D.**
Chief Resident and Trauma Surgeon, Klinik am Eichert, Göppingen, Germany

**Donna D. Ohnmeiss, M.S.**
Clinical Research Scientist, Institute for Spine and Biomedical Research, Plano, Texas

**Michael Osipoff**
Assistant Professor of Medicine, Touro College; Huntington Hospital and St. John's Episcopal Hospital, New York

**Ross Paskoff, M.D.**
Clinical Instructor, Orthopaedic Surgery, SUNY-HSC at Brooklyn, New York

**A. Eugene Pennisi, M.A.**
Clinical Research Assistant, Research Institute International, Inc., Gainseville, Florida

**Bernard A. Pfeifer, M.D.**
Assistant Clinical Professor of Orthopaedics, Boston University School of Medicine; Staff Orthopaedist, Lahey Hitchcock Medical Center, Burlington, Massachusetts

**Malcolm H. Pope, Dr.Med.Sc., P.R.D.**
Professor, University of Iowa; Director, Iowa Spine Research Center, Iowa

**Ramin Raiszadeh, B.S.**
Medical Student, Baylor College of Medicine, Houston

**Nahshon Rand, M.D.**
Instructor, Hebrew University; Senior Orthopaedic Surgeon, Department of Orthopaedic Surgery, Hadassah University Hospital, Jerusalem, Israel

**Kenneth Rohling**
General Electric Corporation Research and Development Center, Schenectady, New York

**Aron D. Rovner, M.D.**
Department of Orthopaedic Surgery
Montefiore Medical Center, New York

**Paul T. Salo, M.D., F.R.C.S.(C)**
Assistant Professor, Department of Surgery, University of Toronto; Staff Physician, Division of Orthopaedics, Toronto Hospital, Toronto, Ontario, Canada

**John Schenck, M.D., Ph.D.**
General Electric Corporation Research and Development Center, Schenectady, New York

**Frank J. Schwab, M.D.**
Associate Attending Spine Surgeon
Director of Orthopaedic Research,
Maimonides Medical Center, New York
Attending Spinal Surgeon
The Hospital for Joint Diseases/NYU

**William O. Shaffer, M.D.**
Associate Professor of Orthopaedic Surgery and Neurosurgery, St. Louis University; Director, Division of Spine Surgery, St. Louis University Hospital, St. Louis

**Steven R. Shaw, M.D.**
Spine Fellow, St. Mary's Spine Center, San Francisco, California

**Harry L. Shufflebarger, M.D.**
Professor, Orthopaedic Surgery and Neurosurgery, University of Miami School of Medicine, Coral Gables, Florida

**James W. Simmons, M.D.**
Clinical Professor of Orthopaedics and Rehabilitation, University of Texas Medical Branch–Galveston; Medical Director, Alamo Bone and Joint Clinic, San Antonio, Texas

**Geoffrey Stewart, M.D.**
Reconstructive Spine Surgeon, The Spine and Scoliosis Center; Clinical Instructor, Orthopaedics, Orlando Regional Healthcare System, Orlando, Florida

**Se-Il Suk, M.D., Ph.D.**
Emeritus Professor, Seoul National University; Professor and Director, Seoul Spine Institute, Inje University, Korea

**Marek Szpalski, M.D.**
Adjunct Assistant Professor of Orthopaedics and Rehabilitiation, Vanderbilt University, Nashville; Consultant, C.H. Molier Longchamp, Brussels

**Samuel P. Thampi, M.D.**
Research Fellow, Spine Service, Montefiore Medical Center, New York

**Christoph Ulrich, M.D.**
Trauma Surgeon and Head of Medical Staff, Klinik am Eichert, Göppingen, Germany

**Alexander R. Vaccaro**
Associate Professor, Thomas Jefferson University; Co-Director of the Delaware Valley Regional Spinal Cord Injury Center and the Rothman Institute, Philadelphia, Pennsylvania

**Gerard P. Varlotta, D.O.**
Clinical Assistant Professor of Rehabilitation Medicine, New York University School of Medicine and Rusk Institute of Rehabilitation Medicine, New York

**Carlos Villanueva, M.D., Ph.D.**
Associate Professor, Universidad Autonoma de Barcelona; Spine Unit Coordinator, Hospital Universitario Traumatologia Vall D'Hebron, Barcelona, Spain

**John C. vom Lehn, M.S.**
General Electric Corporation Research and Development Center, Schenectady, New York

**Kirby Vosburgh, Ph.D.**
General Electric Corporation Research and Development Center, Schenectady, New York

**Denise A. Williams, R.N., B.S.N.**
Perioperative Systems Manager, Kaiser Permanente Fontana Medical Center, Fontana, California

**Patrick Willocx, M.D.**
Eeuwfeestkliniek, Antwerp, Belgium

**Robert B. Winter, M.D.**
Clinical Professor, Department of Orthopaedic Surgery, University of Minnesota; Surgeon, Minnesota Spine Center, Minneapolis

**Kirkham B. Wood, M.D.**
Associate Professor, University of Minnesota; Spine Surgeon, Fairview University Medical Center and Twin Cities Spine Center, Minneapolis

**Hansen A. Yuan, M.D**
Professor of Orthopaedic Surgery and Neurological Surgery, State University of New York at Syracuse, New York

**Michael R. Zindrick, M.D.**
Clinical Associate Professor of Orthopaedic Surgery, Hinsdale Orthopaedics Associates, S.C., Hinsdale, Illinois

**James F. Zucherman, M.D.**
Medical Director, St. Mary's Spine Center and Director, Spine Surgery Fellowship, San Francisco Combined Orthopaedic Residency Program, St. Mary's Medical Center, San Francisco

To Pessi, my partner, and to our wonderful sons: Shaul, Yoni, Adam, and Jeremy with love.
*Yossi*

For Christine, Sam, and Eva, my supportive and beloved family.
*Max*

In reverence to my darling Poeia and gratitude to Frederic, David, and Sarah for their patience and confidence.
*Jeep*

# FOREWORD

Our first thought might be that the failed spine problems are due to ill conceived or performed previous procedures. This is frequently not the case. The spine is a living, dynamic organ system that is ever changing due to stresses, whether they are physical or pathologic. We must understand that there are no surgical procedures that can "stabilize the spine forever." Living bone has the ability to grow, remodel, and heal. At the current state of the art, by using contemporary surgical techniques and planing, we cannot foresee and tailor solutions for an individual patient for his or her next 50 years. We must remember that the spine of an 18-year-old does not look like the spine of a 76-year-old. Moreover, implanted metal that should be a scaffold is actually embedded into the fusion mass. But all metal has a fatigue life and cannot adjust to spine remodeling, so it is forced to migrate, bend, or fatigue fracture. The use of improved metals or other materials may help the prudent surgeon to do procedures previously thought impossible. Yet as long as we do not treat the specific underlying tissue pathology, the concept of fusion, especially long fusion, is like a crude tombstone covering the problem. The fusion mass that has to be hauled by the patient for long time demands its prices in terms of general posture balance and mobility, as well as overloads on the neighboring motion segments.

Only in our preamble is it written that all men are created equal. We have but to look at the child with multiple congenital anomalies to realize this is not true. Nor are we ever all on the same level playing field in real life. During the 20th century, our life expectancies have nearly doubled. Our society has changed from a predominately agrarian through industrial, to presently technological—an automated lifestyle. In general our spines shorten with aging due to diminished disk or vertebral body height. The dorsal spine often goes into increased kyphosis whereas the lumbar spine loses lordosis. Often one level may fail only to be followed a few years later by additional levels. Whether previous surgery was performed or not, we should not feel that this is due to failed surgery but to the aging spine which may require additional treatment.

Who can foresee where will we be 50 years from now? Moreover, who can recommend and execute responsibly individual treatment that will last 50 years? In this sense, the concept of revision spine surgery gets a life of its own and becomes an entity that should be related to separately.

*Charles F. Heinig*

# PREFACE

The growing number of revisions of spine surgery sends an alarming message to the spinal surgery community. If so many cases must be redone, is there something wrong with the indications? Perhaps surgical techniques need to be updated, or perhaps these failures are an inevitable part of the profession.

Historically, the work by Mixter and Barr was considered with the introduction of the Harrington instrumentation as one of the most important milestones in the development of spinal surgery as a subspecialty. Parallel to the general trend in surgical history, one can consider the use of instrumentation as responsible both for great successes and failures in medicine. However, because the long-term failures and the need for revision surgery appears to slowly outnumber the successes, we would like to take a look at the direction of our specialty as surgeons who routinely place spinal instrumentation.

First, we would like to draw attention to the fact that the extent of knowledge accumulated in the last three decades in the field of spine surgery fully justifies the establishment of a formal subspecialty. This may prevent many of the acute failures, which can be contributed to lack of fundamental knowledge in spine surgery on behalf of some people performing spine surgery.

However inexperienced or uneducated, surgeons cannot be blamed for the wave of mid- and long-term failures. Failures do occur even in the hands of experienced and educated surgeons, which means that the state of the art in spine surgery is still in rapid progress. The advent of instrumentation gives us a very powerful tool, and its use needs to be much more clearly defined and refined.

Failures that occur because of poor technique or judgment mistakes, even in the hands of educated surgeons, are not the issue of this text. These should be dealt on the individual level of the surgeon and his or her self-evaluation. We would like to refer to failures of concepts and look to the future to try to avoid these. The best example is the evolution of the understanding of spine balance in light of overzealous corrections that were performed first with Harrington distraction rods and then with Cotrel-Dubousset (CD) derotation maneuver. No one had considered him- or herself overzealous trying to achieve the maximum correction at that time. Yet creating flat backs with Harrington rods or imbalance with CD instrumentation became quite a common result. Our understanding of the spine has considerably evolved and we now pay much more attention to the sagittal balance in deformity surgery.

The most significant portion of conceptual failures may be attributed to either inappropriate balance considerations at the stage of planning the index operation or to bone implant interface problems that have developed during the years afterward. The failures express themselves mostly at the junctions between the fusion mass and the normal tissue as pain and instability, or as progressive imbalance. We are faced with the need to solve these iatrogenic situations.

To prepare ourselves (as surgeons!) for the future we must closely investigate three fields:

**Improving expertise in revisions:** In the next decade or more, we will encounter a growing number of patients who need revisions. These patients were happy with their surgery for decades, but as they reach middle age, their condition begins to deteriorate. We must come up with solutions to the bone quality and bone metal interface problems, as well as to balance problems.

**Performing better primary surgery:** Performing surgeries that will not bring the patients back to the surgeons even in 20 years or more, is a question of significantly better planning and transcendent instrumentation compared with what exists today.

**Developing new concepts of surgery:** Longevity and life expectancy are markedly increased in the last decades. Moreover, the demand for good quality of life is also on the rise, especially among the "baby boomer" generation in America. The demands of the spine as of the rest of the skeleton to "serve" for 8 to 9 decades or more cannot always be fulfilled, and some preventive measures should be employed. The field of osteoporosis research is making small steps forward; however, these are only patches. It seems that no one yet has grasped what is happening conceptually in bone (and spinal column) aging and how to tackle it.

The common denominator of any further developments in the three mentioned fields is the need for new concepts in planning and surgical technologies. As surgeons, however, we must keep our minds open to emerging solutions tangential to our profession—e.g., biochemistry or genetics. These can change the field to the extent that surgery will not be needed altogether, even for trauma, and the patients' problems will be solved in totally different arenas.

As for planing; the future trends encompass the three-dimensional understanding of the spine and its saggital balance. For example, more and more people are focusing on what Dubousset termed the "pelvic vertebra," that "vertebrates" between the femoral heads and the spine. He talks about balanced spine with the pelvis, while considering the balance over the lower limbs. This concept is important when positioning the patient for lumbopelvic fusion. If one fuses in a limited lordotic position, one may end up with a sacrum that is more vertical and hyperextended hips. This certainty is not an ideal situation, especially in degenerative patients in whom hip pathology is present. These kinds of operations require serious "biomechanical" planning. Yet it seems that the suffix bio in the term "spine biomechanics" drives spine biomechanics as far from mechanical sciences as almost art from science. In other words, we have only a very vague idea of what is going on mechanically in the spine. Unlike in general orthopedics, where hip and knee total joint replacements are practiced, based on data currently available, no one can build anything that is even close to the complicated construct of the spinal motion segment. We need much better data acquisition tools, as well as data analyzing instruments. It is essential to develop our understanding of the whole matrix of spinal motion so that exact surgeries can be planned and balance related failures avoided. Hopefully, with the power of the modern computers, this can be materialized.

As for technology, three sections have to be mentioned: surgical techniques, implants and instruments. Along the evolution of surgical techniques, it can be noticed that the breakthrough achievements mostly did not occur in the orthopaedic field, but rather in the neighboring disciplines—e.g., anesthesiology, general surgery, or dentistry. At this time, we are witnessing the introduction of minimal surgery into the spine field. The state of the art fluctuates. We can foresee new types of surgical techniques or approaches emerge, and we should be committed to constantly develop our technical skills.

Instrumentation is getting better by incorporating new technologies into the surgical field. We will see sophisticated computer guided instrumentation with on-line feedback mechanisms. We will see more use of fiber optics and better sets of retractors that allow safe minimal approaches or even stereotactic location of surgical sites.

Materials will also play a major role in the future development. The use of metals as implants is probably almost exhausted. Unless someone develops a revolutionary design of implant that has similar modulus of elasticity to bone, yet has protection capability, the source of materials for new implants will not be in mines. The same goes for cements: the PMMA in use today is far from being satisfactory, let alone the fact that if being introduced today, it would have never obtained an FDA approval. The source of new materials for implants will probably be in the laboratory, in the form of biocompatible biodegradable materials or even genetically engineered pieces of tissues.

The role of bone morphogenic protein (BMP) probably will become more important in the near future of fusion. BMP may lead to less extensive surgery and less solid internal constructs, or even back to short external immobilization. We do hope, however, that together with further developments of BMP, we will be introduced to possible BMP "inhibitors" so that tumors can be treated more efficiently. The long-term future, however, is probably not in fusion. It may be either in other types of mechanical solutions or in nonmechanical, nonorthopaedic fields altogether, such as biochemics or genetics.

In light of this philosophy, we decided to put together a book about revisions. We thought that due to the strict criteria of the good peer-reviewed journals, information and experience about revisions is not properly shared, keeping some very important information from members of our profession. We wanted to provide a stage for thoughts and experiences originating in small series lacking statistical analysis and solutions of large variety of cases that had led surgeons to new thoughts and ideas. We did hope that a volume of about 800 to 900 pages would suffice to cover what is known today about revisions. We learned as we went along, and as always, realized that what we know is like a drop in the sea, and our complete understanding of the spine is far away.

We designed an outline that attempted to define essential issues in spinal revision surgery and outcome studies. We asked for overviews on the various sections of our specialty: general overviews, low back surgery, deformity surgery, cervical spine, and balance considerations in revisions in children. A section discussing anatomic and mechanical aspects of revision, role of fusion and instrumentation, principles of stabilization and correction, and biomechanics of the fusion mass. One of the most important advents, the modern ability to approach the spine through the combined approaches, is covered, followed by a very problematic issue of evaluation and indications. A long list of specific considerations related to pathologic entities such as revision surgery in fractures, revision surgery in degenerative diseases, revision surgery for deformity, and revision of tumor surgery, comprise a significant part of the book. Specific technical considerations in revision surgery and specific problems in revision surgery are two sections that go into the important details of problems we encounter. The major topic of balancing the spine signs the technical section. We believe that rehabilitation is a crucial component to our work, and the topic is covered in the next chapter; the book ends with a chapter on an emerging technique: computer-guided surgery.

Despite the fact that the contributions are outstanding, as mentioned before, it is only the beginning of the long journey into understanding revisions. The last topic in our introduction concerns the political and socioeconomic status of medicine in the western world. On the research and academic level, it seems that the "heavy duty" research will be generated less and less from universities and more and more from research institutions next to huge industrial conglomerates. Experience from our own practices appears to indicate that we cannot rely on universities and university hospitals to carry the heavy financial load of cutting edge research. It looks to us as though modern scientific knowledge will emerge from industry-founded research centers that will be contracted with hospitals, affiliated or not with universities.

As for the clinical medicine, we strongly want to believe that no surgery is being done by any of our colleagues for any reason other than the welfare of the patient. This belief makes any socioeconomic consideration redundant. We do realize that there is a fortune of money involved in spine surgery, be it in surgeons fees, the implant market, or all the periphery of spine surgery. Yet it is morally wrong if these calculations are included in the surgeon/patient relationship, or in indicating specific patients for surgery. Again, economy and costs are important factors, but an individual patient should receive, as individual surgeons, the best available solution. Yet if the future of spine surgery becomes dictated by nonprofessional factors, this would be a great disapointment. Those of us who find it in their hearts to be involved in the political ballgame of our profession, and by that contribute to the profession prosperity, God bless them. We tried to be Socratic and share our thoughts, the basis of the science we have been practicing to date.

*Joseph Y. Margulies*
*Max Aebi*
*Jean-Pierre C. Farcy*

# CONTENTS

# Revision Spine Surgery

# I
# THE PROBLEM OF REVISION

# 1

# REVISIONS: OUTCOME STUDIES

**Ciaran Bolger, Ph.D., F.R.C.S.I.**
**Robert D. Fraser, M.B.B.S., M.D., F.R.A.C.S.**



Increasingly, revision surgery and the management of patients with recurrent low back pain and sciat-ica has come under close scrutiny, particularly with regard to expected outcome. Revision surgery for low back problems is a distinct clinical problem. Reoperation rates for diskectomy vary from 2% to 19%,[13,18,19,22,30,33,37,38,42,46] for decompressive laminectomy from 9% to 17%[6,20,23] and for fusion from 6% to 36%.[4,10,21,27,28] These numbers represent a significant number of individual patients given the numbers undergoing each primary procedure. In contrast to the information available on outcome for these primary procedures, the expected outcome of revision surgery is not clearly established.

The outcome in these reoperated cases would appear to be dependent on a number of factors, some of which are closely related. However, any discussion of outcome necessitates a preliminary evaluation of the literature. Three factors influence the usefulness of the information available: the quality of the studies performed, the measurement of outcome in these studies, and the characteristics of the subjects studied.

## LITERATURE REVIEW

In a recent review of research from 1976 to 1996, there were no prospective studies identified on outcome following repeat lumbar surgery.[3] There were only 20 prospective series from which information on reoperated cases was available. In general, the quality of the published material was low, with few papers examining important criteria in relation to outcomes. Of 106 papers evaluated only 57 had identifiable information in relation to outcome, and of these only 32 studies had a minimum follow-up of more than 6 months and presented results on the basis of more than one outcome measure. Further, only eight studies had more than 20 subjects and provided data on the age and sex of the subjects, previous operations, and compensation status.[2,9,24,25,27,34,40,45] Only four papers considered the effect of a pain-free period since the previous surgery,[2,34,40,45] with only two studies providing data on subjects with psychological problems.[2,45]

The failure to provide even basic demographic information on the study population rendered most of the studies reviewed, while internally valid, worthless in terms of generalizing the results to other populations. The poor quality of outcome studies in relation to revision surgery renders it difficult to analyze outcome and factors that influence that outcome. Weighing outcome in relation to a study characteristic, such as number of subjects, cannot compensate fully for poor study design in the first place.

## OUTCOME MEASURES

It is quite clear that outcome in terms of success or failure depends very much on the way in which it is assessed. A 90% success rate in one series may in fact be the same as a 60% success rate in another. There is a wide variation in what is accepted by different authors as a successful outcome and how that outcome is assessed. Many studies only evaluate one outcome measure such as pain relief.[6,13,14,31,32,36] The lack of uniformity in reporting results is a major source of difficulty in any assessment of outcome.

In addition, inconsistent follow-up and the lack of consensus as to what constitutes an acceptable outcome or even how that outcome is measured greatly affect the value of the published literature and may well bias the results to a significant degree. This is evidenced by the wide range of satisfactory outcome rates reported for almost every characteristic and variable which one that care to examine.[3]

Given these methodological problems, together with publication bias, it is likely that the outcomes reported are an overestimate of the true outcome following repeat lumbar surgery. Further problems are generated by the very nature of the topic itself.

## PATIENT CHARACTERISTICS

Reoperated cases represent a heterogenous population with multiple factors contributing to the final overall outcome of the study. Any attempt to isolate and study individual variables greatly dilutes the number of subjects with any particular factor of interest. For example, the outcome for anterior fusion as a salvage procedure is based on information from only 27 subjects over four studies.[3]

A number of patient characteristics have been demonstrated to be associated with a relatively good outcome for reoperation.[3] Notably, the presence of a symptom-free period of more than 6 months since previous operation, only one previous operation, the absence of psychological problems, the absence of a compensation claim, and, to a lesser extent, the presence of leg pain, may all influence the success rate achievable with reoperation. From the data available, however, it is not possible to decide to what extent each of these factors interact and to what extent the presence of one factor of itself reduces the chances of a satisfactory outcome.

It is because of the profound influence of these confounding factors, with very few of the reports in the literature taking them into account, that any comparison of results reported in the literature is likely to be unreliable.

The flaws described above in relation to the published literature also greatly limit any attempt to develop a comprehensive overview of outcome data or reliable estimates of the influence of various factors and successful outcomes. In particular, it is impossible to perform reliable multivariant analysis that would allow description of the relative contribution of each factor to a successful outcome. The wide range of outcomes reported may to some extent be combined by the use of weighted mean outcomes. However, it is not possible to weight for all the factors that may affect outcome, particularly when basic population details are missing from the majority of studies.

## STANDARDIZING OUTCOME MEASURES

Outcome measures and what constitutes a successful outcome vary widely between studies. In an attempt to overcome this problem in our recent literature synthesis we applied universal outcome measures to each of the studies evaluated.[3,19,44] For the purposes of discussion of outcome in relation to reoperated cases the same universal measure of outcome has been applied:

*Excellent or Good:* Pain absent or occasionally mild; able to work at usual job with minimal or no activity restriction; occasional use of analgesics.

*Fair:* Mild persistent or occasional moderate pain; able to work and perform most normal activities but with restrictions; regular use of analgesics.

*Poor:* Persistent moderate or occasional severe pain with little or no pain relief from surgery or severe activity restriction.

For the purpose of this review excellent or good outcomes are classified as satisfactory. This outcome measure was adopted regardless of the author's ratings. These outcomes were evaluated uniformly across studies,[3,19,44] allowing comparison of different studies using the same basis for measurement of outcome. In addition, studies with less than 6 months' minimum follow-up and studies with only one outcome measure were excluded from consideration for the purposes of this chapter.

## OVERALL OUTCOME

The overall satisfactory outcome in all reoperated cases is approximately 60% (Table 1-1). This combines outcome data on all patients having all reoperations for all types of procedures. However, 60% represents a broad range of satisfactory outcomes reported, from be-

**Table 1-1. Weighted Mean Values for Study Characteristics and Outcome from 32 Selected Studies**

| | Weighted Mean | Range | No. of Studies |
|---|---|---|---|
| Mean follow-up (mos.) | 44.7 | 12–120 | 28 |
| Minimum follow-up (mos.) | 23.6 | 7–120 | 32 |
| Number of subjects | 43.9 | 8–130 | 32 |
| Mean age (yrs) | 43.2 | 37–5 | 22 |
| Interval between operations (yrs) | 4.7 | 0.9–10 | 7 |
| Outcome (good/excellent) | 60.2 | 25–82 | 32 |

**Table 1-2. Satisfactory Outcome and Final Procedure ($n$ = 32 studies)**

| | Weighted Mean (%) | Range | No. of Subjects | No. of Studies |
|---|---|---|---|---|
| Disk (all) | 67.2 | 39–100 | 418 | 12 |
| Same Level | 75.2 | 78–82 | 109 | 4 |
| Different Level | 76.7 | 58–100 | 30 | 4 |
| Scar | 38.9 | 0–55 | 95 | 5 |
| Percutaneous diskectomy | 39 | 39 | 18 | 1 |
| Anterior fusion | 81.5 | 40–100 | 27 | 4 |
| Posterior fusion | 59.8 | 18–84 | 597 | 17 |
| PLIF | 67.4 | 45–76 | 46 | 3 |
| Decompression | 57.6 | 28–100 | 144 | 8 |

tween 25% and 82%, and studies with 8 subjects up to studies with 130 subjects. However, it is a useful starting point for considering any discussion on outcome.

## FACTORS INFLUENCING OUTCOME IN REOPERATED CASES

A number of preoperative factors are now accepted as having a profound influence on the outcome for primary surgical procedures on the lumbar spine. These include psychological disturbance[11] and compensation.[12] In relation to reoperated cases the effect of these factors is less clearly defined. The evaluation of any particular factors influencing outcome in reoperated cases is confounded by the fact that other factors make the study population a heterogenous one. For example, the influence of the number of previous surgeries, the nature of the previous surgeries, and the nature of the current surgery all come into play when trying to evaluate the influence of any one factor.

### NATURE OF FINAL PROCEDURE

A wide range of satisfactory outcomes that depend on the final procedure is reported (Table 1-2). The worst outcome is seen with the excision of scar tissue as a final procedure, with an overall satisfactory outcome of only 39%. This contrasts with an overall satisfactory outcome reported for anterior fusion as a final procedure of 82%. It should be noted, however, that the latter figure is based on only four studies with a total number of 27 subjects.[3]

The overall satisfactory outcome for excision of disk as a final procedure is 67% and it is interesting to note that the outcomes for excision of a disk at the same level as previous surgery or at a different level from the previous surgery is almost identical at 75.2% and 76.7%, respectively.[3] When counselling patients, it should be borne in mind that a number of procedures (including excision of scar tissue, percutaneous diskectomy, posterior fusion, or lumbar decompression), when performed as a final procedure in a multiply operated patient, have satisfactory outcomes of less than 60%. This suggests that these procedures in particular should only be undertaken following careful patient evaluation and with clearly defined technical and clinical goals.

### OUTCOME IN RELATION TO PREVIOUS PROCEDURES

There was a satisfactory outcome rate of approximately 60% when the previous procedure was a diskectomy.[3] However, there was a satisfactory outcome of only 50% in patients whose previous procedure was a fusion. The best outcome (78.6%) was seen when the previous procedure was percutaneous

**Table 1-3. Outcome and Previous Procedure**

| Previous Procedure | Weighted Mean Outcome (%) | Range | No. of Studies |
|---|---|---|---|
| Disk | 59.9 | 25–87 | 22 |
| Fusion | 49.7 | 27–100 | 10 |
| Decompression | 69 | 0–76 | 7 |
| PLIF | 41 | | 2 |
| Percutaneous diskectomy | 78.6 | 73–100 | 3 |
| Chymopapain | 49.3 | 39–100 | 3 |

**Table 1-4. Weighted Mean Outcome for Revision Procedures with Diskectomy As Previous Procedure (*n* = 22 studies)**

| | Weighted Mean (%) | Range | *n* |
|---|---|---|---|
| Overall outcome | 59.9 | 25–87 | 22 |
| Diskectomy | 75.6 | 62–100 | 9 |
| Same | 75.2 | 62–82 | 4 |
| Different | 76.6 | 58–100 | 4 |
| Scar | 41.6 | 0–55 | 4 |
| Percutaneous | 39 | 39 | 1 |
| Anterior fusion | 75 | 75 | 1 |
| Posterior fusion | 57.9 | 35–73 | 9 |
| PLIF | 64.5 | 45–76 | 3 |
| Decompressive laminectomy | 52.1 | 28–79 | 3 |

diskectomy and the worst outcome (41%) was seen when the previous procedure was a posterior lumbar interbody fusion (PLIF).

***Diskectomy as Previous Procedure.*** The overall good and excellent outcome from all secondary procedures was 59.9%, with a range of 25% to 87% (Table 1-3). The outcome in relation to the second procedure when the primary procedure was a diskectomy ranged from 39% when the second operation was a percutaneous diskectomy to 75.6% when the second operation was a second diskectomy.

It should be noted that there is little difference in the weighted average outcome for a second disk procedure whether the disk is at the same or a different level. It should also be noted that there is only one study reporting the use of percutaneous diskectomy for failed open diskectomy[29] and one study reporting an anterior fusion in patients who previously had diskectomy.[37] The outcomes in relation to the final procedure when the previous procedure was a diskectomy are provided in Table 1-4.

***Fusion.*** The overall weighted mean successful outcome from ten studies considering fusion as the primary procedure was 49.7% (ranged of 27% to 100%; Table 1-3). When the primary procedure was a fusion, the mean weighted outcomes ranged from 30% when the second procedure was excision of scar tissue, to 57% when the second procedure was a posterior lumbar interbody fusion. It should be noted, however, that both of these figures are derived from only one study in each case.[2,5] The outcome for secondary procedures when the primary procedure is a fusion is summarized in Table 1-5.

***Lumbar Decompression.*** Seven papers provided a weighted mean outcome of 69% for all secondary procedures performed on patients whose primary procedure was a decompressive laminectomy. A satisfactory outcome varied from 4% for the excision of scar tissue to 76.7% for a posterior fusion with success for this method of fusion ranging from 50% to 74%.[26,35,41,47]

***Posterior Lumbar Interbody Fusion.*** Two studies demonstrated satisfactory outcome in 41% of reoperated PLIF cases. In both studies the second operation was a spinal fusion.[3]

***Percutaneous Diskectomies.*** Three studies reported the weighted outcome of 78.6% with a range of 73% to 100% for second operations in which the primary operation was percutaneous diskectomy. One study reported one patient who had a fusion with a successful outcome.[5] The second study reported two patients who had an open diskectomy with a successful outcome in one of the patients.[29] The third study reported on 11 patients who had a decompressive lam-

**Table 1-5. Weighted Mean Outcome for Revision Procedures with Fusion As Previous Procedure ($n$ = 10 studies)**

| | Weighted Mean (%) | Range | *n* |
|---|---|---|---|
| Overall outcome | 49.7 | 27–100 | 10 |
| Scar | 30 | 30 | 1 |
| Anterior fusion | 50 | 40–100 | 2 |
| Posterior fusion | 50.8 | 0.80 | 8 |
| PLIF | 57 | 57 | 1 |

inectomy following a percutaneous diskectomy with a successful outcome in eight patients.[38]

***Chymopapain Injection.*** Three studies showed combined successful outcome of 49.3% for all procedures following chymopapain injection. One study of 100 patients with diskectomy following chymopapain injection found a successful outcome in 52 patients.[15] One study demonstrated a successful outcome in one patient who had a fusion following chymopapain injection.[5] The third study demonstrated a good or excellent outcome in 13 of 33 patients who had an open diskectomy following chymopapain injection.[3]

It can be seen from the foregoing that the nature of the previous procedure can have a profound effect on outcome for reoperated cases. In relation to patients who have previously had a diskectomy, only 60% of them may expect to have a satisfactory outcome with the second procedure. On the other hand, if the second procedure contemplated is either a diskectomy at the same or different level or an anterior fusion, then 75% of them may be expected to have a satisfactory outcome. However, all other procedures can be expected to have less than 60% satisfactory outcome; in particular, the performing of a percutaneous diskectomy or excision of scar tissue had a satisfactory outcome in only approximately 40% of such patients. If the previous procedure has been a fusion, less than 50% of patients may be expected to have a satisfactory outcome. This is a fairly uniform finding regardless of the nature of the second procedure. Such outcome figures should emphasize the degree of caution that is necessary before recommending further procedures on these patients. A uniform finding across all studies is that surgery solely for epidural scarring or arachnoiditis carries a very low success rate. This does not, however, exclude surgery for a treatable condition that may respond to appropriate surgery, such as recurring disk herniation in the presence of fibrosis.

## PSYCHOLOGICAL FACTORS

Weighted mean outcome analysis of published studies shows a profound influence of psychological factors on outcome for reoperated cases.[3] Patients with a good psychological profile have a satisfactory outcome in 76%, compared to 21% of patients with poor psychological factors. One study found no effect of psychological factors on outcome.[1] Three studies demonstrated a marked effect. In one of these studies, no outcome data was presented but analysis of data from three studies demonstrated a significant effect.[1,2,9,45] This profound effect would suggest that patients who are psychologically disturbed are unlikely to respond to repeat surgery (Table 1-6).

## COMPENSATION

Weighted mean outcome analysis on data from 13 studies also demonstrates the profound effect of compensation on outcome for reoperated cases. In patients in whom there is no litigation or compensation pending, 73% have a satisfactory outcome compared with 35% of patients with ongoing compensation claims. One paper reported an absence of any association between the presence of compensation and satisfactory outcome in repeat diskectomy patients.[7] However, five studies on diskectomy patients showed a significant association between the absence of a compensation claim and a satisfactory outcome.[2,9,17,34,45] A lack of association between a compensation claim and outcome is reported in two studies of fusion patients,[25,27] and a further study in which the nature of the previous surgery was not stated found no association with compensation.[40]

Nevertheless, given the overall weighted outcome from all studies it is likely that compensation plays a significant role in the predicted outcome from reoperated cases (Table 1-6).

## SYMPTOM-FREE PERIOD

Patients who have a symptom-free period of more than 6 months following their previous surgery have a satisfactory outcome of 63%. This compares with a satisfactory outcome of only 38% in patients who do not have a symptom-free period of more than 6 months following their previous surgery.[3] In addition,

**Table 1-6. Patient Characteristics and Outcome**

| | Weighted Mean | Range | No. of Studies | P |
|---|---|---|---|---|
| <6 months symptom-free | 38.3 | 16–82 | 4 | <0.0001 |
| >6 months symptom-free | 62.7 | 50–77 | 6 | |
| 2 operations | 64.5 | 38–84 | 9 | |
| 3 operations | 43.5 | 10–64 | 9 | <0.0001 |
| 4 or more operations | 32.4 | 10–100 | 5 | |
| Psychological + | 21.1 | 10–33 | 2 | <0.0001 |
| Psychological − | 76.3 | 57–88 | 2 | |
| Compensation + | 35.1 | 17–50 | 9 | <0.0001 |
| Compensation − | 73.3 | 43–94 | 8 | |
| Male | 59.6 | 34–74 | 5 | NS |
| Female | 68.4 | 61–83 | 5 | |
| Leg pain | 51.3 | 35–79 | 4 | NS |
| No leg pain | 45.6 | 32–80 | 4 | |
| Smokers | 58.1 | 38–77 | 2 | NS |
| Nonsmokers | 64.1 | 38–83 | 2 | |

two studies claim a significant association with outcome and symptom-free period, although this was not supported with details of outcome.[9,34]

### NUMBER OF PREVIOUS OPERATIONS

From the recent literature review, weighted mean analysis of the number of previous operations and outcome show a dramatic effect on successful outcome as the number of surgeries increases.[3] A satisfactory outcome of the order of 65% was found in patients who have had two operations, but falls to 44% in patients who have had three operations, and to 32% in patients who have had four or more operations. For patients who have had a previous diskectomy, two papers reported no significant association between the number of surgeries and satisfactory outcomes.[9,34] However, no outcome data were provided. Analysis of data from five other diskectomy studies showed a significant association between fewer previous operations and satisfactory outcomes. In diskectomy patients who had undergone two operations, a satisfactory outcome was seen in 60%, compared with 40% in patients who had undergone three operations, and only 23% in patients who had undergone four operations or more.[3]

One study found no effect on the number of previous operations for all reoperated cases.[40] However, given the weighted mean outcome analysis reported above across all studies it is likely that multiple previous operations have a significant effect on patient outcome. In addition, in our literature review, the only factor that had a significant association with outcome on single regressive analysis was the number of previous operations ($t = 0.519$, $P < 0.02$, $n = 21$ studies).[3]

### GENDER

Analysis of data from the published research demonstrates no significant effect of gender on outcome for reoperated cases.[3] Female patients had a satisfactory outcome of 68% compared with 60% in male patients, but this difference was not significant. In diskectomy patients, one study reported a significantly better outcome for repeat surgery in females.[34] However, analysis of data from four other studies concerned with diskectomy demonstrated no such effect.[2,8,17,39]

### PRESENCE OF LEG PAIN

One study found no effect of the presence of leg pain on outcome.[40] Another study claimed that the presence of leg pain had a significant influence on outcome, although no supporting details were provided.[34] Analysis of data from four studies that individually claim a significant effect of leg pain on outcome fails to demonstrate any such association.[2,25,39,45] Weighted mean outcomes for patients without leg pain was 45.6% compared with 51% for patients with leg pain (Table 1-6).[3] However, analysis of data from studies primarily concerned with diskectomy does demonstrate a significant effect at the 0.05 level.[2,39,45]

Patients who have had a diskectomy as a primary procedure and have no leg pain have a satisfactory outcome in 29.6% of cases, whereas patients with leg pain have a satisfactory outcome in 65.7% of cases.[3]

### SMOKING

Two studies report a significantly improved outcome in nonsmokers.[34,41] Contrasting with this, two other studies report no significant association with smoking.[25,43] Analysis of the data from the two studies from which it can be derived shows no significant effect, with smokers having a satisfactory outcome in 64% of cases compared with 59% of cases for nonsmokers.[3,25,41]

## CONCLUSIONS

There is no doubt that there is great difficulty in drawing satisfactory and statistically verifiable conclusions from available published studies. As outlined at the beginning of this chapter, methodological flaws, heterogeneous patient populations, and lack of uniformity in study variables make the combination of results from different studies and the interpretation of the significance of those results difficult. Despite these limitations, it is possible to derive some information that may be useful in the evaluation of patients in whom reoperation is being considered. Clearly, repeat surgery should only be performed when the cause of the patient's symptoms has been accurately determined and when there is a reasonable chance that surgery would be beneficial to the patient. In this regard a number of factors must be considered for each individual patient: the nature of the previous surgery, the nature of the proposed surgery, whether or not the patient has had a pain-free interval, the number of previous surgeries, whether or not the patient is suffering from psychological problems, whether or not there is pending compensation, and when diskectomy is contemplated, whether or not leg pain is present. Only when these factors have been evaluated for each individual patient can a prognosis be given as to the likely outcome following further intervention.

It must be remembered that there is no doubt that repeat surgery in general is associated with a less favorable outcome than for initial procedures, with success rates progressively diminishing with each subsequent operation. The contemporary attitude to informed consent means that the doctor should discuss all reasonable methods of treatment for a particular condition with the patient and, clearly, the reduction in expected success rate depending on what factors individual patients have, together with the risks of surgery, must be considered when advising patients whether or not another operation is appropriate.

In an attempt to aid in the decision-making process and to provide some estimate of the likely outcome for repeated operation we have proposed a prognostic outcome score based on a percentage reduction for a satisfactory outcome when a particular factor is present. It must be stressed that this scoring system is at best a crude measure of the likely outcome. Given the nature of the literature and information available, it is not possible to derive a score from multivariant analysis. While this greatly weakens the strength of the proposed score, we believe it will be useful as a guide to the clinician contemplating reoperation on any individual patient. The scoring method is outlined in Table 1-7. Each factor detailed in the table is given a percentage and the percentage for each individual factor is added together to give an overall outcome reduction estimate. Factors that do not appear on the table are given a score of zero. The total is subtracted from 100% to give the estimated chance of a successful outcome for that patient. For example, a patient who has previously had a fusion and on whom it is proposed to do a further posterior fusion, who has had a symptom-free period of greater than 6 months, but who is undergoing a third operation, has no psychological disturbance, and has pending compensation, would have a total of 70%. That would mean the patient has an estimated 30% chance of gaining a satisfactory outcome from the proposed operation.

This proposed scoring system emphasizes the great care and caution that must be exercised in performing any procedure on a patient who has already undergone lumbar surgery. It is in our interest, and in the interest of our patients, that patients are fully aware and have realistic expectations regarding the likely outcome from any proposed procedure.

**Table 1-7. Prognostic Outcome Score**

| Factor* | Estimated Adverse Effect on Outcome |
|---|---|
| <6 months symptom-free | 20% |
| 3rd operation | 10% |
| 4th or more operation | 20% |
| Psychological disturbance | 20% |
| Compensation | 20% |
| Previous surgery | |
| Disk | 10% |
| Fusion | 20% |
| Proposed surgery | |
| Posterior fusion | 20% |
| Decompression | 20% |
| Scar | 40% |

*Note: All factors must be assessed and the reduction percentage figures added when more than one factor is present, with the total subtracted from 100% to determine the likely successful outcome.

## REFERENCES


1. Bernard TN Jr: Repeat lumbar spine surgery, factors influencing outcome, *Spine* 18:2196-2200, 1993.
2. Biondi J, Greenberg BJ: Redecompression and fusion in failed back syndrome patients, *J Spinal Disord* 3:362-369, 1990.
3. Bolger C, Fraser RD: *Spine* In Press, 1998.
4. Brantigan JW: Pseudarthrosis rate after allograft posterior lumbar interbody fusion with pedicle screw and plate fixation, *Spine* 19:1271-1280, 1994.
5. Brantigan JW, Steffee AD: A carbon fiber implant to aid interbody lumbar fusion, two year clinical results in the first 26 patients, *Spine* 18:2106-2117, 1993.
6. Cavanagh S, Stevens J, Johnson JR: High-resolution MRI in the investigation of recurrent pain after lumbar diskectomy, *J Bone Joint Surg* 4:524-528, 1993.
7. Deburge A, Mazda K, Guigui P, Lassale B: La reintervention dans les echecs du traitement chirurgical des sciatiques, *Chirurgie* 117:545-549, 1991.
8. Fandino J, Botana C, Viladrich A, Gomez-Bueno J: Reoperation after lumbar disc surgery: results in 130 cases, *Acta Neurochirurgica* 122:102-1094, 1993.
9. Finnegan WJ, Fenlin JM, Marvel JP, Nardini RJ, Rothman RH: Results of surgical intervention in the symptomatic multiply-operated back patient, analysis of sixty-seven cases followed for three to seven years, *J Bone Joint Surg* 61-A:1077-1082, 1979.
10. Franklin GM, Haug J, Heyer NJ, McKeefrey SP, Picciano JF: Outcome of lumbar fusion in Washington State workers' compensation, *Spine* 19:1897-1904, 1994.
11. Greenough CG, Fraser RD: Comparison of eight psychometric instruments in unselected patients with back pain, *Spine* 16:1068-1074, 1991.
12. Greenough CG, Fraser RD: The effects of compensation on recovery from low-back injury, *Spine* 14:947-955, 1989.
13. Hanley EN, Shapiro D: The development of low-back pain after excision a lumbar disc, *J Bone Joint Surg* 71-A:719-721, 1989.
14. Hardy RW: *Repeat operation for lumbar disc.* In Hardy RW, editor: *Lumbar disc disease,* New York, 1982, Raven Press, pp. 193-202.
15. Hepner H, Auque GJ, Marchal, H: La chirurgie des hernies discales lombairesapres chimionucleolyse, resultats et analyse. A propos de 100 cas, *Chirurgie* 118:695-699, 1992.
16. Herno A, Airaksinen O, Saari T: Long-term results of surgical treatment of lumbar spinal stenosis, *Spine* 18:1471-1474, 1993.
17. Herron L: Recurrent lumbar disc herniation: results of repeat laminectomy and discectomy, *J Spinal Disord* 7:161-166, 1994.
18. Hirabayashi S, Kumano K, Ogawa Y, Aota Y, Maehiro S: Microdiscectomy and second operation for lumbar disc herniation, *Spine* 18:2206-2211, 1993.
19. Hoffman RM, Wheeler KJ, Deigo RA: Surgery for herniated lumbar discs, *J Gen Int Med* 8:487-496, 1993.
20. Hopp E, Tsou PM: Postdecompression lumbar instability, *Clin Orthop* 227:143-151, 1988.
21. Hutter CG: Posterior intervertebral body fusion, a 25 year study, *Clin Orthop* 179:86-96, 1983.
22. Kambin P, Schaffer JL: Percutaneous lumbar discectomy review of 100 patients and current practice, *Clin Orthop* 238:24-34, 1989.
23. Katz JN, Lipson SJ, Larson MT, McInnes JM, Fossel AH, Liang MH: The outcome of decompressive laminectomy for degenerative lumbar stenosis, *J Bone Joint Surg* 73-A:809-816, 1991.
24. Kim SS, Michelsen CB. Revision surgery for failed back surgery syndrome, *Spine* 17:957-960, 1992.
25. Lauerman WC, Bradford DS, Ogilivie JW, Transfeldt EE: Results of lumbar pseudarthrosis repair, *J Spinal Disord* 5:149-157, 1992.
26. Laus M, Alfonso C, Tigani D, Pignatti G, Ferrari D, Giunti A: Failed back syndrome: a study on 95 patients submitted to reintervention after lumbar nerve root decompression for the treatment of spondylotic lesions, *Chir Organi Mov* LXXIX:119-126, 1994.
27. Lehmann TR, LaRocca HS: Repeat lumbar surgery, a review of patients with failure from previous lumbar surgery treated by spinal canal exploration and lumbar spinal fusion, *Spine* 6:615-619, 1981.
28. Markwalder Th M: Surgical management of neurogenic claudication in 100 patients with lumbar spinal stenosis due to degenerative spondylolisthesis, *Acta Neurochirurgica* 120:136-142, 1993.
29. Mirovsky Y, Neuwirth MG, Halperin N: Automated percutaneous discectomy for reherniations of lumbar discs, *J Spinal Disord* 7:181-184, 1994.
30. Moore AJ, Chilton JD, Uttley D: Long-term results of microlumbar discectomy, *Br J Neurosurg* 8:219-326, 1994.
31. Nakano N: Multiple back operations, *J West Pacific Orthop Assoc* 14:67-75, 1977.
32. Nakano N, Tomita T: Results of surgical treatment of low back pain: a comparative study of the anterior and posterior approach, *Int Orthop (SICOT)* 4:101-106, 1980.
33. Geka NS: Microsurgical lumbar discectomy, clinical analysis of 270 cases, *Neurol Surg* 19:429-434, 1991.
34. Quimjian JD, Matrka PJ: Decompression laminectomy and lateral spinal fusion in patients with previously failed lumbar spine surgery, *Orthop* 11:563-569, 1988.
35. Roy-Camille R, Benazet JP, Desauge JP, Kuntz F: Lumbosacral fusion with pedicular screw plating instrumentation, a ten year follow-up, *Acta Orthop Scand* 64(supp 251):100-104, 1993.
36. Rusu M, Tarasi C: Lumbar spinal stenosis by postdiscectomy hyperostosis, *Revista Medico-Chirurgicala A Societatii De Medici Si Naturalisti Din IASI* 97:235-237, 1993.
37. Sachdev VP: Microsurgical lumbar discectomy: a per-

sonal series of 300 patients with at least 1 year follow-up, *Microsurgery* 7:55-62, 1986.

38. Schaffer JL, Kambin P: Percutaneous posterolateral lumbar discectomy and decompression with a 6.9-millimeter cannula, *J Bone Surg* 73-A:822-831, 1991.
39. Shiraishi T, Crock HV: Re-exploration of the lumbar spine following simple discectomy a review of 23 cases, *Eur Spine J* 4:84-87, 1995.
40. Stewart G, Sachs BL: Patient outcomes after reoperation on the lumbar spine, *J Bone Joint Surg* 78A:706-711, 1996.
41. Thalgott J, LaRocca H, Gardner V, Wetzel T, Lowery G, White J, Cdwyer A: Reconstruction of failed lumbar surgery with narrow AO DCP plates for spinal arthrodesis, *Spine* 16:170-175, 1991.
42. Tria AJ, Williams JM, Harwood D, Zawadsky: Laminectomy with and without spinal fusion, *Clin Orthop* 224:134-137, 1987.
43. Tuite GF, Stern JD, Doran SE, Papadopoulos SM, McGillicuddy JE, Oyedijo DT, Grube SV, Lundquist C, Gilmer HS, Schork MA, Swanson SE, Hoff JT: Outcome after laminectomy for lumbar spinal stenosis. Part 1: Clinical correlations, *J Neurosurg* 81:699-715, 1994.
44. Turner JA, Ersek M, Herron L, et al: Patient outcomes after lumbar spinal fusions, *JAMA* 268:907-911, 1992.
45. Waddell G, Kummel EG, Lotto WN, Graham JD, Hall H, McCulloch JA: Failed lumbar disc surgery and repeat surgery following industrial injuries, *J Bone Joint Surg* 61A:201-206, 1979.
46. Weir BKA, Jacobs GA: Reoperation rate following lumbar discectomy: an analysis of 662 lumbar discectomies, *Spine* 5:366-370, 1980.
47. West JL, Bradford DS, Ogilvie JW: Results of spinal arthrodesis with pedicle screw-plate fixation, *J Bone Joint Surg* 73-A:1179-1185, 1991.

# II
# OVERVIEW

# 2

# REVISION SPINAL SURGERY—AN OVERVIEW

**David W. Amory, Jr., M.D., M.P.H.**
**Ronald L. DeWald, M.D.**



Revision spine surgery, by definition, implies correction of a previously operated spinal problem, be it persistent or new-onset pain, progressive deformity, loss of structural integrity due to failure of the initial procedure, continued degeneration, or the unabated destruction secondary to a neoplastic, inflammatory, or infectious process.

Controversy exists concerning the modes of failure of operative techniques, methods of clinical and radiographic evaluation of the patient, and the indications for reoperation on the spine. In revision surgery certain principles of patient care must be adhered to in order to optimize outcomes.

This chapter serves as an overview of the patient-care philosophy developed over a period of 32 years of clinical practice. This approach to *failed spine surgery* has changed over the years with changes in technology, the innovative ideas and techniques of colleagues, and, mostly, through the unfortunate opportunity of performing surgery to correct surgical interventions that failed.

The term *failed back syndrome* is a misnomer, implying persistence of symptoms as a result of surgery, not despite surgery. By definition, all failed back syndrome patients have undergone spine surgery without improvement. This should not be misconstrued to imply that the operation performed was done incorrectly or inadequately. It is natural to assume that the surgeon is at fault for undertaking an unsuccessful operation. On occasion a surgeon, not sufficiently versed in the intricacies of treating spinal disorders may perform an inappropriate or inadequate procedure. The majority of failed spine surgeries, however, are performed on reasonable surgical candidates by experienced surgeons after an adequate series of nonoperative therapies have failed. Unfortunately, knowledge of the disease of the spine is woefully inadequate considering the complexity of the problem. Despite the technological improvements in the past 20 years, including computed tomography (CT) and magnetic resonance imaging (MRI) scanning, diagnosis remains imprecise and no therapeutic maneuver, including surgery, is uniformly and invariably successful. Revision, like primary spine surgery, should be offered to an informed patient, as a calculated risk, on the reasonable expectation that it may be the optimum mode of therapy for that patient. Therefore, for purposes of our discussion, we refer to the ineffective application of surgery as *refractory back syndrome.*

## MODES OF FAILURE

Spine surgery patients seek help after their initial surgery for several reasons: residual deformity, pain, neuropathy, or implant failure. Failure of spine procedures is caused by an interplay of several factors including a persistence or introduction of spinal deformity from the initial procedure, pseudarthrosis and instability, or the persistence or exacerbation of spinal stenosis or nerve root entrapment. Residual deformity results from either inadequate adherence to appropriate surgical principles, implant failure, or exacerbation of specific disease processes, all of which compromise the structural integrity of the surgically altered spine. Pain and neuropathy often are the result of residual deformity but can also result from implant failure, pseudarthrosis, scarring, or continued degeneration outside the fused segment. Neoplastic, metabolic, rheumatologic, inflammatory, vascular, and genetic conditions can also be present or worsen to cause pain and neuropathy despite adequate initial surgical intervention.

In the clinical evaluation of a patient after a nonresponse to surgery, it is important to determine both the specific physiologic cause of the patient's complaints and the psychosocial factors that may contribute to his/her condition and may inhibit eventual recovery. The history must include a complete account of the patient's preoperative complaints and symptoms, diagnosis, studies performed, conservative modalities used prior to surgery, employment of bracing, and finally procedures performed. The operative reports from previous procedures must be obtained to determine whether intraoperative complications were encountered that may contribute to the patient's condition. An emphasis must be placed on the patient's development of pain, neurologic deficit, or increased deformity postoperatively, specifically with respect to onset and type of symptoms. Early causes of nonresponsive spine surgery include inappropriate preoperative diagnosis and/or patient selection, surgical error or complications, implant failure, and infection. Later causes (greater than 3 months) of nonresponse to surgery can include the above, but are more likely due to degeneration, instability, scarring, or progression of a systemic destructive process.

As in primary spine procedures, the psychosocial status of the patient plays a critical role in outcome in revision surgery.[19,67,73] If present, personality disturbances or chemical dependencies may become exacerbated as a result of the nonresponsive initial surgery. Many authors advise the use of personality examinations to assess the psychologic stability of patients prior to consideration for revision surgery. Wiltse and Rocchio[80] found that hypochondriasis and hysteria scale results on the Minnesota Multiphasic Personality Inventory (MMPI) had the greatest correlation with poor outcome. Careful clinical assessment of a patient usually uncovers psychologic disturbances or substance abuse history that can aid in the choice of conservative or surgical treatment.[59] The patient's expected outcome from previous procedures should be assessed to ensure that unrealistic expectations are not the cause of dissatisfaction. Routine use of psychologic testing does not appear to be necessary, unless the physician believes he/she may need documentation of the patient's psychologic state to justify nonoperative treatment.

The radiographic and laboratory workup should reflect specific clinical suspicion to avoid excess and redundancy. Previous studies must be reviewed thoroughly. In many cases nonresponsive patients will have undergone extensive postoperative studies in an effort to determine the reason for ineffectiveness of the initial procedure.

The indications for surgical intervention in the refractory spine patient are significantly more complex than those for primary spine surgery. The patient's pain, neuropathy, or residual deformity must be weighed against the realistic benefits gained from surgery; the patient's physical and psychologic ability to tolerate a significantly more complex procedure than the one that previously failed and possible complications of that procedure must be taken into account. The best candidates for revision surgery are those who have pain from instability or pseudarthrosis, coronal plane deformity or flat back (sagittal plane deformity), a rib hump, or implant failure. Patients with mechanical pain from persistent or recurrent neurologic compression, discogenic symptoms, nonmechanical causes of pain, or neuropathy are less likely to have optimal results.

The causes of nonresponsive spine procedures can typically be delineated based on the time of onset of symptoms relative to the initial procedures. Specific modes of failure occur in the immediate postoperative period while others occur with time.

## EARLY CAUSES OF REFRACTORY BACK SYNDROME

The most common cause of early failure (within 3 months) after surgical procedures is poor patient selection or an error in the surgical intervention. The initial evaluation should be undertaken with suspicion to first rule out misdiagnosis or the inappropriate surgical patient as cause of failure. An appropriate surgical patient is one with reasonable expectations and working knowledge of the disorder, risks associated with procedures, and alternative therapeutic modalities. Patient expectations from previous procedures should be evaluated to ensure that they were realistic. Previous clinical and radiographic documentation should correlate with the patient's neuropathy, complaints of pain, or deformity.

The clinical and radiographic evaluation can be divided into subgroups in an attempt to elucidate possible causation.

## NEUROLOGIC AND PAIN PROBLEMS

The initial evaluation of a patient who presents with residual pain or neuropathy within 3 months of a spine procedure must begin with a determination of the presence of a pain-free interval or return of lost neurologic function after the initial procedure. If no recovery was experienced postoperatively clinical suspicion should first attempt to delineate whether the appropriate procedure was performed for the patient's complaints and/or whether the patient was an appropriate candidate for surgical intervention. Initial relief of symptoms, followed by gradual recurrence of pain, numbness, or weakness suggest scarring or acute-onset mechanical causes.

Finnegan et al[28] noted that the duration of the pain-free interval can suggest a diagnosis. A history of no pain relief or of postoperative worsening of symptoms suggests that either the wrong diagnosis was made, the wrong operation was performed, or the wrong patient was selected. When temporal onset has been determined, further evaluation should attempt to isolate the specific location of pain or neurologic deficit. The neurologic causes of back pain or dysfunction can differ from causes of limb pain, weakness, or paresthesias.

The differential diagnosis of patients with neck or back pain can be categorized by the temporal onset of symptoms. Common causes of early neck or back pain after previous surgery are wrong or insufficient level of decompression or inadequate decompression at the appropriate level. Failure to recognize lateral recess or foraminal stenosis at the time of decompression leads to immediate or early failure with persistent back and leg symptoms. Graft site pain can also cause nonspecific back pain. Typically, wrong or inadequate decompression can be determined from plain radiographs. Occasionally, MRI with contrast or CT myelogram must be performed if diagnosis can not be determined from plain films. The presence of segmental anomalies necessitates thorough review of the pre- and postoperative films because congenital anomalies are a common cause of technical mistakes. Uncommon early causes of centralized pain or deficit from neurologic causes include cerebrospinal fluid (CSF) leaks and the formation of pseudomeningoceles.

Neck pain after cervical procedures is not uncommon. Bohlman et al[8] demonstrated that more than 20% of successfully treated patients had neck pain. Neck pain is much more common with posterior-cervical procedures or anterior procedures in which a fusion was not performed. Postoperative nuchal or cervicobrachial pain responds well to analgesic medication or application of a soft collar. Severe neck or scapular pain, whether persistent or recurrent in the early postoperative period, is typically due to inadequate removal of spurs, collapse of the decompressed level, and buckling of the posterior longitudinal ligament with pressure on the neural elements in anterior procedures without fusion. In the presence of anterior decompression and fusion, dislodgment of the graft can create instability and compression of the ventral root. Retained hard-disk material compressing the ventral root should be suspected when the initial procedure was performed posteriorly.

Back pain, like neck pain, can be attributed to inappropriate or inadequate decompression in most cases. However, due to the load-bearing characteristics of the lumbar spine, excessive decompression or failure to recognize instability preoperatively can lead to acute symptoms from instability not typically seen in the cervical or thoracic spine. Sacrifice of greater than 50% of both facets or an entire single facet has been shown to lead to subsequent instability.[62] Postoperative dural and nerve root traction may elicit symptoms with lumbar motion in the absence of radiographic hypermobility.

Limb pain and radiculopathy can result from all the previously reviewed causes in conjunction with back or neck pain, but can serve to delineate more specific causes in the absence of centralized pain. Patients with radiculopathy or sciatica complain of radiating pain or paresthesias down the limbs, to the hands or below the knees. Distinct acute causes of postoperative radiculopathy in cervical procedures include sequestered disk fragments that penetrated an unexplored posterior longitudinal ligament, foraminal stenosis that was not adequately decompressed, and recurrent disk herniation or abutment syndrome caused by impingement of instrumentation. Imaging studies show an unchanged root defect if the condition was overlooked during surgery. Lumbar radiculopathy has similar causes with a different incidence than acute cervical pathology. Recurrent disk herniation and acute instability are the most common causes in the lumbar spine area. Typically, patients have a pain-free interval of at least 6 months, if adequate decompression was performed. Absence of a pain-free interval after surgery usually indicates either that the wrong level was approached, the decompression was insufficient, or the wrong procedure was performed. Unrecognized instability and/or dysplastic or acquired spondylolisthesis can cause isolated radicular symptoms and should be considered if the patient's persistent radiculopathy is exacerbated with lumbar motion and flexion-extension radiographs reveal instability (Fig. 2-1).

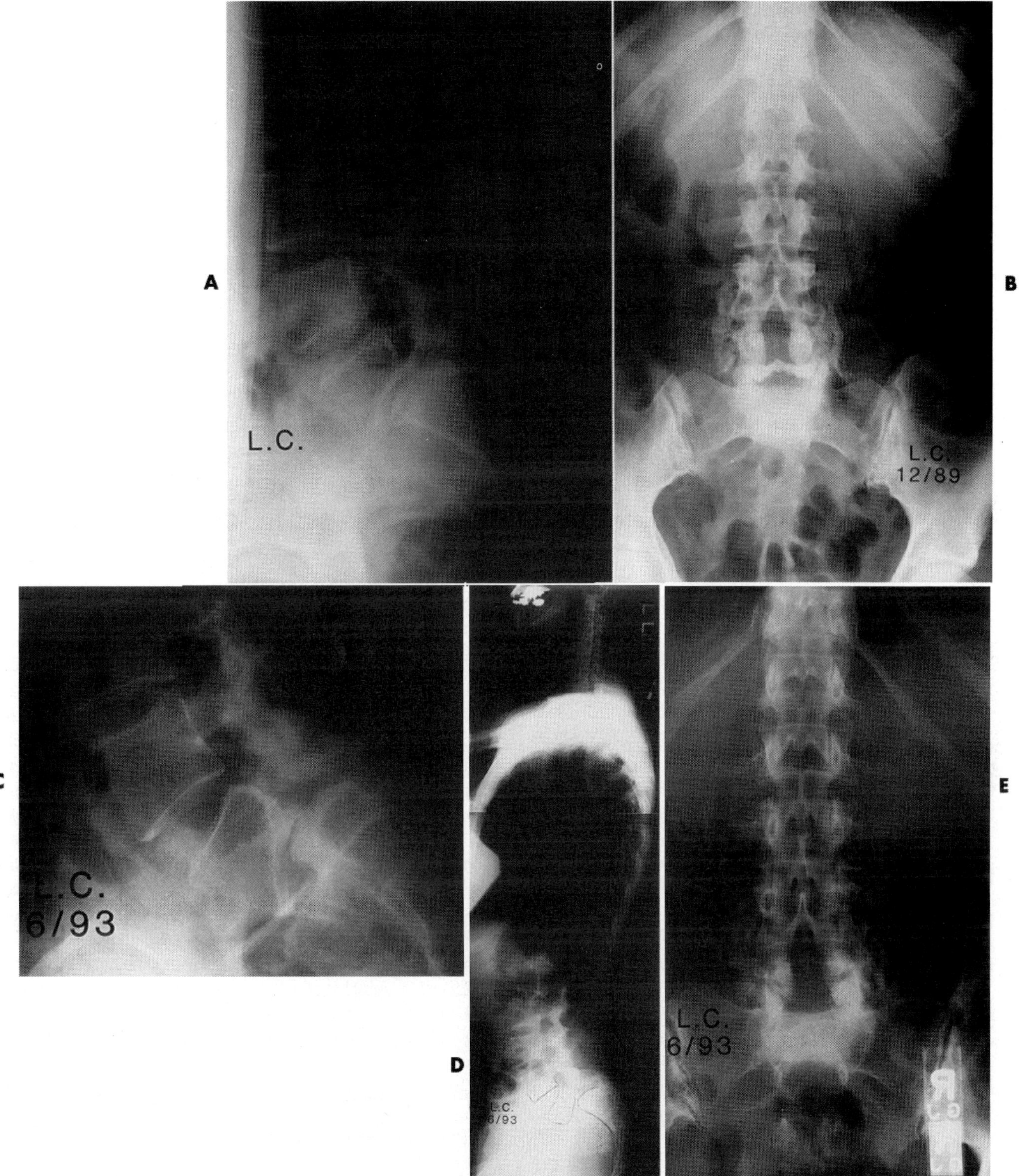


**FIGURE 2-1**

Misdiagnosis. A 52-year-old woman with spondylolisthesis at L5-S1. She underwent a Gill laminectomy at the wrong level, L4-L5 (**A** and **B**). Symptoms persisted and the patient underwent a second operation to decompress the appropriate level, L5-S1 (**C, D,** and **E**).

*Continued*

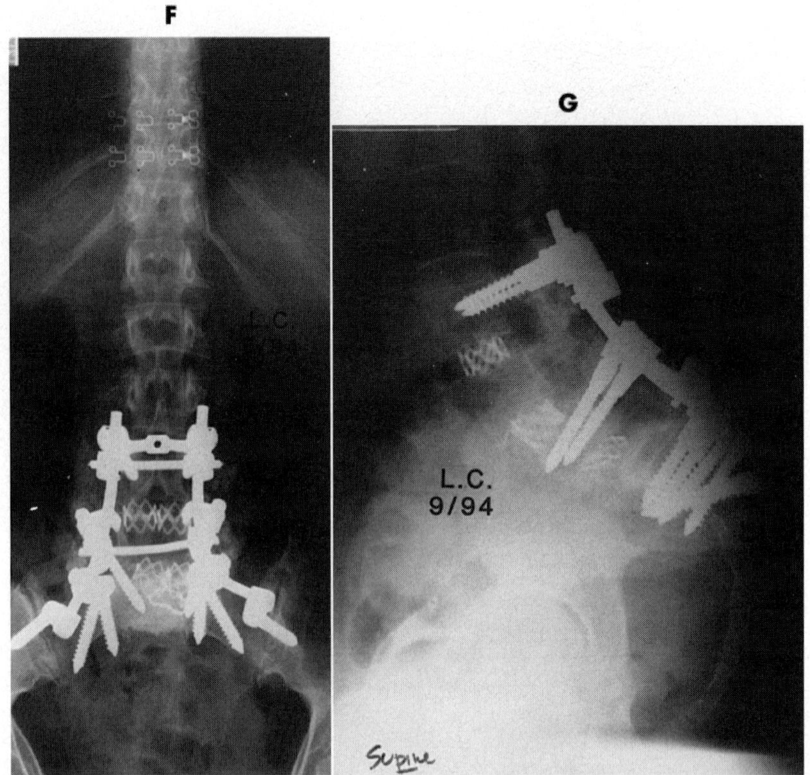


**FIGURE 2-1, CONT'D**

Instability was not addressed. The patient experienced initial pain relief. The spondylolisthesis progressed severely, requiring partial reduction, anterior and posterior fusion with instrumentation (**F** and **G**).

Unintended durotomies occur in approximately 1 out of every 25 lumbar laminotomies and laminectomies[42] and in 1 out of every 6 revision surgeries.[69] The diagnosis of spinal-fluid leak is difficult. Clinical symptoms of nausea, vomiting, and headache—particularly posture related—combined with drainage of clear fluid is suspicious. The best method of diagnosis, if clinically suspected, is injection of technium or iodinated human serum albumin into the cisterna magna (Fig. 2-2).

Cauda equina syndrome, the acute onset of urinary retention with associated saddle anesthesia, severe sciatica, leg weakness, and sensory disturbances in the legs and feet, including the soles, is not uncommon in the early postoperative period. It occurs in approximately 1 out of every 500 diskectomies.[56] The most common cause is postoperative hematoma. If suspected, imaging is emergently indicated with either myelography or MRI to delineate the cause and location of the compression. Andersson[58] has reported an intradural hematoma causing cauda equina syndrome, which would have been missed if prior imaging studies had not been obtained. Immediate exploration of the wound is necessary in almost every case.

Paraplegia is a complication of anterior surgery, particularly with significant deformity correction and in cases of congenital scoliosis. Congenital scoliosis can result in abnormal anatomy. Segmental vessels may not be in a normal position and the vascular supply may be tenuous, particularly in the watershed area of the spine. Several reports have described paraplegia that has resulted from sacrificing segmental vessels in congenital scoliosis.[3] Spine cord monitoring during temporary occlusion of the vessels may help identify those vessels that are contributing to a radicular artery and that should not be sacrificed.[4] Every attempt should be made to preserve segmental vessels when possible.

## DISK PROBLEMS

Herniation or septic inflammation of disks can be a continued source of pain after spine surgery. A long interval of relief with return of function followed by sudden recurrence of symptoms within 3 months is the typical presentation of recurrent disk herniation. No resolution of pain or neuropathy after diskectomy implies residual disk fragments or improper level of decompression. Recurrent disk herniation, requiring additional surgery for pain relief, occurs in approxi-

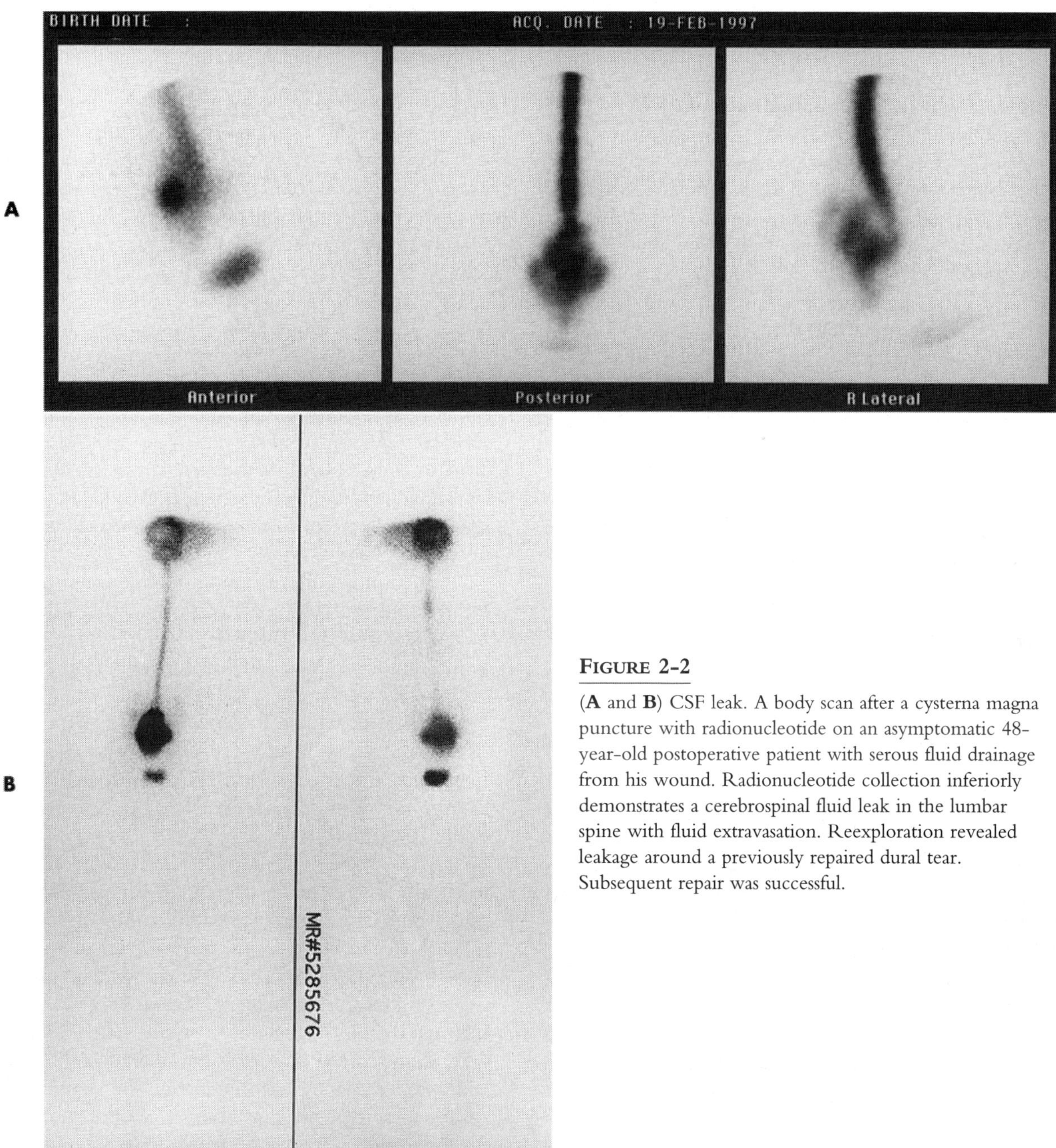


FIGURE 2-2

(**A** and **B**) CSF leak. A body scan after a cysterna magna puncture with radionucleotide on an asymptomatic 48-year-old postoperative patient with serous fluid drainage from his wound. Radionucleotide collection inferiorly demonstrates a cerebrospinal fluid leak in the lumbar spine with fluid extravasation. Reexploration revealed leakage around a previously repaired dural tear. Subsequent repair was successful.

mately 10% to 15% of patients who have primary lumbar disk surgery.[23,34,64] Patients in whom recurrent symptoms develop after a successful diskectomy require careful study to clarify the precise cause of the recurrent symptoms.

Gadolinium (Gd)-enhanced MRI is theoretically the best imaging study to differentiate scar tissue from recurrent disk. In our experience, surgical exploration has not confirmed these findings. If a patient with a recurrent disk herniation does not improve with nonoperative management, then a repeat diskectomy should be performed. If instability is present or more than one herniation occurs in the same spinal unit, anterior or posterolateral fusion are indicated.

## VASCULAR PROBLEMS

One of the most common causes of acute failure of spine procedures is vascular complications. A patient with new or increasing neurologic deficits or pain in the immediate postoperative period should be urgently evaluated for formation of an epidural hematoma or vascular spinal cord injury. Hematoma formation in the lumbar spine or trauma to the artery of Adamkiewicz is postulated to be the most common cause of cauda equina syndrome.[58] Emergent evaluation should include a lateral portable x-ray to assess alignment, which, if normal, should be followed by myelography or CT-myelography. The presence of a hematoma, CSF extravasation, or in some cases retained bone or tissue fragments requires immediate surgical decompression. If these studies reveal no new compression in the operative area, then the patient's injury should be treated as an ischemic vascular spinal cord injury by maintaining adequate blood volume, normal blood pressure, and urinary output.

Vascular complications involving the iliac graft donor sites are not uncommon. The superior gluteal artery exits through the sciatic notch and can be injured in a subperiosteal dissection. Inadvertent penetration has been reported to cause lacerations of this vessel as well as the development of arteriovenous fistula and damage to the ureter.[26] False aneurysms have been reported as a postoperative complication associated with lumbar disk surgery, penetration of the sciatic notch during the harvesting of iliac crest bone graft,[44] and as a result of excessive length of screws eroding vessels.[21] Typical presentation is an unexplained fever, ileus, hematuria, and a palpable mass with or without a bruit. Repair of arteriovenous fistula or false aneurysm is indicated in almost every instance.

Evaluation of the refractory back syndrome must include an elimination of disease processes that can mimic spinal pathology. Vascular claudication and aortic aneurysms have been known to be initially misdiagnosed as spinal pathology and treated operatively. Vascular claudication is usually exacerbated by walking and is worse at night; however, the symptoms can frequently mimic neurogenic claudication in that the pain can be brought on by lying down and decreased by standing or short walks. Cigarette smoking and diabetes are frequently associated with vascular insufficiency. An excellent provocative test to distinguish vascular claudication is to have the patient ride a stationary bicycle; vascular insufficiency is exacerbated while neurogenic claudication is relieved by the flexed riding position. An aortic aneurysm is diagnosed clinically by a large pulsatile mass on abdominal exam with or without bruit. Distal pulses and the ankle brachial index are typically diminished.

## INFECTION PROBLEMS

Early postoperative infection is potentially devastating, particularly when the initial procedure involved instrumentation and fusion. Postoperative infection demands prompt diagnosis and effective treatment to maximize surgical outcome and minimize morbidity. The incidence of postoperative spine infections varies depending on the surgical procedure. Infection rates from lumbar diskectomy are generally less than 1%, but have been reported as high as 5% in patients undergoing microdiskectomy.[24,51,68] Wound infection increases to 25% in patients undergoing deformity surgery for paralytic scoliosis or myelomeningocele.[32]

Clinical suspicion of wound infection must be high in nonresponsive spine patients who present within the first month after their operation. The primary presentation of postoperative spine infection is spinal pain that is disproportional to the physical findings or the usual expected postoperative course, especially in those patients with a persistent low-grade fever. In the early stages, however, the clinical findings can be unremarkable; the patient's only complaint is malaise. Superficial wound infections usually present within the first 5 days postoperatively. Deep wound infections tend to present within the first 2 weeks. Discitis and osteomyelitis tend to present after two weeks and have been known to go undiagnosed for up to 10 months postoperatively.[31]

The diagnosis of postoperative infections is crucial in minimizing the morbidity of associated complications. Diagnostic evaluation should include laboratory, radiographic, radionuclide, and MRI studies as indicated.

The early diagnosis of postoperative infection is crucial in minimizing the morbidity of this complication. Laboratory leukocyte count may be normal. Erythrocyte sedimentation rate (ESR) is elevated although elevation is anticipated in the normal postoperative period. ESR greater than 45 after a week postoperatively has been shown to be consistent with infection.[72] C-reactive protein (CRP) levels are normally high after uncomplicated spine procedures for up to 2 weeks, but respond to an infection within 2 to 3 days thereafter. CRP, however, normalizes faster after successful treatment of an infection. These characteristics make CRP levels more useful than ESR in the early detection of postoperative infection.[31,61]

Postoperative infection can only be definitively diagnosed by a positive aspiration or biopsy, which, in early wound infections, is usually the first and only diagnostic test necessary.

Treatment of early wound infections must be aggressive, if suspected. The operative site must be debrided and lavaged using a pulsatile irrigation system. Intraoperative Gram stains and frozen sections should be obtained to document presence of infection and type of pathogen. Wounds can be closed and hardware left in place. Controversy exists concerning the removal of hardware. Some authors recommend removal in the presence of highly virulent organisms.[71] Hardware removal can compromise the integrity of the fusion. It is difficult to determine when a fusion is solid enough to support the fused segments without instrumentation. The surgeon must be cognizant of the fact that extensor muscles have been deinnervated and no longer effectively stabilize the spine. Removal can cause additional compromise of the fusion mass. As a rule, we do not remove instrumentation in long-fusion segments for at least 2 years or when CT scan documents the formation of contiguous cortical bone throughout the fusion mass. Suction drainage or irrigation systems should be placed and removed only when all drainage has stopped. If long-term intravenous antibiotic therapy is anticipated, placement of a central line should be considered. Postoperatively, the patient's status should be monitored with serial ESR and CRP levels on a weekly basis and attempts should be made to improve the patient's nutritional status.

## IMPLANT PROBLEMS

Instrument failure can be manifested in the immediate or late postoperative periods. Early failure of instrumentation in many cases is due to inappropriate placement, wrong instrumented level, or poor patient selection. Typically, early failure is of bone, not the instruments. The early causes of failure of appropriately placed instruments include hook dislodgement or prominence, screw pullout or rod/plate disengagement due to lamina fracture, osteoporosis or implant failure, which in turn can be caused by poor contouring or excessive distraction/compression on the instruments at implantation.

The cause of instrument failure must be determined prior to revision. It is a mistake to simply reimplant instruments without determining the reason for failure. Revision procedures may require recontouring the rod, adding more points of fixation, or extending the instrumentation to an adjacent level. Zielke[85] described the use of the claw to enhance fixation using two hooks to grasp a segment. Extension of instrumentation is typically required with failed instrumentation that ends at a transitional zone, the thoracolumbar junction, or the apex of the thoracic kyphosis (Fig. 2-3). Proper postoperative external immobilization and avoidance of the prone position may prevent these complications.

Pain associated with prominent instrumentation is an early complication. Bursitis or skin erosions may develop particularly in thin patients. Typically, this can be avoided with removal of bursa or inflammatory tissue, proper rod contour, possible removal, or implantation of prominent hardware at an alternate level.

Anterior instrumentation failure typically occurs as a result of inappropriate placement, poor quality of bone, or hardware fatigue and failure. Anterior cervical plating is commonly used in reconstructive procedures, but carries associated risk of breakage or migration. Failure of this type of instrumentation is particularly prone to failure of purchase in the early postoperative period. Bicortical purchase, however, places the spinal cord at risk during placement. Screw backout can lead to esophageal erosion, which in turn can lead to severe infections.

Posterior cervical instrumentation includes wires, cables, and plates. Lateral mass plating places the cervical roots and vertebral artery at risk. Though pullout is typically less a concern due to solid purchase, neurologic injury, particularly radiculopathy, is more common than in anterior instrumentation. If suspected, CT scanning is the best modality to document nerve root compression.

When these complications occur in the early postoperative period, revision is generally advised regardless of patient symptoms.

The principle of load sharing is essential in the understanding of spinal balance. A spinal column that is not balanced produces stresses and loads that are nonuniform. Biomechanical data have demonstrated that tensile strengths of a posterior rod system are significantly improved if compression is applied across the implant. Posterior distraction places tremendous bending forces on the construct, especially if a deficiency in the anterior column is present. Posterior systems placed in distraction are placed at a higher risk for failure, necessitating stronger implants. Ideal stability is achieved when the anterior column is reconstructed and the posterior column is placed in compression. This reduces the tensile forces on the posterior instrumentation.

Biedermann[6] used a corpectomy model to analyze the effectiveness of posterior instrumentation. He determined that 80% of the forces go through the anterior column and 20% through the posterior column when a small-diameter rod was used in an intact anterior column. When a stiffer posterior implant was used, the forces increased posteriorly to 35% while decreasing anteriorly to 65%. Neither rod failed at more than 5 million cycles under normal physiologic loads. Cunningham[17] tested posterior implants under normal physiologic loads. These loads were determined to be 150% higher than the mean bending strengths demonstrated by the tested implant systems. Findings of both studies reinforce the conclusion that no single one-column posterior implant system can be truly load sharing and is prone to failure.

McLain et al[55] reviewed the early results of short-segment pedicular fixation in 19 patients with unstable thoracolumbar fractures. Early failure was noted in 10 patients. Ebelke et al[23] reported a 33% complication rate associated with instrumentation in patients with short-segment fixation for burst fractures. Those patients with anterior column support showed no failures of the posterior construct. Gurr et al[37] showed a direct correlation between the level of anterior column deficiency and predicted failure rate in 10 of 25 patients.

Anterior deficiency, whether as a result of fracture, disk degeneration, or destructive processes such as in-

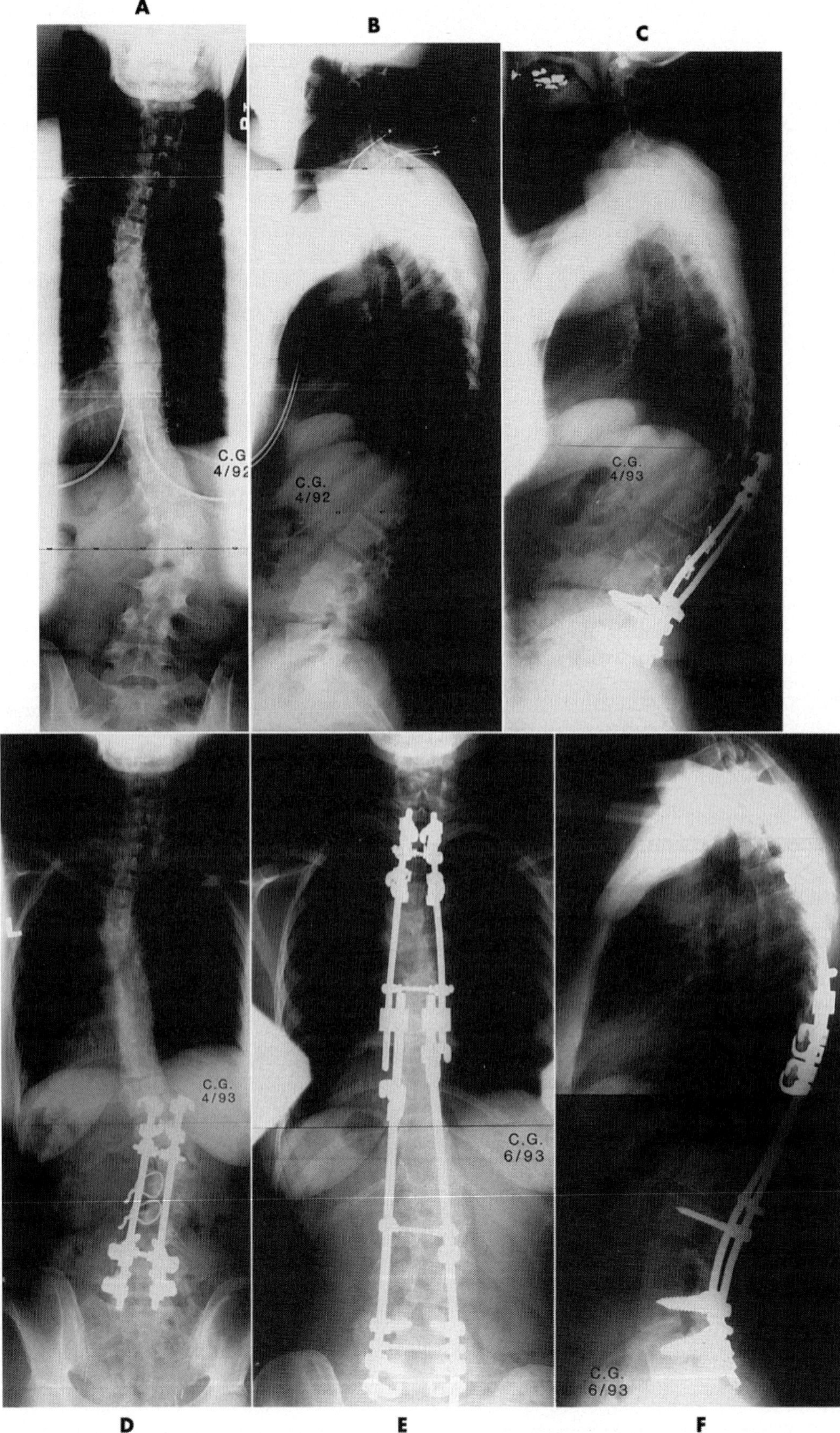


**FIGURE 2-3**

Sagittal balance. De novo scoliosis (**A** and **B**) treated elsewhere with isolated posterior spinal fusion of the lumbar spine to T11, immediately below the apex of the kyphosis (**C** and **D**). Resulting forces lead to a proximal hook pullout three months later and progression of the kyphotic deformity. Implant removal and reimplantation to T1 improved sagittal balance and associated pain symptoms (**E** and **F**). Five millimeter rods in the high dorsal spine prevent metal bulk problems.

fection or neoplasm must be addressed with anterior reconstruction with or without posterior augmentation. The failure of isolated posterior fusion and instrumentation must be addressed with anterior column reconstruction. It is an error to assume that repeat posterior fusion with stiffer instrumentation will alleviate the problem.

### Tumor Problems

A common form of misdiagnosis leading to refractory spine surgery is a failure to recognize spinal tumors. This is typically more common in thoracic conditions. A Mayo Clinic series showed 4% of patients presenting with spine tumors were initially misdiagnosed as having herniated disks.[13] The key to tumor diagnosis is clinical suspicion. Patients with benign intraspinal tumors often sleep more comfortably sitting up while patients with lumbar disk disease almost universally are more comfortable while recumbent. Older patients or those with known or suspected risk factors or a history of malignancy should undergo specific workups to rule out neoplastic causes of their symptoms.

### Rheumatologic Problems

Rheumatoid arthritis, ankylosing spondylitis, and other seronegative spondyloarthropathies can cause neck and back pain and are likely to be misdiagnosed and treated as disk disease. These arthropathies occur in younger patients in which a lack of clinical suspicion allows these entities to be overlooked. The characteristic "double peak" of morning stiffness, relief with activity, and subsequent recurrence of pain with excessive activity should raise suspicion. Arthritis that mimics lumbar disk disease usually causes pain in the lower back or hip, but may be referred to the posterior thigh and may be confused with sciatica. Ankylosing spondylitis can cause pain throughout the entire spine. Osteitis condensans, common in pregnant women or women suffering from endometriosis, can cause low-back pain that mimics spinal stenosis. In younger patients, radiographic changes consistent with degenerative arthritis, spurring, interspace narrowing, and sclerosis of the facet joints may not be present despite pain.

## LATE CAUSES OF REFRACTORY BACK SYNDROME

Nonresponsive spine surgery resulting in symptoms occurring more than 3 months after a procedure are more commonly caused by degeneration, scarring, progressive deformity, or instability. Chronic degeneration and instability can occur within the operative spinal segment, as a result of pseudarthrosis, or, more typically, around a fused segment. As with the early causes, late causes of nonresponsive spine surgery syndrome can be subdivided in an attempt to elucidate causation.

### Neurologic and Pain Problems

Late-onset neurologic and pain problems can typically be attributed to either mechanical or nonmechanical causes. Mechanical causes of pain and neuropathy include degeneration, instability, or progressive deformity. Nonmechanical causes usually can be attributed to scarring.

Mechanical pain syndromes are the most common reason for late-revision spine procedures. Compression of neural elements due to either stenosis of the central canal or lateral recess, instability due to spondylolisthesis or pseudarthrosis, and discogenic causes of back pain are the typical modes of failure. The cause of residual, exacerbated, or new-onset pain resulting from spine surgery is difficult to determine. Many studies[25,81] have documented pain generators associated with deformity and degeneration. Instability after spine procedures generally causes centralized neck and back pain. Patients complain of catching or a sensation of collapse, slipping, or pain with dynamic changes in posture. Instability has specific characteristics when associated with failed spinal decompression for stenosis or after disk excision.

Spinal stenosis either central or lateral, has been documented as the most common cause of nonresponsive spine surgery. Burton, in a review of 725 patients, reported the leading cause of failed spine surgery syndrome was lateral spinal stenosis in 58% and central stenosis in 10% of nonresponsive cases.[10] Typically, this appears to be the result of inadequate initial decompression or decompression of the wrong levels.

Instability can occur after decompression involving sacrifice of an entire facet or 50% of both facets.[1,62] Several studies have documented the development of postoperative spondylolisthesis after posterior decompression.[1,63,66] Patients with postlaminectomy instability have unnecessary pain complaints that involve both the back and the lower extremities. Activity aggravates symptoms, while rest decreases pain. Surgery for this problem should include a posterolateral fusion with instrumentation. A pedicle screw-rod construct works well for patients with multilevel instability.

Instability can occur after diskectomy. Patients typically present with symptoms of low-back pain after a pain-free interval, exacerbated by activity and relieved with rest. In the presence of documented instability posterolateral fusion is indicated.

Spondylolisthesis in the revision candidate usually results from progression of a dysplastic spondylolisthesis (unknown at the initial procedure or inadequately fused) or the development of an acquired spondylolisthesis in the upper segment included in the fusion, the so-called *spondylolysis acquisita*. This type of lesion is common in the presence of a posterior fusion and leads to the development of the posterolateral fusion as a method of preventing this type of lesion. Lytic spondylolisthesis commonly occurs in adjacent segments of long fusions despite uncorrupted anatomy.

Patients who exhibit instability after prior surgical fusions complain of recurrent back and lower-extremity pain after an interval of excellent pain relief. Symptoms though variable in presentation usually occur at an average of 2 years postoperatively. Flexion-extension radiographs reveal gradual deterioration above and below fused segments. This type of degeneration in the segment adjacent to the successful fusion ("transition syndrome") is discussed in a separate section.

The nonmechanical causes of pain or neuropathy in the nonresponsive spine surgery syndrome are caused by neurologic compromise due either to intradural or extradural scarring or processes intrinsic to the spinal cord or peripheral nerve root tissue. LaRocca[47] divided these intrinsic causes of pain into four subtypes of nonresponsive back surgery syndromes: extradural fibrosis, chronic intrinsic radiculopathy, arachnoiditis, and pain centralization of the spinal cord.

***Extradural Fibrosis.*** Cellular activity around the dura postoperatively gives rise to the laminectomy membrane, which can become fibrotic external to the dura and nerve roots in the spinal canal. Fibrous adherence and enlargement around the dura can tether or constrict the dura and ensheathed neural elements leading to chronic compression. If detected early, usually within 3 months, extradural fibrosis may respond to decompression.[47] Extradural fibrosis can usually be delineated on Gd-enhanced MRI.

***Chronic Intrinsic Radiculopathy.*** Chronic compression on neural tissue has been shown both clinically and experimentally to reach a point where irreversible changes take place within the neural tissue. At this point in time, compression-induced ischemia, nutritional insufficiency, or edema renders the nerve permanently damaged and unresponsive to surgical decompression. This entity is difficult to diagnose on MRI and usually requires electromyelographic studies to document severity.

***Arachnoiditis.*** The arachnoid membrane is a thin transparent layer beneath the dura mater, which can become inflamed as a result of spine procedures developing a fibrin exudate that adheres to the nerve roots and thecal sac. Benner and Ehni[5] noted that most cases of arachnoiditis occurred after spine surgery particularly when the procedure had included dural tears, draining wounds, protracted postoperative fever, and excessive bleeding. Wilkinson[79] postulated that unrecognized arachnoiditis may be the primary cause of symptomatology in patients nonresponsive to spine surgery. Nerve root bundling is the characteristic finding of severe arachnoiditis on MRI studies of the lumbar spine.

***Centralization Syndrome.*** This syndrome includes transformations within the spinal cord that become the source of lingering pain. Hyperalgesia, sensitization of nociceptive endings to chemical agents, and deafferentation pain describe different types of centralization syndrome.

## DISK PROBLEMS

Discogenic pain is defined as incapacitating back pain without radicular symptoms, radiographic evidence of neural compression, or segmental hypermobility. Controversy exists about the existence, presentation, and treatment of discogenic back pain. Though the disk itself has no direct innervation, the posterior longitudinal ligament has been shown to be highly innervated. Annular degeneration and bulging is hypothesized to stimulate nociceptors in the posterior longitudinal ligament.

Disk disease can result from progressive degeneration or as a result of an inappropriate choice of fusion levels, incomplete removal of the disk at the time of initial surgery, or reherniation of a treated disk. Weatherley[75] showed five patients with discogenic back pain documented by diskography despite solid posterior fusion. These patients subsequently were relieved with anterior fusion procedures. These results establish the pain-generating capabilities of the nonherniated disk, irritated by motion not completely eliminated by posterior fusion.

Given the inherent debate concerning the existence of discogenic pain, the methods of diagnosis cause similar controversy. Clinically, patients complain of back or neck pain with sclerotomal distribution. Cervical discogenic pain radiates to the superior border of the trapezius, lumbar pain to the buttock and posterior thigh; characteristically, the pain is aggravated by activity or bending.

Several studies suggest that MRI can detect disk disease as accurately as invasive provocative diskography.[32,65] Other studies have documented positive provocative diskograms in patients with a normal MRI.[38,45] A controversial situation exists when the MRI demonstrates a dark disk, indicating decreased hydration and disk degeneration. There is no consensus of scientifically valid studies to guide the physician in the proper treatment. Many authors believe the presence of a dark disk on MRI should be confirmed with diskography.[36,60] Diskography has been a controversial topic since Holt[39] found that 37% of a study group of asymptomatic young men had positive diskograms and concluded that diskography was a nonspecific and unreliable test. Holt's data has recently been challenged particularly in the presence of a pain reproduction criterion, which decreased the false-negative rate of lumbar diskograms to nearly zero in a prospective study of young asymptomatic volunteers.[74] Weatherley et al[75] reported that diskography helped identify the source of symptoms in patients with persistent pain despite posterior and/or later anterior fusion. Byrd noted the importance of diskography to determine if the disk, within a segment to be fused, was symptomatic.[12] He proposed interbody fusion be performed in patients who reported pain after injection. Kostuik reported the role of diskography in the management of adult scoliosis.[46] He believed that diskography played a valuable role in determining if anterior or posterior instrumentation should be used.

Complications associated with diskography include spinal headache, meningitis, discitis, intrathecal hemorrhage, arachnoiditis, severe reaction to accidental intradural injection, and damage to the disk. The rate of complication appears to have declined significantly in recent reports. Authors have expressed concern that diskography may have deleterious effects on the disk itself. Johnson analyzed 80 disks that were injected on two different occasions and found no increased incidence of herniation or annular deterioration.[41] Diskography should be performed only if noninvasive diagnostic tests such as MRI have failed to provide a diagnosis. An MRI should be obtained in a revision candidate to assess the neural canal and disk anatomy. If patients are found to have single level disease no further workup is done. If multilevel disease is encountered then diskography should be undertaken. Diskograms are considered positive if they demonstrate both reproduction and concordant pain and abnormal disk anatomy. Diskography should be viewed as an invasive procedure and should be performed only on patients with symptoms requiring surgery.

Revision surgery for isolated discogenic back pain has been reviewed by several authors. Whitecloud and Seago[72] reported a 70% success rate with anterior cervical interbody fusions for treatment of diskogram-positive cervical pain. Colhoun et al[16] reported an 89% success rate with lumbar fusions for diskogram-positive lumbar pain. Wetzel et al[76] recently reported 46% satisfactory outcome with patients treated with lumbar fusions for discogenic pain. None of these studies were randomized or prospective, and it is unclear whether discogenic pain is best treated with anterior, posterolateral, or circumferential fusion. Our preference is not to perform surgery for perceived discogenic pain until all other conservative modalities have been attempted. Giordano et al[33] documented improvement of discogenic pain with time regardless of treatment. Our experience supports this finding. If surgery is the only remaining treatment and both MRI and provocative diskogram are positive for disk pathology, our preference is to perform circumferential fusion with structural anterior bone or synthetic graft anteriorly and anterior or posterior instrumentation or both.

## Balance Problems

The most common form of dissatisfaction of patients who have undergone surgery to correct deformity is the persistence of the deformity after the first procedure either with or without associated pain. Improper alignment can also be iatrogenic from excessive decompression leading to deformity or improper alignment of previous instrumentation. Residual deformity can typically be explained through specific errors or combinations of errors that precipitate failure. Anatomic spinal alignment is critical as an instrumented or fused segment incorporates more motion segments. Fusions involving one or two segments at noncritical areas of the spine can tolerate improper balance. Improperly aligned fusions over multiple segments, however, lead to increased forces on instrumentation, fusion mass, and adjacent segments.

Scoliosis and kyphosis are problems involving multiple segments, a long column. Curves can be either compensated, with the head centered over the sacrum, or decompensated, with the head not centered over the sacrum. A shift in the center of body mass away from the midline, as occurs in a decompensated spine, introduces a bending moment in addition to the buckling forces described by Euler. The presence of listhesis at individual levels can further complicate spinal balance. Long column imbalance in the revision patient can be due to either inadequate correction during the initial procedure with residual imbalance or progressive decompensation within or around a fusion. Typically, deformity is due to lack of anatomic alignment within the fused segment resulting in a need for the remaining mobile spine to compensate. The most common balance problems requiring revision procedures are progressive kyphosis over a flat lumbar spine fusion, flatback deformity, or degeneration and spondylolisthesis of segments below a fused segment.

To define the pathologic conditions it is necessary to first define normal anatomic balance. Normal coronal alignment is straight. Normal sagittal alignment follows the sagittal vertical axis line (Fig. 2-4). This line falls from C2 in front of T7, behind L3 and across S2 and probably intersects with the trochanteric knee-

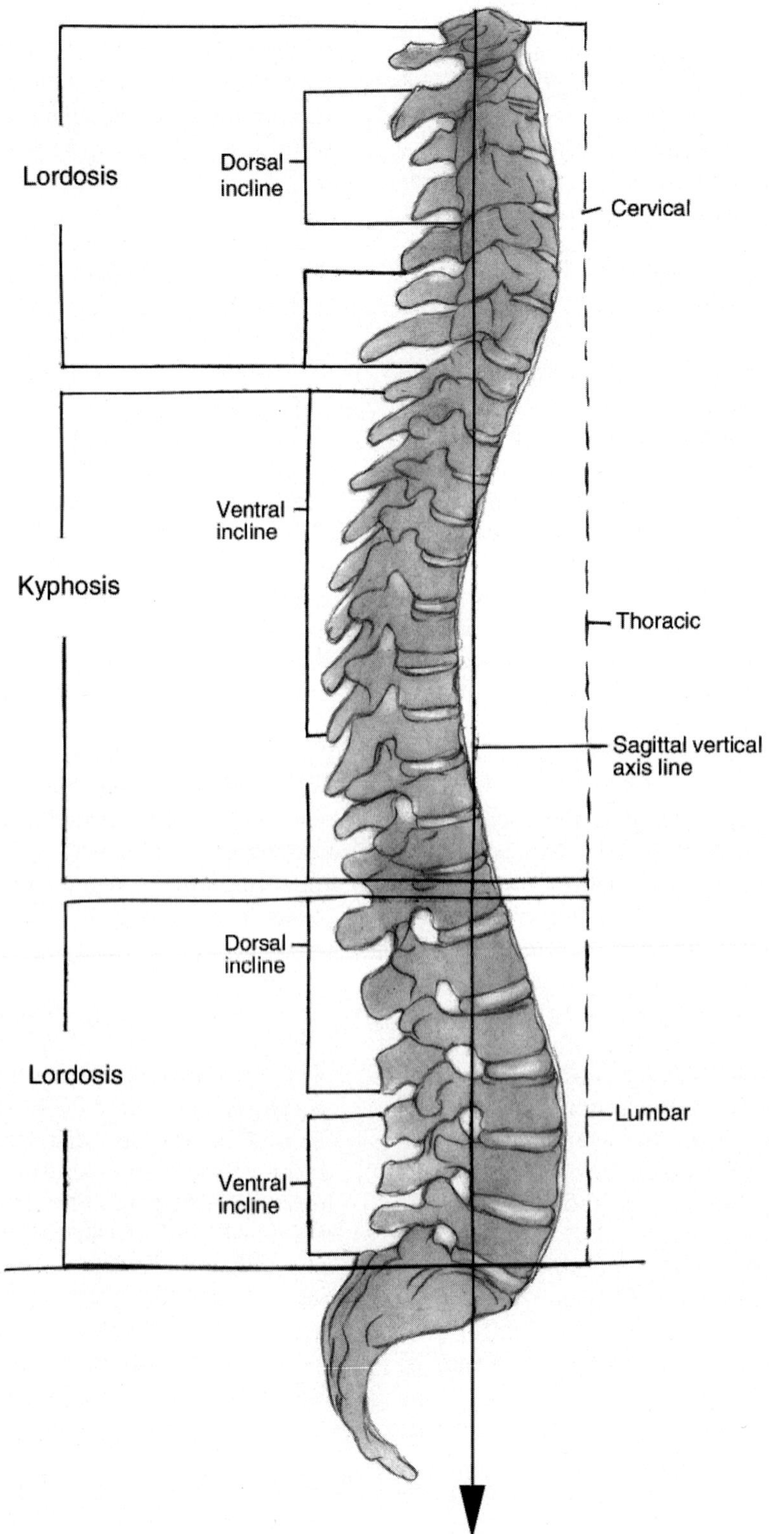


FIGURE 2-4

The sagittal vertical axis line and the orientation of each individual vertebrae. From DeWald RL: Revision surgery for spinal deformity, *Instr Course Lect* 41:236, 1992.

ankle line. In the lumbar spine it is important to note such factors as maximum lordosis (range 32° to 84°; the average is 50°), sacral base slope (range 18° to 66°; the average is 40°), and percent of disk contribution to the maximum lordosis (lumbar disks contribute 80% to maximum lordosis or 47°) (Fig. 2-5).

Specific terminology has been developed to explain specific technical modes of failure causing residual deformity commonly encountered by the revision spine surgeon. These terms describe the iatrogenic causes of nonresponsive spinal surgery:

- **Too-Short Fusion**—This particular situation can occur when the patient has been fused at an early age and the end vertebrae were not correctly identified. The usual result is a decompensated spine with coronal or sagittal plane imbalance.
- **Fallen Over**—This term generally refers to a sudden increase in the scoliotic or kyphotic deformity at the end of the fusion mass. This may be seen when the spine has not been balanced properly and is generally seen in the adult patient in whom the instrumentation did not go above the kyphus.
- **Pseudarthrosis**—Pseudarthrosis represents a failure of fusion. Depending on the location, it may cause increasing deformity with implant failure.
- **Coronal Plane Decompensation**—Coronal plane decompensation generally refers to the dorsal spine not being in line with the midsacral line. In such cases, most of the spine lies outside of the Harrington stable zone.
- **Sagittal Plane Decompensation**—Sagittal plane decompensation is generally seen when the sagittal vertical axis does not fall in front of T7, behind L3, and across S2.
- **Flat Back**—Flat back is a clinical syndrome that results from the loss of lumbar lordosis and normal sacral slope (Fig. 2-6). The patient stays bent forward, the knees are flexed, and the patient complains of pain and fatigue.
- **Rib Hump Deformity**—Rib hump deformity refers to an angular deformity of the ribs on the convex side of the scoliosis.
- **Crankshaft Phenomenon**—Crankshaft phenomenon refers to an increase in the rotation of a growing spine after posterior distraction and fusion caused by isolated anterior spinal growth.
- **Forward Head Thrust**—Forward head thrust is generally seen after kyphosis correction when the cervical lordosis is rigid and cannot spontaneously correct.
- **Wrong Fusion Level Selection**—Wrong fusion level selection generally causes decompensation because the end vertebrae were not in the stable zone.
- **Add-on Phenomenon**—This problem generally occurs in a growing child when the incorrect end vertebrae were selected for the fusion and the scoliosis has progressed above and below the fusion zone. The end vertebrae for fusion are selected conditionally on the posteroanterior radiograph. The end vertebrae must be neutral on the concave bending films, and the disk below should open on both sides on the bending radiographs. The lower end vertebrae must be in the stable zone on the concave bending film and preferably on the standing film. The stable zone is defined by two parallel lines from the lumbosacral facets. The definitive choice of the end vertebrae is determined by the standing lateral radiograph. If the lower vertebrae determined in the frontal plane are at the apex of a junctional kyphosis, the instrumentation must be extended lower, and the hook is reversed to compress the kyphosis to restore the sagittal alignment and avoid decompensation. On the basis of a frontal radiograph, the instrumentation is extended to the next neutral vertebrae.
- **Failure to Recognize the Double Major Curve**—Failure to recognize a double major curve is generally seen when the King classification is used to determine end vertebrae selection for fusion.
- **Failure to Recognize Double Thoracic Curve Pattern**—This situation is generally seen in the upper thoracic curve that does not correct fully on the side-bending radiograph.
- **Wrong Instrumentation Selected**—Generally seen with the use of anterior instrumentation, the spine may fall into kyphosis.

#### FUSION PROBLEMS

Pseudarthrosis is a major cause of late operative failure. Unsuccessful fusion occurs in 3% to 30% of fusions performed, with the incidence directly related to number of levels fused and the type of procedure performed. The incidence of pseudarthrosis in procedures to correct sagittal deformity is low in children and adolescents, but increases with procedures performed on adult patients. Combined anterior and posterior procedures are superior to posterior procedures alone.[11] The pseudarthrosis rate in kyphosis surgery is affected by the degree of deformity. Posterior fusion alone in curves between 50° and 75° results in a 75% pseudarthrosis rate.[82] Strut grafts placed too far anteriorly in contact with the apex or not properly countersunk can fracture or become dislodged. The incidence of pseudarthrosis in primary surgery for spondylolisthesis varies with techniques used, degree of slip, and method of postoperative immobilization. Incomplete disk excision and endplate removal contribute to pseudarthrosis. Although the incidence of pseudarthrosis is high, rigid or loadsharing instrumentation and meticulous surgical techniques including decortication, facetectomies, and autogenous bone graft with growth factor augmentation may lower the incidence.

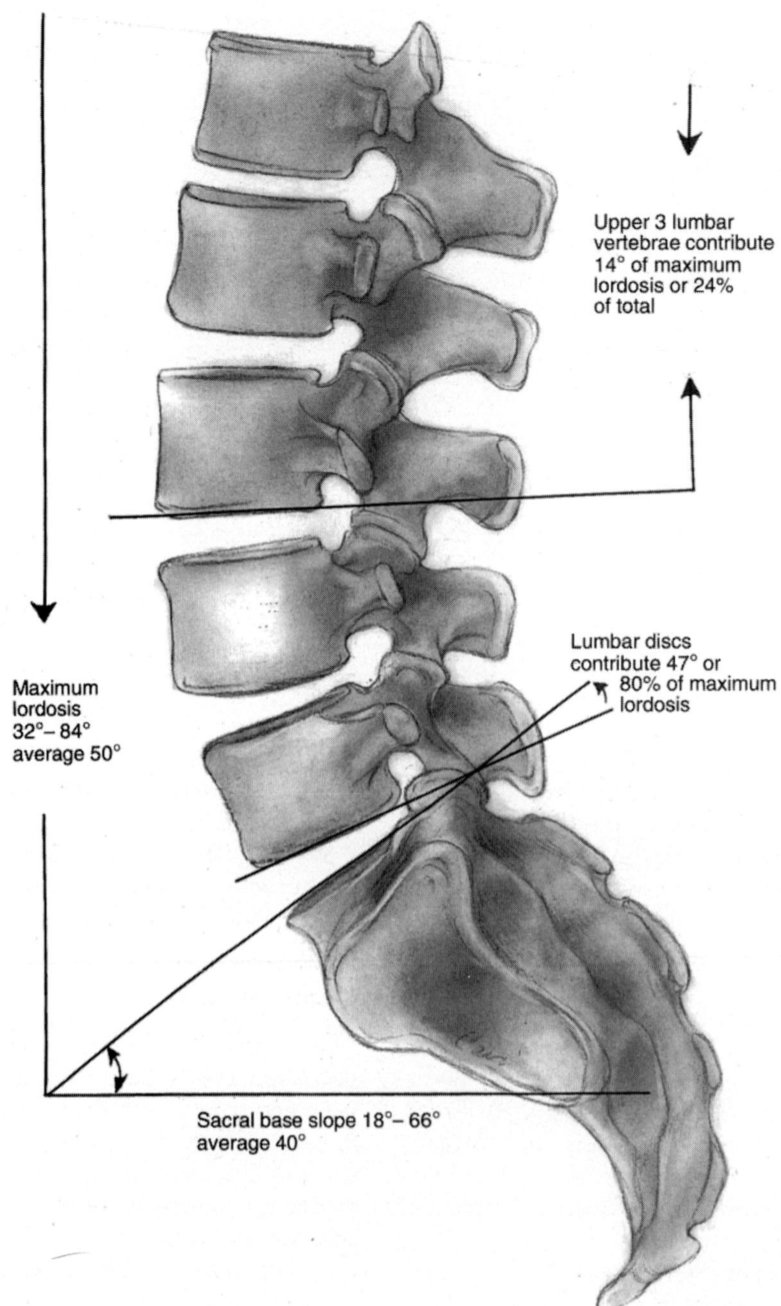


**FIGURE 2-5**

Average maximum lordosis as measured from superior L1 to superior S1; the average sacral slope as measured from superior S1 to the horizontal; the degree the disks contribute to maximum lordosis; and by inference the degrees the vertebral bodies contribute to maximum lordosis. From DeWald RL: Revision surgery for spinal deformity, *Instr Course Lect* 41:240, 1992.

There are multiple risk factors for the development of pseudarthrosis. Cigarette smoking, a history of inadequate postoperative immobilization, a history of previous failed fusion, and the use of allograft should arouse suspicion. Pseudarthrosis is also directly related to the number of levels fused.[14,40] The use of allograft has been shown to be inferior to autograft from posterolateral fusion,[2,43] particularly when autograft was sterilized with ethylene oxide and freeze-dried.

A contribution to the wide discrepancy in the reported incidence of pseudarthrosis is related to the difficulty of diagnosis. Pseudarthrosis is often asympto-

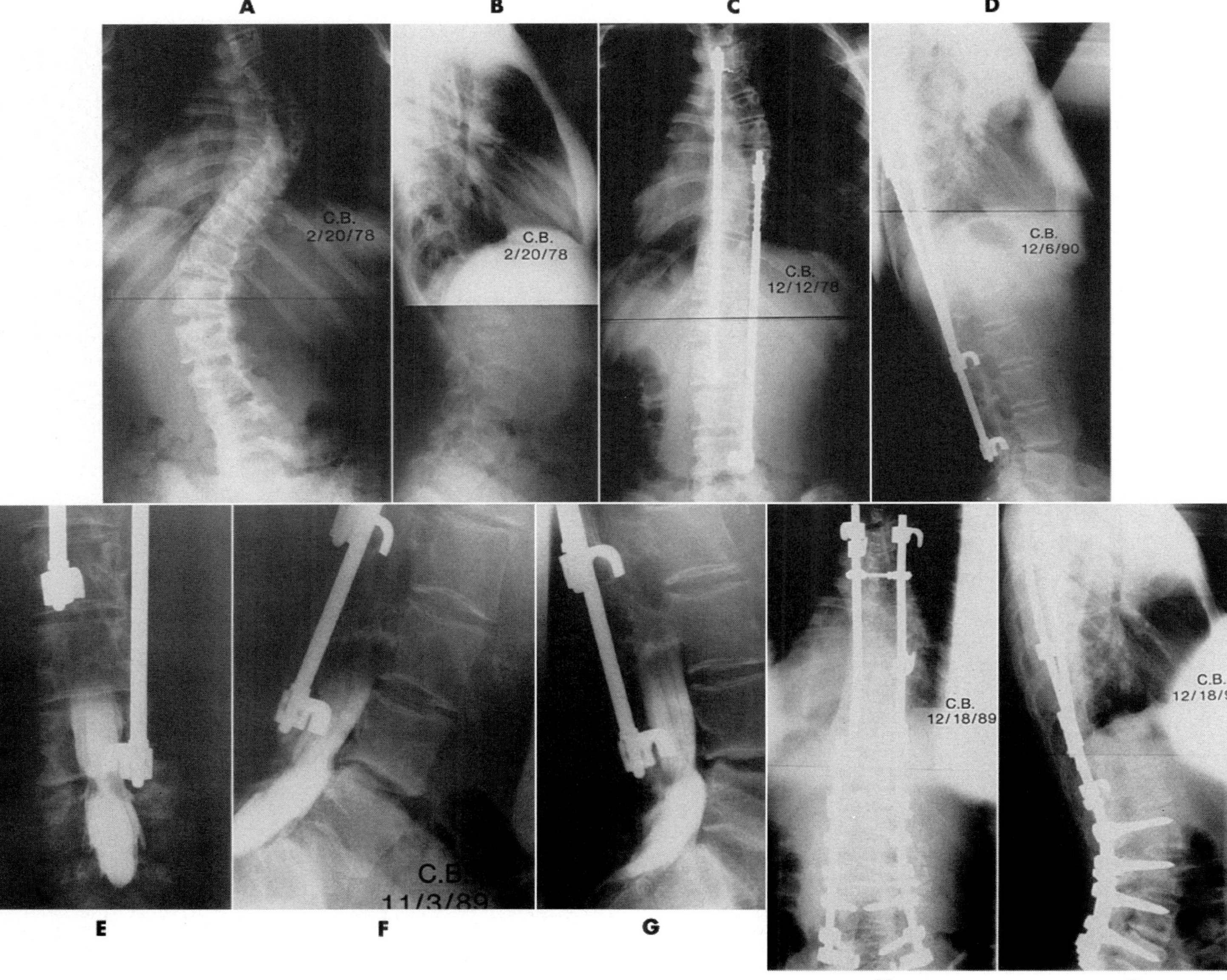


**FIGURE 2-6**

Flat back syndrome. Patient presented (**A–D**) 12 years postoperative, when a pain syndrome developed and myelography (**E**) revealed a defect at L4-L5 below the last fused level. Surgical decompression elsewhere failed to relieve the pain. The flexion-extension myelogram shows instability at L4-L5 (**F** and **G**). Implant removal, oseotomy, and reimplantation were performed (**H** and **I**). Note the restitution of harmonious lumbar lordosis and the proper orientation of the individual vertebrae. L5 was included in this construction because of the instability between L4 and L5.

matic or presents with nonspecific symptoms that vary from vague to disabling pain. Pseudarthrosis is difficult to detect with routine radiographs and imaging is difficult. Many patients remain asymptomatic despite radiographic evidence of pseudarthrosis. The hallmarks of pseudarthrosis are progression of deformity, loss of correction, instrumentation failure, and persistent pain. The incidence of pseudarthrosis in previously instrumented fusions without instrument failure has been reported to be low. Dickson et al[20] conducted a 21-year follow-up on 211 patients treated with Harrington instrumentation. A broken rod was seen in 41% of patients, but the pseudarthrosis repair rate was 17%. Blumenthal and Gill[7] explored the fusion mass in 49 patients undergoing instrumentation removal for one- or two-level posterior or posterolateral lumbar fusions. The overall agreement between radiographic instrumentation failure and surgical findings was 69%. The revision surgeon must always be aware that pseudarthroses may be the presentation of an occult or subclinical infection.

Pseudarthrosis may be detected in 70% of plain radiographs.[48] Radiographic evaluation of suspected pseudarthrosis should include oblique and flexion-extension radiographs. Tomograms, CT, and scintigraphy may be necessary in questionable cases. Tomography increases the rate of diagnosis to 96%.[18] A continuous trabecular pattern traversing the graft segment is consistent with a solid fusion.[70] CT has proven useful in the diagnosis of pseudarthrosis. Direct coronal imaging and the use of three-dimensional CT scanning have been shown to improve the rate of diagnosis over conventional CT.[86] Bone and single photon emission CT (SPECT) scanning in the diagnosis of pseudarthrosis is controversial and has been shown to be accurate in 50% of surgically explored patients.[57]

Techniques for the revision of failed posterior fusions are determined based on the number of levels requiring fusion, the adequacy of posterior element bone stock, and access to the spinal canal through scar tissue. Patients with failed posterior fusion and adequate bone stock who do not require further decompression, should be treated with decortication and augmentation of the posterolateral fusion. Patients with insufficient posterior bone stock should be treated with staged anterior interbody fusion followed by posterolateral fusion augmentation. Patients requiring further decompression can be treated with posterior lumbar interbody fusion (PLIF) if scar tissue can be dissected from the canal or a second-stage anterior lumbar interbody fusion (ALIF) if access can not be obtained. Pseudarthrosis at two or more levels requires interbody fusion, either posterior, if scar tissue can be removed, or anterior if not. Anterior procedures should be reconsidered in the presence of previous abdominal surgery. Instrumentation is recommended when more than two levels require fusion. Patients with pseudarthrosis after anterior fusions in the absence of previous attempts at posterior fusions should undergo revision posterolateral fusion. A failed anterior fusion with a previous posterior fusion should have circumferential fusion with ALIF and augmentation of the posterolateral fusion mass. Anterior procedures in the absence of available structural autograft should be performed with structural allograft supplemented with cancellous autograft. Femoral ring, vertebral body, or synthetic structural fusion grafts or cages can be used. Vertebral body allograft is used at our institution instead of femoral ring allograft. Theoretical advantages of these grafts include better cortical contact and fit due to similar diameter and size and similar material properties to the vertebral body. The efficacy of synthetic materials in augmentation of fusion remains to be determined as does the long-term suitability of various interbody cage devices.

Instrumentation has been shown to enhance fusion rates. Zdeblick,[84] in a prospective study of 253 patients, found enhanced fusion rates in patients undergoing posterolateral fusions compared to patients fused without instrumentation. The study did not differentiate the fusion rates based on specific levels fused or document preoperative instability. The L5-S1 interspace is inherently more stable than the L4-L5 interspace and should as a result have a higher rate of fusion regardless of the use of instrumentation. In lumbar fusion procedures, we uniformly instrument upper-lumbar segments but only add instrumentation at the L5-S1 level when a perceived instability is present. Our threshold for instability, however, is less than the 4 mm reported in the literature. Any perceived motion of flexion-extension films is considered an instability at L5-S1 requiring pedicular instrumentation.

Pseudarthrosis is the most common late complication of fusion procedures in the cervical spine. Pseudarthrosis is common in anterior procedures and less frequent in posterior procedures. Nonunion in multilevel anterior fusions has been reported to be as high as 63%.[83] The risk of pseudarthrosis increases with the number of levels grafted with Robinson-type grafts.[8]

The presence of symptoms associated with cervical pseudarthrosis is approximately 50%. Bohlman et al[8] reported 75% of pseudarthrosis patients were symptomatic. Symptoms typically manifest as radiculopathy. Studies have shown that pseudarthrosis in the cervical spine can coalesce with immobilization up to 1 year later. Unlike lumbar fusion, pseudarthrosis in the cervical spine can typically be diagnosed on plain radiographs, particularly flexion-extension views.

Revision fusion can be done either anteriorly or posteriorly with similar results. Fibular strut grafts have shown lower pseudarthrosis rates. Seating the graft in the vertebral body rather than on the anterior lip[8] or in the notch improves fusion rate. Most authors recommend decompression and fusion. Lateral mass plates can be used to augment a multiple-level fusion. Lowery reviewed three different methods of revision for failed anterior fusions finding posterior fusions with lateral mass plating to be the most effective form of revision procedure.[52] Brodsky et al[9] performed a randomized study comparing revision anterior surgery with posterior fusion and posterior wiring for anterior pseudarthrosis. In the posterior fusion group, they reported 88% good or excellent clinical results with a 94% fusion percentage. In the anterior fusion group they reported 59% good or excellent clinical results with a 79% fusion percentage. Farey et al[27] have noted consolidation of failed anterior fusion mass after successful posterior revision arthrodesis.

## Adjacent-Level Problems

Fusion of the spine shifts the center of motion to levels adjacent to the fusion, putting increased stress on the disk and facet joints. Late onset of back or neck pain in a patient with a fused spine can be caused by degeneration and instability at levels adjacent to the fusion. Frymoyer[29] reported adjacent disk degeneration in 5 of 143 patients treated with disk excision and fusion. Lehman[50] found adjacent level degeneration in 45% of fusion patients. Lee[49] reported on the pathologic facet hypertrophy and spinal stenosis in adjacent segments causing recurrent neck and low-back pain after a lumbar fusion. Disk degeneration and herniation, spondylolisthesis, and spondylolysis also contribute, but are not as common. Degeneration is more common at distal unfused segments but may occur proximally (Fig. 2-7). Deformity, particularly junctional kyphosis, or progression of a curve can occur proximal to the fusion. Cochran et al[15] reported an increasing incidence of low-back pain with fusion below L4, particularly when Harrington rod instrumentation was used without rod contouring. Late onset of back pain may be related to the use of distraction instrumentation in the lower spine. Luk[53] and coworkers studied the effect on the lumbosacral spine of a long-spine fusion in 22 adolescents with idiopathic scoliosis with an average follow-up of 12.8 years. The unfused intervertebral spaces were hypermobile distally, which may be a predisposing factor to degeneration and pain or neuropathy.

Cervical spine degeneration at adjacent levels is less common than in the thoracic or lumbar spine due to more evenly distributed motion among adjacent segments in the cervical spine as compared to the thoracic or lumbar spine where stress is concentrated in those segments immediately adjacent to a fusion.[30] Bohlman and associates[8] showed a 9% incidence of adjacent-level disease in patients who underwent anterior diskectomy and fusion.

In revision surgery the role of diskography is for the assessment of disk integrity above and below previously fused segments, assessment to determine presence of painful pseudarthrosis or symptomatic disks in posterior fused segments, or to determine whether previously decompressed disks require interbody fusion. Diskography should be performed only if noninvasive diagnostic tests such as MRI have failed to provide a diagnosis. Diskography should be viewed as an invasive procedure and should be performed only on patients with symptoms requiring surgery.

Whitecloud[78] reviewed 14 patients who underwent fusions of adjacent levels around previous lumbosacral fusions. Only 5 of the 14 patients had good results. There was a pseudarthrosis rate of 80% in patients treated without instrumentation and 17% in patients treated with instruments. Recommendations were for transpedicular instrumentation when fusing adjacent-level disease.

## Infection

Late postoperative spinal infections are usually considered to occur at least 2 weeks after the procedure and are characterized by a paucity of findings. Patients describe an initial period of decreasing postoperative pain followed by onset of increasing spinal pain, occasionally accompanied by mild to moderate temperature elevations. Pain may often radiate to the abdomen, pelvis, or thigh. Rarely, a patient will demonstrate an acute septic course after surgery. The wound often appears normal, and pain can be elicited with deep palpation or percussion. Physical exam may reveal tension signs and paravertebral muscle spasms.

Postoperative discitis typically presents several weeks to months after the initial procedure. The incidence varies from less than 1% in lumbar discectomy with prophylactic antibiotics to 35% in fusion procedures using instrumentation. Definitive diagnosis of postoperative discitis can be established only by closed-needle biopsy. Cases of late-onset discitis can be treated with antibiotics, bedrest, and immobilization. Indications for surgery in late-onset discitis include the presence of an abscess demonstrating considerable vertebral body destruction and deformity or compression of neural structures. This is particularly true in the cervical spine where the threshold for surgical intervention should be lower than for more caudal elements.

Patients with spinal instrumentation occasionally demonstrate late-onset infection by hematogenous seeding. Typically, a remote infection site or parental violation is identified as the source of infection. Clinical presentation typically demonstrates overt sepsis and occasional spontaneous purulent drainage from a previous surgical site. Medical management is usually unsuccessful and the patient is best treated surgically with aggressive debridement, instrumentation removal, and closure over suction drainage system in the

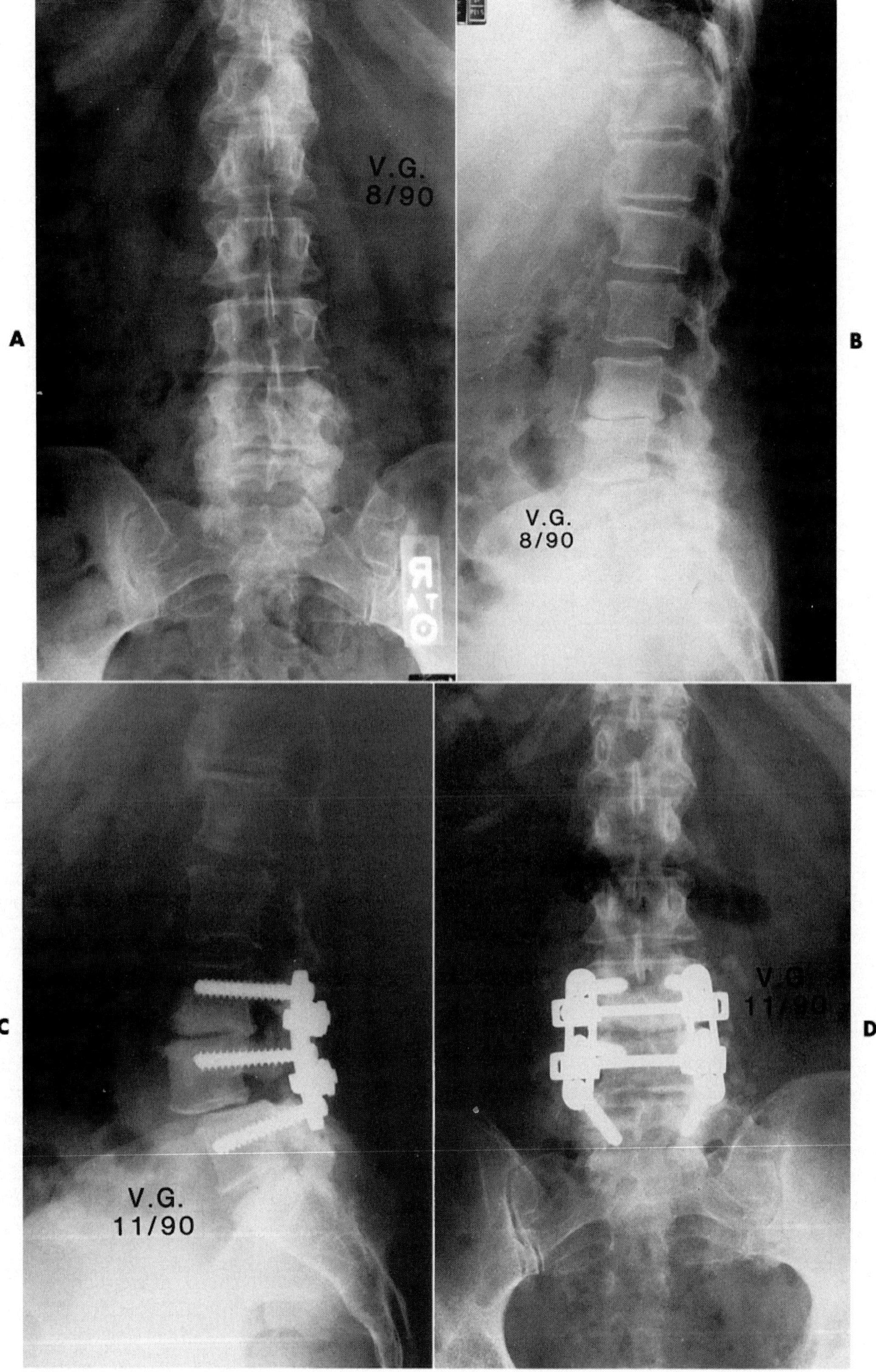


**FIGURE 2-7**

Transition syndrome. L4-L5 spondylolisthesis and disk degeneration at L3-L4 (**A** and **B**) treated with posterior spinal fusion L3 to L5 (**C** and **D**).

*Continued*

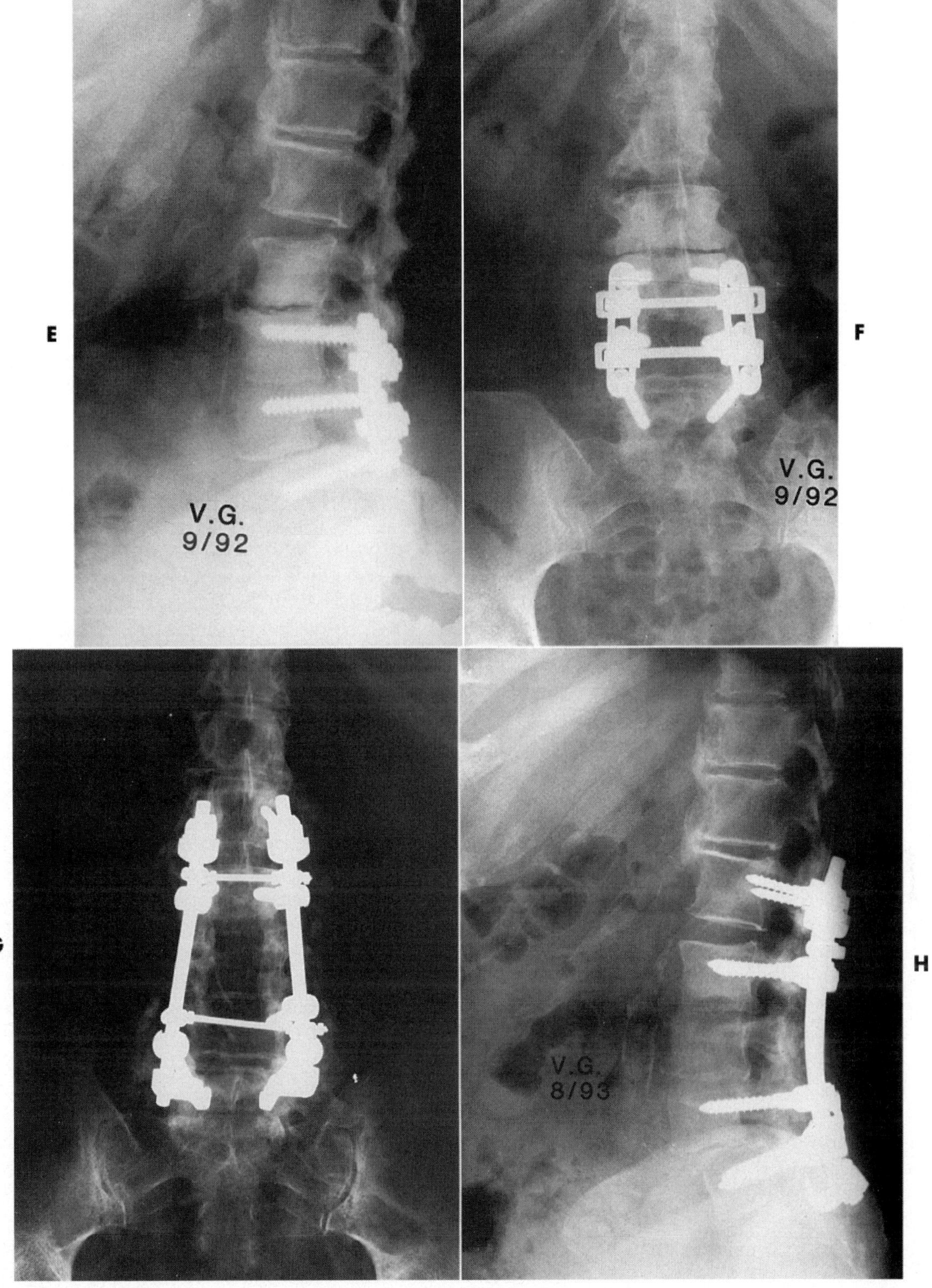


**FIGURE 2-7, CONT'D**

Pain developed three years later (**E** and **F**). Note the collapse of the adjacent disk and nonmarginal syndesmophytes above L1 contributing to the forces transferred across L1-L2 and L2-L3. Fusion of the degenerated disk at L2-L3 would result in similar degeneration at L1-L2. Implant removal and reimplantation to L1 was performed with resolution of symptoms (**G** and **H**).

presence of a solid fuson. If the fusion has failed to heal or a pseudarthrosis exists, a thorough debridement should be performed but consideration should be given to leaving the hardware in place in a hope that the spine will fuse. Augmentation of the fusion site should not be performed until the infection has clinically resolved. Glassman[35] reported on the successful use of antibiotic-impregnated polymethylmethacrylate beads in the treatment of lumbar spine infections without removal of instrumentation in 19 patients.

## CONSIDERATION FOR SURGERY

Once a decision to proceed with revision surgery has been made, extensive preoperative planning is required to ensure as uncomplicated an operative procedure as possible. Fastidious review of the clinical and radiographic information should be performed, if possible in a group setting, so the opinions and criticisms of colleagues can be integrated into the formulation of a plan for surgery that addresses all possible causes of the patient's symptoms and allows consideration of all surgical alternatives.

Diagnosis and prognosis are of extreme importance when considering revision surgery. Clinical and radiographic assessment may provide a clear reason for failure of the initial surgery, but more often than not, the cause of the patient's symptoms are vague or are a combination of several factors requiring that multiple surgical problems be addressed adding to the complexity of the case. Knowledge of the complications associated with specific entities and prognosis with revision procedures are critical in planning the extent of the surgical intervention. Congenital scoliosis is a very rigid defect, is difficult to correct, and carries with it a high risk of neurologic complication. Patients with paralytic scoliosis associated with amyotonia, hypotonia, cerebral palsy, or muscular dystrophy may not be good candidates for revision surgery. A patient with a diagnosis of idiopathic scoliosis usually has an excellent prognosis after revision.

The age and health of the patient must be taken into consideration. The typical revision patient is a chronic pain patient with possible chemical dependency and nutritional problems. It is better to rehabilitate patients physically, mentally, and nutritionally before undertaking revision spine surgery. In some cases, concurrent medical problems can rule out spine surgery.

The number of previous operations is a factor in analyzing the patient's ability to withstand the rigors of spine surgery. Nonresponsive spine patients will endure severe surgical morbidity if they feel it will improve their disfigurement, improve their function, or relieve their pain. The revision patient has been through a spine procedure before and typically has more realistic expectations than for previous procedures. If their expectations are not met, however, depression may ensue. It is thus important to anticipate the patient's expected outcome.

The length of time required for surgery must be considered in planning the number of operations to be done. Surgical team fatigue is a consideration. Same-day surgery is preferred, but to begin the second stage of a procedure after 7 to 8 hours is not in the patient's best interest. Recovery, however, is faster and the patient's nutrition is better[54] with same-day or simultaneous procedures. These judgments must be made during a planning session. If osteotomy and intercurrent traction are required, a staged procedure is indicated. On occasion, simultaneous surgery is necessary. This situation usually arises when both columns are to be osteomized and fused. This procedure is used when the spine is in kyphus and the desire is to place the lumbar segments in lordosis or for vertibrectomies or hemivertibrectomies. An important planning step is to ensure the availability of replacement surgeons in case the procedure becomes involved.

The predicted blood loss is dependent both on the length and type of procedure. Anticipation of expected blood loss is important in planning for the amount of autologous blood that should be donated preoperatively. Correct positioning on a four-poster frame with a free abdomen is valuable for control of blood loss and for correction of the osteotomized spine. The routine use of a cell saver and infusion of autologous fresh frozen plasma also help to decrease the need for blood replacement.

The location of the deformity is an important consideration in preoperative planning. If only the rib hump is a concern, thoracoplasty may be all that is needed. If imbalance is a problem, the surgeon must judge how he can balance the spine. Location of the deformity can be assessed with a bending film. The surgeon should typically not expect to obtain better correction than that seen on the bending films. The choice of type of instrumentation and levels vary depending on the amount of correction that can be obtained. The sagittal plane imbalance is more noticeable than coronal plane imbalance and can usually be improved regardless of the rigidity of the deformity. There is a general consensus among revision deformity surgeons that the more osteotomies performed for rigid deformities the better final correction. If a spine has been fused both anteriorly and posteriorly then both sides must be osteotomized at multiple levels.

Bone quality and availability of bone graft is a consideration. Osteoporosis limits the amount of force that a surgeon can apply to correct the deformity and may influence the decision to use pedicle screws or hooks and the number of levels necessary to ensure stability. Allograft bone is suitable for spine fusions. Irradiation of the graft reduces the risk of human immunodeficiency virus and other infectious processes.

## SURGERY

Revision surgery of the spine is a technically demanding undertaking that requires patience, a solid foundation in anatomy, and extreme caution.

The surgical procedure can be divided into three major parts. The first is careful dissection of the scar tissue, exploration, preparation of the bony surfaces, and removal of hardware. The second is anterior and/or posterior osteotomy of the spine if correction of rigid deformity is required. The third includes harvesting of bone graft and fusion, either anterior, posterior, or both, with or without instrumentation, to correct alignment and ensure stability. A fourth step is the application of intercurrent skeletal traction, especially for rigid coronal plane deformities.

Positioning the patient appropriately prior to the procedure is of greater significance in the revision procedure than in the primary procedure simply because of the increased length of time required for revision. Neurologic complications related to intraoperative positioning (brachial plexus palsy or lateral femoral cutaneous nerve palsy) may be correlated with the length of the procedure.

The surgical exploration of the spine after previous spine surgery is technically difficult and requires patience. Dural tears are common with a history of previous laminectomy and decompression. Instrumentation must be carefully removed because dural adhesions can attach to hooks or wires that traverse the canal. It is not uncommon for the first stage of the procedure to take longer than the second. Exploration of the posterior fusion mass should include periodic attempts to define pseudarthrosis; pressure on the fusion mass or traction using towel clips can usually delineate a pseudarthrosis, even those that could not be diagnosed by radiographic studies. Entrance into the canal should be done in a way to preserve the integrity of the fusion mass, if possible. Calcified disks can be drilled or burred to decompress neural elements. Exploration of the canal and lateral recess with necessary decompression must be performed at appropriate levels.

Osteotomies are used to correct residual deformity in rigid spines that have undergone previous fusion or autofused secondary to degeneration. Kostuik[46] reported on 85 patients with severe rigid deformities requiring osteotomy. Thirty-two patients required intermittent halo-femoral traction and 53 underwent halo-pelvic traction. Forty patients had anterior osteotomies. The degree of correction averaged over 40% with halo-pelvic traction and 32% for halo-femoral traction.

Extensive decompression and pseudarthrosis as well as deformity require fusion. Instrumentation should be considered in patients who smoke, are over 50 years of age, have risk factors for pseudarthrosis, or require correction of deformity. The choice of rigid or load-sharing instrumentation is based on the use of anterior structural bone grafting. Load-sharing pedicle instrumentation is believed to enhance anterior fusion rates. Structural allograft, metal, or carbon fiber cages should be used when alignment requires a rigid anterior structural support and load-sharing constructs are going to be used posteriorly. Deformity correction in revision surgery is best performed using posterior hook and rod constructs for long scoliotic deformities and anterior instrumentation for shorter segment deformity in patients with good vertebral bone stock.

### ANTERIOR SURGERY

If anterior surgery is required for mobilization or circumferential fusion, the standard thoracoabdominal approach is used. The appropriate rib is typically that which leads to the interspace two levels above the most superior vertebrae to be operated upon. The incision extends 3 to 4 cm from the spinous process and follows the rib to the costal chondral junction. The incision then proceeds down the abdomen midway between the umbilicus and the anterior superior iliac spine. It usually ends just caudad to the anterior superior iliac spine unless the L5-S1 disk space is to be included in the procedure. The diaphragm is incised close to its insertion down to the spine. Care is taken to preserve the segmental vessels. Diskectomies are performed with care taken to preserve the endplates that block subsistence of anterior structural graft.

A spine previously fused anteriorly is osteotomized through the previous incision. Anterior implants are usually covered with a bursa and easily removed. Osteotomies are performed back to the posterior longitudinal ligament.

### POSTERIOR SURGERY

The operation begins with excision of the old scar. The usual method is to only expose the lower half of the spine to save blood, if complete dissection is anticipated. Dissections are carried lateral to the spinous process from normal levels into the previously operated segment. This keeps the surgeon lateral to the canal, which is difficult to identify owing to scar tissue and lack of normal anatomic landmarks. Previous instrumentation can also be found in this area and is helpful in identifying spinal levels.

The removal of hardware must be done systematically and with care. Sublaminar wires are typically the most dangerous form of instrumentation and should be removed first. The removal of wires requires removing bone from around the crimp and placing tension on the wire, pulling taut against the anterior surface of the lamina. The wire is then cut close to the lamina while maintaining tension and removed with a smooth even motion. It is important that the wire be freely moveable before it is removed to avoid injuring the dura. Old rods are then cut and removed with the hooks or screws still in place. Sometimes the hooks can become adherent to the underlying dura and should be removed with care. If leaks occur, they must be closed either primarily or with a graft.

If osteotomies are to be performed they are placed in a chevron-type fashion through what were previously the facet joints of the spine. Chevron osteotomies are preferable because they provide medial, lateral, and rotational stability (Fig. 2-8). The actual technique of osteotomy varies depending on the situation. Sometimes it is possible to use a hook site for a beginning or to begin where the sublaminar wires were removed. It is important to use a spreader to obtain ample space to undercut the osteotomy so that the nerve roots are free after correction. It is very important to do as many osteotomies as possible. Usually the lower lumbar spine must be osteotomized, because these vertebrae are the ones that must be moved considerably to correct the sagittal alignment and achieve balance. Positioning the patient on a four-poster frame allows the spine to fall into lordosis after osteotomy.

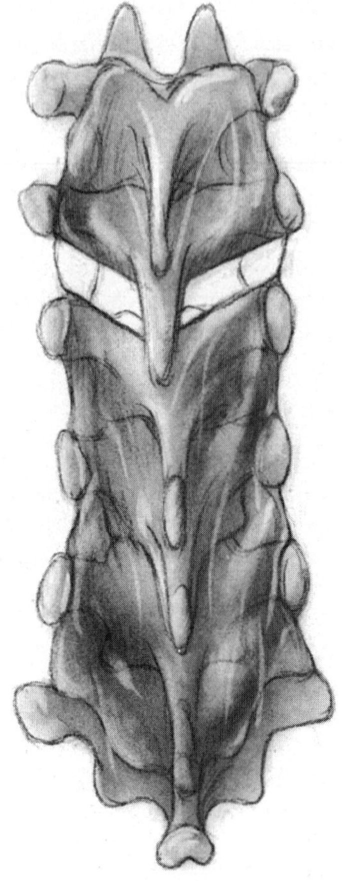

**FIGURE 2-8**

Posterior osteotomy. A posterior spine fusion of a thoracic spine. The osteotomy is outlined and is in the shape of a chevron, with the base inferior and the ends going across the old inferior facet to the intervertebral foramen. From DeWald RL: Revision surgery for spinal deformity, *Instr Course Lect* 41:241, 1992.

If the patient had a previous laminectomy, it is imperative that the surgeon find the pedicles and the roots, because it may be necessary to use pedicle screws for fixation. In the presence of an entrapment syndrome a thorough decompression must be performed. It may be necessary to remove lamina, to remove facet joints, or to extend the instrumentation inferiorly one level. If the lamina is to be removed, a pedicle screw is needed at that level. If the disk is healthy, it is sometimes possible to end the fusion one level higher by performing a facet arthroplasty through the old facet joint. A facet arthroplasty is a technique developed for the facets when the disk above is normal; it is accomplished by removing the fibrous scar and replacing it with fat.

Cotrel-Dubousset instrumentation can be used to rotate the deformity into normal lordosis. Pedicle screws are better than hooks because they place the rotation force more laterally. Reinstrumentation is performed from the last motion segment in the Harrington stable zone with a good disk below to the highest motion segment in the midsacral line above the kyphus. This arrangement balances the coronal plane. In the sagittal plane the amount of thoracic kyphosis must equal the amount of lumbar lordosis to balance the spine.

## COMPLICATIONS

Surgical complications peculiar to revision surgery are typically related to the lack of anatomical landmarks and scarring from the previous procedure. Dural adhesions and tears are significantly more common and difficult to recognize and repair. As a rule, a Valsalva maneuver should be performed prior to closure to ensure that inadvertent durotomy did not occur. Revision patients are at greater risk for neurologic or vascular injury for similar reasons. The deteriorated nutritional and medical status of revision candidates increases the likelihood of wound problems, infection, and continued postoperative medical complications. A common complication after revision surgery, particularly in patients with deformity, is dissatisfaction with regard to cosmesis.

## CONCLUSION

Revision surgery of the spine is demanding, difficult, dangerous, and emotionally draining for both the surgeon and the patient. To achieve the best result, the surgeon must be conscious of the causes of the patient's nonresponsiveness to the initial procedure(s), be suspicious and knowledgeable of alternate diagnoses, meticulous in planning, and must execute a demanding surgical procedure with precision and care.

## REFERENCES

1. Abumi K, Panjabi MM, Kramer K et al: Biomechanical evaluation of lumbar spine stability after graded facetectomies, *Spine* 15:1142, 1990.
2. An HS, Lynch KB, Toth JM: Prospective comparison of autograft vs. allograft for spinal fusion: differences among freeze dried, frozen and mixed grafts, *J Spin Dis* 8:131, 1995.
3. Apel DM, Marrero G, Goldie WD, King J, Tolo VT, Bassett GS: *Avoiding paraplegia during anterior spinal surgery: The role of SSEP monitoring during temporary occlusion of segmental spinal arteries,* Presented at Scoliosis Research Society, Honolulu, HI, 1990, p 363.
4. Bassett GS, Johnson C, Stanley P, Tolo VT: *Spinal angiography vs. SSEP monitoring with temporary occlusion of segmental vessels during anterior spinal surgery,* Presented at POSNA, Memphis, TN, 1994.
5. Benner B, Ehni G: Spinal arachnoiditis. The postoperative variety in particular, *Spine* 3:40, 1978.
6. Biedermann L: Biomechanics of pedicle fixation as related to implant design, Presented at the American-European Meeting on Pedicle Fixation of the Spine and Other Advanced Techniques, Munich, Germany, 1994.
7. Blumenthal SL, Gill K: Can lumbar spine radiographs accurately determine fusion in postoperative patients?, *Spine* 18:1186, 1993.
8. Bohlman HH, Emery SE, Goodfellow DB, Jones PK: Robinson anterior cervical discectomy and arthrodesis for cervical radiculopathy, *J Bone Joint Surg* 75A:1298, 1993.
9. Brodsky AE, Khalil MA, Sassard WR, Newman BP: Repair of symptomatic pseudarthrosis of anterior cervical fusion: posterior versus anterior repair, *Spine* 17:1137-1143, 1992.
10. Burton CV, Kirkaldy Willis WH, Yong-Hung K et al: Causes of failure of surgery of the lumbar spine, *Clin Orthop* 157:191, 1981.
11. Byrd JA, Scoles PV, Winter RB, Bradford DS, Lonstein JE, Moe JH: Adult idiopathic scoliosis treated by anterior and posterior spinal fusion, *J Bone Joint Surg* 69A:843, 1987.
12. Byrd JA III: *The value of diskography for the selection of fusion levels in patients with low back pain,* Presented to the North American Spine Society, Boston, July, 1992.
13. Camissa FP, Glasser D, Lave J et al: Chondrosarcoma of the spina and sacrum, *Orthop Trans* 11:578, 1987.
14. Chow SP, Leong JCY, Ma A, Yau ACM: Anterior spinal fusion of deranged lumbar intervertebral disk—a review of 97 cases, *Spine* 5:452, 1980.
15. Cochran T, Irstam L, Nachemson A: Long-term anatomic and functional changes in patients with adolescent idiopathic scoliosis treated with Harrington rod fusion, *Spine* 18:576, 1983.
16. Colhoun E, McCal :W, Williams L et al: Provocation diskography as a guide to planning operations of the spine, *J Bone Joint Surg Br* 70:267, 1988.
17. Cunningham BW, Sefter JC, Shono Y, McAfee PC: Static and cyclical biomechanical analysis of pedicle screw spinal constructs, *Spine* 18:1677, 1993.
18. Dawson EG, Clader EJ, Bassett LW: A comparison of different methods used to diagnose pseudarthrosis in posterior spine fusion for scoliosis, *J Bone Joint Surg* 67A:1153, 1985.
19. Dhar S, Porter RW: Failed lumbar spine surgery, *Int Orthop* 16:152, 1992.
20. Dickson JH, Erwing WD, Rossi D: Harrington instrumentation and arthrodesis for idiopathic scoliosis (a 21 year follow-up), *J Bone Joint Surg* 72A:678, 1990.
21. Dwyer AF: A fatal complication of paravertebral infection and traumatic aneurysm following Dwyer instrumentation. In: *Proceedings of the Australian Orthopaedic Association, J Bone Joint Surg Br* 61:239, 1979.
22. Ebeling U, Kalbareyk H, Revlen HJ: Microsurgical reoperation following lumbar disk surgery: timing, surgical findings and outcome in 92 patients, *J Neurosurg* 70:397, 1989.
23. Ebelke DK, Asher MA, Neff JR, Krake DP: Survivorship analysis of VSP spine instrumentation in the treatment of thoracolumbar burst fractures, *Spine* 16S:428, 1991.
24. El-Ghindi S, Aref S, Salama M, Andrews J: Infection of intervertebral disks after operation, *J Bone Joint Surg Br* 58:114, 1976.
25. Epstein JA, Epstein BS, Joes MD: Symptomatic lumbar scoliosis with degenerative changes in the elderly, *Spine* 4:542, 1979.
26. Escalas F, DeWald RL: Combined traumatic arteriovenous fistula and ureteral injury. A compilation of iliac bone-grafting, *J Bone Joint Surg* 140:270, 1977.
27. Farey ID, McAfee PC, Davis RF, Long DM: Pseudarthrosis of the cervical spine after anterior arthrodesis, *J Bone Joint Surg Am* 72:1171-1177, 1990.
28. Finnegan WJ, Fenlin JM, Marnel JP, Nardini RJ, Rothman RH: Results of surgical intervention in the symptomatic multiply operated back patient. Analysis of 67 cases followed for three to seven years, *J Bone Joint Surg* 61A:1077, 1979.
29. Frymoyer JW, Matteri RE, Hanley EN, Kuhlmann D, Howe J: Failed lumbar disk surgery requiring second operation. A longer term followup study, *Spine* 3:7-11, 1978.
30. Fuller DA, Kirkpatrick JS, Emery SE, Wilber RG, Davy DT: *A kinematic study of the cervical spine before and after segmental arthrodesis,* Presented at the Cervical Spine Research Society Meeting, New York, New York, December 3, 1993.
31. Gepstein R, Eismont FJ: *Postoperative spine infections.* In Garfin SR, editor: *Complications of spine surgery,* Baltimore, 1989, Williams & Wilkins, p 302.
32. Gibson MJ, Bukley J, Mawwhinney R, Mulholland RC, Worthington BS: Magnetic resonance imaging and diskography in the diagnosis of disk degeneration: a comparative study of 50 disks, *J Bone Joint Surg Br* 68:369-373, 1986.

33. Giordano CP, Neuwirth MG: *Texas Scottish Rite Hospital instrumentation for adult lumbar fusions.* In Bridwell KH, DeWald RL, editors: *The textbook of spinal surgery,* ed 2, Philadelphia, 1997, Lippincott-Raven, p 1645.
34. Goald HJ: Microlumbar discectomy: follow-up of 477 patients, *J Microsurg* 2:95, 1980.
35. Glassman SD, Dima JR, Puno RM, Johnson JR: Salvage of instrumented lumbar fusions complicated by surgical wound infection, *Spine* 21:2163-2169, 1996.
36. Greenspan A, Amparo EG, Gorczyca DP, Montesano PX: Is there a role of diskography in the era of magnetic resonance imaging? Prospective correlation and quantitative analysis of computed tomography-diskography, magnetic resonance imaging, and surgical findings, *J Spinal Disord* 5:26-31, 1992.
37. Gurr KE, McAfee PC, Shih CM: Biomechanical analysis of anterior and posterior instrumentation systems after corpectomy, *J Bone Joint Surg* 70A:1182, 1988.
38. Guyer RD, Collier R, Stith WJ et al: Discitis after diskography, *Spine* 13:1352-1354, 1988.
39. Holt EP Jr: The question of lumbar diskography, *J Bone Joint Surg Am* 50:720-726, 1968.
40. Jackson RK, Boston DA, Edge AJ: Lateral mass fusion. A prospective study of consecutive series with long-term follow-up, *Spine* 10:828, 1985.
41. Johnson RG: Does diskography injure normal disks? An analysis of repeat diskograms, *Spine* 14:424-426, 1989.
42. Jones AM, Stanbough JL, Balderson RA et al: Long term results of lumbar spine surgery complicated by unintended incidental durotomy, *Spine* 14:443, 1989.
43. Jorgenson SS, Lowe TG, France J, Gomez M: *A prospective analysis of autograft versus allograft in posterolateral lumbar fusion in the same patient: a minimum of one year follow-up in 144 patients,* Presented at the North American Spine Society Meeting, San Diego, CA, October, 1993.
44. Kahn B: Superior gluteal artery laceration, a complication of iliac bone graft surgery *Clin Orthop* 140:204, 1979.
45. Kornberg M: Diskography and magnetic resonance imaging in the diagnosis of lumbar disk disruption, *Spine* 14:1368-1372, 1989.
46. Kostuik JP: Decision making in adult scoliosis, *Spine* 4:521-525, 1979.
47. LaRocca H: *Failed lumbar surgery syndromes: causes and correctives.* In Bridwell KH, DeWald RL, editors: *The textbook of spinal surgery,* Philadelphia, 1991, Lippincott, p 719.
48. Lauerman WC, Bradford DS, Ogilvie JW, Transfeldt EE: Results of lumbar pseudarthrosis repair, *J Spinal Disord* 5:149, 1992.
49. Lee CK, Langrana NA: Lumbosacral spinal fusion—a biomechanical study, *Spine* 9:574-581, 1984.
50. Lehmann TR, Spratt KF, Weinstein JN et al: Long term follow-up of lower lumbar fusion patients, *Spine* 12:97-104, 1987.
51. Leung PC: Complications in the first 40 cases of microdiscectomy, *J Spinal Disord* 1:306, 1988.
52. Lowery GL, Swant ML, McDonough RF: Surgical revision for failed anterior cervical fusions, *Spine* 20:2436-2441, 1995.
53. Luk KD, Lee FB, Leong JC, Hsu LC: The effect on the lumbosacral spine of long spinal fusion for idiopathic scoliosis. A minimum 10-year follow-up, *Spine* 12:1996, 1987.
54. Mandlebaum BR, Tolo VT, McAfee PC et al: Nutritional deficiencies after staged anterior and posterior spinal reconstructive surgery, *Clin Orthop* 234:5-11, 1988.
55. McLain RF, Sparling E, Benson DR: Early failure of short segment pedicle instrumentation for thoracolumbar fractures: a preliminary report, *J Bone Joint Surg* 75A:162, 1993.
56. McLaren AC, Bailey SI: Cauda equina syndrome: a complication of lumbar discectomy, *Clin Orthop* 204:143, 1986.
57. McMaster MJ, Merrick MV: The scintigraphic assessment of the scoliotic spine after fusion, *J Bone Joint Surg* 62B:65, 1980.
58. McNeill TW, Andersson GBJ: Complications of degenerative lumbar spine surgery. In Bridwell KH, DeWald RL, editors: *The Textbook of Spinal Surgery,* ed 2, Philadelphia, 1997, Lippincott-Raven, p 1672.
59. McNeill TW, Sinkora G, Leavitt F: Psychological classification of low back pain patients: a prognostic tool, *Spine* 11:955, 1986.
60. Osti OL, Fraser RD, Vernon-Roberts B: Discitis and diskography of annular tears and intervertebral disk degeneration. A prospective clinical comparison. *J Bone Joint Surg Br* 74:431-435, 1992.
61. Peltola H, Varhuaren V, Aalto K: Fever, C-reactive protein and erythrocyte sedimentation rate in monitoring recovery from septic arthritis: a preliminary study, *J Pediatr Orthop* 4:170, 1984.
62. Posner I, White AA, Edwards WT, Hayes WC: A biomechanical analysis of clinical stability of the lumbosacral spine, *Spine* 7:374, 1982.
63. Robertson PA, Groblen LJ, Novotny JE, Katz JN: Postoperative spondylolisthesis at L4-L5, *Spine* 18:1483, 1993.
64. Roaf J: Some observations regarding 905 patients operated upon for protruded lumbar intervertebral disks, *Am J Surg* 97:388, 1959.
65. Schneiderman G, Flanagan B, Kingston S, Thomas J, Dilan WH, Watkins RG: Magnetic resonance imaging in the diagnosis of degeneration: correlation with diskography, *Spine* 12:276-282, 1987.
66. Sienkiewicz PJ, Flately TJ: Postoperative spondylolisthesis, *Clin Orthop* 221:172, 1987.
67. Spengler DM, Loeser JD, Murphy TM: Orthopaedic aspects of chronic pain syndrome, *Instr Course Lect* 29:101, 1980.

68. Stolke D, Sollmann WP, Seifert V: Intra and postoperative complications in lumbar disk surgery, *Spine* 14:56, 1989.
69. Talgot JS, Cotler HB, Sasso RC, LaRocca H, Gardner V: Postoperative infections in spinal implants: classification and analysis: a multicenter study, *Spine* 16:981, 1991.
70. Taylor TKF: Anterior interbody fusion in the management of disorders of the lumbar spine, *J Bone Joint Surg* 52B:784, 1970.
71. Thalgott JS, Cotler HB, Sasso RC, LaRocca H, Gardner V: Postoperative infections in spinal implants, *Spine* 16:981, 1991.
72. Thelander U, Larsson S: Quantification of C-reactive protein levels and erythrocyte sedimentation rate after spinal surgery, *Spine* 17:400, 1992.
73. Tollison CD, Satterthwaite JR: Multiple spine surgical failures. The value of adjunctive psychological assessment, *Orthop Ther* 10:1107, 1990.
74. Walsh TR, Weinstein JN, Spratt KF et al: Lumbar diskography in normal subjects. A controlled prospective study, *J Bone Joint Surg* 72A:1081, 1990.
75. Weatherley CR, Prickett CF, O'Brien JP: Discogenic pain persisting despite solid posterior fusion, *J Bone Joint Surg* 68B:142, 1986.
76. Wetzel FT, LaRocca SH, Lowery GL, Aprill CN: The treatment of lumbar spinal pain syndromes diagnosed by diskography, *Spine* 19:792, 1994.
77. Whitecloud TS, Seago RA: Cervical discogenic syndrome: results of operative intervention in patients with positive diskography, *Spine* 12:313, 1987.
78. Whitecloud TS, Davis J, Olive PM: Operative treatment of the degenerated segment adjacent to a lumbar fusion, *Spine* 19:531-536, 1994.
79. Wilkinson HA: *The failed back syndrome: etiology and therapy,* New York, 1992, Springer Verlag, pp 35-39.
80. Wiltse LC, Rocchio DP: Pre-operative psychological tests as predictors of success of chemonucleosis in the treatment of low back syndrome, *J Bone Joint Surg Am* 57:478, 1975.
81. Winter RB, Lonstein JE, Denis F: Pain patterns in adult scoliosis, *Orthop Clin N Am* 19:339, 1988.
82. Winter RB, Moe JH, Wang JF: Congenital kyphosis. Its natural history and treatment as observed in a study of one hundred and thirty patients, *J Bone Joint Surg* 55A:223, 1973.
83. Zdelblick TA, Ducker TB: The use of freeze-dried allograft bone for anterior cervical fusions, *Spine* 16:726-729, 1991.
84. Zdeblick TA: A prospective, randomized sudy of lumbar fusion, *Spine* 18:983, 1993.
85. Zielke K, Stunkat R, Beaujean F: Ventral derotation spondylodesis (author's translation), *Arch Orthop Unfallchir* 85:257, 1976.
86. Zinreich SJ, Long DM, Davis R, Quinn CB, McAfee PC, Wing H: Three dimensional CT imaging in postsurgical "failed back syndrome," *J Comput Assist Tomogr* 14:475, 1990.

# 3

# REVISIONS IN SPINE SURGERY*

H. V. Crock, M.D., M.S., F.R.C.S., F.R.A.C.S., F.R.C.S. Ed. (Hon)



## HISTORY AND OVERVIEW

In 1947, open heart surgery, joint replacements, and organ transplantations were unheard of. Ten years later, in London, a mechanical heart-lung machine, based on coupling advanced physiological studies with the biomechanics of ventilation and blood flow, was under development. When the pharmacological basis of reversible arrest of cardiac muscle function was established, the first human open heart operation was ready to be performed in England.[15] At the same time, the English surgeon Charnley[5] was developing a technique for total hip joint replacement. His work was based on bioengineering principles with the greater emphasis on mechanics.

While these two revolutionary works were in progress, a young surgeon, named R.Y. Calne, came to Oxford in 1957 to work for 6 months as a house officer in orthopedics. During that time he was preparing to sit for the examinations of the Royal College of Surgeons of England, which lead to the FRCS diploma in general surgery. Within the next 8 years he was to become one of the pioneers in human organ transplantation. In 1965, Calne was appointed to the foundation chair of surgery in the University of Cambridge where he soon established a world-renowned center for renal and liver transplantations. An active research department with expertise in immunology and pharmacology supported his work in tissue transplantation, enabling him to extend its scope to the replacement of multiple organs.

Failures in these three surgical fields (open heart, joint replacement, and organ transplantation) are regarded as accepted hazards, depending, respectively, on factors such as restenosis of arteries due to advancing atheromatosis, loosening of joint prostheses, and immunological incompatibility, and revision operations are not regarded as controversial.[4]

In orthopedics, failures following total joint replacements have reached epidemic proportions. The treatment of many of these patients now rests in the hands of super specialists who often practice only revision surgery. In the second half of the twentieth century, orthopedic practice has been devoted almost exclusively to the use of mechanical solutions for treating joint problems.

Problems in spinal surgery, considered over the same period, have likewise been addressed almost exclusively by mechanical means, with little regard for the physiology of bone, muscle, or nerve. By contrast, problems in cardiac and organ transplant surgery have been solved by blending the use of advances from the sciences of medicine—histochemistry, immunology, and pharmacology—with the long-established mechanical techniques of general surgery.

In 1955, Professor Joseph Barr visited the orthopedic department at St. Vincent's Hospital in the University of Melbourne. He gave a lecture there, based on the paper that he had published with Mixter in 1934.[16] He expressed concern that too much attention was being focused on prolapsed disks. By that time, terms such as disk prolapse and slipped disk had passed into common usage and the cause of sciatica had become inextricably linked in people's minds with disk prolapse. Even so, controversy about the causes of sciatica and back pain was beginning to surface. Dandy[11] had written about concealed ruptured intervertebral disks. Morgan and King[17] drew attention to primary vertebral instability as a cause of back pain and sciatica. In 1970, an attempt was made to change the focus on disk disorders so that the role of disk prolapse as a cause of back pain and sciatica could be placed in a new context alongside other forms of disk pathology that required distinctly different forms of surgical treatment. As a result, terminology was coined to describe two other forms of disk disorders-isolated disk resorption and internal disk disruption.[6]

## ISOLATED DISK RESORPTION

Isolated disk resorption is characterized radiologically by loss of disk height at a single intervertebral level (Fig. 3-1). In advanced forms the distance between the vertebral end plates may be reduced to a few millimeters and a thin black shadow (due to the presence of nitrogen gas) may be seen in the narrowed disk space. This radiological sign was described first by Knutsson[13] in 1942. Sclerotic changes appear in the related vertebral bodies. In contrast to findings in generalized spondylosis, osteophytic formation around the margins of the vertebral bodies is often limited. As the affected disk space narrows, the related facet joints subluxate, narrowing the gaps between the apices of the superior facets of the inferior vertebra and the inferior surfaces of the pedicles of the superior vertebra. The facet subluxations are accompanied by buckling of the ligamentum flavum into the nerve root canals and intervertebral foramina from behind, while the remaining peripheral annular fibers of the resorbed disk bulge like a flat tire into the floor of the spinal canal. Bilateral foraminal and nerve root canal stenoses are thereby established.

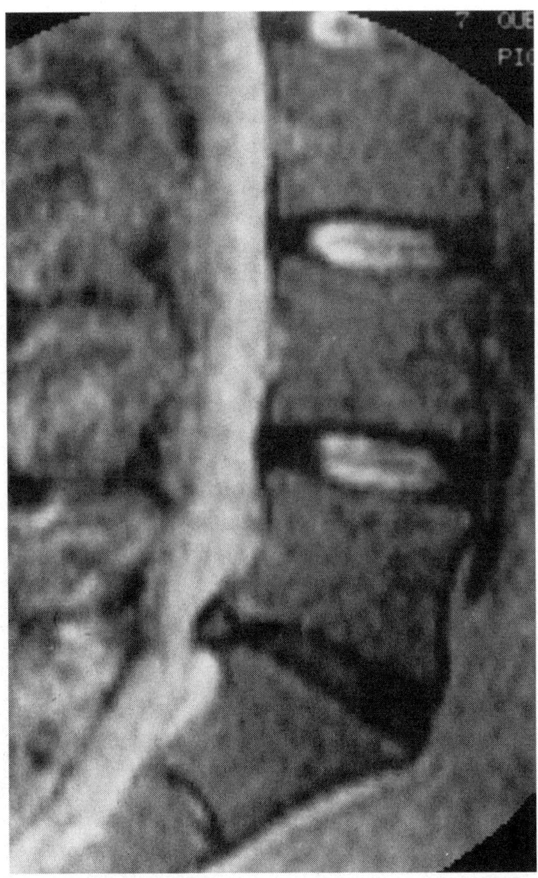

**Figure 3-1**

MRI: A midsagittal image of the lumbar spine of a 45-year-old man showing features of isolated disk resorption at L5/S1 with loss of nuclear signal, decreased disk height, annular bulging, and high signals in the vertebral end plates.

This bulge is frequently reported as a disk prolapse. Removal of this disk tissue by minimal invasive techniques such as microdiskectomy will often lead to recurrent bilateral sciatica due to the unrecognized bilateral foraminal and nerve root canal stenoses, which are the true causes of referred buttock and leg pain in this condition.

Isolated disk resorption at the lumbosacral junction often gives rise to recurrent attacks of disabling bilateral buttock and leg pains. These symptoms are rarely associated with abnormal neurological signs, contrasting with cases of sciatica caused by disk prolapses in which loss of reflexes, motor weakness, and sensory deficits are usually found in the lower limbs.

At the L4/5 level or at the first mobile segment above a segmentation anomaly, acute bouts of painful lumbar scoliosis may occur in association with sciatic pains. Symptoms stemming from either L4/5 or L5/S1 disk resorptions are commonly attributed to vertebral instability, especially if Knutsson's sign is seen on x-rays or CT examinations (Fig. 3-2). However, there are explanations other than instability for the cause of these symptoms and signs. Based on studies of the pathological changes that develop as disk resorption evolves and on the observation of perineural venous obstruction made at surgery during foraminal and nerve root canal decompressions, the symptoms of buttock and leg pains can be ascribed predominantly to circulatory changes in the nerve roots in their stenosed canals.

Venous obstruction of lumbar nerve roots as a cause of sciatica had been hinted at by Putti,[20] however, the importance of relieving perineural venous obstruction by performing bilateral foraminal and nerve root canal decompressions without touching the resorbed disk tissue itself became apparent only gradually in the late 1970s.[10]

Perineural venous obstruction causes nerve root edema and hypersensitivity of its component filaments. During operation, gentle probing of involved

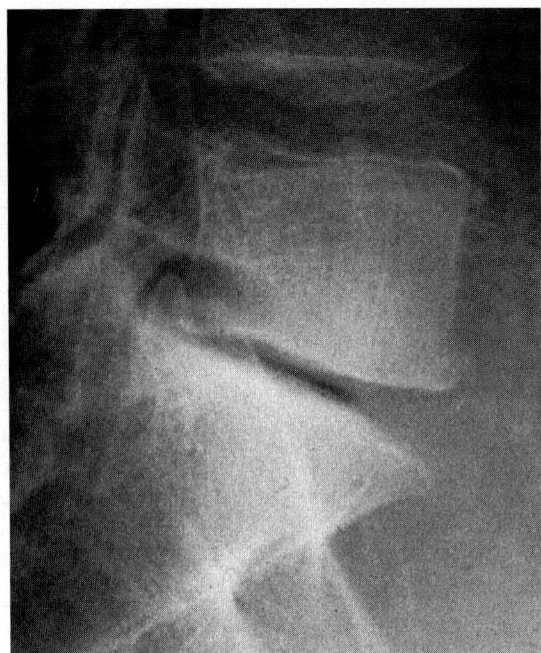

FIGURE 3-2

A lateral radiograph showing classical features of isolated disk resorption at L5/S1. Note Knutsson's gas shadow in the middle of the disk space.

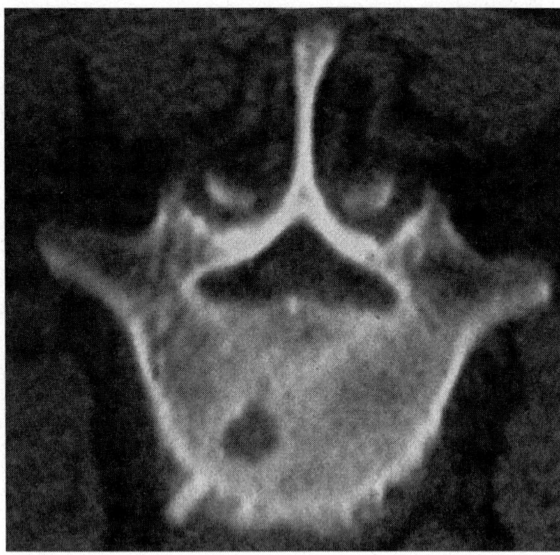

FIGURE 3-3

CT. An axial image showing a punctate lesion in the vertebral end plate of L4 in a 52-year-old woman with isolated disk resorption, causing intractable back pain that was successfully treated by anterior interbody fusion with autogenous bone grafts.

nerves, in situ in their stenotic canals, will produce brisk twitching of the muscles of the buttocks and thighs. These abnormal motor reactions cease within a few minutes as the foraminal and nerve root canal decompressions proceed, until the perineural veins refill. The nerves can then be manipulated without causing muscle twitching in the extremities and, within a few hours of the operation, patients report dramatic relief of their leg pains.

A small number of patients with isolated disk resorption complain of severe localized back pain, without associated referred limb pains. The back pain may become intractable. Its cause is now thought to be due to the punctate lesions that develop in the vertebral end plates (Fig. 3-3). Complex histochemical processes produce these lesions from which nociceptive substances are released, causing the back pain.[1] Contributions to this pain come also from degenerative changes in the related facet joints and from minor degrees of vertebral instability. Spinal fusion is appropriate for treating this very small group.

In long-standing cases of isolated disk resorption, the biomechanical forces transmitted through the lumbar spine are altered, leading to laminal and facet joint hypertrophy at the adjacent vertebral interspace even when the height of that disk space remains normal. Sometimes foraminal and nerve root canal decompressions may also be required at that level.

Surgery is indicated in less than 5% of patients with isolated disk resorption. The vast majority who do require operation will respond well to bilateral foraminal and nerve root canal decompressions at the affected level. Sometimes prolapse of a vertebral end plate cartilage remnant will occur, causing unilateral sciatica. This is best treated by excision of the fragment combined with bilateral foraminal and nerve root canal decompressions.

In patients whose dominant symptoms are back pain, which is usually intractable or frequently recurrent, interbody fusion with autogenous bone grafts will give excellent results. It is important to remember that in the few cases requiring fusion, the great vessels of the lower abdomen (the left common iliac vein especially) may be densely adherent to the anterior margin of the affected disk. Approach to the vertebral interspace is then difficult. Damage to the left common iliac vein in such circumstances may result in catastrophic venous hemorrhage. Therefore, laparoscopic surgery in these cases should be avoided.

## INTERNAL DISK DISRUPTION

Internal disk disruption is a nonprolapsing form of disk disorder often precipitated by trauma. It gives rise to back pain associated with radiating limb pains without abnormal objective neurological findings. These symptoms are aggravated by physical activities and constitutional features of weight loss and easy fatigability are common. Treated by "diskectomy" alone, the patient's symptoms can become dramatically worse. In a Presidential Address delivered to the International

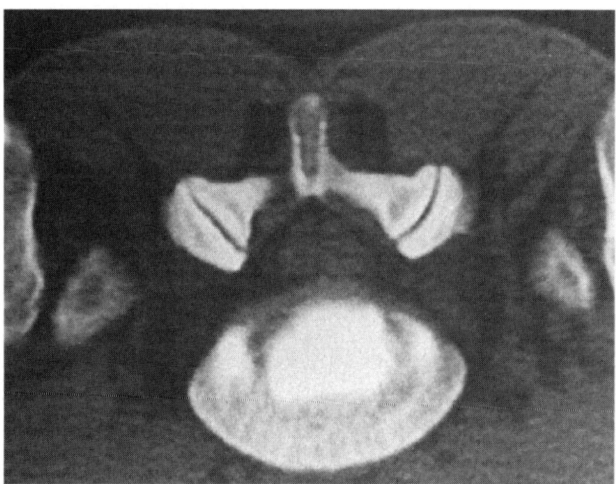

FIGURE 3-4

CT. A diskogram at L5/S1 in an 18-year-old woman showing spread of dye beyond the nucleus into clefts within the annular fibers of the disk. This patient presented with clinical features of internal disk disruption treated successfully by anterior interbody fusion with autogenous grafts.

Society for the Study of the Lumbar Spine in Sydney in 1985 under the title "History Hypothesis and Progress in Clinical Medicine,"[8] the genesis of ideas about this lesion and its treatment were set out (Fig. 3-4). Correlating this clinical syndrome with studies of the nutritional mechanisms of intervertebral disks, based on the arterial supply and venous drainage of the vertebral end plates, the following theory was propounded: nociceptive breakdown products from damaged or abnormal disk tissues leak out of the affected disk via the end plate vessels, passing into the vertebral veins and the perineural venous plexuses to cause back and leg pains. Total disk excision and interbody fusion has restored many of these patients to good health although definitive identification of the chemical substances responsible for causing these pains has not yet been achieved.[8]

Degeneration of disks may also lead to vertebral instability, which can cause back pain and sciatica. Spinal fusion may relieve symptoms in these cases. By contrast, however, the syndrome of internal disk disruption responds poorly to posterior spinal fusion of any type that does not also involve total disk excision.[23]

Although the diagnosis of disk prolapse has been facilitated with CT scanning and magnetic resonance imaging (MRI), in many cases the definition of disk degeneration has become blurred since the introduction of these imaging technologies. The term used to be defined on the basis of changes in the height of the disk spaces with the appearance of marginal osteophytes and asymmetrical narrowing of the vertebral interspaces together with zygapophyseal (facet) joint narrowing, subchondral cysts, and osteophytic formations at the joint margins. Currently, in MRI reports, the term disk degeneration is applied whenever there is loss of nuclear signal on T2-weighted images, even when the vertebral bodies, intervertebral disk heights, and zygapophyseal joints are normal in appearance on plain x-rays. Controversies therefore abound on the question of correlating these MRI images with the patient's clinical complaints.

Before MRI became widely available, diskography was used to identify certain disk lesions. For example, extra foraminal disk prolapses could be outlined clearly in diskograms. In other cases, the injection of radiopaque dye reproduced the patient's pain syndromes, which were then ascribed either to internal disk disruption or, more often, to vertebral instability.

Diskography was introduced in Sweden by Lindblom.[14] Paradoxically, this useful test has been discredited on many occasions, both in public lectures and in print,[19] from the very department in which it was first used. Controversies about its use in association with chemonucleolysis and about the complications of postdiskogram diskitis have continued up to the present time.

While the clinical syndrome of internal disk disruption has attracted widespread interest, its existence as a clinical entity has been challenged recently.[2] By defining the syndrome of internal disk disruption the theory of the mechanical cause of back pain and sciatica was challenged by ideas on causation based on anatomical studies, and on the complexities of protein chemistry. Similarly, by defining isolated disk resorption as an important cause of bilateral buttock and leg pain, the focus of attention is shifted from the adverse mechanical effects of disk bulging to the importance of perineural venous obstruction as the principal cause of the referred leg pain.

Since 1970, the practice of spinal surgery has been influenced profoundly by the introduction of CT, MRI, ultrasonography, and large numbers of devices for spinal fixation. Yet surprisingly, during this period there has been very little change in ideas relating to the causes of spinal disorders.

## TERMINOLOGY

Even the terminology used to describe spinal disorders and their treatment is contentious. Many commonly used terms have no real meaning. For example, the word laminectomy is taken to mean removal of an intervertebral disk prolapse, while the term diskectomy has the same connotation. Patients frequently conclude that their laminectomy or diskectomy operation has resulted in the complete removal of the offending disk, though in fact this is never the case. These terms, used to describe the surgical treatment of disk prolapses, could be replaced with more accurate descriptive terms, such as disk fragment excision.

The term microdiskectomy has been introduced to describe a surgical technique for removing disk tissue. This means that an added tool has been applied to the surgery of disk prolapse allowing the use of a tiny skin incision and removal of the offending disk tissue via a small well-lit portal in the depths of which the disk prolapse stands magnified. It does not mean that there is such an entity as a disk prolapse so small that it requires the use of a microscope. The use of modern operating microscopes, however, has helped to revolutionize a wide range of surgical procedures that include, in particular, surgery of the spinal cord.

In many cases disk prolapses occur in stenosed segments of the vertebral column and the appropriate treatment should include excision of the prolapsed disk fragments and decompression of the foramina and nerve root canals on both sides of the disk space. The use of an operating microscope does nothing to enhance the surgeon's performance of such procedures, though it can provide excellent facilities for photographing perineural venous refilling, which is a key indicator of the adequacy of the decompressions should the surgeon wish to record that phenomenon.

The term disk disruption is now widely used by spinal specialists to describe MRI images with loss of nuclear signal on T2-weighted sequences in cases where plain x-rays of the spine are reported as normal. Diskograms with CT in such cases can provide clear-cut images of internal disk disruption characterized by abnormal patterns of distribution of radiopaque dye within the confines of the disk (see Fig. 3-2). Radiologists, however, rarely use this term when reporting these MR images, preferring to describe the changes as being indicative of disk degeneration. The correlation of both these terms with clinical syndromes remains controversial. For example, some practitioners implicate the changes of disk disruption with clinical syndromes of diskogenic pain or internal disk disruption, in which disk excision and interbody fusion may be indicated, while others regard them as phenomena of normal aging processes in the disk for which no treatment should be offered.

Spinal decompression is another term that is used frequently though it lacks a precise definition. The incidence of spinal stenosis has increased significantly in parallel with increased life expectancy. It is treated most commonly by spinal decompression, which is still performed by many surgeons by excising the spinous process and the central portion of the lamina at an affected level or levels. However, clinical anatomists have drawn attention to the importance of preserving the paraspinal muscles and the lumbodorsal fascia during surgery for decompression of the spinal canal.[3] In contemporary practice, therefore, the operation to relieve lumbar canal stenosis should be performed, in most cases, with preservation of the spinous processes and interspinous ligaments. Following bilateral foraminal and nerve root canal decompressions, the lumbodorsal aponeurosis should be resutured to the midline interspinous ligaments. Hence, spinal decompression should be defined using accurate anatomical terminology to detail individual relevant steps of the operation.

## OBSERVATIONS ON CURRENT PRACTICE

Physicians and surgeons who treat patients with back pain and sciatica still tend to focus their attention predominantly on the entity of disk prolapse. Treatment for it includes a wide range of procedures described with terms such as diskectomy, percutaneous diskectomy, automated percutaneous diskectomy, laser diskectomy, chemonucleolysis, and microdiskectomy. Poor results after disk surgery continue to be blamed on recurrent disk prolapse, scar tissue formation, unrecognized spinal stenosis, or on psychological disturbance in the patient.

Spinal fusion is recommended for treating spinal instability and disk degeneration. It is now performed by a variety of methods using internal fixation devices, ranging from translaminar, transfacet joint screws, to pedicle screw fixation with plates or rods. Some surgeons routinely treat these conditions with interbody fusion cages. A more conservative method for stabilization without fusion has been introduced by Graf,[12] who uses elasticized bands linking adjacent pedicle screws.

Two schools of thought exist on the subject of revisions after spinal operations have failed. One is spearheaded by Nachemson[18] who countenance only a few indications for repeated surgery, restricting these to operations for the treatment of recurrent disk prolapse (which is rare) or to the relief of unrecognized spinal stenosis.

Proponents of the second school subscribe to a wider array of indications. Among this group there are some surgeons who advocate the relentless pursuit of the patient's pain source even if that involves multiple operations using progressively more diverse and complicated procedures (Fig. 3-5). The outcome for patients who follow these surgeons' advice is predictably poor, often leading to physical and mental breakdown compounded by financial ruin. Between these extreme positions of ultraconservatism and repeated complex surgery, there lies a middle road along which useful help can be provided for patients following failed spinal operations.

There are a number of fundamental points to be made that should influence decisions for revision surgery:

1) *Previous history and management.* Indications for the original operation should be analyzed, based on the diagnosis that was given to the patient. Details of

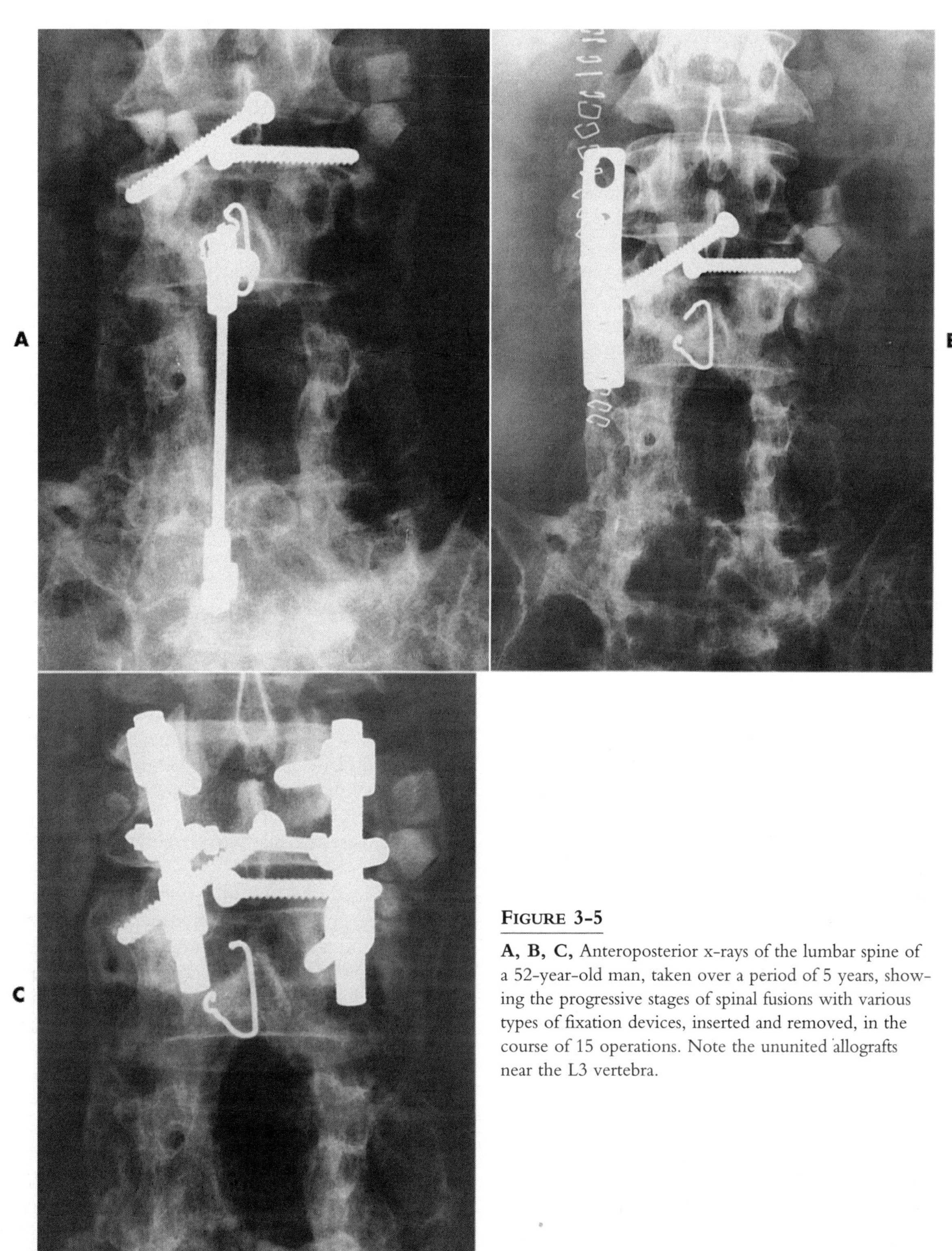


FIGURE 3-5

**A, B, C,** Anteroposterior x-rays of the lumbar spine of a 52-year-old man, taken over a period of 5 years, showing the progressive stages of spinal fusions with various types of fixation devices, inserted and removed, in the course of 15 operations. Note the ununited allografts near the L3 vertebra.

the surgical techniques and of the nature and origin of implanted materials used in the spine should be sought. Many surgeons do not keep accurate accounts of their operative techniques, even failing to record the manufacturer's name of implanted devices. Removal of these devices can only be achieved quickly and safely if the special instruments with which they were inserted are available for their removal. Hence, in planning re-exploration operations, the surgeon must ensure that appropriate instruments, including high-speed drills, are readily available to him. In special cases biological adhesives such as Tisseel may be required if dural damage is likely.

2) *Information from imaging studies.* Information derived even from the most advanced MRI and CT machines still cannot match the accuracy of observations made during the operation by an experienced spinal surgeon. For example, the adequacy of spinal canal decompression cannot always be assessed by radiologic methods.[21] Therefore, in treating patients with persistent disabling sciatica, the surgeon should not necessarily be dissuaded from embarking on reexploration of the appropriate nerve root canal or intervertebral foramen, even if the radiologist's report suggests that there is no recurrent disk prolapse and no evidence of stenosis. The significance of pathological changes in the ligamentum flavum and of laminal and joint thickening along the course of a nerve root canal relating to symptoms, is not easily assessed with imaging studies. Despite the sophistication of modern imaging techniques, a wide gap still exists between the findings at operation and suggested findings based on the interpretation of images from CT, MRI, or ultrasound studies.

   Good quality x-rays of the lumbar spine must always be available before revision surgery is undertaken. These images are vital for assessing spinal segmentation and the changes in the vertebral column that have resulted from earlier surgery. Facilities for obtaining x-ray images during revision operations should always be available in the operating room.

3) *Operative techniques.* Most operations are performed on the lumbar spine by approaches to the spinal canal through interlaminar spaces. The lumbar paraspinal muscles are held against the sides of the spinous processes and the outer surfaces of the laminae by the lumbodorsal aponeurosis. This fascial membrane is attached to the supraspinous and interspinous ligaments. The muscles contain variable quantities of fatty tissues. If the spinous processes and the central segments of the laminae are removed during exposure of the spinal canal, or if the lumbodorsal fascial attachments are permanently disconnected from the midline ligaments, the paraspinal muscles become bowstrung across the roof of the spinal canal. The dead space between the deep surfaces of the muscles and the remnants of the bony roof of the spinal canal or the exposed surface of the dural sac fill with hematoma, in which scar tissue subsequently develops. Varying with the degree of associated paraspinal muscle damage inflicted during the operation, the character of this scar tissue changes. In extreme cases after prolonged, uninterrupted retraction of the muscles, it becomes dense, developing the consistency of solid fibrocartilage in which thin plaques of ectopic bone develop, causing secondary canal stenosis. The development of these changes increases rapidly with repeated operations, particularly if fixation devices such as metal rods fixed to the laminae with encircling wires are used, or after the insertion of pedicle screws with rods or plates. In addition to the muscle damage, intense tissue reactions may be found surrounding the metallic implants. In some cases, after loosening of the devices, hypertrophy of the adjacent zygapophyseal joints and pedicles and related margins of the laminae above the stabilized spinal segment may develop.

Self-retaining retractors applied to the paraspinal muscles act as tourniquets. They should be removed at regular intervals of 30 to 40 minutes throughout the operation.[9] Even those used unilaterally, in the course of microdiskectomies, can produce local muscle necrosis leading to interlaminar scarring and even to interlaminar ossification.

If the paraspinal muscles are replaced in their normal relationship with the roof of the canal by resuturing the lumbodorsal aponeurosis to the midline ligaments, then dense scar tissue is unlikely to cover the dural sac as the epidural fat and the intermuscular fatty tissues prevent its formation. The use of fat grafts is therefore unnecessary. Fat grafts placed on the dural sac may act as foreign bodies and can cause serious neurological damage.

Spinal fusion still retains an important role in the treatment of failed spinal operations. Interbody fusions were usually performed with autogenous bone grafts. In recent years, many other substances have been used as graft materials with the aims of avoiding problems associated with autogenous graft harvesting and of decreasing operating time.

Study of failed interbody fusions in which autogenous cancellous grafts had been used led to the understanding of one mechanism of nonunion. Disk remnants left in the intervertebral space become active after surgery and infiltrate the graft, thereby preventing union between the vertebral bodies.[7]

When autogenous cancellous chips are placed inside metal or carbon fiber cages designed for interbody fusion, this observation may have particular relevance because the bone chips could be infiltrated by reactive tissues from disk remnants, destroying the bony contribution to the interbody fusion. Recalling the outcome after insertion of a Moore's prosthesis into an adolescent hip joint in which the metallic femoral head eventually migrated into the center of the pelvis by eroding the acetabulum, the question of migration of interbody fusion cages must arise. These cages are embedded in cancellous vertebral bodies through which significant mechanical stresses are constantly transmitted. If, after 15 years, a metallic femoral head can migrate through normal acetabular cartilage and its supporting hard compact bone, where are interbody cages likely to end up?

Reexploration operations on the spinal canal are often time-consuming. In elderly patients, posturing in the prone position should be arranged so that the head is not dependent during lengthy procedures. The incidence of postoperative confusional states, which can result from cerebral edema, can thereby be reduced.

With appropriate revision surgery, even some long-standing neurological deficits, such as foot drop, chronic cauda equina lesions, and even paraplegia of nontraumatic origin, may be reversible.[22]

4) *The attending physician's role.* Preoperative and postoperative care administered by a specialist physician is essential for the efficient management of the patient's associated medical problems such as diabetes, high blood pressure, and pain control. Immediately following revision surgery, there is an excellent opportunity for drug withdrawal procedures in those patients who may have become addicted to narcotics for long periods.
5) *Postoperative supervision.* Patients need to be regularly followed up for many months until recovery is complete and they should have ready access to members of the team who have treated them.

## CONCLUSION

The subject of spinal surgery remains engulfed in controversy. The causes of back pain and sciatica and the relevance of particular surgical treatments for them continue to be subject to argument. However, emphasis still rests most commonly on three diagnoses: disk prolapse, spinal instability, and spinal stenosis. In each of these, mechanical factors are implicated as the major cause of symptoms while their treatment continues to be described respectively with such ill-defined terms as: diskectomy, spinal stabilization, spinal fusion, and spinal decompression.

The role of this chapter is to be viewed against this complicated background, bearing in mind that there is no consensus of opinion on diagnosis, the use of terminology, nor on the indications for the use of particular surgical procedures.

There is a current trend in revision spinal surgery toward the use of devices for spinal fixation and for disk replacement with the aim of restoring anatomical normality. The insertion of many of these mechanical aids into the spine usually precludes obtaining tissue samples that might otherwise be used to unravel the complexities of disk and spinal pathology in general. Unless the surgical community recognizes the importance of pursuing such fundamental studies based on specimens obtained at operation, then the outlook for patients with spinal disorders will become increasingly bleak.

The principle of simply modifying spinal pathology to relieve symptoms applies not only at the time of a patient's first operation but also in many instances at the time of revision surgery. This important surgical principle is now widely ignored as spinal surgeons seek ever more sophisticated mechanical solutions to spinal disorders. However, despite seemingly insurmountable problems, revision surgery of the spine is often required and frequently rewarding.

## REFERENCES


1. Brown et al: Sensory and sympathetic innervation of the vertebral endplate in patients with degenerative disc disease, *J Bone Joint Surg* 79(B):147-153, 1997.
2. Blumenthal et al: The role of anterior lumbar fusion for internal disc disruption, *Spine* 13:566-569, 1988.
3. Bogduk N, Macintosh JE: The applied anatomy of the thoracolumbar fascia, *Spine* 9:164-170, 1984.
4. Calne RY: The rejection of renal homografts inhibition in dogs by 6-mercaptopurine, *Lancet* 1:417-418, 1960.
5. Charnley J: Arthroplasty of the hip by the low friction technique, *J Bone Joint Surg* 43:601-606, 1961.
6. Crock HV: A reappraisal of intervertebral disc lesions, *Med J Aust* 1:983-989, 1970.
7. Crock HV: Observations on the management of failed spinal operations, *J Bone Joint Surg* 58B:193-199, 1976.
8. Crock HV: Internal disc disruption: a challenge to disc prolapse 50 years on, *Spine* 11:650-653, 1986.
9. Crock HV, Crock MC: A technique for decompression of the lumbar spinal canal, *Neuro-Orthop* 5:96-99, 1988.
10. Crock HV: Nerve root canal decompression - lumbar perineural venous dilatation as an indicator of its efficacy, *Acta Orthop Scand* 65(2):225-227, 1994.
11. Dandy WE: Concealed ruptured intervertebral discs: plea for elimination of contrast mediums in diagnosis, *JAMA* 117:821-823, 1941.
12. Graf H et al: Instabilité vertébrale: traitement à l'aide d'un systéme souple, *Rachis* 4(2):123-138, 1992.
13. Knutsson F: The vacuum phenomenon in intervertebral discs, *Acta Radiol* 23:173-179, 1942.
14. Lindblom K: Diagnostic puncture of intervertebral discs in sciatica, *Acta Orthop Scand* 17:231-239, 1948.
15. Melrose DG: A heart-lung machine for use in man, *J Physiol* 127:51-53, 1955.

16. Mixter WJ, Barr JS: Rupture of the intervertebral disc with involvement of the spinal canal, *New Engl J Med* 211:210-215, 1934.
17. Morgan FP, King T: Primary instability of lumbar vertebrae as a common cause of low back pain, *J Bone Joint Surg Br* 39:6-22, 1957.
18. Nachemson AL: *Instrumented fusion of the lumbar spine for degenerative disorders, a critical look.* In Szpalski et al, editors: *Instrumented fusion of the degenerative lumbar spine,* Philadelphia, 1996, Lippincott-Raven, p. 307-317.
19. Nachemson A: Lumbar discography, where are we today? Editorial comment, *Spine* 14:555-557, 1989.
20. Putti V: New conceptions in the pathogenesis of sciatic pain, *Lancet* 2:53-60, 1927.
21. Shiraishi T, Crock HV: Lumbar perineural venous obstruction as a cause of sciatica in foraminal and nerve root canal stenosis, *Neuro-Orthop* 17/18:183-189, 1995.
22. Shiraishi T, Crock HV, Reynolds A: Spinal arachnoiditis ossificans: observations on its investigation and treatment, *Eur Spine* J 4:60-63, 1995.
23. Weatherley CR, Prickett CF, O'Brien JP: Discogenic pain persisting despite solid posterior fusion, *J Bone Joint Surg* 68B:142-143, 1986.

# 4

# REVISION, DEFORMITY, AND RECONSTRUCTIVE SURGERY

Robert B. Winter, M.D.



## GENERAL CONSIDERATIONS

Although we would always prefer to do each patient's surgery only once, there are a multitude of situations in which repeat surgery is necessary. If there is any one message I would like to pass along, it would be to analyze the problem very carefully and then to set up a game plan that addresses the problem or problems at hand. Never enter the operating room with the thought that you will invent a solution once you have opened the spine.

### Pain Problems after Deformity Surgery

Pain occurring in the area of the previous surgery is a pseudarthrosis until proven otherwise, even if it takes surgical exploration to solve the issue.

All too often, an assumption is made that the pain is caused by the implants and will be solved by implant removal. The surgeon then removes the implant without adequately exploring the fusion mass and is unpleasantly surprised a few months later when the patient returns with increasing deformity, now requiring a third operation.

Very careful imaging studies, especially oblique views of the fusion and perhaps tomography or high-resolution computed tomography (CT) scans of a suspicious area detect such pseudarthroses, and thus lead to the proper operation and pseudarthrosis repair.

Implants can be painful, especially if prominent, and removal can be appropriate, but never without thorough exploration of the fusion mass integrity first.

### Pain Below a Previous Deformity Fusion

This is almost always due to disk degeneration at the first motion segment, but may involve all of the motion segments distally or just one segment not adjacent to the fusion. I remember vividly a 32-year-old woman who had had a thoracic fusion at T5-L1 as a teenager and came to me with severe, nonradicular low-back pain. A spine surgeon elsewhere had recommended an extension of her fusion to the sacrum. Magnetic resonance imaging (MRI) revealed an isolated disk degeneration (internal disk derangement) at L4-L5. Fusion (anterior and posterior) of this single level gave her complete pain relief and preserved excellent motion.

### Increasing Deformity

Increasing deformity has three possible causes: pseudarthrosis, bending of the fusion mass (crankshafting), and lengthening of the curve. Of these, pseudarthrosis is the most common. Failure to recognize increasing deformity is usually related to inadequate film measurement or failure to appreciate that a scoliotic spine is also developing kyphosis. The treatment of each of these problems is covered in subsequent chapters.

### SUMMARY OF GENERAL PROBLEMS

These are only a few of the many problems that may require further surgery. The skilled surgeon listens to the patient's complaints, does a thorough physical and radiologic evaluation, and then plans the best surgical approach to the problem. Planning is everything.

## REOPERATION OF THE CONGENITAL SPINE

There are a multitude of reasons for reoperation of the congenital spine, some of these being common to spine surgery in general, but others being unique to the congenital patient. The things that are most unique to the congenital spine are the anomalies themselves plus the problems related to abnormal growth.

### REASONS FOR RECONSTRUCTIVE SURGERY IN THE CONGENITAL SPINE

***Pseudarthrosis*** Pseudarthrosis can occur in any spinal fusion operation, and there is no spine surgeon who has not had a pseudarthrosis. This is such a common problem that we should be very suspect of any surgeon who reports a 100% solid fusion rate. Pseudarthroses are failures of the standard knitting process and are, therefore, a biologic event.

The elements of a good arthrodesis that minimize the chance of pseudarthrosis are a) meticulous exposure of the spine with removal of all soft tissues, b) the excision of all facet joints, c) deep decortication of all available posterior elements, d) the addition of adequate amounts of *autogenous* bone graft, and e) secure immobilization of the vertebral elements until union is solid.

In young children, meeting all of these criteria is not easy to accomplish. There may not be adequate autogenous bone graft material. Immobilization is challenging, because instrumentation may not be appropriate, and no matter how snug a cast we apply, the child can wiggle around inside it.

Pseudarthrosis in a congenital scoliosis must be repaired, because progressive deformity will always result. This requires reexploration of the entire fusion mass, vigorous removal of fibrous tissue from the pseudarthrosis area or areas, vigorous decortication around the weak area, the addition of further autogenous bone, and repeat immobilization until absolutely solid.

If there is a significant kyphotic component to the deformity, posterior repairs will continue to fail and an anterior fusion should be added to the program. The appearance of pseudarthrosis after combined anterior-posterior fusion requires that both be redone.

***Lengthening of the Curve.*** This is another very common reason for further surgery. Sometimes it is caused by the failure of the first surgery to be long enough, and sometimes it is caused by unpredictable growth factors. Some fusions need to be lengthened proximally, some distally, and some in both directions. Curve lengthening can be a part of the crankshaft effect or may occur independently. The difference is whether or not there is rotation in addition to the lengthening. Rotation is a key feature of the crankshaft problem.

***The Crankshaft Phenomenon.*** Long before this term was popularized by Dubousset, the phenomenon of fusion mass bending and rotating with increased rib prominence had been discussed by many authors.[4,5]

In patients with idiopathic juvenile or infantile scoliosis requiring arthrodesis prior to the onset of the pubertal growth spurt, crankshafting is virtually universal with posterior fusion alone. The congenital spine is quite different, however, with an incidence of 14% to 20% of patients fused at an early age showing this problem.[2,3,4,5,6] This appears to be related to the absence of healthy anterior growth plates in many patients with congenital problems. (It requires lots of healthy anterior growth plates for crankshafting to occur.)

If a patient does show crankshafting, the necessary treatment is anterior fusion to remove the offending growth plates, posterior exploration to be sure there are no pseudarthroses, osteotomies to achieve recorrection, and thoracoplasty to deal with the too-prominent rib hump.

***Rib Prominence.*** Excessive rib prominence following previous fusion is best managed by thoracoplasty. This can be accomplished posteriorly through the midline incision of the fusion. Dissection is done deep to the trapezius and rhomboid muscles and superficial to the long spinal muscles. The rib is resected from the tip of the transverse process upward to the apex of the prominence, but not the whole prominence. The removed rib is cut into small pieces, which are then placed on the concavity of the fusion mass to thicken it and to fill out the concavity of the curve. Anterior (internal) thoracoplasty can also be done if one has to operate anteriorly for some other reason.

***Another Curve Problem.*** This may be either a compensatory curve below a fused congenital thoracic scoliosis or a second congenital curve.

The compensatory curve below a fused thoracic congenital scoliosis can be a major problem. Despite beginning as a purely compensatory event, this curve can progress severely, far beyond the severity of the original congenital curve. It can show considerable rotation and this is actually a sign that it is becoming a structural curve in and of itself. On two occasions, I applied the concept of instrumentation without fusion to control this curve and still allow for torso growth, because a major portion of the thoracic spine had already been fused at an early age.

A second congenital scoliosis can show progression, particularly during the pubertal growth spurt. This may require extension of the original fusion mass to incorporate the second curve or an entirely separate fusion for the second curve (Figs. 4-1 through 4-6).

***Inadequate Anterior Surgery.*** In my experience, the most common reason for this has been a previous attempt elsewhere to perform an epiphysiodesis or hemivertebra excision via the so-called eggshell approach (transpedicular excavation). This approach is essentially blind and tends to cause inadequate excision of disk and cartilage material as well as inadequate bone grafting. The solution is a formal anterior approach via a thoracotomy with anterior fusion plus exploration and reinforcement of the posterior fusion.

***Paraparesis.*** Paraparesis developing a considerable time after a congenital spine fusion operation usually means that there is a significant kyphosis present and that the previous posterior fusion has a pseudarthrosis (always at the apex of the kyphosis). Neurologic deterioration in a nonkyphotic spine is usually a dysraphic lesion.

To solve this kyphotic problem, an anterior spinal cord decompression must be done at the same time as an anterior fusion. Either under the same anesthetic or a week later, the posterior fusion needs to be redone to repair the weak areas.

***Flat Back Syndrome.*** The flat back syndrome is produced by the use of distraction extending across the

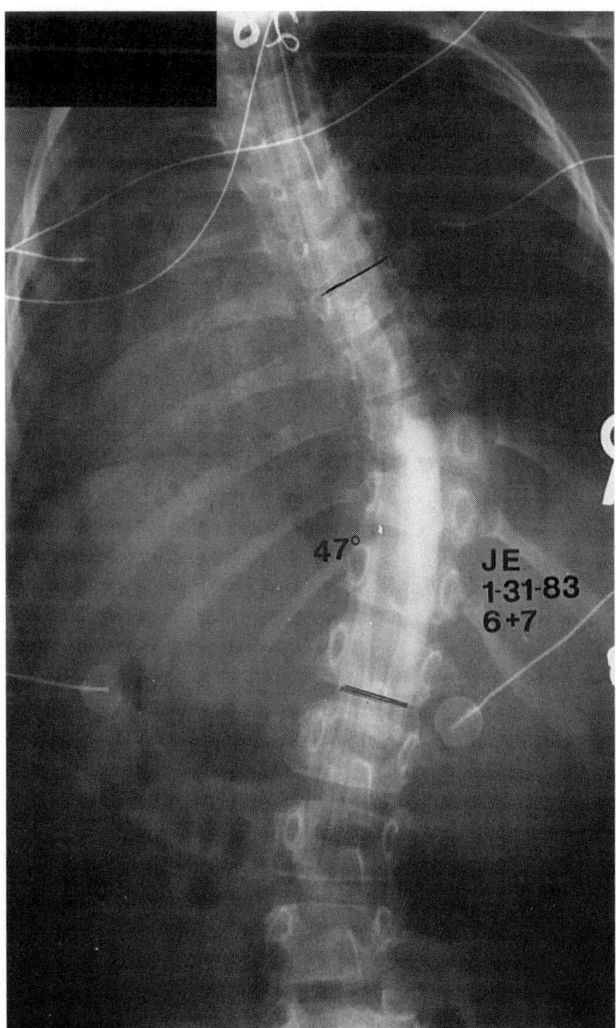


FIGURE 4-1

This 6-year-old girl had a 47-degree congenital scoliosis due to a hemivertebra at T10. A myelogram showed a normal conus level and no dysraphic lesion.

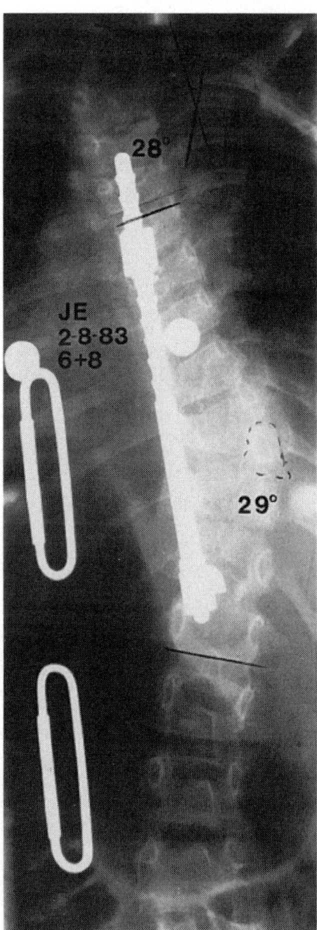


FIGURE 4-2

One month later, a postoperative radiograph shows a Harrington rod T5-T2 with a T5-L1 curve of 29 degrees and a C7-T5 curve of 28 degrees with a left T2 hemivertebra.

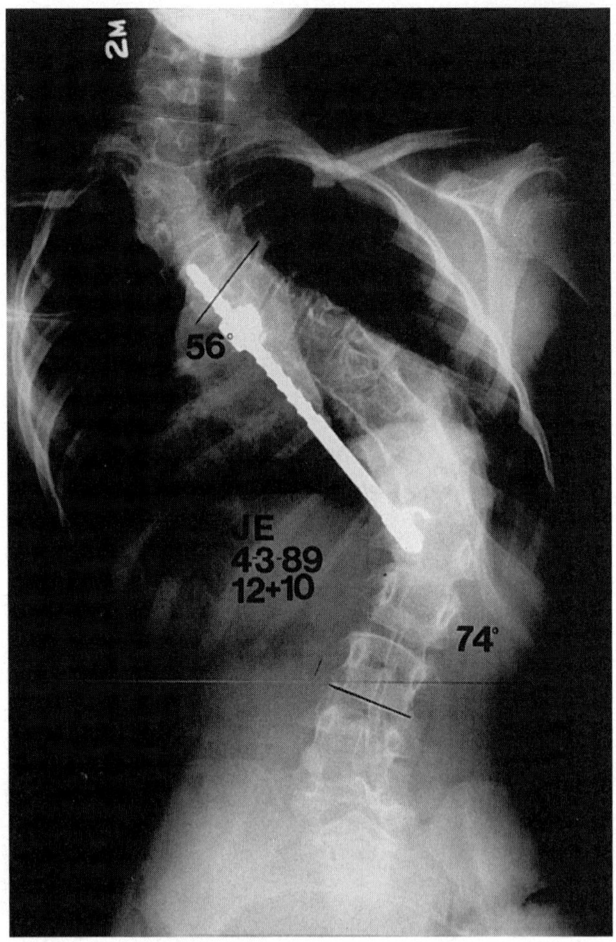


**FIGURE 4-3**

When seen by the author at age 12 years, 10 months, the high T1-T6 scoliosis was 56 degrees and the T6-L3 curve was 74 degrees. This is a mixture of (a) another congenital progressive curve (T1-T6), (b) crankshafting of the original curve, and (c) lengthening of the original curve.

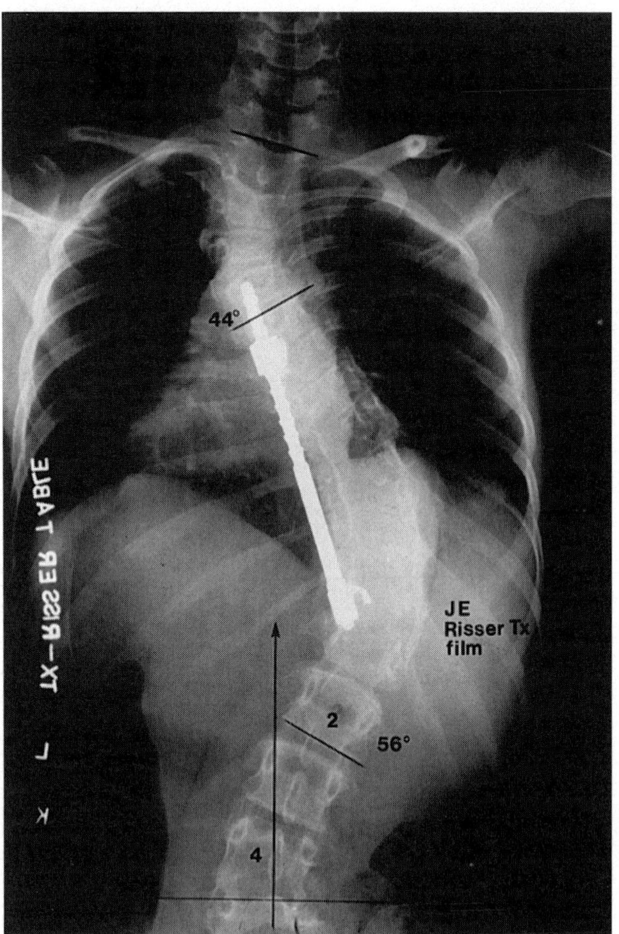


**FIGURE 4-4**

A traction film (supine on a Risser table in maximal traction) shows excellent general realignment of the torso relative to the pelvis.

length of the lumbar spine for treatment of a lumbar scoliosis. Although the scoliosis may be improved, the natural lordosis is eliminated. To treat the flat back syndrome, we first do an anterior diskectomy and fusion in the midlumbar spine, taking care to do a generous resection of the anterior longitudinal ligament and anulus. Autogenous cancellous bone grafts are inserted in the disk spaces.

The patient is then turned prone, the previous fusion mass exposed, the old rods removed, and one or more osteotomies are done in the midlumbar area, corresponding to the levels done anteriorly. After carefully undercutting the osteotomy margins, the osteotomies are closed using compression instrumentation. One must take care not to deviate the spine to one side or the other while closing the osteotomy. Intraoperative radiographs should be done to be sure that decompensation is not being produced.

One helpful trick in doing these osteotomies is to have the patient's hips in full extension. As the osteotomy is completed, the spine tends to sag into a natural lordosis, opening up anteriorly and closing posteriorly. The posterior longitudinal ligament acts as a hinge, preventing instability at the osteotomized level.

Another helpful trick is to slowly close the gap with a midline compression system using the original thin ($\frac{1}{8}''$) Harrington compression rod. This will gradually bend into lordosis as the gap closes. Once the desired correction has been achieved, more stable third-generation hooks and rods can be appropriately bent and secured to the fusion mass.

***Undetected Dysraphism.*** What would you do with the patient who has had a solid fusion for many years, but starts to have neurologic problems? The most likely reason is a previously undetected tethered cord problem. This can be either underneath the previous fusion or remote from it, usually distally.

This requires investigation of the entire spinal canal from head to sacrum by MRI or CT myelography. The lesions one looks for are: Chiari malformation, syringomyelia, diastematomyelia, and tight filum terminale, among others. Appropriate neurosurgical treatment of the lesion is the path to take. I have seen

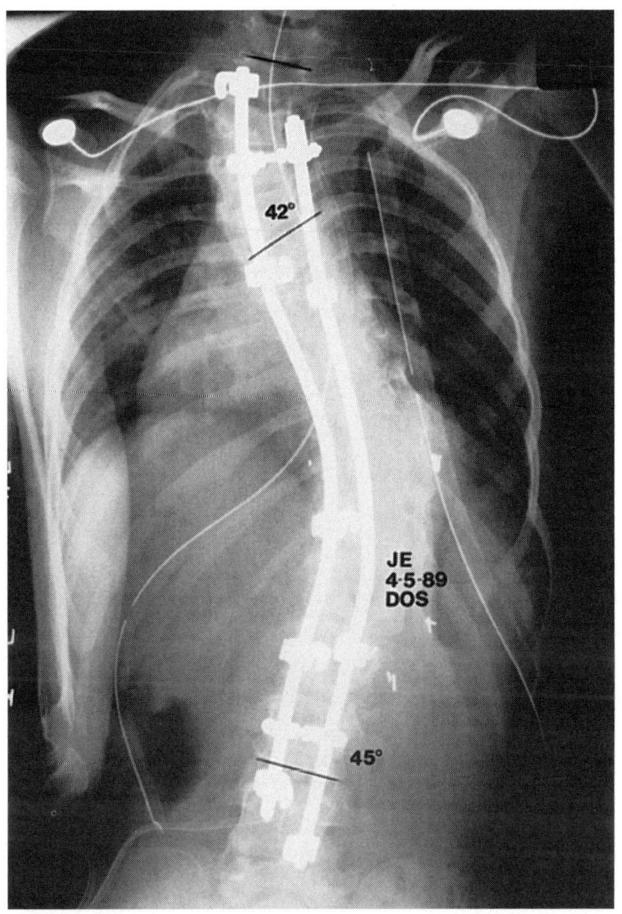


**FIGURE 4-5**

An immediate postoperative radiograph after anterior diskectomy and fusion of T6-L3 and posterior instrumentation and fusion of T1-L4 shows correction of the upper curve to 42 degrees and the lower curve to 45 degrees.

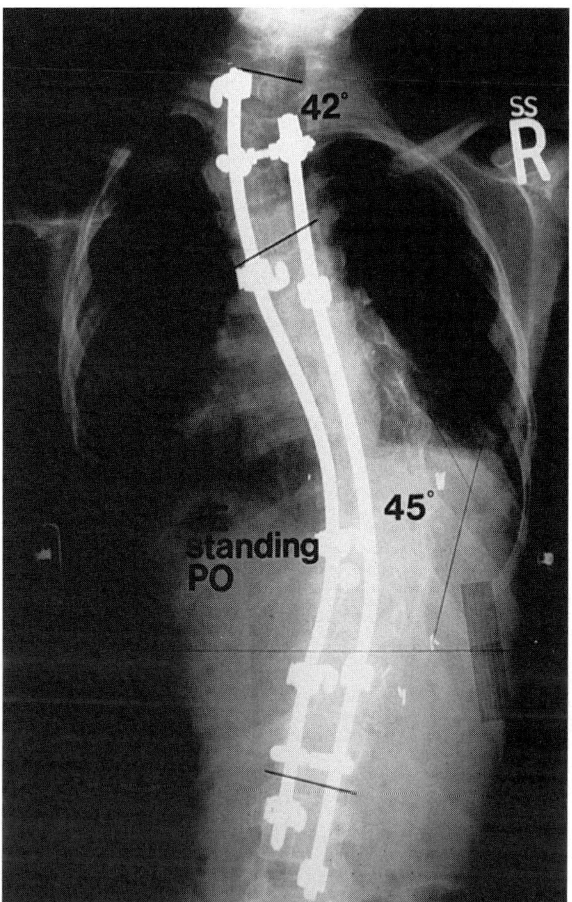


**FIGURE 4-6**

Follow-up radiographs show full maintenance of the achieved correction.

two patients who had all four of these lesions, not an easy problem for the neurosurgeon.

Since the lesion to be removed may lie underneath the old fusion, it is wise to scrub in with the neurosurgeon to make sure that the lateral margins of the fusion mass remain intact and that the removed bone is replaced to reinforce the fusion.

***Junctional Instability.*** Junctional deterioration and/or instability is common after low-back fusions, especially in patients with degenerative disk disease; it is, however, quite rare in congenital spine fusions. We have seen it most commonly in the cervical spine, at the first motion segment proximal to an old cervicothoracic fusion for congenital scoliosis in a patient with associated Klippel-Feil syndrome. This always requires extension of the fusion.

## REFERENCES

1. Onimus M, Manzone R, Michel F, Chirpaz-Cerbat JM: Early operation in congenital scoliosis, *J Pediat Orthop* (B) 1:119-122, 1993.
2. Tello C, Bersusky E, Francheri A: The long-term results of early spine fusion in children with vertebral malformations. Presentation to POSNA (Pediatric Orthopedic Society of North America), May, 1995.
3. Terek RM, Wehner J, Lubicky JP: Crankshaft effect in congenital scoliosis: a preliminary report, *J Pediat Orthop* 11:527-532, 1991.
4. Winter RB, Moe JH: The results of spinal arthrodesis for congenital spine deformity in patients younger than 5 years old, *J Bone Joint Surg* 64A:419-432, 1982.
5. Winter RB, Moe JH, Lonstein JE: Posterior spinal arthrodesis for congenital scoliosis: an analysis of the cases of 290 patients 5–19 years old, *J Bone Joint Surg* 66A:1188-1197, 1984.
6. Winter RB: *Complications in the treatment of the congenital spine.* pp 261-279, In Epps C, Bowen R, editors: *Complications in pediatric orthopedic surgery,* Philadelphia, 1995, J.B. Lippincott, pp 261-279.

# 5

# REVISION CERVICAL SPINE SURGERY

**Vincent J. Devlin, M.D.**
**Paul A. Anderson, M.D.**



Revision cervical spinal surgery requires careful evaluation and planning to achieve a successful outcome. Realization that the initial procedure did not achieve its intended goals may be devastating to the patient and family members. Return to work issues, chronic pain, residual neurologic deficit, litigation, and the unrealistic expectation that "all can be fixed" make management difficult. Unique surgical challenges may present as a direct result of prior procedures and include spinal deformity, compromised bone stock for fixation, persistent neural encroachment, as well as scarring of both the neural elements and associated soft tissues. Preoperative planning must involve a thorough and comprehensive evaluation of the factors that resulted in a less-than-optimal outcome following the initial surgical procedure. If a poor surgical outcome can be attributed to initial errors in surgical strategy or surgical technique with respect to the index procedure, revision surgery may provide a reasonable chance of improved outcome. However, surgical failures attributed to errors in diagnosis or inappropriate patient selection for surgical treatment may not have an improved outcome if further surgery is performed. The purpose of this chapter is to review common causes of failure of cervical spine surgery and to discuss treatment strategies.

## PATIENT EVALUATION

History must be comprehensive when a patient is evaluated for an unsatisfactory result following a cervical procedure. It is critical to obtain a detailed history including the nature and duration of symptoms prior to the index procedure as well as the patient's response to surgery both in the immediate postoperative period as well as over time. The presence or absence of a pain-free interval following surgery should be specifically assessed.[142] The relative contributions of neck pain versus arm pain to the patient's clinical syndrome is important to determine. If neurologic deficit is present, has this improved, worsened, or remained unchanged following surgery? Are the patient's symptoms primarily axial pain, radiculopathy, myelopathy, or a combination of these syndromes? Details regarding prior surgical procedures including operative reports and prior imaging studies should be obtained and reviewed. Consideration of the patient's psychosocial circumstances, expectations regarding treatment, present work situation, as well as the status of possible compensation claims and litigation merit consideration. Tobacco use may be a contributing factor to failure of fusion or progressive disk degeneration and smoking should be discontinued prior to any further surgery.[21]

## PHYSICAL EXAMINATION

Physical examination includes a general neurologic assessment as well as evaluation of the upper extremities to rule out concomitant pathology such as carpal tunnel syndrome, thoracic outlet syndrome, rotator cuff pathology, as well as intrinsic disease of the spinal cord. Cervical range of motion is routinely assessed. Lack of extension may imply significant canal or foraminal stenosis. Painful rotation should lead to careful assessment of the C1-C2 joint. Upper and lower extremity sensory, motor, and reflex function should be documented and the presence or absence of pathologic reflexes noted. Atrophy of specific muscle groups is a worrisome sign.

## IMAGING

Prior imaging studies are reviewed and correlated with the patient's present clinical symptoms. Plain radiographs provide assessment of the extent, level, and type of previous surgery. Important information may be obtained regarding prior laminectomy defects, fusion masses, spinal fixation devices, spinal deformities, and degenerative changes adjacent to previously operated spinal levels. Flexion-extension views may be useful in demonstrating postoperative spinal instability or pseudarthrosis. Comparing measurements of the distance between the tips of spinous processes across fused segments is an accurate measure to determine if a fusion has healed. Arthrodesed segments will show an increase of only 1 to 2 mm on flexion-extension radiographs. Bone scans have a limited role in evaluating the postoperative spine but occasionally may be useful for diagnosing infection, pseudarthrosis, or adjacent-segment degeneration. Esophagrams may be indicated if a patient presents with displaced anterior cervical bone grafts or fixation devices or if direct esophageal injury is suspected.

Magnetic resonance imaging (MRI) or computed tomography (CT) myelography may be indicated depending upon the patient's symptoms, the presence or absence of spinal implants and the specific spinal problem requiring evaluation. MRI provides optimal visualization of spinal cord size and signal intensity as well providing detailed assessment of associated bony and soft tissue structures. Certain pathologic processes may expand the spinal cord (tumor, edema, syrinx) while others may result in decreased spinal cord size (atrophy, myelomalacia) and these findings may alter surgical decision-making. Increased signal intensity within the substance of the spinal cord indicates that there has been some degree of intrinsic damage to the cord.[139] This should alert the surgeon that the particular patient is at increased risk of neurologic complications if further surgery is undertaken. Furthermore, the patient may fail to improve neurologically despite adequate surgical treatment. MRI quality is subject to degradation secondary to metal artifacts that may arise from microscopic metal debris present at the initial surgical site or from spinal implants, especially if the latter are non-titanium implants.[93] CT myelography is of great utility in evaluating the previously operated cervical spine. It provides superior definition of bony detail and provides the ability to successfully image the spine in the presence of spinal implants, which would produce significant artifact on MRI studies. Functional myelography, especially with the neck in extension, may identify dynamic nerve or spinal cord impingement not obvious on supine static studies.

After obtaining a comprehensive history, performing a detailed physical examination, and reviewing imaging studies it may be possible to form an opinion as to the etiology of the patient's initial surgical failure. Frequently encountered problems include poor patient selection for initial surgery, failure to make the correct initial diagnosis, inappropriate surgical indications, and technical problems related to the index procedure. Alternatively, it may be apparent that a poor outcome was due to an unavoidable complication of appropriately performed surgery or that the problem arose due to progression of an underlying disease process. Kostuik[78] has stressed the importance of the time of presentation of the patient's complaints relative to the index surgical procedure. For example, if a patient reports no immediate improvement in symptoms following a procedure, one must consider whether the wrong diagnosis has been made or the wrong procedure has been performed. In the patient who describes immediate relief of symptoms followed by recurrent symptoms within weeks to months after surgery, new pathology or a complication of the index procedure must be considered. In the patient who reports good relief of symptoms for months to years following the index procedure and subsequently presents with recurrent symptomatology, a pseudarthrosis, new pathology, or a problem arising due to a degenerative process occurring adjacent to the previously operated levels should be considered.

## GENERAL PRINCIPLES OF CERVICAL REVISION SURGERY

If the results of a comprehensive diagnostic evaluation suggest that cervical revision surgery is a reasonable and desirable consideration, the indications for surgical intervention will generally fall into one or more of the following categories:

1. *Decompression* may be required to relieve encroachment upon the cervical spinal cord and/or nerve roots that has persisted following prior procedures or has developed subsequent to prior surgery.
2. *Spinal realignment* may be indicated if a spinal deformity is present that requires correction and/or stabilization. Indications for surgery include unacceptable kyphotic deformities, progressive deformities, associated neurologic deficit, and chronic pain.
3. *Spinal stabilization* may be required if pain, deformity progression, or risk of neurologic deterioration is attributed to compromise of the load-carrying capacity of the spinal column. Prior surgical procedures may have been unsuccessful in achieving this goal due to pseudarthrosis, kyphosis, or fixation failure.

Many advances in techniques of cervical spinal surgery have occurred during the past decade, especially in the area of cervical stabilization procedures. Utilizing contemporary methods it is possible to dramatically intervene in select patients and significantly improve their surgical outcome and quality of life. General treatment principles (Box 5-1) include:

1. *Definitive procedures* with the greatest likelihood of successfully addressing all aspects of the patient's pathology should be performed in the revision setting. This may include decompression with fusion and spinal instrumentation either anteriorly, posteriorly, or circumferentially. Our observation is that circumferential procedures are usually the best treatment choice. These are generally performed under the same anesthesia.[89] Patients may need to remain off work or restrict their daily activities for periods up to 6 to 12 months following revision surgery. After this period of time, patients can not easily tolerate additional procedures due to the negative psychological, social, and financial impact an additional extended period of disability would have on their lives while they recover from yet another cervical procedure.
2. *Adequate decompression* procedures should be performed when indicated. Just as decompression without fusion may lead to an unsatisfactory result in certain clinical situations, cervical fusion without adequate decompression may lead to a less-than-optimal clinical outcome.
3. *Stable fixation,* which limits the number of motion segments requiring surgery, increases the likelihood of successful fusion, preserves or restores cervical lordosis, and minimizes the need for external support such as a halo vest is the goal.[8]

**BOX 5-1. BASIC PRINCIPLES OF REVISION CERVICAL SPINE SURGERY**

1. Adequate preoperative assessment
2. Optimization for fusion including smoking cessation
3. Preoperative spinal realignment (with traction if indicated)
4. Perform definitive surgical procedures (combined anterior and posterior procedures often required)
5. Complete neural decompression
6. Restoration of axial height and cervical lordosis
7. Adequate internal fixation
8. Autogenous bone graft used somewhere within the construct
9. Appropriate postoperative immobilization
10. Postoperative rehabilitation

## OCCIPUT-C2 REVISION SURGERY

### OCCIPITOCERVICAL FUSION

Occipitocervical arthrodesis is a rarely performed operation whose indications include deformity secondary to rheumatoid arthritis, trauma, congenital malformation, tumor, and iatrogenic instability. Most clinical series report success regardless of the technique utilized, with fusion rates ranging from 92% to 100%.[9,36,64,69,77,82,86,91,103,110,135] No clinical series specifically addresses revision of failed occipitocervical fusion. In the revision setting, occipitocervical fusion may be the procedure of choice when treating complex craniocervical instabilities and pseudarthroses.

Several surgical techniques for occipitocervical arthrodesis have been described, including onlay bone grafts combined with use of rigid external immobilization,[40] wire-bone constructs used with supplemental rigid external immobilization,[81,128,144] rod-wire or rod-cable constructs[41,44,73,85,109,119,132] used with or without external immobilization (Hartshill-Ransford loop, contoured Steinmann pin, contoured Luque rod), and plate-screw constructs.[59,60,61,117,121,125] Comparative biomechanical analysis[104,137] has shown that plate-screw constructs are stiffer than rod-cable constructs in all testing modes except in flexion in which these techniques are equivalent. Onlay bone graft techniques with prolonged halo immobilization have been reported to be successful in the pediatric population.[40] Wire-bone graft constructs have been used successfully when sufficient bone stock is available posteriorly for wire fixation and if postoperative rigid external immobilization can be tolerated by the patient.[144] Rod-wire techniques were developed in order to provide immediate postoperative stability and possibly eliminate the need for prolonged external immobilization during the process of fusion consolidation. The introduction of flexible multistrand cables has facilitated sublaminar fixation and has increased the strength of the final construct.[130] Rod-plate fixation was developed to address limitations of rod-wire constructs noted in certain complex problems in which the posterior spinal elements are deficient or fractured, complex instability or deformities exist, osteoporosis is present, or resistance to axial settling forces is required. An important advantage of rod-plate fixation is the ability to mobilize the patient postoperatively without rigid external immobilization. Several surgeons have reported excellent results with plate-screw fixation for occipitocervical fusion with no cases of fixation failure, pseudarthrosis, or complications related to the spinal instrumentation.[60,125] However, complications of screw pull-out, screw-failure, plate breakage, and cerebellar subdural hematoma secondary to screw or drill injury have been reported.[22] Recent anatomical studies have focused on identification of optimal sites for screw fixation in the occiput and development of implants to facilitate these fixation strategies.[62,157] Presently, decisions regarding optimal selection of arthrodesis and fixation techniques in this area must be made on a case-by-case basis depending on multiple factors such as the underlying disease process, bone quality, altered surgical anatomy created by prior procedures, availability of specific implants, and the wishes of the patient regarding the need for postoperative immobilization. We recommend using the more rigid forms of fixation such as plate-screw or rod-wire fixation. In the future, more versatile implant systems will be available and permit optimal use of wire, screw, or hook fixation throughout the occipitocervical-thoracic region depending upon the underlying pathologic process.

## REVISION C1-C2 FUSION

In contrast to occipitocervical arthrodesis, pseudarthrosis following atlantoaxial procedures is not uncommon, with reported failure rates ranging from 4% to 60%.[38,58,87,88,97] Excellent fusion success has been reported in traumatic disorders,[29] whereas fusion success in rheumatoid disorders,[27,32,33,83,120,124,158] os odontoideum[46,131] and Down syndrome[38] is problematic. Dickman[37] categorized the reasons for failure in C1-C2 arthrodesis procedures as: metabolic (malnutrition, vitamin deficiency, osteoporosis), pathologic (rheumatoid disease), pharmacologic (steroids, anti-inflammatory medication, cytotoxic agents), biomechanical (inadequate control of C1-C2 motion during bone healing), and technical factors. The technical failures were varied and included failure to use autograft bone graft, failure to use any bone graft, failure to compress the bone graft between C1 and C2, inadequate preparation of the fusion bed especially with respect to decortication of the ring of C1, and failure to use a halo if rigid fixation cannot be obtained or if the bone is osteopenic. Pseudarthroses occurred most commonly at the C1-graft interface and never solely at the C2-graft interface. Spinal fixation failure modes included wire/cable breakage, loosening, or erosion through osteopenic bone. Caution was recommended when utilizing multistrand cables for fixation in osteopenic bone because excess tensioning of these devices may result in these implants cutting through the bone. We recommend limiting tension to twenty pounds or using "washers" such as titanium mesh or cortical bone allografts.

Atlantoaxial arthrodesis has been attempted by a variety of techniques, including bone graft and halo immobilization,[77,116] bone graft and wire fixation (Gallie or Brooks technique) with supplemental external immobilization,[20,50,56,92] bone graft and interlaminar clamp fixation,[100] and bone graft with transarticular screw fixation.[87,88] The biomechanics of fixation at the atlantoaxial joint has been extensively investigated.[30,63,66,98,148] Hanley[65] quantitated the immediate postoperative stability provided by various wiring techniques in an odontoid fracture model. The Brooks technique provided stiffness four times greater than the Gallie technique and five times greater than that obtained from simple midline wiring. Smith[127] analyzed six techniques of C1-C2 fixation: midline wiring, Gallie technique, Brooks technique, Magerl transarticular screw fixation, and the Clark technique both with and without methylmethacrylate augmentation. Only the transarticular screw technique and the augmented Clark technique were able to restore translational stability to the spine in the odontoid fracture model. Grob[57] studied the biomechanics of four fixation techniques: Gallie, Brooks, interlaminar clamps, and Magerl transarticular screw fixation. Results demonstrated that transarticular screws provided the most stable construct and that the Gallie construct was the least effective in stabilizing the injured spinal segment. When feasible, the use of transarticular screw fixation is considered to be the most reliable fixation technique for achieving atlantoaxial arthrodesis.

In revision cases in which the patient presents with persistent symptoms following attempted C1-C2 arthrodesis, thorough clinical and radiographic evaluation to assess for possible pseudarthrosis or persistent neurologic compression is mandatory (Table 5-1). Plain radiography, including flexion-extension views, CT scans, and MRI should be performed as needed to assess four critical factors as a guide to decision-making: C1-C2 alignment, status of the C1 arch, bone stock, and status of the occiput-C1 articulation. First, it is important to assess the relationship of C1 to C2. Is C1-C2 well-aligned or is subluxation present? If subluxation is present, is the displacement reducible with traction or positioning or is the displacement fixed? Fixed C1-C2 displacement is a contraindication

**Table 5-1. C1-2 Revision Fusion Procedures**

| Procedure | Indications |
|---|---|
| Repeat wiring procedure | • Intact C1 arch with adequate bone stock, C1 laminectomy not needed, reducible deformity that permits safe sublaminar wire passage<br>• Aberrant vertebral artery precludes C1-C2 transarticular screw placement |
| Transarticular C1-C2 fixation | • C1-C2 fusion when C1 laminectomy required<br>• Preferred C1-C2 fixation technique (anatomy permitting) |
| Occiput-C2 fusion ± C1 laminectomy | • Basilar invagination<br>• Incompetent C1 arch<br>• Multiple failed C1-C2 fusion attempts<br>• Occiput-C1 instability<br>• Fixed C1-C2 subluxation |

to revision utilizing C1 or C2 sublaminar wires or cable fixation and generally requires C1 laminectomy with extension of fusion to the occiput.[49,128,129] Second, the status of the C1 arch should be assessed on preoperative studies. If the C1 arch is deficient, C1-C2 fixation with transarticular screw fixation is the procedure of choice. Alternatively, an occiput-C2 fusion with rigid fixation is recommended. Third, the status of the bone stock in the C1-C2 region must be assessed. Multiple prior attempts at fusion may leave the posterior bony elements scarred and atrophic. If the remaining ring of C1 is a sclerotic thin remnant of bone then a C1-C2 wiring procedure is not likely to succeed. If transarticular screw fixation is considered, preoperative CT reconstructions of the anticipated screw path are mandatory in order to assess whether screws can be safely placed without violating an anomalous vertebral artery and to ensure that sufficient bone remains to provide secure screw purchase. The fourth factor that must be assessed in decision-making is the status of the occiput-C1 articulation. The presence of basilar invagination or more rarely the presence of occiput-C1 instability would require that fusion be extended to the occiput (Fig. 5-1).

We favor the use of the Magerl transarticular fixation technique for C1-C2 arthrodesis in revision procedures when this technique is technically feasible. Alternatively, a revision Brooks fusion procedure can succeed if remaining bone stock is adequate, an indication for C1 laminectomy is not present, and if the patient will tolerate a period of prolonged external immobilization. However, in situations in which there are deficient posterior elements, severe osteopenia, or if the patient cannot tolerate external immobilization, Magerl transarticular screw fixation is the procedure of choice. If preoperative CT reconstructions of the anticipated screw path show that transarticular screws cannot be safely placed, then consideration should be given to extension of fusion to the occiput with plate-screw fixation and obtaining fixation at C2 with pedicle screws (Fig. 5-2).

## SUBAXIAL CERVICAL SPINE REVISION SURGERY

Evaluation of the patient following failed subaxial cervical surgery is a challenge. The goal of revision surgery is to completely decompress the affected neural elements, correct spinal deformity, and obtain solid arthrodesis. Problems that are potentially correctable with further surgery include pseudarthrosis, persistent nerve root or spinal cord impingement, kyphosis, symptoms due to adjacent-segment degeneration, and problems due to graft migration or displacement of spinal fixation devices.

### PSEUDARTHROSIS

Factors that may influence the rate of pseudarthrosis include graft technique (interbody graft versus strut graft), the source of bone graft (allograft versus autograft), the type of bone graft used (fibula versus ilium), smoking, as well as the use of adjunctive internal fixation and postoperative external immobilization. Radiographic criteria used to assess union of interbody fusions include the presence of bony trabeculae crossing the disk space, absence of radiolucent lines at the graft-host junction and motion less than 2 mm between adjacent spinous processes on flexion-extension views. Radiographic criteria for fusion of strut grafts are similar and include bony trabeculae crossing the superior and inferior junction sites between the graft and vertebra, absence of motion at the junction sites on flexion-extension views, and remodeling of the bone graft. Follow-up of up to 2 years may be required to definitely assess fusion and caution should be exercised prior to this time.

Multiple series describe cervical interbody fusion

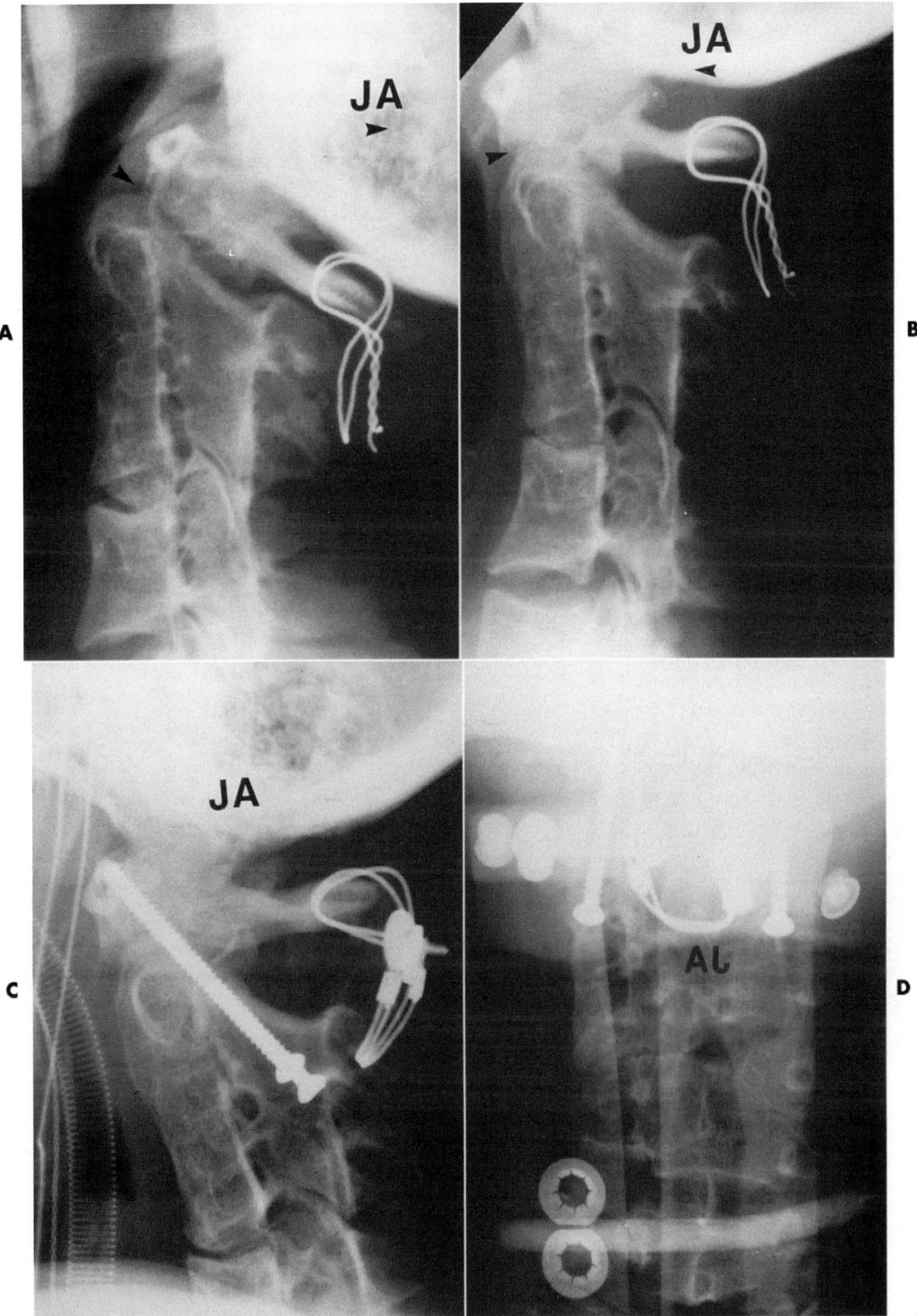


Figure 5-1

Atlantoaxial nonunion. A 23-year-old woman with Klippel-Feil syndrome and os odontoideum treated initially with Gallie technique. Postoperative extension (**A**) and flexion (**B**) radiographs show persistent anteroposterior C1-C2 instability. Revision C1-C2 fusion was performed with transarticular C1-C2 Magerl screw fixation (**C, D**).

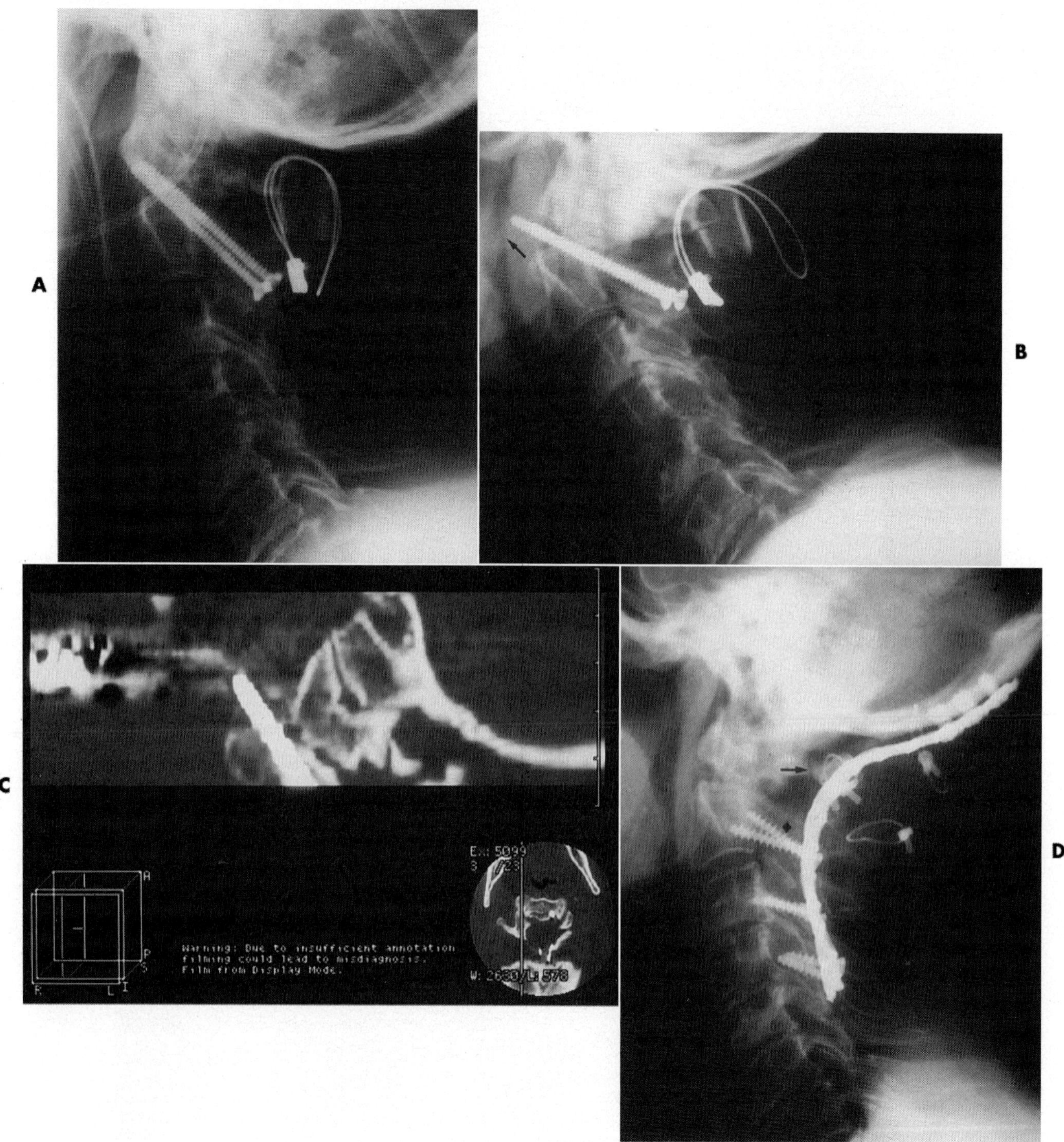


**FIGURE 5-2**

Atlantoaxial nonunion, fixation failure. A 73-year-old man fell and sustained a type 2 odontoid fracture. Postoperative radiograph (**A**) shows that he was treated by Magerl screw fixation. Two weeks postoperatively, the screw migrated through the C1 arch into the retropharynx (**B**). In the critical postoperative radiograph, the screws are angled too low (below the anterior atlantal arch) thereby limiting fixation and leading to fixation failure. CT reconstruction (**C**) shows that the screws are not engaged in C1 and are well anterior in the retropharyngeal space. Fortunately, the screws did not penetrate into the pharyngeal cavity. The patient was referred to our institution and was treated by occiput-cervical fusion with screw-plate fixation (**D**). Fixation at C1 was obtained with a sublaminar wire loop around the C1 lamina (*arrow*) and by C2 pedicle screws (*square*).

using the Smith-Robinson technique with reported pseudarthrosis rates ranging from 3% to 26%.[10,11,31,35,54,111,136,141,145,149] Overall, the pseudarthrosis rate tends to increase as interbody fusion is attempted at more than one level.[48] One recent report cited a 13% overall pseudarthrosis rate with 11% incidence of pseudarthrosis following single-level interbody fusion and a 27% pseudarthrosis rate for two- and three-level fusions using iliac crest autograft.[17] Comparison of iliac crest autograft and freeze-dried iliac graft[155] showed the nonunion rate to be significantly higher in the allograft group (62%) compared to the autograft group (17%) in multilevel fusions, although the nonunion rate was identical in single-level fusions (5%). A recent study has shown that operative correction and early postoperative maintenance of local fusion segment lordosis in multilevel anterior decompression and interbody fusion is important if pseudarthrosis is to be avoided.[25] Reported pseudarthrosis rates for anterior strut grafts range from 0% to 41%.[15,72,146] Fernyhough reported a 27% nonunion rate with autograft fibula strut graft compared to a 41% nonunion rate with allograft fibula strut grafts used to stabilize the multilevel cervical spondylotic spine following multilevel diskectomy and corpectomy.[45] Supplemental external immobilization, supplemental cancellous grafting, and supplemental posterior fixation were advised to improve the likelihood of osseous union. Other series report fusion rates approaching 100% using autogenous fibular strut grafts without supplemental posterior fixation but problems due to loss of axial height (subsidence) and increased postoperative kyphosis were noted (Fig. 5-3).[72]

Although some studies have been unable to correlate the presence of pseudarthrosis with an unfavorable outcome following surgery, several recent studies with long-term follow-up support the relationship between pseudarthrosis and a poor outcome following anterior cervical disk surgery. Bohlman[17] evaluated 122 patients with a mean duration of follow-up of 6 years (range 2 to 15 years) after anterior cervical diskectomy and fusion and noted a significant relationship between pseudarthrosis and postoperative pain in the neck or arm. It was noted that motion and the presence of chondro-osseous spurs at the level of the pseudarthrosis may contribute to residual nerve-root compression. Phillips[106] analyzed the natural history and treatment of anterior cervical pseudarthrosis following anterior cervical diskectomy and fusion with iliac crest autograft. Pseudarthroses were noted in 48 patients over a 14-year period. One-third of the patients had minimal symptoms attributable to the pseudarthrosis at a mean of 5.1 years following surgery. Two-thirds of the patients had symptoms attributable to the pseudarthrosis and 16 of these 32 patients underwent further surgery for pseudarthrosis repair. Among the patients with symptomatic pseudarthroses, one-third had a prolonged symptom-free interval following their initial operation despite radiographic evidence of pseudarthrosis and developed symptoms only after a subsequent traumatic event. This finding suggests disruption of a fibrous union as the etiology of symptoms in this subset of patients. Studies documenting patients with failed fusions who did poorly and subsequently did well after obtaining a solid arthrodesis provide further evidence of the importance of obtaining a successful arthrodesis after anterior cervical diskectomy.[102]

Various surgical approaches have been advocated for the treatment of symptomatic anterior cervical pseudarthroses. Robinson[114] reported four cases with symptomatic nonunions. Two cases underwent successful posterior fusions whereas two patients underwent anterior repair with successful fusion in one case. Brodsky[19] reported a randomized study comparing anterior revision surgery with autograft bone to posterior fusion and posterior wiring and concluded that the posterior approach was more effective (94% fusion rate) than repeat anterior surgery (79% fusion rate). Farey and McAfee[43] reported 100% success in patients with symptomatic anterior pseudarthrosis and radiculopathy treated with posterior nerve root decompression, posterior arthrodesis with autograft, and triple-wire stabilization. However, they cautioned against using the posterior approach in cases of anterior pseudarthrosis with concomitant kyphosis and/or myelopathy because these conditions are best treated with anterior decompression and stabilization. Phillips[106] reported that good results can be obtained with either anterior or posterior approaches for anterior cervical pseudarthroses. All cases treated by the posterior approach achieved successful arthrodesis, whereas 87% of the cases treated by revision anterior surgery achieved arthrodesis. All failed anterior revision procedures were successfully salvaged by posterior arthrodesis procedures. Zdeblick[156] reported successful outcomes in 34 of 35 patients treated for failed anterior cervical diskectomy and fusion procedures. Revision surgery was performed solely by the anterior approach with successful arthrodesis ultimately achieved in 34 patients utilizing autograft. Patients with pseudarthrosis in the absence of significant kyphosis were treated with hemicorpectomy of adjacent vertebral bodies, decompression as needed, and autogenous iliac graft. Patients with pseudarthrosis and significant kyphosis, myelopathy, or with adjacent-level pseudarthroses requiring decompression were treated by corpectomy. Iliac grafts were utilized for one- or two-level corpectomies while fibular graft was utilized if more than two levels were resected. Lowery[84] reported treatment of symptomatic anterior cervical pseudarthroses by three methods: anterior revisions, posterior revisions, and circumferential revi-

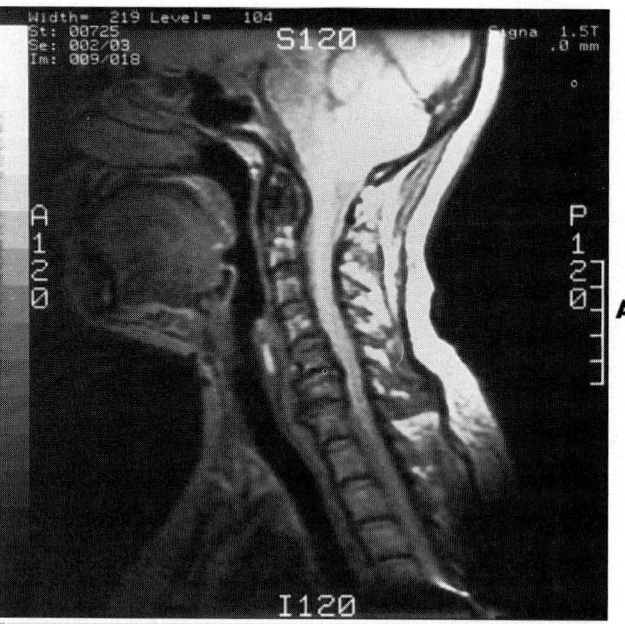


B

C

**Figure 5-3**

Subaxial, anterior pseudarthrosis following strut graft. A 49-year-old woman presented with cervical myeloradiculopathy. **A,** MRI demonstrates stenosis from C4-C5 to C6-C7. This patient was treated with a C5 and C6 corpectomy with C4-C7 fusion and plating with complete relief of preoperative symptoms. Three years following surgery this patient returned with complaints of neck pain and left arm pain. **B,C,** Anteroposterior and lateral radiographs demonstrate fracture of the inferior screws indicating possible pseudarthrosis at C6-C7.

*Continued*

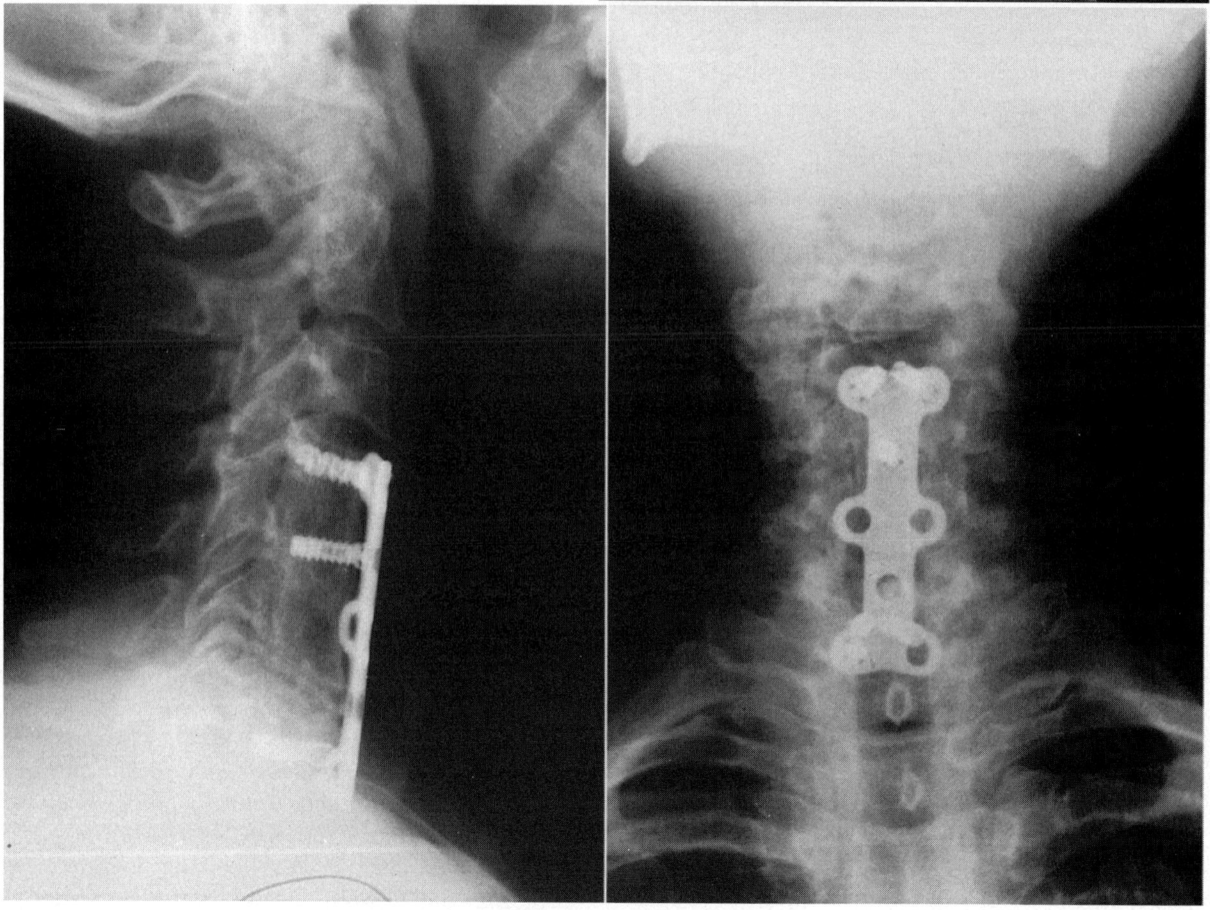

sions. Anterior procedures consisted of resection of the nonunion, regrafting, and anterior cervical plating. Autograft was used in 35% of cases and allograft was used in 65% of cases. A solid fusion was obtained in only 45% of patients after anterior repair alone. Posterior procedures included fixation with articular pillar plating as a supplement to facet fusion with either local bone graft, allograft or autograft, and foraminotomy or laminectomy as required. Solid fusion was achieved in 94% of cases. Circumferential procedures were performed with predominantly allograft anteriorly and predominantly autograft posteriorly, with successful fusions anteriorly and posteriorly in all cases. Recently, Tribus[140] reported solid fusion in

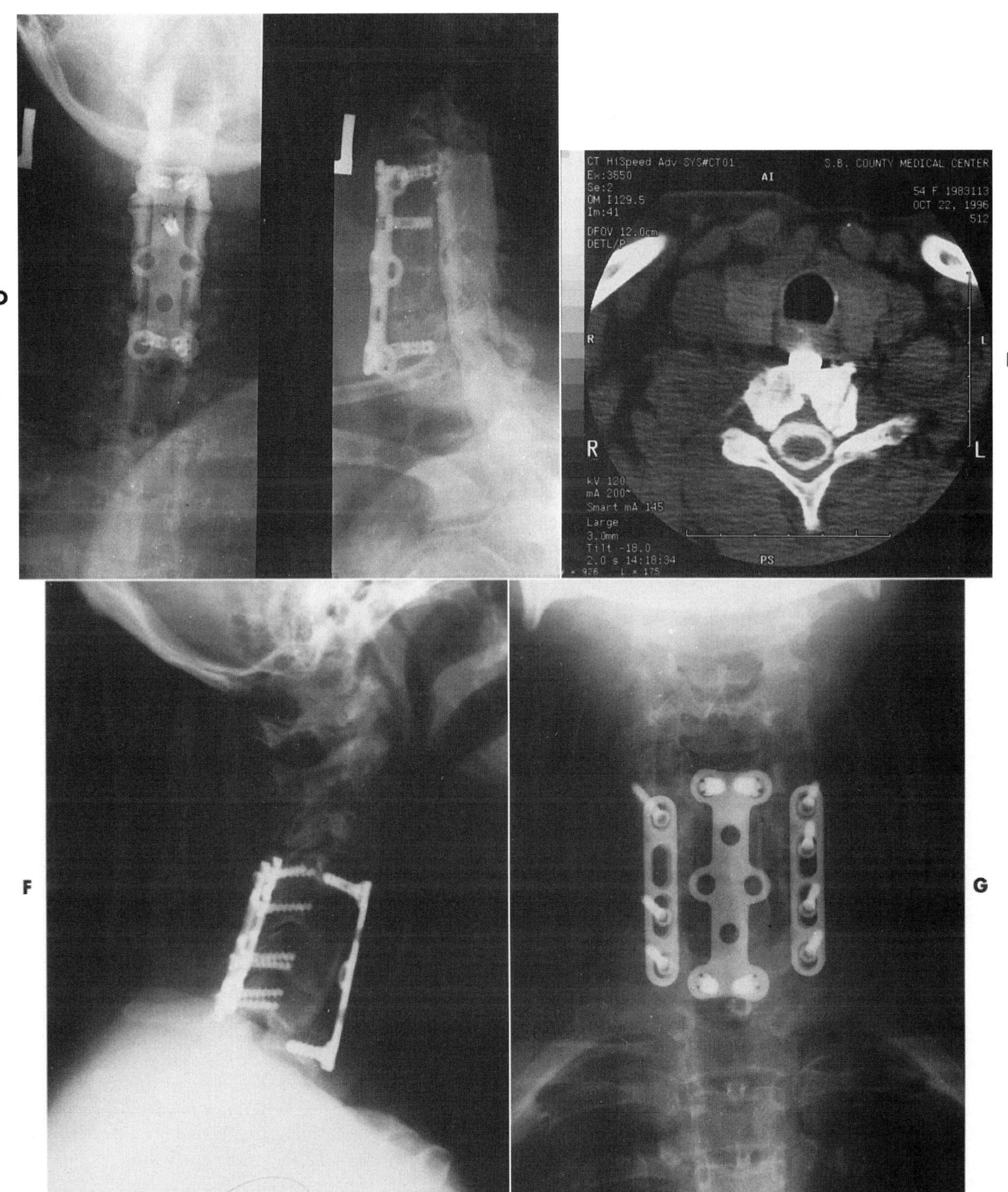


**FIGURE 5-3, CONT'D**

**D,** Cervical myelogram demonstrates poor filling of the C7 nerve roots. **E,** CT following myelography demonstrates significant foraminal stenosis at C6-C7 on the left. This patient underwent an anterior revision procedure with removal of the previous strut graft using tricortical iliac crest autograft. **F,G,** This was followed by posterior cervical plating and fusion C4-C7.

**Table 5-2. C3-7 Revision Procedures for Pseudarthrosis After Interbody Fusion**

| Indication | Procedure |
|---|---|
| Single-level anterior pseudarthrosis with axial pain or radiculopathy | Resection of nonunion by hemicorpectomies, autogenous iliac graft, anterior plating<br>or<br>Posterior foraminotomy, posterior fusion, autogenous iliac graft, internal fixation |
| Single-level pseudarthrosis with kyphosis or myelopathy | Corpectomy (complete vs. partial), autogenous iliac strut graft, anterior plating |
| Multiple-level anterior pseudarthroses | Resection of nonunion with multilevel interbody fusions or corpectomy ± anterior plating combined with posterior fusion with autograft and lateral mass plating or wire fixation |
| Anterior pseudarthrosis following anterior fusion and plating, anterior fixation intact | Posterior fusion with autograft and lateral mass plating |
| Anterior pseudarthrosis following anterior fusion and plating, failure or migration of anterior fixation device | Urgent revision for hardware removal and additional procedures as indicated |

93% of patients following revision of symptomatic pseudarthroses with single-stage anterior autograft and anterior Morscher plate fixation.

Based on review of the literature and our experience, the following treatment recommendations for symptomatic anterior cervical pseudarthroses following attempted interbody fusion are made (Table 5-2). Single-level pseudarthrosis with axial pain with or without radiculopathy can be treated by repeat anterior cervical fusion with resection of the nonunion by hemicorpectomies of adjacent vertebral bodies, decompression as required, autogenous iliac graft, and anterior plating. Alternatively, posterior fusion with autograft and fixation by the triple-wire technique or fixation with lateral mass plates is a valid technique. A posterior foraminotomy should be performed if radicular symptoms are present. However, in the presence of kyphosis, myelopathy or multiple adjacent levels requiring decompression, the anterior approach with corpectomy and autogenous bone grafting is indicated. Anterior plate fixation prevents the development of kyphosis following corpectomy and fusion and avoids the need for halo immobilization, especially when corpectomy is required in the presence of posterior ligamentous laxity or when a prior laminectomy has been performed. Patients who present with anterior pseudarthrosis following anterior interbody fusion and plate fixation can be salvaged with posterior fusion with autograft and fixation with either wires or lateral mass plates if the anterior hardware is intact. If the anterior hardware has loosened, there is imminent danger to the tracheoesophageal structures and an urgent revision procedure should be performed.[126,147] This includes anterior hardware removal and anterior bone grafting followed by posterior fusion with internal fixation. In general, if multiple-level corpectomies and strut grafting are required, a circumferential procedure consisting of anterior strut grafting with or without anterior plating followed by posterior fusion and stabilization usually with plating is our preferred procedure.[96] Anterior plate fixation alone is not considered sufficient to stabilize a long strut graft because screw purchase above and below the corpectomy does not provide segmental fixation for the overall construct and failures have been reported using this fixation technique due to screw breakage and fracture of the vertebrae below the corpectomy.[141]

Anterior cervical diskectomy without fusion is performed by some surgeons in order to avoid graft-related complications. Long-term studies report that this practice may not compromise the overall result of a cervical disk procedure in all patients. However, inferior results for patients treated by diskectomy without fusion have been reported in patients with significant preoperative spondylosis compared to patients with soft disk protrusions.[14,152] Although spontaneous fusion has been reported in up to 70% of patients treated with diskectomy without fusion,[55] the motion segment may settle into a collapsed position with resultant kyphosis and foraminal narrowing. A variable number of these patients develop a discogenic pain syndrome with or without radiculopathy and require revision surgery. There is a paucity of literature to guide revision surgery for this problem. Repeat anterior surgery with interbody grafting using autogenous iliac bone and anterior foraminotomy is a reasonable treatment option (Fig. 5-4). If diskectomy without fusion has been performed over multiple levels and a significant kyphotic deformity is present, anterior cor-

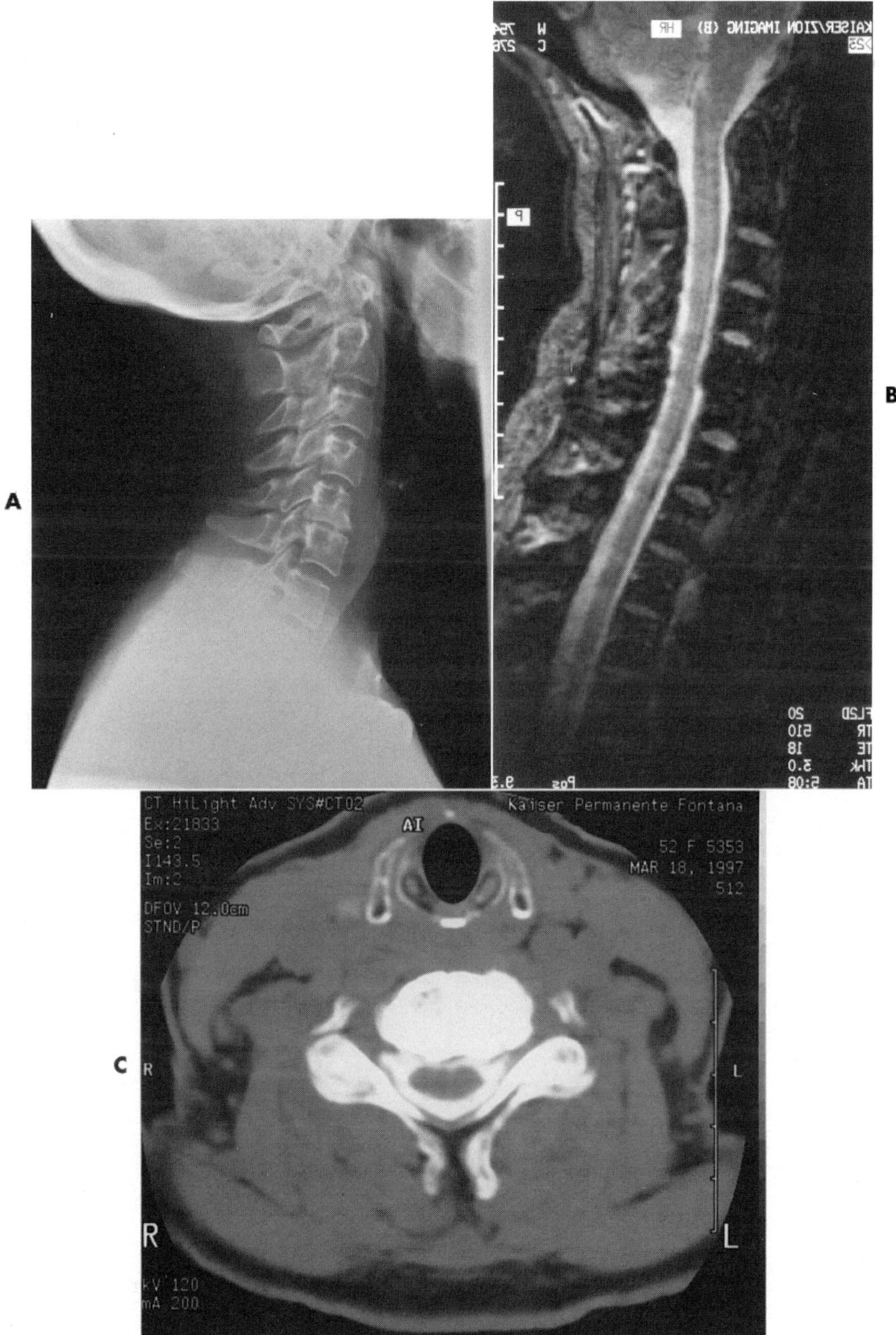


**FIGURE 5-4**

Neck and radicular pain after C5-C6 diskectomy without fusion. **A,** Lateral x-ray of a 52-year-old woman following C5-C6 diskectomy without fusion for cervical and radicular pain. The patient reported only temporary improvement postoperatively and subsequently developed recurrent severe cervical and radicular pain. **B,** Sagittal MRI shows absence of adjacent-segment pathology. **C,** Cervical CT myelogram shows left-sided bony foraminal stenosis.

*Continued*

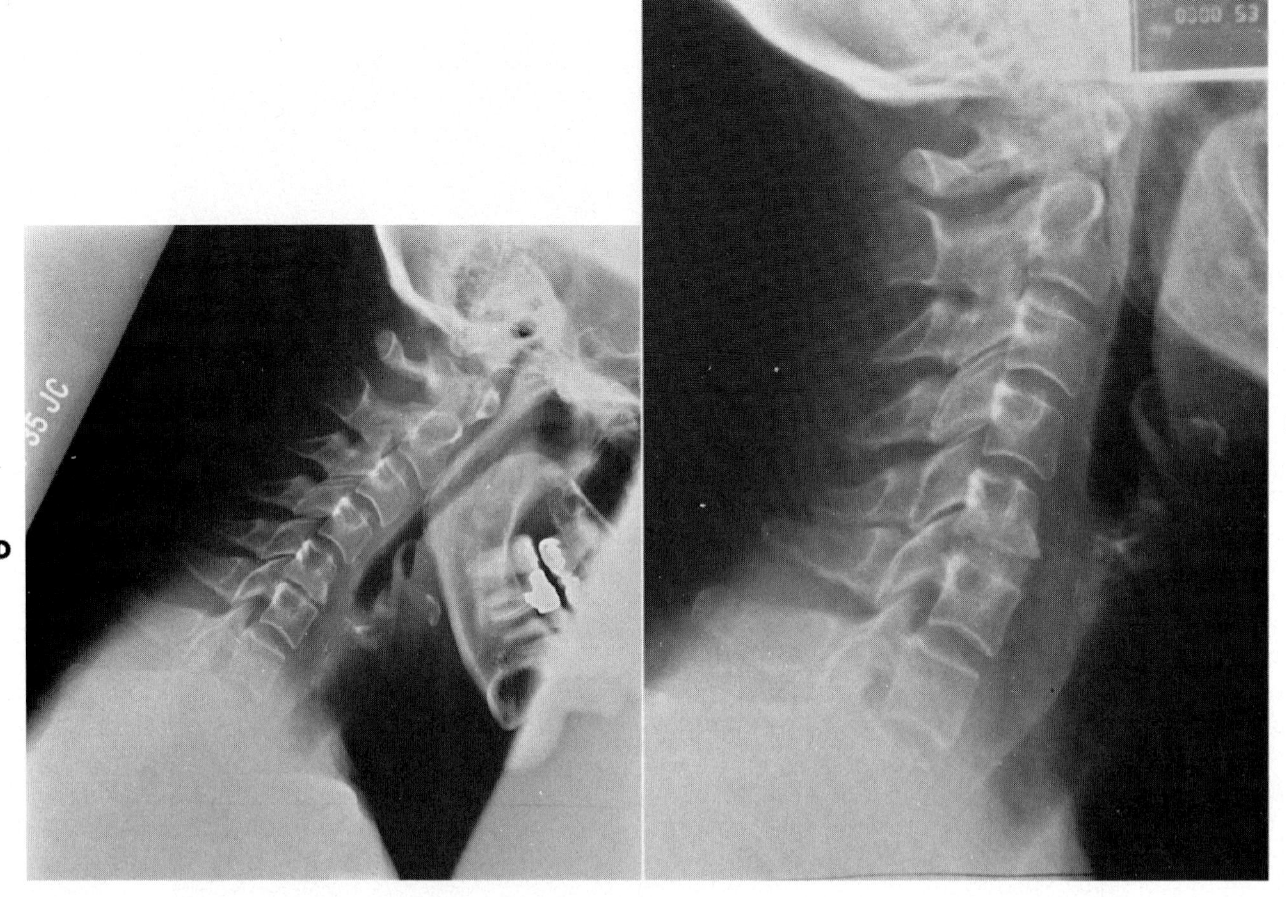

FIGURE 5-4, CONT'D

**D,** Dynamic radiographs show no evidence of abnormal angulation or translation. **E,** The patient had an excellent outcome following revision anterior cervical decompression with anterior foraminotomy and C5-C6 interbody fusion using autogenous iliac crest bone.

pectomy with strut grafting may be required. Alternatively, treatment may be performed through the posterior approach with posterior laminoforaminotomy and instrumented fusion generally with lateral mass plates. A prerequisite for use of the posterior approach alone is achievement of acceptable cervical lordosis with this approach. In cases with severe fixed kyphotic deformity, anterior decompression and strut grafting followed by posterior fusion with lateral mass plating is the procedure of choice.

## RESIDUAL CORD AND/OR NERVE ROOT COMPRESSION

Spinal cord or nerve root impingement may persist or develop following anterior cervical reconstructive surgery (Box 5-2). Neural impingement may be due to retained pathology not adequately decompressed at the initial operation, stenosis due to axial height (subsidence) loss following graft resorption or collapse, stenosis arising at the level of a pseudarthrosis due to bony or soft tissue hypertrophy, malposition of spinal fixation devices, or degenerative changes adjacent to previously fused levels.

### BOX 5-2. INDICATIONS FOR REVISION SURGERY FOR RESIDUAL CORD/ROOT COMPRESSION (C3-C7)

1. Retained pathology not adequately decompressed at initial operation.
2. Stenosis secondary to axial height loss (subsidence) following graft resorption or collapse.
3. Stenosis arising at the level of pseudarthrosis secondary to bony or soft tissue hypertrophy.
4. Malposition of spinal fixation devices with resultant neural impingement.
5. Adjacent-segment degeneration with subsequent neural encroachment.

Persistent radicular pain in the early postoperative period may be due to a sequestered disk fragment that was not removed at the time of surgery or due to inadequate bony decompression. The problem may be diagnosed with repeat imaging studies and treated with revision surgery. Graft-related problems include migration, dislodgement, and fracture. Poor graft sizing, inadequate graft site preparation, and inadequate postoperative immobilization may predispose to early graft collapse. If only mild anterior graft migration is noted, the situation may be salvaged with immediate rigid external immobilization such as that provided by a halo. If the graft becomes dislodged or fractured it will require removal and replacement with a new graft. Anterior plate fixation would be a useful adjunct. Excessive graft height may lead to overdistraction, graft extrusion, or graft fracture and should be avoided. Posterior graft migration with neurologic injury has been reported following fusions performed with the Cloward technique. Significant kyphotic deformities have been noted due to graft collapse or avascular necrosis of the intervening vertebral bodies when multiple levels have been grafted utilizing this technique. Radicular symptoms at a level different from the initial symptoms suggest adjacent-segment pathology and may require additional surgical treatment.

Treatment of residual cord and root compression follows the principles previously outlined for revision cervical surgery. Preoperative assessment should correlate levels of neural compression with levels of possible pseudarthroses, which may require treatment as well. Single-level foraminal stenosis with or without pseudarthrosis can be treated with either an anterior or posterior approach. Patients with kyphosis and/or myelopathy at a single level are best treated with anterior decompression and stabilization. If revision decompression and/or fusion is required at more than one level, combined anterior and posterior procedures are generally preferred (Fig. 5-5).

## ADJACENT-SEGMENT DEGENERATION

Patients with adjacent-segment degeneration may develop symptoms and require surgical treatment for segmental instability, bony stenosis, disk herniation, or facet or disk arthropathy. Patients with adjacent-segment degeneration may present with a range of symptoms including axial pain, radicular pain, or myelopathy. The exact incidence of symptomatic adjacent-segment degeneration is poorly described. A recent study noted that new radiculopathy due to adjacent-segment degeneration following anterior cervical diskectomy and interbody fusion developed in 2% to 3% of patients per year after surgery.[70] No association was noted with fusion length or successful fusion status. Bohlman[17] reported an 8% incidence of adjacent-level disk herniation, spondylosis, or subluxation following anterior cervical diskectomy and interbody fusion after an average postoperative follow-up of 6 years. Satomi[122] reported ten cases of late myelopathy developing as a result of degenerative changes at levels adjacent to prior anterior cervical interbody fusions 4 to 18 years (mean = 10 years) following the initial cervical procedure. Diagnostic evaluation must be tailored to the specific type of adjacent-segment problem suspected as well as guided by the patient's presenting symptoms. If cervical instability is suspected, flexion-extension radiographs are indicated. Radiographic criteria for instability have been defined as sagittal plane translation greater than 3.5 mm or sagittal plane angulation greater than 11 degrees.[142] MRI or CT myelography are indicated if cervical root or cord encroachment are suspected. Precise evaluation of patients with only axial pain is difficult. We find bone scans, facet injections, cervical medial branch blocks, and, occasionally, diskography useful to localize the pain generator.[13,78,141]

The revision surgical procedure is determined by the specific type of adjacent-segment problem requiring treatment (Table 5-3). Surgery generally involves extension of the prior fusion to include the pathologic adjacent segment(s). Strong consideration should be given to the use of spinal instrumentation as an adjunct to fusion due to the concentration of forces on the adjacent level by the lever arm created by the prior fusion mass. Neural decompression may or may not be

**Table 5-3. Surgical Procedures for Adjacent Segment Problems Developing After Prior Cervical Fusions (C3-7)**

| Indication | Procedure |
|---|---|
| Segmental instability (e.g., spondylolisthesis) | Posterior fusion extension with posterior spinal fixation ± decompression as needed<br>or<br>Anterior fusion extension with anterior plate fixation ± decompression as needed |
| Adjacent-level spinal stenosis or disk herniation | Anterior cervical corpectomy and fusion with anterior plate fixation |
| Adjacent-level disk or facet arthropathy | Fusion extension by anterior or posterior approach using spinal instrumentation |
| Adjacent-level instability or stenosis with kyphosis or deficient posterior spinal elements | Combined anterior and posterior fusion extension with spinal instrumentation ± decompression as needed |

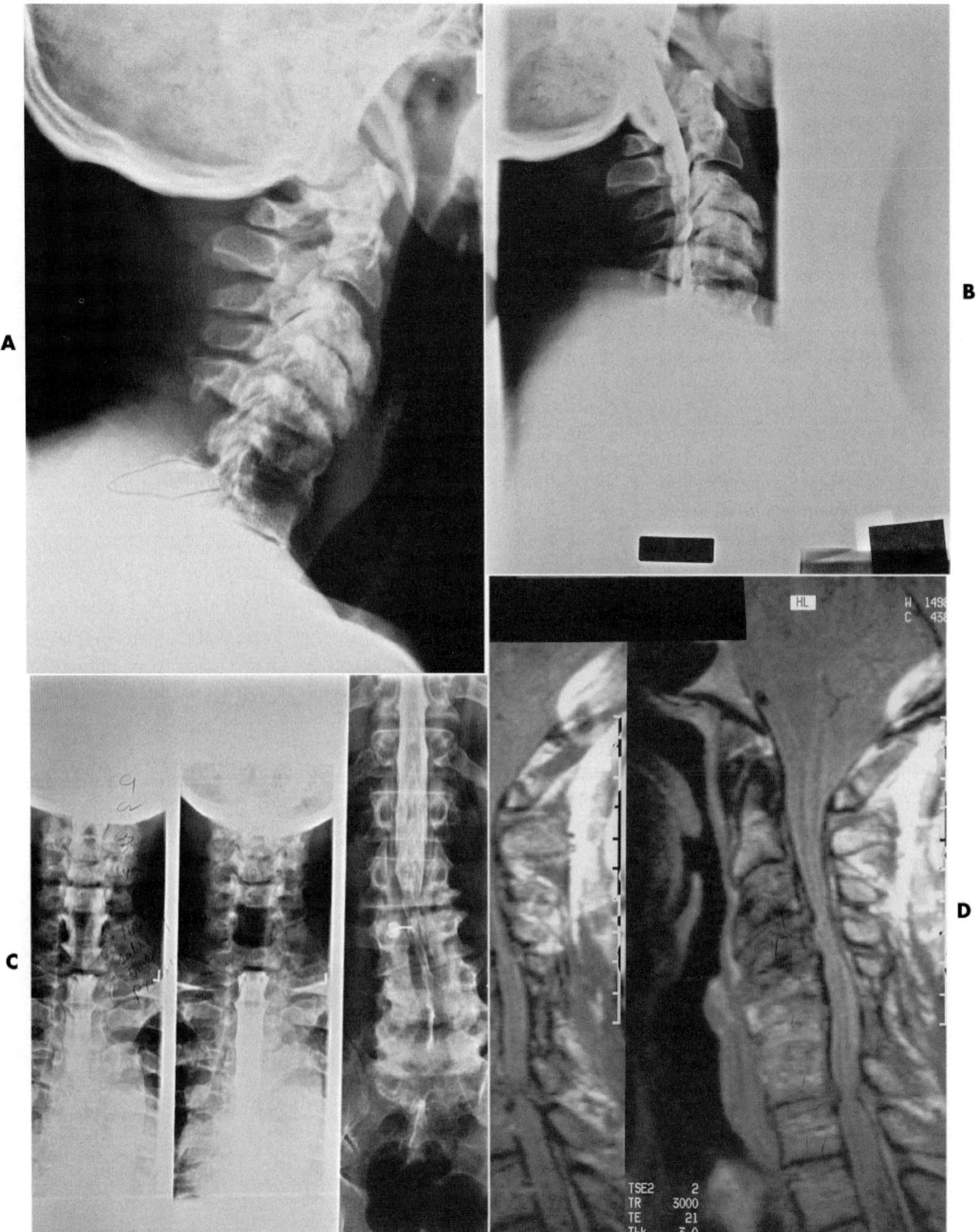


**FIGURE 5-5**

Residual neural compression following cervical laminectomy. A 60-year-old man presented with severe myelopathy, neck pain and ataxia, and a history of prior C6 laminectomy. The patient had been told following his laminectomy that nothing further could be done for his problem. Patient was evaluated at our center with imaging studies in anticipation of cervical surgery, but developed sudden onset of tetraparesis and became confined to a wheelchair. **A,** Lateral x-ray shows prior C6 laminectomy and diffuse hyperostosis throughout the cervical spine. **B,** Lateral cervical myelogram shows multiple level defects in the dye column with stenosis above the prior C6 laminectomy. **C,** Anteroposterior myelogram shows a complete block at C7-T1 below the prior laminectomy as well as co-existent lumbar stenosis. **D,** Sagittal MRI shows cord atrophy and myelomalacia at C3-C4, severe central stenosis and disk protrusion at C7-T1.

*Continued*

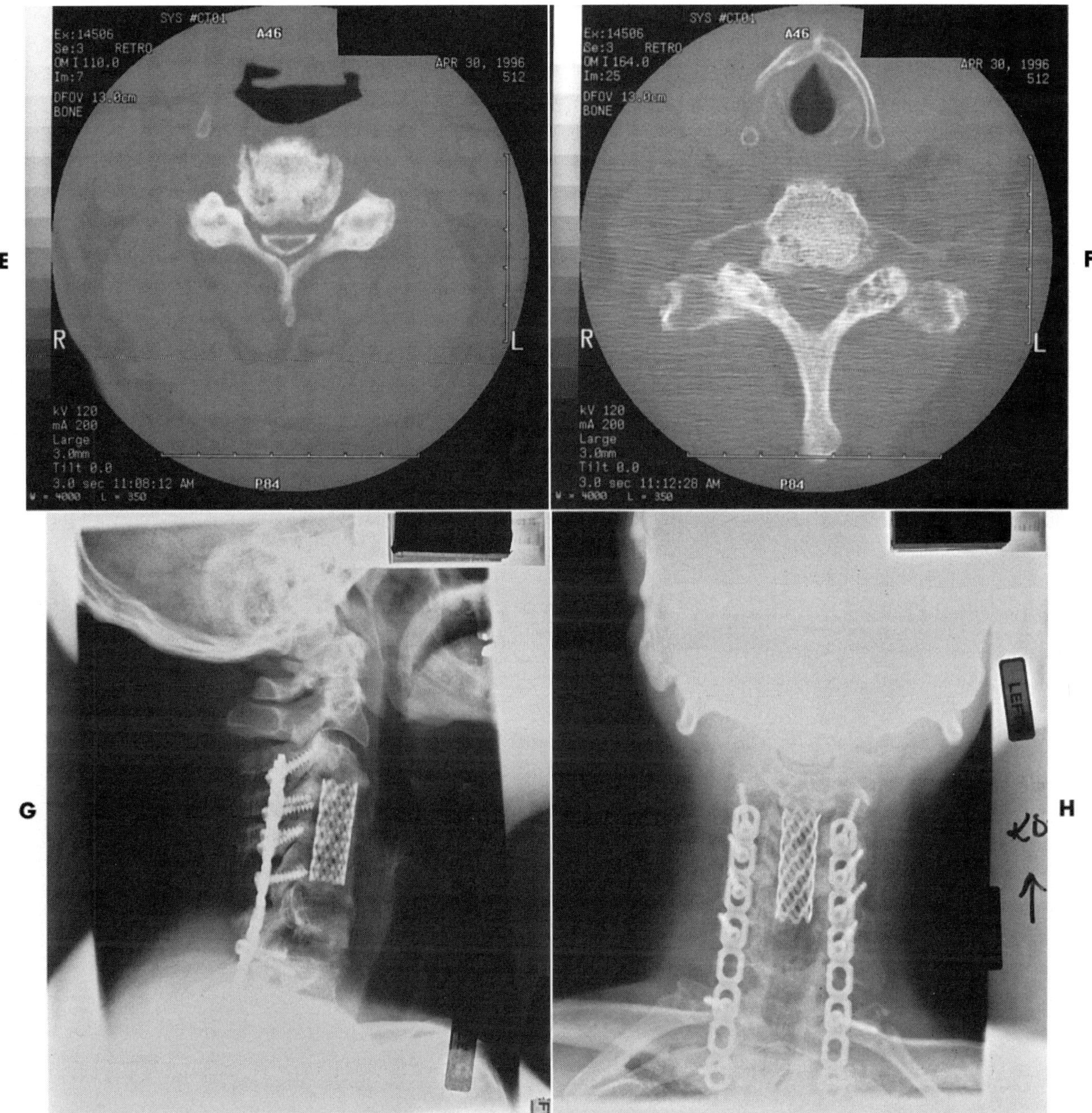


**FIGURE 5-5, CONT'D**

Axial CT (**E**) shows central stenosis at C3-C4 as well as C7-T1 disk protrusion (**F**). Lateral (**G**) and anteroposterior (**H**) x-rays show the surgical reconstruction. First, anterior decompression with corpectomies from C4 through the upper portion of C6 as well as C7-T1 diskectomy were performed. Anterior reconstruction of the corpectomy defect was achieved with titanium mesh and autograft and the C7-T1 level was stabilized with autogenous iliac graft. This was followed by posterior plate fixation C3-T2. Lateral mass screws were used in the cervical spine and laterally directed transverse process-rib screws were used at T1 and T2. When pedicle fixation is problematic and use of a rod-hook system is not desired, screw fixation into the transverse process and rib is feasible at T1 and T2 and may serve as an alternative fixation site.

indicated depending on preoperative evaluation. The decision whether to approach the spine through an anterior or posterior approach should be guided by the location and type of spinal pathology (Fig. 5-6). Segmental instabilities such as spondylolisthesis adjacent to a prior fusion can be treated either by anterior or posterior fusion with spinal instrumentation. Adjacent-level central stenosis or central disk herniations are best treated by anterior decompression and fusion with anterior plate fixation. When anterior cervical diskectomy and fusion is performed adjacent to a prior cervical fusion, the pseudarthrosis rate is higher due to the altered biomechanical situation created by the previously fused segments. One study reported fewer pseudarthroses after anterior cervical corpectomy with fusion than after anterior cervical diskec-

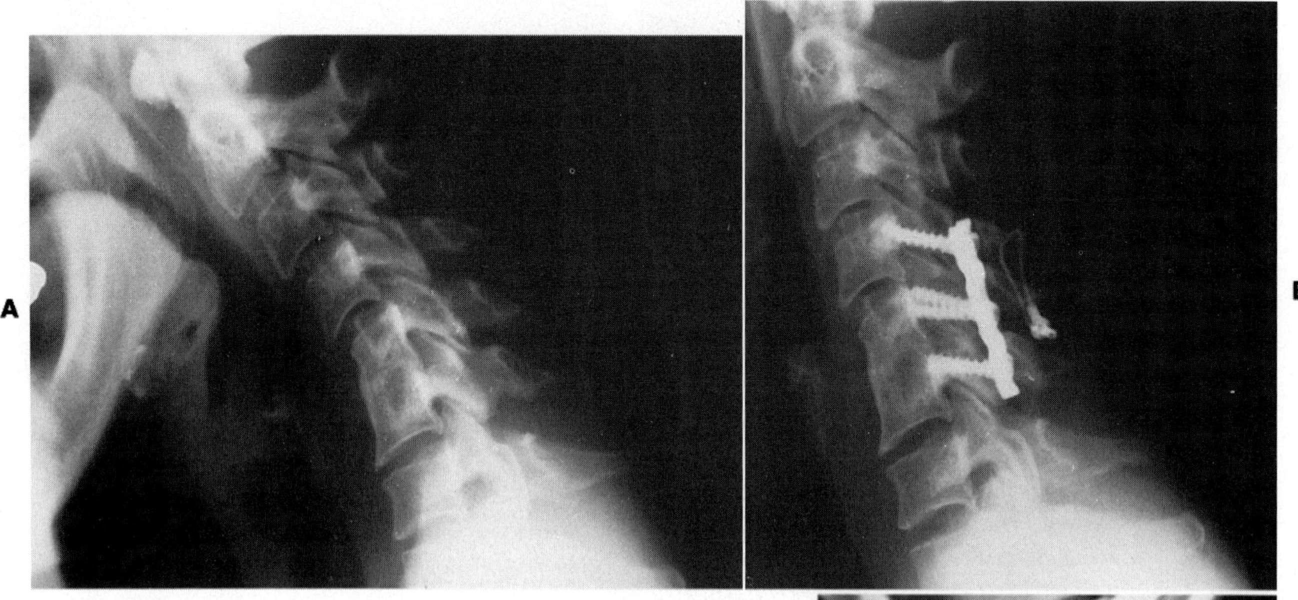


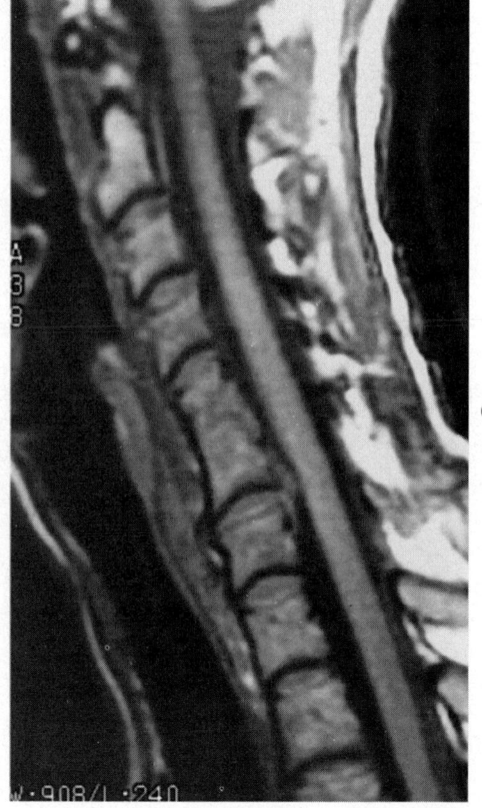


**Figure 5-6**

Adjacent-segment degeneration. A 36-year-old woman developed recurrent neck pain following successful C5-C6 anterior cervical diskectomy and fusion. **A,** Lateral radiograph shows anterior subluxation at C4-C5. Bilateral C4-C5 facet blocks completely relieved her symptoms. **B,** She was treated by posterior C4-C5 cervical fusion with lateral mass plates and autogenous bone graft with excellent outcome. **C,** Eighteen months later she developed acute left-sided C7 radiculopathy secondary to a C6-C7 disk herniation.

*Continued*

tomy with fusion in this situation.[71] Adjacent-segment problems presenting with kyphosis or high-grade instability are generally treated with both anterior and posterior fusion with spinal instrumentation.

## Postsurgical Instability and Kyphosis

Pain, deformity, and neural compression may persist or develop following procedures that compromise the structural integrity of the anterior or posterior spinal columns. Pain may develop due to compromise of the anterior load-bearing capacity of the cervical spinal column such as occurs after collapse of an anterior structural bone graft or after anterior diskectomy without fusion. Cervical laminectomy may lead to translatory or angulatory instabilities. Kyphosis may be localized to a single spinal segment or may be global and involve the entire cervical spine. Neurologic deficit may arise from direct anterior neural impingement or as a result of increased tension in the cord with resultant deleterious effect on cord blood flow as the spinal cord is draped over the apex of a fixed kyphotic deformity. The spinal deformity may be flexible or rigid depending on multiple factors (Table 5-4).

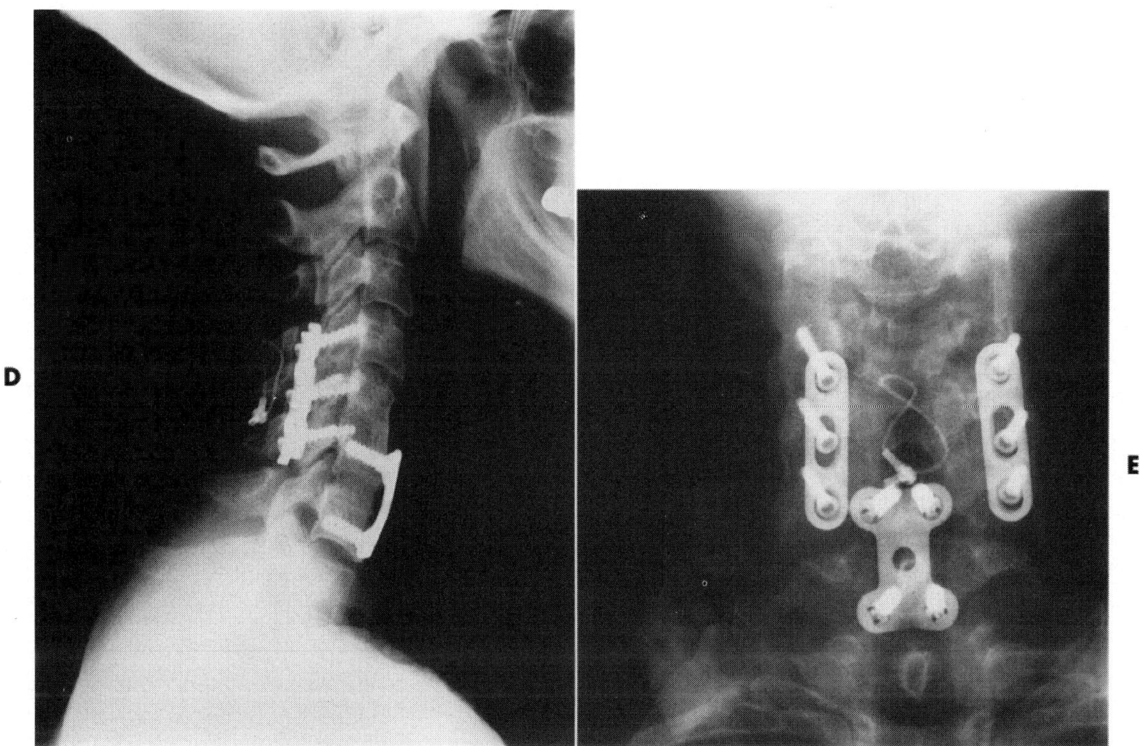


**FIGURE 5-6, CONT'D**

She failed medical management and was treated by an anterior cervical diskectomy and fusion with plate fixation (**D, E**).

Kyphosis following cervical laminectomy is the most common type of kyphotic deformity presenting to spinal surgeons. In the pediatric population the reported incidence of this deformity ranges from 38% to 100% while in adults an incidence ranging from 11% to 17% has been reported following laminectomy for spondylotic myelopathy.[15,47,94] The exact risk for developing a postsurgical deformity is difficult to quantify because of the multifactorial nature of this problem. Variables including patient age, preoperative sagittal alignment, type of spinal pathology, and extent of the index surgical procedure, especially facet resection, may contribute singularly or in combination to the development of postoperative instability.[42,76,108,118,123] The extremely high incidence of kyphosis following cervical laminectomy in children is attributed to the unique characteristics of the immature spine including physiologic hypermobility of the pediatric spine, the greater weight of the head in relation to the trunk in children, as well as the self-perpetuating effect of anterior compression of the cartilaginous vertebral endplates with resultant progressive deformity. In adults, the risk of postoperative deformity is increased in patients with preoperative kyphotic cervical alignment or preexistent segmental spinal instability. Whereas degenerative changes such as osteophyte formation, facet arthrosis, and disk space narrowing are believed to confer a stabilizing effect upon cervical motion segments, a wide mobile disk space adjacent to a severely degenerated motion segment may be at increased risk of postsurgical instability. Once kyphosis develops, progression generally occurs due to the inability of the posterior cervical musculature to resist the flexion moment exerted by the weight of the head. As loss of cervical lordosis occurs, the spinal cord becomes draped over the anterior vertebral bodies and resultant neural compression leads to spinal cord ischemia and resultant myelopathy.

The most efficient treatment for this deformity is prevention. In children, strong consideration should be given to performing a fusion at the time of laminectomy or alternatively performing an osteoplastic laminectomy with reconstruction of the posterior spinal elements.[107] In adults, a laminectomy should be accompanied by arthrodesis if kyphosis or instability are present. Posterior cervical laminoplasty techniques are preferred to laminectomy by some surgeons in the in the initial treatment of adult patients but kyphosis and instability may develop following these procedures as well.

Treatment options for postlaminectomy deformities include posterior procedures, anterior procedures, and circumferential procedures. Surgical decision-making is guided by whether the deformity is flexible or rigid, the presence or absence of neural compression, bone quality, bone stock remaining following prior surgical procedures, as well as biological factors specific to the individual patient.

If the patient presents with a flexible kyphotic de-

**Table 5-4. Revision Procedures for Postsurgical Instability/Kyphosis (C3-7)**

| Indication | Procedure |
|---|---|
| Discogenic pain syndrome ± foraminal stenosis status post anterior cervical diskectomy without fusion (single level) | Anterior fusion with autogenous iliac graft ± anterior foraminotomy |
| Kyphosis, foraminal stenosis status post multilevel anterior cervical diskectomy without fusion | Anterior corpectomy, strut graft, plating<br>or<br>Posterior fusion, foraminotomy, lateral mass plating (if cervical lordosis acceptable)<br>or<br>Anterior decompression and strut grafting, posterior fusion with lateral mass plates |
| Spondylolisthesis status post laminectomy | Posterior fusion, lateral mass plating ± revision decompression |
| Postlaminectomy kyphosis, flexible, no neural compression | Posterior cervical fusion with internal fixation in reduced position ± anterior fusion |
| Postlaminectomy kyphosis, flexible, neural compression present | Realign with traction and repeat imaging studies in reduced position:<br>A) If decompression achieved by realignment, perform posterior spinal fusion with internal fixation in reduced position<br>B) If neural compression persists despite realignment, perform anterior decompression and strut grafting followed by posterior fusion with lateral mass plating |
| Postlaminectomy kyphosis, rigid, neural compression present | Anterior decompression, strut graft followed by posterior fusion with lateral mass plating |

formity and no evidence of neural compression, further surgery may be indicated if the deformity is severe, progressive, or associated with pain. Posterior cervical fusion in the reduced position is the preferred treatment. The fusion should extend from an intact spinous process above the prior laminectomy to an intact spinous process below the laminectomy defect. Preoperative cervical traction is helpful in realigning the spine. Multilevel anterior interbody fusions may be combined with a posterior procedure in the situation in which the remaining posterior bone stock or the patient's healing potential is severely compromised in order to increase the chance of successful arthrodesis. In children, onlay cancellous bone grafting or wiring of rib or iliac grafts to the remaining facet joints combined with halo immobilization has a high success rate. In adult patients, some form of internal fixation is generally used to improve stability, prevent reoccurrence of deformity, and enhance the rate of arthrodesis. Rib or iliac bone graft may be wired to the remaining facet joints or facet wires may be passed around a metallic rod that serves as an internal splint.[23,51] Generally, postoperative immobilization in a halo vest is recommended when these techniques are utilized. Lateral mass screw-plate fixation can provide secure segmental fixation and obviate the need for external immobilization with a halo.[7,67,75,99] If a patient presents with a flexible kyphotic deformity and signs of neural compression, the patient is placed in traction and the spinal canal is imaged to assess whether the neural compression is relieved in the reduced position. If the spinal canal is decompressed by realignment, then posterior stabilization in the reduced position is sufficient. If persistent spinal cord compression is present, then an anterior decompression and reconstruction will be required.

If the patient presents with a rigid postlaminectomy kyphotic deformity and neural compression, posterior surgery alone is generally insufficient. Surgery must address both the spinal cord compression and the kyphotic deformity.[154] Anterior spinal cord compression occurs due to impingement of the cord over the vertebral segments at the apex of the deformity. Anterior diskectomy alone is generally inadequate in removing the midline osteophytes over this region and multilevel corpectomies are generally required to provide adequate decompression. After anterior decompression is achieved, correction of the kyphotic deformity can be achieved through positioning and intraoperative traction and placement of an anterior strut graft. If the strut graft must span two or three disk levels, a tricortical iliac graft provides adequate stability. If the strut graft must span three or more levels, a fibular graft is generally used due to its greater strength. Either fibular autograft or allograft may be utilized. The bone removed during corpectomy is saved and used to supplement the fibular graft and improve the fusion rate, especially when allograft fibula is

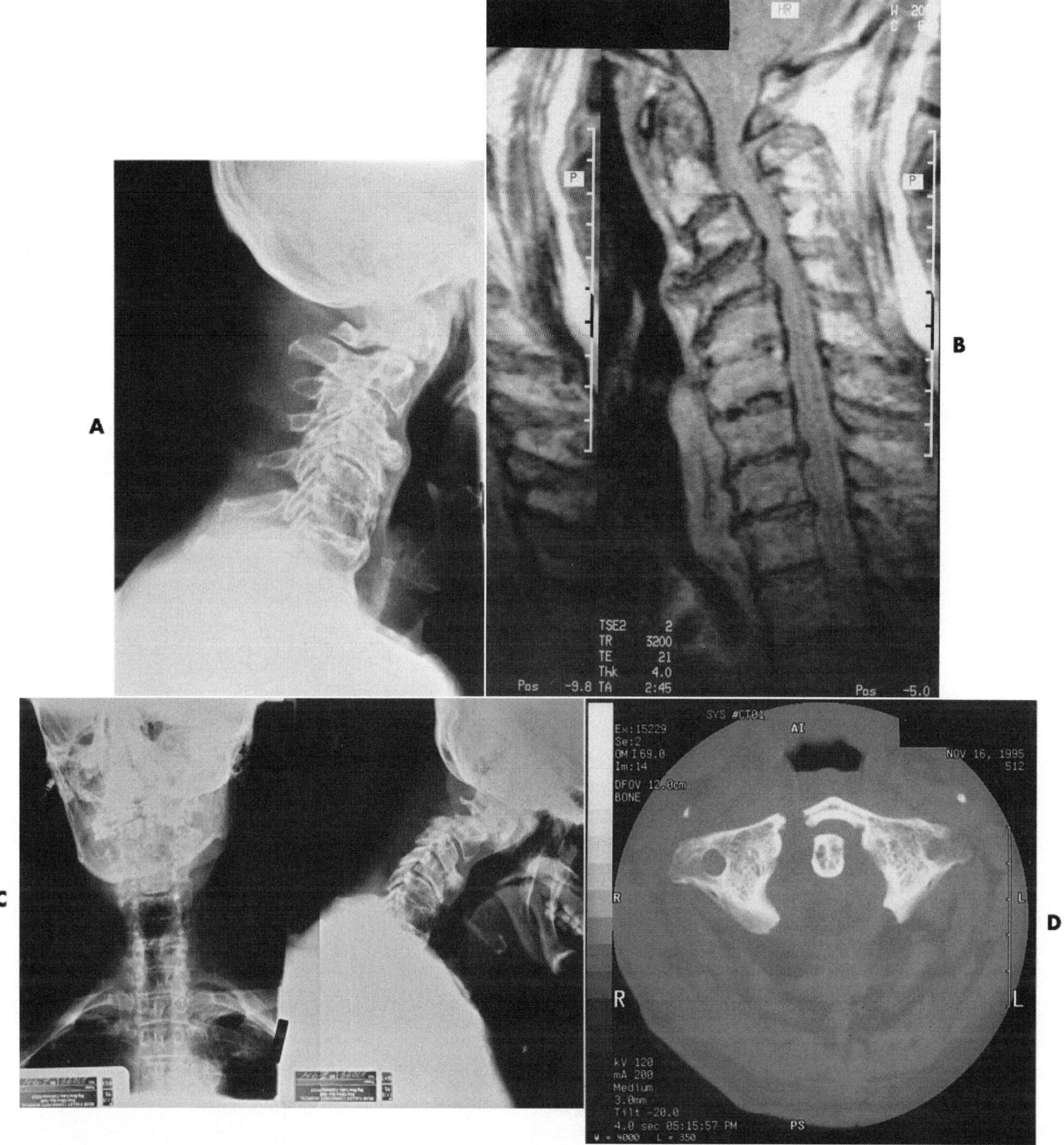


**FIGURE 5-7**

Upper cervical kyphosis, postlaminectomy instability. **A,** Lateral x-ray of an 82-year-old man with severe cervical myelopathy and upper cervical kyphosis. **B,** Sagittal MRI shows severe upper cervical spinal stenosis. Patient was treated by the initial surgeon with C1-C3 laminectomy. After discharge, the patient felt a snap and developed severe upper cervical pain and inability to hold his head erect. **C,** Lateral x-ray shows evidence of prior laminectomy with worsening of the upper cervical kyphosis. **D,** Axial CT shows C1 fracture anteriorly after removal of C1 arch posteriorly. *Continued*

used. Recently, titanium mesh utilized with autogenous iliac bone and local cancellous bone has been used to reconstruct the anterior column following corpectomy. Advantages of these implants include easy customization of mesh to accommodate any corpectomy defect, minimization of graft donor site morbidity, and the improved biomechanical properties of these implants compared with iliac or fibular structural grafts. Titanium mesh increases the torsional stiffness of the overall construct while the sharp edges of the cage provide resistance against shear forces (Fig. 5-7). Disadvantages of titanium mesh include implant cost,

*Text continued on page 76*

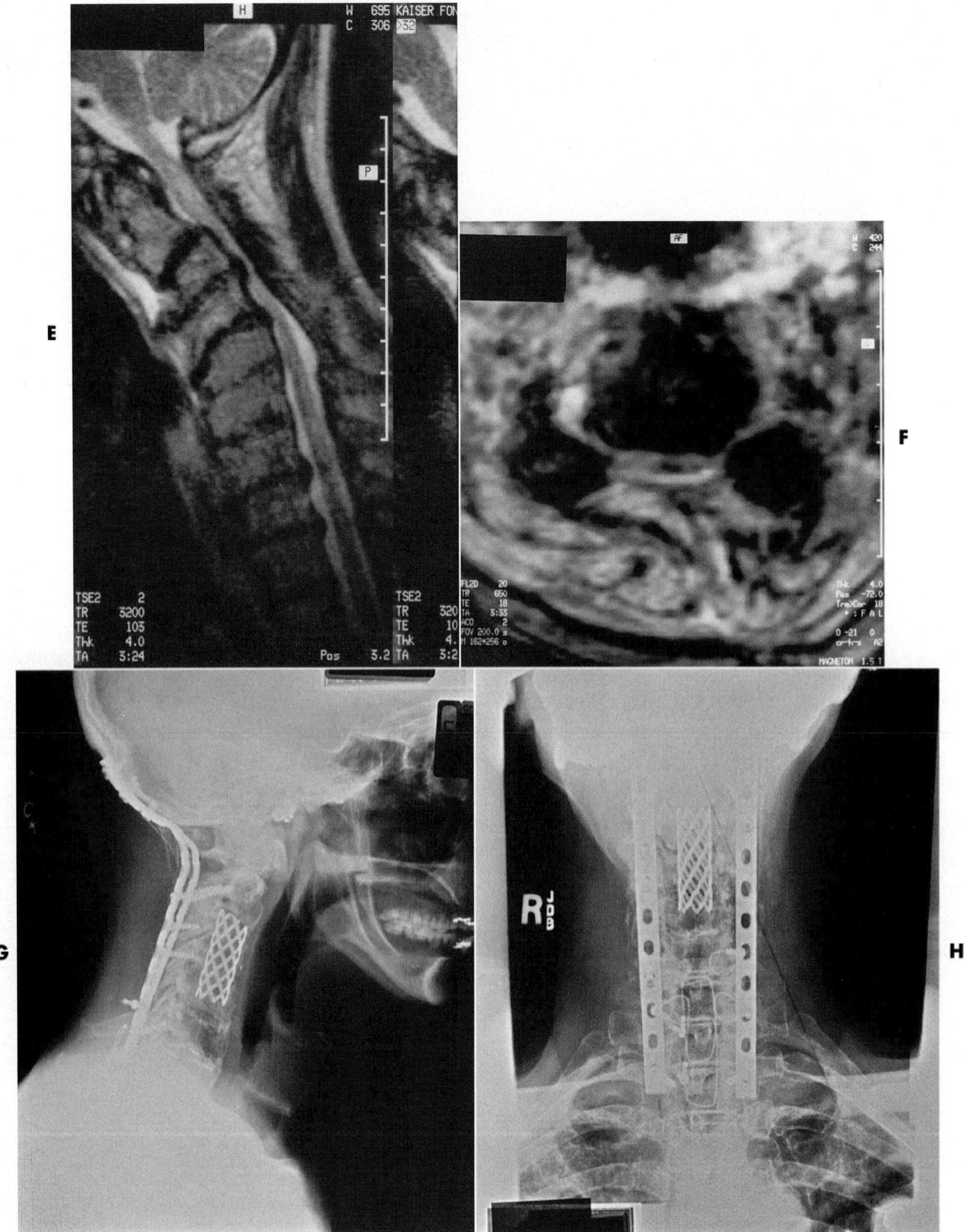


**FIGURE 5-7, CONT'D**

**E,** Sagittal MRI shows persistent cord compression anteriorly over the apex of the kyphosis. **F,** Axial MRI shows severe spinal stenosis due to spondylosis and kyphosis. Lateral (**G**) and anteroposterior (**H**) postoperative x-rays show the result of revision surgery. A preoperative vena cava filter was required due to a history of deep vein thrombosis. First, an extended anterior approach with corpectomies of C3-C5 with reconstruction using titanium mesh and autograft was performed. The patient was frail and could not tolerate same-day anterior-posterior procedures. He was maintained in a halo temporarily and nutritional status was maximized utilizing hyperalimentation until posterior surgery could be performed. He subsequently underwent occiput-T2 fusion with lateral mass plates and cables, autogenous iliac grafting, and removal of the halo. Patient eventually achieved solid arthrodesis with relief of pain.

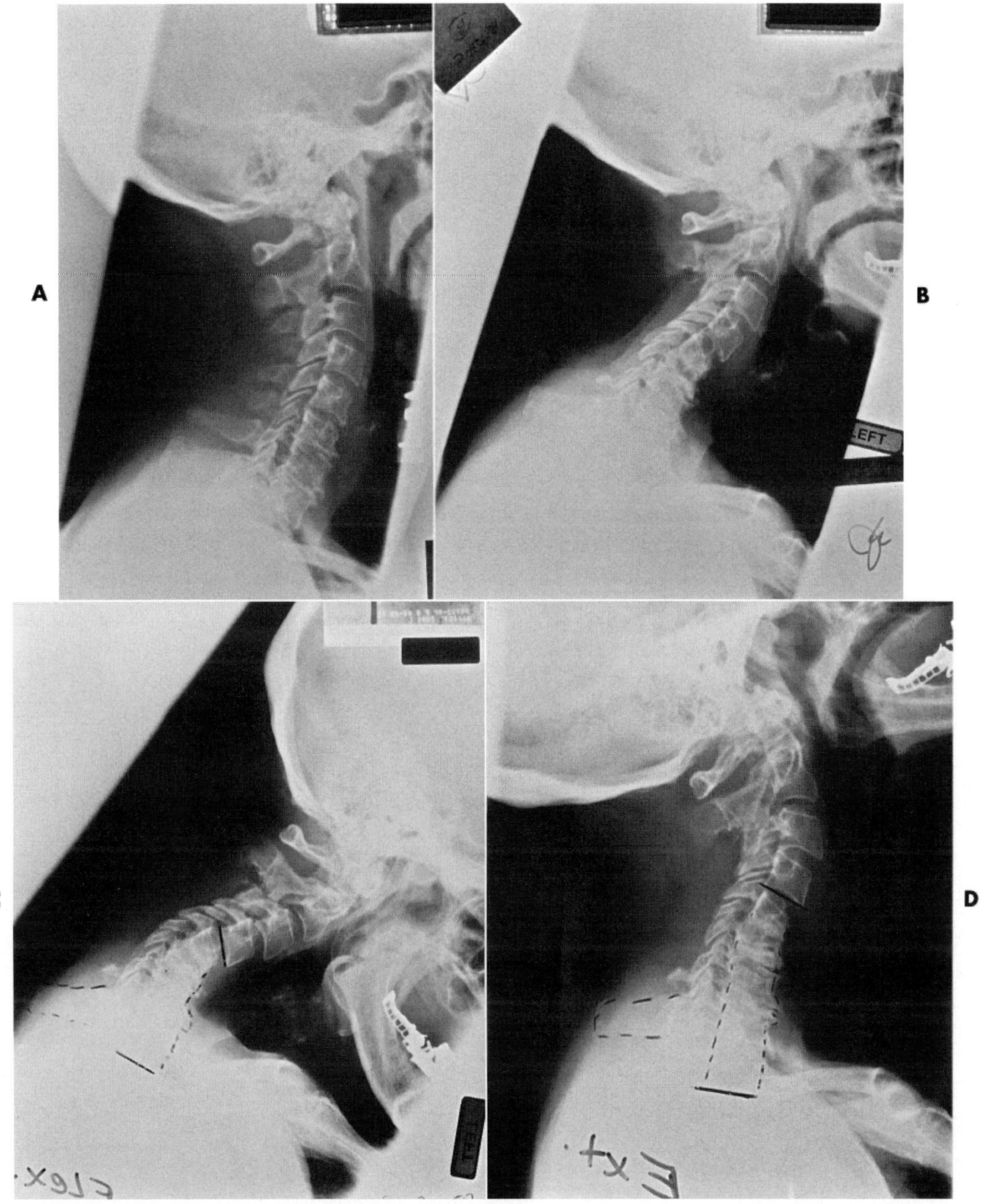


**FIGURE 5-8**

Postlaminectomy cervical kyphosis, subaxial cervical spinal stenosis. A 72-year-old woman underwent C3-C7 laminectomy elsewhere for cervical spinal stenosis. **A,** Lateral preoperative x-ray shows degenerative changes in the lower cervical spine with overall preservation of cervical lordosis. **B,** Postoperative lateral x-ray shows development of a postlaminectomy deformity. The initial surgeon treated the deformity with a single-level allograft interbody fusion procedure, which did not result in successful arthrodesis or significant improvement of kyphosis as shown on postoperative lateral x-rays in flexion (**C**) and extension (**D**). The patient was referred for salvage reconstruction.

*Continued*

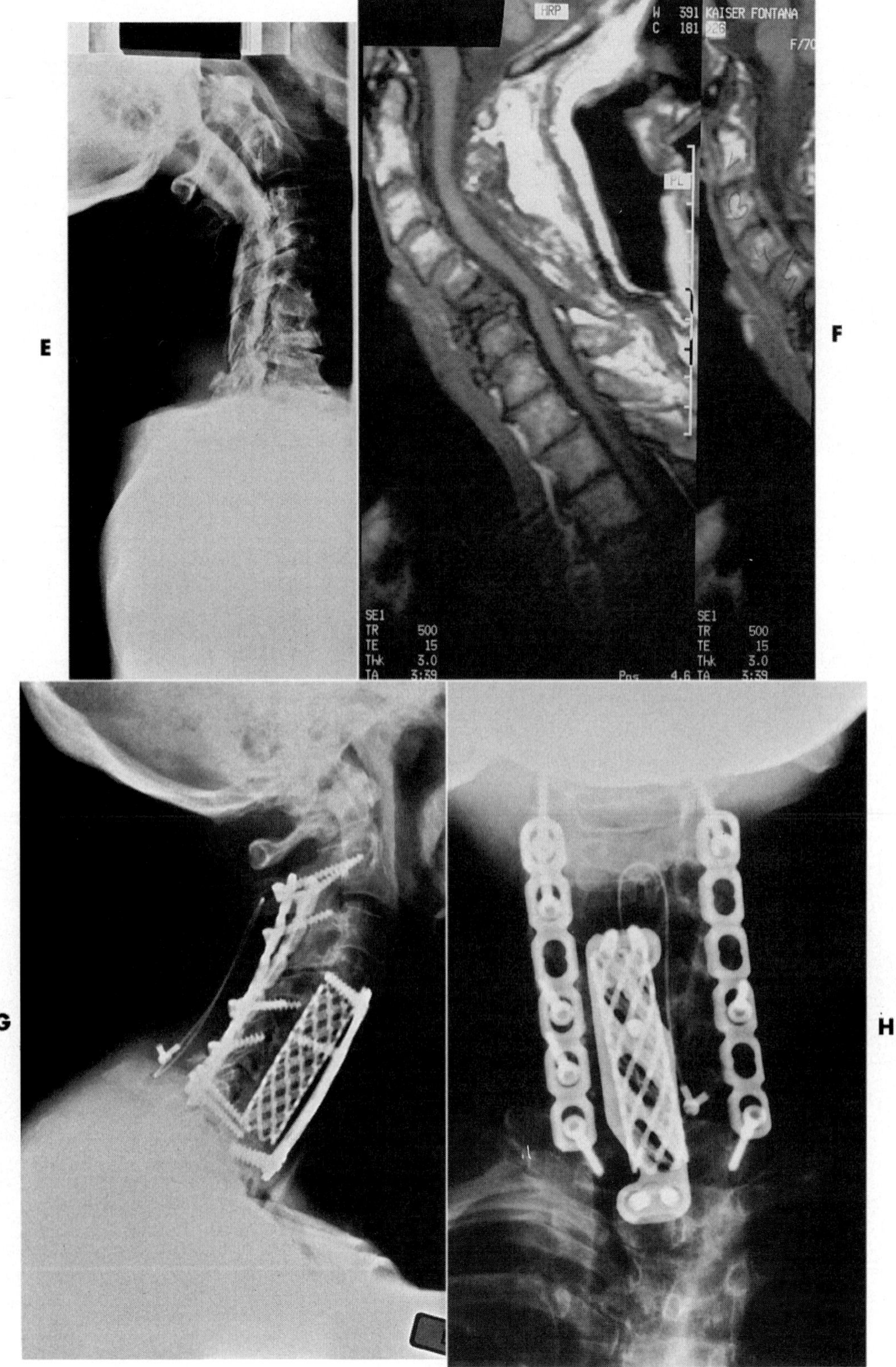


**Figure 5-8, cont'd**

**E,** CT myelography shows flexibility of the kyphotic deformity and residual spinal stenosis at C5-C7. **F,** Sagittal MRI demonstrates cord compression and pseudarthrosis at the site of failed anterior allograft fusion. Lateral (**G**) and anteroposterior (**H**) x-rays show results of cervical reconstruction. Anterior corpectomies C5-C7 followed by anterior reconstruction with titanium mesh filled with autograft bone and anterior plate fixation were performed first with the patient in traction. Then posterior plate fixation was performed from C2-T1. Pedicle fixation was used at C2 and T1. A midline tethering cable was also utilized to provide compression forces to the posterior spinal column.

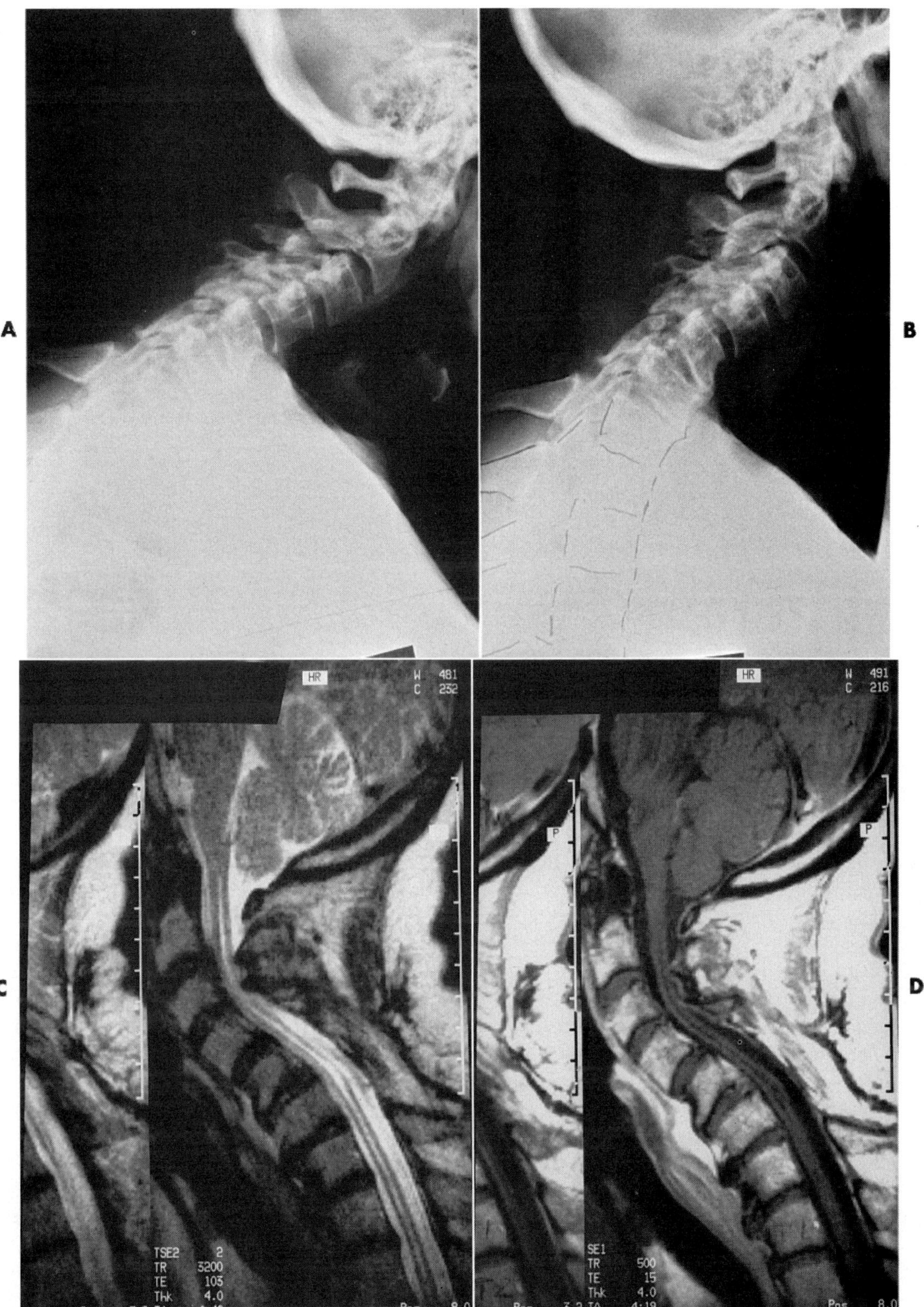


**FIGURE 5-9**

Postlaminectomy cervical kyphosis, myelopathy, syringomyelia. A 56-year-old woman presented with chronic severe neck pain, myelopathy, and cervical kyphosis. She had undergone cervical laminectomy as a teenager following a fracture and the surgical procedure was complicated by a severe neurologic injury. Following this procedure the patient gradually regained her ability to walk and was ambulatory at the time of presentation. **A,** Lateral x-ray shows cervical kyphosis and evidence of prior laminectomy. **B,** Hyperextension lateral x-ray shows minimal correction of kyphosis due to spontaneous autofusion at C5-C6 and C6-C7. **C,D,** Sagittal MRI shows spinal stenosis at C2-C3 and a syrinx within the cervical cord extending from C2-C7.

*Continued*

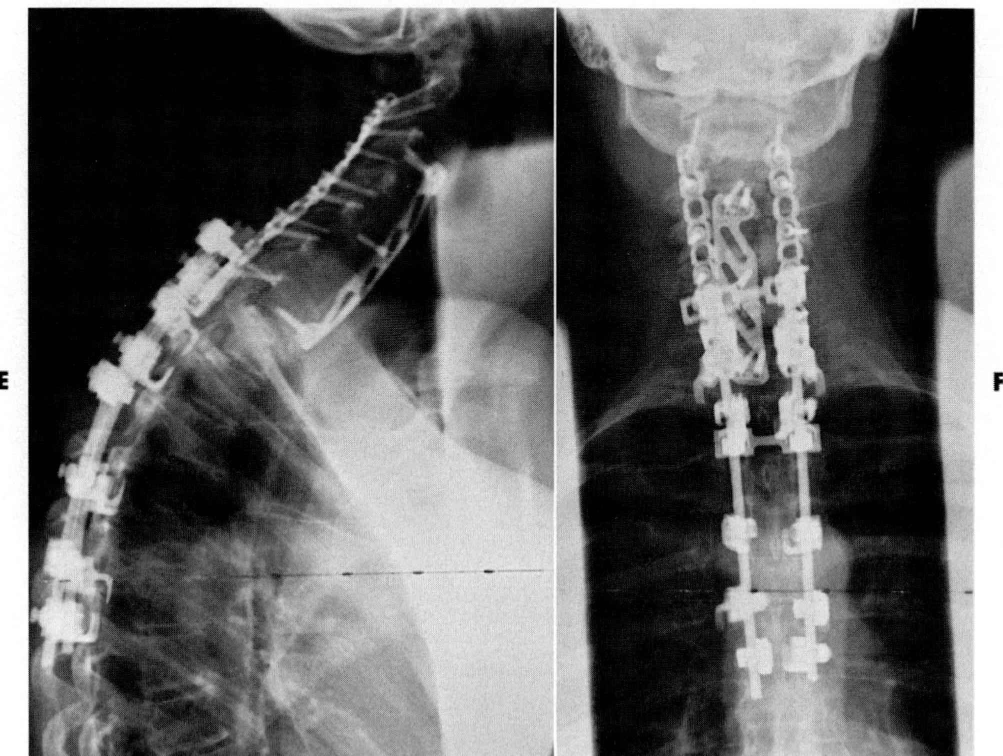


**FIGURE 5-9, CONT'D**

Lateral (**E**) and anteroposterior (**F**) views show the surgical reconstruction. First, anterior cervical fusion C3-C7 and anterior plate fixation were performed. Then posterior fusion and stabilization C2-T6 were performed utilizing a custom rod-plate device that permits lateral mass plates to be connected to a thoracic rod system. This construct provided for equal lever arms above and below the apex of the kyphosis (C7-T1).

potential for subsidence within the cancellous bone of the anterior spinal column, and the technical challenges encountered if revision surgery is required in the future.

It is generally recommended that adjunctive immobilization be used following anterior strut grafting for postlaminectomy deformities in order to decrease the complications of nonunion and graft extrusion. Options include external immobilization with a halo, anterior plate fixation, posterior plate fixation, or some combination of these methods. Halo immobilization is a relatively simple intervention but is not well-tolerated by many patients and has a high rate of complications, although the majority of these complications are minor. Anterior cervical plate fixation has been utilized following multilevel corpectomies in an attempt to avoid external immobilization.[68,96] Anterior plates do not provide true segmental fixation of the spine and rely on fixation into the vertebral bodies at the ends of the anterior construct. Screw/plate pull-out at the inferior end of a long anterior construct due to load concentration at the distal end vertebra is problematic.[141] Furthermore, it has been postulated that an autogenous strut graft must heal with some degree of settling and anterior plate fixation may interfere with this process and actually decrease the rate of fusion. An alternative plating technique utilizing a short anterior buttress plate at the distal end of the graft to prevent extrusion while permitting compressive loading of the anterior strut graft to enhance arthrodesis has been advocated.[52] However, external immobilization with a halo is recommended when this construct is used for treating postlaminectomy deformities. Biomechanical data has shown that posterior cervical fixation is superior to anterior fixation since true segmental fixation of the cervical spine can be achieved.[1,2,53,138] Improved fusion rates are noted when circumferential surgery is compared to anterior fusion and plating in multilevel cervical constructs. Presently, the authors prefer anterior corpectomies and anterior column reconstruction with either allograft fibular strut graft or titanium mesh followed by posterior plate fixation for the treatment of postlaminectomy deformities (Fig. 5-8). Screw fixation in the lateral masses is generally utilized between C3 and C6, whereas pedicle fixation is preferred at C2 and C7 and in the upper thoracic region.[2,12,28,80,95,101,105,150] New hybrid fixation devices permit lateral mass fixation in the cervical region to be connected to a hook-rod system in the thoracic region (Fig. 5-9). Pedicle fixation across the cervicothoracic junction is technically challenging and if pedicular screw fixation is problematic, an al-

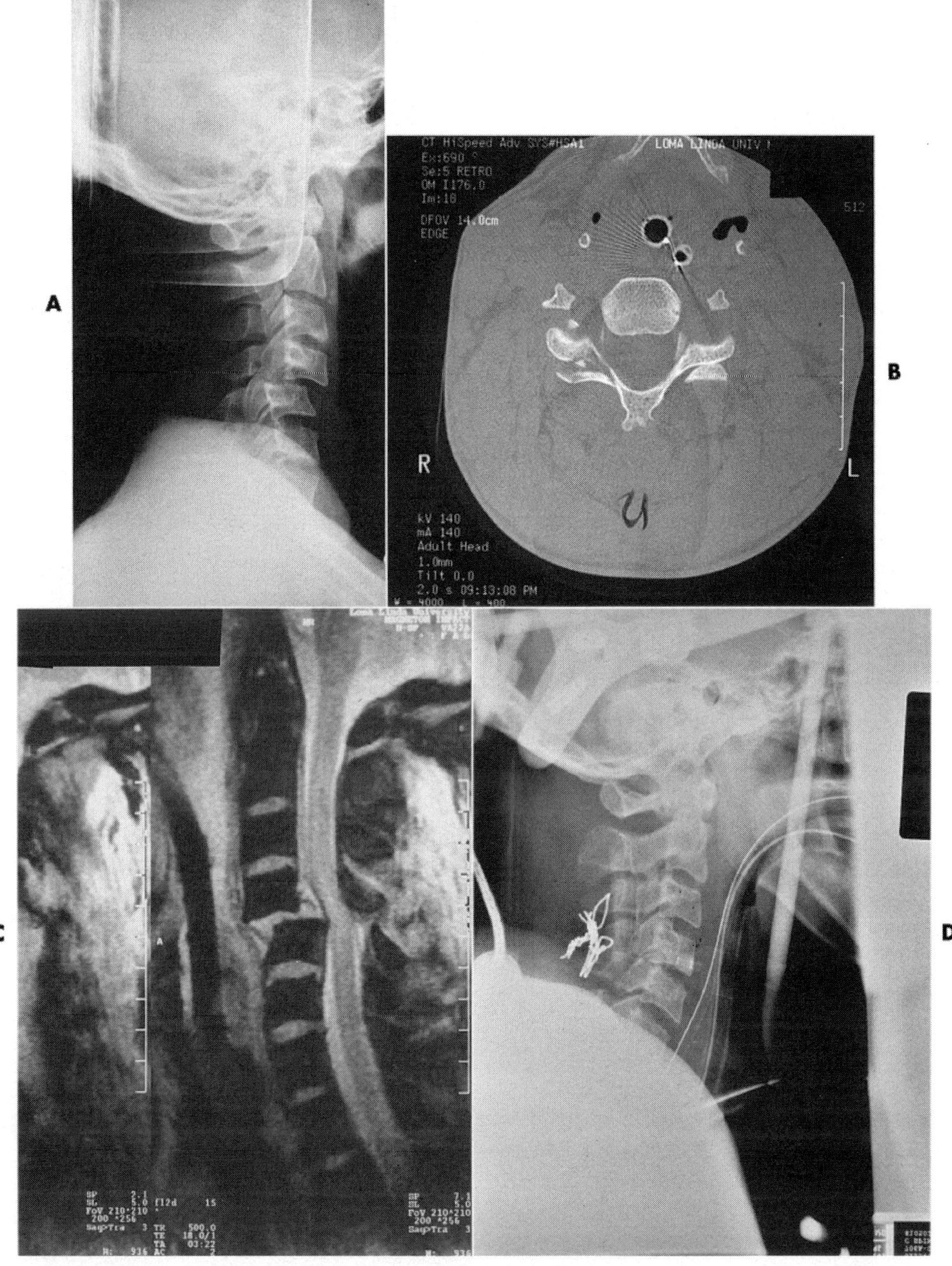


**FIGURE 5-10**

Fracture revision, failure of fixation. A 45-year-old man sustained C4-C5 bilateral facet dislocations with incomplete neural injury. Lateral x-ray (**A**) and CT scan (**B**) depict the injury. **C,** MRI shows cord impingement due to spinal malalignment. The patient was treated at another local hospital with C3-C5 interspinous wiring with allograft and placed in a halo (**D**). *Continued*

ternative fixation site with screw fixation into the transverse process and into the adjacent rib head can be used in the upper thoracic region.

## REVISION SURGERY FOR CERVICAL FRACTURES

Recent advances have improved the prognosis for patients who sustain cervical fractures. Despite improved diagnostic and treatment methods, optimal results are not obtained in all cases. Initial treatment begins with prompt retrieval of the injured patient, assessment of the injury with appropriate radiologic studies, emergent realignment of spinal column displacement, appropriate pharmacologic intervention, and protection of the spinal column from further injury. When surgical intervention is indicated, the goals of treatment are adequate decompression, realignment, and stabilization of the injury to allow maxi-

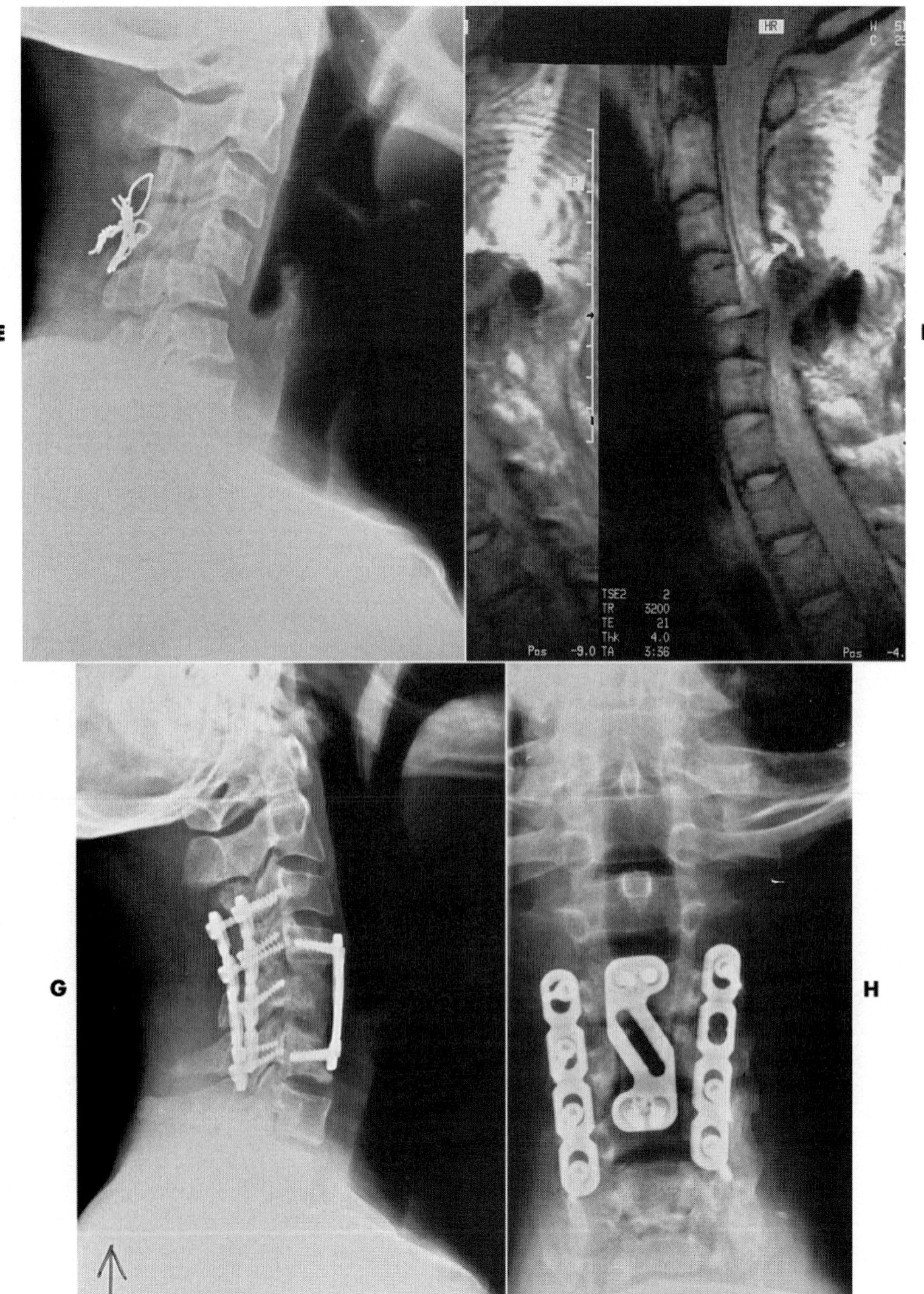


**FIGURE 5-10, CONT'D**

The patient was transferred to a nursing facility and subsequently referred to our facility two months after surgery. Note the recurrence of the deformity at C4-C5 with pull-through of the inferior wire through the spinous process of C5 (**E**). **F,** MRI shows frank cord compression. The patient has persistent neurological deficit including gait problems and upper extremity weakness. Lateral (**G**) and anteroposterior (**H**) x-rays following revision surgery. Revision surgery included C5 corpectomy and reconstruction with autogenous iliac graft and anterior plating C4-C6. Posterior stabilization was performed C3-C6 to incorporate the areas that were treated surgically at the index procedure and included repair of the pseudarthroses noted at each level. *Continued*

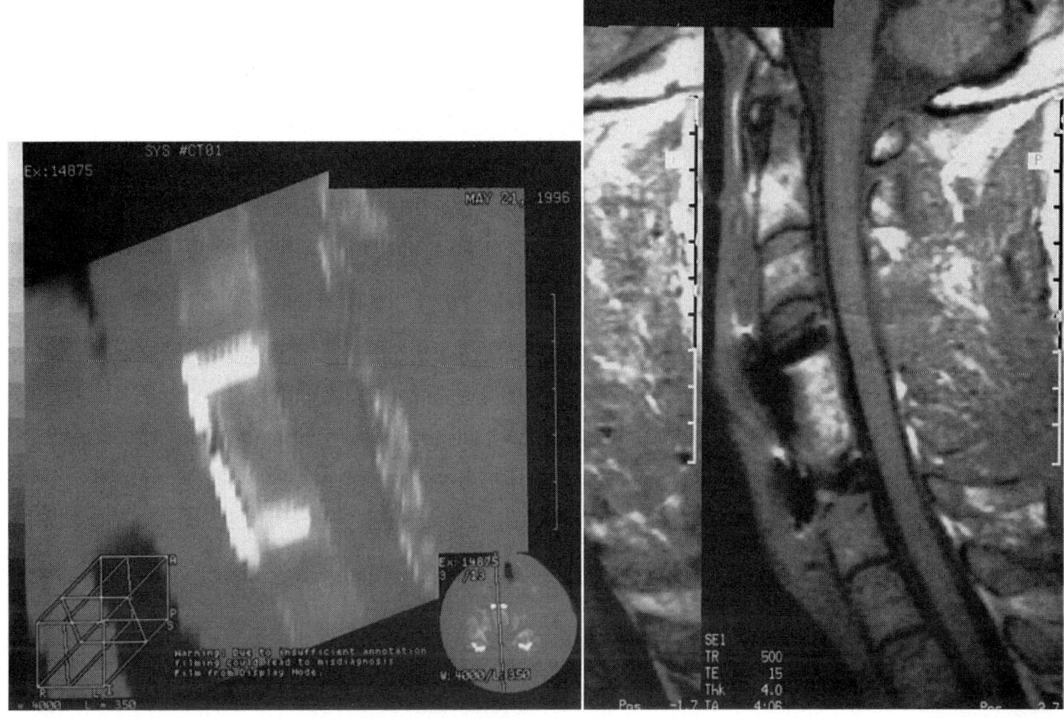

FIGURE 5-10, CONT'D

Postoperative CT (I) and MRI (J) show restoration of spinal canal patency.

mum recovery. Revision surgery may be required due to inadequate or inappropriate initial stabilization or graft technique, residual or recurrent neural compression, or residual spinal deformity.

A variety of cervical fixation techniques are available to the spinal trauma surgeon, including posterior wire/cable fixation,[90,115,133,143] posterior plate fixation,[7] and second generation constrained anterior plate fixation.[79,112] Surgical failures may occur when technically inadequate or inappropriate stabilization or graft techniques are utilized.[151,153] Posterior wire/cable fixation can provide satisfactory stabilization of facet dislocations and ligamentous disruption when the anterior column is intact.[39] Wire/cable fixation alone is inadequate as the sole treatment for rotationally unstable injuries such as fracture-dislocations because recurrence of deformity is likely with this technique. Failure of wiring techniques to provide adequate stabilization following cervical trauma has been documented when three-column cervical instability is present (Fig. 5-10). This type of injury should be suspected when radiographs demonstrate: retrolisthesis and angulation of the superior vertebrae with respect to the subjacent vertebrae, distraction of the posterior interspinous ligaments sufficient to allow subluxation or dislocation of the facets, and distraction of the posterior spinous processes and anterior shear dislocation of one vertebra on another.[34] The selection of anterior plate fixation or posterior plating may be guided by the type of injury.[3,4,5] Factors such as the need to perform an anterior decompression of the spinal cord or the need for a posterior approach to permit reduction may make one approach preferable (Fig. 5-11). However, a randomized study compared anterior fusion and Morscher plate fixation with posterior fusion and lateral mass plate fixation in the treatment of spinal cord injured patients who did not require a specific approach.[18] No significant differences in fusion rates, alignment, neurologic recovery, or long-term pain complaints were noted. Thus, either approach may be chosen depending on surgeon preference and specific indications and conditions of the patient. Anterior strut grafting without internal fixation is not recommended for treatment of unstable cervical fractures due to the high incidence of graft dislodgment and malunion, as well as the potential for possible neurologic injury.[26,134] It is strongly recommended that autogenous iliac graft be utilized and that allograft be avoided.

Occasionally, neural compression may be unrecognized or remain untreated following a significant cervical injury. Alternatively, neural compression may develop as a result of persistent instability, pseudarthrosis, or spinal deformity following a significant cervical bony or ligamentous injury. Anterior decompression and arthrodesis even when performed up to 12

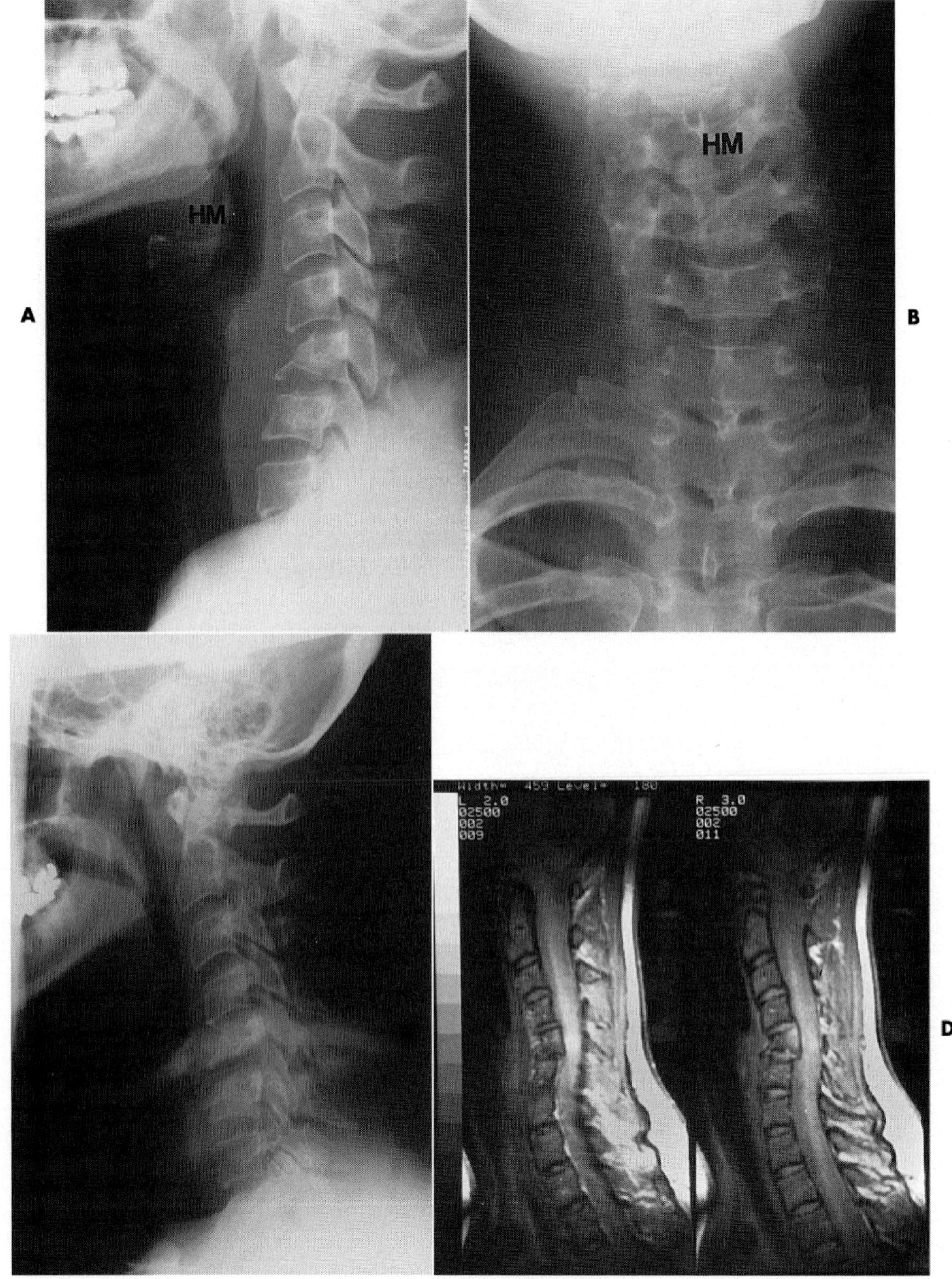


**FIGURE 5-11**

Fracture revision, anterior graft fracture, and failure of fixation. A 31-year-old woman sustained a C5 flexion injury with anterior compression of the C5 vertebral body. Lateral (**A**) and anteroposterior (**B**) x-rays show the initial injury. The patient was initially placed in a halo (**C**) with partial improvement in alignment. **D,** MRI shows C5-C6 retrolisthesis and persistent neural compression. Patient was treated at an outside facility with C5 corpectomy, allograft reconstruction, and anterior plating with a nonconstrained plate system.

*Continued*

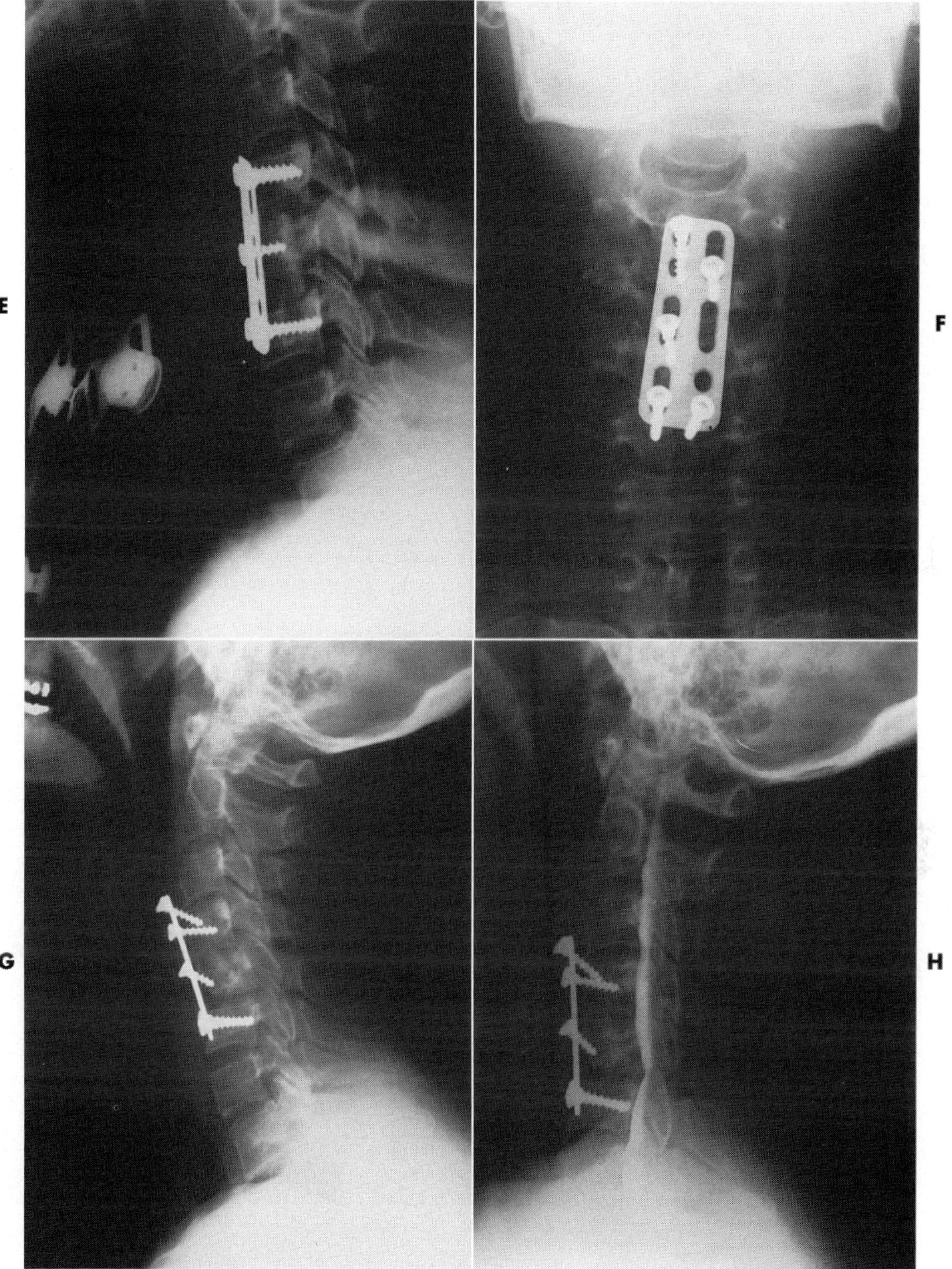


FIGURE 5-11, CONT'D

Postoperative lateral (**E**) and anteroposterior (**F**) x-rays show restoration of spinal alignment. **G,** Subsequent graft collapse and fixation failure were accompanied by the onset of severe neck pain and arm weakness. **H,** Myelogram shows neural compression due to graft displacement.

*Continued*

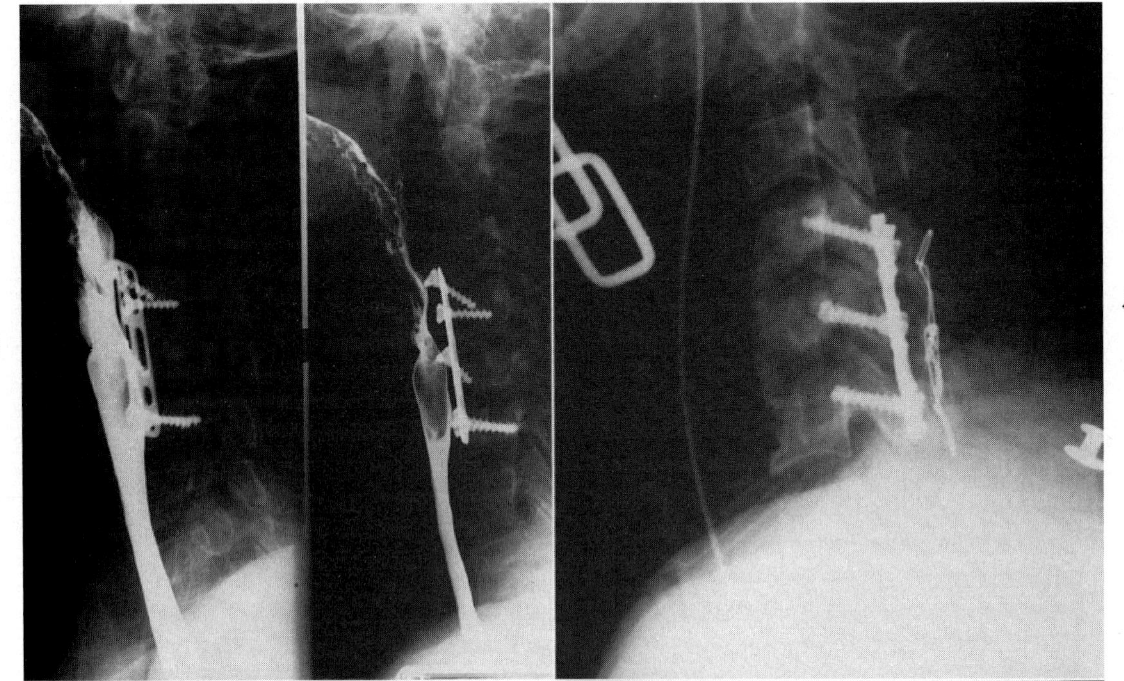


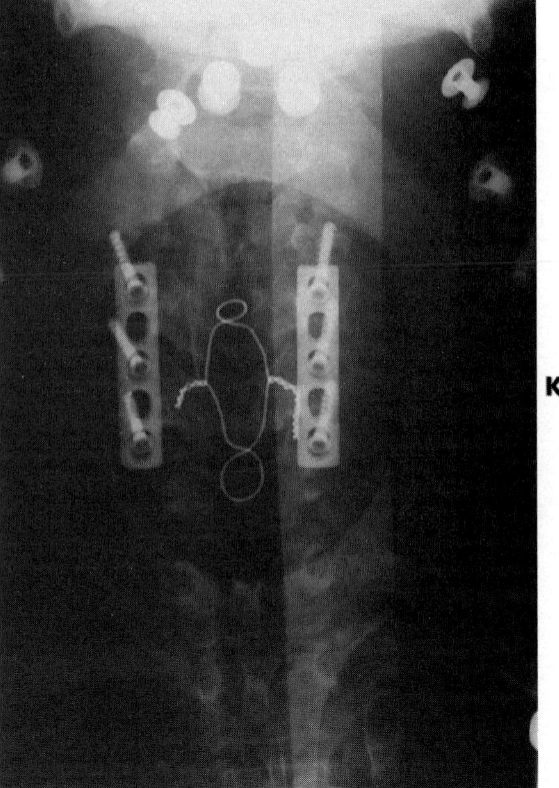


**FIGURE 5-11, CONT'D**

**I,** An esophagram was obtained due to symptoms of swallowing difficulty in order to rule out esophageal injury. Lateral (**J**) and anteroposterior (**K**) x-rays show subsequent revision procedure after referral to our center. The anterior plate and fractured graft were removed and iliac autograft was placed in the corpectomy defect. Then posterior spinal stabilization at C4-C6 with lateral mass plates and interspinous wiring and posterior fusion with autograft was performed.

months after the initial injury can improve neurologic function in both the upper and lower extremities in patients with incomplete quadriplegia due to cervical fractures or dislocations.[16] In patients with complete spinal cord injuries, anterior decompression cannot restore spinal cord function distal to the level of injury. However, decompression may restore motor root function at the level of injury and this may improve upper extremity function and result in improved functional abilities for the patient.[6]

A variety of deformities may result following cervical injuries and may result from neglect, inappropriate treatment, or complications following appropriate intervention. Occasionally, facet dislocations may be unrecognized and present late. In this situation, consideration should be given to obtaining an MRI to exclude the presence of an acute disk herniation associated with the facet injury. Treatment must be individualized to the specific deformity and appropriate decompression, realignment, and stabilization should be performed as indicated. Posttraumatic kyphosis may develop following decompressive laminectomy, following a cervical burst fracture associated with posterior ligamentous injury, or following anterior strut grafting without internal fixation. Anterior corpectomy and anterior plate fixation or circumferential procedures with anterior and posterior stabilization may be required to treat these difficult problems.

## REFERENCES


1. Abitbol JJ, Zdeblick T, Kunz D, McCabe R, Cooke M: A biomechanical analysis of modern anterior and posterior cervical stabilization techniques. Presented at the Twentieth Annual Meeting of the Cervical Spine Research Society, Palm Springs, California, December, 1992.
2. Abumi K, Itoh H, Taneichi H, Kaneda K: Transpedicular screw fixation for traumatic lesions of the middle and lower cervical spine: description of the techniques and preliminary report, *J Spinal Disord* 7:19-28, 1994.
3. Aebi M, Mohler J, Zach GA, Morscher E: Indication, surgical technique, and results of 100 surgically treated fractures and fracture-dislocations of the cervical spine, *Clin Orthop Rel Res* 203:244-257, 1986.
4. Aebi M, Zuber K, Marchesi D: Treatment of cervical spine injuries with anterior plating: indications, techniques, and results, *Spine* 16:S38-S45, 1991.
5. An HS, Gordin R, Renner K: Anatomic considerations for plate-screw fixation of the cervical spine, *Spine* 16:S548-S551, 1991.
6. Anderson PA, Bohlman HH: Anterior decompression and arthrodesis of the cervical spine: long-term motor improvement. Part 2. Improvement in complete traumatic quadriplegia, *J Bone Joint Surg* 74A:683-692,1992.
7. Anderson PA, Henley MB, Grady MS, Montesano PX, Winn HR: Posterior cervical arthrodesis with AO reconstruction plates and bone graft. *Spine* 16S: S72-S79, 1991.
8. Anderson PA, Steinman JC: *Internal fixation of the cervical spine.* In JW Fryomer, editor: *The adult spine: principles and practice,* ed 2, Philadelphia, 1997, Lippincott-Raven, pp 1119-1147.
9. Aronson DD, Kahn RJ, Canady A: Cervical spine instability following suboccipital decompression and cervical laminectomy for Arnold-Chiari syndrome, *Orthop Trans* 13(3):558, 1989.
10. Aronson NI: The management of soft disc protrusions using the Smith-Robinson approach, *Clin Neurosurg* 20:253, 1973.
11. Aronson N, Filtzer DK, Bagan M: Anterior cervical fusion by the Smith-Robinson approach, *J Neurosurg* 29:397, 1968.
12. Bailey AS, Stanescu S, Yeasting RA et al: Anatomic relationships of the cervicothoracic junction, *Spine* 20:1431-1439, 1995.
13. Barnsley L, Chahl J, Lord S, Bogduk N: Diagnosis of cervical zygapophysial pain by double blind differential anesthetic blocks, *Orthop Trans* 8(2):332, 1994
14. Bayley JC, Yoo JU, Kruger DM, Schlegel J: The role of distraction in improving the space available for the cord in cervical spondylosis, *Spine* 20:771-775, 1995.
15. Bell DF, Walker J, O'Connor G: Spinal deformity following multiple level laminectomy in children, *Orthop Trans* 13(3):558, 1989.
16. Bohlman HH, Anderson PA: Anterior decompression and arthrodesis of the cervical spine: long-term motor improvement. Part 1. Improvement in incomplete traumatic quadriparesis, *J Bone Joint Surg* 74A:671-682, 1992.
17. Bohlman HH, Emery SE, Goodfellow D, Jones P: Robinson anterior cervical diskectomy and arthrodesis for cervical radiculopathy, *J Bone Joint Surg* 75A:1298-1307, 1993.
18. Brodke DS, Anderson PA, Newell DW, Grady S et al: Anterior vs posterior stabilization of cervical spine fractures in spinal cord injured patients, *Orthop Trans* 20(2):448, 1996.
19. Brodsky AE, Khalil MA, Sassard WR, Newman BP: Repair of symptomatic pseudarthrosis of anterior cervical fusion, *Spine* 17:1137-1143, 1992.
20. Brooks AI, Jenkins EB: Atlanto-axial arthrodesis by the wedge compression method, *J Bone Joint Surg* 60A:279-284, 1978.
21. Brown CW, Orme TJ, Richardson JD: The rate of pseudarthrosis in patients who are smokers and patients who are non-smokers. A comparison study, *Spine* 11:942-946, 1986.
22. Cahill DW: Occipitocervical fusion with plates and screws: lessons learned from the initial series. North American Spine Society Eleventh Annual Meeting, Vancouver, Canada, October 23-26, 1996.
23. Callahan RA, Johnson RM, Margolis RN, Keggi KJ, Albright JA, Southwick WO: Cervical facet fusion for control of instability after laminectomy, *J Bone Joint Surg* 59A:991-1001, 1977.
24. Callahan RA, Lockwood R, Green B: Modified Brooks fusion for an os odontoideum associated with an incomplete posterior arch of the atlas, *Spine* 8:107-108, 1983.

25. Carlson GD, Phillips FM, Hoyen HA et al: Sagittal alignment: an important factor in anterior cervical interbody fusion. North American Spine Society Eleventh Annual Meeting, Vancouver, Canada, October 23-26, 1996.
26. Caspar W, Barbier DD, Klara PM: Anterior cervical fusion and Caspar plate stabilization for cervical trauma, *Neurosurgery* 25:491-502, 1989.
27. Chan DPK, Ngian KS, Cohen L: Posterior upper cervical fusion in rheumatoid arthritis, *Spine* 17:268-272, 1992.
28. Chapman JR, Anderson PA: Posterior plate fixation of the cervicothoracic junction, *Tech in Orthop* 9(1): 1-2, 1994.
29. Clark CR, White AA: Fractures of the dens: a multicenter study. *J Bone Joint Surg* 67:1340-1348, 1985.
30. Coe JD, Warden KE, Sutterlin CE, McAfee PC: Biomechanical evaluation of cervical spinal stabilization methods in a human cadaveric model, *Spine* 14:1122-1131, 1989.
31. Connolly ES, Seymore RJ, Adams JE: Clinical evaluation of anterior cervical fusion for degenerative cervical disc, *J Neurosurg* 23:431, 1965.
32. Crockard HA: Surgical management of cervical rheumatoid problems, *Spine* 20:2584-2590, 1995.
33. Crockard HA, Calder I, Ransford AO: One stage transoral decompression and posterior fixation in rheumatoid atlanto-axial subluxation, *J Bone Joint Surg* 72B:682-685, 1990.
34. Cybulski GR, Douglas RA, Meyer PR Jr, Rovin R: Complications in three-column cervical spine injuries requiring anterior-posterior stabilization, *Spine* 17:253-256, 1992.
35. DePalma AF, Rothman RH, Lewinneck RE et al: Anterior interbody fusion for severe cervical disc degeneration, *Surg Gynecol Obstet* 134:755, 1972.
36. Dickman CA, Douglas R, Sonntag WKH: Occipitocervical fusion: posterior stabilization of the craniovertebral junction and upper cervical spine, *Barrow Neurol Inst Q* 6(2):2-14, 1990.
37. Dickman CA, Sonntag VKH: Surgical management strategies for atlantoaxial nonunions, *J Neurosurg* 83:248-253, 1995.
38. Doyle JS, Lauerman WC, Kraus D, Wood KB: Complications and long term outcome of upper cervical spine arthrodesis in patients with Down's syndrome, *Orthop Trans* 20(2):448, 1996.
39. Edwards CC, Matz SO, Levine AM: The oblique wiring technique for rotational injuries of the cervical spine, *Orthop Trans* 10:455, 1986.
40. Elia M, Mazzara JT, Fielding JW: Onlay technique for occipitocervical fusion, *Clin Orthop* 280:170-174, 1992.
41. Ellis PM, Findlay JM: Craniocervical fusion with contoured Luque rod and autogenic bone graft, *Can J Surg* 37:50-54, 1994.
42. Fager CA: Results of adequate posterior decompression in the relief of spondylotic cervical myelopathy, *J Neurosurg* 38:684-692, 1973.
43. Farey ID, McAfee PC, Davis RF, Long DM: Pseudarthrosis of the cervical spine after anterior arthrodesis: treatment by posterior nerve-root decompression, stabilization and arthrodesis. *J Bone Joint Surg* 72A:1171-1177, 1990.
44. Fehlings MG, Errico T, Cooper P et al: Occipitocervical fusion with a five millimeter malleable rod and segmental fixation, *Neurosurgery* 32:198-208, 1993.
45. Fernyhough JC, White JI, LaRocca H: Fusion rates in multi-level cervical spondylosis comparing allograft fibula and autograft fibula in 126 patients, *Spine* 16S:561-564,1991.
46. Fielding JW, Hensinger RN, Hawkins RJ: Os odontoideum. *J Bone Joint Surg* 62A:376-382, 1980.
47. Fielding JW, Tolli TC: Surgical management of postlaminectomy kyphosis, *Semin. Spine Surg* 1:271-275, 1989.
48. Fisher JR, Emery SE: Higher incidence of pseudarthrosis and poor outcomes for three-level anterior cervical diskectomy and fusion, North American Spine Society Eleventh Annual Meeting, Vancouver, Canada, October 23-26, 1996.
49. Fraser AB, Sen C, Casden AM et al: Cervical transdural intramedullary migration of a sublaminar wire: a complication of cervical fixation, *Spine* 19:456-459, 1994.
50. Gallie WE: Fractures and dislocations of the upper cervical spine, *Am J Surg* 46:495-499; 1939.
51. Garfin SR, Moore MR, Marshall LF: A modified technique for cervical facet fusions, *Clin Orthop* 230:149-153, 1988.
52. Ghanayem AJ, Rapoff AJ, O'Brien TJ, Zdeblick TA: Anterior plate stabilization of multilevel cervical corpectomies: a biomechanical analysis of alternative plating techniques. North American Spine Society Eleventh Annual Meeting, Vancouver, Canada, October 23-26, 1996.
53. Gill K, Paschal S, Corin J et al: Posterior plating of the cervical spine: a biomechanical comparison of different posterior fusion techniques, *Spine* 13: 813-816, 1988.
54. Gore DR, Sepic SB: Anterior cervical fusion for degenerated or protruded discs: a review of one hundred forty-six patients, *Spine* 9:667-671, 1979.
55. Grisoli F, Graziani N, Fabrizi AP et al: Anterior diskectomy without fusion for treatment of cervical lateral soft disc extrusion: a follow-up of 120 cases, *Neurosurgery* 24:853-858,1989.
56. Griswold DM, Albright JA, Schiffman E et al: Atlanto-axial fusion for instability, *J Bone Joint Surg* 60A:285-292, 1978.
57. Grob D, Crisco J, Panjabi M, Dvorak J: Biomechan-

ical evaluation of four different posterior atlanto-axial fixation techniques, *Spine* 17:480-490, 1992.

58. Grob D, Jeanneret B, Aebi M, Markwalder TH: Atlanto-axial fusion with transarticular screw fixation, *J Bone Joint Surg* 73B:972-976, 1991.
59. Grob D, Panjabi M, Froehlich M, Hayek J. Posterior occipitocervical fusion: a preliminary report of a new technique, *Spine* 16(suppl):S17-S24, 1991.
60. Grob D, Dvorak J, Panjabi MM, Antinnes JA: The role of plate and screw fixation in occipitocervical fusion in rheumatoid arthritis, *Spine* 19:2545-2551, 1994.
61. Grob D, Dvorak, Panjabi MM et al: Posterior occipito-cervical fusion, *Spine* 16:S17-S24, 1991.
62. Haher TR: Occipital screw pullout strength: a biomechanical investigation of occipital morphology, *J Spinal Cord Med* 19:118-122, 1996.
63. Hajek PD, Lipka J, Hartlin P et al: Biomechanical study of C1-C2 posterior arthrodesis techniques, *Spine* 18:173-177, 1993.
64. Hamblin DL: Occipito-cervical fusion. Indications, technique and results, *J Bone Joint Surg* 49B:33-45, 1967.
65. Hanley EN, Harvell JC: Immediate postoperative stability of the atlanto-axial articulation: a biomechanical study comparing simple midline wiring, and the Gallie and Brooks procedures, *J Spinal Disord:* 5:306-310, 1992.
66. Hanson PB, Montesano PX, Sharkey N, Rauschning W: Anatomic and biomechanical assessment of transarticular screw fixation for atlanto-axial instability, *Spine* 16:1141-1145, 1991.
67. Heller JG: Complications of posterior cervical plating, *Semin Spine Surg* 5:128-138, 1993.
68. Herman JM, Sonntag VK: Cervical corpectomy and plate fixation for postlaminectomy kyphosis, *J Neurosurg* 80:963-970, 1994.
69. Heywood AWB, Learmonth JD, Thomas M: Internal fixation for occipito-cervical fusion, *J Bone Joint Surg* 70B:709-711, 1988.
70. Hilibrand AS, Carlson GD, Palumbo MA, Bohlman HH: Radiculopathy due to degeneration of segments adjacent to cervical fusions. North American Spine Society Eleventh Annual Meeting, Vancouver, Canada, October 23-26, 1996.
71. Hilibrand AS, Yoo JU, Carlson GD: The outcome of anterior cervical fusions adjacent to prior fusions. North American Spine Society Eleventh Annual Meeting, Vancouver, Canada, October 23-26, 1996.
72. Hughes SS, Pringle T, Phillips FM, Bohlman HH, Emery SE: Multilevel cervical corpectomy and fibular strut grafting: intermediate clinical and radiographic followup, *Orthop Trans* 20(2):432, 1996.
73. Itoh T, Tsuji H, Katoh Y, Yonezawa T, Kitagawa H: Occipital cervical fusion reinforced by Luque's segmental spinal instrumentation for rheumatoid disease, *Spine* 13:1234-1238, 1988.
74. Jeanneret B, Magerl F: Primary posterior fusion of C1-2 for odontoid fractures: indications, techniques, and results of transarticular screw fixation, *J Spinal Disord* 5:464-475, 1992.
75. Jonsson H, Rauschning W: Anatomical and morphometric studies in posterior cervical spinal screw-plate systems, *J Spinal Disord* 7:429-438, 1994.
76. Katsumi Y, Honma T, Nakamura T: Analysis of cervical instability resulting from laminectomies for removal of spinal cord tumor, *Spine* 14:1172-1176, 1989.
77. Koop SE, Winter PR, Loinstein JE: The surgical treatment of instability of the upper part of the cervical spine in children and adolescents, *J Bone Joint Surg* 66A:403-411, 1984.
78. Kostuik JP: *The surgical treatment of failures of laminectomy and spinal fusion.* In Anderson GBJ, McNeil TW, editors: *Lumbar spinal stenosis,* St Louis, 1992, Mosby, pp. 425-469.
79. Kostuik JP, Connolly PJ, Esses SI: Anterior cervical plate fixation with the titanium hollow screw plate system, *Spine* 18:1273-1278, 1993.
80. Kotani Y, Cunningham BW, Abumi K, McAfee PC: Biomechanical analysis of cervical stabilization systems: an assessment of transpedicular screw fixation in the cervical spine, *Spine* 19:2529-2539, 1994.
81. Kraus DR, Peppelman WC, Agarwal AK et al: Incidence of subaxial subluxation in patients with generalized rheumatoid arthritis who have had previous occipital cervical fusions, *Spine* 16:S486-S489, 1991.
82. Letts M, Slutsky D: Occipitocervical arthrodesis in children, *J Bone Joint Surg* 67A:592-597, 1985.
83. Lipson SJ: Cervical myelopathy and posterior atlanto-axial subluxation in patients with rheumatoid arthritis, *J Bone Joint Surg* 69A:833-836, 1987.
84. Lowery GL, Swank ML, McDonough RF: Surgical revision for failed anterior cervical fusions, *Spine* 20:2436-2441, 1995.
85. MacKenzie AI, Uttley D, Marsh HT, Bell BA: Craniocervical stabilization using Luque/Hartshill rectangles, *Neurosurgery* 26:32-36, 1990.
86. Malcolm GP, Ransford AO, Crockard HA: Treatment of non-rheumatoid occipitocervical instability: internal fixation with the Hartshill-Ransford loop, *J Bone Joint Surg* 76B:357-366, 1994.
87. Marcotte P, Dickman CA, Sonntag VK et al: Posterior atlantoaxial facet screw fixation, *J Neurosurg* 79:234-237, 1993.
88. Magerl F, Seemann PS: *Stable posterior fusion of the atlas and axis by transarticular screw fixation.* In Kehr P, Weidner A, editors: *Cervical spine.* Berlin, 1987, Springer-Verlag, pp 322-327.
89. McAfee PC, Bohlman HH. One-stage anterior cervi-

cal decompression and posterior stabilization with circumferential arthrodesis: a study of twenty-four patients who had a traumatic or neoplastic lesion, *J Bone Joint Surg* 71A:78-88, 1989.

90. McAfee PC, Bohlman HH, Wilson WL: The triple-wire fixation technique for stabilization of acute fracture-dislocations: a biomechanical analysis, *Orthop Trans* 9:142, 1985.

91. McAfee PC, Cassidy JR, Davis RF et al: Fusion of the occiput to the upper cervical spine-a review of 37 cases, *Spine* 16(10S): S490-S494, 1991.

92. McGraw RW, Rusch RM: Atlanto-axial arthrodesis, *J Bone Joint Surg* 55B:482-489, 1973.

93. Meeks L, Goodrich A, Toro V et al: Magnetic resonance imaging artifacts after anterior cervical diskectomy and fusion: a cadaveric study, *Orthop Trans* 8(2):329, 1994.

94. Mikawa Y, Shikata J, Yamamuro T: Spinal deformity and instability after multilevel cervical laminectomy, *Spine* 12:6-11,1987.

95. Misenhemer GR, Peek RD, Wiltse LL, Rothman SLG, Widell EH: Anatomic analysis of pedicle angle and cancellous diameter as related to screw size, *Spine* 14:367-372, 1989.

96. Mitchell DW, Betcher RA, Littlejohn SG et al: Biomechanical pull-out strength of the CSLP anchor screws. Presented at the Twenty-Third Annual Meeting of the Cervical Spine Research Society, Santa Fe, November 30-December 2, 1995.

97. Mitsui H: A new operation for atlanto-axial arthrodesis, *J Bone Joint Surg* 66B:422-425, 1984.

98. Montesano PX, Jauch EC, Anderson PA et al: Biomechanics of cervical spine internal fixation, *Spine* 16:S10-S16, 1991.

99. Montesano PX, Jauch E, Johnson H: Anatomic and biomechanical study of posterior cervical plate arthrodesis: an evaluation of two different techniques of screw placement, *J Spinal Disord* 5:301-305, 1992.

100. Moskovich R, Crockard HA: Atlantoaxial arthrodesis using interlaminar clamps. An improved technique, *Spine* 17:2612-2617, 1992.

101. Mueller ME, Allgoewer M, Schneider R, Willenegger H: Manual of internal fixation. Techniques recommended by the AOASIF Group, ed 3, Berlin, 1991, Springer-Verlag, pp 666-669.

102. Newman M: The outcome of pseudarthrosis after cervical anterior fusion, *Spine* 18:2380-2382, 1993.

103. Newman P, Sweetman R: Occipital cervical fusion, *J Bone Joint Surg* 51B:423-431, 1969.

104. O'Brien MF, Sutterlin CE III: Occipitocervical biomechanics: clinical and biomechanical implications for posterior occipitocervical stabilization and fusion, *Spine: State of the Art Reviews* 10(2):281-313, 1996.

105. Pait G, Arnautovic KI, Borba LAB, Van Hemert RL: Pedicle screw fixation of C7, T1, T2: articular shelf concept. North American Spine Society Eleventh Annual Meeting, Vancouver, Canada, October 23-26, 1996.

106. Phillips FM, Carlson G, Emery SE, Bohlman HH: Anterior cervical pseudarthrosis-natural history and treatment. North American Spine Society Eleventh Annual Meeting, Vancouver, Canada, October 23-26, 1996.

107. Raimondi AJ, Gutierrez FA, DiRocco C: Laminotomy and total reconstruction of the posterior spinal arch for spinal canal surgery in childhood, *J Neurosurg* 45:555-560, 1976.

108. Raynor RB, Pugh J, Shapiro I: Cervical facetectomy and its effect on spine strength, *J Neurosurg* 63:278-282, 1985.

109. Ransford AO, Crockard HA, Pozo JL, Thomas NP, Nelson IW: Craniocervical instability treated by contoured loop fixation, *J Bone Joint Surg* 68B:173-177, 1986.

110. Rea GL, Mullin BB, Mervis LJ, Miller CL: Occipitocervical fixation in nontraumatic upper cervical spine instability, *Surg Neurol* 40:255-261, 1993.

111. Riley LH Jr, Robinson RA, Johnson KA et al: The results of anterior interbody fusion of the cervical spine: review of ninety-three consecutive cases, *J Neurosurg* 30:127-133, 1969.

112. Ripa DR, Kowall MG, Meyer PR, Rusin JJ: Series of ninety-two traumatic cervical spine injuries stabilized with anterior ASIF plate fusion technique, *Spine* 16:S46-S55, 1991.

113. Roberts A, Wickstrom J: Prognosis of odontoid fractures, *J Bone Joint Surg* 54A:117-121, 1972.

114. Robinson RA, Walker AE, Ferlic DC et al: The results of an anterior interbody fusion of the cervical spine, *J Bone Joint Surg* 44A:1569-1574, 1962.

115. Rogers WA: Treatment of fracture-dislocation of the cervical spine, *J Bone Joint Surg* 24:245-248, 1942.

116. Roy L, Gibson DA: Cervical spine fusions in children, *Clin Orthop* 73:146-151, 1980.

117. Roy-Camille R, Mazel C, Saillant G: *Treatment of cervical spine injuries by posterior osteosynthesis with plates and screws.* In Kehr P, Weidner A, editors: *Cervical Spine,* Berlin, 1987, Springer-Verlag, pp 163.

118. Saito T, Yamamuro T, Shikata J, Oka M, Tsutsumi S: Analysis and prevention of spinal column deformity following cervical laminectomy. 1. Pathogenetic analysis of postlaminectomy deformities, *Spine* 16: 494-502, 1991.

119. Sakou T, Kawaida H, Morizono Y: Occipitoatlantoaxial fusion utilizing a rectangular rod, *Clin Orthop Rel Res* 239:136-144, 1989.

120. Santavirta S, Slatis P, Kankaanpaa U, Sandelin J, Laasonen E: Treatment for the cervical spine in rheumatoid arthritis: *J Bone Joint Surg* 71A:189-195, 1989.

121. Sasso RC, Jeanneret B, Fisher K, Magerl F: Occipitocervical fusion with posterior plate and screw instrumentation, *Spine* 19:2364-2368, 1994.

122. Satomi K, Ishii Y, MiyasakaY et al: Late myelopathy after anterior cervical interbody fusion, *Orthop Trans* 8(2):362, 1994.
123. Sim FH, Svien HJ, Bickel WH, Janes JM: Swan-neck deformity following extensive cervical laminectomy. A review of twenty-one cases, *J Bone Joint Surg* 59A:564-580, 1974.
124. Slatis P, Santavirta S, Sandelin J, Konttinen YT: Cranial subluxation of the odontoid process in rheumatoid arthrits, *J Bone Joint Surg* 71A:381-392, 1989.
125. Smith MD, Anderson P, Grady MS: Occipitocervical arthrodesis using contoured plate fixation: an early report on a versatile fixation technique, *Spine* 18:556-571, 1993.
126. Smith MD, Bolesta MJ: Esophgeal perforation after anterior cervical plate fixation: a report of two cases, *J Spinal Disord* 5:357-362, 1992.
127. Smith MD, Kotzar G, Uyoo J, Bohlmann HH: A biomechanical analysis of atlantoaxial stabilization methods using a bovine model, *Clin Orthop* 290:285-295, 1993.
128. Smith MD, Phillips WA, Hensinger RN: Fusion of the upper cervical spine in children and adolescents-an analysis of 17 patients, *Spine* 16:695-701, 1991.
129. Smith MD, Phillips WA, Hensinger RN: Complications of fusion to the upper cervical spine, *Spine* 16:702-705, 1991.
130. Songer MN, Spencer DL, Meyer PR Jr, Jayaraman G: The use of sublaminar cable to replace Luque wires, *Spine* 16:8S:418-421, 1991.
131. Spierings ELH, Braakman R: The management of os odontoideum-analysis of 37 cases, *J Bone Joint Surg* 64B:422-427, 1982.
132. Stambough JL, Balderston RA, Grey S: Technique for occipito-cervical fusion in osteopenic patients, *J Spine Disord* 3:404-407, 1990.
133. Stauffer ES: Wiring techniques of the posterior cervical spine for the treatment of trauma, *Orthopaedics* 11:1543-1548, 1988.
134. Stauffer ES, Kelly EG: Fracture dislocations of the cervical spine: instability and recurrent deformity following treatment by interbody fusion, *J Bone Joint Surg* 59A:45-48, 1977.
135. Stevens JM, Kendall BE, Crockard HA, Ransford A: The odontoid process in Morquio-Brailsford's disease. The effects of occipitocervical fusion, *J Bone Joint Surg* 68B:350-356, 1986.
136. Stuck RM: Anterior cervical disc excision and fusion: report of two hundred consecutive cases, *Rocky M Med J* 60:25-29, 1963.
137. Sutterlin CE: *Occipitocervical and upper cervical methods of fusion and fixation.* In Bridwell KH, DeWald RL, editors: *Textbook of spinal surgery,* ed 2, Philadelphia, 1997, Lippincott-Raven, pp 1039-1053.
138. Sutterlin CE, McAfee PC, Warden KE et al: A biomechanical evaluation of cervical spine stabilization methods in a bovine model: static and cyclical loading, *Spine* 13:795-802, 1988.
139. Takahashi M, Yamashita Y, Sakamoto Y, Kojima R: Chronic cervical compression: clinical significance of increased signal intensity on MR images, *Radiology* 173:219-224, 1989.
140. Tribus CB, Corteen DP, Zdeblick TA: The efficacy of anterior cervical plating in the treatment of symptomatic pseudoarthrosis of the cervical spine, *Orthop Trans* 20(2):433, 1996.
141. Vaccaro AR, Abraham D, Cotler J et al: Failure of multilevel anterior unicortical cervical plate instrumentation [poster]. Presented at the Twenty-Third Annual Meeting of the Cervical Spine Research Society, Santa Fe, November 30-December 2, 1995.
142. Vaccaro AR, Mirkovic S, Bauer RD, Garfin SR: *Revision lumbar and cervical degenerative spine surgery—indications and techniques.* In Bridwell KH, DeWald RL, editors: *Textbook of spinal surgery,* ed 2, Philadelphia, 1997, Lippincott-Raven, pp 1457-1494.
143. Weiland DJ, McAfee PC. Posterior cervical fusion with the triple-wire strut graft technique: 100 consecutive patients, *J Spinal Disord* 4:15-21, 1991.
144. Wertheim SB, Bohlman HH: Occipitocervical fusion, *J Bone Joint Surg* 69A:833-836, 1987.
145. White AA III, Southwick WO, DePonte RJ et al: Relief of pain by anterior cervical spine fusion for spondylosis: a report of sixty-five cases, *J Bone Joint Surg* 55A:525, 1973.
146. Whitecloud TS, LaRocca SH: Fibula strut graft in reconstructive surgery of the cervical spine, *Spine* 1:33-43, 1976.
147. Whitehill R, Sirna EC, Young DC, Cantrell RW: Late esophageal perforation from an autogenous bone graft, *J Bone Joint Surg* 67A:644-645, 1995.
148. Wilke HJ, Fischer K, Kuger A, Magerl F, Claes L, Worsdorfer O: In vitro investigations of internal fixation systems of the upper cervical spine II: stability of posterior atlanto-axial fixation techniques, *Eur Spine J* 1:191-199, 1992.
149. Williams JL, Allen MD Jr, Harkess JW: Late results of cervical diskectomy and interbody fusion: some factors influencing the results, *J Bone Joint Surg* 50A:277-281, 1968.
150. Xu R, Ebraheim NA, Yeasting R et al: Anatomy of C7 lateral mass and projection of pedicle axis on its posterior aspect, *J Spinal Disord* 8:116-120, 1995.
151. Yablon IG, Foster T, Spoo J et al: Fixation failure in the cervical spine. Presented at the Tenth Annual Conference of the North American Spine Society, Washington, DC, October 18-21, 1995.
152. Yamamoto I, Ikeda A, Shibuya N et al: Clinical long-term results of anterior discectomy without interbody fusion for cervical disc disease, *Spine* 16:272-279, 1991.
153. Zdeblick TAA: Complications of anterior spinal instrumentation, *Semin Spine Surg* 5:101-107, 1993.

154. Zdeblick TA, Bohlman HH: Cervical kyphosis and myelopathy. Treatment by anterior corpectomy and strut-grafting, *J Bone Joint Surg* 71A:170-182, 1989.
155. Zdeblick TA, Ducker TB: The use of freeze-dried allograft bone for anterior cervical fusions, *Spine* 16:726-729, 1991.
156. Zdeblick TA, Hughes SS, Riew KD, Bohlman HH. Failed anterior cervical diskectomy and arthrodesis, *J Bone Joint Surg* 79A:523-532, 1997.
157. Zipnick RI, Merola AA, Gorup J, Kunkle K, Shin T, Caruso S, Haher TR: The occiput-anatomic considerations for internal fixation, *Spine: State of the Art Reviews* 10(2):269-274, 1996.
158. Zoma A, Sturrock RD, Fisher WD, Freeman PA, Hamblen DL: Surgical stabilization of the rheumatoid cervical spine: a review of indications and results, *J Bone Joint Surg* 73B:851-858, 1991.

# 6

# BALANCE CONSIDERATIONS IN REVISIONS IN CHILDREN

**Jean Dubousset, M.D.**



Treatment failures for spinal deformities include mechanical problems, functional compromise, pain, and cosmetic discontent. Most of these occur after treatment that involves surgical correction, and are in direct relation to problems of balance and subsequently imbalance. This imbalance may already exist prior to surgery and may not have been addressed, or insufficiently corrected. Occasionally, the malalignment problem was absent before surgery and resulted entirely from the surgical treatment itself.

Historically, when surgical treatment of spinal deformities was done only by fusion and postoperative cast immobilization, postoperative imbalance was rarely noted. With the development of instrumentation, particularly with Harrington instrumentation and segmental spinal instrumentation, the incidence of imbalance problems increased dramatically. This also applies to the increasingly rigid newer segmental instrumentation systems that apply multiple rods, hooks, and pedicular screws. These problems of imbalance are in relation to errors of strategies for correction, the technique of correction, and absence or impossibility to get a good perioperative radiograph, and with the fact that perioperative radiographs are performed in a recumbent position and imbalance appears mainly in a standing position.

It is my impression that when dealing with revision surgery for spine, the three-dimensional balance for the long-term result is the most important factor to be considered, far more significantly than the percentage of Cobb angle correction.

## BASIC PRINCIPLES OF BALANCE OF THE BODY IN HUMANS

### The Principles

The first concept is that we must consider the spine as a whole, in which the entire head (4.5 to 5.5 kg) is the first vertebra and the entire pelvis is the last vertebra (called the pelvic vertebra).

This pelvic vertebra has a much greater mobility than the 1.5° existing inside the sacroiliac joint.[2] In fact, this pelvic vertebra is an intercalary bone between the trunk and the lower limbs. It has an important role in the standing and sitting posture. For example, when the pelvic vertebra tilts forward to recover balance, the lumbar spine goes into lordosis and, conversely, when the pelvic vertebra tilts backward, the lumbar spine becomes kyphotic. This way, head and trunk are maintained in an erect posture (Fig. 6-1).

The erect posture, as well standing or sitting, is the definition of the human species (*Homo sapiens erectus*). The two feet delineate a surface that represents the *sustentative polygon*. A plumb line dropped to the center of this basement polygon determines the central coordinate system for the human body. This plumb line also represents the axis of gravity at the cross-section of the coronal and sagittal reference planes. From an anatomical point of view, the axis of gravity (seen

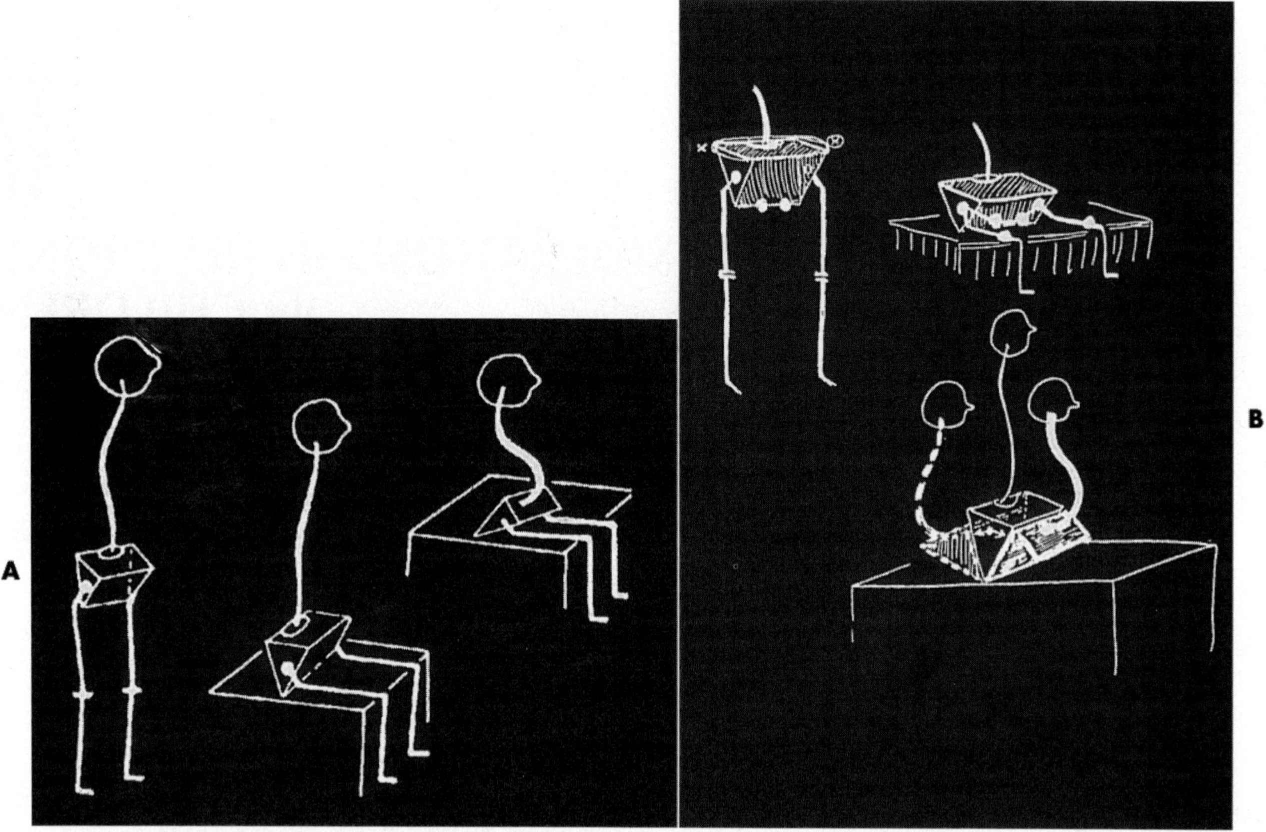


**FIGURE 6-1**

**A, B,** The head and pelvic vertebra concept. The entire head is the first vertebra. The entire pelvis is the last vertebra intercalary between trunk and the lower extremities. This is essential as a link in standing and sitting positions.

sagittally) coincides with a plumb line dropped down from the tragus.

When the patient is sitting, the basement polygon is defined by a surface limited by the pressure points of both ischial tuberosities and the posterior surface of both thighs. The center of this polygon is more difficult to define; the crossing point of the sagittal plane with a frontal plane passing just in front of the line that links together both ischial tuberosities is a reference point for this center.

Thus, balance is the status of the patient standing or sitting in an erect posture with his body aligned to a gravity line passing through the center of the basement polygon. Clinically, this status is correlated with a minimum of muscular strain. To describe this, I would like to use the structure of the Eiffel Tower as an analogy: the Eiffel Tower is well balanced because each one of the four basement pillars has an elastic behavior perfectly adapted to bending stresses such as wind.

Balance in regard to the spine is economy of energy. Indeed, a whole skeleton may simply be placed in a stable standing posture if you reproduce an anterior iliofemoral ligament with a resistant rubber band and if you replace the gastrocnemius with an inextensible cord.

This simple experiment is to be correlated with scientific barycentremetric studies.[1] These studies are based on a device that determines the center of gravity of successive horizontal slices of the human body. The studies confirm an empirical idea that the sagittal gravity line axis of the patient passes through the odontoid process and lies just behind the center of the femoral head in front of the sacral promontory.

These are the underlying data to my concept of the *cone of economy* (Fig. 6-2): If the spine is located inside of such a cone, the patient can stand up with almost no muscular energy expenditure. In such a situation the stress loads on the spinal processes are minimal, if not absent. If fusion is the goal, it is almost always successful in this situation even when no instrumentation is used. This is one practical example in which three-dimensional balance must be considered for successful outcome. The principle of three-dimensional analysis should be a basic rule in the treatment approach for spinal pathology.

In regard to static balance, coronal balance corresponds to a good arrangement (or distribution) of the stresses surrounding the spine, with almost equal stresses on the right and left half of the patient. Sagittal balance is realized if the center of gravity line follows

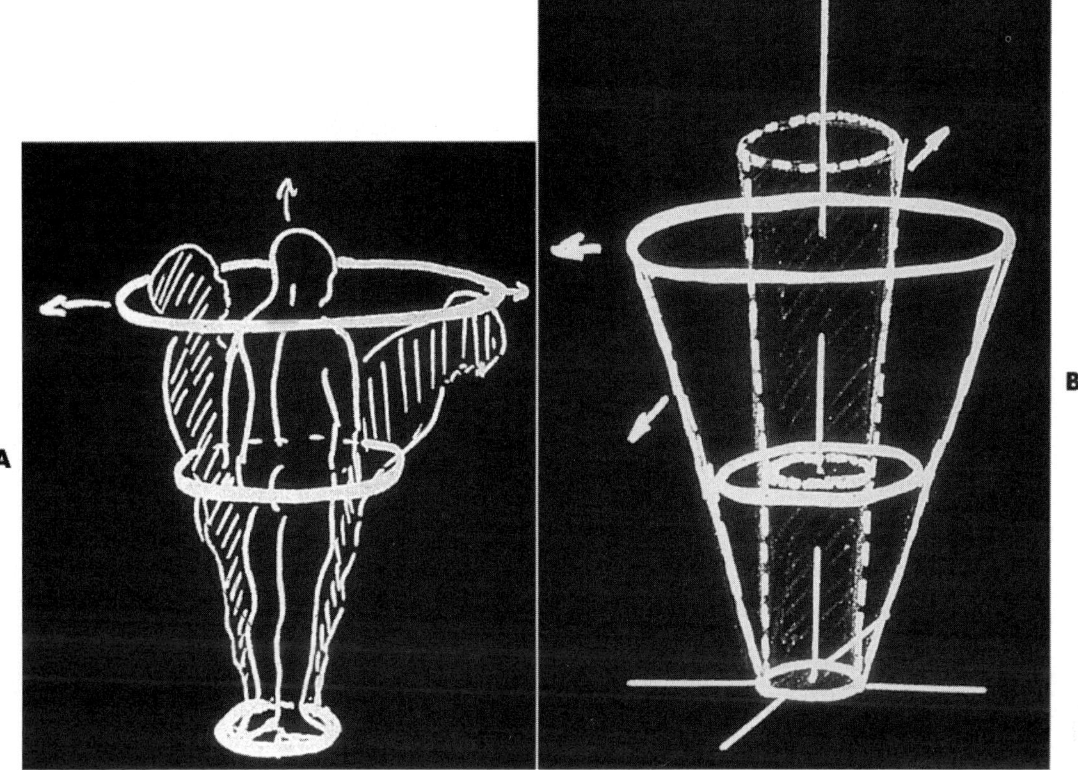


FIGURE 6-2

**A, B,** The cone of economy concept, in which inside the small cone of economy almost all muscle function is at rest around the spine. When permanently outside of this cone, permanent stresses occur on the spinal structures and this can lead to failure of structures, including a fusion and instrumentation.

the line from the odontoid process down to the center of the basement polygon. Finally, to accomplish horizontal balance, the lower disk of the instrumented spine must be placed in the center of the gravity line.

Even more important than static balance is the concept of *dynamic balance.* Dynamic balance should be analyzed by testing the motion of the spine in the three dimensions (e.g., frontward-backward to explore the sagittal plane, right-left to explore the coronal plane, and rotating right-left to look at the horizontal balance). If the excursion of the spine is symmetrical in these three planes, good balance is more likely to be achieved.

For example when the first motion segment under fusion mass has a symmetrical motion in the three planes it is in dynamic balance. Therefore, we might consider this segment to be in the ideal position for long-term function (Fig. 6-3).

The goal of spinal surgery as well as primary revision surgery is to replace the spine inside of the *cone of economy* with a perfect static and dynamic three-dimensional balance, not to obtain deformity reduction in only the coronal or sagittal plane.

Another factor closely related to balance is stability. It is very important to consider this concept for primary and revision surgery. Immediate instability is defined by dynamic x-ray findings. For example flexion-extension or right and left side-bending films may demonstrate a range of motion between two adjacent segments that is beyond the normal range of motion, especially with the loss of alignment of the points of reference.

Potential instability is more tenuous and treacherous because no abnormal motion may be detected on dynamic x-rays. However, an abrupt malalignment in the continuity of the points of reference may be present (e.g., in the spinal canal). Instability may occur either progressively with a malalignment increasing with time, or suddenly secondary to a minor trauma with sometimes dangerous consequences for the nervous or spinal cord structures.

## MEASUREMENT OF BALANCE AND IMBALANCE

***Static Measurement.*** In a standing or sitting patient in a relaxed posture, the analysis is based on a plumb line, dropped down from the tragus for the sagittal plane or from T1 for the coronal plane. For sagittal balance, this gravity line should lie just behind the hip joint. For coronal balance, the plumb line going down from T1

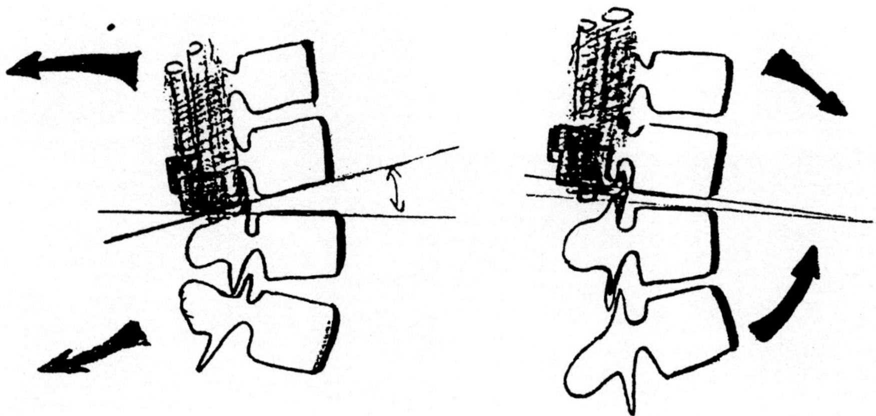

FIGURE 6-3

The goal of any instrumentation and fusion of the spine is to leave the mobile disk space and segments (including pelvis) below the fusion balanced in three dimensions. For example, here in the sagittal plane as excursion in front as in back. This concept applies equally in the coronal and in the horizontal plane.

must follow the intergluteal crease if the two lower limbs are of equal length.

For revision surgery, this knowledge is fundamental in the attempt to recover coronal as well as sagittal balance. One cannot overemphasize the importance of replacing the spine inside the cone of economy. If the spine remains outside of this cone, you may anticipate a failure no matter how much instrumentation is placed on the spine. This failure will occur by fatigue fracture of the fusion mass or the implant itself.

***Dynamic Measurement.*** Spinal mobility should be checked before surgery, and then again two or three months after surgery. Personally, I very closely observe the excursion of the body above the first nonfused motion segment. I check to see whether the patient has symmetrical forward and backward bending as well as right and left bending. If the amplitude of motion is quite symmetrical, I anticipate a good dynamic balance. In my opinion, there should be a rather good outcome at long-term follow-up. If, on the contrary, a clear asymmetrical dynamic motion is detected (e.g., 0° or 5° of lateral right bending as opposed to 25° or 30° of lateral left bending), an early deterioration of the remaining motion segments can be anticipated.

***Imaging Investigations.*** The previous clinical examination can be done with dynamic x-ray. However, to check many levels with x-ray is very invasive and should not be used in a routine way. Magnetic resonance imaging (MRI) can be a good tool to detect signs of disk space degeneration, especially for revision surgery under a previously operated segment. MRI will also permit an analysis of the condition of the posterior muscles below or around a previous posterior fusion and detect cases in which the muscles are completely degenerated. Such a finding should be anticipated by careful physical examination of the paraspinal muscles looking for contracture. A simple useful test is an alternative paraspinal muscle relaxation in successive right and left monopodal positions. If there is any doubt upon the quality of a disk space, we recommend that it be checked with diskography or arthroscan. Based on the radiological findings and clinical symptomatology, a decision is made whether or not to include this spinal level into the planned fusion.

When dealing with clinical dynamic measurement, data variability is very important. This is why we try to improve the quality of this measurement with a motion analysis equipment based on an optoelectronic data analysis system.[3] This method allows the quantification and study of the static and dynamic balance of the spine including pelvis, head, and the lower limbs.

## ETIOLOGIES OF POSTOPERATIVE IMBALANCE

We can subdivide the causes of postoperative imbalance according to the three planes (sagittal, coronal, and horizontal), whatever the cause may be (e.g., scoliosis, kyphosis, fractures, tumors, etc.).

### SAGITTAL PLANE

***Inside the Instrumented Area.*** Improper bending of the rod or a bad hook pattern may lead to imbalance, especially when, after rotation of the rod or translation of the spine, the first free motion segment remains outside of the cone of economy or when the rod remains flat or pushes the spine too much anteriorly. In

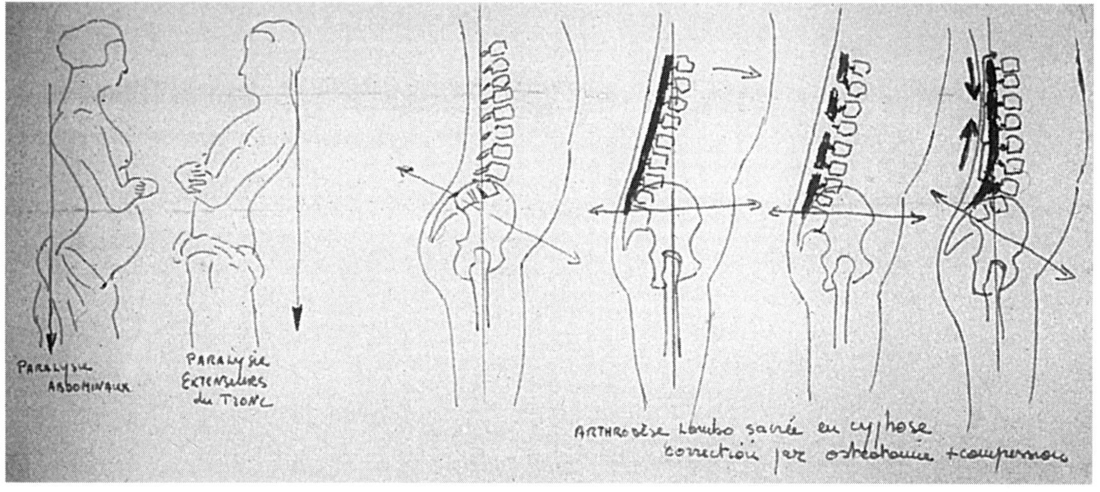


**FIGURE 6-4**

Compared to the original Duchenne drawings on the left, the postoperative *flat back* must be corrected by osteotomies and posterior compression to reestablish balance.

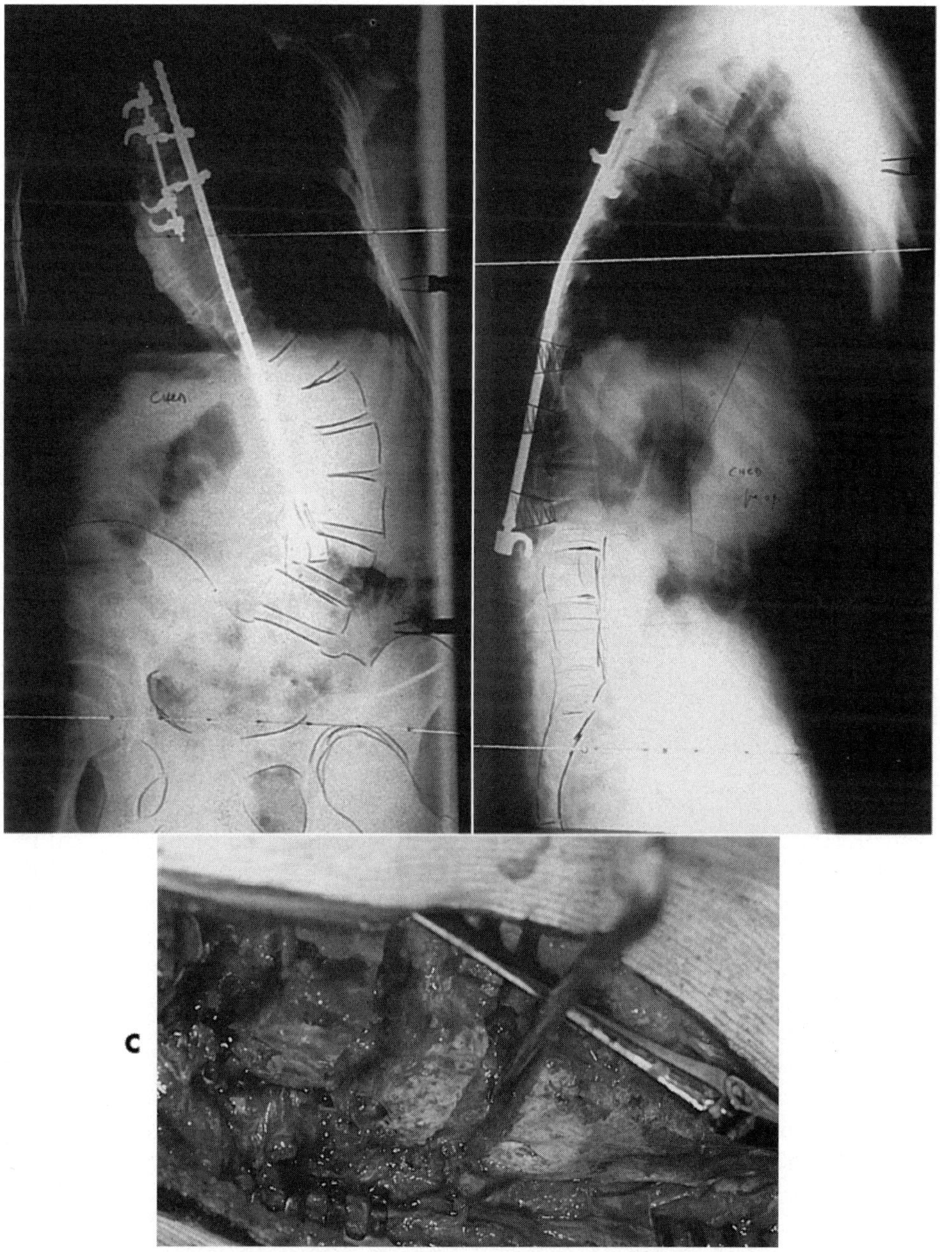

**FIGURE 6-5**

**A, B,** Preoperative old fusion performed for scoliosis with thoracolumbar kyphosis. Significant imbalance is now present in both planes. **C,** Posterior osteotomies of the fusion mass.

*Continued*

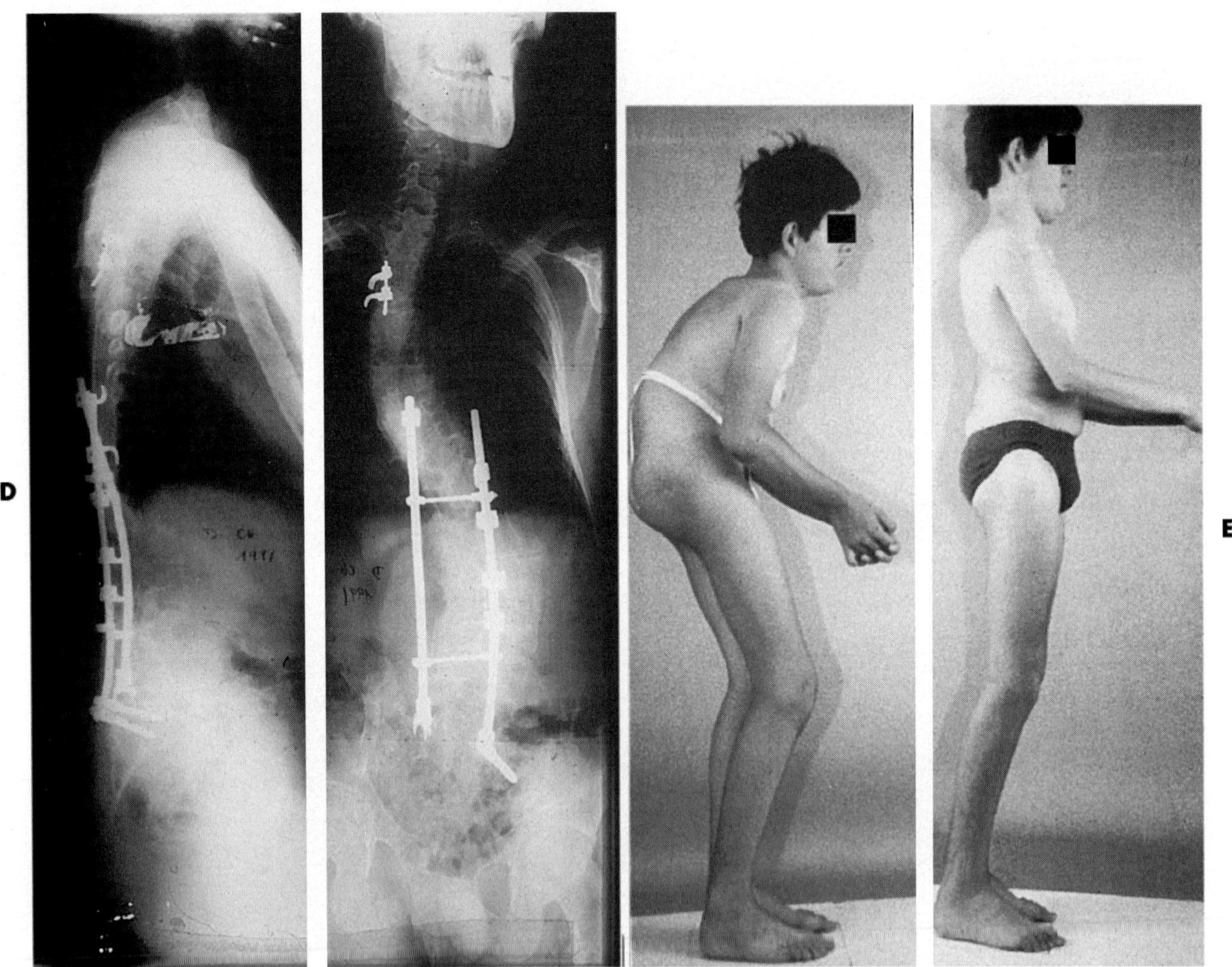

FIGURE 6-5, CONT'D

**D,** Posterior instrumentation with compression and fusion, reestablishing balance. **E,** Preoperative and postoperative clinical appearance.

such cases, it is necessary to remove posterior instruments (sometimes partially), and to perform posterior osteotomies and reinstrumentation with proper bending of the rods down to the correct levels of instrumentation (Fig. 6-4). One should be aware of the coupling effect of the rotation of the rod on the free motion segments below the fusion.

An example of this is the *flat back* observed with the old Harrington instrumentation, in which the spine was instrumented down to the lower lumbar region. The flattening of the physiologic lumbar lordosis created a hyperextension in remaining free motion segments below the fusion mass. Thus, the entire instrumented spine was pushed anteriorly. In such cases, whatever the instrumentation used previously, it is necessary to perform one or more posterior osteotomies (Fig. 6-5). Subsequently, the spine must be reinstrumented with the rods contoured into sufficient lumbar lordosis (Fig. 6-6). In some cases, combined approaches are necessary. Timing of the procedure depends on the particular type of imbalance present.

In all cases, especially for adult or paralytic spinal problems, it is very important to analyze precisely the motion of the hip joints based on the concept of the pelvic vertebra as an intercalary bone.

Finally, in some cases, a previous fusion down to the pelvis created an overcorrection of the lumbar hyperlordosis (Fig. 6-7). This creates a forward tilt of the trunk. Revision can be performed by removal of instruments, posterior lumbar osteotomies, and reinstrumentation. Another less aggressive possibility may be to perform a bilateral supra-acetabular pelvic osteotomy (Fig. 6-8). An anterior opening wedge restores a gravity line behind the femoral heads in the sagittal projection. For such osteotomies it is necessary to open slowly and, in some cases, progressively with an external fixator in order to prevent too much stretching of the femoral nerve.

Ignoring the three-columns concept of the spine in trauma, leaving an anterior gap after posterior surgery, or correction of kyphosis creating an anterior empty space are potential situations for failure of the poste-

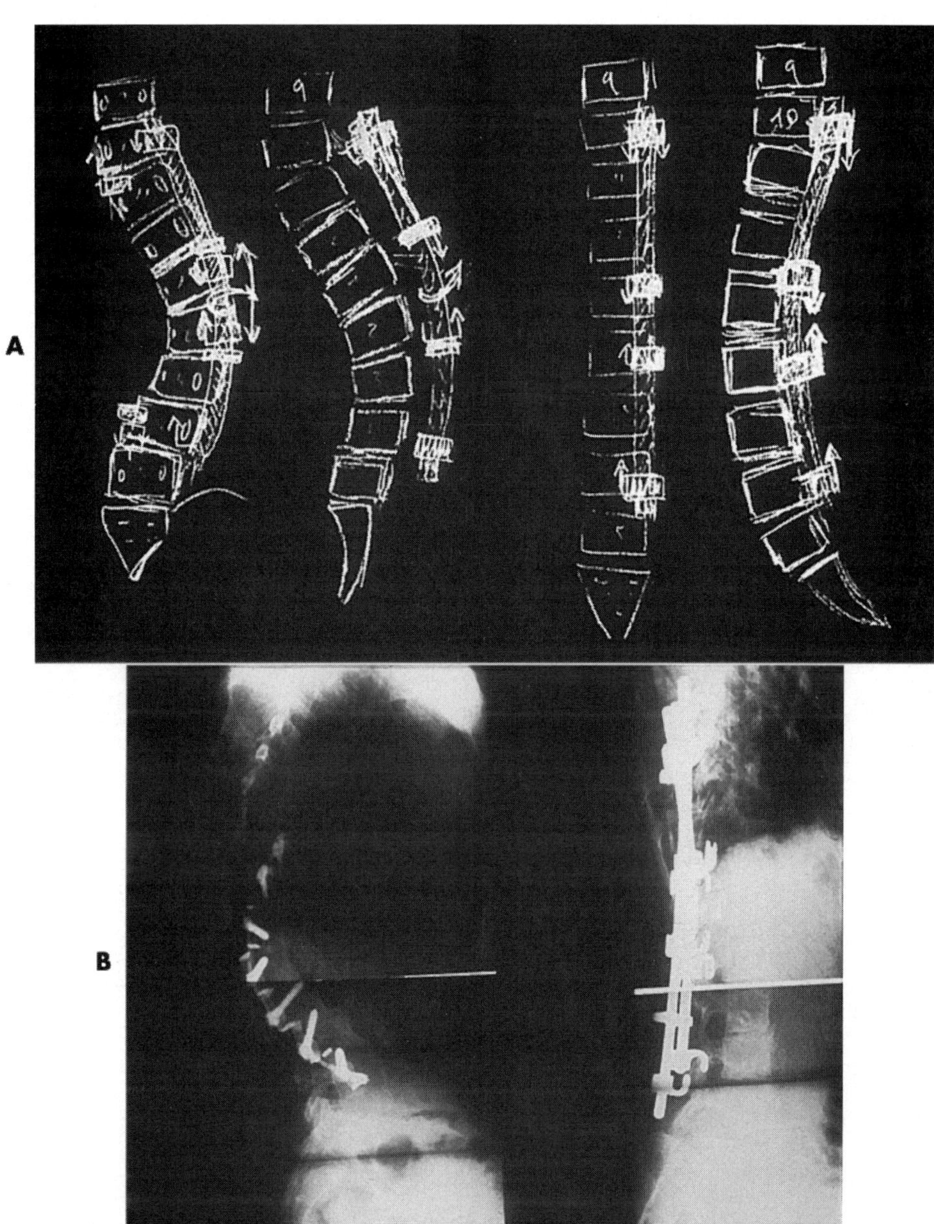


FIGURE 6-6

**A,** Principle of correction of lumbar deformity by rotation of a pre-contoured CD rod attached to the posterior aspect of the spine with hooks or screws. **B**, Results obtained on a patient treated previously with Dwyer instrumentation.

rior fusion and instrumentation. Even if a good balance is achieved primarily, ignorance of the three-columns concept leads to weakness of the anterior column and failure.

The treatment of such a case is based on the concept that one should remove the posterior instruments, and then follow this with posterior osteotomy, traction, anterior fusion, and posterior instrumentation and fusion.

***Imbalance Above the Instrumentation Area.*** Imbalance above the instrumented fusion is mostly a kyphotic deformity arising above an instrumented area when previous surgery stopped at the level of the apex of thoracic kyphosis. This problem can arise in patients in whom poor postural tone exists (cerebral palsy and neuromuscular disease) or in patients with good muscle tone but when the correction of a thoracolumbar spine did not recover sufficient lordosis or created too much of lower thoracic lordosis. To recover balance of the head and horizontal lateral eye line vision the spine bends forward above the previous fusion. In such cases it is necessary to extend the fusion above and to link to the previous one with connectors and linking

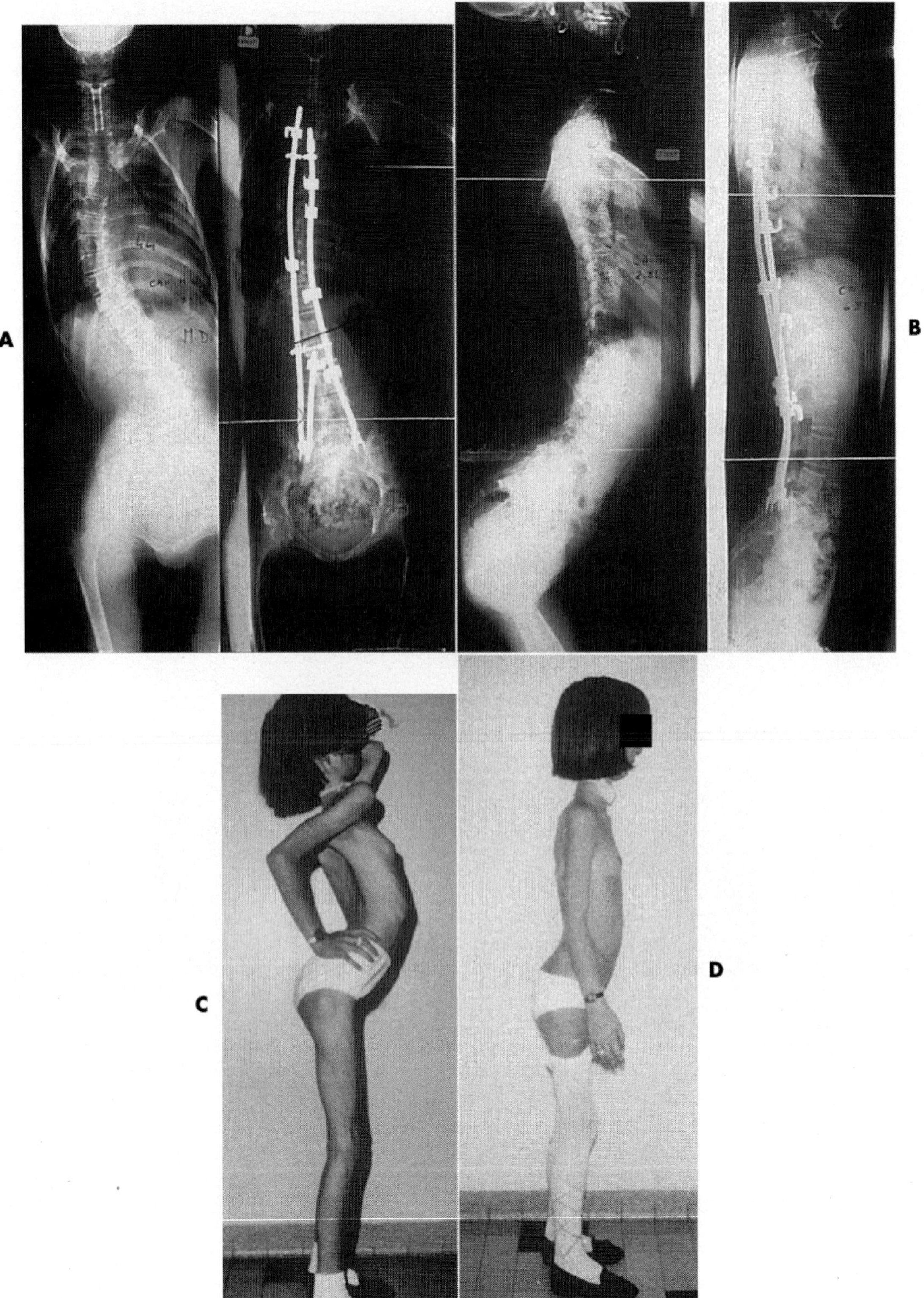

FIGURE 6-7

**A, B,** Central core disease in a patient with tracheostomy and thoracic as well as lumbar lordoscoliosis treated with posterior CD instrumentation. **C, D,** Preoperative and postoperative clinical results. Prior to surgery, the head required constant support by hand. Excellent balance and stability were achieved surgically.

A

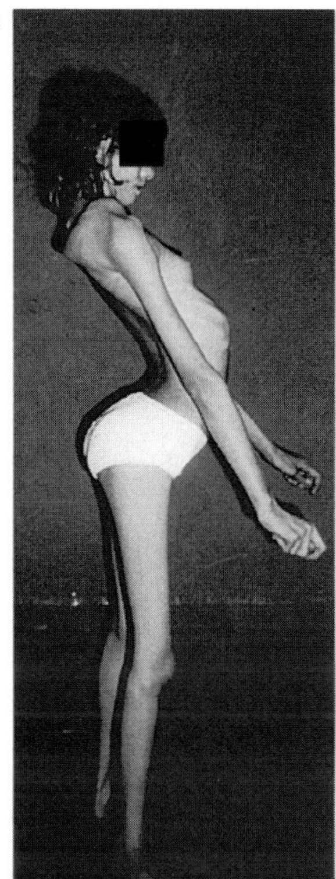

**FIGURE 6-8**

Fascioscapulohumeral congenital myopathy. **A,** Preoperative clinical status. **B,** Preoperative and postoperative radiographic images illustrating pelvic fixation. **C,** Imbalance obtained with excessive lordosis correction. *Continued*

B

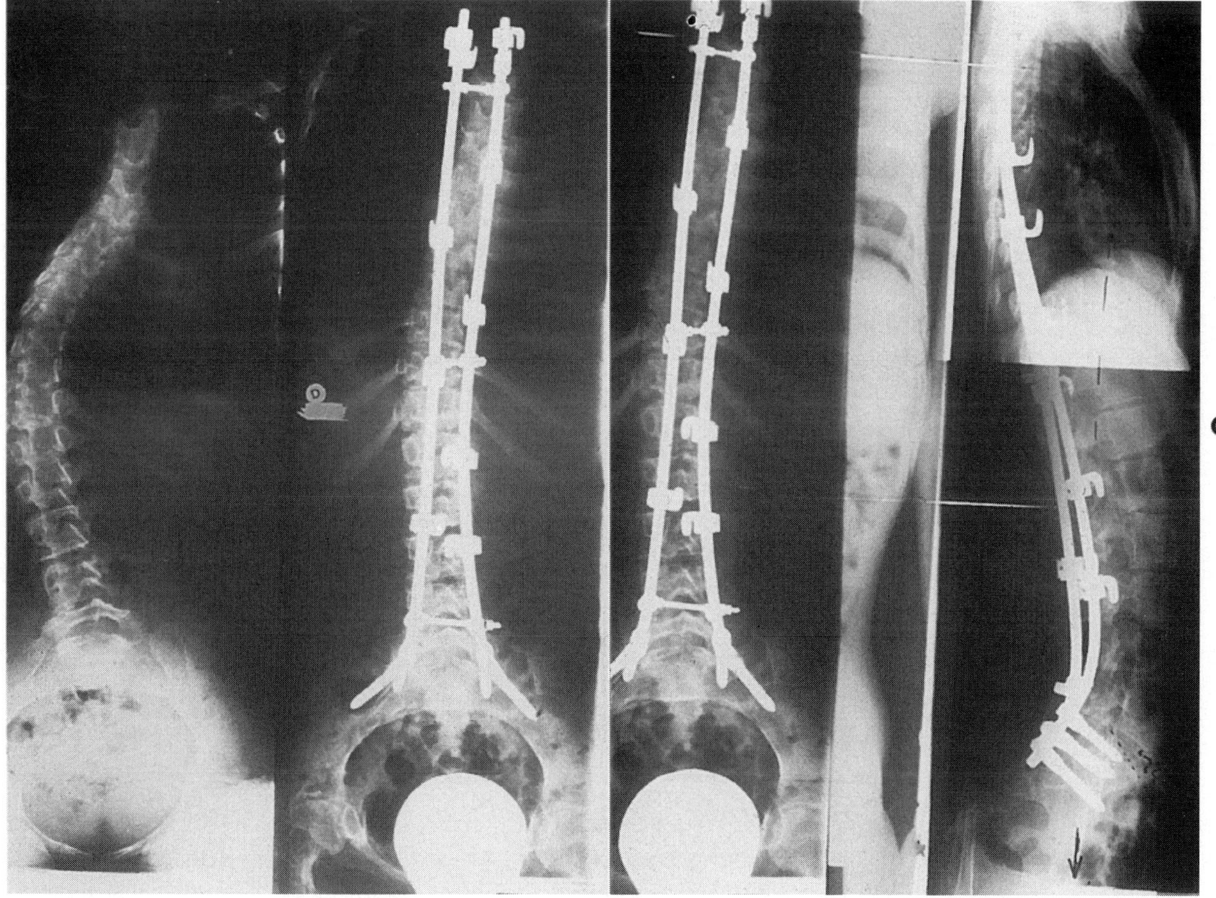

C

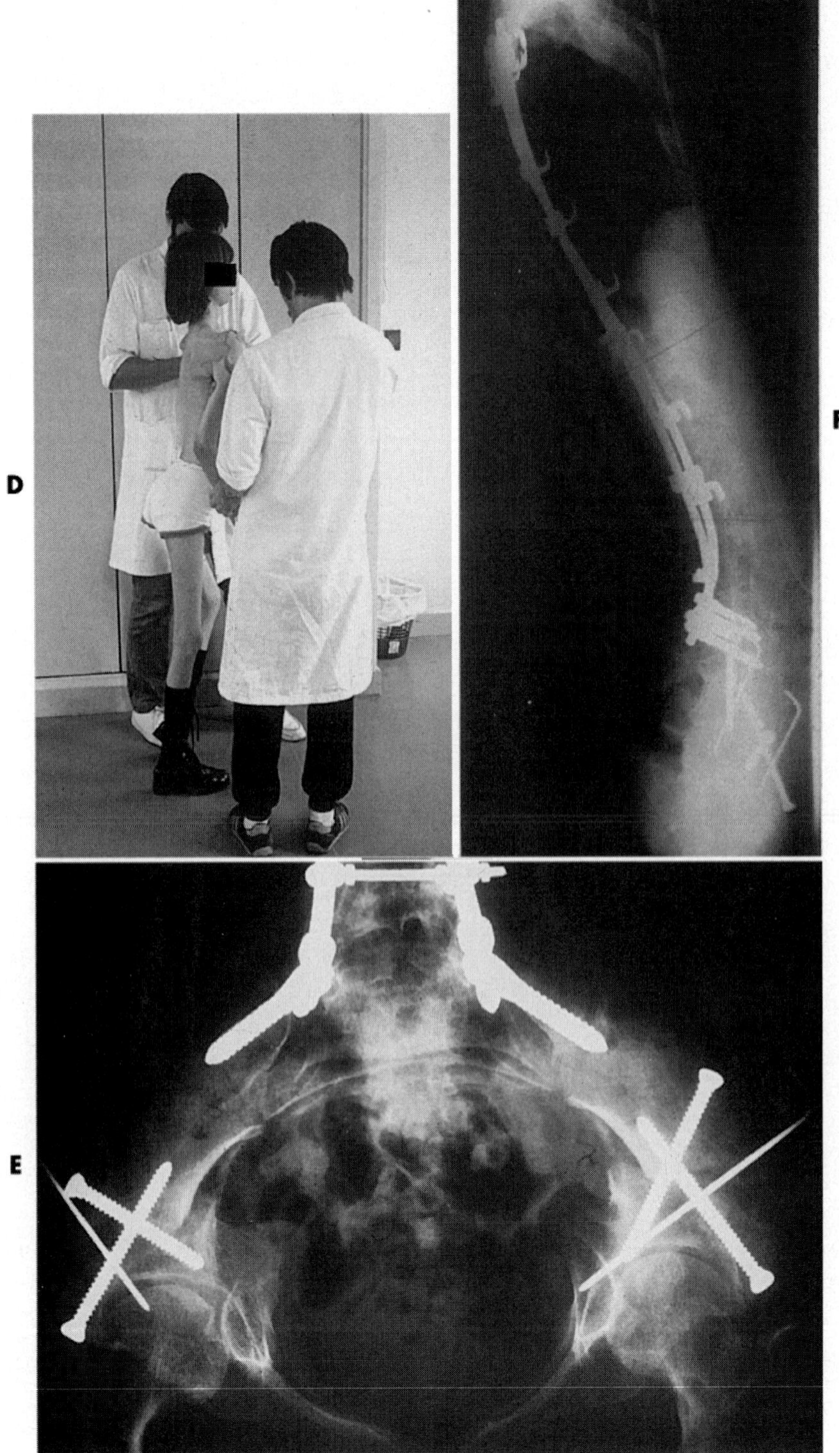


FIGURE 6-8, CONT'D

**D,** Patient standing with help (postoperative picture). **E,** Bilateral supra-acetabular pelvic osteotomies. **F,** Final x-rays showing balanced spine with gravity line falling behind the femoral head axis.

devices. Particular care is necessary to achieve a meticulous fusion at the level of linkage of the two instrumentations; don't hesitate to do an anterior fusion if an anterior empty space exists.

***Below the Instrumented Area.*** The most frequent reason for revision is junctional kyphosis arising below an instrumentation and fusion of the thoracic spine. This usually is a thoracic deformity coexisting with a mild but structural lumbar curve. The previous instrumentation was too short and left the spine going into an anteriorly directed posture above and below the junction, thus creating a junctional kyphosis. Even with a multiple hook-rod system, this coupling effect occurs if the length of instrumentation ignores the junctional zone. This may also occur if, in a dystrophic or postlaminectomy spine, the previous fusion stops inside of the pathological zone (e.g., in order to save one disk). In fact, because of lack of postoperative sagittal balance, it is sometimes necessary in these cases to extend the fusion down and sometimes to the sacrum.

Failure below the instrumented fusion can also occur in a paralytic patient when the exact level of paralysis is disregarded. When a fusion is stopped short of the sacrum in order to preserve, theoretically, the ambulation capacity of a paralyzed patient, the lack of muscle function between spine and pelvis leads to forward falling of the trunk. Extension of the fusion and instrumentation down to the sacrum, thus treating the patient and not the x-rays, reestablishes good stability and may even allow the recovery of some ambulation possibilities.

LOCALIZED HYPERLORDOSIS. When a deformity occurs into lordosis, it occurs below the instrumented area, much like kyphosis occurs above the instrumented area. Localized hyperlordosis permits the recovery of a satisfactory positioning of the pelvic vertebra in the space and in the sagittal plane. In some cases, this is well tolerated in patients that are relatively young. However, facet syndrome and facet degeneration during adulthood may occur later. This may require extension of fusion down to the sacrum.

I have seen one case in a patient with osteorenal dystrophy and double major curve fused with Cotrel-Dubousset (CD) instrumentation from T4 to L4 with a very good result in which a bilateral spondylolysis L5-S1 below the fusion developed six months postoperatively, only to recover a correct sagittal balance after this hyperlordosis. At the 10-year follow-up this patient still had good results, but it is not known whether the patient will suffer back pain at a later time. I suspect, though, that the lysis of the elongated pars has spontaneously fused so that the patient may never have problems with back pain.

SPONDYLOLISTHESIS. An elongation of the pars of the vertebra above the fusion mass without any lysis has been seen in some children with congenital spondylolisthesis and adolescents with persistent lumbosacral kyphosis. The spinal balance concept is very important for the treatment of spondylolisthesis with a vertical sacrum. If lumbosacral kyphosis exists and posterior tilting of the pelvic vertebra has not been reduced, the result is very often cosmetically and functionally not satisfactory. This may occur in some cases after in situ fusion.

To recover good function and cosmesis it is mandatory to recover a good sagittal balance. Therefore it is necessary to recover a normal lumbosacral angle. Posterior osteotomies may be required to bring the pelvic vertebra into hyperextension. One should focus on the correction of the lumbosacral kyphosis. Complete correction of the slippage is dangerous for the nerve roots. Restoring the sagittal balance of the spine will assure a stable result.

This is exactly the way we reduce primarily severe spondylolisthesis. A posterolateral fusion through the Wiltse approach is sufficient to maintain the reduction if the gravity line is normal and the lumbosacral angle (posterior wall of S1-S2-superior plateau of L5 on a sagittal projection) is around 110 degrees. In such a position the patient is absolutely inside the so-called cone of economy and if the anterior interbody (L5-S1) empty space may be corrected by remaining growth, the anterior fusion is not necessary. On the contrary, if the patient is an old adolescent it is preferable to fill the anterior empty space with an anterior L5-S1 fusion.

## CORONAL PLANE

***Trunk Asymmetry or Lateral Tilting.*** Trunk asymmetry or lateral tilting can be observed, for example, in a double curve predominant in the lumbar region in which a perfect surgical correction of the lumbar curve has been done in the coronal plane with an anterior instrumentation. Unfortunately, such correction may represent an overcorrection for the residual stiff thoracic curve.

Sometimes the tilting is increased by too much wedging of the first disk below the fusion. When symptomatic, because of pain or imbalance, at this level we believe that a revision has to be done with realignment along the gravity line by compression on the convex side of the wedged disk below the previously fused area. The instrumentation should moreover include a fusion of the stiff thoracic curve in order to rebalance the spine toward the gravity line. Bending films below and above the previously instrumented area helps to choose the correct levels. In some cases it may be necessary to perform some wedge osteotomies in the fusion mass to save some motion levels and improve the correction.

***Coronal Decompensation.*** Coronal decompensation occurs particularly in true double major scoliotic curves. Most at risk are those curve patterns with a major thoracic and a less important lumbar curve, the so-called King II curve. In both cases there is a junctional zone between the two curves. The junctional zone contains 1 disk and 2 vertebrae or 2 disks and 4 vertebrae linking together the 2 lordotic curves (one thoracic the other lumbar). The junctional zone represents an unstable spinal segment with potential kyphosis and torsion. Significant curve progression may be observed if spinal instrumentation stops exactly above this unstable segment. Whatever the correction maneuver may be, the fusion mass and instrumentation will tilt toward the concave side of the instrumented curve, thus producing a coronal decompensation. To correct or prevent this, it is necessary to extend the fusion one level below the junctional zone. A claw configuration including the last two lower vertebrae may be helpful. The hook pattern of this claw should allow for compression on the convex side and distraction back to back hooks on the concave.

Another etiology for coronal decompensation in double major curves are spinal fusions ending exactly at the apex of the lumbar curve. To restore the spinal balance in this curve, extensive surgery may be necessary. A new fusion should be performed including the entire lumbar curve. In severe decompensation this may not be sufficient. Appropriate osteotomies through the previous fusion mass may be necessary for sufficient correction.

***Shoulder-Level Asymmetry.*** The main causes of shoulder-level asymmetry are pitfalls in preoperative planning. Most often the stiffness of the upper thoracic curve has been underestimated, thus the lower thoracic curve has been overcorrected. Revision in such cases requires extension of the instrumentation up to T1. Very significant correction is usually necessary. If such a correction cannot be realized with the remaining segments above the fusion mass and if an osteotomy of the fusion mass is not feasible for any reason, then a compensatory correction may be obtained by extending the fusion one level below the previous fusion. Appropriate unilateral compression may allow restoration of the shoulder alignment, which was not completely achieved by the extension above the previous fusion. Prevention of this pitfall is based on a good preoperative analysis of the double thoracic curve pattern by bending films. The resulting imbalance occurring after correction of the lower thoracic curve alone may be appreciated through the difference of two maximum correction angles: the angle of maximum correction of the entire upper correction up to T1, and the angle of maximum correction formed by the apical vertebra of the lower curve and its most cephalad vertebra. These angles are measured on appropriate bend films. The difference between these two angles represents an estimation of the imbalance occurring after correction of the lower thoracic curve alone.

***Pelvic Obliquity.*** Pain as well as cosmetic aspects in pelvic obliquity may lead to revision surgery. A combination of osteotomy of the graft with or without extension of the fusion down to the sacrum may be necessary to recover the coronal balance.

Pelvic obliquity may occur in cases of idiopathic scoliosis when corrective surgery was stopped on L3 instead of L4. After surgery, the L3-L4 disk space remains twisted and shifted laterally. The resulting coronal decompensation may even be aggravated by the rotation of the rod necessary to recover the lumbar lordosis. In such a case it is necessary to extend the instrumentation and fusion down to L4. Prevention is done by a careful study of the preoperative bending film. One should appreciate the rehorizontalization of the first free motion segment under the planned fusion. An almost symmetrical movement should be observed on the left-right side-bend film. Moreover, it is important to observe an almost complete detorsion of the last vertebra included in the fusion on the corrective bend film. This phenomenon is due to the coupling effect of torsion and detorsion resulting from the lateral inclination of this last vertebra. On the corrective lateral bend film the last vertebra must be inside the stable zone defined by Paul Harrington.

## HORIZONTAL PLANE

***Decompensation and Imbalance.*** Decompensation and imbalance may be secondary to the previously described coupling effect. The same procedures that are used for coronal decompensation apply for prevention and correction.

***Progressive Imbalance.*** The second reason for horizontal plane decompensation is progressive imbalance and decompensation due to the *crankshaft phenomenon*. This phenomenon occurs when a posterior fusion has been performed before the end of the growth period with significant remaining growth potential. Ongoing growth of the anterior part of the spine combined with a solid posterior fusion moves the spinal segments away from the gravity line in the horizontal plane.

The treatment of such a disorder needs three staged surgical procedures that may be performed during the same session in some cases. These procedures are multiple posterior osteotomies of the fusion mass, anterior release and fusion, and posterior reinstrumentation. The extension of the posterior fusion depends on the level of correction that may be obtained through the previous osteotomies and, consequently, how many supplementary motion segments should be included to obtain the expected balance.

## SUMMARY

The reasons for imbalance after previous spinal surgery come from ignorance or incomplete consideration of the sagittal gravity line axis, the cone of economy concept, the pelvic vertebra concept, and the junctional zone concept.

There is an obvious relation with a lack of preoperative three-dimensional analysis. Moreover, there is a lack of consideration for the fourth dimension, which is time and growth. Careful segmental as well as global analysis will prevent these problems and guide revision treatment.

When established, postoperative imbalance may be corrected through (1) extension of the instrumentation above and/or below the previous fusion and instrumentation; (2) partial or total removal of the previous instrumentation followed by one or more posterior osteotomies; combined anterior and posterior osteotomies may be necessary in some cases; (3) osteotomies outside of the spine like a pelvic osteotomy for sagittal imbalance in selected cases (bilateral combined supra-acetabular osteotomies); (4) anterior hemiepiphysiodesis to prevent or cure crankshaft phenomenon; and (5) proper consideration for anterior column insufficiency especially in tumor or trauma problems in which anterior fusion and instrumentation may be necessary.

Along with thorough preoperative planning, it is important to control perioperatively the effect of corrective maneuvers on the spinal balance. To appreciate the coronal balance, place 2 pins in symmetrical points of the posterior iliac crest, thereafter we place a perforated semicircular protractor over these pins and we draw a plumb line coming down from the spinous process of C7 or T1. The angle of lateral inclination obtained by this method is comparable in our experience to the postoperative clinical measurement with a standard error of approximately 5°. Perioperative control of the sagittal balance is much more difficult to achieve.

In order to improve our control over these factors, we are currently performing a research project applying optoelectronic methods of pre-, peri-, and postoperative spinal contour analysis. These methods derive from the gait analysis control principles. They may help us to define the ideal balance for the individual patient before surgery and the precise amount of correction may thus be estimated. Applied to corrective intraoperative maneuvers, these methods should provide us more control over what we are really doing to the spinal geometry during surgery. Eventually, these methods may help us to measure more precisely the functional postoperative result and how our patient will experience the changes in his spinal balance after surgery during his daily living activities. These perspectives are only a research axis at the present time, but with the explosion of computer technology, they will certainly invade the operating room one day leading to improved care of patients.

## REFERENCES

1. Duval-Beaupère G, Schmidt C, Cosson P: A barycentremetric study of the sagittal shape of the spine and pelvis: the conditions required for an economic standing position, *Ann Biomed Eng* 20(4):451-462, 1992.
2. Miller JA, Schultz AB, Anderson GB: Load-displacement behaviors of sacroiliac joints, *J Orthop Res* 5:92, 1987.
3. Ployon A et al: In-vivo experimental research into the pre- and post-operative behavior of the scoliotic spine, *Hum Movement Sci* 16:2-3, 1997.

# III

# ANATOMIC AND MECHANICAL ASPECTS OF REVISION

# 7

# REVISION SURGERY: THE ROLE OF FUSION AND INSTRUMENTATION—PRINCIPLES OF STABILIZATION AND CORRECTION

**Joseph Y. Margulies, M.D., Ph.D.**



## REVISION SURGERY

The need for decompression, stabilization, and/or alignment brings the patient back to the surgeon with the *failed back* diagnosis. This is a mechanical diagnosis that expresses the fact that the previously surgically treated spine does not fulfill its mechanical function. Pain per se is only one presentation of this failure, and by itself is only a symptom. Regardless of the specific indication, unless the patient needs decompression, stabilization, and/or alignment, or any combination of these, surgery is not necessary. Unless pain is translated and related to an anatomical origin, surgery is a shot in the dark.

A fusion is necessary when an unstable spinal segment or segments need to be stabilized. This instability can be caused either by the underlying pathology or by the surgeon when decompressing or realigning. The common pathway to achieve stability is to create a fusion. Fusion, however, does not have much to do with the basic etiology and pathophysiology of the underlying disease. Most of the time fusion does not even address the source of the phenomenon. It is a crude mechanical means that practically covers the problem with a *tombstone* of fusion mass.

In addition, the type of stability spine surgeons want to achieve is actually a state of *stable equilibrium,* rather than an *unstable equilibrium,* which is the way we were created. That is, we actually function in an unstable equilibrium. Thus the role of fusion is to be a sarcophagus that holds in it a bunch of devils that we can not control in any other way at the present state of our art, yet it is the best solution we have.

What is the role of instrumentation? The first role of instrumentation is to help achieve fusion. No matter how fancy the instrumentation, it does not mean much without solid bony fusion. Most experts agree that instrumentation can facilitate fusion by splinting the unstable segments until bone healing occurs. The second role of instrumentation is to help in correction, reduction, or any other maneuver that is needed. This concept, that the instrumentation has a role in correction, is the reason for so many systems in the market. Historically, the Harrington instrumentation yields 95% of fusion, much of what came later was done rather to facilitate correction. There are various ways to correct a curve; the implants and the ancillary instrumentation are designed to execute the philosophy of correction.

## REVISION ALGORITHM

The spine can be unstable due to anterior column deficiency, posterior column deficiency, or a combination of both. Stabilization of the spine can be done by anterior approach, posterior approach, and by combined anterior and posterior approach. The logical mechanical way is to approach the lesion from the same direction; using the anterior approach for anterior lesions and using the posterior approach for posterior lesions. The clinical considerations are somewhat more convoluted (Fig. 7-1).

### POSTERIOR APPROACH

If the anterior column is intact, a cantilever implant for posterior fusion is sufficient to provide stability in axial compressive and torsional modes. If the anterior column is deficient, a structural graft or devices such as the Harms cage has to be used for the load-sharing role; this can still be done from the back. The addition of a separate cantilever implant in the front adds to torsional rigidity but necessitates additional anterior approach.

### ANTERIOR APPROACH

When the posterior column is intact and can take part in its tension band and load-sharing effect, recon-

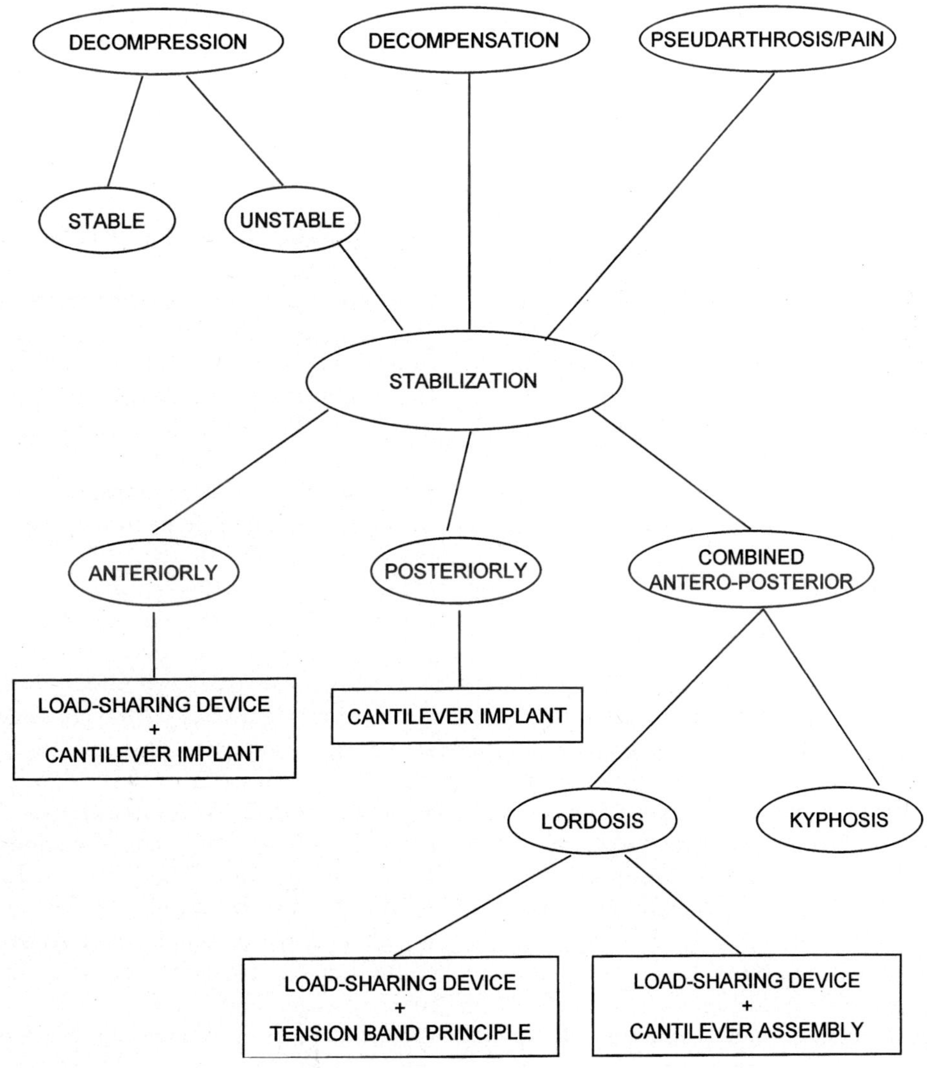


**FIGURE 7-1**

Algorithm for revision procedures.

struction of the anterior column and a cantilever implant instrumented anteriorly is sufficient to provide axial compressive and torsional stability.

### COMBINED ANTERIOR AND POSTERIOR APPROACH

In the lumbar spine, the principle of load sharing of the anterior column and tension band of the posterior spinal column needs to be considered. The anterior column is subjected to compressive forces, whereas the dorsal column is subjected to distractive forces. The posterior spinal muscles play an active role as a tension band to maintain the alignment of the spine. Thus in the lumbar region, in situations of vertebrectomy, the use of spacer is important for the load sharing, and the use of a rod-based system as a tension band is important to maintain the lumbar lordosis. Thin rods are used as tension bands (4-5 mm), compared with the conventional cantilever implants, which are thicker (6 mm and greater).

Load-sharing spacers are also used in anterior column disruptions of the thoracic region of the spine, with or without anterior cantilever implant to control the rotations. Here, the use of a posterior tension band construct may affect adversely by obliterating the kyphosis.

Spinal revision surgery may be required to treat a variety of problems such as pseudarthrosis, coronal or sagittal decompensation, or deterioration of motion segments adjacent to a prior fusion. Extension of the fusion, pseudarthrosis repair, as well as osteotomies may be indicated depending on the underlying problem. The reconstructive spinal surgeon must design internal fixation constructs that create a stable environment for fusion to occur in balanced alignment with adjacent spinal motion segments.

## THE ROLE OF FUSION

The decision to perform spine surgery is valid if the patient's problem can be defined anatomically and can be solved by neural decompression, tumor excision, correction of deformity, stabilization of unstable segments, or a combination of these procedures. The indications to perform surgery in certain lumbar degenerative disorders is made more difficult because of the frequent poor correlation between imaging studies and clinical symptomatology as well as the absence of a universally accepted clinical definition of lumbar spinal instability. In any spine procedure, the last step before closing the incision is to evaluate and treat possible spinal instability, which may be obvious or occult. Although certain procedures are performed to correct instability, other procedures, such as extensive decompressive procedures, may create instability. In any case, the spine must be stabilized prior to closing the incision. Fusion is the most popular means of stabilization. Theoretically, methods other than fusion can be used to treat instability (e.g., muscle strengthening or implanting artificial disks or ligaments). The existence of a surgically performed fusion in a patient, however, is evidence that a surgeon encountered a prior instability. Fusion can be employed to treat a single motion segment or the entire spine, depending on the length of the unstable section and considerations of spinal balance. The instability may be of an acute nature, arising from trauma, or it can be caused by surgical decompression. Instability can be chronic, as caused by a degenerative process, or it can be a postural instability, as evident in deformities. In general, fusion is a comprehensive solution to instability, as it eliminates pathological motion between neighboring elements. The fusion mass consolidates and includes spinal elements between which a "fracture situation" has been created, and bone surfaces are permitted to heal into a single unit. It is important to understand that a fusion cannot correct a deformity and that a fusion cannot provide decompression of the spinal canal. A fusion is only a consolidation of the existing situation at the end of a surgical procedure.

## THE ROLE OF INSTRUMENTATION

There is a consensus that the main role of instrumentation is to facilitate bone healing by splinting the fusion site. However, there is no consensus regarding the practice of correcting deformities using instrumentation. There is also no consensus regarding noninstrumented in situ fusions that address spinal pathology without attempting anatomic realignment or reduction. The role of instrumentation as a splinting device to provide stable fixation until fusion occurs is well established. Instrumentation permits realignment of the spine during surgery and minimizes spinal motion that may decrease the success of fusion. The various aspects of the role of instrumentation are depicted in Figure 7-2. These are stages in a variation on a surgical sequence for apical overcorrection popularized by Mills et al.[1] The rod and screws are used as an instrument during surgery to overcorrect the scoliosis apex and to rotate the spine from kyphotic to lordotic position. Then it is used as a scaffold on which the disk height is restored by a spreader and maintained by titanium mesh cages. On the same scaffold, the vertebral bodies are compressed over the inserted cages, and, finally, it is used a splint to hold the whole construct together as a buttressing device until bone healing occurs. This type of instrumentation also demonstrates the two options of anterior column augmentations: the rods and screws can cre-

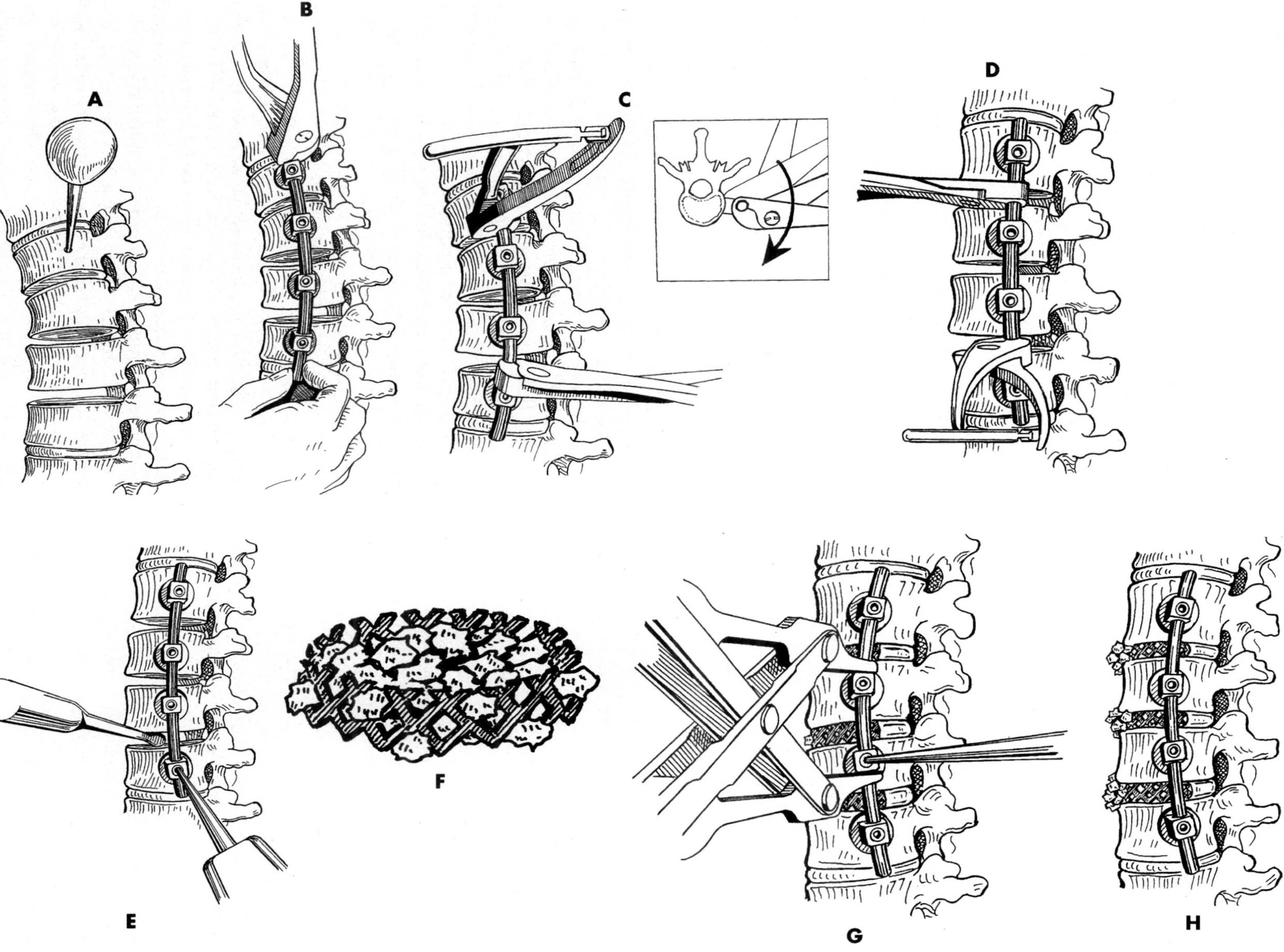


FIGURE 7-2

Surgical sequence demonstrating the dual role of instrumentation: an instrument for correction and a device for stabilization until fusion occurs. **A,** Insertion of screws. **B,** Passing the rod. **C, D,** Rotating the rod and forcing the segment to change its position. **E,** Restoring disk height. **F,** Titanium mesh cages filled with bone graft. **G,** Compressing. **H,** The final situation. (Drawings by Vladimir Golyakhovsky, M.D., Ph.D.)

ate a cantilever-type system for load transferring. In combination with the cages, which are load-sharing devices, the rod and the screws can take part in the load sharing, but are also a buttressing device that keeps the whole construct together.

## SPINAL STABILITY

The stability of the spine can be predicted if the mechanical behavior is known. The determinants of mechanical behavior vary among individuals. Therefore, the prediction of response to abnormal loading is impossible. A universal definition of instability that includes all variables of mechanical behavior does not exist. The stability of the spine is affected by restraining structures that, if damaged or lax, will lead to altered equilibrium and ultimately instability.[2,3] A spinal column that is able to maintain alignment when subjected to physiological loads in any plane while protecting the neural elements is considered stable. If displacement of the spinal column is likely to occur, then the spinal column is considered unstable.[4] Most definitions of stability allude to the effect of dynamic loading as well as the presence of deformation over time.[5] Unfortunately, there is no way to restore any kind of dynamic stability at the level of the motion segment. Common practice is to fuse the affected motion segment, sacrificing its mobility altogether, so as to restore the function of the entire spinal column.

## PRINCIPLES OF STABILIZATION

Surgical stabilization of the spine may be considered to occur in two stages. In the first stage, a *fracture situation* is created during surgery in which adjacent bone surfaces are decorticated, bone graft is applied, and spinal instrumentation or external mobilization is utilized to decrease mobility at the surgical site. The different bones are "cheated" to fuse into one continuous bone. The second stage begins after surgery and consists of the cascade of events involved in the poorly understood biologic process of fusion consolidation. The surgeon's influence over this process includes the use of meticulous operative technique, selection of the location for fusion (anterior or posterior), as well as the selection of appropriate spinal implants that will adequately support the spine until fusion occurs. The act of stabilization starts at an unstable stage that is caused either by the underlying pathology or by the surgeon. The unstable site constitutes a gap in the continuity of a normal functional structure and must be treated in a way that permits growth of a bony bridge across this region. Understanding the mechanics of the spine is crucial in determining exactly where this gap exists. Haher demonstrated that a localized site of mechanical damage to one of the columns of the spine changes the location of the instantaneous axis of rotation.[6] The existence of an axis of rotation in an abnormal location is a sign of instability and may warrant correction. Regardless of how one defines the spinal columns, it is important to augment the unsound columns and thus regain the mechanical stability of the spine. Modern surgical technique and technologically advanced implants permit short fusions localized to the unstable columns.

## PRINCIPLES OF CORRECTION

Although many revolutionary ideas can be found in Harrington's writings,[7-10] the posterior system he introduced was designed to treat deformities in the coronal plane. The scoliotic spine was fixed at the end vertebrae with hooks and distraction was applied through a ratcheted rod, which stretched the spine between these hooks. The rod and hooks served as an internal splint until fusion occurred and the construct was generally supplemented by external immobilization with a cast or brace. In an attempt to improve on problems with hook dislodgment and eliminate the need for postoperative external immobilization, Luquė[11,12] developed the sublaminar wiring technique. This technique provided correction in the coronal and sagittal planes via segmental control with wires. It provided for multiple points of fixation that enhanced deformity correction and decreased the risk of fixation failure. Hybrid methods that combined the techniques of Harrington and Luque evolved and included the Wisconsin construct with or without Drummond buttons as well as the use of square-ended rods and special hooks as introduced by Moe.[13] Although Wisconsin or "Harri-Luque" techniques were safe in most hands, the fear of potential neurological injury by wires and the lack of positive reports in the literature led to a search for alternative methods. Since its introduction in 1984,[14] Cotrel-Dubousset (CD) instrumentation has become the gold standard for posterior spinal fixation. It provides for multiple points of fixation with hooks and avoids the need to place sublaminar wires. CD instrumentation permits correction in the coronal and sagittal planes. It permits kyphosing-distraction and lordotic-compression forces to act along the same rod as a means of simultaneously controlling coronal and sagittal deformities. The premise that the derotation maneuver proposed by Cotrel and Dubousset[14] realigns the deformed coronal spine into normal sagittal posture was not uniformly accepted. Subsequent studies have shown that the transverse plane derotation achieved with this system is more global than segmental in nature. This led to the development of alternative approaches to achieving curve correction. The principle of maximum control over each affected segment is paramount in the operative correction of spinal deformities. The goal is translation of each vertebra into its desired position by connection to a rod, which is prebent to the appropriate sagittal contour. Techniques of segmental fixation have evolved through the use of combinations of hooks, wires, and ultimately pedicle screws. Adequate ancillary instruments may provide efficient lever arms to augment the correction maneuver. The AcroMed Isola[15] and Synthes Universal Spine Systems[16] best represent this approach.

Another way is to place strong, stiff, but ductile rods on the spine and use the technique of in situ bending to bring the spine to the "normal" contour. This technique accentuates placing the rods in such a way that, at the end of the correction maneuver, the center of rotation of the whole assembly, which is now in the rods, is as close as possible to the normal center of rotation. The ductility of the rod is crucial to the success of this kind of correction. Jackson promotes this approach.[17]

Anterior approaches are also utilized for the correction of spinal deformities. In anterior approaches, correction is achieved first through obtaining flexibility as the spine is released via diskectomy or osteotomy and subsequently realigned with implants. Global curve derotation as a correction maneuver is possible with the anterior approach. Local curve derotation may be better achieved with the anterior approach than with the posterior approach. Recently, rigid anterior implant systems have been introduced in order to be used as a tool in surgery for derotation, improve fixation strength, and to decrease instrumentation failure and pseudarthrosis rates. Control over deformities may be achieved by resection of disk or bone in order to change the relative length of the spinal columns. Shortening the anterior column produces kyphosis. Elongating the anterior column produces lordosis. Resection or insertion of a wedge can be utilized to align scoliosis or enhance correction of sagittal plane deformities. Structural grafts or implant spacers can be used to restore anterior column height and reestablish the normal relationship between vertebrae. If performed properly, restoration of disk space height provides indirect opening and decompression of neural foramina. Posterior lumbar interbody fusion (PLIF), anterior lumbar interbody fusion (ALIF), or a posterior maneuver utilizing a pedicular screw-based construct can restore disk height. The success of posterior pedicle screw-based constructs depends upon the presence of adequate anterior column structural support.

In certain spinal disorders, combined anterior and posterior techniques are required in order to achieve sufficient deformity correction, provide for adequate spinal canal decompression and increase the likelihood of successful arthrodesis. Harms[18] advocates the combined approach as the most efficient method to treat a wide variety of spinal problems based on the concepts of the posterior tension band and anterior load-sharing principles. A relatively thin posterior compression implant, combined with a solid anterior spacer, creates a construct in which 80% of the load is applied to the anterior column and 20% of the load is applied to the posterior column. The logical application of this concept is the correction of kyphotic deformities. A variation of the combined approach consists of an interbody fusion, which may be accomplished as either a PLIF or ALIF and stabilized by posterior instrumentation. In this approach, the purpose of the posterior fixation is to stabilize the interbody graft or cage and a formal posterior fusion is not performed. In the most extreme and severe deformities, resection and decancellation procedures as advocated by Luque and Bradford[19] may be required. These procedures create circumferential instability and permit subsequent spinal correction through shortening the spinal column. Such techniques permit correction of deformities, which are not adequately treated by any other approach. Heinig[20] has applied this concept of creating iatrogenic instability solely through the posterior approach in order to correct severe deformities and has termed this the eggshell procedure.

## FUSION TECHNIQUES

### NONINSTRUMENTED FUSION

Noninstrumented fusion techniques may be classified as spinous process-related fusions, interlaminar fusions, posterolateral fusions, or interbody fusions. The indications for noninstrumented fusion at the L5-S1 junction are limited, due to limited success.[21,22] Adherence to the technical aspects of these procedures, specifically meticulous bone graft "carpentry" is crucial to the success of this type of procedure. In the future, the need for internal fixation may be diminished, especially in cases in which anatomic alignment is not the primary concern, if bone morphogenetic protein (BMP) and other agents for bone induction and conduction prove efficacious.

### INSTRUMENTED FUSION

Modern posterior spinal fixation systems consist of three basic elements: (1) implants attached to the posterior spinal elements; (2) implants attached to the sacrum or pelvis; and (3) longitudinal members connecting the posterior implants. There are three basic options for gaining purchase upon the posterior elements of the spine: hooks, wires or cables, and screws. A single hook permits control in one plane, in either a distraction or compression mode. Once the hook is engaged in a construct and combined with other hooks, various corrective forces can be applied to the spine across the entire instrumented segment. The introduction of hook claws has greatly improved upon the fixation achieved by single hooks. Claw fixation combines up-going and down-going hooks across a single or adjacent level to achieve strong mechanical interlock that greatly exceeds the fixation strength achieved by single hooks. Wires may be placed through the spinous process, underneath the lamina or in the sub-pars position. The amount of force that can be applied to a wire is less than can be applied to a hook due to the smaller area of contact of the wire with the bone.[6] The introduction of flexible cables as an alternative to wires offers superior mechanical properties and provides a margin of safety due to their ease of placement. Pedicle screws permit control of the spine in all planes and permit control of all three spinal columns from a single posterior approach.

Distal fixation options when fusion includes the sacrum are more varied. Hooks and wires are of limited value and are not widely used for sacral fixation. Various types of screw fixation techniques using either single or multiple screws to achieve purchase in the sacrum are the most commonly used techniques to achieve distal fixation. Sacral screws may be placed laterally into the sacral ala or medially into the sacral body toward the promontory to reach the upper end plate of the sacrum. When maximal distal fixation is necessary, methods to enhance sacral fixation include Galveston fixation, the Jackson technique, and iliosacral screw fixation. The Galveston method engages the ilium in the construct by utilizing a post, which may consist of either a smooth rod or a screw. The post extends within the ilium and is placed in the column of bone located just above the sciatic notch. The Jackson technique enhances S1 screw fixation utilizing the concept of the iliac buttress.[23] The distal end of the rods pass through medially directed sacral screws and into the sacrum between its two cortices and under the wings of the ilium. Iliosacral screws are placed from the ilium into the body of the sacrum and engage at least three cortices in their path, thereby constituting a strong foundation for a spinopelvic construct. In most instrumentation constructs, the rods on each side of the spine are linked together with transverse devices in order to convert the unilateral rods to a quadrilateral construct of increased overall strength and rigidity. It is crucial to realize that the goal of the procedure is to achieve a successful fusion and that the spinal instrumentation construct will fail if fusion does not occur.

Anterior spinal fixation options are varied. Selection of the appropriate technique depends upon a variety of factors that include the type and location of spinal pathology, the number of levels requiring surgical treatment, the integrity of the anterior and middle spinal columns, and the goals of the surgical procedure. The modern anterior spinal fixation options include interbody spacers, intervertebral spacers, screw-plate fixation systems, and screw-rod fixation systems. ALIF has been reported to have a significant incidence of nonunion when iliac bone graft alone is utilized without supplemental spinal fixation. In an attempt to improve the success rate of interbody fusion and possibly eliminate the need for adjunctive posterior fixation, a variety of interbody spacers have been introduced. These include allograft femoral rings, cylindrical fusion cages such as the BAK device, Moss titanium fusion cages, as well as carbon fiber anterior fusion devices. This is a rapidly emerging field and many of these devices have shown great promise in early studies.[24-30] When an entire vertebral body requires replacement, options include autograft, structural allograft, fusion cages, or polymethylmethacrylate (PMMA). Such constructs are generally used with supplemental spinal fixation anteriorly, posteriorly, or in a combined anterior-posterior fixation construct. Anterior fixation options include both screw-plate and screw-rod devices. Anterior screw-plate devices (e.g., Synthes locking plate, Z-plate, CASP system) permit in situ spinal fixation. Anterior screw-rod devices (e.g., Kostuik-Harrington, anterior TSRH, Kaneda) are more versatile and permit both distraction and compression as well as deformity correction and can be more easily adapted to fixation over multiple levels than screw-plate systems. Placement of bulky fixation devices across the L5-S1 junction is generally discouraged due to the proximity of vascular structures to the implant device.

## IMPLANT MATERIALS

The chief implant materials used in spinal surgery are stainless steel and titanium alloys. They provide strength, can be contoured to match bony surfaces, and are biocompatible. Stainless steels are alloys composed mainly of iron (more than 58%), chromium (17%–20%), and nickel (13%–16%). As a class of alloys, they are favored because of the inexpensive nature of their base elements as well as the wide range of structural and mechanical properties that can be achieved by varying the constituent ratios. Pure titanium is a good material for orthopedic use because of its low density, high ductility, and magnetic resonance imaging/computed tomography compatibility. Its chief drawback, however, is its low modulus of elasticity. As a result, titanium is usually combined with aluminum and vanadium to produce an alloy that has a greater tensile and fatigue strength than stainless steel. Although the modulus of elasticity of this alloy is greater than that of pure titanium, it is still less than the modulus of stainless steel. As a consequence, larger hardware must be used to provide comparable rigidity if titanium is used. The structural properties of titanium alloys are approximately half those of stainless steel alloys.[31] PMMA is sometimes used as an adjunct to internal fixation. PMMA is stiffer than cancellous bone but less stiff than cortical bone. It is used primarily in cases in which bone quality compromises fixation. Several authors have demonstrated the efficacy of PMMA in enhancing screw fixation.

## SPECIAL PROBLEMS

### SPINAL DECOMPENSATION

Normal spinal balance exists when the head is centered over a level pelvis and shoulders in the coronal and sagittal planes. In the sagittal plane, the normal lordosis of the lumbar spine permits the head to be balanced over the pelvis with the hips in full extension.[32] Spinal decompensation is the result of any condition in the coronal and/or sagittal plane that alters this normal alignment. The effects of spinal decompensation on the patient are significant. Complaints associated with decompensation include apparent leg length discrepancy, gait abnormalities, back pain, spinal fatigue, decreased standing tolerance, pelvic obliquity, difficulty with sitting, cosmetic deformity, and degenerative changes in adjacent motion segments. The flat back syndrome is an example of spinal decompensation in the sagittal plane. This problem arises following a lumbar fusion, which results in a loss of lumbar lordosis with subsequent forward inclination of the trunk and an inability to stand erect without hip or knee flexion. It is generally seen in the adult who has undergone surgical fusion extending below L3. In young patients in which the sacrum is not part of the fusion, decompensation may occur at the last level of the mobile spine, with a corresponding acute hyperextension that can cause nerve root impingement. Additional spinal reconstructive surgery to restore lumbar lordosis through osteotomy procedures is frequently required to treat this disabling condition.

### PEDIATRIC DISORDERS

The unique aspects of the pediatric spine that must be taken into consideration are the potential for further growth, the difference in elasticity of ligaments compared to adults, the differences in osseous tissue (thicker, biologically more active periosteum), and the relatively smaller size of the spinal elements. Because pediatric bone has not yet achieved its peak bone mineral density and deforms at lower peak forces, it can absorb more energy to ultimate failure. Vertebral body and sacral growth characteristics may have direct consequences for the disease process, as in spondylolisthesis progression, or may affect treatment, as in the crankshaft phenomenon occurring following posterior fusion.

### OSTEOPOROSIS

Metallic constructs implanted in osteopenic bone cannot be expected to provide solid mechanical support. This situation poses a serious challenge in the treatment of osteoporotic patients. The number of osteopenic (mainly osteoporotic) patients has grown markedly in the United States and Europe and the treatment of mechanical insufficiency in this population remains a great challenge. The weak purchase of screws in osteopenic bone precludes application of forceful corrective maneuvers. It has been demonstrated that hook claws on the laminae may provide for a better grip than screws.[33] In other studies, cement or bone graft were utilized to augment screw purchase in osteopenic vertebrae.[34]

### SACROILIAC JOINT FUSION

The nature and significance of movement in the sacroiliac joint as well as the relationship of the sacroiliac joint to lumbar pain symptomatology remain controversial. Overlapping innervation and referred pain phenomenon make the diagnosis of pain emerging from the sacroiliac joint difficult. The basic role of the sacroiliac joint is to absorb, with minimal movement, the loads of the axial skeleton. All biomechanical loads, whether they are due to sitting, standing, or walking, must pass through the sacroiliac joint. Surgical fusions for sacroiliac dysfunction are rarely performed except for sacroiliac dysfunction following a major traumatic injury. However, recent studies have demonstrated painful incompetence of the sacroiliac joint by radiographically controlled injections and surgical arthrodesis of the sacroiliac joint has been reported to provide satisfactory pain relief in select cases. Another related area of ongoing investigation is the consequence of fusion of the spine to the sacrum in relation to sacroiliac function and sacroiliac pain symptomatology.

## FUTURE DIRECTIONS

Although spinal arthrodesis is widely practiced and is constantly being perfected, it should be appreciated that fusion is a crude solution to the malfunction of sophisticated anatomic mechanisms. While restoration of function of the patient can be accomplished by eliminating motion at the affected level, restoration of normal function of a pathologic motion segment is not possible utilizing present technology. Future approaches may abandon fusion altogether and seek other means of treating painful deformity or instability. Restoration of motion is the objective of reconstructive surgery in other areas of orthopedic surgery. Artificial disks and ligaments may become the state of the art in futuristic orthopedics in the next century.

## REFERENCES

1. Mills MB, Hey LA, Diminick MJ, Hall JE: *Long-term follow-up of patients with short segment anterior instrumentation in the treatment of adolescent idiopathic thoracolumbar scoliosis,* Rosemont, Ill, 1994, Scoliosis Research Society.
2. Gertzbein SD, Seligmen MD, Holtby R et al: Centrode pattern and segmental instability in degenerative disc disease, *Spine* 10:257, 1985.
3. Nachenson A: Lumbar spine instability: a critical update and symptoms summary, *Spine* 10:290, 1985.
4. Purcell GA, Markolf KL, Dawson EG: Twelfth thoracic-first lumbar vertebral mechanical stability of fractures after Harrington rod instrumentation, *J Bone Joint Surg* 63A:71, 1981.
5. Haher TR, Tozzi JM, Lospinuso MF et al: The contribution of the three columns of the spine to spinal stability: biomechanical model, *Paraplegia* 27:432, 1989.
6. Haher TR, Felmly WT, Welin D et al: The IAR as a function of the three columns of the spine, Amsterdam, Netherlands, September 17, 1989, Proc Scoliosis Research Society.
7. Harrington PR: Treatment of scoliosis: Correction and internal fixation by spine instrumentation, *J Bone Joint Surg* 44A:591-561, 1962.
8. Dickson JH, Harrington PR: The evolution of the Harrington instrumentation technique in scoliosis, *J Bone Joint Surg* 55A:993-1002, 1973.
9. Harrington PR, Dickson JH: The development and further prospects of internal fixation of the spine, *Israeli J Med Sci* 9:773-778, 1973.
10. Harrington PR: Instrumentation in structural scoliosis, *Mod Trends Orthop* 5:95-123, 1967.
11. Luque ER: Segmental spinal instrumentation for correction of scoliosis, *Clin Orthop* 163:192-198, 1982a.
12. Luque ER: The anatomic basis and development of segmental spinal instrumentation, *Spine* 7:256-259, 1982b.
13. Moe JH: *Present trends in the successful treatment of scoliosis: The iatrogenic loss of lumbar lordosis.* Xth Congress Latino-Americano de Ortopedie y Traumatologica, Rio de Janeiro, Brazil, July 1997.
14. Cotrel Y, Dubousset J, Guillaumat M: New universal instrumentation in spinal surgery, *Clin Orthop* 227:10, 1988.
15. Asher MA: Isola instrumentation: In Brown CW, editor: *Scoliosis Research Society Instrumentation Manual,* 1993.
16. Aebi M: Correction of degenerative scoliosis of the lumbar spine, *Clin Orthop* 232:80-86, 1988.
17. Jackson RP: *Intrasacral fixation with C-D.* In Brown CW, editor: *Spinal instrumentation technique,* Rosemont, Ill, 1994, Scoliosis Research Society.
18. Bohm H, Harms J, Donk R, Zielke K: Correction and stabilization of angular kyphosis, *Clin Orthop* 258:56, 1990.
19. Luque ER, editor: *Segmental spinal instrumentation,* Thorofare, NJ, 1984, Slack.
20. Heinig C, Kostuik J: Laminoplasty. In Frymoyer J, editor: *Adult spine,* vol 2, New York, 1991, Raven Press, pp 1811-1849.
21. Apel DM, Lorenz MA, Zindrick MR: Symptomatic spondylolisthesis in adults: Four decades later, *Spine* 14:345, 1989.
22. Riley PM, Gillespie R, Koneska J: Severe spondylolisthesis and spondyloptosis: Results of posterolateral fusion in children and adolescents, *J Bone Joint Surg* 68B:856, 1986.
23. Jackson RP, McManus AC: The iliac buttress. a computed tomographic study of sacral anatomy, *Spine* 18:1318, 1993.
24. Ali MS, French TA, Hasting GW, et al: Carbon fibre composite bone plates: Development, evaluation and early clinical experience, *J Bone Joint Surg* [BR] 726:586-591, 1990.
25. Bagby G, Kuslich S: Arthrodesis of the lumbar spine utilizing a rigid housing containing bone graft: The BAK interbody fusion method. In Thalgott J, editor: *Manual of internal fixation,* New York, 1994, Raven Press.
26. Brodke D, Dick J, Zdeblick T, et al: *Biomechanical comparison of posterior lumbar interbody fusion including a new threaded titanium cage.* Presented at the annual meeting of the International Society for the Study of the Lumbar Spine, Marseilles, France, 1993.
27. Brantigan J, Steffee A, Geiger J: A carbon fiber implant to aid interbody lumbar fusion: Mechanical testing, *Spine* 16:5277-5282, 1991.
28. Brantigan J, Steffe A: A carbon fiber implant to aid interbody lumbar fusion, *Spine* 18:2106-2117, 1993.
29. Leong JCY, Chow MS, Yan ACM: Titanium-mesh block replacement of the intervertebral disk, *Clin Orthop* 300:52-63, 1994.
30. Matthis W, Biedermann L: *Biomechanical analysis of the*

*load-sharing principle using TSRH and the MOSS device.* Poster presented at International Meeting on Advanced Spine Techniques. München, Germany, June 1994.

31. *Metals handbook,* ed 8, vol 10, Metals Park, Ohio, 1975, American Society for Metals, pp 10-26.
32. Lenke LG, Bridwell KH, O'Brien MF, Baldus C, Blanke K: Recognition and treatment of the proximal thoracic curve in adolescent idiopathic scoliosis treated with Cotrel-Dubousset instrumentation, *Spine* 19:1589, 1994.
33. Coe JD, Warden KE, Herzig MA, McAfee PC: Influence of bone mineral density on the fixation of thoracolumbar implants: A comparative study of transpedicular screws, laminar hooks, and spinous process wires, *Spine* 15:902, 1990.
34. Zindrick MR, Wiltse LL, Widell EH et al: A biomechanical study of intrapeduncular screw fixation in the lumbosacral spine, *Clin Orthop* 203:99, 1986.

# 8

# IMPLANTS: MODES OF FAILURE

**Thomas R. Haher, M.D.**
**Andrew A. Merola, M.D.**
**Steven A. Caruso, M.Eng.**
**Ross Paskoff, M.D.**



"The object of engineering design is to anticipate failure and to design against it."[10]

Henry Petroski

What is the definition of failure? Does it have the same meaning to metallurgists, clinicians, engineers, and manufacturers? The relevant definition of failure must be explored in different settings. First, in the microscopic setting, the relationship of shifting atomic planes and crystal lattices may affect the mechanical properties of the material. Cracks may then propagate through the structure as a result of this change. In the macroscopic world, failure can be defined using the relationship between load and deflection or stress and strain. Failure may be defined as the ultimate tensile stress with discontinuity of the material or in the ductile portion of the curve with an unacceptable and permanent change in the shape of the material. The goal of this chapter is to explore the many definitions of failure and study the theories of failure as well as the techniques used in the analysis of failure. Specific examples of failure analysis will be conducted in spinal constructs.

The function of spinal implants is twofold: (1) To achieve stability. The implant imparts correctional forces onto the spine by utilizing force anchors. The anchors attach to the bony spine. These anchors are hooks, screws, and wires. (2) Application of forces to the spine. Forces may be applied to the spine via two methods, linear and rotation. Linear force application includes compression, or tensile force application. Rotational forces may be applied through a moment or a torque. By the application of these forces implants can be used to achieve derotation or translation or to apply tensile forces resulting in distraction or compressive forces resulting in compression.

The surgeon may apply any of the above forces to the spine using implants. The spine will react to these force applications by creating an equal and opposite force. This reaction force acts upon the implant; therefore, forces are applied to the spine by the implant and an equal and opposite reaction force is transmitted from spine to the implant. The combination of the instrumentation force combined with the spinal reactive force creates internal stress in the implant.

Other complex forces exist secondary to spinal motion in normal activities of daily living. These forces impart external implant stresses. This combination of internal and external stress is additive. When these stresses become too great for the equilibrium thus established, failure will result. Once again failure may be defined in two ways: (1) When maximum normal stress reaches the ultimate tensile stress the implant will fracture. This is defined as Coulomb's criteria. (2) Increased stress may also result in functional failure if plastic deformation occurs. With plastic deformation, the implant and its anchors will no longer be able to transmit or apply the desired force to the spine. Therefore the implant may be intact in functional failure although permanent plastic deformation (failure) has occurred.

## GEOMETRY OF MICROSTRUCTURE: RELATIONSHIP TO MATERIAL PROPERTIES OF IMPLANTS

The clinician, design engineer, and manufacturer all require knowledge of the material properties of an implant to predict its mechanical behavior. Implant behavior can be viewed on several levels. The atomic level dictates the material properties, whereas the macroscopic geometric arrangement governs the structural properties.

The spinal surgeon may be interested in a material that is able to withstand large loads prior to fracture (strong), that possesses the ability to permanently deform (ductile), and has a high applied load to resulting deformation ratio (stiff). These material characteristics will allow intraoperative shaping of the implant while assuring proper load-sharing or load-transferring properties. The design engineer may require fasteners of specific clearances with appropriate mechanical characteristics to assure the necessary strength. He/she must work within dimensional constraints as dictated by the geometry of the biological substrate, i.e., low profile, implant bulk, fiddle factor, etc. The manufacturer must be responsible for the feasibility of implant production. Is the implant material available at a reasonable cost? Is it able to be placed and worked in a lathe or mold? Is it able to be extruded or cold worked? What is the overall fabricability of the alloy? All of the above concerns reflect the atomic structure of the element or alloy.

### MAKING AN IMPLANT

The first step in making an implant is to choose the element or alloy that possesses the characteristics desired. This could be iron or an alloy of iron called steel. Materials have a distinct atomic array or a specific spatial relationship of the atoms. The relationship of these atoms to each other is called a unit cell (Fig. 8-1). The position and the regularity of the atoms/molecules influence the mechanical properties of the implant. The arrangements of the atoms within the unit cell are a matter of choice of the design engineer. The different arrays of the atoms will have a direct effect on the desired structural and mechanical properties. The next

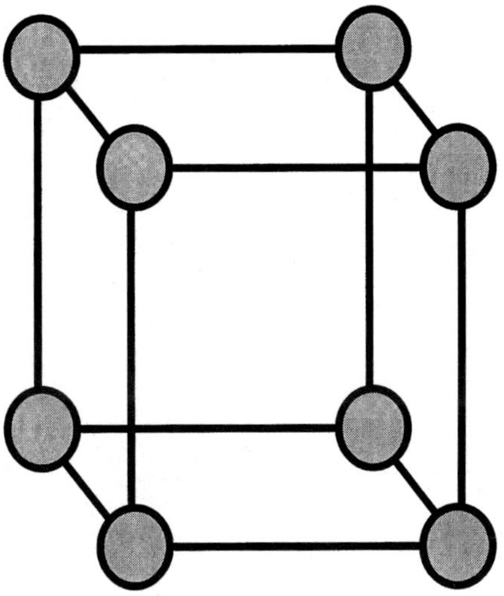

FIGURE 8-1

A unit cell is the basic arrangement of the atoms in a crystal.

step is to grow these atomic arrays or unit cells of atoms or molecules. This step takes place when molten or liquid metal is cooled. When a transformation temperature is reached, the liquid becomes a solid. This occurs as a result of the coalescence, or joining, of the unit cells to each other. These initial solid structures are called dendrites. An example of a dendrite would be a snow crystal forming on a hard surface such as a window. The site of the growing solid is called a nucleation site. There are usually many nucleation sites in the process of forming a solid. The existence of these multiple sites allows the existence of many regions of solidification or crystallization. As these regions, called *grains,* continue to grow, they will eventually meet one another. The areas where the crystals meet are called the grain boundary (Fig. 8-2).[3] A grain boundary is defined as a surface imperfection that separates crystals of different orientations.[6]

As a result of the independent growth of crystals or grains, the spatial relationships are unique with respect to adjacent grains. The result is a difference in the reflection of light for each grain. This allows a visual identification of grains within a solid. The size of the grain may vary with the rate of cooling, as well as other factors. The size of the grain is important because it is directly related to the propagation of a crack and subsequent failure of the structure. In order for an implant to fail, the crack must propagate from one side of the implant to the other past a critical dimension. The grain boundary is the path of least resistance for the crack. What is a grain boundary again? A grain boundary is that area between or among grains, or the mutual interference planes between the grains. It is the result of growing crystals hitting or bumping into one another. The grain boundaries may also be a repository for materials that do not fit into the unit cell.[9] As the crystal

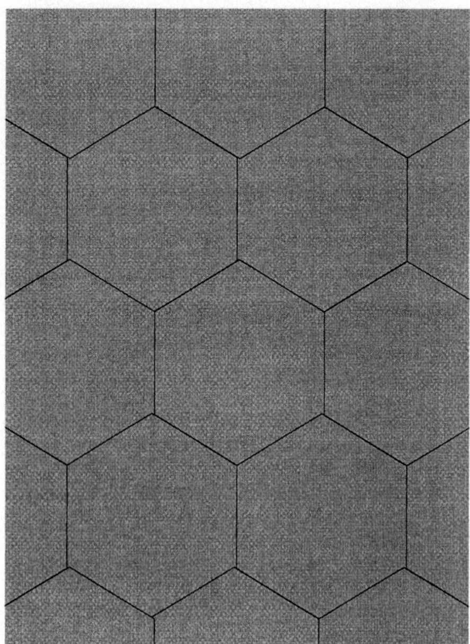

**FIGURE 8-2**

Grain boundaries. A crystal grows from different nucleation sites forming a grain. When different grains enlarge and abut one another a boundary is formed. This boundary is visible as a result of the different orientations of the crystals within each grain.

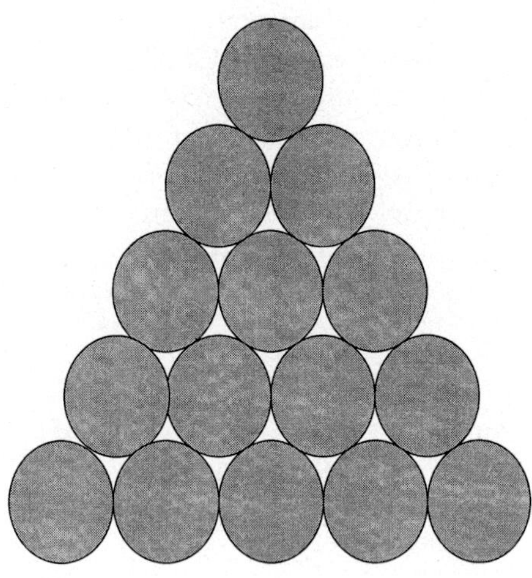

**FIGURE 8-3**

Atoms of a crystal arranged in stacking order with symmetry throughout. This arrangement requires the lowest energy state.

grows, particles that do not comprise the atomic array are pushed aside while the crystal is being formed and growing. The foreign material is deposited in the grain boundaries. As a result, grain boundaries can be seen as distinct lines on a cut surface of a metal. The crystal lattice or architecture found in a grain does not exist in the grain boundary and therefore the forces holding the grains together are far less than the energy holding the atoms together in the crystal. The energy needed to propagate a crack through the crystal would be far greater than the energy needed to grow a crack through the grain boundary. Therefore, the grain boundary is the path of least resistance for crack propagation. How does the size of the grain affect strength? Because the grain boundary is the "path of least resistance," as the number of grain boundaries increases so too does the energy needed for the crack to move through the increased number of boundaries. Consider a material composed of two grains with one boundary between the grains. A crack would not have a difficult time moving through this single grain boundary to reach the other side of the implant, causing failure. Now consider a material composed of millions of grains with millions and millions of grain boundaries. If a crack were to propagate through this material it would follow a convoluted path composed of a maze of boundaries. Crack propagation would be significantly more difficult, resulting in a stronger material.

## PURITY OF THE MATERIAL

As the metal cools from the liquid to the solid state, the unit cells attach to one another, forming the solid. This process follows a strict geometrical format, fitting together the various atoms or molecules as if they were parts of a puzzle. If impurities are present during this process, they cannot fit into the growing crystal. The impurities are pushed aside and are deposited in the grain boundaries. This process increases the weakness of the already-compromised grain boundary. The presence of impurities in the material therefore may render the material weaker.

## DISLOCATION THEORY

Irregularities in the crystal may make the material stronger. When the material transforms from a liquid to a solid there is an orderly pattern, or arrangement, of the atoms or molecules. The pattern resembles cannon balls in a stockpile or kernels of corn on the cob (Fig. 8-3). Under specific conditions, the rows or layers of atoms are able to slide over one another. This sliding of crystalline planes within a solid is called a dislocation (Fig. 8-4). A dislocation is a local discontinuity in the lattice or crystal accompanied by slightly different spacing in adjacent sections.[3] The presence of dislocations changes the mechanical properties of the material by making the material more brittle. Dislocations cause deformation of the crystal. Stresses are generated by this deformation and the resulting interaction between dislocations is called *work-hardening.*[6] An example of this phenomenon may be seen with the repeated bending of a paper clip. As the paper clip is subjected to repeated bending beyond its elastic limit, dislocations are produced within the crystal

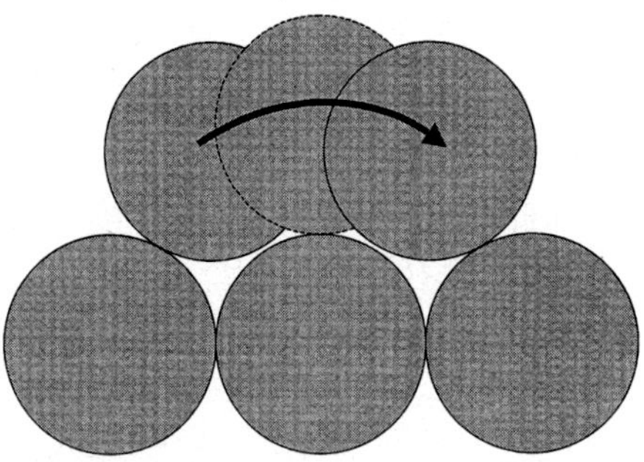

FIGURE 8-4

Dislocation theory. Atoms within a crystal are able to slide over one another. Additional energy is required and results in a change in the mechanical behavior of the material. The material becomes brittle.

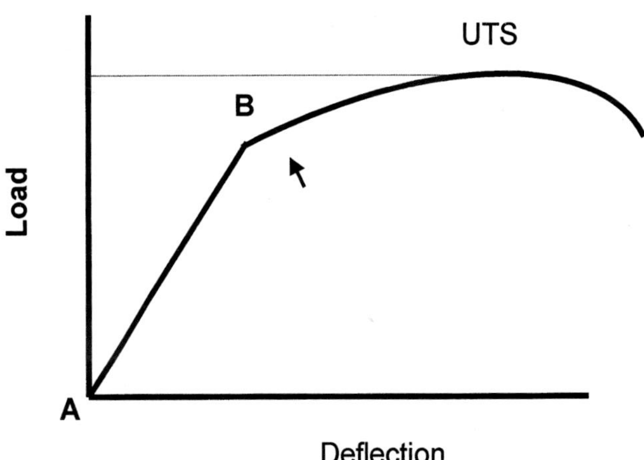


FIGURE 8-5

Load-versus-deflection curve. The relationship of an applied load to a resulting deformation of the specimen. The linear region is defined as the elastic region in which removal of the applied load will result in a proportionate decrease in deformation with no resulting permanent deformation. The plastic region is defined as a state of permanent deformation when the load is removed. The load-deflection will vary with the dimensions of the specimen.

structure. The material becomes brittle and finally reaches its ultimate strength, resulting in failure. Assume that a number of paper clips are given to a number of people. The people are asked to bend the paper clips until they break or failure results. The number of bends needed to cause failure is tallied. It becomes apparent that the number of bends needed to cause failure is not the same. Why? The paper clips may not be equally strong and not every person bends the clip in the same manner. This is the first lesson in failure. Failure by fatigue is not a precisely predictable event.[10]

## LOAD-DEFLECTION AND STRESS-STRAIN CURVES

Engineers perform mechanical and structural tests on implants and constructs in order to ascertain knowledge about the in vivo performances of the structures. Application of a monotonic force to a structure, such as an implant, results in a corresponding displacement. Graphical representation of this relationship reveals several distinct points and regions. These points and regions define the mechanical behavior and failure of the implant.[7] Figure 8-5 shows a load versus deflection curve for a material loaded in uniaxial, monotonic, concentric tension. Region *AB* of Figure 8-5 is the elastic region, in which a linear relation between applied load and corresponding linear displacement exists. The constant of proportionality between the load and displacement in this region (i.e., the slope of the linear portion of the graph) is known as the axial stiffness, a structural property of the implant. Engineers and surgeons are interested in this property because it defines the amount of elastic deformation an implant can expect when subjected to a given load. It is the stiffness of a system that either allows load sharing or promotes stress shielding. Stiffer implants conduct more load and allow less to transfer through the remaining anatomic structures or bone graft-type reconstructive elements. The ideal implant seems to be one that is stiff enough to prevent excessive motion while allowing enough motion to promote bony fusion.[2]

The relationship between the load applied to a material and the resulting deformation can be normalized based on geometry to achieve a stress-versus-strain curve. Normalization means that the curve will reflect the material properties of the implant regardless of the dimensions, geometry, or other extrinsic qualities. An example of a stress-versus-strain curve is shown in Figure 8-6. The slope of the linear, elastic region of the curve is called the modulus of elasticity, or Young's Modulus. Young's Modulus is the capacity of the material to resist deformation in the elastic region of the stress-strain curve.[1] Young's Modulus is similar to stiffness, as found in the elastic region of a load-versus-deformation curve, however, the load-versus-deflection curve does not take into account variations in cross-sectional area or the change in length with respect to the original length. Young's Modulus, therefore, is a material property, whereas stiffness is a structural property. The use of the stress-strain curve is the standard technique for evaluating material properties.[1]

The first deviation from stress/strain linearity is the proportional limit, or elastic limit. This is the first point on the curve at which removal of the applied load will not result in full recovery of deformation. Progression past *point B* signifies that the material has entered the plastic region. Unloading of the material within this region will result in the production of marked permanent axial deformation. The yield point (*point C*) is verbally defined somewhat ambiguously as "the point on the curve at which a marked increase in deformation occurs without a significant increase in load."[13] Depending on the material, this may or may not occur soon after the elastic limit is reached. Engineers therefore often use a specific test result to define yield stress; it is that stress that results in a permanent strain of 0.2% (Fig. 8-6). *Point B* separates the linear, elastic region from the nonlinear, plastic region. Engineers and surgeons are concerned with this property, as they desire an implant that has a yield stress larger than that which is expected to be produced in vivo, thereby avoiding unwanted permanent deformations. In addition, they often desire the ability to contour the implant to a patient's lordosis or kyphosis, so the implant must have the ability to permanently deform with the use of special instruments.

As shown in Figure 8-5 (load-versus-deformation curve) and Figure 8-6 (stress-versus-strain curve), a material that possesses the ability to permanently deform is called a ductile material. The opposite, a brittle material, fails with little or no deformation in the plastic range. 316-stainless steel implants are relatively ductile, while those constructed of titanium are more brittle. This characteristic is important in spine surgery, because in situ bending is often required. It is important for the surgeon to understand that permanent deformation of any kind has several effects on the structural properties of the implant. The yield stress and resilience are increased, while the toughness is decreased. For orthopedic surgeons and implant design engineers, energy absorption is much more important than stress or strain, therefore the effects on resilience and toughness are of special importance. Graphically, energy absorption at any point on the stress-versus-strain or load-versus-deflection curve is equal to the area beneath that portion of the curve. Figure 8-7 illustrates a linearly elastic, perfectly plastic material. Resilience, which is the area under the elastic region of the curve, illustrates the threshold energy required to cause permanent deformation. Toughness is the energy to failure, and is graphically depicted by the area under the entire curve. Prebending of a stainless steel (or other ductile material) plate or rod increases the resilience by increasing the yield stress, but decreases the toughness. Titanium implants should not be contoured, because titanium is a brittle material and any prebending achieved will make the implant even more brittle.

Continued application of increasing load beyond the yield stress (Fig. 8-6) will result in progression along the plastic region until the ultimate tensile strength (UTS) is achieved. This is the largest force the implant will permit. After reaching the UTS, the structure will undergo increased deformation with decreasing force until failure occurs. For orthopedic implants, the UTS is not as important as the fatigue strength, because implants rarely fail as a result of monotonic force application. Implants fail due to repetitive loads, which are often significantly lower than the yield stress. Engineers can determine the endurance limit by subjecting several identical implant samples to cyclic loading with constant frequency (usually 5 cycles per second) but varying amplitudes. As the loading amplitude decreases, the fatigue life increases logarithmically. At a certain load, the number of cycles to failure will reach a limit, whereas the structure can theoretically survive an infinite number of cycles at the given frequency. For orthopedic implant design, "infinity" is defined as $1 \times 10^8$ cycles.[13] This represents the amount of time that the implant is designed to survive before bony fusion inherits the role of primary stabilizing structure.

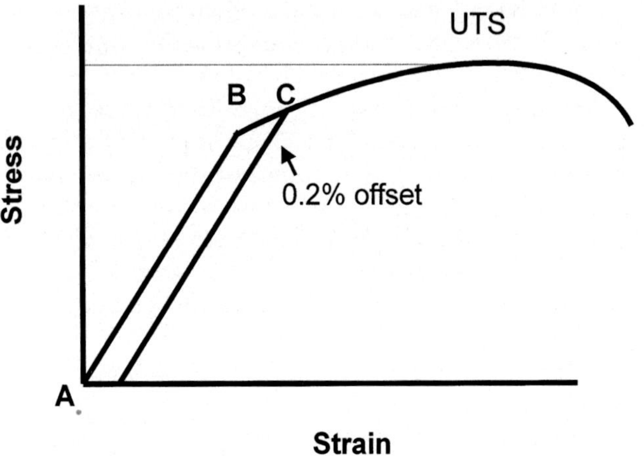


**FIGURE 8-6**

The relationship of stress to strain is not a function of the dimensions of the specimen. The stress and strain are normalized to account for the specimens of different dimensions.

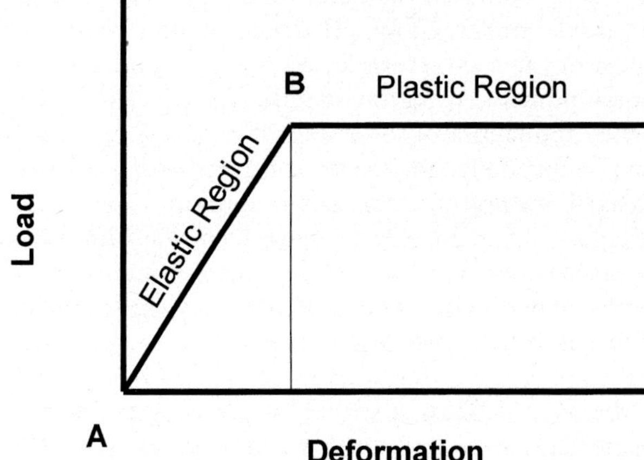


**FIGURE 8-7**

Stress-versus-strain diagram for a linearly elastic, perfectly plastic material. The area under the elastic region is the resilience, whereas the area under the entire curve (to failure) is the toughness.

As stated above, repetitive loading and unloading of a material may result in failure. The loads required for this type of failure are less than the UTS or even the yield strength. How can this be possible? We have defined failure by the stress-strain curve with failure occurring when the stress exceeds the UTS. However, in fatigue failure the stress needed is considerably less. Why?[14] Is it crack propagation or a brittle fracture? When the yield point of a material is exceeded, permanent or plastic deformation results. This is also known as work hardening. Work hardening alters the properties of the material by increasing the yield strength at the expense of lower ductility and toughness. Refer to the stress-strain diagram (Fig. 8-6). Loading beyond the yield strength produces a plastic or permanent deformation. This in turn reduces ductility since the ability of the material to deform has been reduced. The stiffness or the modulus of the material does not change significantly because the linear portion of the stress-strain remains constant. The yield stress, however, for the next cycle of loading has increased. The work to failure on reloading has decreased. Thus, work hardening has reduced toughness because the area under the stress-strain curve has been reduced. All of the above may take place with loads lower than the UTS.

## DESIGN CRITERIA

When designing an implant based on known stress-strain analysis, the following should be considered:

1. How accurate are the predicted operating loads?
2. How refined is the mathematical and in vitro analysis of load applications to the implant and bone?
3. Has sufficient testing been performed according to American Society for Testing and Materials (ASTM) formats?
4. How closely will test data represent the general behavior of the implant?
5. Will sufficient quality control be present during manufacturing?
6. What will be the effect of time (fatigue and corrosion) on implant life?
7. What will be the consequence of implant failure on the spine?

When uncertainties exist as to the above questions (as they inevitably do), a Factor of Safety (FS) is introduced into the implant design. This assures implant longevity and function by defining a design stress that is greater than the predicted failure stress.

$$\text{Design Stress} = \text{Failure Stress} \times \text{FS} \qquad \text{Eq. 1}$$

The factor of safety is always greater than one.

Failure may have many definitions based on the previously discussed terms. If failure reflects a permanent deformation of a part manufactured under crucial specifications then the plastic deformation as reflected by the plastic region of the curve will show the point of failure. This is referred to as yielding and may occur in a fastener or connector. Over-tightening of the inner screw that locks a rod to a hook or screw may result in plastic deformation in the U-shaped rod holder portion of the hook or screw. This would result in failure of the system without breaking the rod or hook. Failure may be defined as a discontinuity of the material as it would be in the case of the plate or screw breakage. The region of interest in the stress-strain curve would be the UTS. This would reflect the breaking of the rod, plate, screw, etc. Thus, failure may be defined from yielding to fracture.

## ANALYSIS OF A FRACTURE

In the investigation of a fractured implant the following questions should be asked:[14]

1) *Inspection of the surface of the fracture.* How many fracture sites are there? What is the relation of the fracture site to the expected or known regions of loading? Is the origin of the fracture site visible? Is there evidence of corrosion?
2) *Surface of the part.* What is the contact pattern of the implant? Has loading during its life deformed the surface or has it been deformed after fracture? Is there evidence of the surface from manufacturing or assembly?
3) *Geometry and design.* Are there regions of stress concentrations present such as a hole in a plate or in the region of a thread of a screw? Was the implant designed to be rigid, load sharing, or load bearing? Was it intended to be loaded in tension, torsion, or compression? Was the design sound or was the implant used as it was intended to be used? How does the assembly work? Was the implant dimensionally correct?
4) *Manufacturing and processing.* Did stress concentrations within the implant cause the failure? If wrought metal was used, were the seams, inclusion bodies, or forging problems inspected? If the implant was a casting, were shrinkage cavities present?
5) *Properties of the implant.* Are the material properties of the implant within specifications? Are the metals similar? Are multiple parts present?
6) *Adjacent parts.* The fractured part may not be the part responsible for failure. It may be damaged due to the abnormal load of another adjacent part. Were all fasteners tight? A loose inner screw or nut may transmit loads to another part in the construct.
7) *Assembly.* Is there evidence of misalignment in the construct? Are the parts machined well, avoiding

increased stress? Did the construct deflect excessively under stress? An example would be a 3.2-mm ventral derotation spondylodesis (VDS) rod in an anterior or posterior construct.

8) *Environmental reactions.* Is the implant inert with respect to in vivo conditions? A critical corrosive environment may cause cracking under load known as stress corrosion cracking.

The reason for failure of an implant should be explored. By understanding the mechanism of failure the clinician may be able to understand if the implant was used as it was designed or if there were intrinsic flaws in the implant resulting in breakage.[13]

## ANALYSIS OF FAILURE IN SPINAL IMPLANTS

### EFFECTS OF MACROSCALE GEOMETRY ON DESIGN, STRENGTH, AND FAILURE

Spinal implants do not fail as a result of pure axial forces (neither compression nor tension). Implants fail as a result of bending loads, which are produced by forces acting eccentrically to the implant's neutral axis. The moment produced, which is impure because it causes the generation of a reaction force, is defined by the resultant load that the implant experiences multiplied by the moment arm. The moment arm is defined as the perpendicular distance from the line of action of the force to the distance to the "pivot point", regardless of the state of motion.[13] In the case of internal stress analysis, the pivot point is that point on the structure where the internal moment is to be calculated.

Failure due to bending is especially true in the case of pedicle screw constructs. The pedicle screw is a three-column fixation system; it is inserted in the posterior column and transverses the middle column, extending into the anterior column. Although a majority of the compressive load experienced by the spine is located in the anterior column,[4] the screws are connected via rods or plates at the posterior column. A considerable moment arm is produced and, thus, the cantilevered screw experiences a bending moment. This moment is greatest at the screw/rod or screw/plate connection, as this is the point where the moment arm is greatest (Fig. 8-8).

The normal stress distribution that the screw experiences is related to the applied moment and to the area moment of inertia ($I$), which is a function of the cross-sectional geometry of the member. $I$ is the ability of a member to resist bending and is thus a static property. It depends not only on the cross-sectional area of the member but on the distribution of that area about the neutral axis. Like an I-beam, distribution of a member's cross-sectional area away from the neutral axis increases flexural stiffness and strength. The neutral axis (NA) is the plane of zero normal stress. For a cantilever screw experiencing a downward force due to body weight, those fibers above the NA are in tension whereas those below it are in compression. The equation relating normal stress at any point in a member to moment and moment of inertia is:

$$\text{Stress} = My/I \qquad \text{Eq. 2}$$

The maximum normal stress occurs at the fibers farthest from the neutral axis, at a distance denoted c (Fig. 8-9). For a symmetrical cross-section, such as a rod or plate, $c = h/2$. The geometric properties of the section may be summed up using the Section Modulus (S), which is equal to $I/c$ (Fig. 8-10). Plugging the section modulus into Equation 2 yields an equation

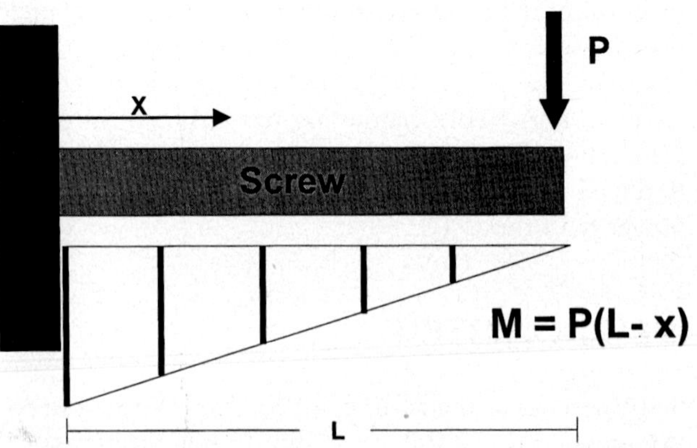


**FIGURE 8-8**

Cantilever beam (screw) loaded at the distal end, with the resulting moment diagram pictured below. Note that the maximum bending moment occurs at the screw-rod junction.

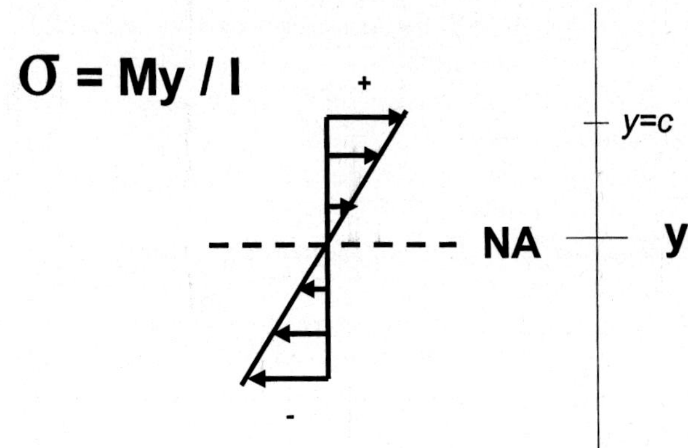


**FIGURE 8-9**

Cantilever beam (screw-rod construct) with constant cross-sectional geometry. The resulting normal stress diagram is shown below, illustrating the relation between internal bending moment and normal stress distribution.

for the maximum normal stress of a structure, illustrating the role of cross-sectional geometry as a constant of proportionality between applied moment (M) and incurred maximum normal stress (sigma). Thus, the design engineer, knowing the approximate loading scenario that an implant is to expect, can design the cross-sectional geometry such that the loads experienced are within acceptable limits. These limits are governed by the ultimate tensile strength of the material and the factor of safety. Therefore, given that the largest moment experienced by a cantilever screw is at the connection to the plate or rod, some manufacturers taper their screws such that the cross-sectional geometry varies according to internal moment, thus controlling the normal stress distribution. Figure 8-11 shows the resulting normal stress distributions at three points on a cantilever beam of constant cross-sectional geometry. Note that the normal stress distribution increases as the moment area increases. Figure 8-12 illustrates how a tapered screw controls normal stress distribution by increasing the beam's Section Modulus (S).

The stiffness of a rectangular cross-sectioned implant, such as a plate, is proportional to the cube of the height, while the strength is proportional to the square of the height (Fig. 8-13). For a circular cross-sectional member, such as a rod or roughly a screw, the stiffness and strength are proportional to the radius to the fourth power and third power respectively (Figs. 8-14, 8-15, 8-16, and 8-17).[12] In structural engineering, beams and columns are designed according to the loading they are expected to experience. Similarly, in the design of orthopedic implants, it is advantageous to design an implant such that the area moment of inertia varies according to the loading. As Equation 1 demonstrates, such that the maximum normal stress ($\sigma_u$) does not exceed the ultimate strength of the material.

The stress distributions and calculations for implant strengths discussed above assume homogeneous, im-

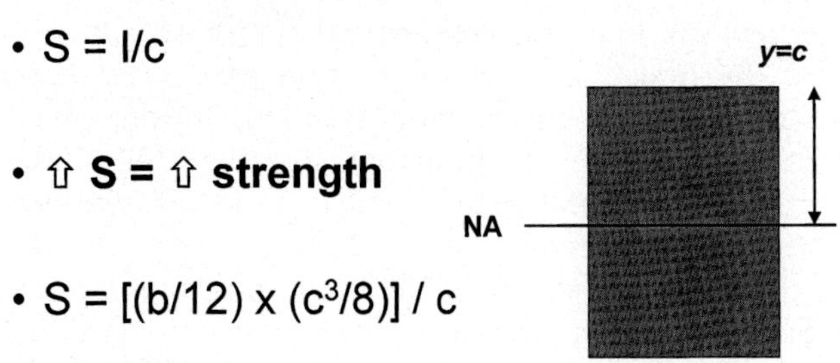


FIGURE 8-10

The Section Modulus (S) is equal to the area moment of inertia divided by the distance from the neutral axis to the farthest fiber (*c*). Given a known loading situation, engineers use the section modulus to design a structure within allowable stress limits.

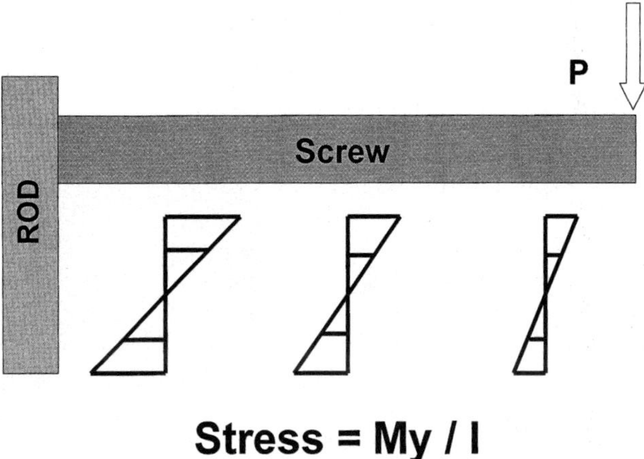


FIGURE 8-11

A screw-rod construct behaves much like a cantilever beam. For a resultant load at the distal aspect of the screw, the bending moment varies as does the moment arm. Therefore, the greatest bending moment occurs at the screw-rod junction. The stress diagrams below the screw illustrate the increase in tensile as well as compressive normal stresses proximal to the force application.

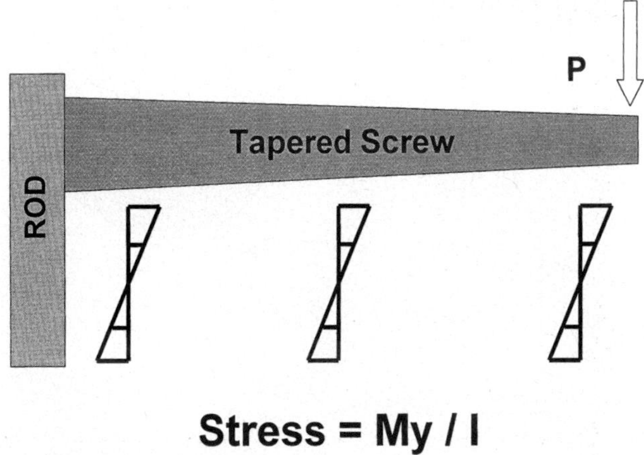


FIGURE 8-12

Tapered cantilever beam. Resulting normal stress diagram illustrates the ability to control normal stress distributions by appropriately designing the cross-sectional geometry (i.e., the Section Modulus).

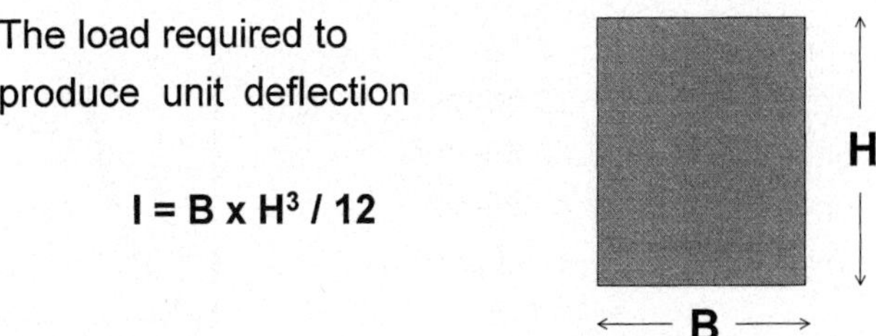


FIGURE 8-13

For a rectangular cross-section, the bending rigidity is linearly proportional to the length of the base and proportional to the cube of the height.

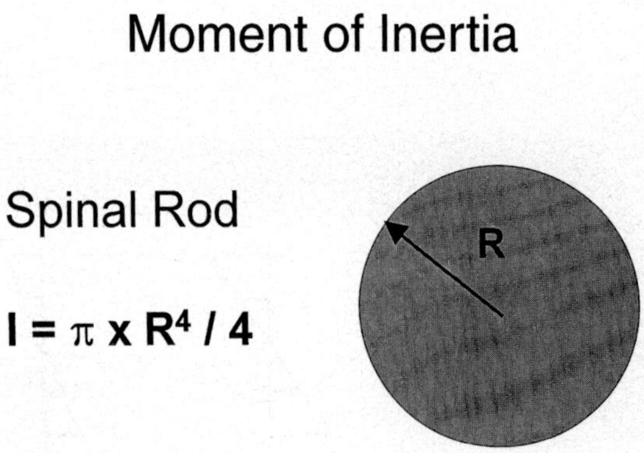

Moment of Inertia

Spinal Rod

$I = \pi \times R^4 / 4$

R

FIGURE 8-14

The bending rigidity of a rod (circular cross-section) is proportional to the radius-to-the-fourth power.

Strength of a Rod

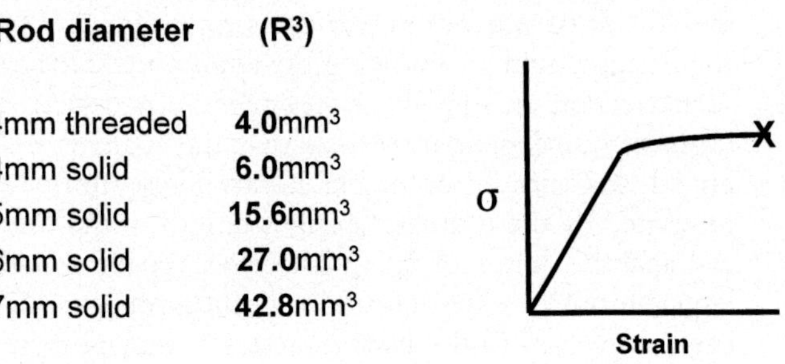

| Rod diameter | ($R^3$) |
|---|---|
| 4mm threaded | 4.0mm³ |
| 4mm solid | 6.0mm³ |
| 5mm solid | 15.6mm³ |
| 6mm solid | 27.0mm³ |
| 7mm solid | 42.8mm³ |



FIGURE 8-17

The bending strength is proportional to the area moment of inertia divided by the radius.

Moment of Inertia

4mm threaded rod

$I = 5.14mm^4$

4mm solid rod

$I = 12.6mm^4$

5mm solid rod

$I = 30.6mm^4$

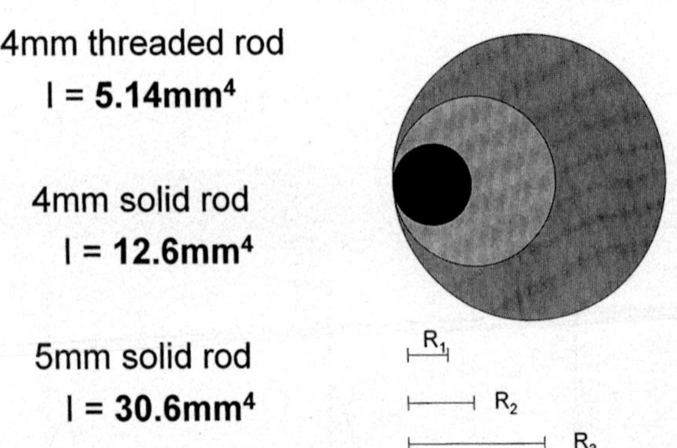



FIGURE 8-15

A graphical as well as mathematical illustration of the area moments of inertia of three spinal rods. The bending rigidity is proportional to the area moment of inertia.

Resistance to Bending

| Rod diameter | I |
|---|---|
| 4mm threaded | 5.14mm⁴ |
| 4mm solid | 12.56mm⁴ |
| 5mm solid | 30.60mm⁴ |
| 6mm solid | 63.50mm⁴ |
| 7mm solid | 118.0mm⁴ |

I

$y=x^4$

R

Stiffness $\alpha$ I

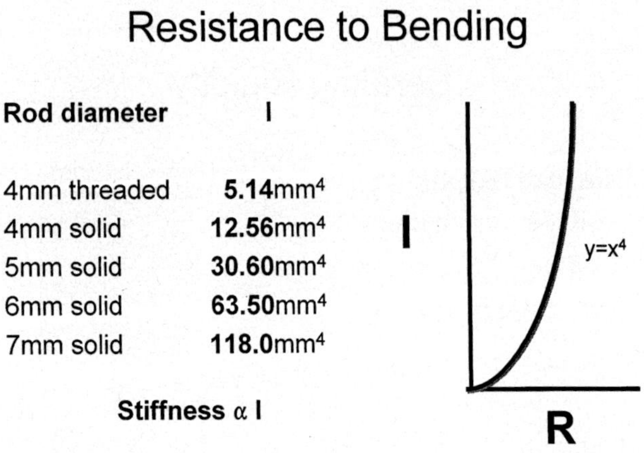

FIGURE 8-16

A graphical as well as mathematical illustration of the area moments of inertia of five spinal rods. The bending rigidity is proportional to the area moment of inertia.

perfection-free conditions. A structure will begin to exhibit permanent deformation and eventually fail at the first point where its yield stress and ultimate tensile stress are exceeded, respectively. Under normal bending loading conditions, this occurs at the structural plane farthest from the neutral axis (C). Often stress concentrations exist due to discontinuities, such as imperfections, abnormalities, holes, sharp angles, notches, grooves, or other changes in geometry. Manufacturing or design errors can cause these stress concentrations, called stress risers, as can surface scratches or abrasions incurred during surgical implantation of hardware. The structural result of a stress riser is a nonlinear and often nonexpected stress distribution (up to four times the local stress field that would otherwise exist), which can lead to failure at loading well below the design load.

Orthopedic implant companies attribute part of the cost of their products to intense quality control programs that aim to ensure homogeneous, defect-free implants. Once in the surgeon's hands, it is his/her responsibility to employ care so as not to create any intraoperative stress risers. Screws, by the general nature of their design, have discontinuities in their structures where the inner diameter meets the thread. One job of the design engineer is to minimize stress risers without compromising purchase strength. Some manufacturers have incorporated filet-type transitions from inner diameter to thread in order to minimize stress concentrations

Spinal implants rarely fail as a result of monotonic force application; they occur from repetitive loading, which is often within the elastic region. This is the main reason that monotonic screw pull-out data is criticized at research conferences and in publications. Since fatigue failure will inevitably occur in spinal implants if given enough time, the goal of instrumentation is to stabilize the spine until bony fusion can mature and relieve the implant of its load-carrying responsibilities. Orthopedic spine surgery is thus a race between fusion and failure.

The American Society for Metals defines fatigue as the phenomenon leading to fracture under repeated or fluctuation stresses having a maximum value less than the tensile strength of the material. Fatigue fractures are progressive, beginning as minute cracks that grow under the action of a fluctuation stress.[8]

## CLINICAL EXAMPLES OF IMPLANT FAILURE WITH ANALYSIS

"... it is easier to draw lessons from examples of poor performance than from good performance."

ANTON TEDESKO[11]

## CASE STUDIES

### CASE 1

A 12-year-old boy presented with low back pain, S1 radicular pain to the lower extremities with hamstring tightness. Serial radiographs (Figs. 8-18 and 8-19) revealed progressive slipping (spondylolisthesis) of L4 on L5. The patient underwent a posterior spinal fusion with instrumentation of L4-L5 without anterior fusion (Figs. 8-20 and 8-21). The patient had a benign postoperative course. His symptoms were relieved. On subsequent routine follow-up, he was asymptomatic, however, radiographs showed failure of all four pedicle screws.

#### Analysis

Pedicle screws experience cantilever-bending forces, as the loads applied to the distal end result in bending moments throughout the implant. The internal bending moment that the screw experiences is a result of the force magnitude multiplied by the distance to the point of interest. The greatest internal bending moment, therefore, is located at the screw-plate interface, as this location is farthest from the resultant force application point. Normal stress is equal to the internal moment ($M$) multiplied by the distance from the neu-

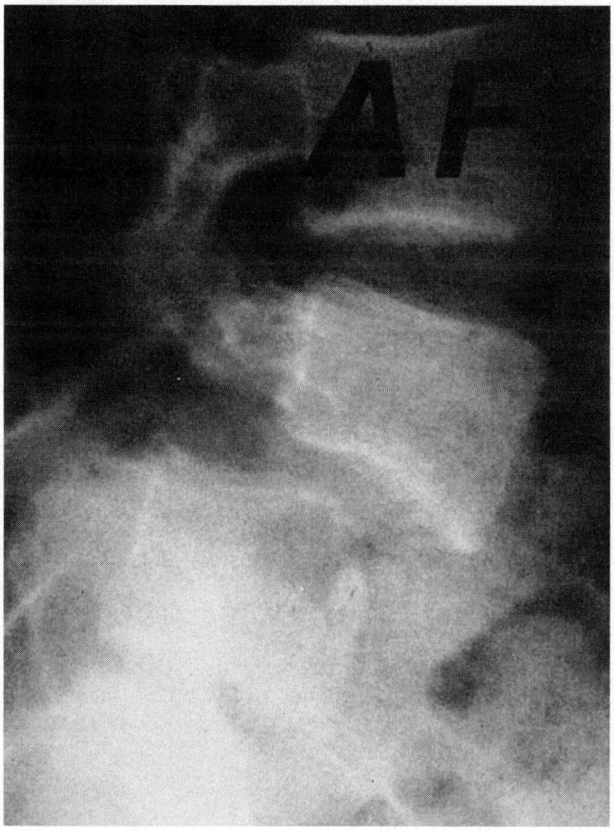

**FIGURE 8-18**

Lateral plane radiograph of 12-year-old boy presenting with a grade 3 spondylolisthesis at L4-L5.

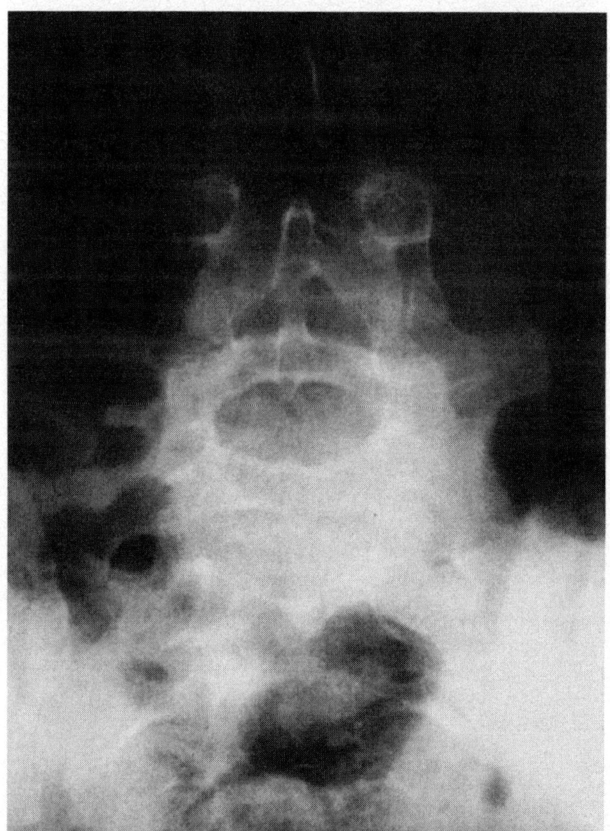

**FIGURE 8-19**

P-A plane radiograph of 12-year-old boy presenting with a grade 3 spondylolisthesis at L4-L5.

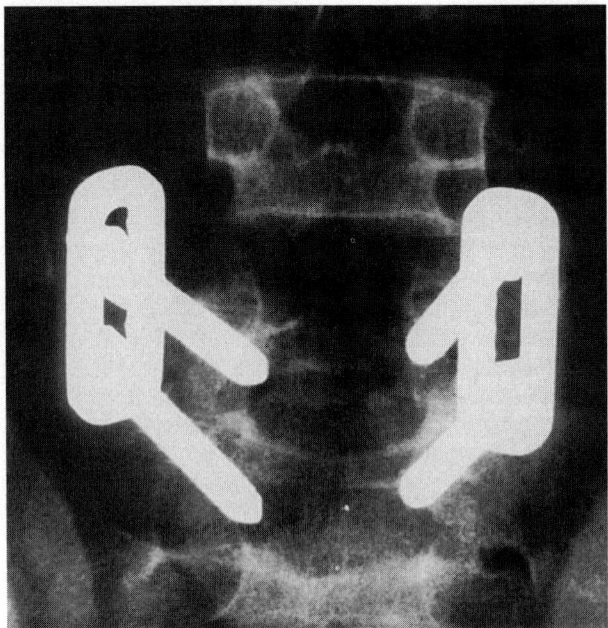

**FIGURE 8-20**

Posteroanterior postoperative plane radiograph of 12-year-old boy with a grade 3 spondylolisthesis at L4-L5 reduced with posterior screws and plates only.

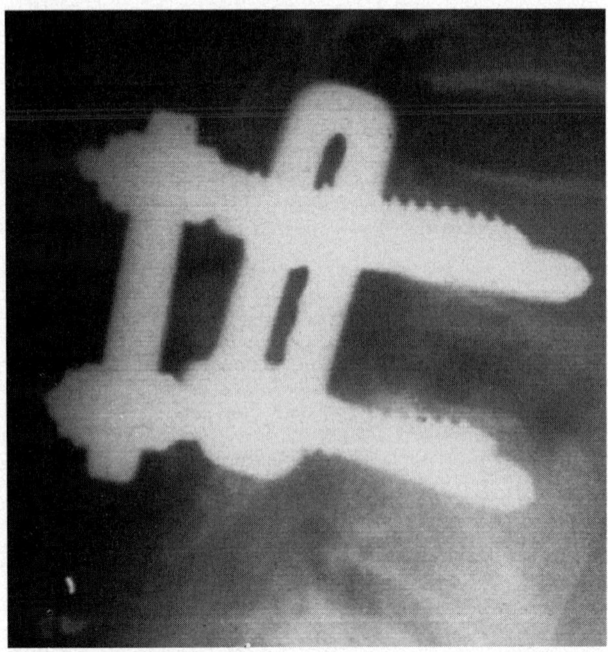

**FIGURE 8-21**

Lateral postoperative plane radiograph of 12-year-old boy with a grade 3 spondylolisthesis at L4-L5 reduced with posterior screws and plates only.

tral axis ($y$) divided by the area moment of inertia ($I$). Therefore, the greatest normal stress exists at the screw-plate junction. It is for this reason that some manufacturers design their screws in a conical manner,

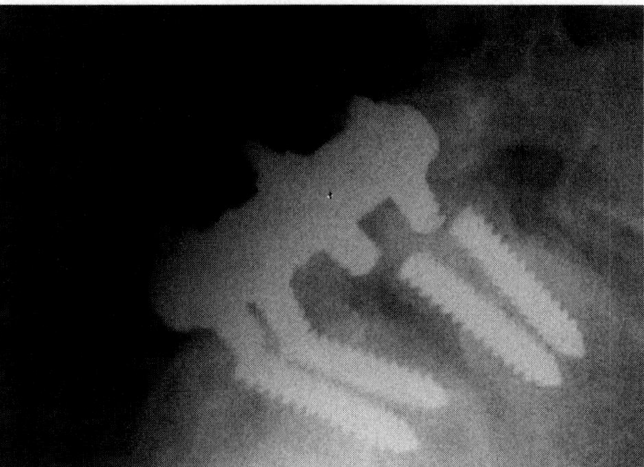

**FIGURE 8-22**

Eighteen months postoperative: lateral view shows four fractured pedicle screws and some loss of reduction.

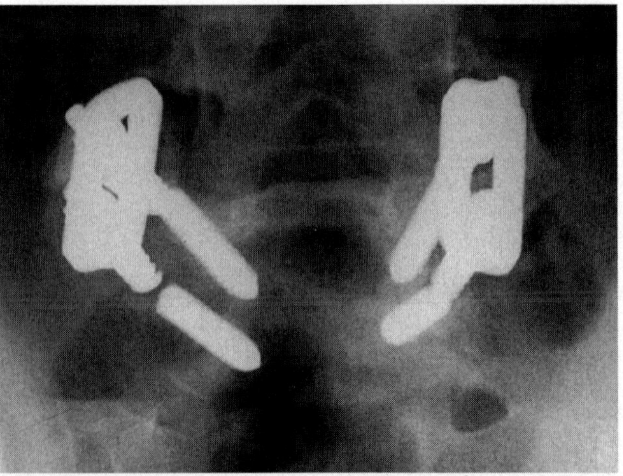

**FIGURE 8-23**

Eighteen months postoperative: posteroanterior view clearly shows three fractured pedicle screws.

such that the area moment of inertia increases as does the internal moment, thereby distributing the normal stresses farther away from the neutral axis.

Posteroanterior (PA) and lateral radiographs obtained 18 months postoperatively (Figs. 8-22 and 8-23) show proximal failure of all four screws, although the patient's spondylolisthesis has not significantly regressed as compared to the immediate postoperative films (Figs. 8-20 and 8-21). The patient was asymptomatic at the time of the post-fracture radiographs. Notice that the screws fractured not at the screw-plate junction, but slightly distal to that intersection. These factors indicate that the bony fusion is solid. Bony fusion is visible proximal to the fracture. In this case, the point of highest bending moment existed at the junction of the fusion mass and the distal screw, thus fracture occurred there.

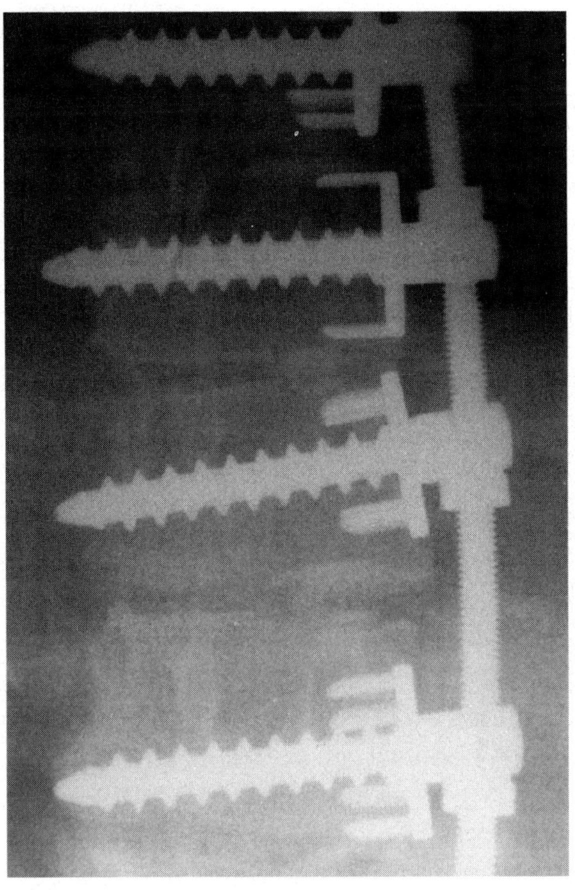

FIGURE 8-24

A 13-year-old girl who presented with severe thoracic scoliosis was instrumented with an anterior screw-rod system to control and correct the curve. Postoperative posteroanterior film shows over-correction between the third and fourth screws, placing the rod in extreme tension.

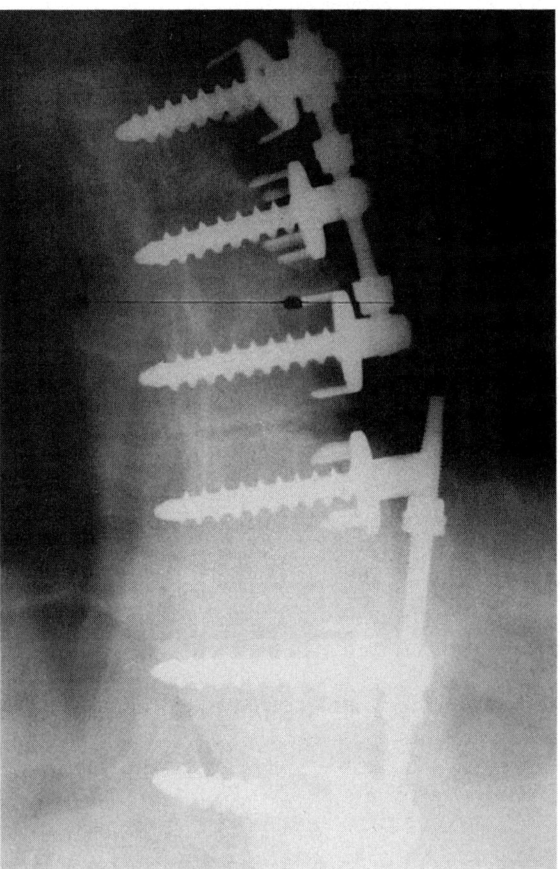

FIGURE 8-25

Posteroanterior view at 30-month follow-up shows rod fracture between the third and fourth screws at the middle of the construct.

## CASE 2

A 13-year-old girl presented with severe progressive thoracic scoliosis. The curve was too large and the patient was too mature for brace containment. Surgery was indicated to control and correct the curve. The patient underwent an anterior thoracic fusion with instrumentation. A 4-mm threaded rod was used with 6-mm vertebral body screws (Fig. 8-24). The patient was braced postoperatively. On subsequent follow-up two years after surgery, radiographs revealed a fractured rod (Fig. 8-25). The fracture was between the third and fourth screws of a six-screw construct.

### Analysis

Prefailure and postfailure radiographs are presented for review. The prefailure films show over-correction of the affected spinal segment, as seen by the divergence of the screws as well as by the production of a slight concavity where a convexity existed preoperatively. Also note that the contralateral disk space is under tension. Load sharing is reduced or nonexistent because most or all loads are transferred to the spinal rod. The rod is under tension, as shown by the compression of the ipsilateral disk space. The moment is greatest at the rod-screw junction as shown in Figure 8-8. The rod failed at this site due to fatigue in the region of the highest moment.

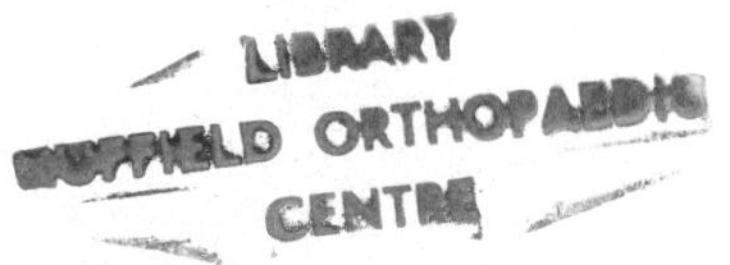

## CASE 3

A 53-year-old man with rheumatoid arthritis and myelopathy involvement who underwent a revision occipitocervical fusion. One year postrevision surgery he presented with severe occipital pain and progressive myelopathy. The lateral radiograph is seen in Figure 8-26.

**Analysis**

Zipnick et al[15] demonstrated that the thickest part of the occiput is the occipital protuberance, the intersection of the superior nuchal line (SNL) and the midline. Forty-five percent of the overall thickness at this region was outer cortical shell, whereas the inner cortical shell accounted for only 10%. Based on this data, they recommended that occipitocervical screws be placed at or near the occipital protuberance. My colleagues and I, in a follow-up study, performed monotonic axial pull-out tests at 21 locations above, below, and lateral to the occipital protuberance.[5] Our findings agreed with those of Zipnick, and found that the weakest location caudal to the protuberance was near the foramen magnum. Quantitatively, I found that the pull-out strength for unicortical screws decreased by 14% per 1.5 cm away from the protuberance above the SNL, and by 53% per 1.5 cm away from the protuberance below the SNL.[5]

In the current case, the most cephalad screw is too far away from the occipital protuberance. Cyclic flexion and extension of the head, either passive or active, causes fatigue at the bone-screw interface. To my knowledge, no study currently exists that demonstrates a correlation between monotonic pull-out strength and bone-screw interface fatigue failure, the latter of which is believed to be the common mode of failure in this situation. A correlation of some degree seems intuitive.

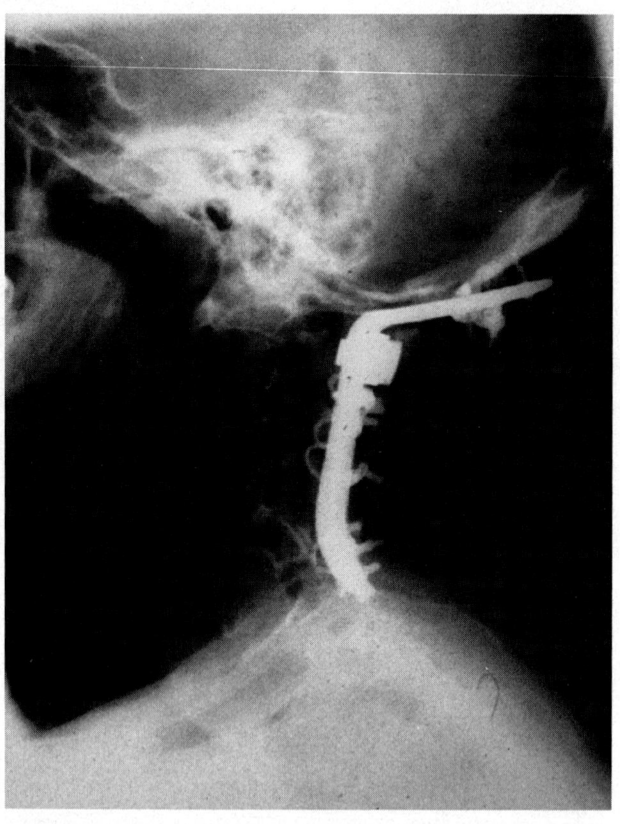

**FIGURE 8-26**

Failed revision occipitocervical fusion. Cortical screw pull-out occurred at the most cephalad screw, most likely as a result of cyclic motion.

## REFERENCES


1. Ashby MF, Jones DRH: *Engineering materials I: an introduction to their properties and applications,* Oxford, 1980, Pergamon Press, p 29.
2. Caruso SA, Margulies JY, Merola AA, Zipnick RI, Gorup JM, Haher TR: *Instrumented fusions of the lumbosacral spine: a technical overview.* In Margulies JY, editor: *Lumbosacral and spinopelvic fixation,* Philadelphia, 1996, Lippincott-Raven, p 199.
3. D'Isa FA: *Mechanics of metals,* Reading, MA, 1968, Addison-Wesley, p 9.
4. Haher TR, O'Brien M, Dryer JW, Nucci R, Zipnick R, Leone DJ: The role of lumbar facet joints in spinal stability. Identification of alternate paths of loading, *Spine* 19:2667-2670, 1994.
5. Haher TR, Yeung AW, Caruso SA, Merola A, Shin T, Gorup JM, Zipnick RI: Occipital screw pullout strength: a biomechanical investigation of occipital morphology, *Spine,* In Press.
6. Hayden HW, Moffatt WG, Wulff J: *The structure and properties of materials,* vol 3, New York, 1964, John Wiley and Sons.
7. Litsky AS, Spector M: Biomaterials. In Sheldon R, Simon, MD, editors: *Orthopaedic basic science,* American Academy of Orthopaedic Surgeons, 1994, p 447.
8. *Metals Handbook, ed 8, vol 10,* American Society for Metals, 1975, pp 134-153.
9. Moffatt WG, Pearsall GW, Wulff J: *The structure and properties of materials, vol 1,* New York, 1964, John Wiley and Sons, p 90.
10. Mow VC, Flatow EL, Foster RJ: Biomechanics. In Sheldon

R, Simon, MD, editors: *Orthopaedic basic science,* American Academy of Orthopaedic Surgeons, 1994, p 459.

11. Petroski H: To engineer is human: the role of failure in successful design, New York, 1992, Vintage Books, p 22.
12. Basic concepts in biomechanics of fracture and fixation. In Tencer AF, Johnson KD, editors: *Biomechanics in orthopaedic trauma*, Philadelphia,1994, Lippincott-Raven, pp 6-11.
13. Van B, Cochran G: A primer of orthopaedic biomechanics, New York, Churchill Livingstone, p 19.
14. Wulpi DJ: *Understanding how components fail,* Metals Park, Ohio, American Society for Metals, 1985, p 2.
15. Zipnick RI, Merola AA, Gorup JM, Kunkle K, Shin T, Caruso SA, Haher TR: Occipital morphology: an anatomic guide to internal fixation, *Spine* 21:1719-1724, 1996.

# IV

# ANATOMIC CONSIDERATIONS IN APPROACHES TO REVISION SURGERY

# 9

# POSTERIOR APPROACH AND ANATOMIC POSTOPERATIVE ALTERATIONS

**Michael R. Zindrick, M.D.**
**Alexander J. Ghanayem, M.D.**



There are two considerations in achieving the pain-relief goals of revision surgery: decompression and stabilization. A thorough understanding of these two goals must be mastered in revision spine surgery. Consideration of what anatomy currently exists and what anatomy will result after the required procedure is performed are paramount to success. In this chapter, the authors' goals are to review the principles and concepts of how to approach the previously operated spine. The odds of a successful postoperative outcome will be maximized with a well-organized preoperative, intraoperative, and postoperative treatment plan.

## PREOPERATIVE EVALUATION AND CONSIDERATIONS

Proper patient selection remains the most important element in successful spinal surgery. Unrealistic expectations, significant psychological overlay, secondary gain, and numerous other factors are major impediments to a successful outcome. There are many very thorough texts concerning these aspects of patient selection and we would refer the reader to them because a thorough review of this aspect of spinal surgery is beyond the scope of this chapter. It is assumed that the above issues are clarified and understood prior to the decision to proceed with another surgical procedure. Often, the reason the prior surgical procedure failed is due to initial poor patient selection. In such a case another procedure will only compound the patient's problems. Clearly defined spinal pathology that was either not initially addressed in the first surgical procedure, is now a result of the first surgical procedure, or has developed subsequently must be identified.

### DIAGNOSTIC STUDIES

Careful preoperative evaluation is a mandate for those surgeons performing revision posterior spine surgery. This process requires a clear understanding of the clinical problem and relevant anatomy, spinal stability, bone and soft tissue quality, and general patient health. The majority of this evaluation is performed with plain radiographs and other neuroimaging studies.

Plain radiographs are the simplest and least expensive spinal imaging study but they provide a wealth of information. Whenever possible, standing (as opposed to supine) anteroposterior and lateral radiographs should be obtained. This will provide information regarding sagittal and coronal balance, subluxations, or other instability patterns. Supine radiographs, while technically easier, may not reveal malalignment or instability problems. Supine radiographs may allow the radiology technician to utilize other exposure techniques to help to better define and evaluate posterolateral fusion masses, especially in larger patients. A supine anteroposterior radiograph of the lumbosacral junction (30° cephalad angulation of the x-ray source) will better visualize the posterolateral gutters between L5 and the sacrum. Oblique radiographs are performed supine and used to assess the integrity of the pars interarticularis.

Standing lateral flexion and extension radiographs can be used to assess additional subluxation, possible reduction of a spondylolytic segment, accentuate a subtle or suspicious instability pattern, and evaluate motion through a fusion mass.

Finally, because radiographs can be repeated in the operating room, normal structures, areas of laminectomy defects, and resected spinous processes should be clearly identified. Intraoperative radiographs with reference metallic markers will help serve as a guide to the regional anatomy when used in comparison to the preoperative studies.

The use of CT myelography and/or magnetic resonance imaging (MRI) scans depend on the underlying revision problem. Revision decompression procedures require clear identification of regions of central, lateral recess, and foraminal stenosis. High-quality MRI scans, usually with gadolinium contrast enhancement, can define these areas. MRI scans that are nondiagnostic, poor quality scans, or the presence of spinal instrumentation may require the addition of CT myelography. Patients with significant deformity from degenerative or postsurgical scoliosis may be imaged better with CT myelography as opposed to MRI. The final decision as to which study or studies to obtain rests with the treating physician. He or she must be confident as to the presence or absence of neurocompressive lesions and with the surgical planning addressing this pathology. The authors feel both to be helpful.

Revision fusion procedures, usually with instrumentation, require thorough knowledge of the remaining posterior elements. This includes pedicle width (medial-lateral and superior-inferior), length including available length to the anterior cortex of the vertebral body, and the pedicle angle, both sagittal and coronal. The relative position of the transverse process, mammary body, and the pedicle should be noted during preoperative planning. CT scans or high quality MRI can delineate these bony landmarks. The pars interarticularis should also be identified and evaluated for defects or stress fractures. Alterations of normal anatomy must be evaluated and understood. In revision fusion procedures, fusion bone can still be present and may overlie the pars, pedicle start point, or transverse process. This should be noted to avoid unnecessary dissection of the soft tissues in search of these structures and direct the physician to the location of the pseudarthrosis to be repaired (Fig. 9-1).

Other special tests that can be used include bone scan and diskography. Bone scans can be used to evaluate a fusion mass for consolidation. This test, however, can yield both false-positive and false-negative results. The test can be false positive when performed within 1 to 2 years of the initial surgery. Increased uptake in the posterolateral gutter can raise the level of suspicion of a pseudarthrosis. However, the lack of uptake is not always indicative of a solid arthrodesis. It is possible for a posterolateral fusion mass to consolidate to the transverse processes without uniting the two processes together. A space would remain between the two masses of bone that would not be a true pseudarthrosis and would appear cold (no uptake) on a bone scan.

The role of diskography has not clearly been defined in both primary and revision surgery. Diskography may be helpful to assess the disk adjacent to previously fused levels or an unfused segment. This segment should be evaluated for both extent of degeneration and as a possible source of pain generation. Diskography has also been suggested to be useful in determining if a disk space within a posterior fusion is still a pain generator, either due to pseudarthrosis of this level or excessive motion despite posterior bony union. Diskographic results need to be interpreted with caution. It is essential that the individual performing the diskography be skilled in the technical and interpretative aspects of the procedure to minimize patient discomfort. It is also mandatory that the patient is cooperative. Valuable information can be gained during diskography. Should a patient complain inappropriately of excessive pain at the time of subcutaneous local anesthetic infiltration, patient pain threshold and degree of pain behavior and magnification are better appreciated. Conversely, the test may be very valuable if a patient cooperates throughout the procedure and only responds appropriately to pain stimuli when an abnormal disk is injected while the patient has no pain when a nondegenerative central disk is injected.

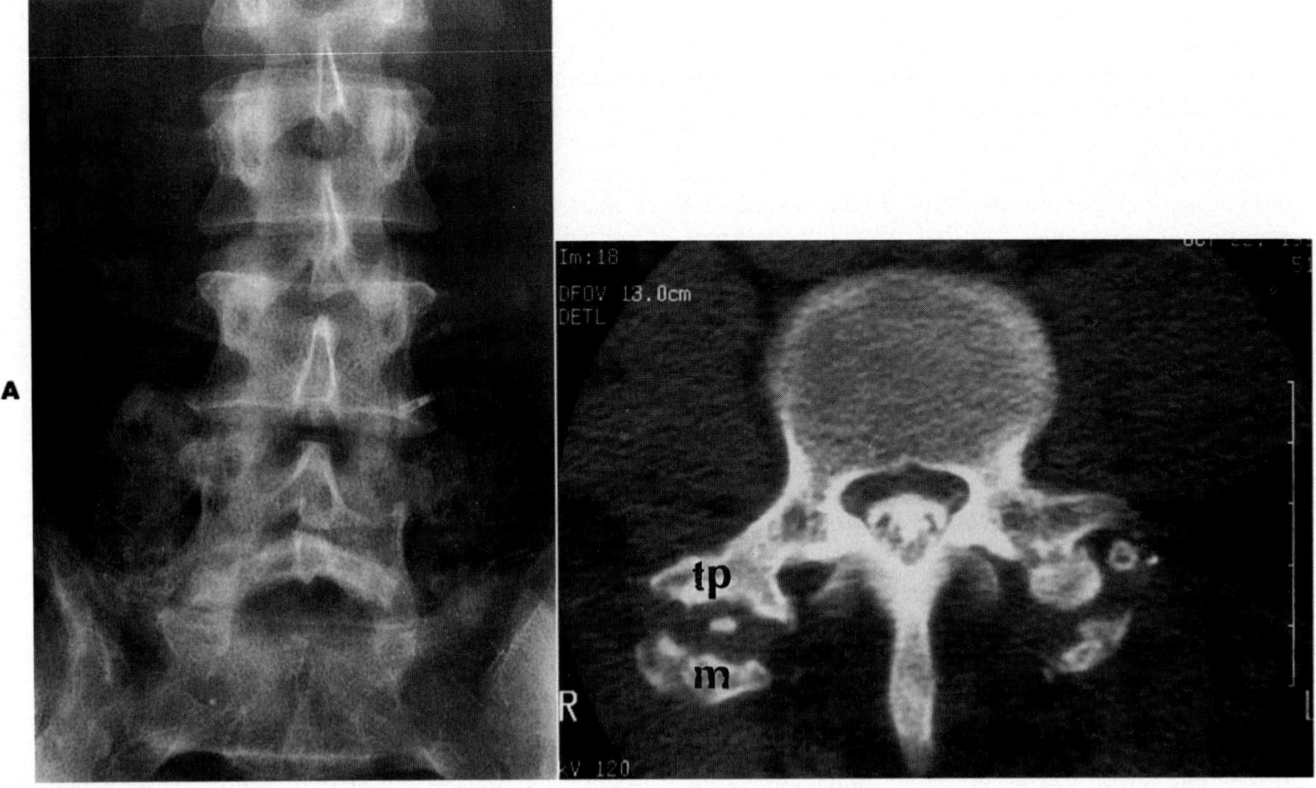


**FIGURE 9-1**

Despite the appearance of adequate fusion bone seen on the anteroposterior lumbar radiograph (**A**), the axial CT scan (**B**) reveals failure of the posterolateral bone mass (*m*) to unite with the underlying transverse process (*TP*).

## EVALUATION OF SPINAL STABILITY

Spinal stability or instability should be ascertained in the preoperative planning period. Standing lateral radiographs, with or without flexion and extension views, are usually sufficient to diagnose instability in the sagittal plane (i.e., spondylolisthesis or retrolisthesis). Standing anteroposterior radiographs will usually highlight lateral listhesis and degenerative scoliosis. Evidence of pars defects and resected facet joints should also raise suspicion of instability despite the lack of significant motion or translation on plain radiographs. In cases of severe stenosis, supporting structures such as the pars or facet joints may be resected intraoperatively. These potential situations should be noted and a contingency plan devised to stabilize the spine if necessary.

## TISSUE QUALITY

The status of the soft tissue envelope surrounding the spine as well as bone quality should be noted. Patients with multiple previous procedures, prior posterior wound infections, radiation dermatitis, and thin paraspinal musculature (i.e., in the elderly) may be at risk for soft tissue deficiency when trying to close the back after a major reconstructive procedure. On the other hand, it may be difficult to obtain adequate spinal exposure in obese patients or in patients with thick paraspinal musculature.

Bone quality should also be assessed. Osteoporosis greatly diminishes the purchase of pedicle screws and bone hooks. This may result in loss of fixation, especially when trying to correct spinal deformity or in cases of significant instability.

## GENERAL PATIENT HEALTH

More focus has been placed on the general health of patients undergoing spine surgery over the past ten years. Cigarette smoking has resulted in lower fusion and higher infection rates. Diabetics have impaired healing potential and immune responses, especially when diabetes is poorly controlled. Patients with neoplastic processes or prior irradiation to the spine also have impaired healing potential and are at increased risk for postoperative infections. Preoperative nutritional status has been shown to be predictive of postoperative infections and should be optimized in patients at risk. Preoperative cardiac clearance and medical evaluation should be obtained when appropriate.

## FORMULATING THE SURGICAL GAME PLAN

### DECOMPRESSION

The need for spinal decompression must be evaluated preoperatively. Was an adequate decompression performed in previous surgeries? Has new pathology developed subsequently, such as a junctional stenosis? Will the required decompression involve the central canal, the lateral recesses, or the foramen and require further destabilization of the spine? Will decompression only be adequately achieved by reducing a malalignment of the spine in either the sagittal or coronal plane?

A game plan for decompression can be established preoperatively by understanding the above concepts and identifying what normal anatomic structures still remain and where the normal and abnormal anatomy interface. Evaluating the existing anatomy with CT scans, plane radiographs, and MRI can aid in identifying this transitional area. Surgically approaching the abnormal anatomy from the area of normal anatomy is a safe method by which to enter the area of scarring. Once in the area of scarring, remaining close to bone structures allows the surgeon to safely develop a plane for dissection. The value of understanding which bone structures exist preoperatively becomes obvious then for safe dissection in the area of previous surgery.

The authors have found the use of sharp curettes of assorted sizes to be the safest and most expedient tools for developing this anatomic plane of dissection. Varying sizes of angled rongeurs are helpful. Long instruments allow for greater leverage and control. All tools should be sharp and well-maintained.

### STABILIZATION

The other major concern after decompression is stabilization. The spine may be unstable to begin with or have the potential to become unstable after the required decompression. In either situation, the surgeon needs to consider spinal stability and address it in an appropriate fashion. We can separate stability into two types: macroinstability, such as those that are obvious radiographically, including scoliosis, spondylolisthesis, and retrolisthesis, and microinstability, which is not as easily detected radiographically. Pain in such a motion segment is produced in a pathologic fashion under normal physiologic loads. The presence of microinstability can be suggested on T2-weighted MRI images or/and confirmed with diskography.

Another consideration regarding stability is the potential need for restoration of anatomic alignment. Spinal malalignment in either the coronal or sagittal plane needs to be evaluated for the need for correction. Restoration of malalignment can prevent further deterioration of remaining motion segments and resultant realignment can produce the needed decompression of neural structures. The latter is often seen in cases of degenerative scoliosis in the concave neural foramen.

## SURGICAL TECHNIQUE

### THE INCISION

The multiply operated back will often have multiple scars in the skin. The revision procedure should be performed through a generous incision that allows for ample exposure. The previous scar can be excised at the time of surgery to allow for healthy, well-vascularized skin-to-skin wound edge healing.

### THE FASCIA AND MUSCLE

Often, to identify landmarks, the incision needs to be extended both cephalad and caudal to expose existing spinous processes and lamina. Once these structures are identified dissection can be carried down through the fascia to existing lamina. In the area of previous laminectomy, dissection should be made initially in the midline and then slope laterally to expose the existing lateral facet and lamina. This will prevent inadvertent entering of the previous laminectomy site and dural incision. Once the lateral structures are located, further cleaning of existing bone structures is performed with Cobb elevator, curette and rongeur (Fig. 9-2). With retractors in the paraspinal muscles the scar can now be removed from the previous laminectomy. Understanding the posterior margins as outlined by the existing lamina above and below, and the location of the facet joints laterally, one can then excise scar to this level. Further scar resection is performed by developing the plane along the lateral and cephalad margins of the existing lamina.

To prepare the fusion bed, dissection laterally over the facet joints can next be performed, thus exposing the transverse process, lateral face of the superior facet joints, and remaining pars interarticularis. Decortication can be performed at this time of the lateral face of the facet joint with a curette.

### DECOMPRESSION

Every experienced surgeon has techniques that help when working around scar. The goals are to free the dural sac and nerve roots of scar enough to allow required resection of bone or soft tissue that is causing any neural compression. This is accomplished with the least amount of trauma to the neural structures, avoiding a dural tear or root injury. General principles are

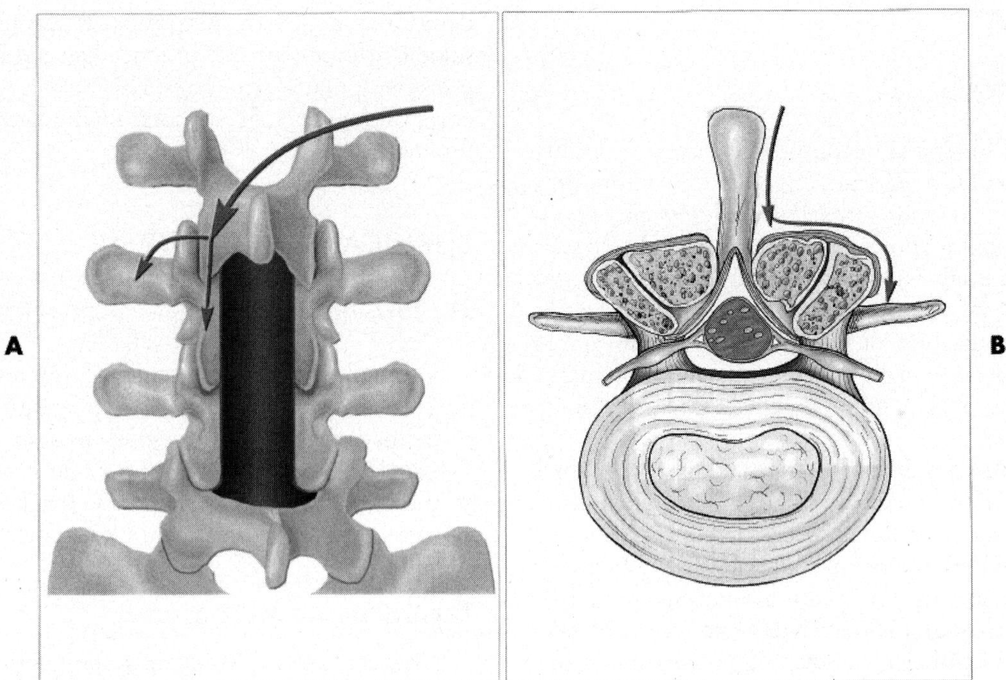


**FIGURE 9-2**

Posterior (**A**) and axial (**B**) view of the technique and approach of locating the junction between unresected or residual lamina and scar. Once the lamina bone is located, the surgeon should proceed laterally toward the remaining portions of the resected lamina thus defining the lateral margins and the wound depth to the spinal canal. Removal of postsurgical scar and spinal canal decompression can now safely be performed.

to use the bone as the margin to develop a plane between it and the dural scar. Numerous tools can accomplish this task safely. The authors find sharp curettes to be very effective and safe to separate scar and dura from bone. The cutting edge is used on the bone surface while the blunt cup of the curette protects the neural structures and gently pushes them out of harm's way. Once margins are developed, Kerrison rongeurs can be utilized to remove offending lamina, facet joints, facet joint capsule, and ligamentum flavum. High-speed burrs are also popular for this purpose. When used, however, the dura should always be protected. Early intraspinal landmark identification prevents injury to nerve roots and dura. Locating the pedicle and disk space early defines for the surgeon the location of the foramen and lateral margin of the spinal canal. The nerve root can be located medial to the pedicle and tracked laterally and distally through the foramen.

Decompressing the nerve root through the foramen can be difficult in cases of severe disk space collapse with or without spondylolisthesis. When a fusion with spinal instrumentation is to be performed, the authors have found that inserting the pedicle screws above and below the foramen allows the surgeon to then distract the disk space or reduce a spondylolisthesis so as to safely decompress the nerve root in the lateral recess and foramen (Fig. 9-3).

Should a dural tear be encountered it should be repaired in a watertight fashion. Great care must be exercised to prevent inadvertent suturing of rootlets to the undersurface of the dura at the time of repair. Using an interrupted stitch to retract and raise the dura on either side of the tear will allow the neural structures to fall back into the dura and away from the area of repair and suture line.

## Locating and Cannulating the Pedicle

Locating the pedicle above and below an area of previous surgery should not be difficult. Pedicles within an area of previous laminectomy can be identified laterally by finding the transverse process and from within the canal. Should a previous posterolateral fusion attempt have been made either successfully or not, locating the pedicle becomes more difficult. Tricks to find the pedicle in this case include locating the pedicle above and below to establish the lateral line the pedicle should be found within, locating the medial border of the pedicle within the spinal canal with maximum radiographic assistance using either a fluoroscope or multiple intraoperative plain radi-

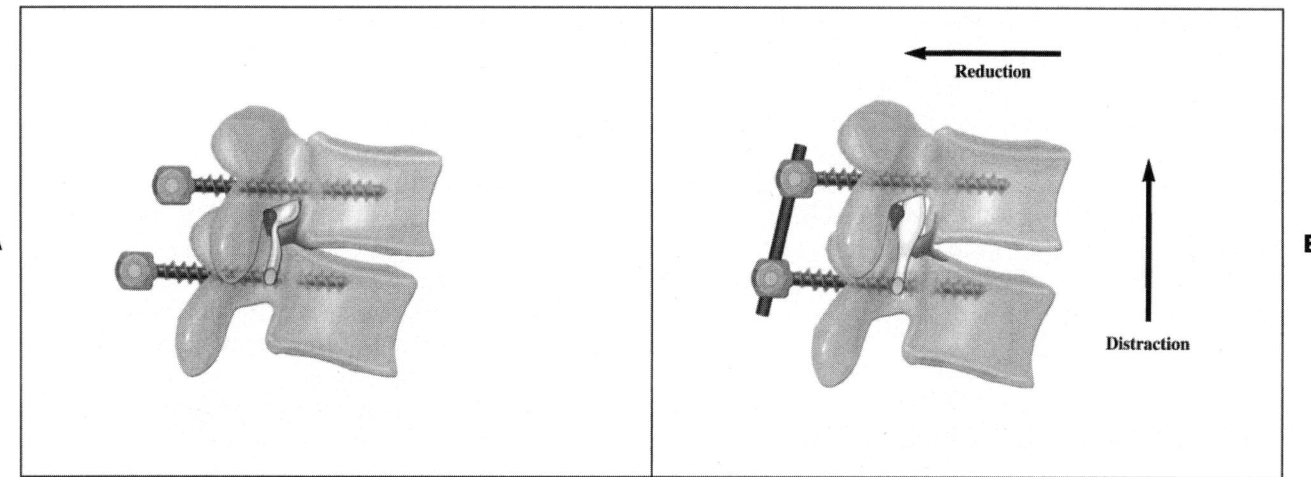


FIGURE 9-3

**A,** Sagittal view of a nerve root being severely compressed in the neural foramen. Pedicle screws have been inserted. **B,** Reduction of the spondylolisthesis and slight distraction of the disk space allows for safe passage of a Kerrison rongeur into the foramen to decompress the root.

ographs with radiopaque markers (Fig. 9-4). Visualization from multiple planes gives the surgeon the greatest chance for successful screw insertion in difficult cases.

## ILIAC CREST BONE GRAFT HARVESTING

If fusion has already been attempted, the surgeon should know preoperatively which crest was previously harvested. This may be apparent from scars or may require evaluation of the previous operative report. As a general rule, the graft should be harvested from a virgin iliac crest to guarantee the best quality bone. If both crests have been harvested previously, the anterior crests can be used. This technique requires the operation to begin with the patient supine and graft harvesting from the anterior lateral iliac crests. Bilateral harvesting may be required. The patient is then turned prone for the index procedure after graft harvesting.

## FUSION

If the goal of the procedure is to obtain a solid fusion either for the first time or in the case of a pseudarthrosis repair, the fusion bed has to be prepared by meticulously decorticating the transverse processes, facet joints, pars interarticularis, and lateral face of the facet joint. Old bone grafts not adherent to these structures should be resected in cases of pseudarthrosis. Generous amounts of good quality cancellous and corticocancellous bone graft is then packed into the fusion bed area. Attention to detail during this phase of the operation can make the difference between a successful outcome and another failed surgical adventure for the patient.

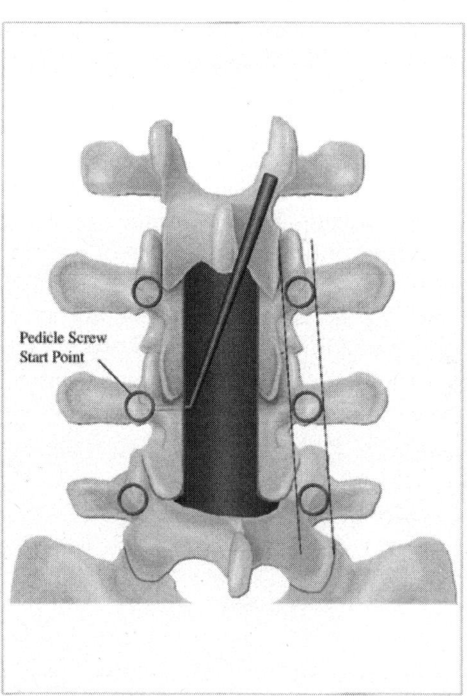


FIGURE 9-4

Identifying the pedicle in revision cases can be aided either by defining its borders from within the canal using an angled probe or by locating the transverse process at the level and then the pedicles above and below. The latter establishes medial and lateral borders in which the pedicle in question should be found.

## WOUND CLOSURE

Intraoperatively, periodic release of retractors minimizes muscle trauma and ischemia. Devitalized muscle and tissue should be resected at the time of wound closure. The wound is closed in layers balancing the need to eliminate as much dead space as possible while preventing excessive tension on the tissues. Layers closed are the fascia, subcutaneous layer, and skin. Draining the deep layer is preferable to prevent excessive hematoma collection and pressure upon the exposed dura. If a large subcutaneous dead space is present, draining this space is also desirable. The subcutaneous margins may need to be undermined to mobilize the skin edge for closure if scar resection was performed at the time of initial incision.

## POSTOPERATIVE CONSIDERATIONS

### NUTRITION AND GENERAL HEALTH

As in the preoperative period, good nutritional balance should be maintained and supported if necessary. This is especially important in those patients with prior infections, neoplastic disorders, trauma, and in the elderly. Diabetics should be more vigilant in maintaining control of blood sugars and smokers should not resume smoking.

### BRACING

The role of bracing depends on the procedure performed and the confidence in quality of surgical fixation achieved. Braces can be used for postoperative comfort or to provide additional stability after a reconstructive procedure. Rigid thermoplastic braces are best at providing stability. Abdominal binders or corsets provide support to the abdomen and help encourage good posture thus providing postoperative comfort.

### REHABILITATION

Technically perfect revision spine surgery usually will not obtain optimal results without some sort of postoperative rehabilitation. In decompressive procedures, formal therapy may not be necessary in the patient motivated to walk and maintain trunk stability and strength. Patients undergoing more intensive procedures may require more aggressive rehabilitation after a period of healing. This rehabilitation usually includes abdominal and paraspinal muscle strengthening, trunk stabilization and flexibility exercises, and general cardiovascular reconditioning.

## SUMMARY

The previously operated patient challenges the health care profession with many complex and difficult issues. Multiple problems are compounded by depression and other psychological conditions exacerbated by chronic pain and an often hopeless outlook relayed by previous health care professionals. Definite addressable pathology must be identified in a well-selected patient if any chance of success is to be gained by another surgical procedure. An organized game plan formulated after careful and thorough preoperative evaluation of the patient can result in a beneficial secondary procedure when combined with careful patient selection.

## SUGGESTED READING


1. Biondi J, Greenberg B: Redecompression and fusion in failed back syndrome patients, *J Spinal Disord* 3:362-369, 1990.
2. Crock HV: Observations on the management of failed spinal operations, *J Bone Joint Surg Br* 58:193-199, 1976.
3. Johnsson KE, Redlund-Johnell I, Uden A, Willner S: Preoperative and postoperative instability in lumbar spinal stenosis, *Spine* 14:591-593, 1989.
4. Klein JD, Hey LA, Yu CS et al: Perioperative nutrition and postoperative complications in patients undergoing spinal surgery, Burlington, VT, June 1996, International Society for the Study of Lumbar Spine Annual Meeting.
5. Krag MH: *Spinal fusion: overview of options and posterior internal fixation devices.* In Frymoyer JW, editor: *The adult spine: principles and practice,* New York, 1991, Raven Press.
6. Lauerman WC, Wiesel SW: The failed back: an algorithm, *Semin Spine Surg* 8:208-220, 1996.
7. Lorenz MA, Patwardhan AG, Zindrick MR: *Instability and mechanics of implants and braces for thoracic and lumbar fractures.* In Errico TJ, Bauer RD, Waugh T, editors: *Spinal trauma,* Philadelphia, 1991, JB Lippincott, pp 271-280.
8. Mirkovic S, Abitol JJ, Steinman J, Edwards CC, Schaffler M, Massie J, Garfin SR: Anatomic consideration for sacral screw placement, *Spine* 16(suppl 6): 289-294, 1991.
9. Stambough JL: Causes of failed back syndrome, *Semin Spine Surg* 8:165-176, 1996.
10. Spengler DM, Freeman C, Westbrook R, Miller JW:

Low-back pain following multiple lumbar spine procedures. Failure of initial selection, *Spine* 5:356-360, 1980.

11. Whitecloud TS III, Davis JM, Olive PM: Operative treatment of the degenerated segment adjacent to a lumbar fusion, *Spine* 19:531-536, 1994.
12. Zindrick, MR, Wiltse LL, Doornik A, Widell EH, Knight GW, Patwardhan AG, Thomas JC, Rothman SL, Fields BT: Analysis of the morphometric characteristics of the thoracic and lumbar pedicles, *Spine* 12:160-166, 1987.

# 10

# ANTERIOR APPROACH TO THE SPINE

**Mohammad E. Majd, M.D.**
**James W. Harkess, M.D.**
**Richard T. Holt, M.D.**
**Kurt Madsen, D.O.**
**John Mahan, M.D.**



The anterior approach to the spine provides direct vision and access to the vertebral column. A sound understanding of the three-dimensional anatomy of the spine and a well-considered, organized surgical plan are paramount. These enable the spine surgeon to choose an approach or a combination of approaches that permits direct access to the deformity or lesions and accommodates any need for extensive exposure.

This approach allows the spine surgeon to manage rigid deformity due to congenital or acquired disease, disk herniation, infection, tumor, and fracture, permitting better curve correction and fixation; by this means, the natural height and sagittal plane alignment of the spine can be restored. A fundamental concept in the field of surgery is that the easiest approach with the lowest complication rate is facilitated by adequate knowledge of the relevant anatomy.

Indications for the anterior approach to the thoracic, thoracolumbar, and combined thoracic and thoracolumbar spine are predicated on the need to correct deformity directly by the release of soft tissue contractures, or by manipulation of the major weight-bearing axial forces on the spine to obtain a reduction and final alignment. This approach may leave a scar that is unacceptable to the patient and a postoperative course that is more painful. Similarly, the demands on the surgeon are more complex (relating to chest tube care and intensive care unit (ICU) management; however, the anterior approach provides an unrivaled exposure and potential for curve correction. Some of the procedures that are facilitated are annulectomy, diskectomy and anterior longitudinal ligament release, rib head resection, thoracoplasty, and finally corpectomy. Access to the anterior column is advantageous and, at times, critical to the success of major spinal procedures.

The indication for anterior spine surgery to the lower lumbar and lumbosacral joint is multifaceted, and without any clear consensus as to the approach. In our experience, the treatment of a pseudarthrosis at that level is best accomplished by an anterior interbody fusion. Patients at increased risk for pseudarthrosis, such as smokers, diabetics, and patients on steroids, should be considered for interbody fusion at the time of the initial surgery.[1] Treatment of tumors or infection of the lumbosacral area, although infrequent, typically requires an anterior approach because of the involvement of the anterior column. An anterior approach should also be considered in patients who have previously had a posterior decompression. The rationale for this is that after posterior decompression, it is extremely difficult to retract the dura adequately to facilitate a posterolateral interbody fusion.

Several factors must be taken into account in evaluating a patient for a possible anterior approach. First and foremost, is the patient physically fit to undergo such an extensive procedure, with its longer operating time and antecedent risks? In other words, is the risk-benefit ratio low enough to subject the patient, especially one with a diminished life expectancy (e.g., elderly patients), to this relatively high-risk procedure? A relative contraindication to anterior surgery is a previous anterior approach. Typically, scarring enhances the risk of vascular injury to the point at which even the most experienced surgeon may have difficulty in gaining access to the spine. Furthermore, the scarring impedes the blunt dissection so critical to a careful, bloodless exposure. Another relative contraindication is previous retroperitoneal surgery or abdominal surgery that makes entering the retroperitoneal space difficult if not impossible.[2] A good example would be a patient who has had a ruptured appendix treated by open packing of the wound.

Overall, the indications for anterior spine procedures are multiple and include vertebral tumor, fracture-dislocation, disk herniation, deformity, infection, osteotomy, decompression, corpectomy, anterior spinal release, and pseudarthrosis.

There is no absolute contraindication for the anterior approach but previous anterior surgery or pathology are relative contraindications.

## ANTERIOR APPROACH TO THE UPPER THORACIC SPINE T3-T5

### PERTINENT ANATOMY

In this area, because of the site of the incision, the surgeon must be familiar with the anatomy of the latissimus dorsi, the rhomboid muscles, the trapezius, and the long thoracic nerve. On the left side of the thorax, cephalad to the aortic arch (at the level of T4), the thoracic duct, the esophagus, and subclavian artery are close to the spine. The esophagus is located posteriorly and the aorta is located to the left side of the midline anterior to the vertebral body. The thoracic duct is present on the right side of the midline and the

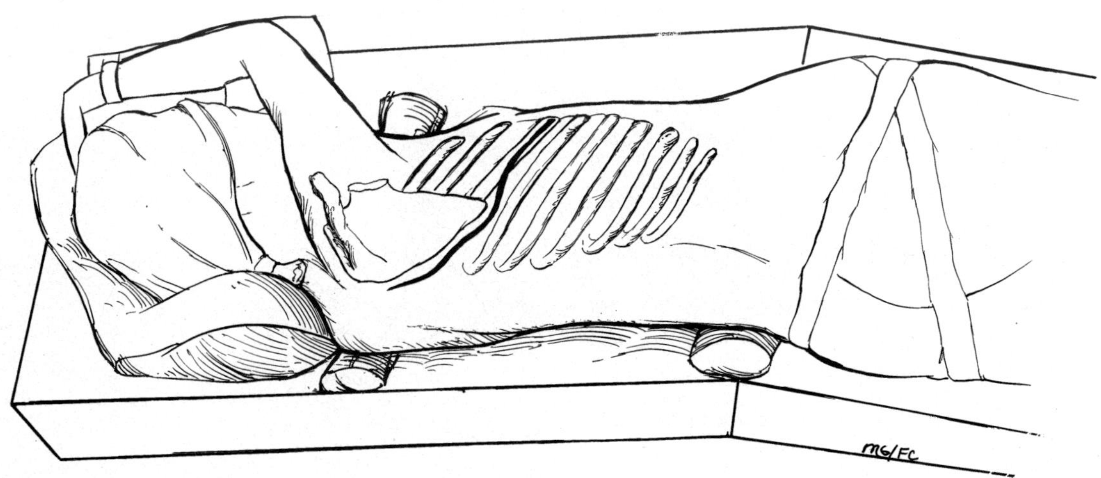


**FIGURE 10-1**

Positioning of the patient. For upper and midthoracic spine approach.

superior vena cava, azygos vein, and brachiocephalic vein are also located in the right hemithorax.[3]

## POSITIONING

The operation is performed with the patient in the lateral decubitus position. If deformity is present, place the incision on the convexity. If there is no deformity, the surgery may be performed from either side. For better visualization and increased extension of the operative field, flexing the table or placing a padded roll cephalad to the ileum is helpful. A well-padded roll in the axilla is crucial for protecting the brachial plexus. Normally we tilt the patient forward and cross tape over the greater trochanter to hold the patient in a lateral position. An adjustable arm holder is a convenient device to hold the arm as far from the chest as possible (Fig. 10-1).

## INCISION

The incision for the upper thoracic spine is hockey-stick-shaped and starts at the level of scapular crest and exactly parallels the medial border of scapula and curves around the inferior angle of the scapula to the midaxillary line (Fig. 10-1). The lower part of the trapezius muscle is divided, and the latissimus dorsi and rhomboid muscles detached from the medial border and inferior angle of scapula to facilitate the elevation of the scapula for rib counting. This leaves a 0.5 inch of muscle at the medial border to facilitate the repair of muscles (Fig. 10-2). The scapula is then retracted so that the surgeon's hand may be passed under the scapula to palpate the uppermost ribs. Normally the highest rib that is palpated in this position is the second, because the first rib is inside and in front of it. Owing to the attachment of the muscles to the second rib, palpation of the first rib is difficult. Another important guide is to check the interspace between the ribs. Normally the interspace between the second and the third ribs is the widest interspace.[4] The serratus anterior muscle is likewise transected as far caudally as possible to space the long thoracic nerve.

It is easy to access the vertebral body by following the direction of the ribs (the fourth rib may be followed to the costotransverse articulation of the fourth vertebral body).

## RIB RESECTION

After the appropriate rib is selected, electrocautery is used to detach the periosteum along the cephalad edge of the rib. By the continued use of electrocautery, the periosteum is detached from the caudal edge, being careful to preserve the intercostal neurovascular bundle. We strip the rib subperiosteally using a smooth motion with an Alexander elevator from anterior to posterior along the upper border first, then along the caudal portion of the rib. Complete elevation of periosteum is thereby achieved. Careful attention to the intercostal neurovascular bundle in this maneuver minimizes postoperative intercostal neuralgia (Fig. 10-2).

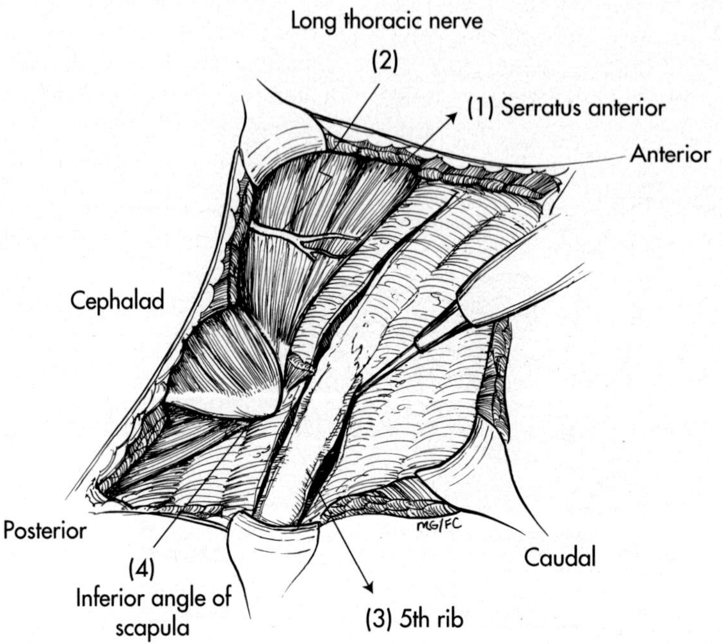


**FIGURE 10-2**

The incision. (*1*) Serratus anterior; (*2*) long thoracic nerve; (*3*) fifth rib; (*4*) inferior angle of scapula.

To expose two motion segments, the posterior third of the rib is excised. A double-action rib cutter is used to cut the rib at the posterior angle. Following the removal of the rib, the underlying parietal pleura is exposed and incised with Metzenbaum scissors or a finger to open the thorax. The wound edges are protected with moist pads. A Charnley hip retractor is then inserted, which allows greater exposure with less prominence than with rib spreaders. We also use a moist sponge to retract and protect the lung and we do not use a double lumen intubation for deflating the lung at the surgical site. The reason for this is to decrease the rate of postoperative atelectasis and subsequent pneumonia. The use of a malleable retractor shaped into a U is a good way to retract and protect the lung (Fig. 10-3).

## INTRATHORACIC PROCEDURE

When the anterior part of the spine at T3-T5 is exposed, the parietal pleura is divided with scissors and is dissected from the underlying tissue. The segmental vessels then come into view at the vertebral body site (Fig. 10-3). To facilitate division of the vessels, the first ligature should be anterior and close to the aorta to preserve the anastomosis at the neural foramen, and the second tie made posteriorly (see the description of the "banjo technique" in the "Anterior Approach to the Midthoracic Spine" section of this chapter). A Cobb elevator is used to raise a U-shaped flap of anterior longitudinal ligament and periosteum. The assistant should protect the important anatomic structures with a malleable retractor while the surgeon raises the flap with a Cobb elevator (Fig. 10-4). We believe this flap development is critical in preventing a chylothorax. Some operators divide the pleura and develop a subpleural plane over the major vessels and thoracic duct without elevating them en masse with a soft tissue flap of periosteum, anterior longitudinal ligament, and annulus. Bony bleeding is controlled by Gelfoam moistened with thrombin. Reapproximating or closing of this flap is helpful to cover the hardware and the graft. This closed flap also contains the hematoma, decreases the amount of bleeding and drainage following surgery, promotes the rate of bone healing, and consequently, vertebral fusion.

## POSTOPERATIVE MANAGEMENT

After completing the procedure, the flap is sewn back by suturing the periosteum and anterior longitudinal ligament to pleura, and pleura to pleura, in two layers. Normally we use a number 28 or 32 French chest tube to exit through the anterior axillary line at the 8th to 9th interspace. The drainage is monitored

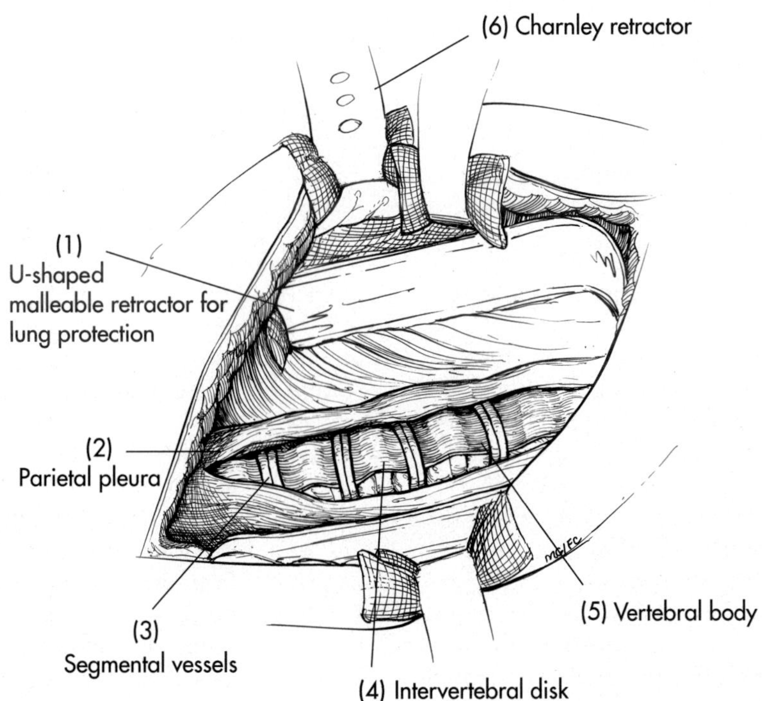


**FIGURE 10-3**

Rib resection. (*1*) U-shaped malleable retractor for lung protection; (*2*) parietal pleura; (*3*) segmental vessels; (*4*) intervertebral disk; (*5*) vertebral body; (*6*) Charnley retractor.

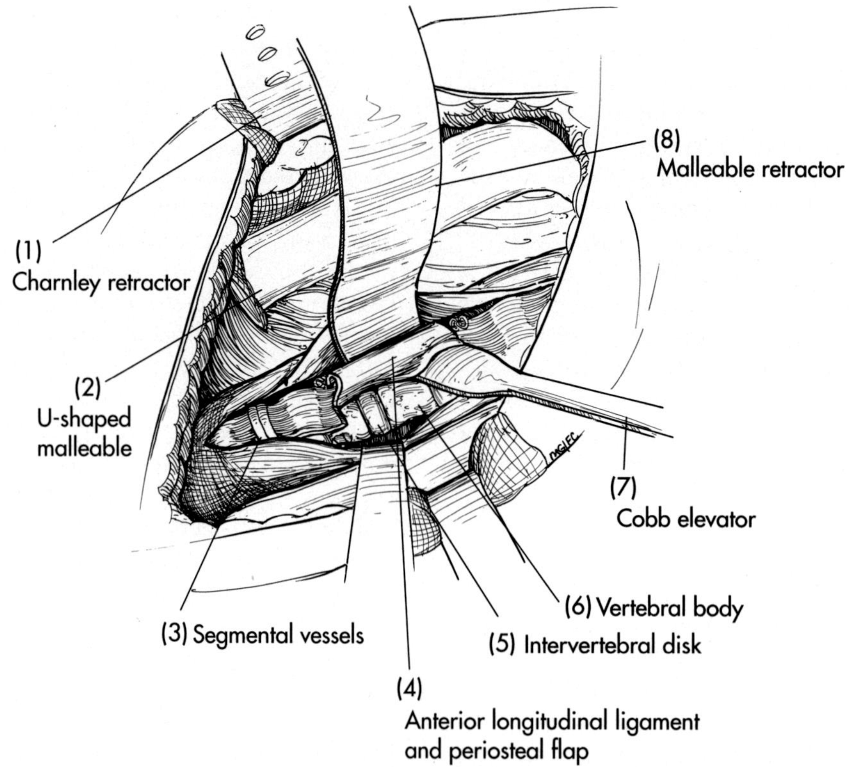


**FIGURE 10-4**

Intrathoracic procedure. (*1*) Charnley retractor; (*2*) U-shaped malleable; (*3*) segmental vessels; (*4*) anterior longitudinal ligament and periosteal flap; (*5*) intervertebral disk; (*6*) vertebral body; (*7*) Cobb elevator; (*8*) malleable retractor.

by the nurses on each shift, and when the drainage slows down to 25 to 30 ml per shift, the chest tube is removed and a chest x-ray is taken to verify the amount of pneumo- or hemothorax.

## POTENTIAL PROBLEMS

Possible problems are thoracic duct injury, injury to great vessels, spinal cord ischemia, and/or esophageotracheal injury.

***Thoracic Duct Injury.*** The thoracic duct is on the left side of thorax cephalad to the aortic arch (at the level of T4), and it follows the course of the aorta on the right side. There is a variation in the course of the thoracic duct in patients older than 70 years when the duct tends to stay on the left side of the aorta in 83% of the cases.[5] Injury to the thoracic duct during exposure of the vertebra should be avoided because a chylothorax may result. Repair of the injured thoracic duct or by packing with Gelfoam soaked in thrombin is useless. The best way to treat chylothorax is by the prolonged use of a chest tube.

***Injury to Great Vessels.*** The superior vena cava, the proximal portion and entry part of the azygos vein, and the right brachiocephalic vein are located in close proximity to the T3, T4, and T5 vertebral bodies. The brachiocephalic artery and right vagus nerve are also in close contact to the above-mentioned bodies. Injury to the venous, arterial, and nervous structures during exposure of the vertebral body should be avoided. Veins are very fragile and susceptible to trauma during the act of sweeping soft tissue from the anterior aspect of the vertebral body. Such venous injury can often be easily repaired by hemoclips. Arterial and nerve injuries are very rare, but, if they occur, they should be repaired directly.

***Spinal Cord Ischemia.*** The blood supply to the spinal cord is of special importance in spine surgery and is variable. The spinal cord is supplied by one anterior and two posterior spinal arteries. The anterior radicular arteries from the vertebral arteries between C6 and C2 leave the foramen transversarium and enter the neural foramina at inconstant levels. The anterior spinal artery is derived at its apex from the vertebral arteries in the foramen magnum.

The spinal cord is also supplied by branches of the posterior radicular arteries at inconstant levels of the cervical spine. These vessels in turn are derived from the vertebral, ascending, and deep cervical arter-

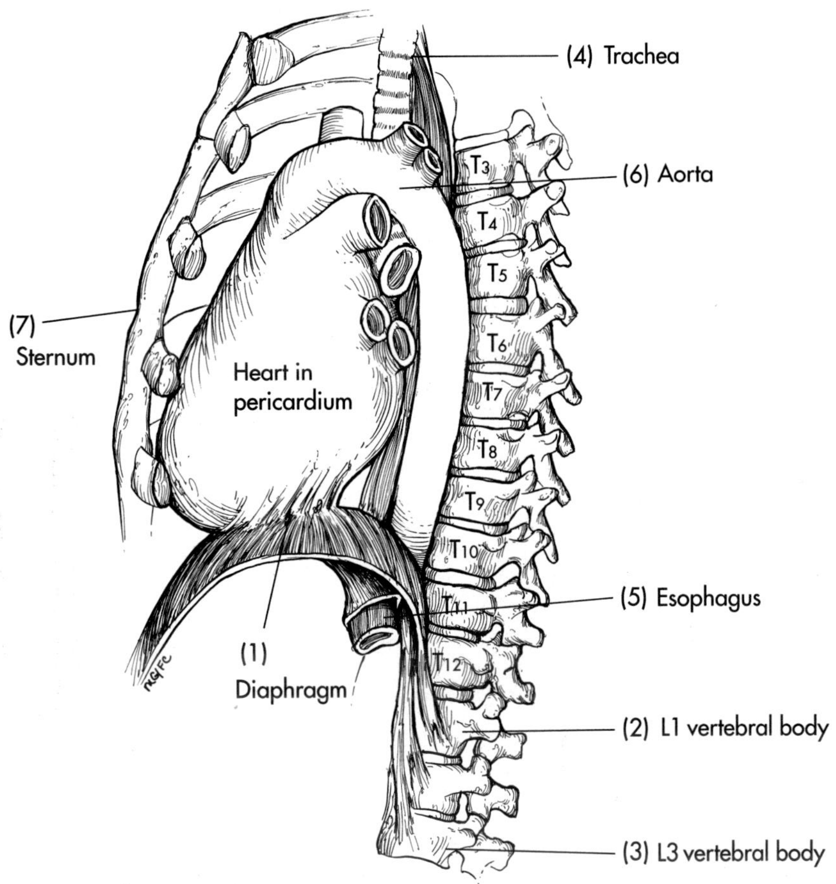


**FIGURE 10-5**

Pertinent anatomy in the anterior approach to the midthoracic spine. (*1*) Diaphragm; (*2*) L1 vertebral body; (*3*) L3 vertebral body; (*4*) trachea; (*5*) esophagus; (*6*) aorta; (*7*) sternum.

ies. In the thoracic spine, the blood supply to the spinal cord is derived from the posterior intercostal arteries branching into anterior and posterior radicular arteries. These supply the anterior spinal artery and posterior spinal arteries via inconstant segmental levels. These vessels are tenuous and small in caliber. Most of the anatomic texts refer to the artery of Adamkiewicz as a major anterior radicular artery coming from one of the posterior intercostal arteries; however, in our practice, we have never identified this large caliber artery and we doubt its existence.

The lumbar blood supply comes from segmental lumbar arteries leaving the aorta and forming anastomotic loops posteriorly, cauda equina arteries following the segmental nerves, and also anastomotic loops anteriorly. The middle sacral artery gives segmental branches to the cauda equina and terminal dural tube.[6]

***Tracheoesophageal Injury.*** The esophagus is located posterior to the aortic arch and is on the left side of the spinal column. The trachea is located anterior to the esophagus and the right main bronchus branches are located at the level of T6-T7. In general, injury to the tracheoesophageal complex is extremely rare.

## ANTERIOR APPROACH TO THE MIDTHORACIC SPINE T6-T10

### PERTINENT ANATOMY

The parietal pleura lies immediately subjacent to the periosteal envelope of the rib and is entered immediately upon incising this tissue. The heart in its pericardium and the arch of aorta match the T3-T9 vertebral bodies. The bronchus descends no lower than T5 but the esophagus, aorta, and inferior vena cava are all intimate anteriorly with the vertebral bodies from T6-T10 (Fig. 10-5). The azygos vein drains intercostal vessels on the right side from T5 and sometimes lower. The sympathetic chain with its segmental ganglia rests extrapleurally and just anterior to the costovertebral junction. The splanchnic nerve and its seg-

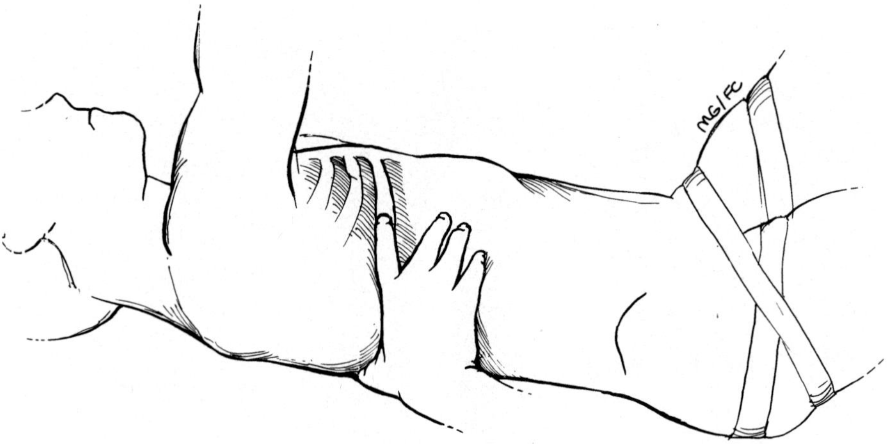


**FIGURE 10-6**

Selection of correct rib for excision in patients with deformity. The surgeon's thumb is placed on the most deformed spinus process, and the index finger touches the rib that should be removed.

mental tributaries run in the interval between the azygos vein and the sympathetic chain.

## POSITIONING

The patient is placed in the lateral decubitus position on his or her left side with the right side up. An approach from the right avoids the aortic arch and the heart; during the approach to the thoracic disks, the aorta and arch are further away, and the segmental vessels may be more prominent and easier to ligate. The feet are dropped with the upper knee held extended to facilitate gapping and stretching of the spine. The kidney rest is centered on the flank, the table dropped, and a pillow placed between the legs. The axilla and all pressure points are padded, the arm is elevated above the shoulder and rested on an arm holder. Ideally, the area of convexity or greatest deformity should be uppermost so that a right convex midthoracic curve is placed left side down. Finally the surgeon stands behind or posterior to the patient.

## INCISION

The incision for the midthoracic spine (T6-T10) must be performed with the relevant pathology kept in mind. It is best to make a rib incision two levels proximal to the vertebral body to be approached. Some surgeons may prefer to make a curvilinear incision a fingerbreadth below the tip of the scapula and curve toward the inframammary crease. In deformity surgery, our technique places great importance on locating the area of greatest deformity along the posterior thoracic spine with the surgeon's thumb and then moving the index finger perpendicularly toward the midaxillary line, palpating the underlying rib (Fig. 10-6). The incision thus follows the outline of this rib, so that sharp dissection with the knife incises the periosteum and allows resection of the proper rib and exposure of the apical vertebra. In choosing the appropriate rib when deformity is not an issue (e.g., in thoracic disk herniation and discitis), remember to count the ribs carefully preoperatively and then, if necessary, use an intraoperative marker to identify the disk space. Removal of the T8 rib and a small portion of the ninth rib head makes it easier to see the T8-T9 disk space. This dissection does not exploit an internervous plane but rapid exposure and streamlining of the surgical technique is enhanced by using a Charnley retractor and by laparotomy sponge packing of the wound margin in lieu of cauterizing the capillary bleeding.

The rib resection should be effected by electrocautery as described in the prior section on exposure of T3-T5. The cautery is used cephalad to caudad making it possible to preserve the periosteal bed. An Alexander elevator should be used by the same pattern to detach the rib musculature into the axilla of its attachment. Once again, the chondral end of the rib is held by a Kocher clamp and the rib resected from the costal cartilage anterior to the angle of the rib posteriorly. The parietal pleura is then opened by Metzenbaum scissors. Charnley retractors keep the chest cavity in full view and a band retractor, shaped in a semicircle, protects the lung. The aorta and other sensitive ventral structures may be protected by placing a "sausage roll" of wet lap sponges and a "sweetheart retractor." A retractor is kept between the surgeon's tool and the vital structures, especially with flap elevation.

When the thoracotomy has been completed, the segmental vessels are ligated as they are encountered during raising of the soft tissue flap. The parietal pleura intimately covers both the sympathetic and splanchnic

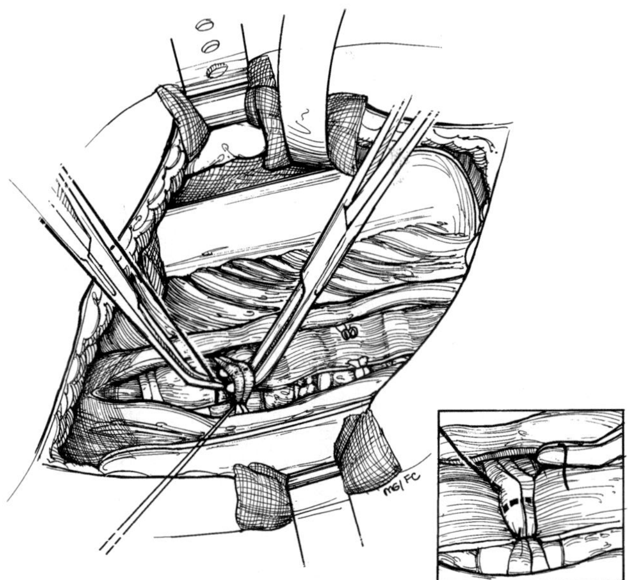

**FIGURE 10-7**

Banjo technique. Ligation of segmental vessels.

nerves overlying the vertebral body and intervening disk, but speed of exposure and streamlining of technique is enhanced by using Charnley retractors and packing the wound margin with laparotomy pads rather than cauterizing the capillary bleeding. The so-called "banjo technique" consists of placing sequential ligatures on the vessels at the periphery of the vertebral body to be exposed. Right-angle hemostats are used first to expose and then to elevate the vessels. The elbow of the instrument is placed against bone, the tip elevated away from the operator, and the opposing long right angle with silk tie should be placed within the teeth of the hemostats and thread held parallel to the shanks of the instrument. The tips of these instruments are opposed in a rectangular fashion, the silk grasped by the operators, first hemostat and then ligature completed. Once this suture is tied, a second suture is passed by elevating the vessel with the previous suture and passing the second right angle in a similar fashion. The first ligature must be anterior and medial to be close to the aorta. This preserves the anastomotic blood supply to the cord and avoids segmental ischemia. The second tie is placed as far posterior as possible to facilitate division of the vessels and exposure of the field (Fig. 10-7). When this is accomplished, elevation of the periosteal and anterior longitudinal ligament flap, which begins at the center of vertebral body field, is started and proceeds toward the mid ventral aspect of the body and if possible, beyond (see Fig. 10-4). We do not use bone wax because this inhibits osteogenesis and bone fusion. Hemostasis is therefore obtained by thrombin-soaked Gelfoam being rubbed into the interstices of the bleeding bone. Flap closure is achieved by a #1 running absorbable suture (Vicryl) and anterior longitudinal ligament stitched to the pleura and pleura to the pleura. We use #2 Vicryl as intercostal stitches to approximate the ribs and #0 Vicryl to suture the rib musculature, periosteal bed, and subcutaneous layer; the skin is closed by a subcuticular #000 suture.

The chest is drained by a 28 French chest tube placed into the pleural space and posterior gutter two interspaces away from the incision. The tube is removed when the drainage is less than 25 ml per shift. At this point, active pulmonary toilet support, elevation of the head of the bed to allow dependent drainage, and decreased postoperative atelectasis is recommended. The patient is mobilized by physical therapy on the first postoperative day.

### POTENTIAL PROBLEMS

Injury to various anatomic structures in close physical proximity to the plane of dissection is possible including the thoracic duct, the great vessels such as aorta and azygos vein, the heart, spinal cord ischemia, the esophagus-bronchus, and finally the diaphragm.

All the major complications of thoracic surgery may occur, such as atelectasis, pneumonia, airway obstruction, and congestive heart failure; pulmonary edema may also occur if fluid replacement is excessive. Direct injury to the heart is less probable when the right-sided approach in the midthoracic spine is used; however, vigorous or overzealous retraction and flap elevation might damage the heart on operating from T4-T9.

Diaphragmatic injury can occur at the caudal end of the exposure but formal diaphragmatic take-down normally is necessary during the thoracoabdominal approaches to the T11-L2 areas but not to the midthoracic spine.

## ANTERIOR APPROACH TO THE THORACOLUMBAR JUNCTION T12-L2

### PERTINENT ANATOMY

In the thoracolumbar region, there are several anatomical features to be considered. It is important to be familiar with the attachments of the diaphragm. The diaphragm is a muscular structure that has curved attachments to the lateral thorax. The aorta, esophagus, and vena cava pass it posteriorly and these structures are anterior to the spine (see Fig. 10-5). In taking down the diaphragm, the surgeon must be cognizant of its curved attachment and its position relative to the spine, to avoid vascular and esophageal injuries at the T12-L1 disk space.[6] The spleen is located retroperitoneally and is susceptible to injury from forceful retraction in this area. Within and beneath the psoas muscle are the roots of the femoral, obturator ilio inguinal, and genitofemoral nerves. Thus, the psoas muscle, when necessary, should be gently mobilized from its medial aspect. The sympathetic ganglia are anterolateral to the spinal column and directly susceptible to injury, which is often unavoidable.

## POSITIONING

The patient is positioned in the lateral decubitus position with the left upper extremity and apex of the deformity facing upward. The lowermost axilla is padded by a roll to prevent neurapraxia, and the patient is centered over the break in the operating table. The arm facing upward is placed on a separate padded arm holder. Avoid the use of a Mayo stand whenever possible. An arm holder attached to the table, such as a Krause arm holder, is better and allows the intraoperative adjustment of the table position. The upper leg is extended and the legs are padded with foam and secured to the table with adhesive tape. We do not use a bean bag because it impinges the abdomen and thereby impedes retroperitoneal dissection. The bean bag also precludes flexing of the operating room table and obscures any intraoperative radiographic investigation. The bed is then tilted backward at an angle of approximately 15°. The break in the table is opened to accentuate any deformity facing upwards. The entire flank is draped from the axilla cephalad to the anterior superior iliac spine caudally and from the umbilicus anteriorly to below the spine posteriorly (Fig. 10-8).

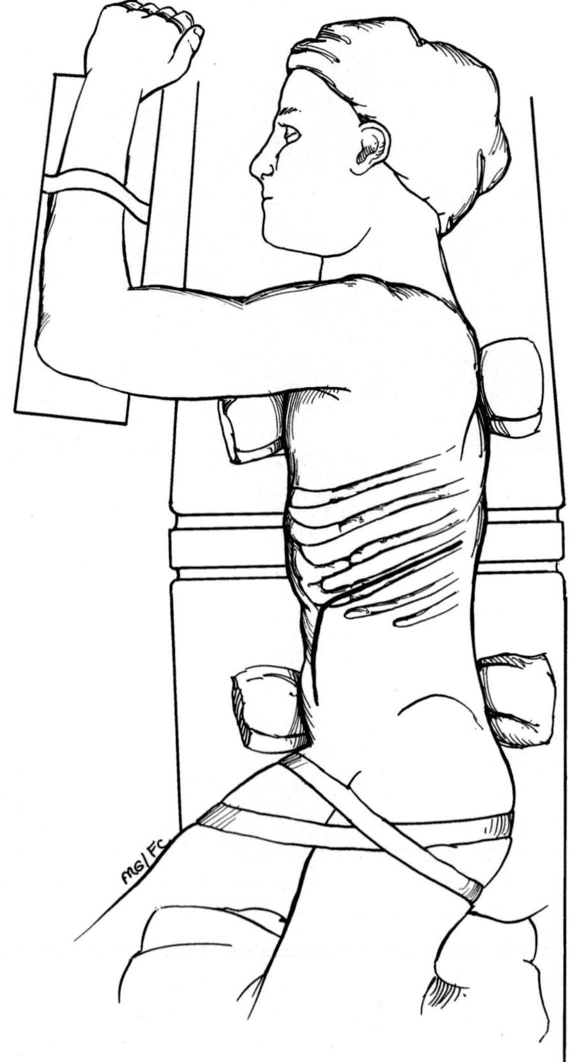

**FIGURE 10-8**

Positioning of the patient for thoracolumbar spine approach.

## INCISION

The incision for the approach to the thoracolumbar junction begins in the midaxillary line in the thoracic area and curves anteriorly over the tenth rib toward the lateral border of the rectus abdominus (see Fig. 10-8). The tenth rib may be identified by counting upward from the lowermost rib cage and is usually the highest rib that is not attached anteromedially to chondral cartilage.

## RIB RESECTION

Tenth-rib resection gives the most reliable exposure to the diaphragm and also affords the most consistent access to the thoracolumbar junction. Once the incision is made, dissection begins in the thoracic region to expose the rib. The electrocautery is employed to incise the overlying muscle to minimize blood loss, and the rib is exposed subperiosteally, cephalad and caudally with an Alexander elevator. A rib cutter is then used to cut the tenth rib close to the cartilage margin medially and as far posteriorly as the dissection permits at this point. The chest is then entered by cutting through the underlying pleura beneath the exposed periosteum. The resected rib is morselized for later use as bone graft and placed under a moist lap pad on the back table. The remaining portion of the rib attached to the cartilage is grasped with a Kocher clamp and held with upward tension while the opposite hand retracts the chest cavity with opposing counter traction. This maneuver permits blunt dissection to begin behind this region in the retroperitoneal fat. Blunt dissection is continued circumferentially to expose the retroperitoneum by separating the parietal peritoneum from the abdominal muscles anteromedially, continuing this dissection posteriorly toward the diaphragm and psoas muscle. It is important to begin this dissection anteromedially in the area of the transversalis fascia because this facilitates the entire exposure at a later point. Further incision of the abdominal musculature medial to this point also increases the exposure.

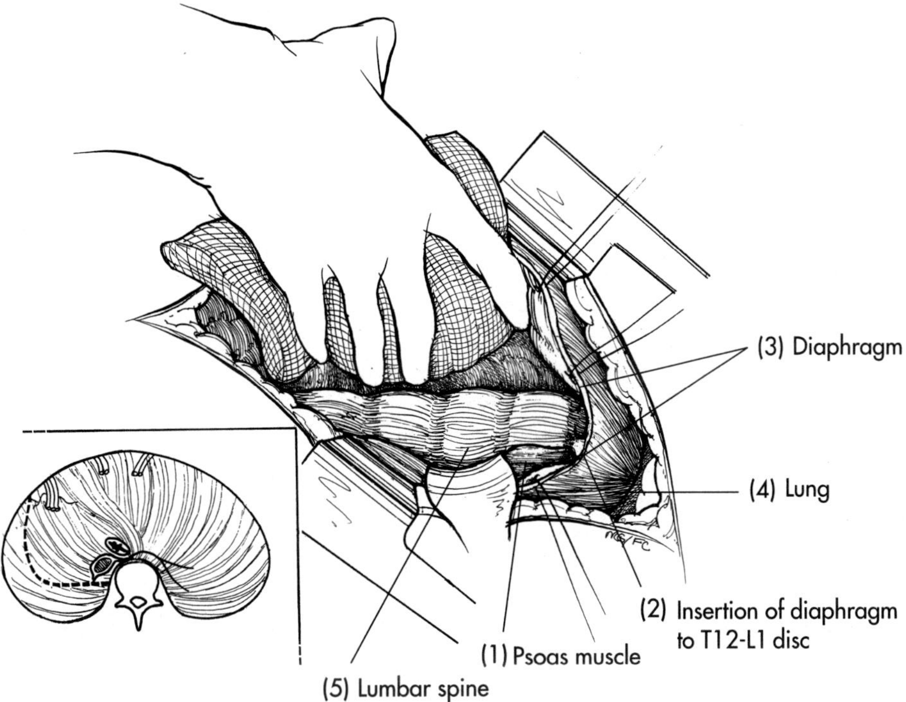


FIGURE 10-9

Division of diaphragm with preservation of all structural tissue under it, to its insertion to the T12-L1 disk space. (*1*) Psoas muscle; (*2*) insertion of diaphragm to T12-L1; (*3*) diaphragm; (*4*) lung; (*5*) lumbar spine.

## DIAPHRAGM INCISION

At this point in the dissection, the thoracic spine is clearly visible within the chest cavity. The diaphragm, psoas, and crural ligaments are also visible. The diaphragm is separated by the use of electrocautery preserving a 1-cm cuff of tissue by a curved incision that follows the lateral contour of the diaphragm and the underlying rib medially to its ultimate attachment to a vertebra or intervertebral disk (Fig. 10-9). It is best to continue this incision to an avascular part of the spine (i.e., a disk space). The psoas is then cleared of the overlying retroperitoneum. The segmental vessels are meticulously ligated in succession to facilitate the mobilization of the great vessels away from the anterior spine. These vessels are located midway between the disks, which are more prominent than the bodies. Once the first ligature is tied, it is used to elevate the vessel so that a second suture may be passed and tied, ("the Banjo technique"; see Fig. 10-7). A flap of the anterior longitudinal ligament and periosteum is created by incising a rectangle of periosteum and the anterior longitudinal ligament from the lateral aspect of the vertebral column. This flap is carefully developed with a Cobb, elevator paying particular attention so that the continuity of its length is preserved. A malleable retractor is then placed within this flap, affording an additional layer of tissue protecting vital organs from inadvertent injury (see Fig. 10-4). Closure of this periosteal flap at the conclusion of the procedure covers any hardware, and also helps to contain the formation of hematoma in this area and further promote bone healing. The elevation of this flap and the dissection and ligation of segmental vessels may precipitate vigorous bleeding, particularly from vertebral nutrient vessels. This type of bleeding is best addressed by packing the site with thrombin-soaked Gelfoam while dissection is continued in another area. At this point, the thoracolumbar junction is now adequately exposed and the dissection continues toward the specific goals of the procedure. At the conclusion of the procedure, the periosteal flap is closed by a running Vicryl suture. The anterior longitudinal ligament and periosteum are sewn back to the psoas aponeurosis and muscle. In some patients after instrumentation, closure of the flap is not practical but approximation is possible. The diaphragm is closed with a running Vicryl #1 suture. A chest tube is brought out proximally through a separate stab incision and later tied loosely to the skin with a silk tie. In our series, there have not been any complications from the use of this type of suture. An assistant holds the diaphragm with Babcock forceps while the surgeon sutures the diaphragm. The chest portion of the intercostal incision is closed with an interrupted #2 costal suture to approximate the ninth and eleventh ribs. Each muscle layer of the abdominal portion of the incision is closed separately with a running suture. The subcutaneous layer and skin are then approximated with a continuous Vicryl suture. The chest tube is attached to a Pleurevac drainage and the incision dressed.

### POTENTIAL PROBLEMS

Most of the problems encountered with this approach result from an unfamiliarity with the pertinent anatomy. The great vessels are vulnerable to injury, and in the absence of specific indications, the left-sided approach is to be preferred to avoid injury to the venous structures along the right side of the spinal column. The abdominal viscera are also susceptible to injury by excessive force during retraction. We do not routinely deflate the ipsilateral lung and this has not been a problem. The use of a malleable retractor placed in the chest cavity following incision of the diaphragm normally protects this lung from injury (see Fig. 10-3). By keeping the ipsilateral lung inflated, the problems associated with postoperative atelecstasis may be avoided, but this potentially exposes the lung to injury. Finally, bleeding problems should be approached systematically. Oozing blood from exposed bone is best managed by thrombin-soaked Gelfoam and gauze. If this fails to stop the blood loss, a bleeding segmental vessel on the opposite side of the dissection may be the culprit. In this event the vessel is clamped by a hemostat and a second right-angle clamp is applied more proximally with the elbow portion of the clamp. The vessel is then ligated. Pressure applied medially from the point of the spine at the hemorrhage is helpful in controlling the vessel.

A familiarity with basic vascular techniques is important in allowing the spinal surgeon to effectively undertake this approach. It should also be noted that the sympathetic ganglia are often encountered in the thoracolumbar area and these too are susceptible to injury. This should be avoided if at all possible, but injury to the sympathetic ganglion is frequently unavoidable in gaining adequate access to the anterolateral portion of the thoracolumbar junction. It follows that the patient should be warned preoperatively of the sequelae of this injury in addition to other possible complications. Diaphragmatic and retroperitoneal hernias are possible and best prevented by careful closure of the diaphragm, chest, and abdominal muscular layers. In our experience we have not seen a single case of diaphragmatic hernia following this type of closure. Weakness of the hip flexor due to detachment of the psoas muscle may be seen in some patients; this weakness gradually improves.

### AFTER CARE

The patient is usually kept on a patient-controlled analgesia device for at least the first 24 hours. Since intercostal pain is significant and interferes with pulmonary toilet, we recommend routine intercostal blockade with Marcaine and epidural anesthesia after operating proximal to the tenth rib level. This is especially helpful in patients with compromised pulmonary function. The chest tube is routinely removed when the Pleurevac output falls below 20 to 30 ml per shift.

Postoperative ileus is possible even with the indirect manipulation of the abdominal contents and may preclude feeding the patient. Clear liquids are given initially, and the diet is advanced according to subsequent bowel activity. In most cases the patient is ambulatory 1 or 2 days postoperatively and narcotic analgesia may be administered by mouth after the chest tube has been removed and the patient is tolerating a regular diet.

## ANTERIOR APPROACH TO THE LUMBOSACRAL JUNCTION

### PERTINENT ANATOMY

Successful anterior approach to the lumbosacral area can be accomplished only by a team that is thoroughly conversant with the method. It is a great advantage to rehearse the entire procedure with the anesthesiologist and nursing staff before attempting such a procedure. It is also critical to educate surgical assistants about the role they will play. Everyone must function efficiently to create a less stressful environment for the surgeon, to maximize the surgeon's efforts, and to minimize risk to the patient. The surgeon must be completely familiar with the anatomy of the rectus abdominus muscle, its fascia and neurovascular bundle. The nerve supply to the rectus abdominis enters the muscle from the lateral side so that a surgical exposure of the muscle from the lateral side jeopardizes the innervation of the muscle. The rectus muscle is enclosed in the rectus sheath. The anterior sheath is formed by the aponeurosis of the external oblique, which is fused to the anterior lamina of the internal oblique, split to embrace the rectus muscle. The posterior wall of the sheath is formed by fusion of the posterior lamina of the internal oblique and the transversus abdominis. This posterior wall is defective inferiorly and ends midway between the umbilicus and pubis. The lower border of the posterior wall is thickened and is known as the arcuate ligament and the inferior epigastric artery passes underneath this ligament to enter the sheath. Below the arcuate ligament the rectus lies on the transversalis fascia. It is important to identify the arcuate ligament because immediately below it is the entrance to the retroperitoneal space. Anterior to the lower lumbar and lumbosacral spine are the psoas muscle, iliac vessels, and ureter. The level of the bifurcation of the aorta varies, but normally it bifurcates at the L4-L5 disk space or at the upper part of L5 vertebral body. However, it might vary from L4 to S1. When the bifurcation is high, the surgeon should work between the iliac artery and vein. When low, the surgeon should work on the side of the aorta and the vena cava. In both situations careful attention to the ureter is mandatory. Ligation of the fifth lumbar artery and iliolumbar vein facilitates exposure of the L4-L5 disk and the midsacral vessels that bisect the L5-S1 disk should be ligated to operate on the lumbosacral disk. Prior to operation, the patient should be given prophylactic anticoagulants and antibiotics and should have an indwelling Foley catheter and tracheal intubation.

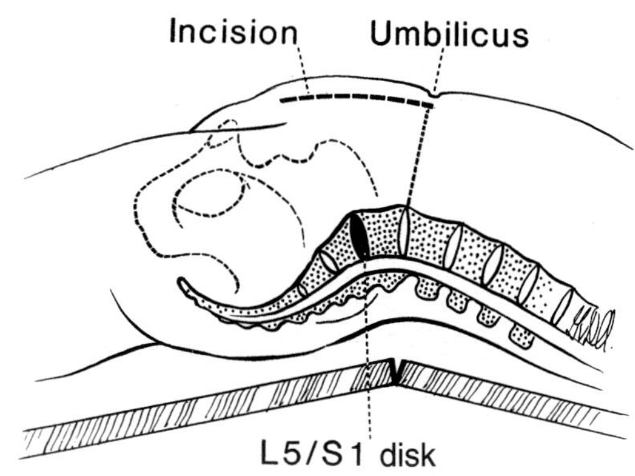


**FIGURE 10-10**

The operating room table is "broken" to facilitate hypoextension of the lumbar spine. In determining the level of the incision, the L4-L5 disk space is level with the umbilicus.

## POSITIONING

The patient is positioned supine on the operating table with the lumbar area overlying the break in the table. The table is then broken to allow hyperextension of the lumbar spine (Fig. 10-10). This tends to open the disk spaces and facilitates placement of an interbody graft. The abdomen should be shaved, avoiding the groin area. The operative area is circumscribed by disposable adhesive drapes prior to skin preparation. To help determine the level of the incision, remember that the L4-L5 disk space is at the level of the umbilicus (Fig. 10-11). The incision is made 2 cm lateral to the midline on the left side just cephalad to the umbilicus and continued to three fingerbreadths above the pubis (see Fig. 10-11). The incision is then carried sharply down to the fascia overlying the rectus muscle. The need to coagulate the fat may be obviated if there is effective compression on the skin edges. If the patient is not obese, it is best to tunnel just superficial to the fascial layer to the anterior iliac crest to avoid a second incision to obtain a bone graft (Fig. 10-12, *A*).

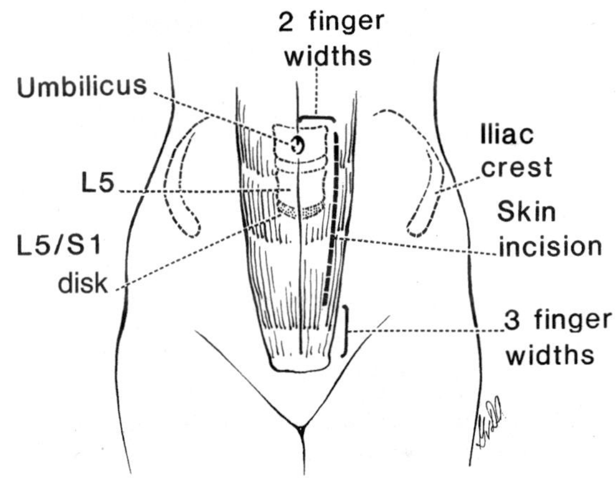


**FIGURE 10-11**

The incision is made 2 cm lateral to the midline on the left side, just cephalad to the umbilicus and continued to 3 fingerbreadths above the pubis.

To harvest bone for grafting, we use a method attributed to Harms, which preserves the upper border of the iliac crest. This method appears to alleviate some of the discomfort experienced by patients. The first step is to divide the fascia with electrocautery at the intermuscular line overlying the anterior crest starting 1 cm posterior to the anterior superior iliac spine and continuing posteriorly for 4 to 5 cm (Fig. 10-12, *B*). A subperiosteal dissection of the inner table with a Cobb elevator is then performed and the elevator left in place to serve as a retractor. A straight 0.5-inch osteotome is used to lift off a cortical window, beginning just deep to the top of the iliac crest (Fig. 10-12, *C*). The cancellous bone is harvested with a curette and ronguer (Fig. 10-12, *D*). At completion, Gelfoam is packed into the site and the fascia closed. We suture the subcutaneous fat to the fascia, thereby closing the dead space.

After taking the graft, the surgeon should stand on the patient's left side at the level of the knees. One assistant should be positioned next to the surgeon at the level of the chest and a second assistant on the right side (Fig. 10-13). A longitudinal incision is made through the fascia overlying the rectus muscle exposing the muscle body (Fig. 10-14, *A*). At this time a decision is made whether to go medially or laterally to the rectus muscle. Going laterally is technically easier but places the innervation of the muscle at a higher risk with the chance of hernia. For a medial exposure, the medial leaf of the fascia is grasped by a hemostat to allow dissection between fascia and muscle. We typically use a peanut or a finger, gently sweeping the muscle free from the undersurface of the posterior sheath. Occasionally, perforating vessels in the muscle are seen; these should be coagulated with cautery.

Once the most medial edge of the muscle has been reached, a sponge stick is used to sweep the transversalis fascia from the undersurface of the muscle. The

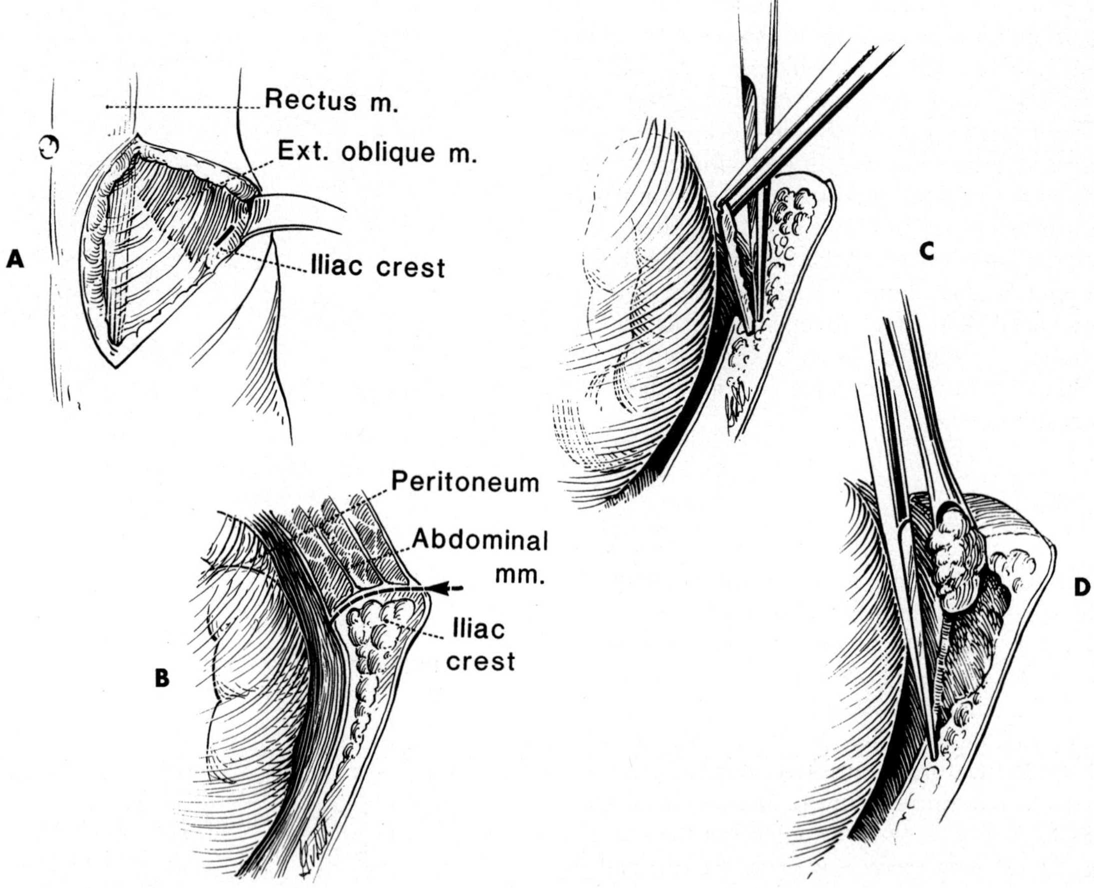


**FIGURE 10-12**

**(A)** The incision on the fascia of the rectus abdominus. It is tunneled just superficial to the fascial layer of the anterior iliac crest, thus avoiding a second incision to obtain a bone graft. **(B)** Dividing the fascia at the intermuscular line overlying the anterior crest.

epigastric vessels must be left attached to the undersurface of the muscle. The surgeon continues laterally until a point is reached where it appears the fascia is "stitched" into the lateral side. The arcuate ligament is then identified, marking the point of entrance to the retroperitoneal space.[7] In women this is a much more recognizable landmark. Using a sponge stick just caudad to the ligament in a gentle sweeping motion, the surgeon pushes downward and toward the midline, freeing the retroperitoneal fat from under the fascia. Because the peritoneum is more intimately attached to the fascia medially, it is necessary to keep the dissection lateral to avoid tears (Fig. 10-14, *B*). At this time the ligament can clearly be seen and should be divided at its attachment to the lateral wall. The surgeon continues to release cephalad 4 to 5 cm, always staying as far lateral as possible to avoid entering the peritoneal cavity. Care should be taken that the peritoneum and fat have been swept away from the undersurface before cutting the ligament. On releasing the ligament and fascial attachment the peritoneum can now be swept medially and cephalad. A large Deaver retractor is placed into the wound to help retract the abdominal contents. The handle of the retractor should always be pointing at the patient's right shoulder. A small Deaver retractor is used to retract the peritoneal contents in the more caudal area. This retractor is directed perpendicular to the long axis of the patient's body.

At this time the psoas muscle, iliac vessels, and ureter should be identified. If they can not be seen, the surgeon is dissecting posterior to the psoas and consequently putting the nerve roots at risk. Traction must never be applied to the ureter, and, before proceeding with the next step, all fat must be dissected clear from the vessels. The spine should now be palpated and the L5-S1 disk space located (Fig. 10-15, *A*). It is typically the most prominent point of the spine. At this juncture a radiograph should be taken to confirm the level. Now a small Deaver retractor should be used to retract the fat from this area, exposing the disk space. The retractor should be dipped so that the flat edge of the Deaver retractor is parallel to the spine. Dissection of

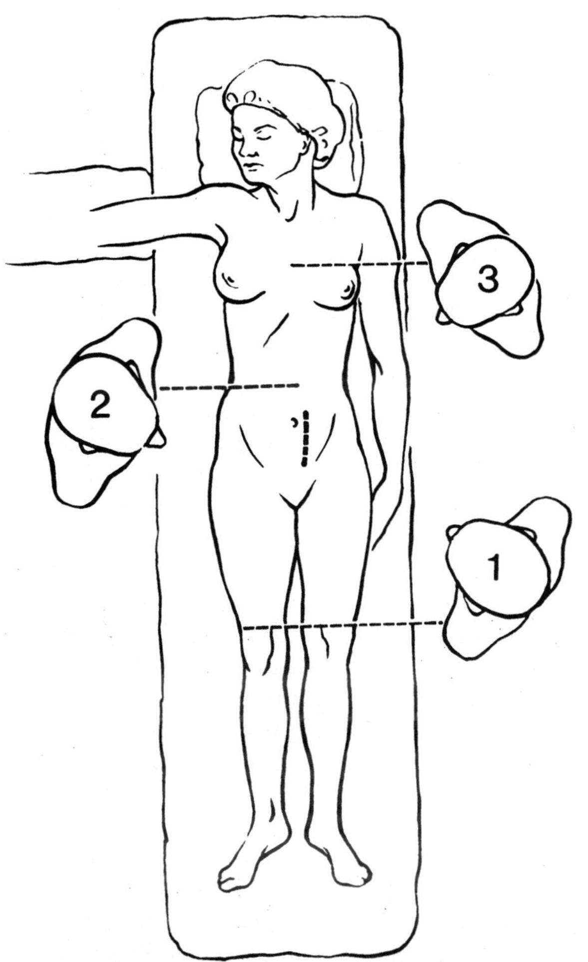


**FIGURE 10-13**

The surgeon should stand to the left side of the patient at the level of the knee (*1*). An assistant is on the patient's right side (*2*), and the other assistant is positioned next to the surgeon at the level of the patient's chest (*3*).

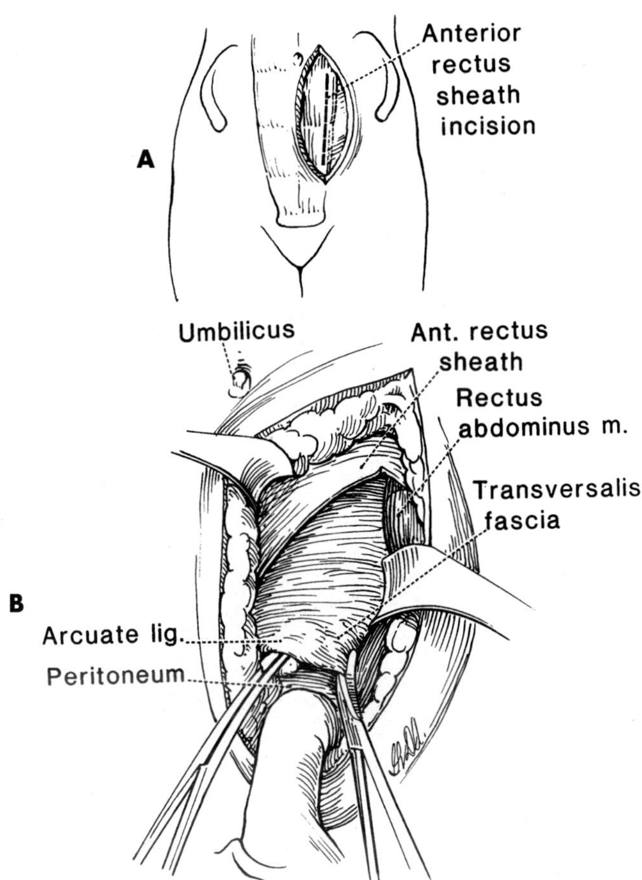


**FIGURE 10-14**

**(A)** A longitudinal incision is made through the fascia overlying the rectus muscle to expose the muscle belly. **(B)** The arcuate ligament marks the point of entrance to the retroperitoneal space. Using a sponge stick caudad to the ligament in a gentle sweeping motion, the surgeon pushes down and toward the midline to free the retroperitoneal fat from under the fascia.

any remaining soft tissue overlying the disk space is affected by dissection with a peanut and Yankauer suction to keep the field clear of blood. The soft tissue is peeled by the peanut while placing the soft tissue under traction with the reverse suction. This dramatically improves visualization and is important for placing the retractors. After clearing the soft tissue, a small vessel will remain. This is the middle sacral vessel and should be ligated at this time (Fig. 10-15, *B*).

To enter the disk space successfully, all intervening soft tissue must be retracted to avoid inadvertent injury to the iliac vessels. There are several different methods, including Deaver retractors, Steinmann pins, and Schmidt retractors. We use Schmidt retractors because they offer the greatest protection and typically ease the physical requirements of the assistants (Fig. 10-16, *A* and *B*). We place the right retractor first (Fig. 10-16, *C*). The soft tissue needs to be teased as far superiorly, inferiorly, and to the right prior to placing the retractor. The superior point is placed superior to the disk space into L5 and tapped into place. The retractor is rotated, keeping the inferior point against bone to avoid soft tissue entrapment, to a point where it is below the disk space and overriding the S1 body. The retractor is soundly tapped into position, and the small Deaver retractor is removed. This procedure is now repeated for the left side. Finally the large Deaver retractor is allowed to rest against the superior aspect of the retractors keeping the peritoneal contents behind it. A large malleable retractor is used in a similar fashion inferiorly to protect the bladder.

At this time, the annulus may be raised as a flap or may be completely resected. The advantage of a flap is that it holds the graft in at the end of the procedure and also assists in retraction of the vessels. The flap is created by making an H-type incision into the annulus with the long arms running parallel to the end plates. Sutures are placed into the flaps on either side

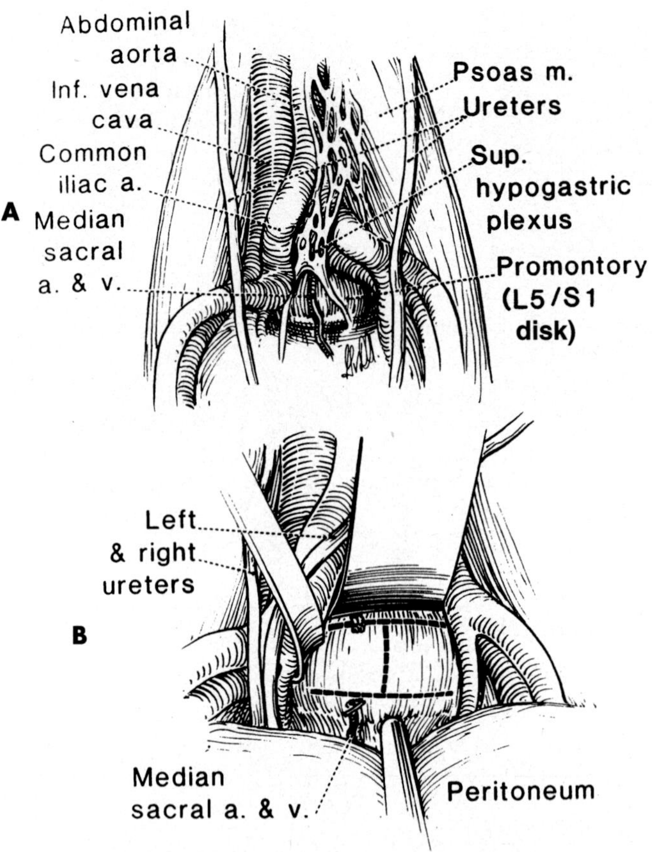


**FIGURE 10-15**

**A,** The psoas muscle, iliac vessel, and ureter should be identified. All fat must be dissected clear from the vessels. The spine is palpated and the L5-S1 disk space is ligated. **B,** A peanut and Yankauer suction is used to dissect any remaining soft tissue overlying the disk space. After the soft tissue is cleared, a small vessel will remain. This is the middle sacral vessel; it should be ligated.

and tagged. Retraction is facilitated by placing gentle traction on the suture ends (Fig. 10-16, *D*). The disadvantage of creating a flap is that it is a difficult technique and the flaps are often friable and tear easily with retraction. Alternatively a right- or left-side base flap is feasible. We generally resect the annulus in toto and have had no complications if all soft tissue has been completely retracted beforehand.

Once the annulus has been retracted, the disk space is evacuated. Using a large Cobb elevator, the end plates should be stripped off as far posterior as possible. Typically a posterior lip similar to that on an oil can may be used as a stopping gauge. The disk is removed completely using a ronguer and curette. It is important to never grasp anything outside the disk space. It is equally important that the curettes are kept within the disk space to obviate the risk of injuring a vessel. The end plates should be completely stripped of all soft tissue leaving the cortical end plate intact to support the interbody graft.

After placement of the graft, the wound is well-irrigated. The retractor on the right should be removed first. This should be done quickly and safely to avoid scraping along the vessels. At this point, bleeding should be checked. If no bleeding is present, the left retractor is removed. If using a Schmidt retractor, the surgeon must make sure that the soft tissue is swept from the tips of the retractor before removal.

The same approach is applicable to L4-L5 and L3-L4 disks. At these levels, the approach is much easier than L5-S1. We repair the transversalis fascia and rectus fascia by a running absorbable suture. We do not routinely place a drain in the wound.

Complications from this approach fall into five categories. The first, which is almost unavoidable, is that patients often are sympathectomized on the left. This is interpreted by the patient and family as a colder right foot. In actuality, the left foot is warmer because of the vasodilatation associated with the sympathectomy.

The second and most worrisome complication is vascular injury. The old adage that "an ounce of prevention is better than a pound of cure" certainly applies here. If enough of these procedures are performed, eventually a vascular injury occurs. When it does, it is best to attempt to ligate the vessel by a suture. If the tear is small enough, a hemoclip will suffice.

The third complication is often overlooked but equally important: injury to the ureter. The best advice is to be knowledgeable of the anatomy. If such an injury occurs, a consultant urologist is the best ally. Occasionally, in retroperitoneal surgery, especially with repeat dissections, there is a question of the integrity of the ureter. The ureter can be tested interoperatively for leakage. The technique is to inject 5 cc of methylene blue intravenously. Within 5 to 10 minutes, the methylene blue begins to concentrate in the urine. The ureter can be observed to turn blue. If there is a urine leak from the ureter, the blue color is evident in the wound.

The fourth complication is thromboembolic disease, which is prevented by having the patient wear compressive stockings during and after the procedure and ambulation as early as possible.

The fifth complication is incisional hernia resulting from closure of the flank wounds. This is especially likely to occur in older patients or patients with poor muscle mass. A way to help prevent the herniation is to place a piece of Marlex on the most superficial layer of muscle. After closure of the muscle, a strip of Marlex is laid over the incision overlapping 3 to 4 cm on either side of the incision. The Marlex is then sewn to the fascia with interrupted stitches to hold the Marlex down smooth and tight to the fascia. After wound closure, the fibrous tissue grows into the Marlex, reinforcing the incision.

In considering an anterior approach to the lumbosacral area, the principles involved must be under-

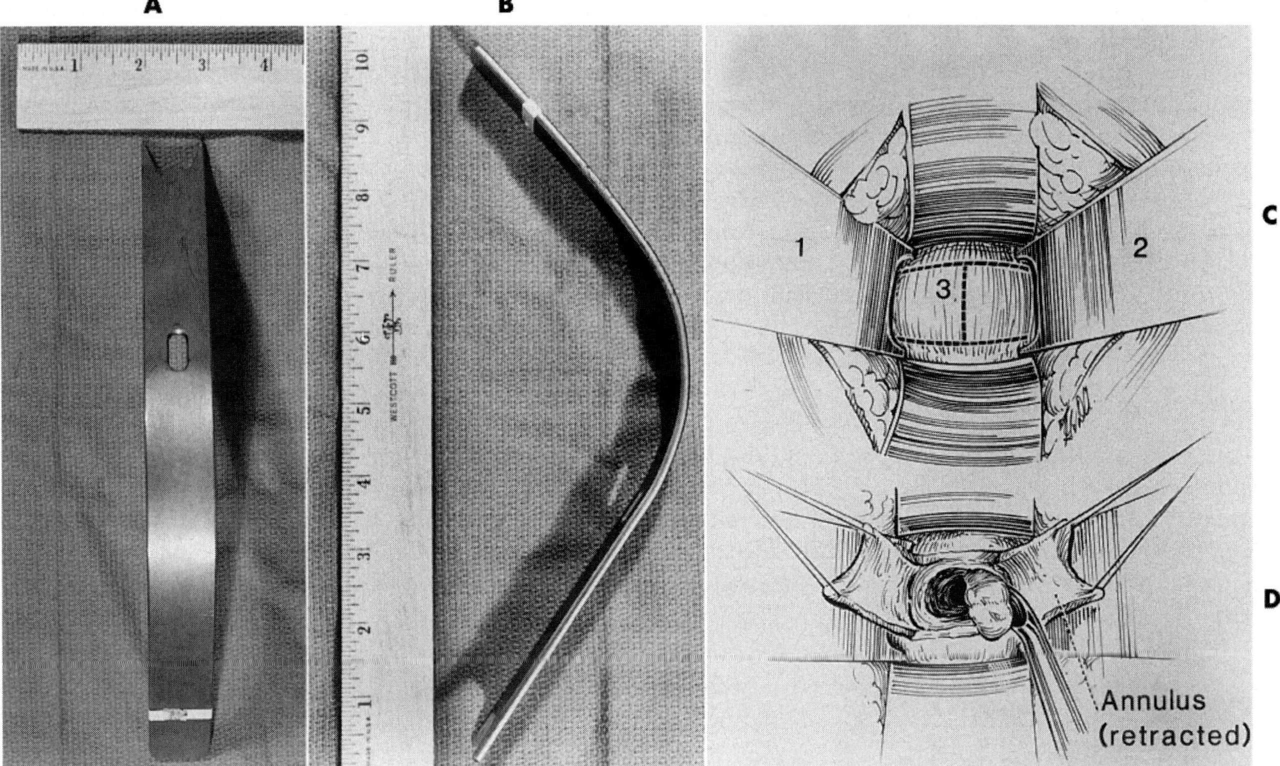


FIGURE 10-16

Schmidt retractor. **A,** Anteroposterior view. **B,** Lateral view. **C,** The retractors are placed. **D,** The flap is created by making an H-shaped incision into the annulus with the long arm running parallel to the end plates. Retraction is facilitated by placing gentle traction on the suture ends.

stood. A qualified spine surgeon with proper training can master this approach. It is important that, prior to the procedure, the surgeon has prepared the team to accomplish the approach. In addition, during the procedure, the focus must be on the patient and not on extraneous activities within the operating room. The surgeon needs to avoid distractions, have arrangements made for all the necessary equipment, and have the confidence to deal with any complication that might arise. The anterior approach to the lumbosacral joint, although difficult, is not unmanageable and the benefits of such a procedure far outweigh the risks.

## EXTENSILE APPROACH TO THE ANTERIOR SPINE

A longer portion of anterior spine may be exposed by combining the individual approaches described as continuous segments. This extensile incision combines the incisions of the approaches described and is tailored to the desired goals of an individual anterior procedure. It would be unlikely to conceive of a procedure requiring the exposure of the entire anterior spine and thus the concept of extensile exposure is offered to emphasize the continuity of the anterior approaches we have discussed. The individual approaches are by design sequentially conterminous for the ultimate purpose of continuity.

### POSITIONING

Positioning is similar to that of the exposure of the thoracolumbar area and the entire chest, flank, and abdomen are draped out.

### INCISION

The incision includes those of individual approaches that, when combined, afford the surgeon with the exposure necessary to perform a given procedure. As an example, the exposure of the anterior spine from T4 to L4 is described to illustrate important features of the extensile approach. A continuous incision is made from the scapula, curving over the thorax and abdomen anteriorly and inferiorly. Following subcutaneous dissection, a *thoracotomy* is performed in the upper thorax with rib removal as needed to permit exposure of the corresponding segment of the anterior spine. Further subcutaneous dissection inferiorly exposes the lower ribs. The thoracolumbar junction is then exposed as previously described. The inferior aspect of the thoracolumbar incision may be extended through the abdomen in continuity with the proximal portion of the lumbosacral approach as previously discussed. The spine is now exposed from T4 to L4 and the intrathoracic portion of the procedure takes place alternatively between the two "windows" in the thoracic cavity, namely, the upper rib thoracotomy and tenth rib thoracotomy (Fig. 10-17). At the conclusion of the procedure, a chest tube is placed through a separate stab incision and the wound is closed in layers.

## COMPLICATIONS

In addition to the potential complications discussed, exposing a larger segment of the anterior spine with the extensile approach presents additional concerns. A larger bleeding surface and longer operative time may contribute to excessive blood loss requiring transfusion. Every effort should be made to perform those portions of the procedure that have the greatest potential for blood loss, such as corpectomies, toward the conclusion of the procedure when feasible to minimize ongoing blood loss. Liberal use of Gelfoam, thrombin, and gauze packing help to minimize sanguineous oozing from exposed bone. The length of the exposure and longer operative times can also lead to wound desiccation, which predisposes tissues to surface necrosis and subsequent infection. At frequent intervals, the superficial areas of skin and adipose tissue should be liberally moistened with saline irrigation. Retractors should be released periodically when not in use. Hypothermia may result from a large exposure open for an extended time. Every effort should be made to use warm irrigation, room temperature control, and a Bair Hugger device. Preoperatively, the operating room temperature should remain elevated and the patient kept covered until the time comes for positioning and

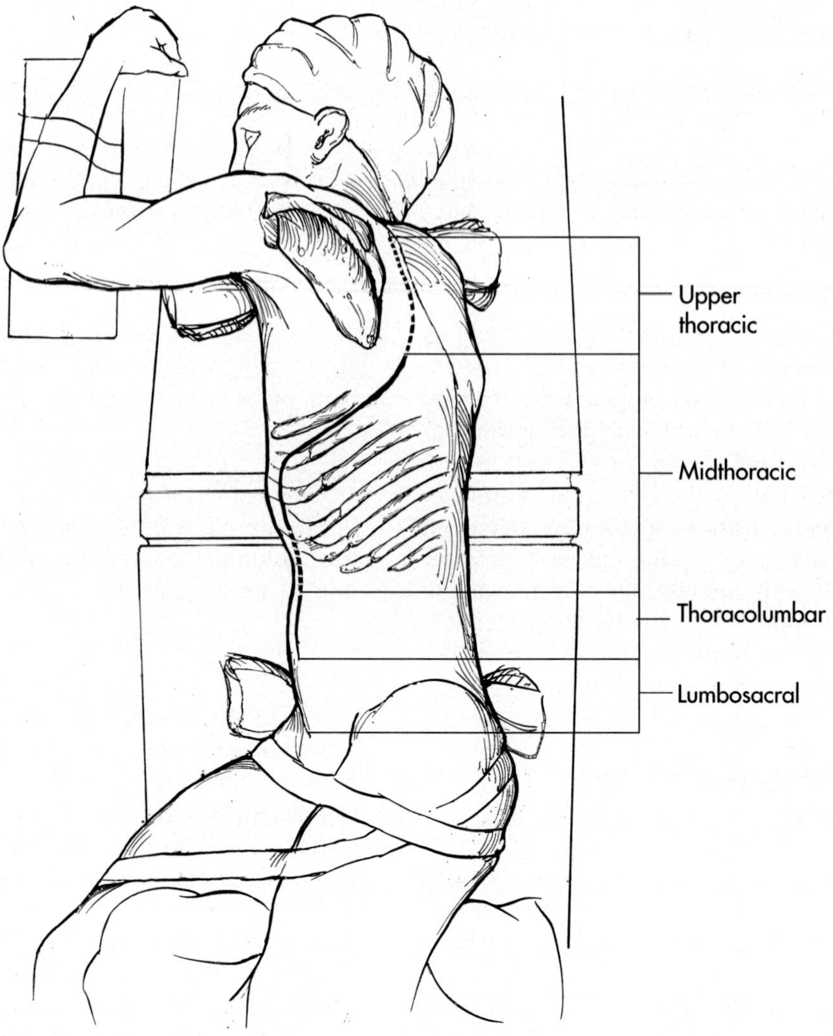


**FIGURE 10-17**

Extensile approach for exposure of the upper, midthoracic, thoracolumbar, and lumbosacral spine.

skin preparation. Hypothermia contributes to coagulation abnormalities, which are often life threatening. Finally, the preparation and training of the operating room staff, the preoperative checking of instrumentation, and efficient cooperative teamwork are noble precepts important to any surgical endeavor, but these cannot be overemphasized in the performance of an extensile anterior procedure. The surgeon's confidence in his own ability is crucial to its success and this is engendered by his awareness of and commitment to the important details of the technique, and rehearsal in his/her mind prior to the procedure.

## REFERENCES

1. Grob D, Scheier HJ, Dvorak J, Siegrist H, Rubeli M, Joller R: Circumferential fusion of the lumbar and lumbosacral spine. *Arch Orthop Trauma Surg* 111:20-25, 1991.
2. Freebody D, Bedall R, Taylor RD: Anterior transperitoneal lumbar fusion, *J Bone Joint Surg* 53B:617-627, 1971.
3. Perry J: *Surgical approaches to the spine.* In Pierce D, Nichol V, editors: *The total care of spinal cord injuries,* Boston, 1977, Little, Brown, pp 53-81.
4. Winter RB, Lonstein JE, Denis F, Smith MO: *Atlas of spine surgery,* 1995, Philadelphia, WB Saunders Co.
5. Watkins RG: *Surgical approaches to the spine,* Saunders, NY, 1983, Springer Verlag.
6. Hodgson AR, Yau ACMC: *Anterior surgical approaches to the spinal column.* In Apley AG, editor: *Recent advances in orthopaedics,* Baltimore, 1964, Williams & Wilkins, pp 289-323.
7. Harmon PH: Anterior extraperitoneal lumbar disc excision and vertebral bone fusion. *Clin Orthop* 16:169-198, 1963.

# 11

# SALVAGE OF SEVERE FLEXION DEFORMITIES OF THE THORACOLUMBAR SPINE

**Marc A. Asher, M.D.**



Loss of sagittal plane alignment into a severe fixed flexion deformity, either hyperkyphosis or hypolordosis, may occur following attempted treatment of almost any spinal disorder. The principal two causes for this are failure to achieve normal sagittal plane alignment during surgery and loss of sagittal plane alignment following surgery, such as from posterior column weakening following laminectomy, fusion mass pseudarthrosis, end instrumented vertebra angulation, or adjacent segment add-on. The patient's chief complaint is usually back pain, typically at the apex of maximum loss of sagittal plane alignment, but occasionally remote from it, principally at the lumbosacral junction. In addition, patients are usually unhappy with their appearance. Neurological compromise may occur, but is uncommon.

Reconstruction involves the problems associated with the need to simultaneously shorten the posterior column, lengthen the anterior column, and provide stabilization posteriorly and quite often, structural graft anteriorly. In addition, corpectomy is occasionally needed.

Farcey has been a leading proponent of a simultaneous exposure approach to these problems, with positioning the patient in the orthogonal (90° ) lateral decubitus position and on the edge of the side of the table so that the teams working posteriorly and anteriorly can proceed at the same time. The advantages of this approach in Farcey's hands are an excellent reconstruction and an operative time similar to that of only one approach.[1,5] The disadvantages are that it requires two fully trained surgical teams and implant placement, decompression, and posterior osteotomy may be more difficult in the lateral decubitus position than in the prone position.

A possible solution is a sequential-simultaneous procedure in which the patient is first operated in the prone position on a four-poster frame, with as much of the operation as possible done in this more comfortable operating position. Then the patient is turned to a 90° lateral decubitus position, and the operation is completed with both anterior and posterior columns exposed. Thus, two experienced surgical teams are unnecessary, and much of the posterior surgery is easier. The trade-off is a longer operative time.

The purposes of this chapter are to describe the sequential-simultaneous technique, providing examples and a preliminary report on experience to date.

## PATIENT AND SURGEON PREPARATION

The patient must have trunk deformity and pain of such a degree that the surgeon is comfortable recommending reconstruction. The patient must understand the possible severe complications, including death (be it ever so unlikely), paralysis of varying degrees, infection, pseudarthrosis, implant-related problems, and chronic pain. Also, any patient should understand that there is a 20% incidence of reoperation and that usually their pain will not be totally resolved. While trunk alignment will be greatly improved, a patient will have some rather long incisions.

Preoperative planning includes a complete analysis of the patient's spine deformity, including standing 36-inch posteroanterior and lateral radiographs, as well as cross-table lateral with bolster at the apex of the flexion deformity radiographs. Normal sagittal plane alignment is now well-known and provides the goal of realignment (Fig. 11-1).[3,4,6]

A careful preoperative assessment will address possible levels of posterior osteotomy, instrumentation levels, type of instrumentation to be used posteriorly, side of anterior approach, surgery necessary from the front (diskectomy or corpectomy), levels to be operated, and type of graft to be used (allograft, autograft, or a combination and whether structural or nonstructural).

For thoracic hyperkyphosis and thoracolumbar kyphosis, the extent of treatment is dependent upon the preoperative sagittal plane configuration of the spine. In the absence of thoracic hyperkyphosis preoperatively, that is hyperkyphosis above the area of pathological kyphosis, a short segment reconstruction can be done, usually two vertebrae above and two below the involved vertebra.

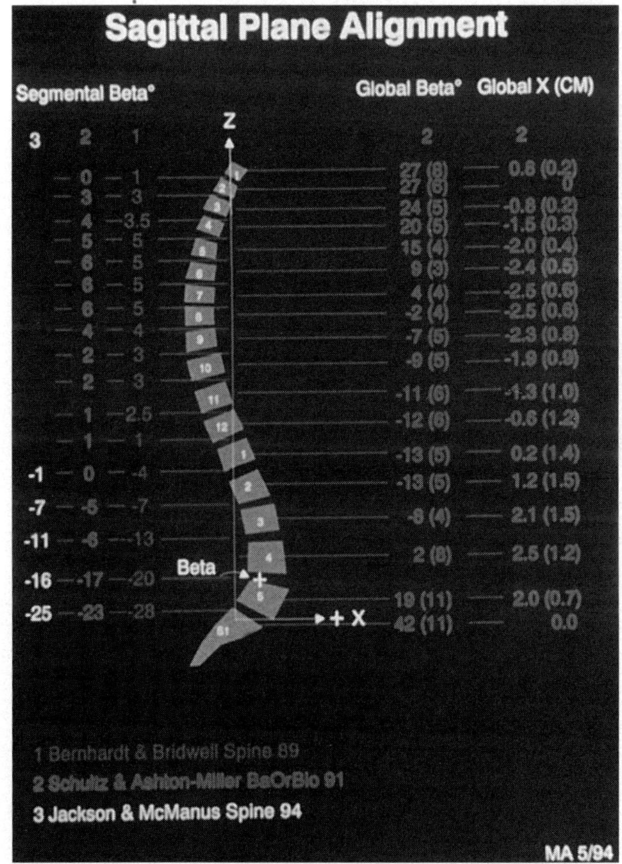


**FIGURE 11-1**

Normal sagittal plane alignment of the thoracolumbar spine. (Beta is in degrees; see References 3,5, and 6.) (From Asher M: Isola spinal instrumentation system for scoliosis. In Bridwell KH and DeWald RL, editors: *The textbook of spinal surgery,* ed 2, Philadelphia, 1997, Lippincott-Raven.)

In the presence of preexisting hyperkyphosis, the upper instrumented level should extend to a level of normal spine alignment, usually above T10 and below T1.

The lowest instrumented level, assuming pedicle screw anchorage is used, is generally the vertebra above the first normally sagittally aligned motion segment caudal to the hyperkyphosis/kyphosis deformity.

Posterior instrumentation consists of an upper and a lower foundation. A foundation is defined as two or more anchors stable and strong to the point that corrective loads can be delivered and deforming loads resisted. For thoracic hyperkyphosis and thoracolumbar kyphosis, the upper instrumented foundation anchors are usually hooks placed in claw configurations, either intrasegmental transverse process facet claws or intersegmental supralaminar-sublaminar staggered claw foundations. An alternative in the high thoracic spine is multiple fully segmental double sublaminar wires. For lumbar hypolordosis, the upper foundation is formed with pedicle screws.

In virtually all instances (e.g., thoracic hyperkyphosis, thoracolumbar kyphosis, and lumbar hypolordosis), the lower foundation is formed of pedicle screws that are as large, long, and as triangulated as possible. Four are usually adequate; six are always adequate. The only exceptions are those patients whose pedicles are simply too small to accept pedicle screws. In these instances, intersegmental laminar hook claws are recommended, generally requiring an extension of the instrumentation one vertebral segment distally.

With lumbar hypolordosis, especially in the lower lumbar spine, an instrumented long-fuse short procedure can be planned with care during the surgery to preserve the integrity of the facet joint and its capsule at the motion segments. The anterior approach is generally performed from the right for thoracic hyperkyphosis and from the left for thoracolumbar kyphosis and lumbar hypolordosis. The level entered is generally one level above the upper vertebral body to be operated on.

## SURGICAL TECHNIQUE

General considerations include all those associated with major spine surgery, which have been thoroughly detailed recently.[2]

Operating table preparation includes the means for obtaining lateral x-rays of the patient in the 90° orthogonal position at the edge of the table. This involves adding a platform to the operating table, such as a three-quarter inch plywood board and transversely placed two-by-fours (Fig. 11-2). The four-poster frame is set on this, and the patient positioned on the

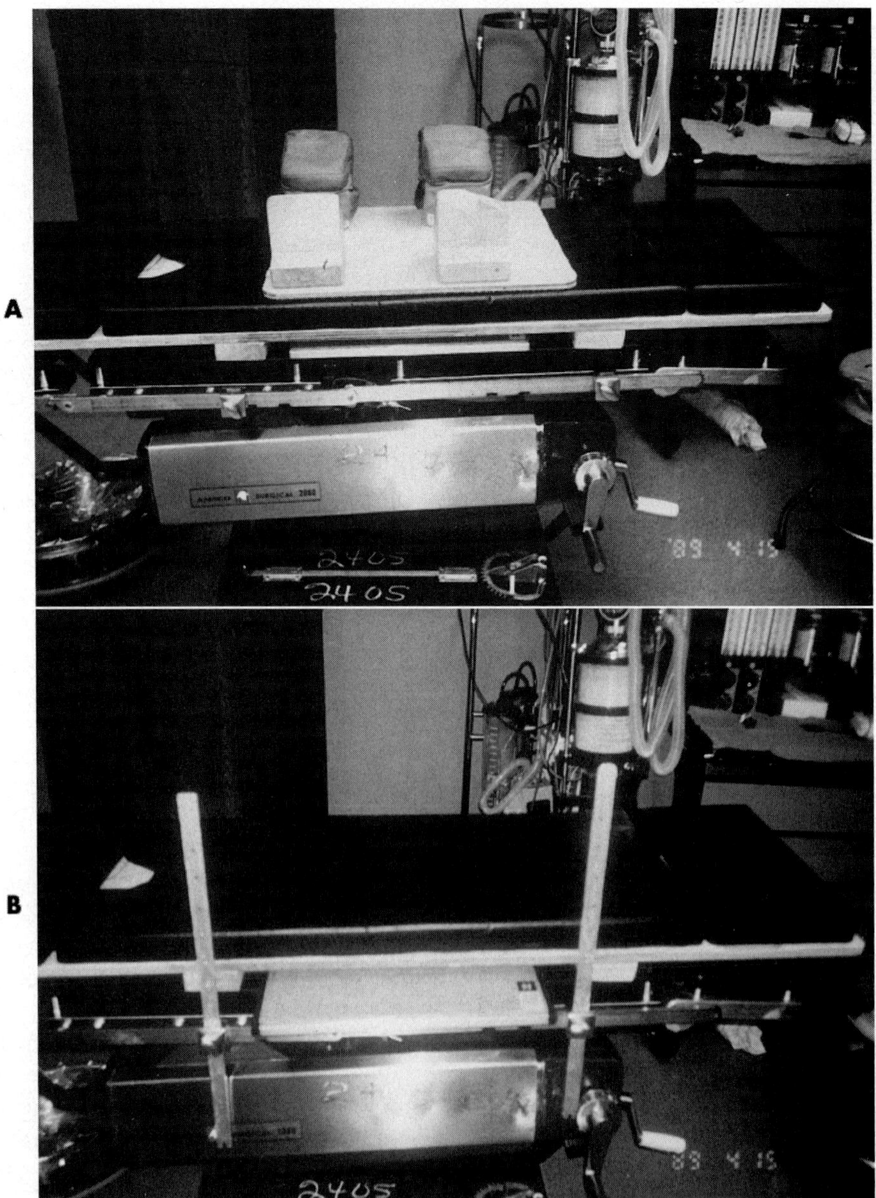

**FIGURE 11-2**

Operating table set-up showing $\frac{1}{4}$-inch (6.35 mm) plywood riser and four-poster frame partially prepared for patient's prone position (**A**) and partially prepared for the patient's 90-degree orthogonal lateral position (**B**). The vertical posts allow the patient to be positioned at the edge of the table, which is necessary to permit access to the posterior incision. The plywood riser enables lateral radiographs to be taken with the patient at the edge of the operating table.

four-poster frame in the usual manner with all the precautions previously described.[2] A larger-than-usual surgical preparation and draping of the back is done for the posterior incision. Adhesive drape is placed after the existing surgical scars have been marked and all the other drapes have been placed.

The posterior procedure is conducted in the standard manner with placement of the anchors of the upper as well as the lower foundation, followed by osteotomy and decompression as necessary, and longitudinal member placement into the upper anchors, including placement of the transverse connection. This creates the upper cantilever foundation. A facet fusion is done prior to creation of this foundation, as it is in the lower foundation area as well. Slotted connectors are placed on the rod and brought down onto the posts of the variable screw placement (VSP) screws with nuts placed to hold as much reduction as possible.

For short segment kyphosis, it is necessary to use short post screws, at least adjacent to the kyphotic deformity, in order for the slotted connectors to feed over the screws. An alternative that may be considered in the low thoracic spine is closed head screws for the upper foundation and open connection screws for the lower. If this option is chosen, care should be taken in placing the screws to be sure that the connections line up with each other. Markers are quite helpful for this, with placement of end markers before intermediate markers and end screws before intermediate screws.

Once the posterior procedure has been advanced as far as it can, the incision is packed with kidney tape and the skin closed with interrupted heavy duty temporary stitches. The Vi-Drape surface is rinsed and thoroughly dried and covered with two additional layers ofVi-Drape. At this point the scrub nurse moves his/her material away and all draping is removed, except the Vi-Drape adherent to the skin. Using a minimum of six lifters (the anesthesiologist for the head, a person for both legs, and two people on either side of the trunk), the patient is lifted directly off the table. A seventh person removes the four-poster frame and places the bean bag on the padded table. The patient is then rotated into the appropriate left or right lateral decubitus position.

Various precautions are taken when placing the patient in the lateral decubitus position. The patient is moved directly to the edge of the table and secured there in the 90° orthogonal lateral position not only with the bean bag but also with posterior uprights at the shoulder and buttocks levels. The reason the patient must be at the edge of the table is to provide surgical access to the posterior incision.

## THE ANTERIOR PROCEDURE

The patient's trunk is surgically prepared and sterilely draped, including previously placed adhesive Vi-Drape over the posterior incision. The anterior approach is made in the routine manner, entering through the rib one or sometimes two levels above the upper operated disk space. The appropriate diskectomies and corpectomies are performed. At this point, the Vi-Drape over the posterior incision is incised, and the temporarily placed sutures are removed, thus re-exposing the posterior operative site.

Cantilever reduction of the sagittal plane deformity is continued by further approximating the caudal ends of the rod to the caudal anchors. As this occurs, the opening anteriorly is monitored. In order to obtain full advantage of the simultaneous approach, it is essential that the contouring of the rods be accurate to restore sagittal plane alignment. Because there is some elastic deformation of the rods, it is generally desirable to overbend them by 5° to 10°

Choice of graft material anteriorly is dictated by the level and extent of the deformity. If multiple level diskectomies are being done and the lowest instrumented motion segment disk is intact, a thorough packing of the disk spaces with nonstructural autograft from the approached rib is appropriate. If added bone graft is needed, a nonadjacent rib can be partially removed.

The posterior instrumentation is completed along with placement of graft posteriorly. Recommended tightening sequences of the instrumentation are carefully followed. A second transverse connection is placed distally.

In the presence of large disk defects in the upper lumbar spine and particularly when the lowest instrumented motion segment has had a large anterior void created with diskectomy, a structural bone graft such as femoral or humeral allografts filled with autograft rib or crest bone is recommended. Careful shaping with a power burr is necessary to obtain the tightest fit possible. In the presence of a corpectomy defect, a structural graft is essential. In the mid and upper thoracic spine this can be accomplished with three or four appropriate length autologous rib pieces bundled together with two separated heavy silk ties and carefully shaped for a tight fit with a power instrument. At the thoracolumbar junction and in the lumbar spine, carefully shaped, bundled autologous fibula or allograft femoral or humeral cortical shafts thoroughly packed with autograft may be used. Prior to closure, the wounds are thoroughly irrigated with warm saline. In addition, the posterior incision is thoroughly irrigated with an antibiotic solution using a pulse lavage delivery.

Closures are done in the standard manner. The most difficult closure is posterior because of the awkward position. Great care is taken to secure the deep fascia to any remaining midline spinous processes with interrupted permanent sutures or in the absence of midline spinous processes with suture passage under the spinal implants. A midline running hemostat locking absorbable suture is then placed. During closure of the deep subcutaneous tissue with running non-locking suture, frequent passage of the needle through the deep fascia is done to further close the dead space. A subcutaneous Hemovac exiting near the upper/cephalad end of the incision is recommended. Skin closure posteriorly is almost always done with staples, whereas the anterior lateral incision may be closed with subcuticular suture.

## PATIENT EXAMPLES

Thoracolumbar hyperkyphosis with one or two motion segments is best corrected with two-vertebra fixation above and below and structural graft as shown in Figure 11-3. When the hyperkyphosis extends over many segments, nonstructural autograft is appropriate.

In the lower lumbar spine, it is best to keep instrumentation and fusion as short as possible but sometimes instrumentation long-fusion short is appropriate as shown in Figure 11-4.

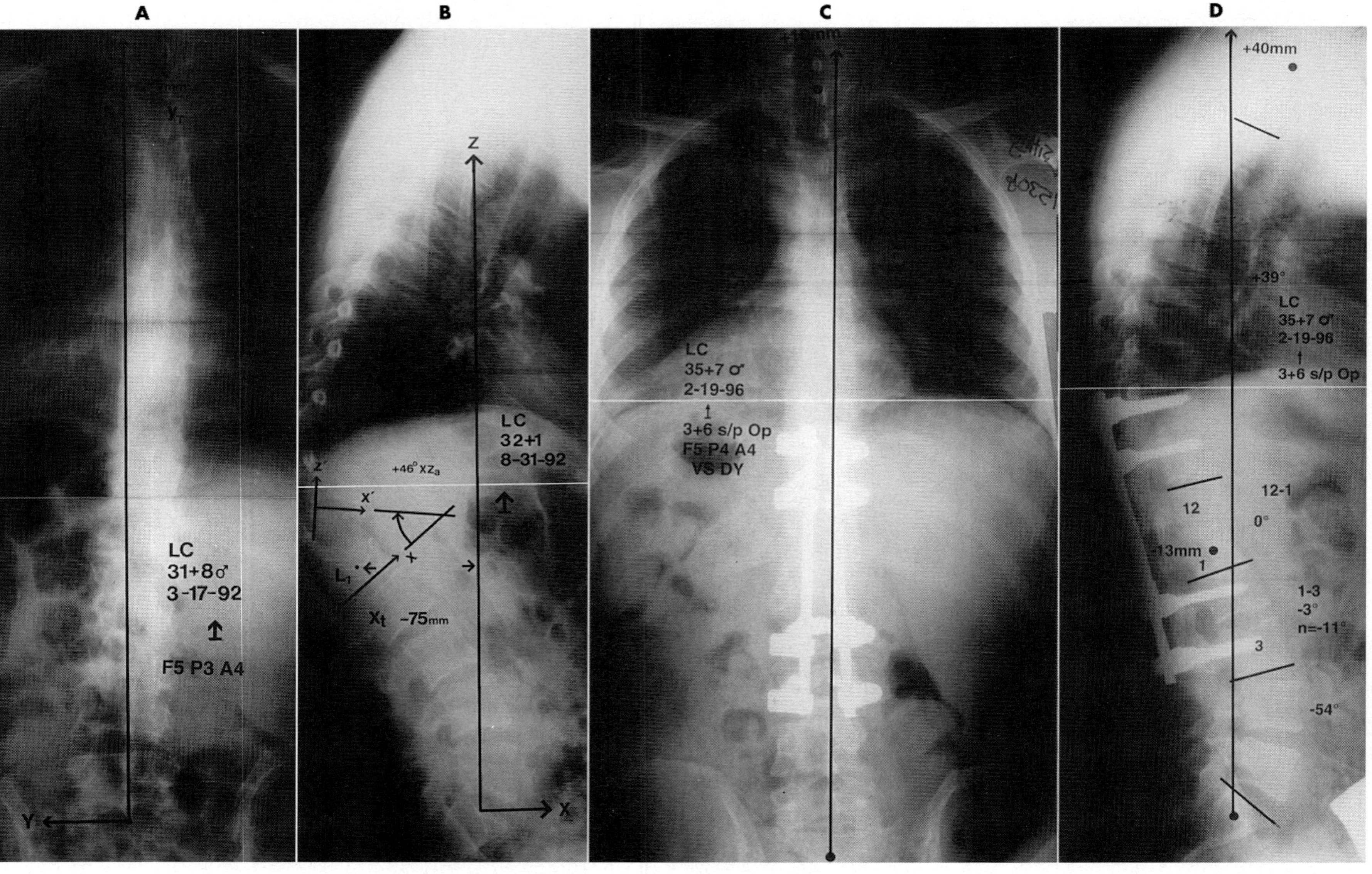


**FIGURE 11-3**

Thirty-one-year-old man with posttraumatic hyperkyphosis who had previously been operated. Preoperative posteroanterior (**A**), lateral (**B**), and most recent follow-up posteroanterior (**C**) and lateral (**D**) radiographs are shown.

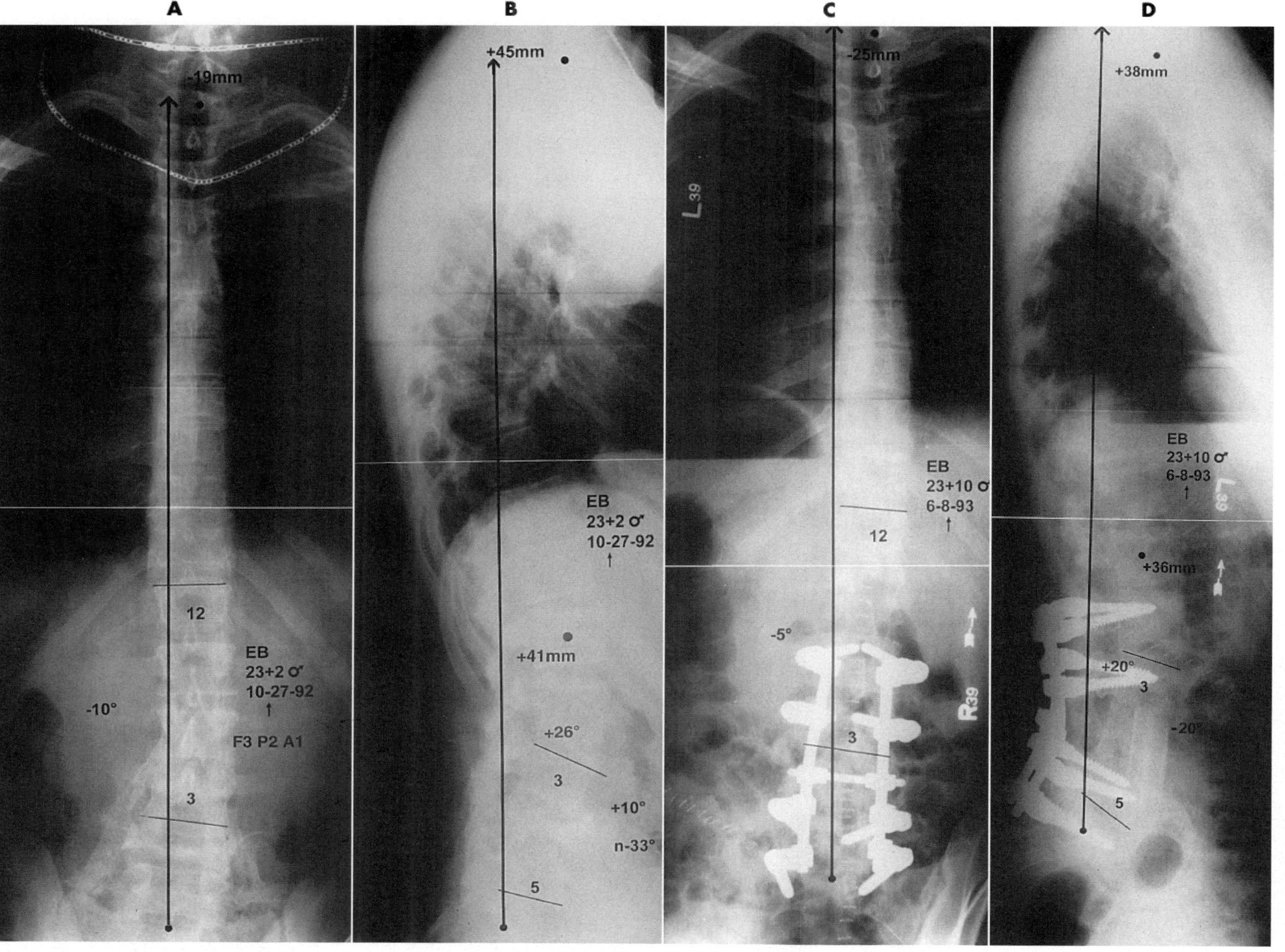


## FIGURE 11-4

A 23-year-old man, who sustained an L4 burst fracture and had previous posterior instrumentation and fusion with subsequent hypolordosis. Standing preoperative posteroanterior (**A**) and lateral (**B**) radiographs illustrate the hypolordosis. In an effort to save critical motion segments, he was initially instrumented long, L2 to sacrum (**C** and **D**), and subsequently shortened to L3-L5 (**E**), in spite of the fact that he had had a previous L5-S1 fusion attempt but with pseudarthrosis and intact facet joints.

*Continued*

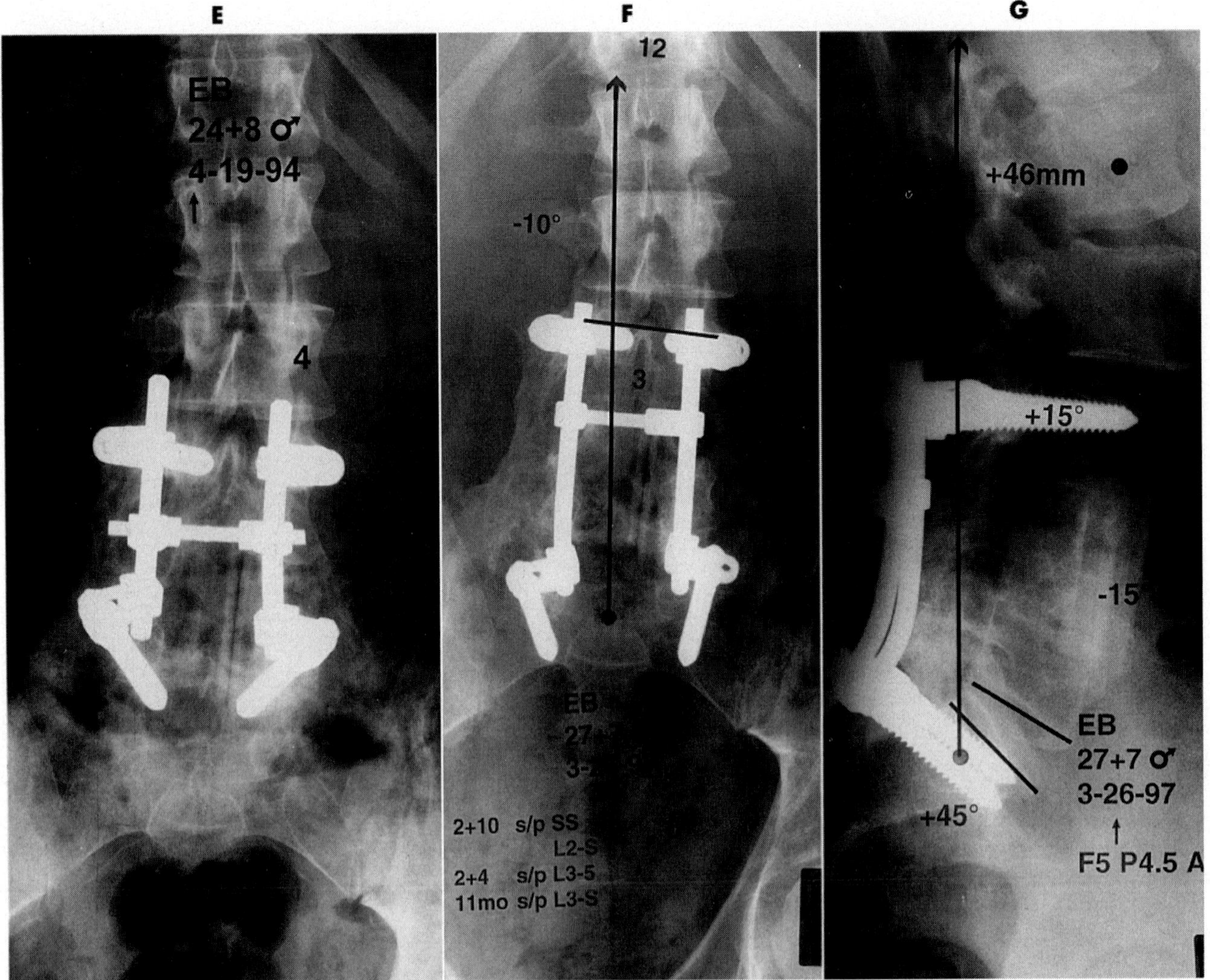


**Figure 11-4, cont'd**

He subsequently developed dynamic L5 radicular pain and instrumentation. Fusion was extended with satisfactory resolution of symptoms. His latest standing posteroanterior (**F**) and lateral (**G**) radiographs show satisfactory sagittal plane alignment and no suggestion of degeneration of the previously instrumented L2-L3 motion segment.

Sequential-simultaneous surgery of the thoracolumbar spine is useful in the salvage of nontraumatic disorders. An example of idiopathic scoliosis salvage is shown in Figure 11-5 and of degenerative disk disorder salvage in Figure 11-6.

## CASE SERIES

From 1992 through 1997, 17 patients (9 males, 8 females) ranging in age from 14 years to 48 years were operated. The index diagnoses were posttraumatic hyperkyphosis (10), adolescent idiopathic scoliosis salvage (1), chondroplasia (1), metastatic cancer (1), spondyloepiphysiodysplasia (1), Scheuermann's kyphosis (1), Scheuermann's kyphosis salvage (1), and degeneration (1).

Ten patients had had prior surgery (average of 2.3 prior surgeries). Their average operative time was 700 minutes, blood loss was 2200 cc, and hospital stay was 8 days. There were no deaths, neurological complications, acute or delayed wound infections, or acute instrumentation failures in these ten salvage patients or in the seven primarily operated patients.

Of the ten salvage patients, three have required reoperation. One was reoperated for pseudarthrosis and an osteotomy of the posterior fusion mass done with compression applied. There was satisfactory healing. One patient has recently required reoperation for what is believed to be pain related to implant soft tissue irritation. This outcome is pending. One had planned construct shortening with the subsequent need to re-add the L5-S1 motion segment, the site of a previous arthrodesis attempt, but pseudarthrosis.

*Text continued on page 166*

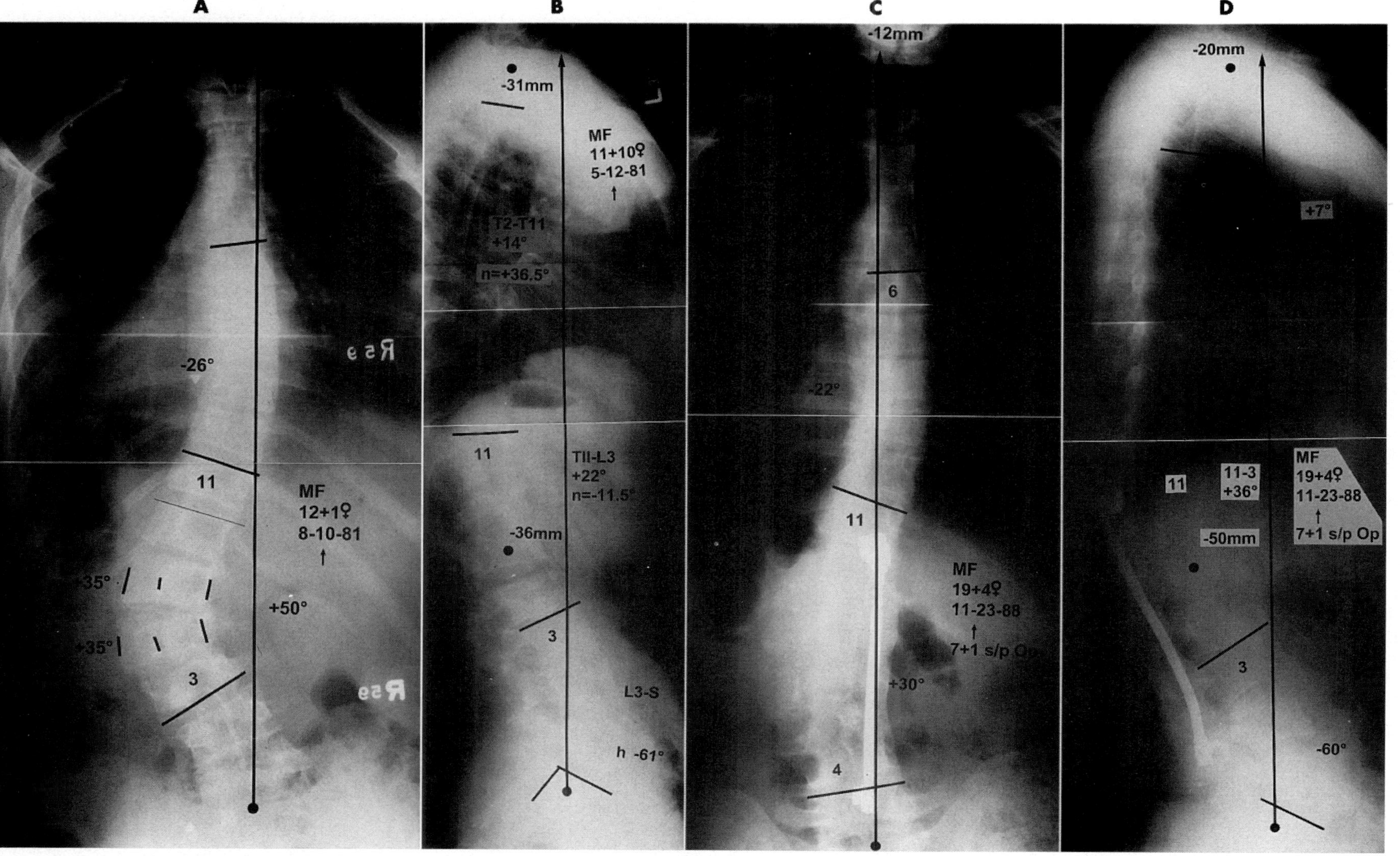


**FIGURE 11-5**

Preoperative posteroanterior (**A**) and lateral (**B**) radiographs of a 12-year-old girl with idiopathic scoliosis who was originally operated with Harrington distraction instrumentation for her lumbar scoliosis. Seven years later she presented with low back pain. Her standing posteroanterior (**C**) and lateral (**D**) radiographs show thoracolumbar kyphosis.

*Continued*

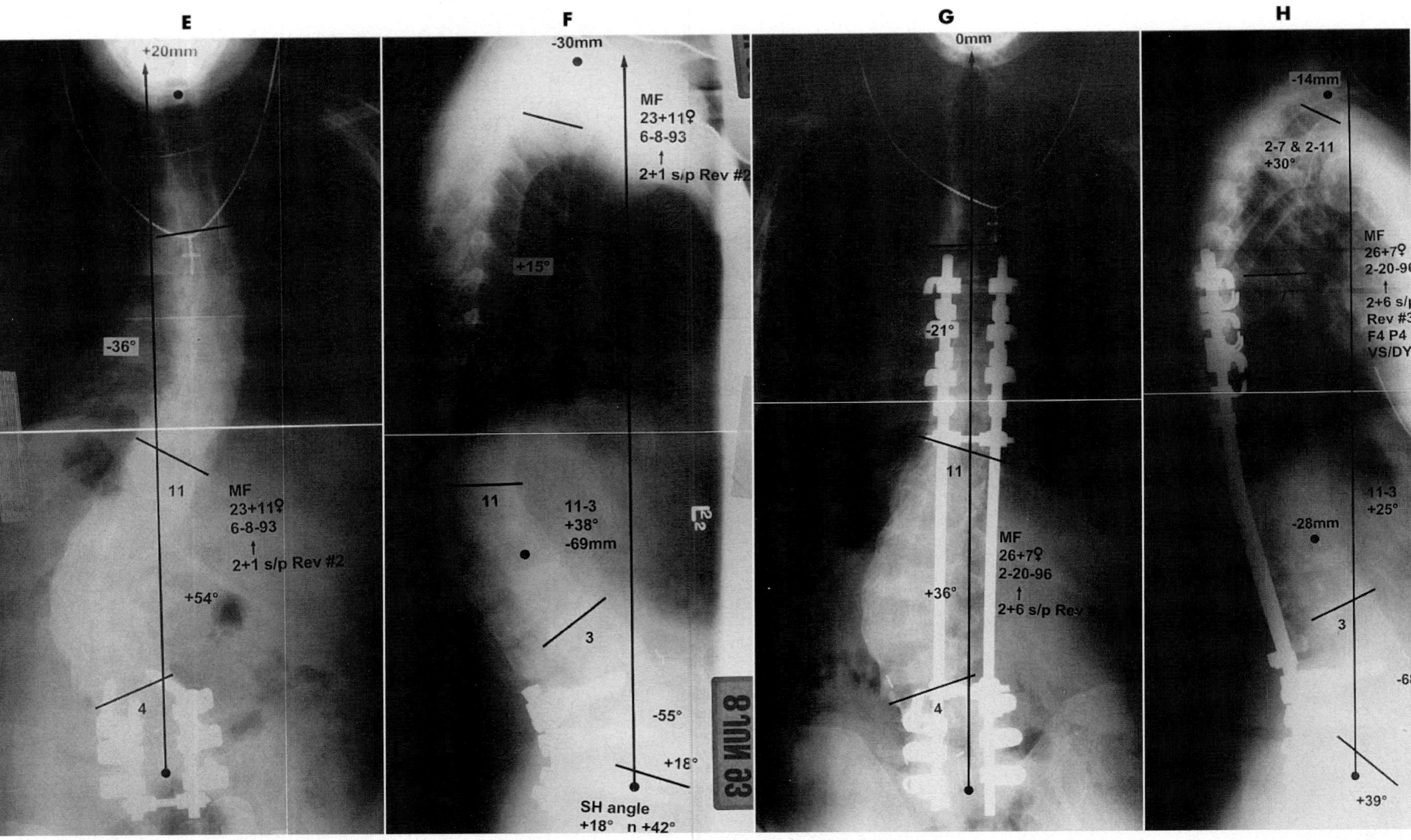


**FIGURE 11-5, CONT'D**

Lumbosacral fusion relieved her lumbosacral pain. (**E** and **F**), only to incapacitate her with thoracolumbar junction pain. Sequential-simultaneous realignment of the thoracolumbar junction (**G** and **H**) has provided her with satisfactory pain relief.

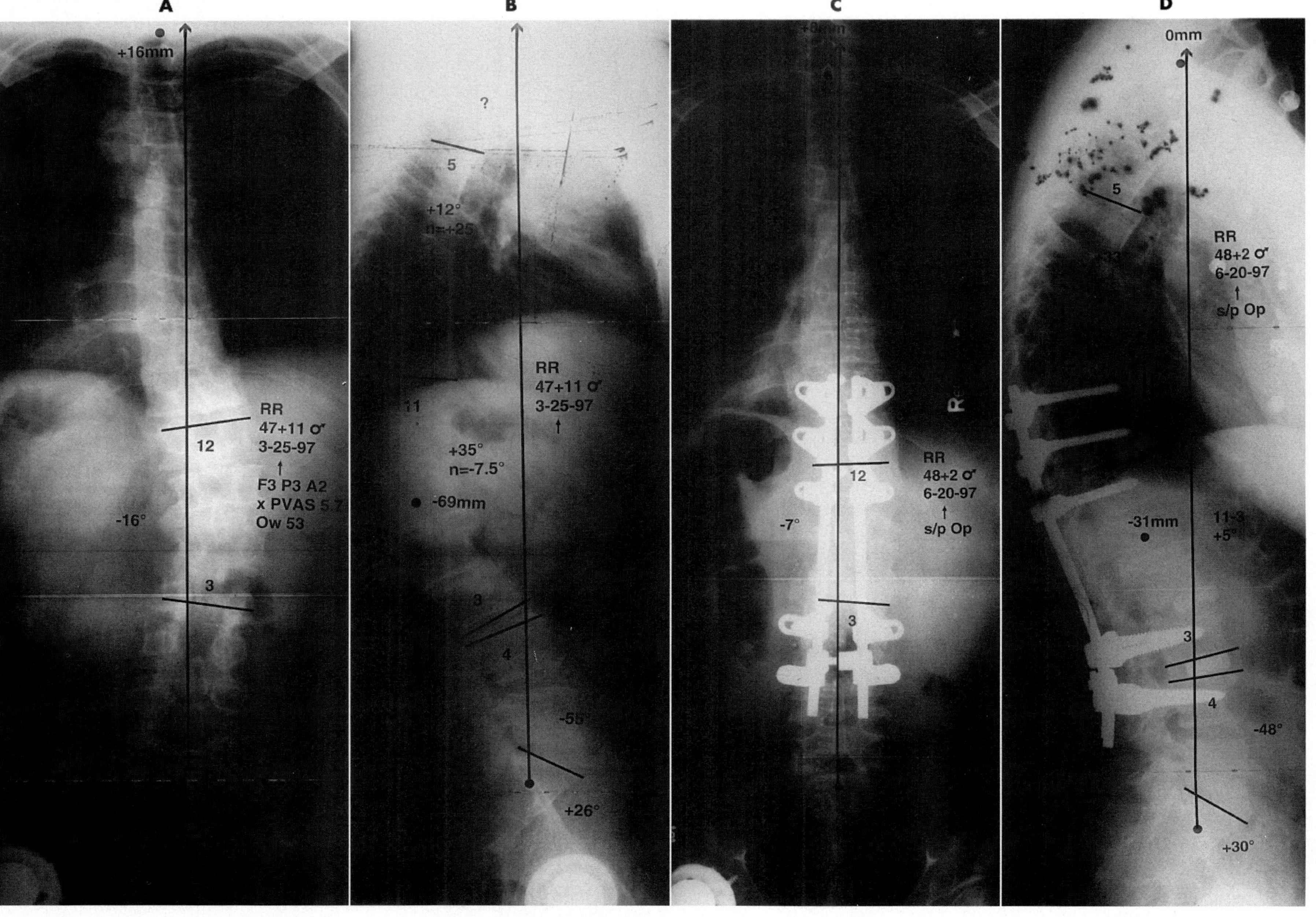


**FIGURE 11-6**

A 47-year-old man with upper lumbar degenerative disk disease who had previously undergone three upper lumbar procedures without relief of symptoms and worsening deformity. Standing posteroanterior (**A**), lateral (**B**), and postoperative standing posteroanterior (**C**) and lateral (**D**) radiographs are shown. The anterior column reconstruction involves structural femoral rings of the lower two disk space levels without which a longer instrumentation would have been necessary.

Nine of the ten salvage patients were eligible for 12 or more months of follow-up, and all considered their surgery to have been either satisfactory or very satisfactory. All would at least probably undergo the same procedure again if they were faced with the same problem.

## DISCUSSION

Most patients requiring anterior and posterior surgery for thoracolumbar spinal disorders can be operated in a sequential or staged manner. The patient most suited to a simultaneous approach is one with stiffening of the spinal column, both anteriorly and posteriorly, and especially one requiring structural bone graft anteriorly. The simultaneous approach is probably not appropriate for L5-S1 flexion deformity. This is probably best approached with either a sequential posterior-anterior-posterior or posterior lumbar interbody approach.

The principal drawbacks of sequential-simultaneous surgery are a longer operating time and the need to change the patient's position intraoperatively. The principal advantage is a better working position for posterior osteotomy and instrumentation.

## CONCLUSION

The sequential-simultaneous approach to stiff thoracolumbar spine deformities provides the optimum working conditions for posterior osteotomy and instrumentation, while offering the advantages of simultaneous approach in which cantilever correction of the deformity can be achieved from posterior instrumentation and structural bone graft placed anteriorly.

## REFERENCES


1. Acaroglu ER, Schwab FJ, Farcy JP: Simultaneous anterior and posterior approaches for correction of the late deformity due to thoracolumbar fractures, *Euro. Spine J* 5:56-62, 1996.
2. Asher MA, Fox DK: *Anesthesia for patients undergoing spine surgery for thoracolumbar spine deformity*. In Porter S, editor: *Anesthesia for surgery of the spine,* New York, 1995, McGraw-Hill, pp 171-198.
3. Bernhardt M, Bridwell KH: Segmental analysis of the sagittal plane alignment of the normal thoracic and lumbar spines and thoracolumbar junction, *Spine* 14:717-721, 1989.
4. Jackson RP, McManus AC: Radiographic analysis of sagittal plane alignment and balance in standing volunteers and patients with low back pain matched for age, sex, and size: a prospective controlled clinical study, *Spine* 19:1611-1618, 1994.
5. Rawlins BA, Weidenbaum M, Farcy J-P: Simultaneous anterior and posterior procedures for short segment spine pathology. Presented at Annual Meeting of the North American Spine Society, paper #69, Boston, MA, July 9-11, 1992.
6. Shultz AB, Ashton-Miller JA: *Biomechanics of the human spine*. In Mow VC, Hayes WC, editors: *Basic orthopaedic biomechanics,* New York, 1991, Raven Press, pp 337-374.

# 12

# SIMULTANEOUS ANTERIOR AND POSTERIOR APPROACHES TO THE SPINE FOR REVISION SURGERY: CURRENT INDICATIONS AND TECHNIQUES

**Frank J. Schwab, M.D.**
**John R. Klein, M.D.**
**Jean-Pierre C. Farcy, M.D.**



Due to the complex pathology that is often present in failed spinal surgery, revision surgery frequently is required to address both the anterior and posterior portions of the spine. Thus, the surgical technique applied during revision surgery must permit access and intervention to all portions of the spine. In order to address this challenging task, numerous surgical approaches have been proposed: posterior alone (with transpedicular subtraction or osteotomy),[4,9,12,24] anterior with a later stage posterior surgery,[18,23] anterior combined with second stage (same sitting) posterior,[10] or even anterior (for release, osteotomy) followed by posterior (osteotomy and fixation) and again anterior surgery (anterior grafting). More recently simultaneous anterior and posterior spinal approaches have been developed.[11,22]

Anterior and posterior approaches are frequently required in revision spinal surgery to adequately address the deformity.[4,7,13] Indirect intervention, such as transpedicular techniques may limit access to an abundant anterior bony column (large callus, malunion). Adherent vascular structures in the anterior soft tissue scar may also be endangered without direct visualization. Direct visualization of the anterior spinal column is thus desirable in procedures that require correction of deformity and stabilization of the spine.

Among those who advocate various anterior-posterior approaches there has been much discussion regarding performing surgery in one sitting (sequential or simultaneous) or two (staged).[18,20,21,23] Staged procedures permit a period of recovery between the two interventions. However, a statistically higher complication rate has been noted in staged procedures when compared to sequential procedures.[2,3,6,8,14,16,17,19,20,22] Sequential procedures still carry the disadvantage of requiring multiple patient repositionings intraoperatively. This can significantly increase the anesthesia time and the neurologic risk due to manipulation of the patient with acute instability of the spine. An example would be a patient with kyphotic malunion of the spine who has been instrumented in the past. To address this surgically would require an instrumentation removal posteriorly followed by an anterior osteotomy and then a posterior osteotomy with reinstrumentation.

A simultaneous approach is defined as two teams operating at the same time approaching the spine from the front and back. In revision spinal surgery, the simultaneous approach is the only technique that permits complete and constant control of the anterior and posterior columns of the spine during the entire surgery. This advantageous aspect is a significant consideration when planning revision surgery on the spine.

## INDICATIONS FOR SIMULTANEOUS ANTERIOR-POSTERIOR APPROACHES TO THE SPINE

Currently, a simultaneous anterior and posterior approach to the spine is best indicated for short segment revision pathology (such as fracture malunion), or short segment intervention (anterior-posterior osteotomy for flat back). The following is a brief outline of current indications for a simultaneous surgical intervention on the spine.

### COMPLEX PSEUDARTHROSES

Pseudarthrosis of the spine in high-risk patients (smokers or patients who have had previous revision for pseudoarthroses) may warrant anterior and posterior approaches to the spine in order to increase fusion surface area and to benefit from the high vascularity of the anterior column.

Malunions of the spine are rigid, short segment deformities that frequently require one or several closely placed osteotomies anteriorly and posteriorly. Often, the kyphotic deformity requires partial or total anterior corpectomies in order to safely achieve correction of deformity. Posteriorly these complex cases require chevron osteotomies. The combined anterior and posterior resections permit safe shortening of the spine and simultaneous correction.

The flat back deformities can only truly be corrected by simultaneous approaches to the spine. Because of the significant sagittal plane deformity, multilevel anterior and posterior osteotomies are necessary. The crucial realignment in three dimensions is optimized with direct visualization of both columns. The simultaneous technique also permits constant graft visualization anteriorly and avoids the transitional instability in sequential surgery. Although transpedicular posterior approaches have been developed, we reserve these for cases when an anterior approach may be contraindicated (respiratory compromise or problems related to previous anterior surgery).

## PREOPERATIVE PLANNING

Prior to undertaking a simultaneous anterior-posterior surgery, detailed preoperative planning is essential. The exact level of anterior and posterior osteotomies must be planned as well as which levels of the spine need to be instrumented. The level and orientation of each screw, hook, and rod-rod connector should be anticipated. The sequence of surgical progression between anterior and posterior teams is carefully anticipated preoperatively.

## ANESTHESIA

The patient is placed under general anesthesia. Although a selective intubation may be more convenient for the surgeon when a thoracotomy is involved, it is not mandatory and increases the risk for postoperative atelectasis. Significant blood loss should be anticipated and the use of a cell saver is essential. Predonation or cross-matching of banked blood for 3 to 4 units is required. During the operative procedure somatosensory evoked potential monitoring (SSEP), as well as motor evoked potentials (MEP) are used.

## PATIENT POSITIONING

The patient is placed on the operating table in the lateral decubitus position. The back of the patient is straight from shoulders to the pelvis and is placed as close as possible to the side of the table. A special table has been recently designed in order to facilitate the positioning of the patient and permit adjustments during the surgery in order to alternatively optimize operative exposure for the anterior or posterior operating team (Fig. 12-1). This table thus provides optimum patient accessibility compared to traditional tables. At any time during the surgical procedure the table can be positioned (rotated) to be completely prone or supine depending upon the need of the surgical teams. This table is easily attached to the Jackson table frame and positioning intraoperatively is controlled by the nursing and anesthesia teams. The patient is draped circumferentially for easy access to back, flank, chest, and abdomen. The surgical team consists of two spine surgeons and two assistant surgeons. Two nursing teams and separate instrumentation setups are required.

## SURGICAL APPROACHES

The usual posterior midline approach and standard anterior approach are performed simultaneously by the two teams. The posterior surgical team works in the sitting position. Performing the posterior approach

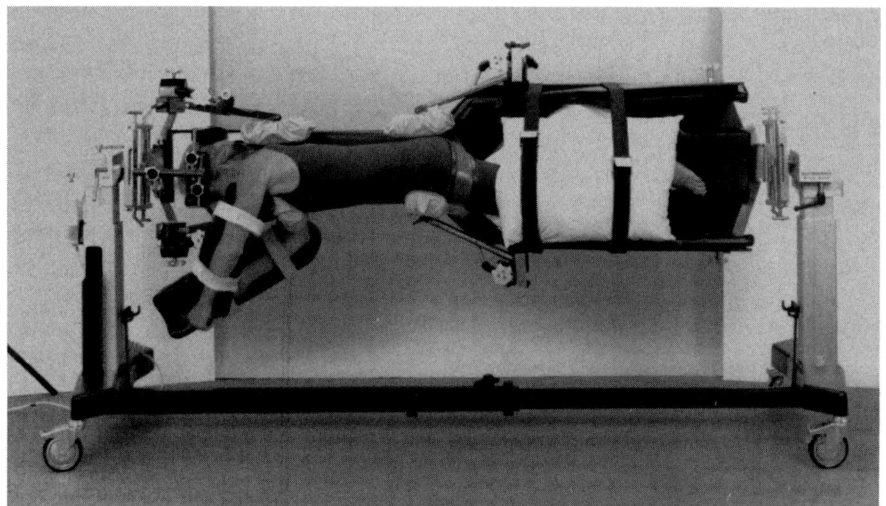

FIGURE 12-1

Patient positioned on special table attachment for simultaneous anterior-posterior approach. Patient can be rotated 90 degrees to the prone or supine position intraoperatively, providing better exposure to each surgical team alternatively as necessary during the surgery.

in the lateral position is initially uncomfortable and requires some adjustment. The skin incision is centered at the level of the deformity.

The anterior approach can be one of the three standard approaches to the thoracic and/or lumbar spine: a thoracotomy for a thoracic spine approach, a thoracophrenolaparotomy for the thoracoabdominal junction, and a retroperitoneal approach for the lumbar spine. In revision surgery of the thoracic spine particular caution is required in the thoracic approach. Pulmonary adhesions may considerably complicate the approach to the spine. Malunion as a late complication of fracture is frequently associated with pleural adhesions of the lung. This is due to bleeding and pleural injury at the time of initial injury. Meticulous dissection is thus required to avoid pleural injury during revision surgery. Once the proper spinal level has been exposed and dissection completed, the planned osteotomy (or osteotomies) can be performed at the level of the apex of the kyphosis.

It is recommended that for simultaneous (as also in sequential) approaches to the spine that a bridge of tissue between the two incisions be maintained. This distance should be at least 5 centimeters.

## REALIGNMENT TECHNIQUE

When both anterior and posterior aspects of the spine have been exposed, spinal realignment can proceed. The basic technique can be applied to thoracic and lumbar revision surgery, although the anatomic level clearly dictates variations in the anterior approach and the posterior fixation. Critical points to consider are, firstly, the need to place adequate posterior instrumentation prior to any anterior manipulation so that the spine is not completely unstable at any time during the surgery. Secondly, posterior osteotomy is required prior to anterior reduction in order to avoid elongation or injury of the neural elements. The concept of spinal shortening is essential to this technique. Any sagittal plane correction must involve a shortening osteotomy, not simply a corrective sagittal osteotomy. In our experience two different instrumentation and reduction techniques can be applied for the simultaneous anterior and posterior correction of deformity. The two-rod and four-rod techniques that we employ are discussed in detail below.

The ideal level for osteotomy is selected preoperatively based upon the level of deformity, level of the conus, and degree of deformity. However, intraoperatively, the direct vision of the deformity is helpful in selecting the exact site of correction. After careful exposure of the anterior spine out to the edge of the foramen, careful retraction of vascular structures is performed with malleable retractors. Once protection of soft tissue structures is ensured, a set of straight and curved 0.5-inch osteotomes is selected. One of the straight osteotomes is then gently introduced into the middle of the selected vertebra, perpendicular to the deformity. Without going beyond the opposite (posterior) wall of the vertebrae, the osteotome is introduced to a depth of approximately 4 cm in the vertebra. The contact of the opposite cortex can be felt as an increase in resistance against the osteotome tip. A change in tone can also be appreciated as the osteotome advances against the opposite cortical wall. A second curved osteotome is then introduced, the convexity in touch with the straight osteotome. The osteotomy is then achieved by breaking the callus with a gentle movement between the two osteotomes. It should be noted that in some cases of fracture malunion despite abundant anterior callus formation, disks can still be identified. These remnant disks should be utilized to gain access by dissection to the posterior longitudinal ligament. This will permit a safer retraction and protection of the dura during the corpectomy.

## TWO-ROD TECHNIQUE OF POSTERIOR INSTRUMENTATION

The two-rod technique relies upon a right- and left-sided posterior construct that consists of proximal hooks firmly attached to rods that are gradually brought down upon a set of double-threaded pedicle screws. This construct is particularly applicable in revision cases in which the regional kyphosis is not extreme. It is essential to follow a predetermined surgical sequence for this technique.

1. Installation of posterior instrumentation, not tightened (double-threaded screws with incomplete seating of clamp);
2. Posterior osteotomy of the spine, shortening;
3. Anterior osteotomy/corpectomy, shortening of spine;
4. Closure of posterior osteotomy by gentle reduction;
5. Placement of anterior strut or cage; and
6. Compression of posterior instrumentation, complete osteotomy closure.

The two-rod technique is ideal for short segment pathology such as fracture malunion. The most frequently used instrumentation construct is a hook claw, which is placed such that the inferior (upgoing) hook is one or two levels above the deformity and a pedicle screw at the first mobile level below the deformity. The claw should encompass two vertebral levels. A set of pedicle screws (double-threaded if significant kyphosis) are implanted bilaterally at the first intact vertebra below the region of pathology. Two rods are selected and contoured to the desired sagittal spine alignment and secured with the hooks above and the double-threaded screws below without an initial reduction (Fig. 12-2). The inferior portion of the construct is not completely set at this stage; however, partial stabilization is achieved. As outlined above, a posterior chevron osteotomy is then performed in the callus at the involved level. It is critical that an adequate posterior osteotomy precede any anterior reduction so that the neural elements are not stretched over an elongated posterior column. If there is a frontal plane deformity associated with the sagittal plane kyphosis, then modification of the chevron can be performed in order to correct the spine three-dimensionally (uneven resections on each side of the chevron).

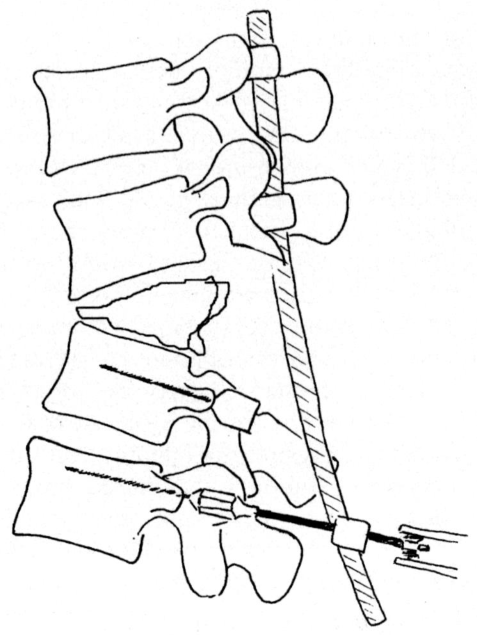

**FIGURE 12-2**

Illustration of the two-rod technique. Posterior osteotomy and placement of instrumentation. The double-threaded screw is partially tightened after which the anterior corpectomy can proceed.

During the posterior approach, the anterior approach to the spine is also performed. The anterior osteotomy is not begun until the posterior instrumentation is in place and preliminary assembly is achieved. The anterior procedure then proceeds with a total or subtotal corpectomy. Upon completion of the anterior resection, gradual reduction of deformity can proceed. The rods on each side are slowly brought into contact with the pedicle screws, applying the machine thread on the bilateral double-threaded screws. Simultaneous assistance can be given anteriorly with use of a distractor in the corpectomy site. A controlled reduction/realignment thus occurs with gradual closure of the posterior osteotomy. Visual control, both anteriorly and posteriorly, allows for maximal protection of the neural structures during the procedure. As the deformity is carefully reduced continuous SSEP and MEP monitoring is performed. The posterior construct is then preliminarily tightened when the rods are firmly seated into the pedicle screws. The distal construct can be supplemented with laminar hooks to augment pull-out strength.

After reduction the prepared anterior graft is seated (Fig. 12-3). Tricortical autologous iliac graft, allograft, or cages can be used and placed anteriorly.[2,5] The iliac crest can usually be reached either through the anterior or posterior incision by subcutaneous dissection to avoid an additional scar. Only the surgeries of the thoracic spine will require a second incision for bone graft harvest. Following placement of the anterior graft (or cage filled with cancellous bone) the posterior construct can be given a final compression in order to firmly engage the anterior graft (or cage) and close the posterior chevron osteotomy.

The two-rod technique can also be performed with a variety of the new instrumentation systems that may not have double-threaded screws. Some systems offer tools that can be applied to create a gradual reduction of a seated pedicle screw to the rod. The key is to ensure a controlled reduction at all times, particularly when an unstable spine is created by the anterior and posterior osteotomies (Fig. 12-4, *A* and *B*)

## Four-Rod Technique of Posterior Instrumentation

The four-rod technique is a modification of the two-rod technique that we find particularly useful in complex three-dimensional revisions such as those performed for malunion and the flat back deformity. The interruption of continuous rod on each side by implementing a pair of ascending and descending rods has multiple advantages (Fig. 12-5). The four-rod technique permits the creation of two solid foundations, one cephalad, one caudad, across the deformity. By first establishing these foundations increased control is possible during the destabilizing aspects of the revision surgery. Furthermore, once osteotomies and realignment have been performed, the interlocking of the foundations requires no further excess leverage across any particular screw or hook and final tightening and assembly occur across the two sets of rod-rod connectors (dominoes), and closure can begin on the case. By having placed all instrumentation prior to any osteotomy minimal blood loss is incurred. The osteotomy can then be performed with the knowledge that prolonged bleeding with poor visualization is minimized because wound closure begins shortly after the final instrumentation is interlocked and compressed. A further advantage of the four-rod technique is the added freedom in translating the two foundations with respect to one another. A frontal plane deformity with offset between the cephalad and caudal levels of the spine can be corrected by adjustments between the upper and lower foundations through the rod-rod connectors and individual rod contouring as well as final compression/distraction maneuvers.

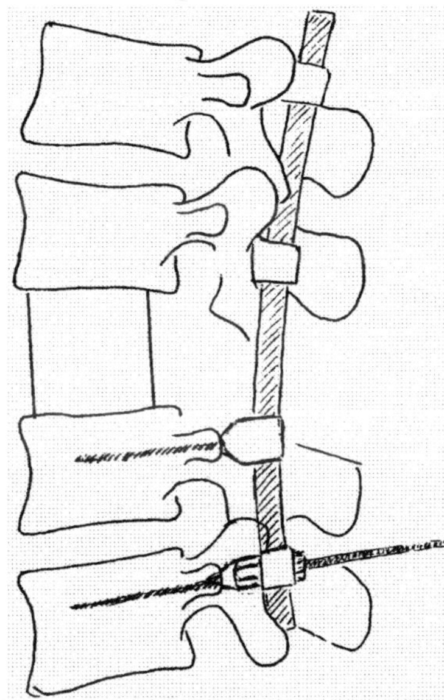

**Figure 12-3**

Illustration of the reduced spine by the two-rod technique. The anterior bone graft has been placed into the vertebrectomy defect. Posterior instrumentation is then tightened after slight compression of the graft.

In the four-rod technique the anterior and posterior surgical teams can progress with greater independence from one another. The posterior instrumentation can be temporarily connected even during the osteotomy thus avoiding any significant instability of the spine.

When anterior and posterior teams are progressing simultaneously it may be desirable to connect one set of rods (right or left) posteriorly via a rod-rod connector and leaving the other side open. This permits sufficient sliding of the inferior rod on the free side distally (while still engaged with the pedicle screws) allowing for sufficient exposure of the pars and inferior facet regions at the desired osteotomy site. The chevron osteotomy can thus be started, after which the inferior rod on that side is gently eased back into position, firmly connected to the pedicle screws, and linked to the descending rod on that side with a rod-rod connector. Subsequently, the opposite rod con-

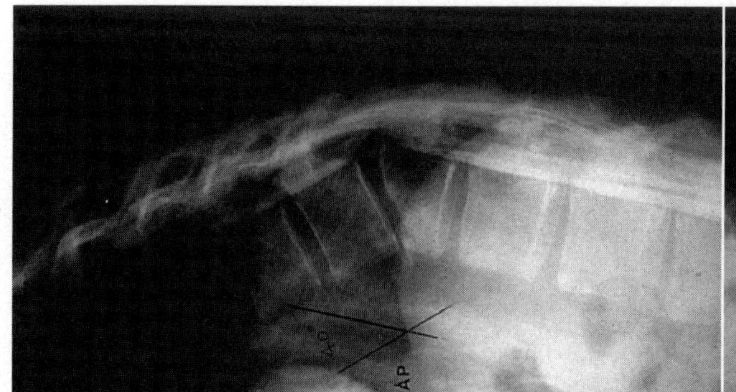


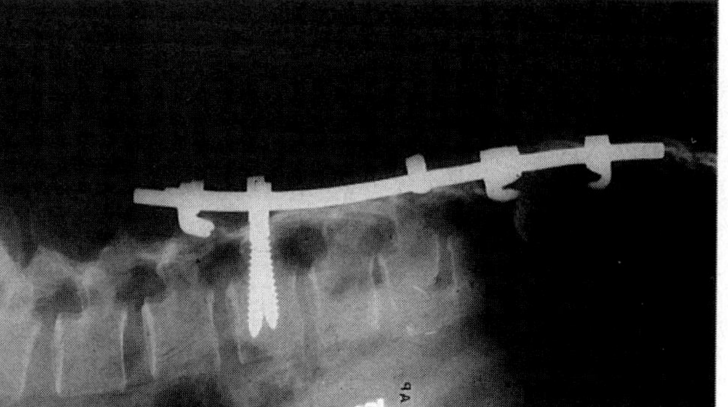


**Figure 12-4**

**A,** Lateral myelogram demonstrating a malunion with significant canal compromise. Patient demonstrated progressive neurological impairment after injury. **B,** Follow-up radiograph demonstrating the two-rod technique. The anterior graft that was compressed by the posterior instrumentation has consolidated. Sagittal contour has been restored and maintained.

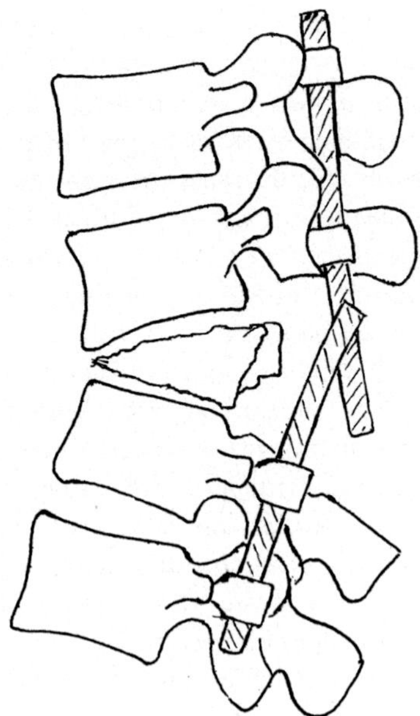

FIGURE 12-5

Illustration of the four-rod technique. Posterior osteotomy and placement of instrumentation has been performed. Following this stage anterior decompression/vertebrectomy can proceed.

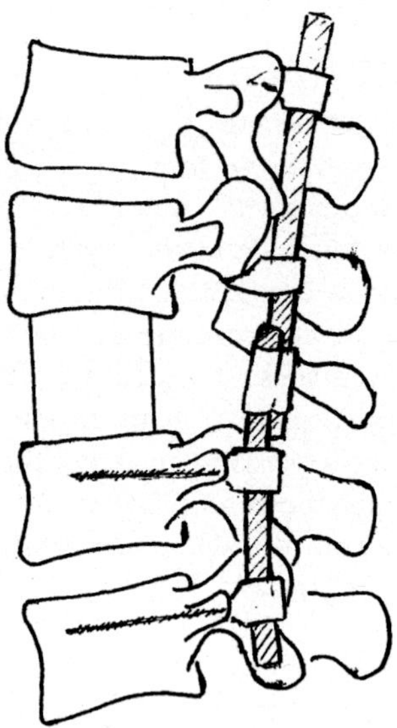

FIGURE 12-6

Illustration of reduced spine with placement of anterior strut graft. Posterior instrumentation is firmly tightened after slight compression of the anterior graft.

nection is loosened in order to proceed with completion of the chevron osteotomy. Following this, the loosened rods are reconnected and final adjustments of the construct can proceed in order to reduce the deformity if the anterior osteotomy is complete.

When anterior osteotomy/release is completed it is important to proceed with placement of the anterior grafting or cage placement prior to final adjustments in the posterior instrumentation (Fig. 12-6). Tricortical autologous iliac graft, allograft, or different types of cages, can be used and placed anteriorly. The iliac crest can usually be reached either through the anterior or posterior incision by subcutaneous dissection in order to avoid an additional scar. Only the surgeries of the thoracic spine will require a second incision for bone graft harvest.

After anterior grafting, posterior reduction of the deformity can proceed in a gradual and controlled manner. Once the proximal and distal foundations are connected via the rod-rod connectors, a sequence of gentle adjustments will permit reduction of the deformity and closure of the posterior osteotomy. The maneuvers consist of compression across the rod-rod connectors, translation of rods with respect to one another by rotating the connectors, and in situ rod contouring. Simultaneous anterior and posterior visual control allows for maximal protection of the neural structures during the procedure. Continuous monitoring with SSEP and MEP is necessary to ensure the safety of neurologic structures. After final tightening, cross-links can be applied to the posterior instrumentation and a posterior or posterolateral fusion is performed, using autologous bone graft, following decortication.

For anterior approaches that violate the thorax, a chest tube is placed and the thoracotomy closed. A multilayer closure is performed and a closed suction drainage system is placed for both the bone graft donor site and posterior wound.

## POSTOPERATIVE CONSIDERATIONS

Adequate pain relief postoperatively will include opiates as tolerated. We have preferred to limit the use of patient-controlled analgesia (PCA). Patients are encouraged to get out of bed with assistance on the first postoperative day, and may begin ambulation with a therapist as soon as the chest tube has been removed (usually within 3 days). Use of a brace is rarely necessary because of the stability achieved with internal fixation.

## ADVANTAGES AND PITFALLS OF SIMULTANEOUS SURGERY

Revision surgery is associated with longer operating times and higher blood losses than primary surgery. However, compared to staged procedures, the simultaneous anterior and posterior approach is associated with significantly decreased operating time, blood loss, and hospital length of stay.[1,7] This technique, while technically demanding, provides advantages. It combines the advantages of a solid posterior instrumentation with the benefits of an anterior decompression and circumferential grafting. This technique may be neurologically safer than any other technique. Absence of manipulation of the patient throughout the entire procedure eliminates the risk of acute instability during the two stages. The progressive, slow, electrophysiologically supervised and directly visualized reduction by the posterior instrumentation avoids any distraction of the spine. Furthermore, permanent control of the anterior graft during the compression of the posterior instrumentation provides protection against dislodgment. Simultaneous anterior and posterior visual control allows for an optimal alignment of the spine in both the frontal and sagittal planes after osteotomy.

## CONCLUSIONS AND RECOMMENDATIONS

Simultaneous approaches to the spine can be applied for a variety of pathologies, however, it seems particularly suited for revision surgery. Revision spinal surgery for complex pseudarthrosis, malunion with significant deformity, and sagittal plane malalignment syndromes (e.g., flat back, lumbosacral fusions) are ideally addressed by simultaneous anterior and posterior surgery.

Simultaneous approaches to the spine require two well-trained and experienced spinal surgery teams. This procedure requires continuous and close coordination between both teams. As in all spine surgery, there is a learning curve that affects not only the surgeon, but also the anesthesia and nursing staff.

With the continuous advances seen in all aspects of medicine, it is inevitable that significant progress will occur in the instrumentation systems and ancillary equipment involved with the simultaneous spinal techniques. The development of the simultaneous access operating table represents one of these already-achieved advances. In the near future, the use of minimally invasive endoscopic techniques will most likely play a role in simultaneous anterior and posterior surgery (Mangione P, personal communication, 1997).[15]

## REFERENCES


1. Acaroglu ER, Schwab FJ, Farcy JP: Simultaneous anterior and posterior approaches for correction of late deformity due to thoracolumbar fractures, *Eur Spine J* 5:56-62, 1996.
2. Bradford DS, Ganjavian S, Antonious D, Winter RB, Lonstein JE, Moe JH: Anterior strut grafting for the treatment of kyphosis, *J Bone Joint Surg* 64A:680-690, 1982.
3. Bradford DS, Winter RB, Lonstein JE, Moe JH: Techniques of anterior spinal surgery for the management of kyphosis, *Clin Orthop* 128:129-139, 1977.
4. Bradford DS, Tribus CB: Current concepts and management of patients with fixed decompensated spinal deformity, *Clin Orthop* 306:64-72, 1994.
5. Bridwell KH, Lenke LG, McEnery KW, Baldus C, Blanke K: Anterior fresh frozen structural allografts in the thoracic and lumbar spine. Do they work if combined with posterior fusion and instrumentation in adult patients with kyphosis or anterior column defect? *Spine* 20:1410-1418, 1995.
6. Dick J, Boachie O, Wilson M: One stage vs. two stage anterior and posterior spinal reconstruction in adults: comparison of outcomes including nutritional status, complication rates, hospital costs, and other factors, *Spine* 17(suppl 8):310-316, 1992.
7. Farcy JP: Simultaneous anterior and posterior procedures for short segment spine pathology. American Academy of Orthopaedic Surgeons. Videotape #23112.
8. Fountain SS: A single staged combined surgical approach for vertebral resections, *J Bone Joint Surg* 61A: 1011-1017, 1979.
9. Gertzbein SD, Hornis MB: Wedge osteotomy for the correction of posttraumatic kyphosis: a new technique and a report of three cases, *Spine* 17:374-379, 1992.
10. Kostuik JP, Maurais GR, Richardson WJ, Okajima Y: Combined single stage anterior and posterior osteotomy for correction of iatrogenic lumbar kyphosis, *Spine* 13:257-266, 1988.
11. Kozak JA, O'Brien JP: Simultaneous combined anterior and posterior fusion : an independent analysis of a treatment for the disabled low-back pain patient, *Spine* 15:322-328, 1990.
12. Lehmer SM, Keppler L, Biscup RS, Enker P, Miller SD, Steffee AD: Posterior transvertebral osteotomy for adult thoracolumbar kyphosis, *Spine* 19:2060-2067, 1994.
13. Malcolm BW, Bradford DS, Winter RB, Chou SN: Post traumatic kyphosis: a review of forty-eight surgically treated patients, *J Bone Joint Surg* 63A:891-900, 1981.
14. Mandebaum BR, Tollo VT, McAfee PC, Bursest P: Nutritional deficiencies after staged anterior and posterior spinal reconstructive surgery, *Clin Orthop* 234:5-11, 1988.
15. Mangione P, Bernard P, Senegas J: Retroperitoneoscopic bone grafting with posterior osteosynthesis for unstable L3, L4 and L4-L5 spondylolisthesis, a report of 6 cases, *Second Central European GICD Forum*. May 28-30, 1997.
16. McAfee PC: Complications of anterior approaches to

the thoracolumbar spine. Emphasis on Kaneda instrumentation, *Clin Orthop* 306:110-119, 1994.

17. McBride GG, Bradford DS: Vertebral body replacement with femoral neck allograft and vascularized rib strut graft: a technique for treating post-traumatic kyphosis with neurologic deficit, *Spine* 8:406-415, 1983.
18. McDonnell MF, Glassman SD, Dimar JR, Puno RM, Johnson JR: Perioperative complications of anterior procedures on the spine, *J Bone Joint Surg* 78:839-847, 1996.
19. O'Brien JP, Dawson MHO, Herrod CW, Monbarger G, Speck G, Weatherly CR: Simultaneous combined anterior and posterior fusion: a surgical solution for failed spinal surgery with a brief review of the first 150 patients, *Clin Orthop* 203:191-195, 1986.
20. Powell ET, Krengel WF, King HA, Lagrone MO: Comparison of same day sequential anterior and posterior spinal fusion with delayed two-stage anterior and posterior spinal fusion, *Spine* 19:1256-1259, 1994.
21. Schufflebarger HL, Grimm JO, Bui V, Thompson JD: Anterior and posterior spinal fusion: staged vs. same day surgery, *Spine* 16:930-933, 1991.
22. Spencer DL, DeWald RL: Simultaneous anterior and posterior surgical approach to the thoracic and lumbar spine, *Spine* 4:29-36, 1979.
23. Whitesides TE: Traumatic kyphosis of the thoracolumbar spine, *Clin Orthop* 128:78, 1977.
24. Wu SS, Hwa SY, Lin LC, Pai WM, Chen PQ, Au MK: Management of rigid post-traumatic kyphosis, *Spine,* 21:2260-2266, 1996.

# 13

# POSTERIOR-ANTERIOR-POSTERIOR SEQUENCE IN REVISION SPINAL SURGERY

Harry L. Shufflebarger, M.D.



Revision spinal surgery may be indicated for several reasons. These include pseudarthrosis, failure of spinal instrumentation, and imbalance. Imbalance may take several forms. Coronal plane imbalance in scoliosis is easily recognized. Sagittal plane imbalance occurs in many conditions. Examples of sagittal plane imbalance may include lumbar flat back syndrome, posttraumatic kyphosis, postlaminectomy conditions, and failed procedures for degenerative conditions. Junctional zone problems are an increasingly frequent indication for revision surgery. A common factor of nearly every condition requiring revision surgery is kyphosis. Rarely is lordosis a feature of revision spinal surgery.

Combined anterior and posterior approaches in revision surgery have been employed in the same day successfully for the past decade.[1,3,6] The general sequence has been first anterior and then posterior. This sequence usually involves anterior release and grafting, either with nonstructural or structural grafts. The sequence of posterior and then anterior has also been employed, with the posterior portion identifying and repairing the necessary levels. The anterior portion then addresses anterior grafting at the defective levels.

Simultaneous approach to both the anterior and posterior has also been recommended for revision spinal surgery.[4,8] This approach is attractive from theoretical considerations to be discussed. But, the simultaneous approach is technically difficult. In simultaneous approaches, there are anatomical limitations imposed by the necessary lateral decubitus position, particularly approaches to the sacrum. Lower lumbar and sacral exposures are best accomplished either from an oblique position or supine position.

The sequence of posterior-anterior-posterior (BFB for back-front-back) favorably lends itself for reconstruction of the spine in conditions requiring revision surgery. The theoretical considerations or principles supporting this approach will be considered. From this can be derived indications for the approach. Personal experience, logistics, and complications will be presented.

## THEORETICAL CONSIDERATIONS

Spinal revision problems are problems in kyphosis. It follows that the goal of revision surgery is to produce more lordosis than is present prior to the revision. Using Scheuermann's kyphosis as a prototype (recognizing that this is not a revision situation initially), the usual approach has been anterior release followed by posterior instrumentation with one of the multiple hook-screw-rod systems. This prototype is only utilized to demonstrate the significant anterior column defect that can be produced by a sufficient anterior release in conjunction with the posterior shortening procedure and powerful posterior instrumentation. A high rate of failure of distal implants in Scheuermann's disease (10% to 15%), has been recently reported.[4] The reason for the failure may be multifactorial. One of the prime factors is the significant anterior column deficit produced by the combination of anterior diskectomy and the posterior lordization (correction of kyphosis). Figure 13-1 demonstrates the marked anterior disk space opening produced by this sequence of surgery (anterior release and posterior segmental instrumentation). Failure

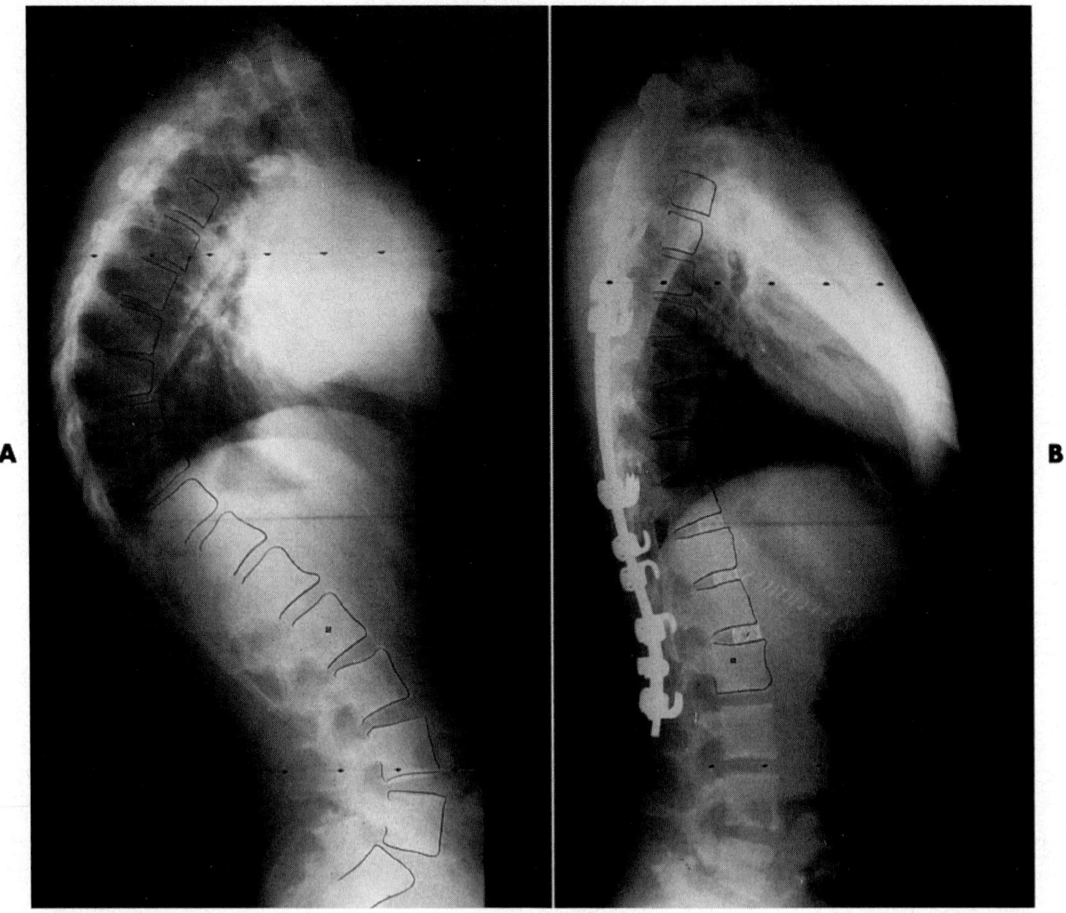


FIGURE 13-1

**A, B,** This Scheuermann's kyphosis was treated with anterior release with nonstructural grafts above thoracic 11, and structural intradiskal grafts distal to thoracic 11. Note the marked anterior opening of the several disk spaces proximal to thoracic 11. The long segment instrumentation above and below these levels with anterior column deficit alleviates the transfer of load to the posterior instrumentation. Note the load sharing structural grafts in the distal portion of the instrumentation.

would be most likely at the ends, where protection is not provided by a long posterior instrumentation or by structural anterior support as demonstrated here.

In order to produce lordosis in revision surgery, the posterior column must be shortened and the anterior column lengthened. If the anterior approach is performed first, a release is accomplished. The interbody graft may be morselized autogenous bone or a structural graft (cadaver femoral ring, fibula, or prosthetic-type device supplemented with morselized autogenous bone). Lordosis is produced by distraction of the disk space. The amount of lordosis attainable by the anterior first approach is limited by the posterior anatomic situation (pseudarthrosis, fusion, fibrosis). It follows that the posterior portion will increase the lordosis attained by the anterior procedure, causing loosening of the structural or nonstructural graft. An anterior column deficiency is created, and the anterior graft is no longer under compression. Anterior compression is desirable to promote the anterior arthrodesis. Whereas maximum correction may be obtained by this approach, the biomechanical situation produced is less than optimum. If anterior instrumentation is placed, this will either limit the posterior correction or fail when the posterior correction is accomplished. Figure 13-2 presents a diagrammatic explanation of the mechanics.

The second possible approach is posterior and then anterior. The posterior portion usually includes exploration of the spine, removal of existing instrumentation if present, and a posterior shortening procedure. The posterior shortening may include excision of pseudarthrosis, osteotomy, segmental mobilization, or extension of a previous fusion. Posterior instrumentation is a usual feature at this time. This posterior first approach does have the advantage of identifying the exact levels of pseudarthrosis, thus defining the anterior levels to be treated for pseudarthrosis. A disadvantage of posterior first is that the amount of posterior shortening (and thus lordosis) produced is limited by the anterior structures. The anterior approach follows the posterior approach and consists of diskectomy (or corpectomy) and grafting of the space created. Here, the posterior instrumentation limits the amount of interspace distrac-

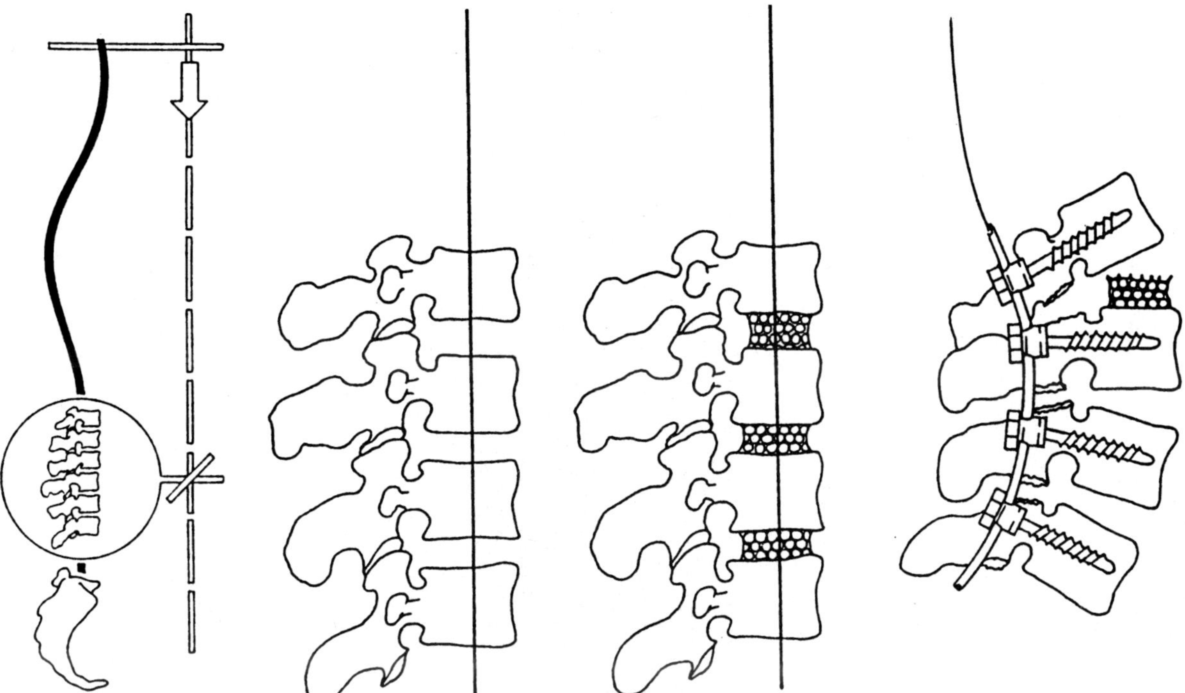

FIGURE 13-2

This diagram shows the mechanics and anatomy of the anterior first then the posterior sequence. A relative lumbar kyphosis is present. The anterior procedure accomplishes structural anterior graft (placed at every level, but illustrated at only one level) but the amount of lordosis attainable is limited by the posterior structural changes. After placement of the posterior instrumentation bent to increase the lumbar lordosis, the anterior structural graft is unloaded. This creates an anterior column deficit, unloads the anterior graft, and may contribute to failure of the arthrodesis.

tion and thus, lordosis that can be produced by the anterior approach. It is also difficult to distract the space and to insert the graft under compression (Fig. 13-3).

There are several biomechanical and anatomical goals of revision spinal surgery. Maximum correction of lordosis, secure posterior instrumentation, and structural anterior column support under compression load are all desirable. The posterior first approach accomplishes posterior column shortening via either excision of pseudarthrosis, osteotomy, or segmental mobilization. Stopping at this point will permit maximum correction from the anterior approach, as well as placement of a structural anterior graft under compression (either by disk space or interbody distraction). In the case of only interbody grafts, anterior instrumentation is not necessary. With corpectomy and longer anterior graft, anterior instrumentation may be desirable to prevent graft displacement during either the position change or third stage. With maximum correction attained by the combination of posterior shortening and anterior distraction and grafting, the posterior wound is reopened and instrumentation placed. Compression forces are then applied posteriorly, which may further increase the correction. The additional correction relative to lordosis is achieved by posterior compression with an anterior fulcrum (Fig. 13-4). Additional compression posteriorly will be transferred to the anterior column, providing more graft stability and favoring bony healing. In practice, placement of the spinal anchors (hooks or screws) during the initial posterior approach facilitates the second posterior approach (by now many hours into the procedure). Figure 13-4 shows a diagrammatic representation of the mechanics of the BFB approach. The BFB approach for pseudarthrosis has the additional advantage of positive identification of the levels of pseudarthrosis, permitting the accurate anterior levels for the revision procedure.

As Figure 13-4 illustrates, an additional mechanical event occurs with this technique (Lebwohl, personal communication). The structural anterior graft places the fulcrum for correction in the anterior column of the spine. Contrast this to the more usual situations. Without a structural anterior column graft, posterior compression relies upon an intact middle column as the fulcrum to effect lordosis. This produces a much shorter lever arm for production of lordosis than is present with the fulcrum in the anterior column. The longer lever arm is much more effective in producing lordosis as well as compression in the anterior column. Jackson[2] advocates in situ bending of a rod connected to the spine by bone screws. No anterior surgery is recommended. Jackson's technique places the fulcrum of sagittal angulation (lordosis production) at the rod-screw interface. This is even more posterior, and transfers a significant stress to the bone-screw interface. The

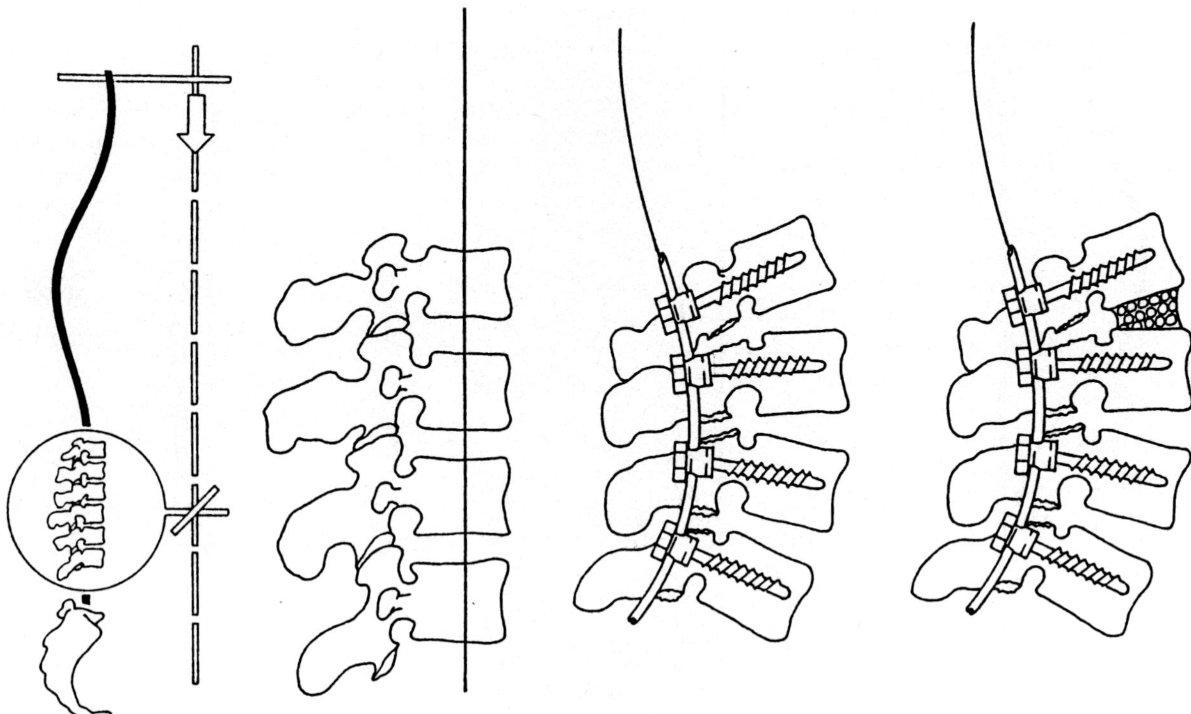

FIGURE 13-3

The mechanics and anatomy of the posterior first, then anterior sequence is illustrated. A relative lumbar kyphosis is present. The posterior first procedure accomplishes shortening of the posterior column and placement of the posterior instrumentation. The anterior procedure follows, with placement of a structural interbody graft (performed at every level, but illustrated here at only one level). In this instance, it is not possible to increase the lordosis as it is fixed by the posterior instrumentation. Also, it is not possible to compression-load the anterior graft because the posterior instrumentation is fixed. While an anterior column deficit is not absolutely produced, a relative anterior deficit is present due to the inability to load the anterior column with compression.

lever arm in this technique is mechanically much less efficient than in the method with the fulcrum in the anterior column. The addition of a structural anterior graft positions the fulcrum for lordosis forces as anterior as possible and assures the longest lever arm possible for production of lordosis. Mechanically, this is the optimum position for the fulcrum for the production of lordosis.

The simultaneous anterior and posterior approach to the spine permits application of the same mechanics and anatomical alterations to the spine as does the BFB sequence. The author employed this approach for the treatment of short fixed kyphosis problems many years ago. The sequence in the simultaneous approach is simultaneous exposure and placement of posterior spinal anchors. The necessary anterior procedure is then performed. The posterior longitudinal member or rod is then placed. The posterior compression is accomplished with the anterior graft under direct vision. The main advantage of this technique is that only one set up is required. The other advantage involves saving time, because the anterior and posterior approaches are done simultaneously. Another advantage is that the placement and integrity of the anterior structural graft is assured by direct vision.

There are several disadvantages to this procedure. The awkward position for the posterior approach is the most objectionable. The problems presented are the need to perform the posterior portion while seated, the inability for adequate surgical assistance, the difficulty in blood salvage for cell saver, and the difficulty in placing implants, particularly screws in the down side of the spine. Image intensification is difficult at best, and frequently impossible, during simultaneous procedures. The approach to the distal lumbar spine and sacrum is difficult in the lateral decubitus position required for the simultaneous approach. While accomplishing the mechanical and anatomic requirements of revision surgery, the simultaneous approach has significant limitations.

The BFB sequence accomplishes the mechanical and anatomic needs of revision spinal surgery. Posterior exploration and identification of pseudarthrosis (if the indication for the revision), posterior shortening procedures (pseudarthrosis repair, osteotomy, segmental mobilization) and placement of spinal anchors are accomplished during the initial posterior procedure. Iliac bone graft can be taken at this stage if required. The anterior procedure follows, permitting anterior release (diskectomy or corpectomy), anterior column distraction (lordosis producing), and anterior column structural grafting under compression. After closure, the

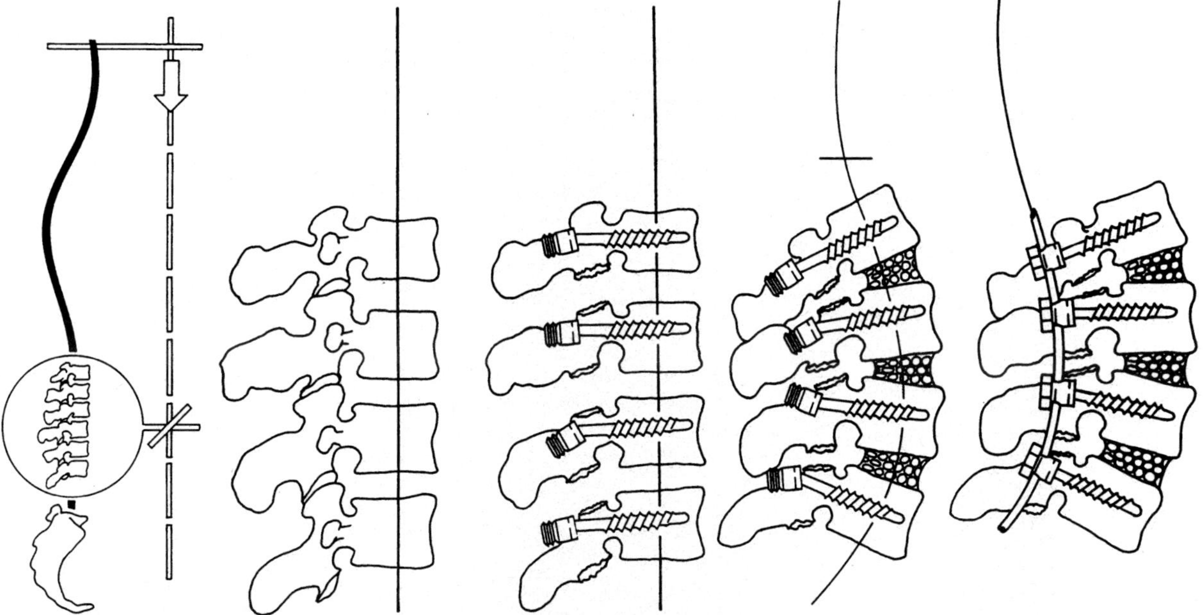

FIGURE 13-4

The mechanics and anatomy of the posterior-anterior-posterior sequence. A relative lumbar kyphosis is present. The initial posterior procedure is shortening. Depending upon the pathology, this may include segmental shortening by facetectomy, excision of pseudarthrosis, or osteotomy. Posterior implants are placed. The anterior procedure follows, with structural interbody grafts at every level. These grafts are placed with distraction of the disk space, providing compression of the graft after the disk space distraction is released. The next phase is placement of the rod in the previously placed posterior implants, and the application of compression forces to the posterior rods. This imparts additional compression to the anterior construct. This sequence permits maximum mobility, maximum opening of the anterior space, placement of the anterior graft under maximum compression, and posterior compression of the anterior graft.

posterior wound is opened, and the rods placed applying additional compression. If additional correction is produced by the bend in the rod, anterior column deficit is not produced as compression is applied to the construct, and this is transferred to the anterior grafts. Figure 13-5 illustrates the method of correction. It is well-demonstrated in this degenerative scoliosis that the majority of corrections are attained by the posterior release and the anterior multilevel structural interbody graft. The addition of the rods posteriorly did not appreciably change the correction.

## INDICATIONS

The BFB sequence is the method of choice for this author for revision spinal surgery. Both long and short segment revision surgery are applicable to this technique. This includes pseudarthrosis for short and long segment instrumentations, sagittal plane malalignment of any etiology, and extension of previous fusion. Examples in various diagnostic categories demonstrate the wide application of this sequence.

Figure 13-6 demonstrates repair of multilevel pseudarthrosis as well as extension of the instrumentation to the sacrum. Here, Harri-Luque instrumentation was employed for correction of adult scoliosis. Spondylolisthesis was present distal to the distal level of the instrumentation. The sequence was posterior removal of the instrumentation and taking down the multiple levels of pseudarthrosis. Segmental release (facetectomy, interspinous ligament, and ligamentum flavum) of the unoperated levels was done. Posterior shortening was accomplished at every level. Spinal anchors were placed and iliac graft taken. The anterior approach followed, with diskectomy and structural interbody grafting below the diaphragm from lumbar 2 to the sacrum. Finally, the rods were placed posteriorly.

Figure 13-7 demonstrates an example of postlaminectomy kyphosis. Laminectomy was done for arteriovenous malformation with neurologic deficit. Two years later, the progressive kyphosis was corrected by the BFB sequence. The technical details are as previously described. Figure 13-8 demonstrates revision for posttraumatic deformity. Here, cord compression and partial neurologic deficit required corpectomy and decompression. The sequence was posterior release and spinal anchor placement, followed by anterior corpectomy and structural graft placement augmented with anterior instrumentation, followed by posterior compression. Resolution of neurological signs followed.

Complex pseudarthroses are well-suited to the BFB sequence. They can be defined as long segment

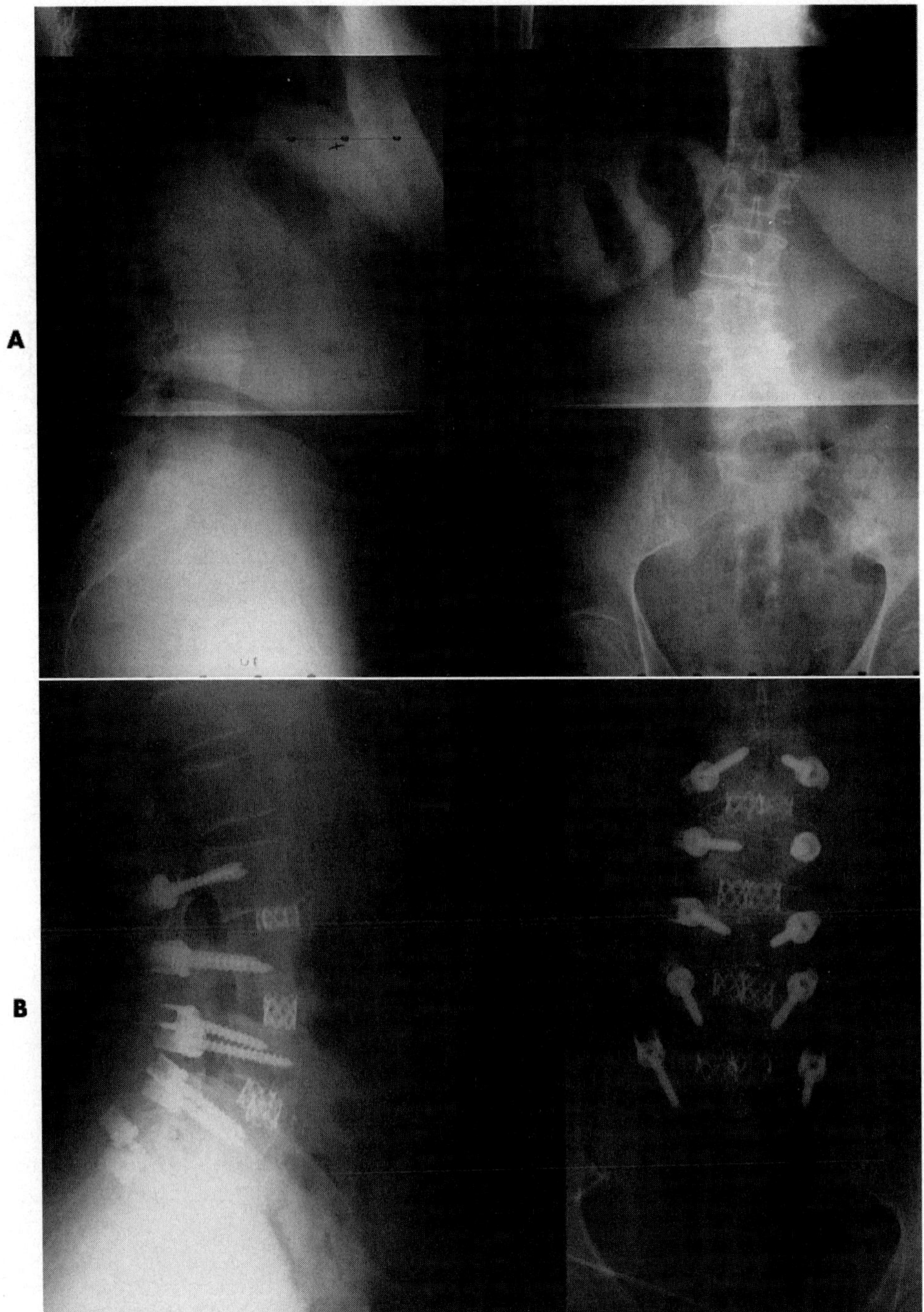

FIGURE 13-5

**A,** Degenerative lumbar scoliosis is present, with loss of lumbar kyphosis. **B,** Posterior release and placement of screws has been accomplished. In addition, the second stage of anterior placement of structural interbody grafts has been completed. Note the correction of the coronal and sagittal deformities by the release and anterior grafts. No rods have been placed.

*Continued*

pseudarthrosis, usually with multiple levels, and as those requiring extension of fusion and/or osteotomy. Posterior first permits identification of pseudarthrosis levels and removal of instrumentation, posterior shortening procedures, and placement of spinal anchors. The anterior lengthening and structural graft placement is then accomplished, achieving maximum lordosis with compression. Posterior compression forces are then applied. Figures 13-6 and 13-9 demonstrates such a complex pseudarthrosis.

A series of 20 cases of complex pseudarthrosis with 2-year follow-up was recently presented.[4] All patients received three-stage same-day surgery. This group was consecutive for the procedure. No surgeries were abandoned or staged due to intraoperative problems. No significant complications requiring extended hos-

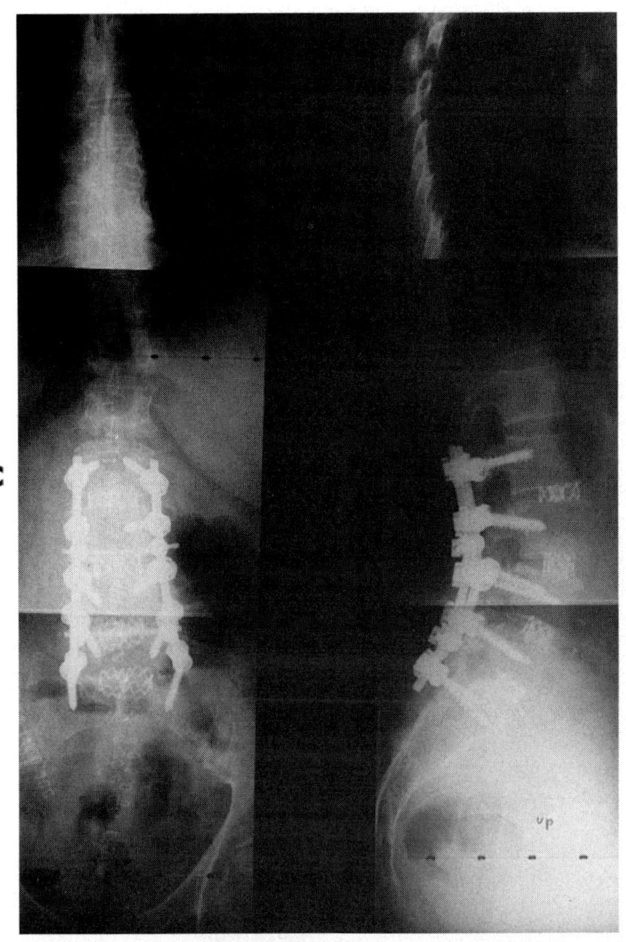

**FIGURE 13-5, CONT'D**

**C,** The rods have been placed, achieving only posterior compression of the anterior grafts.

pitalization or reoperation were encountered. This group verified the efficacy and safety of the BFB sequence in difficult salvage spinal problems.

## LOGISTICS

Revision spinal surgery is a major undertaking, particularly when approaching both sides of the spine. A well-planned team approach to two- and three-stage spinal surgery is mandatory for satisfactory outcome and patient safety. The safety and efficacy of two-stage same-day surgery is well established.[1,3,6,8] Going from two- to three-stage spinal surgery should not be difficult.

Successful and timely execution of a three-stage spinal procedure requires an excellent and experienced operating room staff in addition to an experienced surgical team and anesthesiology physicians. As an example, the logistics and staff employed at the University of Miami-affiliated hospitals, Miami, Florida, will be described.

The surgical set-up is critical to successful and timely two- and three-stage spinal surgery. The set-ups for both the anterior and posterior portions are opened at the same time. This requires a large enough operating room to hold the two set-ups, the surgical area, and all ancillary equipment (spinal monitor, cell saver, perhaps C-arm for a portion), and anesthesia machine. Two operating tables are desirable. I use the Jackson frame for the posterior approach, and a regular table for the anterior approach. The patient is turned from table to table.

Excellent aseptic technique is required with such a large sterile area (two set-ups, as well as the draped surgical area). There may be a theoretical objection to having both set-ups open for a 6-hour, or longer, procedure. It should be remembered that many procedures are done from the same set-up lasting much longer than 10 hours, without thought of changing the set-up after a given period of time. During change of position time, it is helpful to appoint an observer to ensure that all sterile areas remain free of contamination. In over 15 years of doing two- and three-stage spinal procedures as described, there has not been a single acute infection.

Instruments and bone grafts are frequently passed from the posterior to the anterior set-up, or vice versa. Again, an observer of sterile technique during these passages is desirable. The advantage of opening everything at the start is obvious. The time saved during turnover from back to front to back is apparent. My average time from application of dressings to one wound and making the incision on the next stage is less than 15 minutes. Separate counts of sponges and needles for each set-up is mandatory. Countable items for the posterior portions should be retained in the room until the procedures are complete. Countable items for the anterior portion of the procedure may be removed from the room after the anterior portion, but should be retained in the immediate area if further verification is required.

Two scrub nurses and two circulating nurses make the opening of instruments and supplies efficient, as well as setting up these. This is accomplished prior to bringing the patient in the room. The anesthesiologist prepares the patient with necessary lines in the holding area, and the neurophysiologic technician applies appropriate monitoring electrodes and stimulators. When the set-up is ready the patient is brought into the room and anesthesia is induced. The patient is then turned from the stretcher onto the Jackson table.

The first posterior approach is accomplished. All necessary procedures are performed. These may include removal of instrumentation, exploration of spine, repair of pseudarthroses, osteotomy, segmental mobilization, placement of spinal anchors, and taking of iliac bone graft. The wound is then closed using running sutures on the deep fascia and subcutaneous tissue. The skin is not closed. Sterile dressings are applied. Care must be taken to limit the width of the dressing and taped area so as to not impinge on the planned anterior incisional area. All drapes are re-

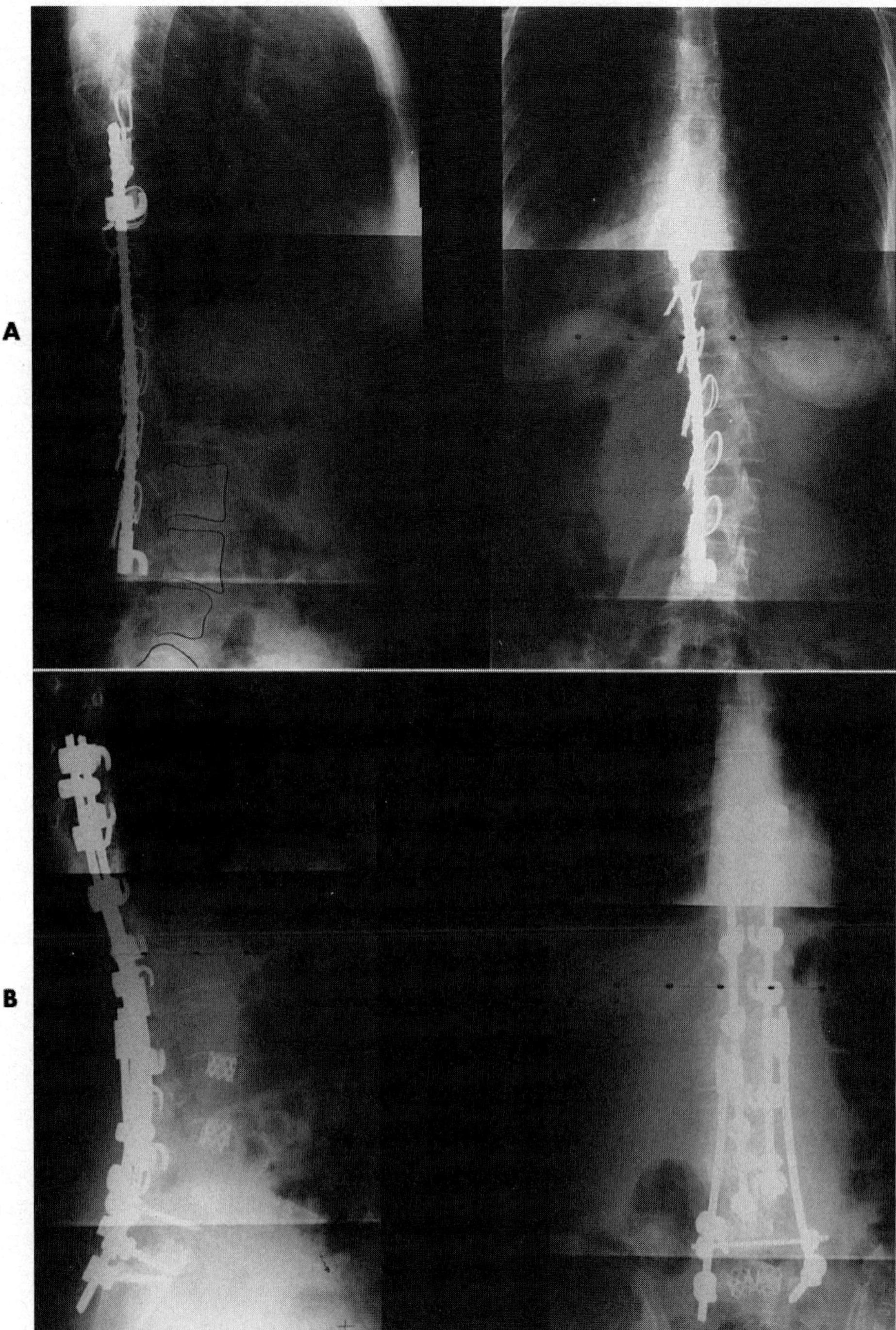


FIGURE 13-6

**A,** Harri-Luque correction of an adult with idiopathic scoliosis. Note the presence of spondylolisthesis distal to the distal instrumented level and the lumbar flat back. **B,** The back-front-back sequence was employed to correct the lumbar flat back and extend the fusion distal to include the spondylolisthesis and the MRI-demonstrated degenerative lumbosacral joint. Pseudarthroses were present at every level previously instrumented.

moved, and the set-up for the posterior procedure (including Mayfield overbed table) is removed to a remote area of the room. Care must be taken to preserve the sterility of the posterior set-up at this stage. An observer is most helpful for the few minutes of this stage. The patient is then turned onto the regular surgical table and positioned for the anterior procedure. This is usually supine for procedures below the diaphragm, oblique for thoracoabdominal approaches, and lateral for thoracic approaches. For anterior approaches involving the lumbar spine, it is helpful to place a large bolster (two 1-liter bags of intravenous fluids taped to-

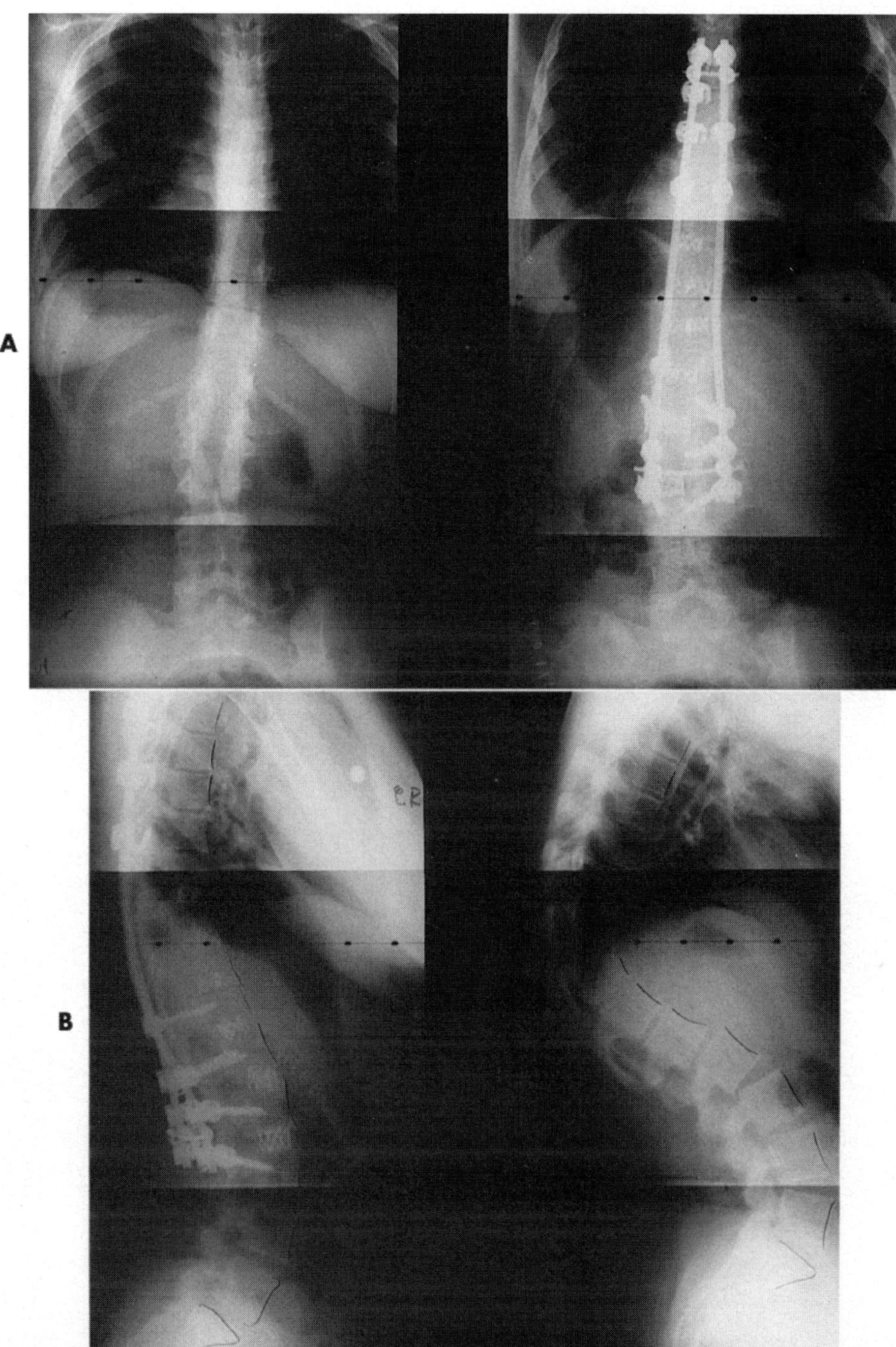

**FIGURE 13-7**

The before and after coronal views **(A)** and the after and before sagittal views **(B)** of a post-laminectomy kyphosis. Two years previously, thoracolumbar laminectomy had been performed for arteriovenous malformation. The progressive kyphosis was corrected by the back-front-back sequence, with the provision of anterior column support at all levels distal to the apex.

gether) under the lumbar spine to assist in creation of lordosis. The anterior set-up is brought into the field after the patient is prepped and draped.

The anterior procedure is then performed. A general, vascular, or thoracic surgeon usually performs the anterior exposure and closure, preserving the spinal surgeon for the spinal surgery. The anterior portion includes diskectomy and/or corpectomy, anterior distraction, and anterior structural graft placement. Harms' titanium cages filled with autogenous bone obtained during the posterior portion of the procedure have been used for the past 5 years for the structural graft. Prior to this, cadaver femoral rings were used. Decortication and graft placement anterior to

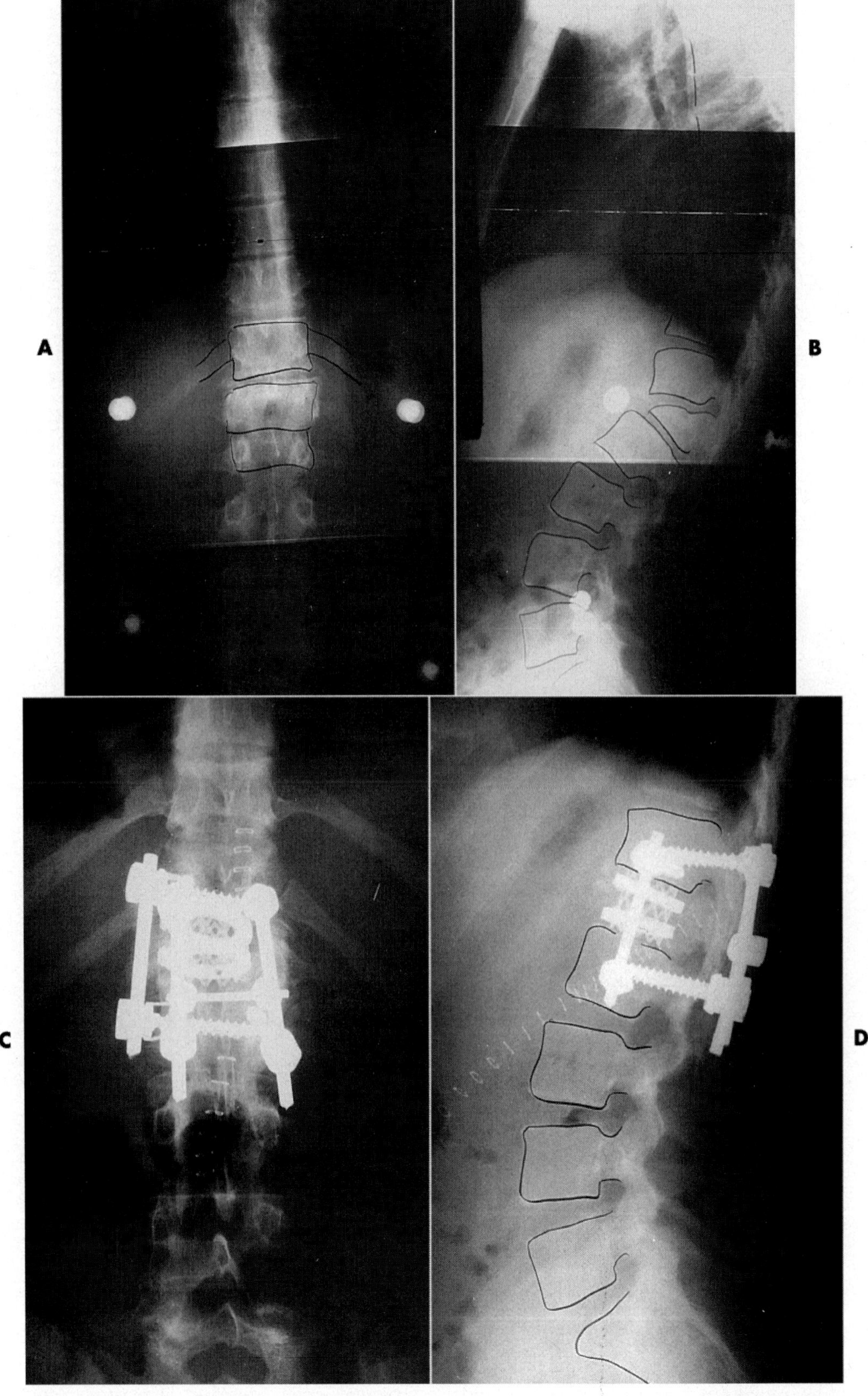


**FIGURE 13-8**

**A, B,** Posttraumatic kyphosis is presented. **C, D,** This has been corrected by the back-front-back sequence. The first posterior approach accomplished segmental release and placement of screws. The anterior portion accomplished corpectomy and interbody graft, stabilized by anterior screws. The second posterior approach afforded additional anterior compression via placement of the rods. Canal decompression and normalization of the sagittal contour is attained.

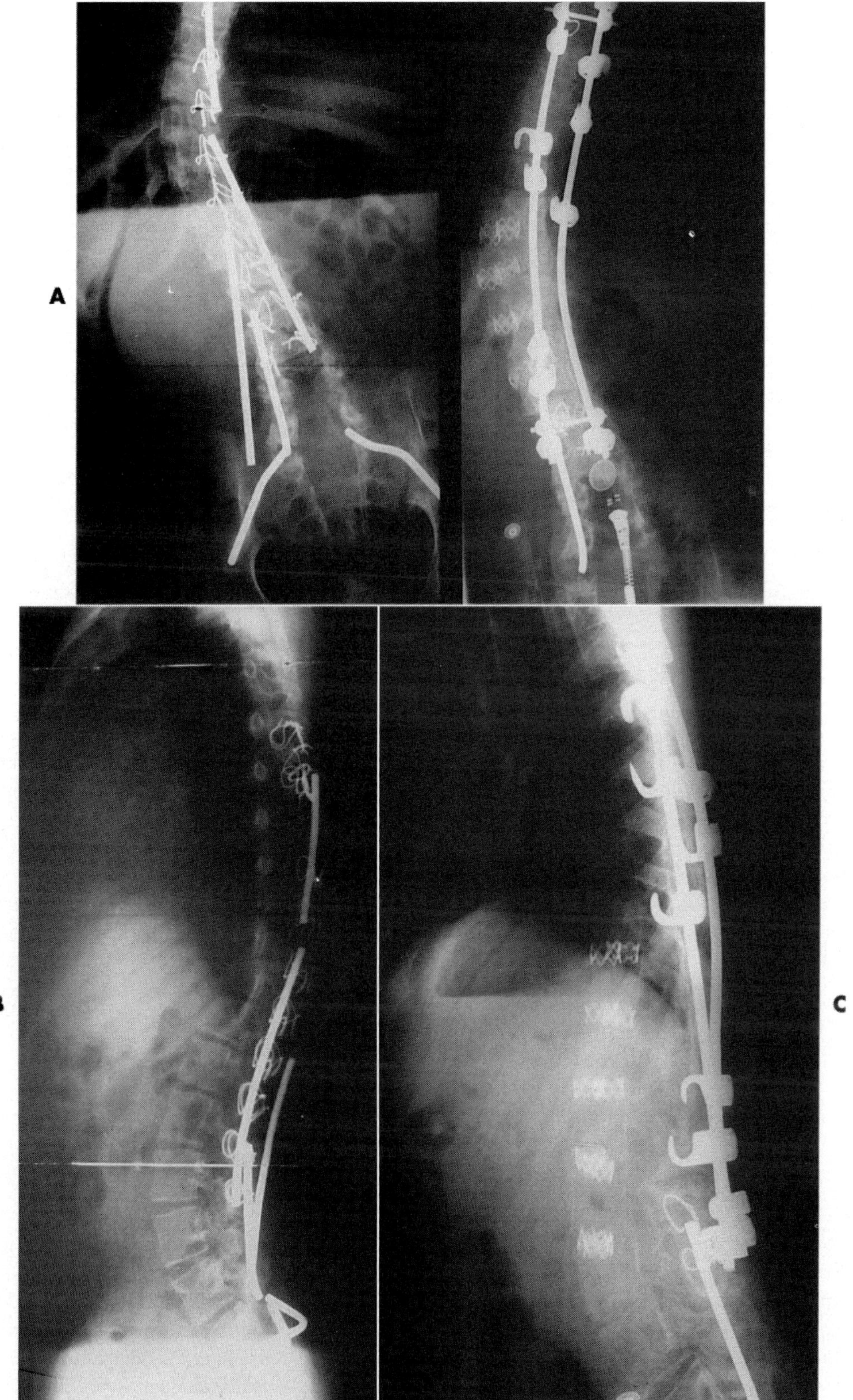


FIGURE 13-9

**A,** The coronal views of a complex pseudarthrosis in a patient with myelodysplasia is seen. **B, C,** Sagittal views. The back-front-back sequence allows the levels of pseudarthrosis to be identified, mobilized, and anteriorly grafted. Then, posterior compression of the anterior graft is achieved. A portion of the Luque trolley is embedded in the fusion mass and was not removed.

the cages are routine parts of the procedure. The anterior wound is then closed and dressings applied. The anterior set-up can then be removed from the operating room. Again, an observer is invaluable during the position changes. The patient is then repositioned on the Jackson frame. After preparation and draping, the posterior set-up is again positioned. The posterior wound is then reopened. The rods are placed and usually compression forces applied. Decortication and grafting is accomplished prior to closure. The posterior wound is then closed, and the patient turned onto his bed and transferred to recovery after demonstration of movement of the lower extremities.

After surgery, the patient is usually extubated, and treated in the intensive care unit. Ambulation without external support is usually possible on the second or third postoperative day. Discharge is usually on the 7th to 10th day. Three-stage spinal surgery on the same day is a major undertaking, particularly in the complex multilevel previously operated patient. With an experienced nursing staff and ancillary personnel, three-stage surgery can be safely accomplished in a timely manner.

## REQUIREMENTS FOR PROCEDURE

The editor of this text requested a list of necessary equipment to accomplish this procedure in a hospital unknown to me. The following would be the minimum. I have done this procedure in many places in the world, without a great deal of difficulty.

1. Anesthesiologist familiar with hypotensive anesthetic techniques (systolic approximately 75-90 mm Hg) and wake-up test.
2. Two surgical tables.
3. Two scrub nurses and two circulating nurses.
4. Separate set-ups for the anterior and posterior procedures, both to be opened at the same time before the start of surgery.
5. Blood recovery system and spinal cord monitoring are desirable but not mandatory.

The specific instruments to accomplish the various portions of the procedure are available at most hospitals that perform spinal surgery. Usually not many instruments are required, and few if any exotic instruments are required. The instruments available with the Harms' cages are useful. The instruments supplied with spinal instrumentation (posterior or anterior) are necessary.

## CONCLUSIONS

Same-day three-stage (anterior-posterior-anterior) spinal surgery can be safely and efficaciously accomplished. An adequately sized room to permit opening all instruments and equipment prior to surgery and an experienced team minimizes down time.

Revision spinal surgery is generally a problem in kyphosis. Posterior correction creates an anterior column deficit that should be filled. Anterior grafts require compression forces for optimum healing.

BFB surgery fulfills the requirements of revision spinal surgery. These include: (1) first posterior approach: posterior shortening (pseudarthrosis repair, osteotomy, segmental release), posterior placement of spinal anchors, and taking of bone graft; (2) anterior approach: disk removal or corpectomy, anterior distraction to create lordosis with structural grafting under compression; and (3) second posterior approach: placement of rods and application of posterior compression forces.

## REFERENCES


1. Harms JG, Beele BA, Bohm H et al: *Lumbosacral fusion with Harms' instrumentation.* In Margulies JY et al, editors: *Lumbosacral and spinopelvic fixation,* Philadelphia, 1996, Lippincott-Raven, pp 529-538.
2. Jackson RP: *Jackson sacral fixation and contoured spinal correction techniques.* In Margulies JY et al, editors: *Lumbosacral and spinopelvic fixation,* Philadelphia, 1996, Lippincott-Raven, pp 357-379.
3. Kostuik JP, Maurais GR, Richardson WJ et al: Combined single stage anterior and posterior osteotomy for correction of iatrogenic lumbar kyphosis, *Spine* 13:257-266, 1988.
4. O'Brien JP, Dawson MHO, Heard CW et al: Simultaneous combined anterior and posterior spinal fusion, *Clin Orthop* 203:191, 1986.
5. Scoliosis Research Society, M & M Report, presented at Annual Meeting, Asheville, 1995.
6. Shufflebarger HL, Grimm JO, Bui V, Thomson JD: Anterior and posterior spinal fusion: staged vs. same day surgery, *Spine* 16:930-933, 1991.
7. Shufflebarger HL. Complex pseudoarthrosis: posterior/anterior/posterior sequence using Harms' cages and Moss Miami instrumentation. Presented at WPOA Spine Section, Annual Meeting, Kochi, Japan, 1996.
8. Spencer DL, DeWald RL: Simultaneous anterior and posterior surgical approach to the thoracic and lumbar spine, *Spine* 4:29-36, 1979.
9. Wright M, DeWald RL: *Flat back syndrome.* In Margulies JY et al, editors: *Lumbosacral and spondylo-pelvic fixation,* Philadelphia, 1996, Lippincott-Raven, p 698.

# V
# EVALUATION AND INDICATIONS FOR REVISION SURGERY

# 14

# IMAGING OF THE POSTOPERATIVE SPINE PATIENT: AN ALGORITHMIC APPROACH

**David Lamb, M.D.**
**Scott D. Boden, M.D.**



The primary goal in the evaluation of a symptomatic patient who has had previous spine surgery is to efficiently arrive at a correct diagnosis for the persistent, recurrent, or new pain. The secondary goal is to determine if this patient can be helped with additional surgery or if he/she would best be managed with nonoperative treatment. The frequency and cost of persistent pain and disability from prior failed spine surgery is staggering. Waddell reports that 15% of the 300,000 patients undergoing de novo laminectomies annually in the U.S. may continue to be disabled.[32]

The potential reasons for this failed spine surgery are multifactorial (Table 14-1). Potential factors include the accuracy of the preoperative indications for the index procedure, host medical and psychosocial factors, and cognitive technical errors in surgical technique.[7] The task of the revision spine surgeon is to distinguish surgically treatable from nonsurgical entities. Some etiologies that account for failed spine surgery that are potentially amenable to surgical treatment include: recurrent or residual herniated disk material, iatrogenic spinal instability (spondylosis or pseudarthrosis), stenosis (lateral, central, junctional), and discitis. In contrast, some symptomatic entities are usually not amenable to surgical treatment. These include intradural and extradural scarring as seen with arachnoiditis and epidural fibrosis, psychosocial instability, and symptomatic metabolic disease.

Management of many of the surgically treatable entities is based on diagnostic and treatment algorithms similar to those used for their analogous primary counterparts. In this chapter, our first goal is to review the role of plain films, bone scans, computed tomography (CT), and magnetic resonance imaging (MRI) in the postoperative spine patient. Our second goal is to focus on the most common imaging abnormalities unique to the symptomatic postoperative spine patient, namely, recurrent disk herniation, pseudarthrosis, junctional stenosis, and discitis. Lastly, based upon the strengths and weaknesses of specific imaging modalities in conjunction with their corresponding clinical symptomatology, an algorithm for diagnosis and a guide to treatment of the symptomatic postoperative spine patient are proposed.

## IMAGING MODALITIES FOR EVALUATING THE POSTOPERATIVE SPINE PATIENT

We start by focusing on each specific imaging technique and its diagnostic- and treatment-based value. Plain radiographs serve as an excellent initial diagnostic tool for evaluating gross instability of the spine in either the frontal or sagittal plane. Degenerative instability above or below an old fusion or iatrogenic instability secondary to previously destabilizing procedure can often be demonstrated with dynamic radiography (Fig. 14-1). Standing weightbearing lateral flexion and extension views must be assessed for any evidence of abnormal motion. Although controversial, relative sagittal plane translation of greater than 4 mm

**Table 14-1. Differential Diagnosis of the Multiply Operated Spine**

| History, Physical Examination, Radiographs | Original Disk Not Removed | Recurrent Disk at Same Level | Recurrent Disk at Different Level | Spinal Instability | Spinal Stenosis | Arachnoiditis | Epidural Scar Tissue | Discitis |
|---|---|---|---|---|---|---|---|---|
| Painfree interval | None | > 6 months | > 6 months | | | > 1 month but < 6 months | > 1 month, gradual onset | |
| Predominant pain: radicular vs axial | Radicular | Radicular | Radicular | ± Axial | Axial + Radicular | Axial + Radicular | Axial and/or Radicular | Axial |
| Tension sign | + | + | + | | | May be positive | May be positive | |
| Neurologic examination | + Same pattern | + Same pattern | + Different level | | + After stress | | | |
| Plain films | + Wrong level | | | | + | | | ± |
| Lateral motion films | | | | + | | | | |
| Metrizamide | + But unchanged | + Same level | + Different level | | + | + | + | |
| CT scan | + | + | + | | + | | + (IV contrast) | + (IV contrast) |
| MRI | + | + | + | | + | + | + (Gadolinium contrast) | + |

Modified from Boden SD, Wiesel SW, Laws ER Jr, Rothman RH: The Aging Spine. Philadelphia, W.B. Saunders, 1991.

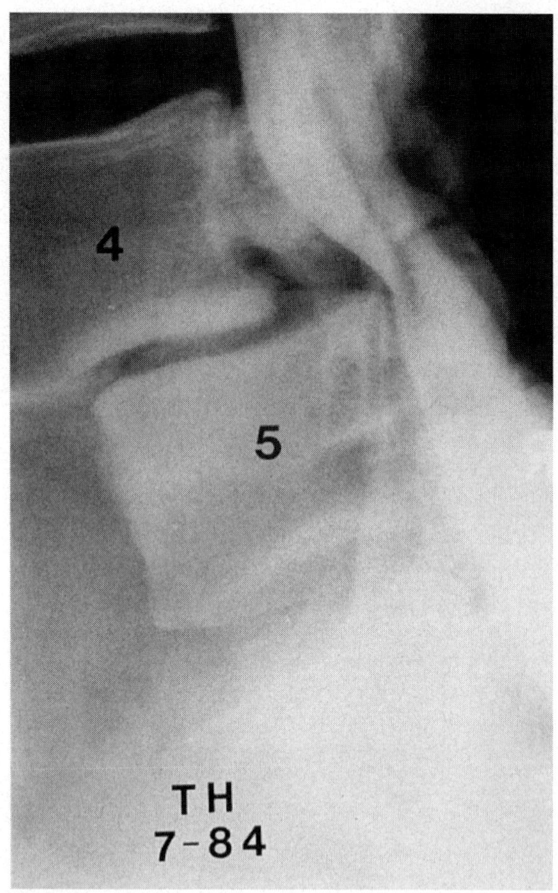


FIGURE 14-1

Lateral myelogram shows iatrogenic spinal stenosis due to anterior slippage following a previous laminectomy.

or 12% of the anteroposterior diameter of the vertebral body and relative rotation of greater than 11° between segments are commonly cited guidelines for instability of the spine (Fig. 14-2). At the lumbosacral junction the criteria are slightly higher, with greater than 25% translation or rotation greater than 19° tolerated.

In addition to instability, plain films should be evaluated for the extent and level of previous laminectomies or for evidence of spinal stenosis and facet arthropathy. The site of surgery should correspond with anatomic pathology in the preoperative radiographs and with the patient's index clinical symptomatology. Broken or loose hardware from previously attempted fusions should be noted, as it suggests the probability, although not the absolute existence, of pseudarthrosis (Fig. 14-3). Although much information can be ascertained from static and dynamic radiography, plain films alone are unreliable for detecting pseudarthrosis and a high clinical suspicion must be present.[15,17,18,19,29]

In the postoperative spine patient the bone scan has been shown to be of some value for detecting pseudarthrosis. The anatomically complex nature of pseudarthrosis often makes radiographic detection quite difficult. The frequent use of metallic fixation devices further complicates radiographic detection and may limit the use of CT and MRI. With pseudarthrosis there is continued motion with impact loading on adjacent bone surfaces, resulting in activated osteoblast and increased uptake of $Tc^{99}$ diphosphonate compounds. Pronounced uptake at a site of a spine fusion more than 1 year following a surgical procedure is highly suspicious for pseudarthrosis. The overlapping distribution of osteoblastic and osteoclastic activity in a large and anatomically complex bone structure (such as a fusion mass) favors the use of single photon emission tomography (SPECT) over an ordinary bone scan. This technique separates, by cross-sectional plane, the areas of interest from underlying and overlying distributions of osseous activity, thus providing three-dimensional positional information. Compared to planar imaging, SPECT produces approximately a 20% to 50% increase in nonunion detection in the lumbosacral spine.[27]

Water-soluble myelography, when followed by computed tomographic scanning, is of value in the postoperative spine patient. Information concerning the size of the spinal canal, extradural compression, surgical defects, and hypertrophied bony changes causing stenosis are all readily obtained. Although a sensitive test for demonstrating the changes of arachnoiditis, myelography falls short in distinguishing between disk material and epidural scar tissue.

MRI is the most useful diagnostic tool in distinguishing recurrent or residual disk herniation from epidural scar tissue. Intravenous contrast medium enhancement with gadolinium (Gd) or other paramagnetic contrast materials helps to identify scar tissue because it is relatively vascular. A herniated or recurrent disk, however, is avascular and therefore does not enhance. Postsurgical changes and resolving hematoma following successful lumbar decompression present a mass effect on MRI and preclude interpretation of recurrence prior to 6 months. Thus, caution should be used when evaluating MRIs too soon after the index surgery. Finally, the MRI scan is useful for the detection of other processes that may cause continued symptoms after previous back surgery. These include various metabolic abnormalities, infections, and tumors in the spine.

## ABNORMALITIES SPECIFIC TO POSTOPERATIVE IMAGING

At the outset, the evaluation of a postoperative imaging study is subject to the same caveat as any imaging study, specifically, the prevalence of plain film, myelogram, CT, or MRI abnormalities in approximately 33% of asymptomatic populations.[3,14,30,33] This high prevalence of incidental abnormalities underscores the importance of clinical correlation to avoid further errors in decision making and treatment.

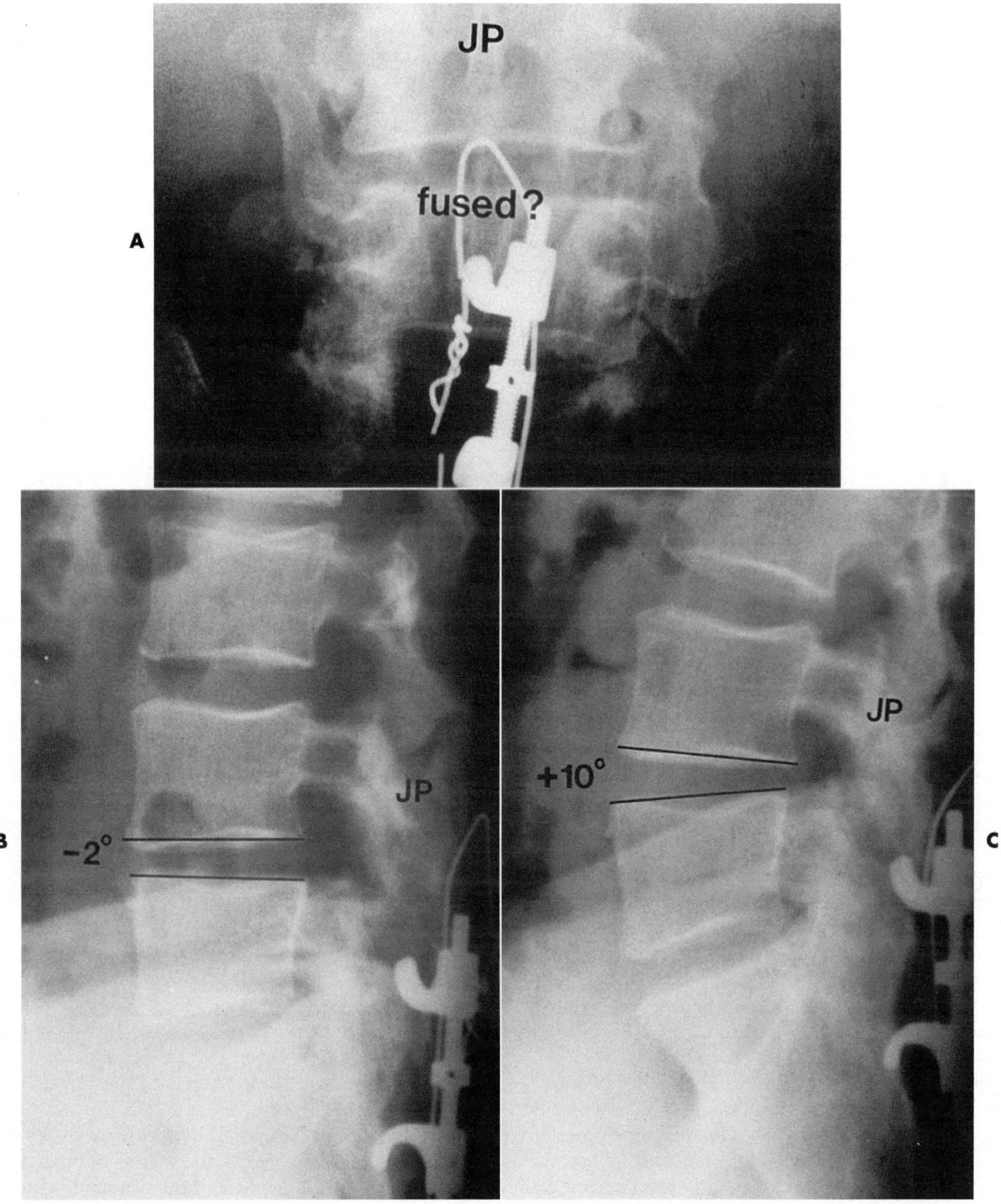


FIGURE 14-2

**A,** This is an AP radiograph of a patient with persistent low back pain (axial) following a lumbar decompression and attempted posterolateral fusion with instrumentation. Note the failed fixation and wispy bone graft. **B, C,** Flexion/extension films demonstrate motion at L4 to L5 motion segment.

*Continued*

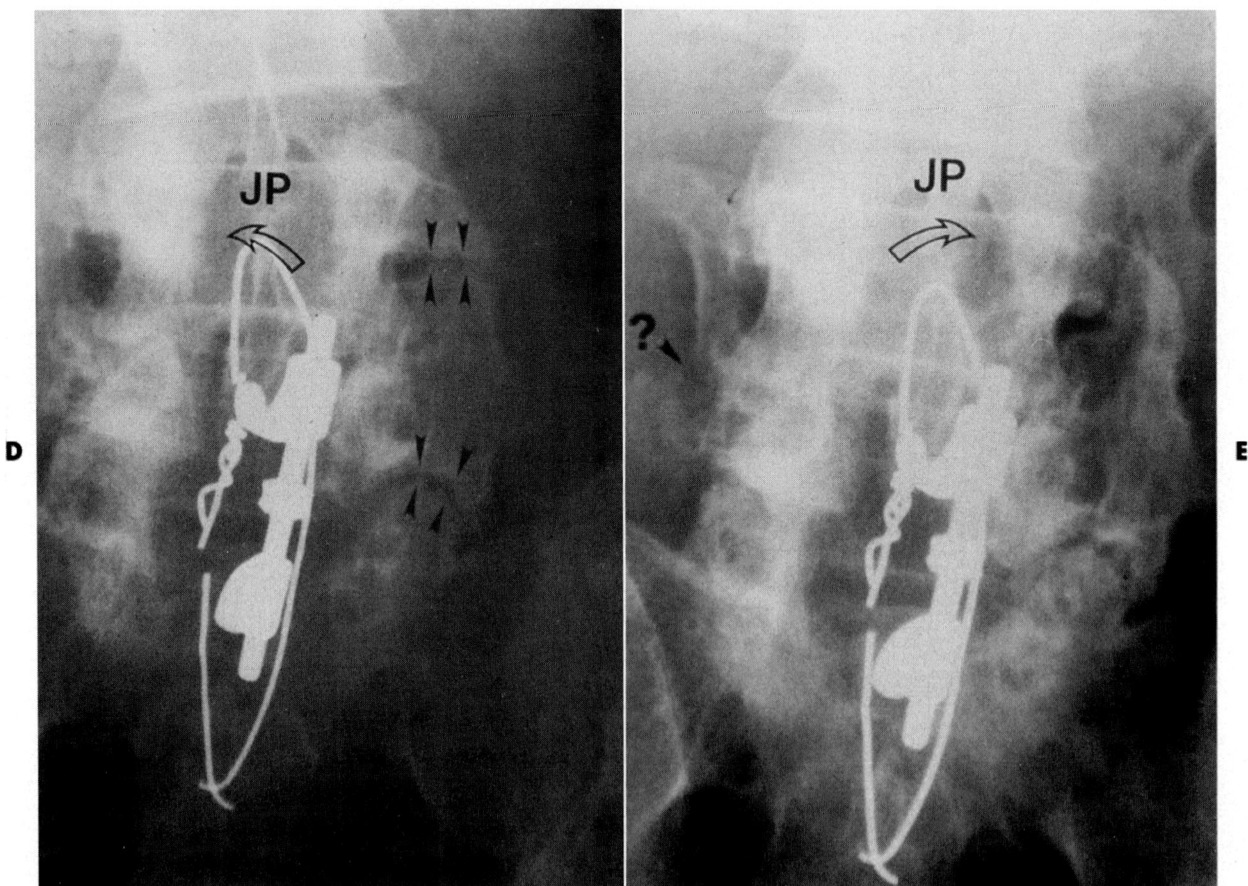


**FIGURE 14-2, CONT'D**

**D, E,** Side-bending films (*open arrows show direction*) suggest a site of pseudarthrosis (*arrowheads*).

With the knowledge of the presence of asymptomatic lesions and normal degenerative findings in various imaging modalities, the clinician can focus upon some common clinical entities responsible for failed spine surgery. Often the symptomatic spine patient is referred, already "worked up" with numerous postoperative imaging studies. It then becomes the responsibility of the revision spine surgeon to interpret these images and ascribe a diagnosis. Some of the more common causes of failed spine surgery include pseudarthrosis, instability, recurrent or residual stenosis, discitis, and recurrent disk herniation.

Pseudarthrosis or nonunion at the site of an attempted spinal arthrodesis is common. The reported incidence ranges from 7% to 45% depending upon the index pathology, region of the spine, use of internal fixation, choice of bone graft, and host inhibitory factors (smoking, steroids, diabetes, etc.).[29] The presence of asymptomatic nonunions further complicates the diagnostic problem. Presently the "gold standard" for detection of pseudarthrosis is surgical exploration, which exceeds the accuracy of most imaging modalities. Plain radiographs (including oblique, flexion, and extension views) are of limited accuracy in documenting spinal motion.[6] Three recent papers demonstrate the accuracy of radiographs in detecting a solid lumbar arthrodesis confirmed at surgical exploration to range from 62% to 68%.[2,9,23] In short, plain radiographs and tomography may be useful in the observation of trabecular bone patterns in a fusion mass; however, they often can not serve as a definitive diagnostic tool (Fig. 14-4).

Computed tomographic analysis of the solidity of lumbar fusion (Figs. 14-5 and 14-6) offers only a marginally higher rate of correlation with surgical exploration (70%).[25] This can be improved with coronal and sagittal reconstructions.[13] The evaluation of a fusion mass is more difficult with the presence of metallic internal fixation devices that generate MR and CT artifacts, which, in turn, tend to obscure the fusion mass. The current literature offers little to support the role of MRI in determining the solidity of fusion mass in the lumbar spine, and its use is limited with the presence of metallic implants.

In the cervical spine there is some evidence to support the utility of MRI in evaluating the status of a fusion after anterior cervical diskectomy and interbody fusion with instrumentation. In a persistently symptomatic patient with questionable radiolucent zones present on plain radiography or tomography, a continuous hyperintense signal found on T1-weighted images between adjacent motion segments may suggest a

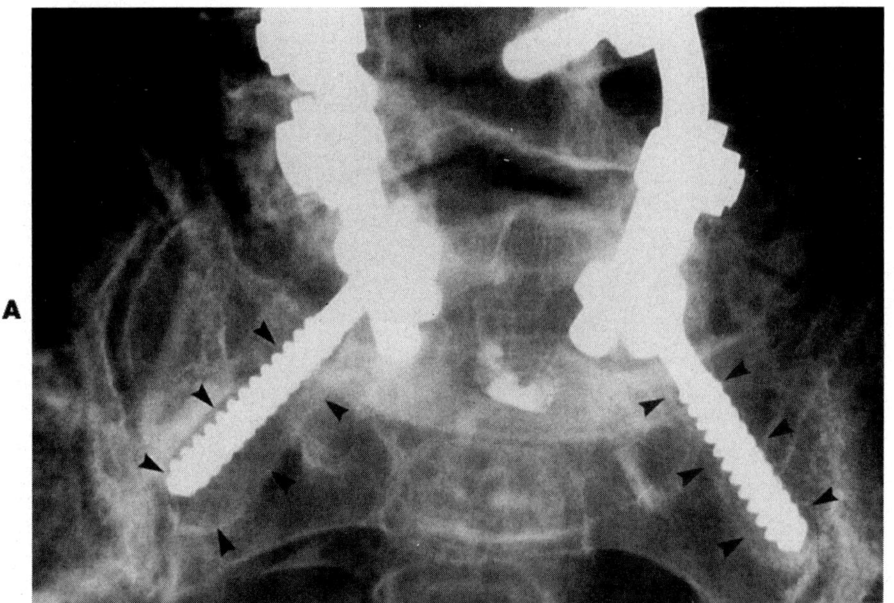

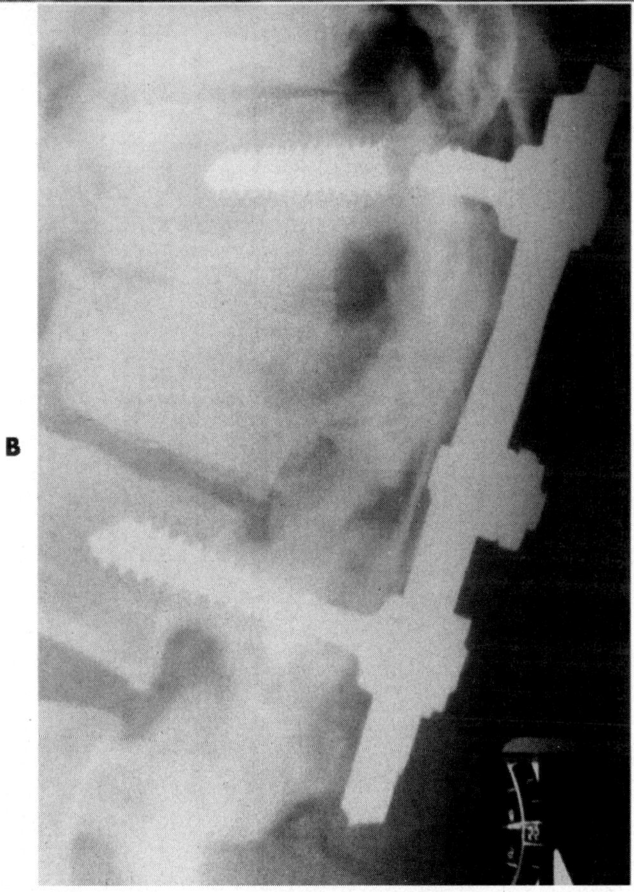

**FIGURE 14-3**

**(A)** AP radiograph demonstrating failure of segmental hardware fixation by loosening; *small black arrows* show windshield wiper effect of loose hardware. **(B)** Lateral radiograph from a patient with catastrophic failure of pedicle screws.

solid fusion with remodeling and fatty-marrow replacement occurring.[1]

A less common but potentially serious reason for persistent back pain after spine surgery is infection. In the acute setting the clinical signs of fever, leukocytosis, and wound infection most often obviate the need for diagnostic imaging; however, these symptoms may be present in less than 50% of patients with infections. In the absence of overt signs of systemic infection, the diagnosis of discitis should be considered in a patient who fails to improve after uncomplicated diskectomy. The imaging challenge becomes to distinguish between normal postoperative changes after an uncomplicated diskectomy and changes of a postoperative infection in the disk space. Plain films rarely offer insight into the process acutely (first 2 weeks) and may be of value only after end-plate erosion and vertebral body involvement have occurred. A characteristic pattern

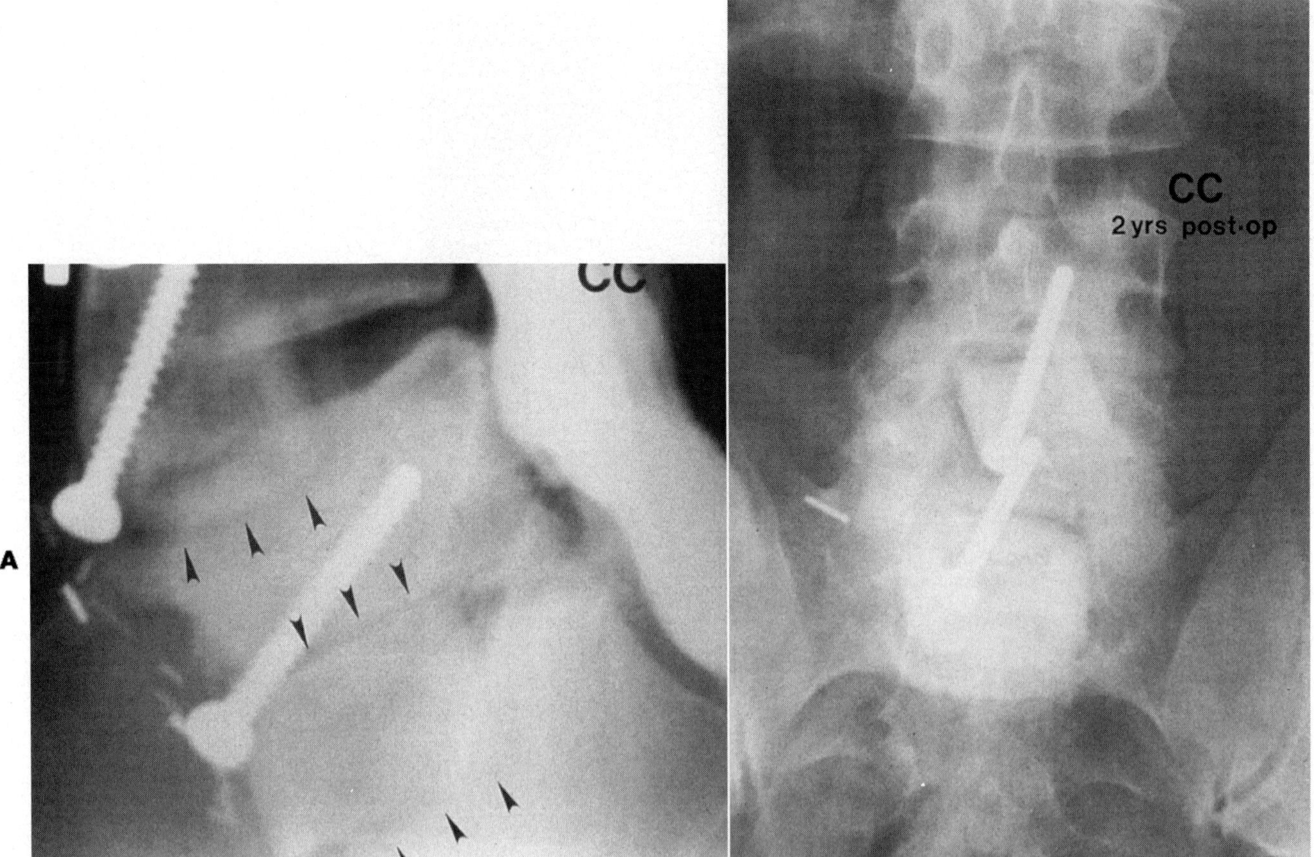


FIGURE 14-4

**A, B,** Attempted anterior allograft fusion with radiolucent zones typical of a nonunion.

predictive of postoperative discitis is described in Gd-enhanced MRI (Table 14-2).[5] This triad includes enhancement of adjacent vertebral bone marrow on each side of the affected disk space, decreased marrow signal on unenhanced T1-weighted sequences, and increased signal on T2-weighted sequences.

In addition to pseudarthrosis and discitis, perhaps the most common cause of leg pain after previous spine surgery is stenosis. Residual or new spinal stenosis can result from inadequate index decompression, missed lateral foraminal encroachment, or junctional stenosis above or below the fusion mass. Plain radiography offers little insight into residual spinal stenosis or neuronal compression. The main stay of diagnosis rests in the proper interpretation of CT and MRI findings with their anatomic correlation. Specifically central and paracentral stenosis are readily apparent when studied with contrast-enhanced CT. CT myelography is better than MRI in distinguishing persistent stenosis because of the ability to discern superior articular facet hypertrophy from residual ligamentum flavum and bulging posterior disk margins. These three structures are often indistinguishable in T1-weighted images.

Persistent radicular pain despite apparently decompressed foramen should lead the revision spine surgeon to scrutinize both the pre- and postforaminal zones of the exiting nerve root. Nerve root irritation can be caused by lateral recess stenosis cephalad to the inferior pedicle. This is best seen with CT myelography. In the extraforaminal zone (far lateral) nerve root irritation is best detected with parasagittal Gd-enhanced MRI.

The goal of postoperative imaging in the failed spine surgery patient is to distinguish scar tissue from potentially treatable causes of nerve root compression. This is especially important when deciding between recurrent herniated disk and scar as a cause of leg pain. Postoperative studies in which CT was used have shown that approximately 40% of asymptomatic patients have persistent mass effect consistent with a herniated disk, which is indistinguishable from changes seen in symptomatic patients postoperatively.[12,22,26] Unenhanced CT can distinguish scar tissue from disk material in 43% to 60% of these patients.[8,16] With intravenous injection of a contrast agent the likelihood of correct diagnosis increases to 70% to 83%.[8,10,16,24,28,31] Unenhanced MRI has been reported to have an accuracy of 76% to 89%, comparable with that of enhanced CT.[10,11,20,21,28] The diagnostic accuracy of contrast-enhanced MRI approaches 96% to 100%.[12,21] However, the physician must be aware of the normal spectrum of postoperative MRI changes that occur during the first 3 to 6

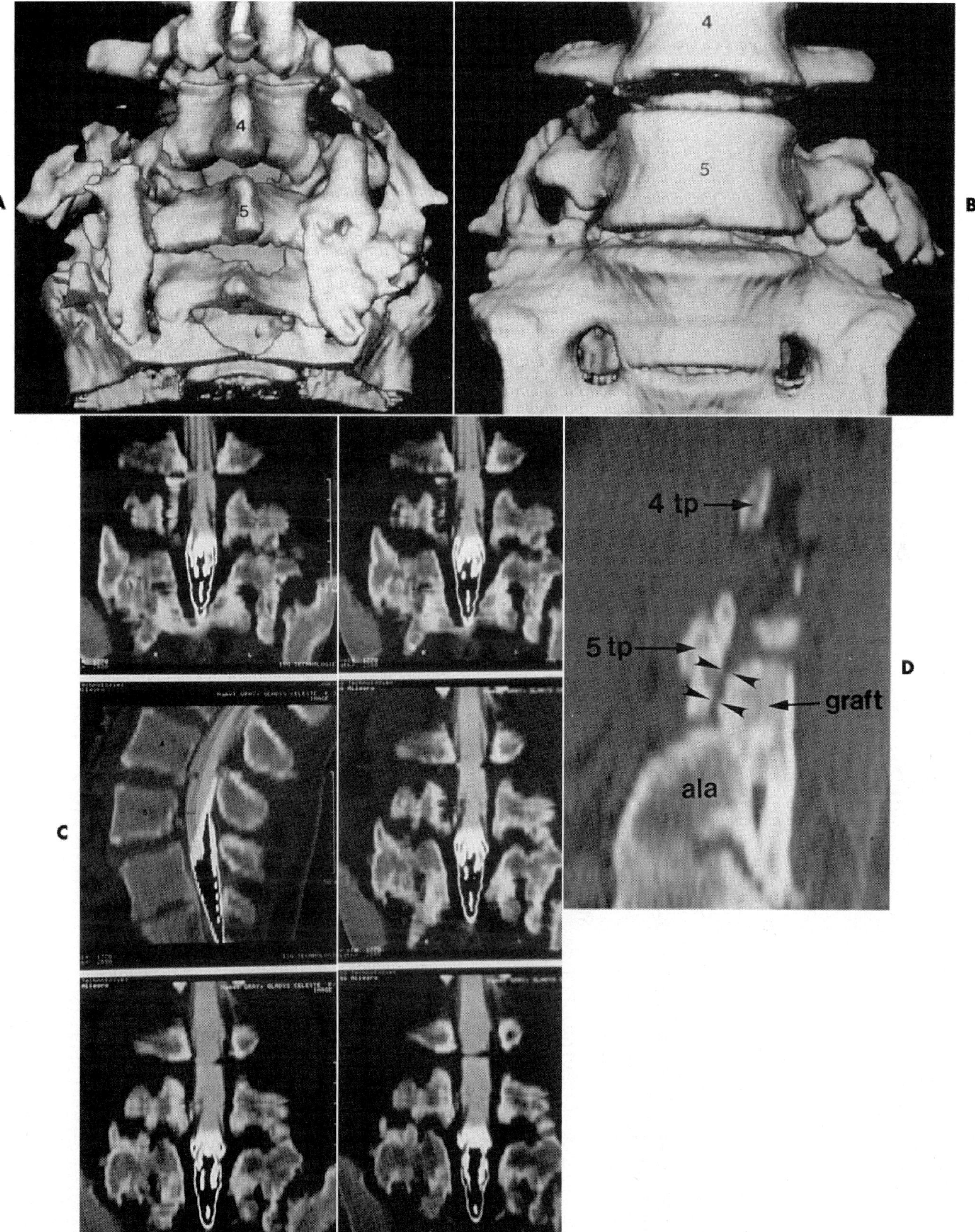


**FIGURE 14-5**

**A, B,** Three-dimensional reconstruction of lumbosacral area of a symptomatic patient following L5 to the sacrum fusion with suspected pseudarthrosis. **C,** Sagittal and coronal reconstruction suggest a hairline pseudarthrosis at L5-S1. **D,** Parasagittal CT view confirms the suspected diagnosis.

**Table 14-2. Magnetic Resonance Imaging Signal Characteristics of Degenerative Intervertebral-Disk Disease and Discitis**

| | Marrow | | | Central Portion of Disk | | |
|---|---|---|---|---|---|---|
| | T1-Weighted Images | T2-Weighted Images | T1-Weighted Images with Gadolinium | T1-Weighted Images | T2- Weighted Images | T1-Weighted Images with Gadolinium |
| Degenerative disk disease | | | | | | |
| Type I | Hypointense | Hyperintense | Hyperintense | Isointense/ hypointense | Hypointense | Isointense/hyperintense |
| Type II | Hyperintense | Isointense/ hyperintense | Isointense | Isointense/ hypointense | Hypointense | Isointense/hyperintense |
| Type III | Hypointense | Hypointense | Isointense | Isointense | Hypointense | Isointense |
| Discitis | Hypointense | Hyperintense | Hypointense | Hypointense | Hyperintense | Hyperintense |

From Boden SD: Current Concepts Review: The use of radiographic imaging studies in the evaluation of patients who have degenerative disorders of the lumbar spine, *J Bone Joint Surg* 78-A:114–124, 1996.

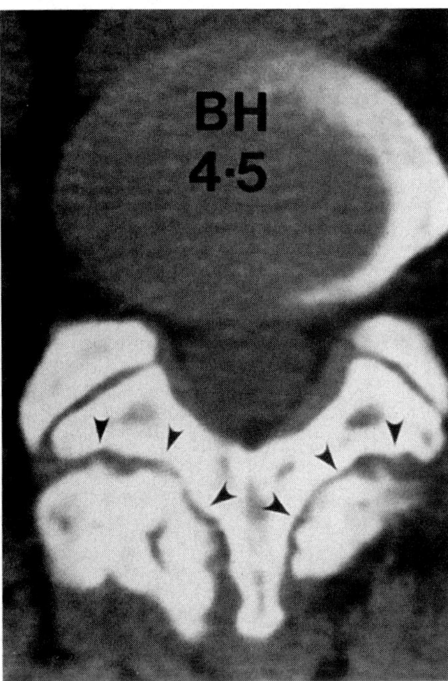


**FIGURE 14-6**

Axial CT shows poor incorporation of bone graft following an attempted interlaminar fusion. This gap was easily missed by plain films but was obvious with CT.

months, which can mimic pathology.[4] Thus, for a patient who has had a previous operation on the spine, MRI should always be performed with use of an intravenous injection of paramagnetic contrast medium (Fig. 14-7). If MRI is contraindicated, myelography followed by CT is the next best choice of imaging modalities to detect nerve root compression.

## AN IMAGING ALGORITHM

Lastly, we present an algorithm as a guideline for the radiographic evaluation of the symptomatic previously operated spine patient (Fig. 14-8). This algorithm is based on the premise that radiographic studies serve only to confirm a diagnosis suggested by history and physical exam. Stage I consists of a medical and psychosocial evaluation to rule out systemic disease or *supratentorial* pathology. Stage II begins with a thorough history and physical examination focusing on previous surgery, pain-free intervals, and symptomatology. The goal of stage II is to classify the pain into one of three categories: predominately axial, predominately radicular, or mixed axial and radicular pain. Stage III addresses each of these categories by guiding the selection of

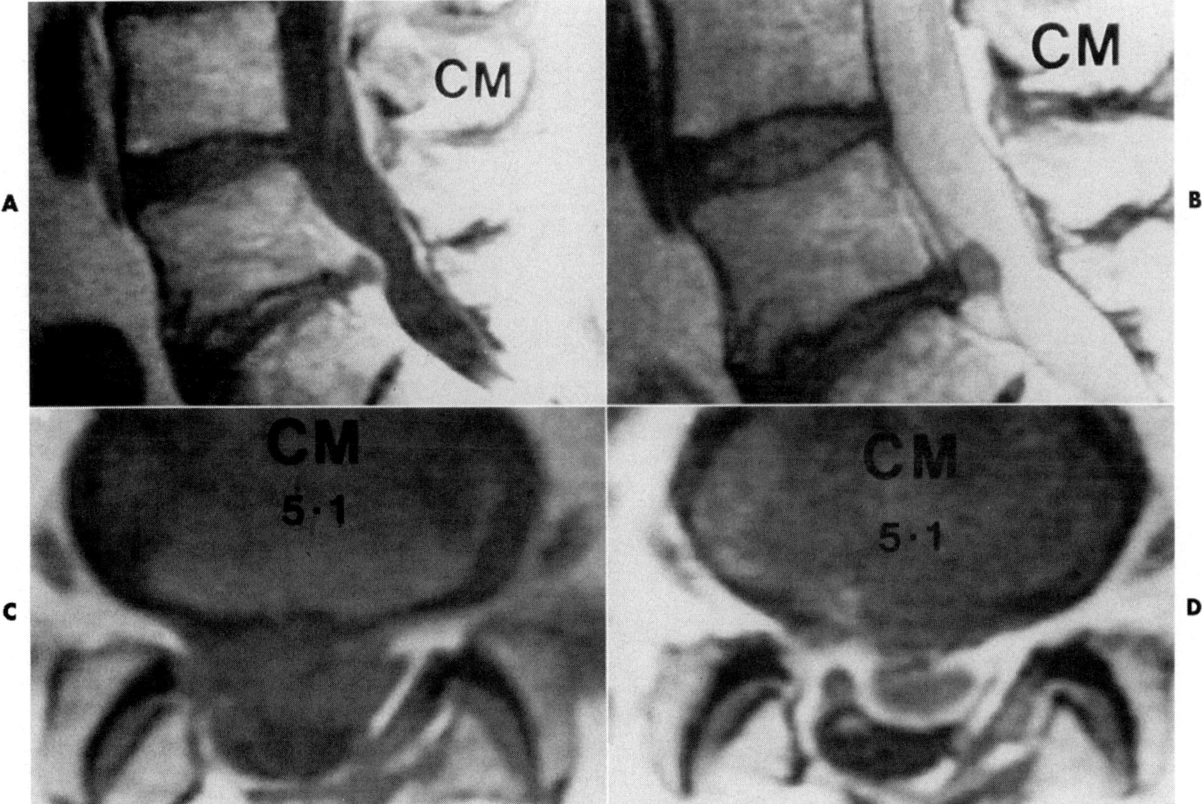


**FIGURE 14-7**

**A,** Patient with recurrent radiculopathy following L5-S1 diskectomy with a good pain-free interval. **B, C,** Unenhanced axial and sagittal MR scans suggest possible compression due to scar, disk, or hematoma. **D,** Gd-enhanced MR scan clearly demonstrates herniated disk recurrence with characteristic "pea sign" of a peripheral rim of enhancement.

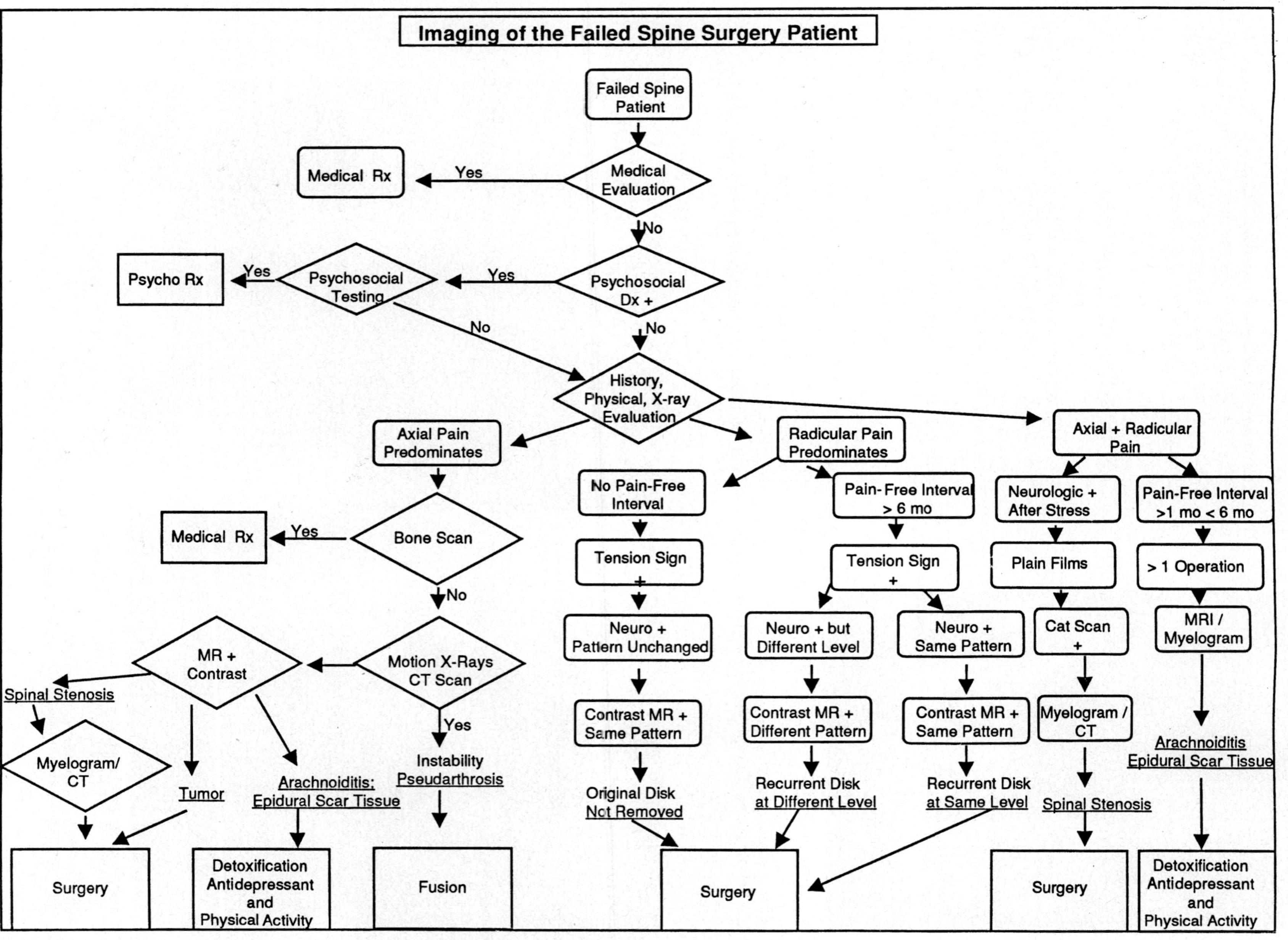


FIGURE 14-8
An algorithm guideline for the radiographic evaluation of the patient undergoing revision spine surgery.

confirmatory imaging based on a presumptive diagnosis. For example, recurrent radicular pain after diskectomy with a pain-free interval of greater than 6 months with correlating neurologic pattern is most likely a recurrent herniation. This patient's pathology is best confirmed with Gd-enhanced MRI.

## CONCLUSIONS

In summary, we have reviewed the common imaging modalities used in the evaluation of postoperative spine patients. To facilitate a more informed interpretation of these studies the various strengths and weaknesses of each imaging option must be considered. Patients must be separated into categories of either problems that are surgically treatable or those that are not. An organized and focused approach minimizes overuse and improves the success of revision spine surgeries.

## REFERENCES


1. Albert TJ, Lamb DJ: MRI evaluation of fusion mass incorporation after anterior cervical fusion, *Jeff Ortho J* XX:18-21, 1991.
2. Blumenthal SL, Gill K: Can lumbar spine radiographs accurately determine fusion in postoperative patients? Correlation of routine radiographs with a second surgical look at lumbar fusions, *Spine* 18:1186-1189, 1993.
3. Boden SD, Davis DO, Dina TS, et al: Abnormal magnetic resonance scans of the lumbar spine in asymptomatic subjects: a prospective investigation, *J Bone Joint Surg* 72:403-408, 1990.
4. Boden SD, Davis DO, Dina TS, Parker CP, O'Malley S, Sunner JL, Wiesel SW: Contrast-enhanced MR imaging performed after successful lumbar disk surgery: prospective study. *Radiology* 182:59-64, 1992.
5. Boden SD, Davis DO, Dina TS, Sunner JL, Wiesel SW: Postoperative diskitis: distinguishing early MR imaging findings from normal postoperative disk space changes, *Radiology* 184:765-771, 1992.
6. Boden SD, Wiesel SW: Lumbosacral segmental motion in normal individuals: have we been measuring instability properly? *Spine* 15:571-576, 1990.
7. Boden SD, Wiesel SW: Errors in decision making following radiographic investigations of the spine, *Sem Spine Surg* 5:90-100, 1993.
8. Braun IF, Hoffman JC Jr, Davis PC, Landman JA, Tindall GT: Contrast enhancement in CT differentiation between recurrent disk herniation and postoperative scar: prospective study, *AJR: Am J Roentgenol* 145:785-790, 1985.
9. Brodsky AE, Kovalsky ES, Khalil MA: Correlation of radiologic assessment of lumbar spine fusions with surgical exploration, *Spine* 16(suppl):S261-S265, 1991.
10. Bundschuh CV, Modic MT, Ross JS, Masaryk TJ, Bohlman H: Epidural fibrosis and recurrent disk herniation in the lumbar spine: MR imaging assessment, *AJR: Am J Roentgenol* 150:923-932, 1988.
11. Bundschuh CV, Stein L, Slusser JH, Schinco FP, Zadaga LF, Dillon JD: Distinguishing between scar and recurrent herniated disk in postoperative patients: value of contrast-enhanced CT and MR imaging, *AJNR: Am J Neuroradiol* 11:949-958, 1990.
12. Cervellini P, Curri D, Bernardi L, Volpin L, Benedetti A: Computed tomography after lumbar disc surgery: a comparison between symptomatic and asymptomatic patients, *Acta Neurochir* 43:44-47, 1988.
13. Chafetz N, Cann CE, Morris JM, Steinbach LS, Goldberg HI, Ax L: Pseudoarthrosis following lumbar fusion: detection by direct coronal CT scanning, *Radiology* 162:803-805, 1987.
14. Collier D Jr, Fogelman I, Brown ML: Bone scintigraphy. Part 2. Orthopedic bone scanning, *J Nucl Med* 34:2241-2246, 1993.
15. DePalma AF, Rothman RH: The Classic: the nature of pseudoarthrosis, *Clin Orthop* 284:3-10, 1992.
16. Firooznia H, Kricheff II, Rafii M, Golimbu C: Lumbar spine after surgery: examination with intravenous contrast-enhanced CT, *Radiology* 163:221-226, 1987.
17. Frymoyer JW, Hanley EN Jr, Howe J, Kuhlmann D, Matteri RE: A comparison of radiographic findings in fusion and nonfusion patients ten or more years following lumbar disc surgery, *Spine* 4:435-440, 1979.
18. Heggeness MH, Esses SI: Classification of pseudarthroses of the lumbar spine, *Spine* 16:S449-S454, 1991.
19. Heggeness MH, Esses SI, Mody DR: A histologic study of lumbar pseudarthrosis, *Spine* 18:1016-1020, 1993.
20. Hochhauser L, Kieffer SA, Caqcayorin ED, Petro GR, Teller WF: Recurrent postdiskectomy low back pain. MR-surgical correlation, *AJR: Am J Roentgenol* 151: 755-760, 1988.
21. Hueftle MG, Modic MT, Ross JS, Masaryk TJ, Carter JR, Wilber RG, Bohlman HH, Steinberg PM, Delamarter RB: Lumbar spine: postoperative MR imaging with Gd-DTPA, *Radiology* 167:817-824, 1988.

22. Ilkko E, Lahde S, Koivukangas J, Jalovaara P: Computed tomography after lumbar disc surgery, *Acta Radiol* 29:179-182, 1988.
23. Kant AP, Daum WJ, Dean SM, Uchida T: Evaluation of lumbar spine fusion: plain radiographs versus direct surgical exploration and observation, *Spine* 20:2313-2317, 1995.
24. Kieffer SA, Witwer GA, Cacayorin ED, Schell GR, Modesti LM, Yuan HA: Recurrent post-discectomy pain. CT-surgical correlation, *Acta Radiol* 369(suppl): 719-722, 1986.
25. Laasonen EM, Soini J: Low back pain after lumbar fusion: surgical and computed tomographic analysis, *Spine* 14:210-213, 1989.
26. Montaldi S, Fankhauser H, Schnyder P, de Tribolet N: Computed tomography of the postoperative intervertebral disc and lumbar spinal canal: investigation of twenty-five patients after successful operation for lumbar disc herniation, *Neurosurgery* 22:1014-1022, 1988.
27. Slizofski WJ, Collier BD, Flatley TJ, Carrera GF, Hellman RS, Isitman: Painful pseudarthrosis following lumbar spinal infusion: detection by combined SPECT and planar bone scintigraphy, *Skeletal Radiol* 16:138-141, 1987.
28. Sotiropoulous S, Chafetz N, Lang P, Winkler M, Morris JM, Weinstein PR, Genant HK: Differentiation between postoperative scar and recurrent disk herniation: prospective comparison of MR, CT, and contrast-enhanced CT, *AJNR* 10:639-643, 1989.
29. Steinmann JC, Herkowitz HN: Pseudarthrosis of the spine, *Clin Orthop* 284:80-90, 1992.
30. Torgenson WR, Botter WE: Comparative roentgenographic study of the asymptomatic and symptomatic lumbar spine, *J Bone Joint Surg* 58-A:850-853, 1976.
31. Tullberg T, Grane P, Rydberg J, Isacson J: Comparison of contrast-enhanced computed tomography and gadolinium-enhanced magnetic resonance imaging one year after lumbar discectomy, *Spine* 19: 183-188, 1994.
32. Waddell G: Failures of disc surgery and repeat surgery, *Acta Orthop Belgica* 53:300-302, 1987.
33. Wiesel SW, Bell GR, Feffer HL, et al: A study of computer-assisted tomography: I. The incidence of positive CAT scans in an asymptomatic group of patients, *Spine* 9:549-551, 1984.

# 15

# PAIN EVALUATION, INVASIVE DIAGNOSTIC RADIOLOGY, AND PATIENT SELECTION

**Richard D. Guyer, M.D.**
**Donna D. Ohnmeiss, M.S.**



Diagnosing symptomatic structural pathology in chronic low back pain patients is very difficult. The issue becomes even more challenging in patients who have persistent or recurring pain after surgical intervention. While the results of surgery are greatly varied, the incidence of patients failing to experience long-term relief following spine surgery is estimated to be at least 15%.[15] Also, as a group, the chance of having a good result following subsequent operation is generally reduced.

Pain in patients who have had previous spine surgery can arise from one of several sources or combinations thereof. Possible causes for postoperative symptoms include: recurrent disk herniation, symptomatic pseudarthrosis, iatrogenic instability, failure to address symptomatic pathology at the initial surgery (wrong spinal level or failure to address all pathology), symptomatic disk within a fused segment, fibrosis, arachnoiditis, nerve damage, reflex sympathetic dystrophy, hardware-related problems (hardware failure, painful hardware, migration onto neural tissue, or inappropriate placement), pathology developed at an adjacent level, sacroiliac joint problems, stenosis at the level adjacent to a fused segment, or facet problems. In this chapter, issues related to pain evauation, the role of invasive radiographic imaging in the previously operated patient, and patient selection for subsequent surgery are discussed.

## PAIN EVALUATION

As with any patient, the first step in evaluation is carefully taking the history and performing a physical examination. In patients who have previously undergone spine surgery, the history needs to be more in-depth than in other patients and must include a careful review of the patient's medical chart. Particular attention should be paid to the operative notes, discharge notes, and the office notes from the period after surgery. These can help define the clinical development of the current episode. Also, they may reflect items the patient did not feel were important enough to comment on or that have changed with memory. Additional items to be investigated are the symptoms and diagnostic evaluation findings that led to the initial surgery, the type of surgery performed, if there were any perioperative complications, if the patient experienced any period of significant pain relief following the initial procedure, and if psychological screening was performed before intervention.

### COMPARISON OF PRESENT PAIN TO ORIGINAL SYMPTOMS

One of the most important components of the patient's history is careful assessment of the presenting pain complaints. This needs to be conducted from several aspects. First, the presenting symptoms need to be evaluated as a comparison to the pain for which surgery was initially performed. Also, it needs to be determined if the patient experienced either pain relief or significantly reduced symptoms following the surgery and if so, for what period of time. The third component of the pain assessment is the pain location with respect to back versus leg pain and if the pain is in a diffuse pattern or if it is well localized. These three pieces of pain information combined can provide helpful insight as to the origin of the current symptoms.

Assessing current symptoms with respect to those previously experienced can provide important information in determining if the pain is the old problem unresolved or recurring, or if a new problem has developed. Pain in the previously operated patient may be experienced in several fashions compared to previous symptoms. Each may be associated with one or more suspected origins. Pain that is the same as before the surgery with no period of pain relief after the operative intervention is an indication that symptomatic pathology was not adequately addressed with the procedure performed. If the pain is similar to that experienced prior to surgery, but the patient did have a period of pain relief afterward, then one should suspect recurrent pathology. This is particularly true if the patient underwent a decompressive procedure. Patients presenting with pain different from their initial symptoms have a wide variety of possible problems. This may be related to newly developed pathology such as postdecompressive instability, pathology at different spinal levels (particularly those adjacent to the operated segment, including the sacroiliac joint), infection, scarring, facet joint pathology, or stenosis developed at the adjacent level. Another possible, less frequent cause of pain in previously operated patients is related to abnormalities of the autonomic nervous system. Sachs et al reported on a series of 11 patients with reflex sympathetic dystrophy after lumbar spine surgery (incidence of 1%).[49] All patients had burning pain, vasomotor dysfunction, and dystrophic changes in at least one of the lower extremities. Symptoms appeared in a range of 4 days to 20 weeks after surgery. Taking into consideration the length of time between surgery and the occurrence of pain complaint can help to delineate the origin of the symptoms.

### PAIN-FREE PERIOD

If the patient failed to enjoy any period of pain relief after surgery, one needs to suspect that the initial surgery failed to address the source of the patient's symptoms. This may be due to either misdiagnosis or failure to adequately address the problem during the surgical procedure (for example, not removing a free extruded disk fragment that is compressing a nerve root or, in the case of fusion, failing to address disk pathology or symptomatic pathology at the level adjacent to that operated). If the patient experiences pain after an initial period of relief, one needs to determine the length of time symptoms subsided. If the time period was less than 6 months one should suspect arachnoiditis, scarring, reflex sympathetic dystrophy, discitis, or other infection. If the patient enjoyed pain relief for more than 6 months, one should suspect the development of a new source of symptoms or a recurrent disk herniation if the symptoms are similar to those initially experienced. Other sources of new pain include disk herniation at a different lumbar level or on the opposite side from the first, breakdown of a lumbar level adjacent to an operated segment or of the sacroiliac joint, facet hypertrophy, stenosis, or damage done to posterior musculature during surgery.

### PAIN LOCATION

Great care should be taken in investigating the patient's pain location. This should be recorded in terms of back versus leg pain and if leg pain is present, is it unilateral or bilateral. The type of pain should be recorded. If significant leg pain is present and is in well-defined patterns, then one needs to investigate the possibility of nerve root compression due to herniated disk material, scar, boney compression, donor site pain, or misplaced spinal instrumentation such as pedicle screws compressing the nerve root or threaded fusion cages pushing disk or endplate fragments onto the nerve root. In the case of leg pain related to the graft donor site, the pain typically originates in the lateral crest where the graft was taken and radiates into the buttock and thigh. Although these are the primary causes of leg pain following spine surgery, other sources should not be overlooked. These include primarily the possibility of pain referred from the facets, sacroiliac joints, disks, ligaments, or other spinal structures. Kostuik described causes of leg pain following lumbar fusion with respect to the length of time between surgery and symptom onset.[32] He attributes early onset of leg pain to fixation impinging a nerve root. Leg pain arising months after surgery was associated with accelerated disk degeneration or loosening of fixation, and pain arising late after surgery was attributed to donor site pain, disk pain associated with pseudarthrosis, or stenosis or disk pain at the level adjacent to the fused segment.

If the patient's pain is primarily limited to the low back and associated with particular motions, mechanical instability should be suspected.[33] This may arise following decompressive procedures or a failed fusion that has allowed excessive motion in the previously operated region. Hopp and Tsou reported a 17% reoperation rate for instability created by decompressive procedures for lumbar spinal stenosis.[21] Kostuik has attributed back pain arising early after fusion to infection, wrong level(s) fused, or psychological distress. Back pain arising months after surgery may be associated with pseudarthrosis, disk disruption, accelerated degeneration of a disk adjacent to the fused segment, or lack of conditioning. The potentially detrimental effects of surgery on spinal musculature has recently been investigated.[28,50] This, combined with the patient's reduced activity due to pain, supports the need for comprehensive rehabilitation following low back surgery. Back pain appearing long after surgery was associated with late pseudarthrosis, instability, spondylolysis, or compression fracture.[32] Other items to investigate with respect to pain are the type of pain present. Radicular numbness may be more likely related to nerve root compression. Burning pain or hyperalgesia in the lower extremity may be related to postoperative reflex sympathetic dystrophy.

## PHYSICAL EXAMINATION

The physical examination should include routine sensory and motor evaluation. These results should be compared to the results of the same examinations performed before and shortly after the previous surgery to determine if there has been any change. The physical examination findings are less valuable if the preoperative information is not available so that it can be determined if this is a new problem, a recurrent one, or one that was not resolved with the previous intervention. Root tension signs are also tested. However, one must keep in mind that the interpretation of these tests may be more difficult in the operated patient because they may be effected by scar tissue or arachnoiditis. In addition to the evaluations discussed above, Jönsson and Strömqvist have recently described clinical characteristics of patients with recurrent sciatica.[27] They found that patients with recurrent disk herniation were significantly more likely to have at least two of the three following characteristics present as compared to patients whose problems were associated with fibrosis: pain when coughing, pain with a straight-leg raise at less than 30°, or a greatly reduced walking capacity. They also commented that patients with recurrent herniation tended to have had a longer pain-free period following surgery than did patients whose pain was associated with scar.[27]

## CONSIDERATION FOR ADJACENT-LEVEL PATHOLOGY

Although not as common as patients who have previously undergone diskectomy, some patients do return with symptoms following decompression for stenosis. Pain in such patients may have one of several causes. In such patients one needs to determine if there is boney regrowth at the previously operated level, symptomatic instability created by the surgery, scar formation in the operative area, or symptoms arising at a new location in the spine. Hopp and Tsou found that 17% of patients who underwent decompression for stenosis later required reoperation for instability.[21]

One of the possible reasons for a patient presenting with symptoms following lumbar spine surgery is that the level adjacent to the fused segment may be painful. If the presentation is shortly after the initial fusion surgery, it may be that the initial operation did not address pathology at all the affected spinal levels. If the presenting symptoms arise some time after the initial surgery, it may be that the patient has developed new pathology. Intuitively, the concept is appealing that stabilizing one or more lumbar segments causes increased load or alters the mechanics of the adjacent segment resulting in accelerated degeneration. In a cadaveric study, Lee and Langrana found that lumbar sacral fusion generated increased stresses at the adjacent levels, particularly the facet joints.[35] In a later clinical study, Lee noted accelerated degeneration of the disk adjacent to a posteriorly fused segment and associated facet joint degeneration.[34] A study from Australia found that there was no significant increase in adjacent-segment degeneration following anterior lumbar interbody fusion in a group of patients being evaluated a minimum of 10 years after surgery.[45] In a more recent presentation, Chapman et al reported that a risk factor for developing problems at the level adjacent to a fusion is related to surgically creating a hyperlordotic or kyphotic lumbar spine.[10] Other factors they found to be related to this problem were older age, obesity, osteoporosis, being a female smoker, multiply operated spine, and multiple other health problems.

In a study using single photon emission computed tomography (SPECT) scanning to evaluate patients who had undergone spine fusion, investigators found that 63% of patients had lesions in the free-motion segment adjacent to a fused segment.[12] The rate was greatest in patients who had a circumferential fusion (67%). The lesions were seen in 28% of patients with posterior fusion and 46% of posterolateral fusions. In postfusion patients there is the possibility of developing spinal stenosis at the adjacent level. The incidence of this following posterior fusion has been reported to be 30%.[37] This problem was found in only 2.5% of a population being followed after anterior lumbar fusion.[45]

One generally overlooked possible source of pain in patients who have previously undergone lumbar spine fusion is that of pain arising in the sacroiliac joint. Although pain arising from lumbar spinal levels adjacent to a fused segment is considered, the possibility of pain arising from the sacroiliac joint following surgery has received relatively little consideration. However, the mechanics of spine fusion forcing more stress onto this joint after fusion may be similar to mechanics thought to be related to the stresses at adjacent segments. Pain arising from the sacroiliac joint may present similarly to that associated with other spinal structures and is typically referred into the groin, upper posterior thigh, and buttock.[3,30,31] Pain arising in the sacroiliac joint may be unilateral or bilateral, but is rarely referred below the knee. In many patients, it is present in combination with other spinal pathologies.[3] It will likely not be similar to the patient's initial pain, if the patient has enjoyed a pain-free period following the initial surgery. With the current trend to use more rigid internal fixation systems with rods and cages, this may result in a greater incidence of sacroiliac joint problems postoperatively.

## INVASIVE RADIOLOGY

As in the evaluation of any patient presenting with low back and/or leg pain, noninvasive imaging modalities are the first used in the evaluation process. However, interpretation of studies are especially difficult in patients with previous surgery. Special problems encountered in this population are scarring, metallic instrumentation distorting the images, and imaging of asymptomatic abnormalities. The high rate of imaging disk abnormalities in asymptomatic subjects is well documented.[7,8,24] Although these studies were performed in subjects with no previous back surgery, they still indicate the high prevalence of imaging abnormalities not associated with symptoms. It is likely that the problem is also common in previously operated patients and thus must be interpreted with caution. Frymoyer et al found that there was a significantly greater occurrence of traction spurs and facet subluxations in patients who had undergone fusion than among those who had not.[16] However, these changes were not clearly related to developing symptoms. Lehman reported that 30 or more years after fusion, 50% of patients had abnormalities demonstrated on radiographs, but these were unrelated to developing symptoms, and 85% of the patients were pleased with their results.[37] These studies bring out the importance of not relying too heavily on imaging findings when diagnosing the previously operated patient. If noninvasive assessment yields equivocal results or more information is required in the contemplation of further surgical intervention, invasive radiographic procedures such as myelography and diskography can be helpful in delineating the source of pain. As with any patient, the results of imaging evaluations must be considered in combination with the patient's history, location of pain complaints, and physical examination findings, in order to avoid misinterpretation of the value of the image findings. In patients presenting with pain after lumbar spine surgery, this may be even more important because the potential sources of the problem have become greater when considering the possibility of scar, infection, iatrogenic instability, arachnoiditis, pseudarthrosis, and painful or misplaced hardware. With the added complexity of potential problems in this population, more indepth diagnostic workup may also be necessary. In evaluating a series of symptomatic previously operated patients using magnetic resonance imaging (MRI), intrathecally enhanced computed tomography (CT), myelography, diskography, and CT diskography, Bernard found that only 61% of patients could have been fully diagnosed using one test.[1] Among the 45 patients, 19 had more than one diagnosis confirmed at the time of surgery.

Byrd et al reported that in the evaluation of the symptomatic postoperative spine, among plain films, myelography, CT, epidural venography, intravenously enhanced CT, and tomography, the evaluations that were the most helpful were plain films and enhanced CT scans.[9] The pathologies most frequently found were granulation tissue, spondylosis, recurrent or residual disk herniation, and arachnoiditis.

In the case of the patient who is presenting with radicular pain following diskectomy, the first diagnostic imaging study is typically MRI. In postoperative patients this test should be performed with and without gadolinium (Gd) enhancement. This method allows better differentiation of scar from possible recurrent disk material. The enhanced scan should be performed soon after the introduction of the contrast, so that it has infiltrated scar tissue, but not yet infiltrated the more dense disk tissue. Milette et al have warned that the results of postdiskectomy MRI should be used cautiously when planning future intervention.[39] He reported that even though MRI was effective for differentiating recurrent herniation from scar, the imaging results did not correlate with clinical outcome.

### MYELOGRAPHY

In the workup of the postoperative patient, myelography has a role in the detection of arachnoiditis, misplaced internal fixation, and other compressive symptomatology. Postmyelography CT scanning can provide useful information in the diagnosis of pain arising from arachnoiditis or misplaced hardware. Arachnoiditis is difficult to identify based on clinical examination. It is generally associated with radicular pain in nonspecific patterns. It is usually identified by myelography or CT myelography. The condition is not common following current methods of myelography. Arachnoiditis is typically identified based on an irregular appearing thecal sac that is shortened and the nerve roots appeared thickened or clumped together.

Although mechanical pain associated with iatrogenic instability is often identified by plain radiographs, including flexion and extension views, myelography may also be helpful in making this diagnosis, particularly if flexion and extension radiographs are taken with the myelographic contrast present. This may be particularly helpful if the patient typically experiences pain with these motions.

Myelography does have some shortcomings. Hiltselberger et al reported on myelographic imaging abnormalities in patients with no pain.[20] Also, myelography is limited only to identifying compression of the thecal sac or exiting nerve roots. It does not provide a good means of differentiating between recurrent disk herniation and scar tissue. Irstam reported on the use of myelography to evaluate recurrent disk herniation in a series of 44 patients who underwent myelography and reoperation after surgery for disk herniation.[22] He found that myelography could help identify the extent of the lesion, but was not helpful in distinguishing scar from recurrent disk herniation.

## DISKOGRAPHY

Although controversial since its introduction, diskography remains the only examination that provides a pain provocation component. This part of the examination may be particularly helpful in the previously operated patient in the presence of the difficulty of interpreting many of the imaging evaluations. Although the accuracy of the combined imaging and pain provocation diskographic evaluation is high,[56] this evaluation may be difficult to perform in patients with posterior fusion in which the fusion mass blocks the optimal needle approach to the disk to be investigated.

Several investigators have reported on the use of diskography in previously operated patients. Several have reported on using diskography in patients presenting with radicular symptoms following diskectomy.[2,17,47] These authors found that diskography can differentiate disk pathology from scar even in patients where Gd-enhanced MRI yielded equivocal results. Also, the pain provocation component of the exam can be pursued to determine if the visualized disk abnormality is related to the patient's presenting symptoms. This part of the examination may be particularly helpful in light of Milette's report that while MRI could be used to differentiate scar from disk herniation, it was not related to clinical outcome.

Jackson et al have reported the results of comparing several diagnostic imaging methods including diskography, CT diskography, myelography, CT myelography, and CT.[23] In the subgroup of patients they investigated who had previously undergone lumbar spine surgery, they found that CT diskography was the most accurate single test. It was the most sensitive at 100% and also the most specific (87.5%) in the identification of recurrent herniated disk.

Pain following lumbar spine fusion can arise from any one of several sources or from more than one source. One of first suspected origins is painful pseudarthrosis. However, this condition may be difficult to diagnose given the poor evaluation methods to determine if solid boney union has been achieved. Also, some patients with clear nonunion do not have significant symptoms. Likewise, in some patients in whom a solid fusion has been achieved, significant symptoms are present.

Johnson and Macnab reported that diskography is helpful in identifying pseudarthrosis later confirmed at the time of surgery.[25] Simmons described a case of a patient who presented with pain following posterior fusion surgery from L4 to the sacrum.[52] The patient underwent diskography from L3-L4 to L5-S1 disks. The L4-L5 was very painful and the other two levels were not clinically painful. During reoperation, pseudarthrosis was noted at the L4-L5 level. The level was refused and the patient's symptoms resolved. Perhaps one of the more difficult and frustrating patients to evaluate and treat is the one who has pain although a solid posterior fusion has been achieved. Although it may be tempting to some to attribute such persistent symptoms to the patient's mental condition or desire for secondary gains, one must consider that the original surgery may not have adequately addressed the patient's symptomatic pathology. In a small series of patients, Weatherley described painful disk disruption in the disk within a solidly fused segment.[57] In these patients, subsequent anterior fusion provided pain relief. Symptomatic disk within a fused segment has also been noted by other authors.[25] Rolander had earlier described motion under a fused segment.[48] Lee and Langrana also reported motion in the anterior column following posterior fusion.[35] These studies suggest that if a patient has the clinical entity that Crock described as "internal disk derangement,"[11] posterior fusion may not be an adequate treatment because it does not directly address the disk pathology. The limited motion allowed in the anterior column following posterior fusion may be enough to continue to irritate nerve endings in the disk annulus and provoke pain. Such a problem may best be identified by diskography. It was recently reported that these internal disk ruptures that are not associated with deformation of the outer annular wall can be related to lower extremity pain.[43]

One additional use of diskography is to investigate the disk adjacent to a previously fused segment. Johnson and Macnab found diskography helpful in differentiating whether the previously operated levels were producing the patient's symptoms or if pain was related to the level above the fused segment.[25] Diskography can be used to determine if the patient's pain is reproduced at the adjacent level during the injection and if the CT diskographic image demonstrates correlative pathology.

One potential drawback of diskography is the interpretation of the pain responses during disk injection. Most diskographers prefer to inject at least one level in which the patient does not report significant pain provocation. Block et al reported that patients who tend to report pain upon the injection of a nondisrupted disk were significantly more likely to have elevated scores on the hysteria and hypochondriasis scales of the Minnesota Multiphasic Personality Inventory (MMPI).[5] In a similar study, Ohnmeiss et al found that patients indicating pain in unusual patterns on pain drawings were more likely to report pain upon the injection of nondisrupted disks.[44]

Recently, the North American Spine Society published indications for lumbar diskography.[18] Indications that may be applicable to previously operated patients include: 1) further evaluation of a disk that has been found to be abnormal or investigation of the relationship of the imaged abnormalities to clinical symptoms. This may include recurrent disk herniation and lateral disk herniation; 2) patients with persistent symptoms in whom other tests have not confirmed a suspected disk as a source of pain; 3) assessment of patients who have persistent pain after a fusion procedure. Diskography may help identify painful pseudarthrosis or a symptomatic disk level under a solid posterior fusion; 4) assessment of disks prior to the carrying out of a planned fusion to determine if the disks in the planned fusion segment are painful and to determine the condition of the adjacent disks.

## PATIENT SELECTION

As with any spine surgery, the most important issue in achieving a successful treatment result is proper patient selection. One must exercise particular caution in patients with previous spine surgery in whom the results of further surgery are typically worse than for initial procedures. In such a population, one should carefully consider the patient's history, physical examination findings, radiographic evaluation results, and psychological screening results. These combined factors can help to provide indications as to whether further surgical intervention is warranted. Several investigators have identified issues related to a particularly good, or conversely poor, outcome of repeat spine surgery. Biondi and Greenberg reported factors related to a poor outcome for subsequent surgery were: Workers' Compensation, a pain-free interval of less than 6 months' duration, male gender, history of psychiatric illness, and primary diagnosis of perinural fibrosis.[4] Finnegan et al also found that patients receiving compensation or patients with psychological problems tended to do more poorly after repeat surgery than patients without such factors present.[13] North et al reported that factors associated with a good outcome from repeat spine surgery were younger age, female gender, a history of good results from previous spine surgery, absence of epidural scar, and prevalence of radicular pain.[40] In a series of patients undergoing fusion with pedicle screw fixation in patients with postlaminectomy instability, Lee reported that factors related to a poor outcome were osteoporosis, concomitant disk herniation, and persistent stenosis at or adjacent to the operated level.[36] Bernard reported that age, number of previous operations, and psychological status were not related to the outcome of repeat surgery. However, he found that a noncompensatable injury, return to work, a negative history of litigation, and attaining a solid fusion were significantly related to a good outcome of repeat surgery.[1] Quimjian and Matrka reported factors related to good outcome following repeat spine surgery were unilateral radicular pain pattern, a pain-free interval of 1 year after the initial surgery, and myelography indicative of recurrent disk herniation.[46] Yaksich reported that the optimum patient to submit for repeat spine surgery has leg pain rather than back pain, has a recurrent or residual disk herniation associated with stenosis, and is highly motivated to improve.[59]

With respect to patients who specifically are presenting with symptoms following diskectomy, repeat surgery has been found to be beneficial to patients whose symptoms are related to recurrent disk herniation, but results in those with symptoms related primarily to scar are not as good.[26,27,51]

Silvers et al reported on 38 patients with true recurrent disk herniation, that is, herniation at the same level and on the same side as what had been operated previously.[51] They found that 64% were satisfied with the outcome of the subsequent surgery, only 22% returned to work, and 27% returned to activity. These figures were worse than for patients who were undergoing a subsequent diskectomy for problems at different levels or on the other side. Herron noted poorer results of reoperation for patients with litigation or work-related issues.[19] Waddell et al had reported that a pain-free interval of at least 6 months was associated with a good result of repeat surgery.[55] Other factors they identified as related to good results were predominant complaints of leg pain rather than back pain, and a primary diagnosis of recurrent disk herniation.

Strömqvest reported that recurrent sciatica due to fibrosis was not an indication for fusion.[54] However, instability following facetectomy responded well to fusion.

Bernard reported that in a series of 45 patients undergoing repeat spine surgery, factors that were associated with a good outcome were noncompensatable injury, return to work after surgery, no litigation, and achieving a solid fusion.[2]

Kim and Michelsen reported that the factor most strongly related to a successful result from repeat spine surgery was pseudarthrosis repair.[29] Whitecloud et al reported on a series of 14 patients who underwent neural decompression and fusion at a segment adjacent to a previous fusion.[58] They found that osteoporosis and a period of less than 3 years between the initial and subsequent surgeries were associated with a poor outcome. They also recommended that internal fixation be used when extending a fusion to include an additional level.

Patients in whom an internal fixation system has been used may have pain associated with the hardware. The more simple case of this is the thinner patient who feels the hardware and finds it uncomfortable. The incidence of the hardware itself being painful independent of nerve root impingement or problems related to broken hardware is still debatable. One of the few studies addressing this issue was performed in a patient with local pain over the hardware. McCullen et al reported that removal of hardware improved pain complaints in only one-third of the patients undergoing this procedure, approximately one-third were unchanged, and the remaining reported being made worse by the removal.[38] The fact that some patients do experience relief following hardware removal may make this a worthwhile consideration; however, it is obvious that work needs to be done to determine if indications can be defined for those patients who can benefit from this procedure. Hardware injection may be helpful in some of these cases.

## PSYCHOLOGICAL EVALUATION

There is a strong tendency to rely on imaging studies in the evaluation of surgical candidates; however, one must consider not only the visualization of pathology, but also the patient's personality and psychological state. Spengler et al found that psychological evaluations were a better predictor of surgical outcome than were imaging studies, which were better related to operative findings.[53] Their study did not specifically address previously operated patients, but did bring recognition to the importance of the patient's personality in surgical outcome. A preoperative psychosocial screening package for spine surgery candidates has been developed and preliminary results are promising in screening out those patients whose personality makes them poor surgical candidates.[6] It incorporates many of the factors that have been reported to be related to surgical outcome including the hysteria and hypochondriasis scales of the MMPI, coping skills, depression, previous surgery, work and lifestyle stability, job satisfaction, concomitant health conditions, and other factors. Each assessment has a weighted score and from this an overall evaluation is derived. It is suggested to the surgeon that the patient is clear for surgery, clear for surgery but needs therapy, needs therapy prior to being cleared for surgery, or the patient is not a good candidate and surgery should not be pursued.

If it appears that everything was done appropriately during the first surgery (i.e., correct procedure, appropriate levels and approach, and no iatrogenic pathologies developed) but the patient reports no pain relief, one may be more suspect of psychological or personality problems. This may be particularly true if the patient did not go through psychological screening prior to the initial surgery. However, until a full diagnostic workup has been performed and a psychologist has screened the patient to identify psychological problems, the patient's continuing pain complaints should not be automatically attributed to personality and the patient's problems simply ignored.

Some patients fail to meet selection criteria for routine intervention such as repeat decompression or fusion. These patients may have pain arising from problems such as scar or nerve damage. In such patients for whom traditional spine salvage surgery is not indicated, spinal cord stimulation (SCS) may be considered. This procedure is reserved primarily for patients who have chronic intractable pain that has not been helped by conservative care and who do not have a lesion thought to be associated with structural pathology such as stenosis, adjacent-level pathology, facet degeneration, instability, recurrent disk herniation, or other such defined pathology. Spinal cord stimulation candidates should undergo a psychological screening by a person well experienced in dealing with back pain patients. One particular group of patients who may benefit from SCS are those with pain arising from epidural fibrosis. This condition does not respond well to traditional surgery and is often made worse by it. Fiume et al reported good results with SCS for epidural fibrosis.[14] They found that female gender and radicular pain were associated with good outcome. Ohnmeiss et al recently reported significant improvement in pain and function in a group of patients with chronic intractable pain after at least one spine surgery and who were not considered candidates for traditional spine surgery.[42] In a recent randomized study comparing spinal cord stimulation to conventional spine surgery in the treatment of previously operated patients, SCS provided statistically better results.[41]

One area that has not received much attention with respect to spine surgery is that of expectations. If the patient's expectations for future surgery are too great, he/she should not be considered a good surgical candidate until expectations are realistic. Prior to further surgical intervention, expected results need to be fully discussed. This may be particularly important in patients who have already had a poor result after surgical intervention. These patients need to understand that an additional surgery may or may not help their condition, and may in fact make it worse. In any case, the patient needs to understand that total pain relief and full return to activities or to be "good as new" is extremely unlikely. It is also important that the patient understand that he/she has been in a state of reduced activity for some time, and to return to usual activity level, participation in a rehabilitation program following surgery is needed. The patient should clearly understand that surgery is not in and of itself going to "fix" all their problems. It may be helpful to have the patient see a psychologist to address depression or other emotional problems that may be associated with the failure of the initial surgery and the lack of guarantees of the outcome of the second. Participation of the patient's family in the discussion of expectations can also be beneficial so that all understand what the patient is expected to do to achieve maximal results, but that return to prepain onset condition is not likely.

## DISCUSSION

Typically, results of repeat surgery are not as good as those from initial procedures; however, as described previously in this chapter, investigators have identified factors that are related to clinical outcomes in repeat surgery. When contemplating repeat surgery many things need to be considered: the factors described earlier in this chapter as related to outcome, the patient's history, careful evaluation of their pain complaints, period of pain relief following the previous surgical intervention, correlation of history and physical examination findings to radiographic imaging, and expectations. Technically the surgery is typically more difficult due to scarring from previous surgery, which also increases the chances of a dural tear. Another technical factor to consider is the use of instrumentation that may improve the fusion rate but is not advised in patients with osteoporosis.

If the patient meets well-defined selection criteria, surgery should not be withheld simply because the patient has previously had surgery, and there is fear that a bad result will be obtained from further intervention. However, the desire to help the patient must be tempered with resisting temptation to do something to try to help, even if the indications for further intervention are not clear. In patients who are not likely to benefit from traditional surgery, in particular those with pain related to epidural fibrosis or ill-localized pain, SCS may be helpful.

One must carefully assess the patient's condition and determine an appropriate course of treatment. The decision to subject the patient to additional surgery should not be undertaken lightly. Unless there are indications for surgery and a clinical history and physical examination findings that correlate with radiographic findings, and clearance by a psychologist, additional surgery should not be pursued. Likewise, if the patient does present with well-defined indications for surgery, one should not be overly hesitant to pursue this course simply because the patient has had prior surgery.

## REFERENCES

1. Bernard TN Jr: Repeat lumbar spine surgery: factors influencing outcome, *Spine* 18:2196-2200, 1993.
2. Bernard TN Jr: Using computed tomography/discography and enhanced magnetic resonance imaging to distinguish between scar tissue and recurrent lumbar disc herniation, *Spine* 19:2826-2832, 1994.
3. Bernard TN Jr, Cassidy JD: *The sacroiliac joint syndrome: pathophysiology, diagnosis, and management.* In Frymoyer JW, editor: *The adult spine: principles and practice,* Philadelphia, 1997, Lippincott-Raven Publishers, pp 2343-2366.
4. Biondi J, Greenberg BJ: Redecompression and fusion in failed back syndrome patients, *J Spinal Disord* 3:362-369, 1990.
5. Block AR, Vanharanta H, Ohnmeiss DD, Guyer RD: Discographic pain reports: influence of psychological factors, *Spine* 21:334-338, 1996.
6. Block AR, Ware D, Ohnmeiss DD, Guyer RD, Pladjewitz C: Initial results from a psycho-social screening package for spine surgery candidates. Presentation at the International Society for the Study of the Lumbar Spine. June, 1996; Burlington, Vermont.
7. Boden SD, Davis DO, Dina TS, Patronas NJ, Wiesel SW: Abnormal magnetic-resonance scans of the lumbar spine in asymptomatic subjects, *J Bone Joint Surg* 72-A:403-408, 1990.
8. Boos N, Reider R, Schnade V, Spratt K, Semmer N, Aebi M: The diagnostic accuracy of MRI, work per-

ception and psychological factors in identifying symptomatic disc herniations, *Spine* 20:2613-2625, 1995.

9. Byrd SE, Cohn ML, Biggers SL, Huntington CT, Locke GE, Charles MF: The radiographic evaluation of the symptomatic postoperative lumbar spine patient, *Spine* 10:652-661, 1985.
10. Chapman MP, Bridwell KH, Lenke LG, Hamill CL, Baldus C, Blanke K: Risk factors for transition syndromes above or below solid fusions. Presented at the Annual Meeting of the North American Spine Society. Washington, D.C., October, 1995.
11. Crock HV: Internal disc disruption: a challenge to disc prolapse fifty year on, *Spine* 11:650-653, 1986.
12. Even-Sapir E, Martin RH, Mitchell MJ, Iles SE, Barnes DC, Clark AJ: Assessment of painful late effects of lumbar spinal fusion with SPECT, *J Nucl Med* 35:416-22, 1994.
13. Finnegan WJ, Fenlin JM, Marvel JP, Nardini RJ: Salvage spine surgery, *J Bone Joint Surg* 61-A:1077-1082, 1979.
14. Fiume D, Sherkat S, Callovini GM, Parziale G, Gazzeri G: Treatment of the failed back surgery syndrome due to lumbo-sacral epidural fibrosis. Acta Neurochir Suppl (Wein) 64:116-118, 1995.
15. Frymoyer JW: *Magnitude of the problem.* In Weinstein JN, Wiesel SW, editors: *The lumbar spine.* Philadelphia, 1990, Saunders, pp 32-38.
16. Frymoyer JW, Hanley EN, Howe J, Kuhlmann D, Matteri RE: A comparison of radiographic findings in fusion and nonfusion patients ten or more years following lumbar disc surgery, *Spine* 4:435-440, 1979.
17. Guyer RD, Ohnmeiss DD, Hochschuler SH, et al: The use of CT/Discography to identify recurrent disc herniation not visualized by gadolinium enhanced MRI. Presented to the Federation of Spine Associations. March, 1991; Anaheim, California.
18. Guyer RD, Ohnmeiss DD: Contemporary concepts in spine care: lumbar discography. Position statement from the North American Spine Society Diagnostic and Therapeutic Committee. *Spine* 20:2048-2059, 1995.
19. Herron L: Recurrent lumbar disc herniation: results of repeat laminectomy and discectomy, *J Spinal Disord* 7:161-166, 1994.
20. Hiltselberger WE, Witten RM: Abnormal myelograms in asymptomatic patients, *J Neurosurg* 28:204-208, 1968.
21. Hopp E, Tsou PM: Postdecompression lumbar instability, *Clin Orthop* 227:143-151, 1988.
22. Irstam L: Differential diagnosis of recurrent lumbar disc herniation and postoperative deformation by myelography. An impossible task, *Spine* 9:759-763, 1984.
23. Jackson RP, Cain JE Jr, Jacobs RR, et al: The neuroradiographic diagnosis of lumbar herniated nucleus pulposus: I. A comparison of computed tomography (CT), myelography, CT-myelography, discography, and CT-discography, *Spine* 14:1356-1361, 1989.
24. Jensen MC, Brant-Zawadzki MN, Obuchowski N, Modic MT, Malkasian D, Ross JS: Magnetic resonance imaging of the lumbar spine in people without back pain, *New Engl J Med* 331:69-73, 1994.
25. Johnson RG, Macnab I: Localization of symptomatic lumbar pseudarthrosis by use of discography, *Clin Orthop* 197:164-170, 1985.
26. Jönsson B, Strömqvist B: Repeat decompression of lumbar nerve roots: a prospective two-year evaluation, *J Bone Joint Surg* 75-B:894-897, 1993.
27. Jönsson B, Strömqvist B: Clinical characteristics of recurrent sciatica after lumbar discectomy, *Spine* 21:500-505, 1996.
28. Kawaguchi Y, Matsui H, Tsuji H: Back muscle injury after posterior lumbar spine surgery. Part 2: Histologic and histochemical analyses in humans, *Spine* 19:2598-2602, 1994.
29. Kim SS, Michelsen CB: Revision surgery for failed back surgery syndrome, *Spine* 17:957-960, 1992.
30. Kirkaldy-Willis WH, Hill RJ: A more precise diagnosis for low-back pain, *Spine* 4:102-109, 1979.
31. Kleiner JB, Weingarten P: Sacroiliac joint dysfunction as a complication of spinal fusion. Presented at the annual meeting of the North American Spine Society. Washington, D.C., October, 1995.
32. Kostuik JP: *Failures after spinal fusion.* In Frymoyer JW, editor: *The adult spine: principles and practice,* Philadelphia, 1997, Lippincott-Raven Publishers, pp 2277-2326.
33. Lauerman WC, Wiesel SW: The failed back: an algorithm, *Semin Spine Surg* 8:208-220, 1996.
34. Lee CK: Accelerated degeneration of the segment adjacent to a lumbar fusion, *Spine* 13:375-377, 1988.
35. Lee CK, Langrana NA: Lumbosacral spinal fusion: a biomechanical study, *Spine* 9:574-581, 1984.
36. Lee TC: Transpedicular reduction and stabilization for postlaminectomy lumbar instability, *Acta Neurochir (Wein)* 138:139-144, 1996.
37. Lehmann TR, Spratt KF, Tozzi JE, et al: Long-term follow-up of lower lumbar fusion patients, *Spine* 12:97-104, 1987.
38. McCullen GM, Yuan HA, Frederickson BE: The removal of posterior lumbar instrumentation to relieve localized discomfort over the hardware. Presented at the Annual Meeting of the North American Spine Society. Washington, D.C., October, 1995.
39. Milette PC, Fontaine S, Lepanto L, Dery R, Breton G: Clinical impact of contrast-enhanced MR imaging reports in patients with previous lumbar disc surgery, *AJR Am J Roentgenol* 167:217-223, 1996.
40. North RB, Campbell JN, James CS, Conover-Walker MK, Wang H, Piantadosi S, Rybock JD, Long DM: Failed back surgery syndrome: 5 year follow-up in 102 patients undergoing repeat operation, *Neurosurgery* 28:685-690, 1991.
41. North RB, Kidd DH, Lee MS, Piantodosi S: A prospective, randomized study of spinal cord stimulation versus reoperation for failed back surgery syndrome: initial results, *Stereotact Funct Neurosurg* 62:267-272, 1994.

42. Ohnmeiss DD, Rashbaum RF, Bogdanffy GM: Prospective outcome evaluation of spinal cord stimulation in patients with intractable leg pain, *Spine* 21:1344-1350, 1996.
43. Ohnmeiss DD, Vanharanta H, Ekholm J: Disc disruption and lower extremity pain, *Spine* 22:1600-1605, 1997.
44. Ohnmeiss DD, Vanharanta H, Guyer RD: The association between pain drawings and CT/discographic pain responses, *Spine* 20:729-733, 1995.
45. Penta M, Sandhu A, Fraser RD: Magnetic resonance imaging assessment of disc degeneration 10 years after anterior lumbar interbody fusion, *Spine* 20:743-747, 1995.
46. Quimjian JD, Matrka PJ: Decompression laminectomy and lateral spinal fusion in patients with previously failed lumbar spine surgery, *Orthopaedics* 11:563-569, 1988.
47. Rappoport LH, Pravda J, Leipzig JM, et al: The role of discogram/CT in assessing postoperative disc herniations. Presented to the International Society for the Study of the Lumbar Spine (poster). Chicago, IL; May, 1992.
48. Rolander SD: Motion of the lumbar spine with special reference to the stability effect of posterior fusion. *Acta Orthop Scand* 90(suppl):1-143, 1966.
49. Sachs BL, Zindrick MR, Beasley RD: Reflex sympathetic dystrophy after operative procedures on the lumbar spine, *J Bone Joint Surg* 75-A:721-731, 1993.
50. Sihvonen T, Herno A, Paljarvi L, Airaksinen O, Partanen J, Tapaninaho A: Local denervation atrophy of paraspinal muscles in postoperative failed back syndrome, *Spine* 18:575-581, 1993.
51. Silvers HR, Lewis PJ, Asch HL, Clabeaux DE: Lumbar diskectomy for recurrent disk herniation, *J Spinal Disord* 7:408-419, 1994.
52. Simmons EH, Segil CM: An evaluation of discography in the localization of symptomatic levels in discogenic disease of the spine, *Clin Orthop* 108:57-69, 1975.
53. Spengler DM, Ouellette EA, Battie M, Zeh J: Elective discectomy for herniation of a lumbar disc. Additional experience with an objective method, *J Bone Joint Surg* 72-A:230-237, 1990.
54. Strömqvist B: Postlaminectomy problems with reference to spinal fusion, *Acta Orthop Scand* 251(suppl): 87-89, 1993.
55. Waddell Kummel EG, Lotto WN, Graham JD, Hall H, McCulloch JA: Failed lumbar disc surgery and repeat surgery following industrial injuries, *J Bone Joint Surg* 61-A:201-207, 1979.
56. Walsh TR, Weinstein JN, Spratt KF, et al: Lumbar discography in normal subjects: a controlled, prospective study, *J Bone Joint Surg* 72-A:1081-1088, 1990.
57. Weatherley CR, Prickett CF, O'Brein JP: Discogenic pain persisting despite solid posterior fusion, *J Bone Joint Surg* 68-B:142-143, 1986.
58. Whitecloud TS III, Divis JM, Olive PM: Operative treatment of the degenerated segment adjacent to a lumbar fusion, *Spine* 19:531-536, 1994.
59. Yaksich I: Failed back surgery syndrome: problems, pitfalls, and prevention, *Ann Acad Med Singapore* 22(suppl 3):414-417, 1993.

# 16

# GENERAL ASPECTS OF PATIENT SELECTION

John Dove, F.R.C.S.



This chapter relates only to the selection of patients for revision surgery for low back pain. I have previously published the principles of my approach to the selection of patients for primary low back pain surgery.[2,9] I have also previously published details of my technique for primary low back pain surgery.[1,3] As far as revision low back pain surgery is concerned, I coauthored an algorithmic approach to such cases.[13]

## THE SURGEON

The surgeon who intends to undertake revision low back pain surgery must be fully familiar with the complexities of this difficult condition and fully aware that careful assessment of such patients is required. He or she needs to know that the mere fact that an abnormality can be pointed out, for example on the magnetic resonance imaging (MRI) scan, does not of itself mean that the patient is a candidate for surgery. It is assumed that the surgeon is fully familiar with the writings of experts such as Waddell and Main regarding the understanding of the behavior and psychology of patients with low back pain.[7,12] From a technical point of view, it is crucial that the surgeon be experienced in the practice of primary low back pain surgery.

## THE PATIENT

The patient needs to be warned from the beginning that the more back pain operations he has previously had, the less likely it is that any subsequent such operation will be successful. It has been shown statistically that a second operation has only a 50% chance of success and if the patient has had two operations or more, then it is likely that following any further surgery the patient will be worse rather than better.[5]

For any consideration to be given to surgery, the patient must be clear that the pain has been bad enough for long enough and all appropriate nonoperative modalities must first have been tried.

The patient should, as part of the assessment, be required to complete a pain drawing and scientifically validated questionnaires. In my unit, I routinely use the Oswestry Disability Questionnaire[4] together with a modified version of the Zung questionnaire[14] and the modified somatic perception questionnaire.[6] It must be appreciated that if patients have a positive score on psychological testing and exhibit nonorganic features on examination, this does not of itself mean that they are deliberately exaggerating or malingering. Nor does it mean that these patients do not have a genuine pain problem. Many of these patients are very genuinely and very severely disabled. It is probable, however, that further surgery would be unsuccessful and they are more likely to be worse off.

It should be noted that disability and psychology questionnaires may be geographically specific. The questionnaire that the surgeon uses must be validated for patients in the region that he or she is dealing

with. For example, questionnaires validated for use with North American patients do not apply to patients in England. These are real differences in the patient populations and not mere semantic nuances.

## HISTORY

In addition to the various questionnaires, a detailed history is required. This takes time, so these patients must be allocated sufficient time for their consultations. Not less than half an hour is likely to be necessary for the evaluation of such patients.

It needs to be established as to whether the onset of the pain was gradual or whether it was sudden. If it was sudden and if there was an injury, then it must be established as to whether there is any compensation claim in relation to that injury. It is well-established that the results of low back pain surgery in patients with ongoing compensation claims are less good than in other patients. The reasons for this are multifactorial.

Specific details must be sought of their previous surgery and in this regard a very useful summary is provided by Porter.[10] The patient's main symptoms prior to surgery and whether the symptoms were relieved by that surgery needs to be established. One also needs to establish whether the pain that the patient suffers now is similar in nature and site to the pain that they had prior to surgery or quite different. Details of the relevant operation notes and the original preoperative investigations are also necessary whenever possible.

For example, it is quite insufficient to state that a particular patient still has back and leg pain despite low back surgery. In such a patient, a number of potential and quite different scenarios could be presented:

1. The patient who had back and right leg pain prior to surgery might continue to have exactly the same pain following surgery without relief even for a short time. In these circumstances one would have to be suspicious that the surgery had not addressed the patient's problem. For example a diskectomy might have been carried out at the inappropriate level.
2. The patient might have the same back and leg pain after surgery that they had before surgery but might have been pain free following surgery for many months or longer. In such circumstances one would need to look into the possibility of recurrent nerve root compression. If the pain had suddenly come on again after the patient had been pain-free for several months, one might suspect a recurrent disk lesion, whereas if the pain had come on gradually one might be suspicious that the root pain was the result of extradural scarring.
3. The patient might have pain in the back and same leg after operation that they had before operation but the leg pain might be quite different in nature with, for example, dysthesiae. Then one might be suspicious that there may have been some intraoperative nerve root damage.
4. Following surgery with, for example, internal fixation, the patient might still have back and leg pain but the pain might be in the other leg and severe in nature. In these circumstances, urgent investigation to exclude nerve root compression as the result of misplaced internal fixation would be required.
5. The patient might still have the same back pain following surgery when a fusion for mechanical instability was carried out but might have been pain free for a year or two in between. In these circumstances one would investigate the patient on the basis that they might have developed a pseudarthrosis. In other words very precise details are required of the nature and site of the pain before and after operation and as to whether or not there was a pain-free interval following surgery.

## EXAMINATION

In addition to having completed the appropriate questionnaires outlined above, note is made of how the patient presents himself during the taking of the history and it should be noted if family members attend with the patient (e.g., if an essentially fit middle-aged man attends with his wife this needs to be noted). It does not mean that the patient does not have a genuine pain problem but it does say something about how that particular couple approaches their difficulties. One has however of course to be reasonable and it may well be that the family member is attending merely because the patient is not in a position, because of his pain problem, to drive himself.

Specific examination is made for Waddell's nonorganic signs.[11] Note needs to be made of the nature of any surgical scars and as to whether they are well healed, nonadherent, and nontender or otherwise. The neurological examination will need to look for specific evidence of nerve root damage.

## INVESTIGATIONS

If, as is the position in many cases, following the history and examination, it is quite clear that the patient is not a candidate for surgery then the surgeon should resist the temptation to investigate the patient. This may involve taking considerable time with the patient to explain to them why they are not suitable for surgery and why investigations are likely to be counter-productive.

For example, if following the history and examination the surgeon has decided that the patient is not suitable for surgery but allows himself to be tempted into ordering an MRI scan, he may find well localized degenerative change in one specific disk and is then tempted to carry out surgery even though it is likely that the result of such surgery will result in the patient being no better or even worse. Patients must understand that there is a very real chance of their being made worse by inappropriate revision low back surgery. The response of the patient is often then to say "But what am I going to do? I can not go on like this." The patient needs to know that the surgeon is sympathetic toward their ongoing pain problem and arrangements must be made for the patient to have appropriate nonsurgical pain relief methods. It must be explained to the patient that although he or she has a major pain problem and the surgeon is sympathetic to this, the pain alone is not an indication for carrying out major surgery that is more likely to make the patient worse rather than better.

In those very few patients in whom, following the history and examination, it seems that surgery might be appropriate, then investigations are required to establish whether there is a well-localized pain source that is suitable for surgery. The investigation will depend on the type of problem with which the surgeon is faced:

1. If a pseudarthrosis is suspected then one might require plain lateral flexion/extension x-rays, possibly together with plain tomography of the fusion mass.
2. If nerve root compression is suspected then an MRI scan is likely to be required and in revision surgery in which there has been previous scarring this is likely to need to be supplemented with contrast.
3. If nerve root compression in the presence of metallic internal fixation is suspected, then a CT radiculogram may well be more informative than an MRI scan.
4. If there is significant leg pain then, in addition to the imaging studies, supportive evidence of specific nerve root involvement may be sought, either from neurophysiological studies, a selective nerve block, or a combination of the two.

## COUNSELING

Following the various investigations, whether or not surgery is going to be discussed with the patient, detailed counseling will be required.

If, as will be the case in the majority of patients, the investigations do not show a clear-cut surgically treatable pain source that fits in with the patient's pain pattern, the patients must not be offered surgery. It will be necessary, however, for the surgeon to take some time to explain to the patient why surgery is not appropriate. If this is not done the patient may misinterpret why the surgeon has not offered an operation and may seek help elsewhere, when surgery may be offered for the wrong reasons all too often with the wrong results. It is the author's practice in addition to verbal counseling to write to the patient with a copy to the referring surgeon and general practitioner explaining the detail of the assessment and why surgery is likely to be counter-productive.

In those very few patients in which the investigations do show a clear-cut surgically treatable pain source that fits in with the patient's pain pattern, it is of course reasonable to offer the patient surgery. They need to be warned that in revision surgery the surgery itself is technically more difficult and the risk of intra-operative nerve damage, for example, is therefore higher than in primary surgery. The patient needs to be warned of specific risks but it is particularly important that the patient be warned that even if the surgery proceeds uneventfully and without complications, there can be no guarantee that the pain relief would be as good as the patient would like.

It is my practice to counsel the patient verbally in detail and then to send a written explanation of exactly what the surgery will involve and its attendant risks and possible rewards. The patient is asked to discuss matters in general with either the referring surgeon or the general practitioner. The patient is thereafter invited to submit any further questions, either at a further consultation or by letter. The patient is advised that if he wishes to proceed with surgery that he should write saying that he wishes to proceed and only at that point is the patient listed for surgery.

## SUMMARY

Surgery for low back pain and for revision low back pain in particular is a minefield. The surgeon must be very experienced in primary low back pain surgery and very careful assessment of the patient is required, the majority of patients not being suitable for surgery. In those few cases in which the patient has pain that is bad enough and has gone on for an unacceptably long length of time and who following a detailed assessment with a history and examination including scientifically validated questionnaires proves to be a possible suitable candidate for surgery and if subsequent investigations reveal a localized surgically treatable pain source that fits in with the patient's pain pattern, then it is reasonable to offer the patient surgery but they need to be counselled in detail about the potential risks and rewards and they need to know that even if the surgery proceeds uneventfully satisfactory pain relief cannot be guaranteed.

In the last 20 years, considerable expertise has been developed to help us identify those patients who will not do well with low back surgery. It is important to use this expertise to identify the likely failures and the surgeon must then resist the temptation to operate on such patients. All too often surgery is carried out essentially because the surgeon feels sorry for the clearly genuinely disabled patient but without having any clear plan as to what the surgery is likely to achieve. The assumption of the surgeon and patient in such cases is that at least they cannot be any worse off. That is not the case; failures of revision low back surgery are often very much worse off and are some of the most disabled of all our patients.[8] Revision low back surgery must be reserved for those very few patients with precise indications.

## REFERENCES

1. Dove J: Internal fixation of the lumbar spine: the Hartshill rectangle, *Clin Orthop* 203:135, 1986.
2. Dove J: *Surgery for chronic low back pain.* In Findlay G, Owen R, editors: *Surgery of the spine,* 1991, Blackwell, p 775.
3. Dove J: *The Hartshill system for the back of the lumbosacral spine.* In Marguiles JY et al, editors: *Lumbosacral and spinopelvic fixation,* Philadelphia, 1996, Lippincott-Raven, p 351.
4. Fairbank JCT et al: Oswestry disability questionnaire, *Physiotherapy* 66:271, 1980.
5. Finnegan et al: Results of surgical intervention in the symptomatic multiply-operated back patient, *J Bone Joint Surg* 61A:1077, 1979.
6. Main CJ: The modified somatic perception questionnaire, *Psycho-somatic Res* 27:503, 1983.
7. Main CJ: Psychological approaches to management and treatment in the lumbar spine and back pain. In Jayson MIV, editor: *The lumbar spine and back pain,* 1987, Churchill Livingstone, p 436.
8. O'Brien JP: The role of fusion for chronic low back pain, *Orthop Clin North Am* 14:639, 1983.
9. Porter R, Dove J: *Spinal fusion - indications and methods.* In Porter RW, editor: *Management of Back Pain,* 1993, Churchill Livingstone, p 277.
10. Porter RW: *Repeat spinal surgery.* In Porter RW, editor: *Management of back pain,* 1993, Churchill Livingstone, p 317.
11. Waddell G et al: Non organic physical signs in low back pain, *Spine* 5:117, 1980
12. Waddell G: *Understanding the patient with backache.* In Jason MIV, editor: *The lumbar spine and back pain,* 1987, Churchill Livingstone, p 420.
13. Wiesel et al: *Multiply operated lumbar spine: algorithmic approach.* In Weinstein JN, Wiesel SW, editors: *The lumbar spine,* Philadelphia, 1996, Saunders, p 1106.
14. Zung WWK: A self-rating depression scale, *Arch Gen Psychiat* 12:63, 1965.

# 17

# AN ALGORITHMIC APPROACH TO INVESTIGATION, TREATMENT, AND COMPLICATIONS

**Alexander G. Hadjipavlou, M.D.**
**J. Walt Simmons, M.D.**
**Malcolm H. Pope, Dr. Med Sc, Ph.D.**



In his presidential address to the 1986 annual meeting of the International Society for the Study of the Lumbar Spine in Dallas, Texas, Mooney[155] raised the question, "Where is the pain coming from?" Although considerable progress has been made since then, no conclusive evidence exists to clearly identify the pathoanatomical origin of back pain, which remains controversial and has generated scathing debates. Nachemson[162] has referred to this collection of symptomatology as "low back pain syndrome."

While different spinal disorders, such as spinal stenosis, degenerative disk disease, spinal deformities, failed back surgery syndrome, etc., are highly associated with low back pain, the actual structural origin of the pain remains unresolved. In this context, although some of the concepts of the origin of low back pain as pain generators are not widely accepted, such as "facetogenic," "discogenic," "sacroiliac," "myofascial," etc., they cannot be discarded outright for they may provide useful and potentially critical information as to the potential source of low back pain. The laboratory investigation of low back pain depends largely upon the availability of imaging resources. The use of the tests depends upon the philosophy of the investigator to recognize these controversial concepts.

Algorithmic approaches for diagnosis and management of low back pain have been designed by several investigators.[86,96,154,215,222,239] However, the overall laboratory investigation of low back pain has not been systematized in an algorithmic approach.[86] For this reason, we designed a series of algorithms encompassing most of the currently discussed low back pain tests, especially diskography and facet blocks for specific diagnoses.

According to Holmes and Rothman,[96] an algorithm is an instrument that "epitomizes therapeutic effects by basing decisions on well-delineated rules rather than emotion and intuition." Such a conventional-wisdom approach permits definition, simple decision, and a piecemeal solution to problems using a predetermined path. The specificity, sensitivity, and accuracy have not

Reprinted with permission from Hadjipavlou AG et al: An algorithmic approach to the investigation, treatment, and complications of surgery for low back pain, *Seminars in Spine Surgery* 10(2):193-218, 1998.

yet been established for all of these tests, especially diskography and other provocative tests that remain controversial. However, the problems or temporary solutions in the algorithm can be scrutinized and improved as knowledge and technology advance. Without such a comprehensive approach we might never be able to provide data for successful epidemiological study, the recognized basis of health care planning.

The algorithms used here were initially published and presented[86,215] and subsequently updated as new diagnostic imaging and therapeutic modalities were implemented. They were developed in two clinical settings—The University of Texas Medical Branch at Galveston, Department of Orthopaedics, Division of Spine Surgery, and Alamo Bone and Joint Clinic, San Antonio, Texas—that deal primarily with difficult back problems, especially patients with worker's compensation injuries. Both white and blue collar workers are treated, with the great preponderance being blue collar manual laborers. A multidisciplinary approach to the patient's problem is stressed by the involvement of orthopedic surgeons, neurosurgeons, neurologists, anesthesiologists, physician assistants, nurses, physical and occupational therapists, and psychologists. An algorithm permits each member of the team to understand the approach to each patient, and adherence to the protocol helps to prevent a missed diagnosis or an inappropriate treatment. An algorithmic approach also permits a team member to rationally assess the benefit of a particular modality of evaluation or therapy as comparative data is available for a large number of patients.

Our purpose was to design a logical, step-wise investigation that included all possible and potential origins of low back pain. The algorithms are based on diagnosis made through descriptive symptomatology and confirmed either by invasive or noninvasive imaging sources. The use of an open-ended approach in the design means that the investigation does not end until some sort of diagnosis is established. Entry into the algorithm begins with the assumption that a group of symptoms or signs is suggestive of a specific structure as a pain generator, and therefore is accordingly tested. If the results of the test are conclusive for a specific diagnosis, treatment is initiated and the treatment outcome is correlated with the test. If the results of the test are not suggestive of any specific diagnosis or if the treatment fails, the algorithm guides the user down a signposted path where a new decision is analyzed piecemeal until a final diagnosis is made with some certainty.

Pathoanatomical and physiological studies combined with clinical patterns of low back pain indicate that the facets and intervertebral disks (three-joint complex) are likely major pain generators.[112] Pathoanatomical studies have shown that the degeneration of these structures is interrelated. Pain potentially may have multifactorial origins with varying proportion and intensity contributed by varying structures; it also is conceivable that one structure may contribute disproportionately to the clinical manifestation of pain at a particular point in time.

## EVALUATION FOR LOW BACK PAIN GENERATORS

Figure 17-1 represents the patient's entrance into the algorithm. The initial evaluation can be performed by a mid-level practitioner, after which an orthopedic surgeon or neurosurgeon completes the history and physical exam and proceeds piecemeal with the diagnosis according to the appropriate algorithm.

According to the U.S. government guidelines from the Agency for Health Care Policy and Research for Acute Low Back Problems in Adults,[4] the Oklahoma Physician Advisory Committee's Low Back Pain Treatment Guidelines,[173] and the Quebec Task Force on Spinal Disorders,[187] most patients are likely to return to work within four to six weeks, while a minority remain symptomatic longer than four weeks. The guidelines state that it seems acceptable and cost-effective not to proceed with radiologic evaluation during this period. Routine radiographic studies may be obtained if low back pain persists after four to six weeks of conservative treatment. However, if the history and clinical examination raises concerns or "red flags"—such as major trauma, suspicious history of cancer (night pain) especially under age 20 or over 50, constitutional symptoms suggestive of infection, or suspicion of cauda equina—urgent imaging would be appropriate.[4]

## DIAGNOSTIC MODALITIES

### PERSONALITY, PSYCHOLOGICAL, AND PSYCHOSOCIAL EVALUATION

According to the Oklahoma Treatment Guidelines,[173] these evaluation procedures are well-accepted, especially for the subacute or chronic pain population who exhibit delayed recovery and recurrent conditions. They are best implemented if a patient has not made the expected recovery within 8 to 12 weeks of conservative therapy. Screening should be performed by a Ph.D. level psychologist or an M.D. trained in psychiatry. Finneson[60] provides an excellent report on the psychology of low back pain dysfunction, which is recommended to all providers who take care of low back pain patients. He states that "proper patient management of a suspected nonorganic backache demands a thorough and, in some instances, an exhaustive evaluation." Hospitalization may be indicated for the purposes of this evaluation. He warns against labeling a patient as neurotic before exhausting all avenues to rule out organic disease. A doctor-patient relationship should be established to help treat the patient and permit the patient to receive treatment.

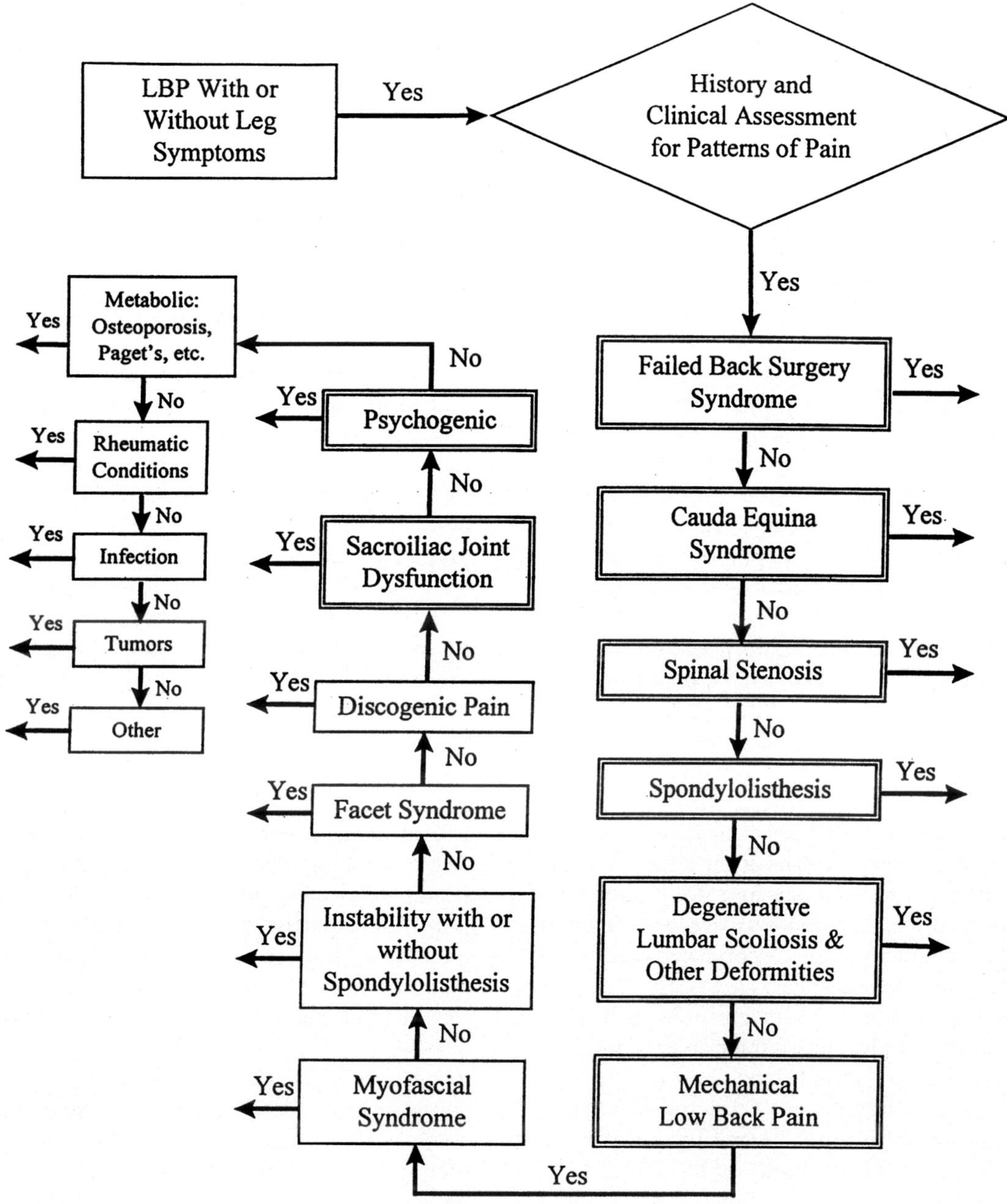


FIGURE 17-1

Initial patient evaluation for low back pain (LBP). Rectangular shapes indicate *diagnosis;* oval shapes indicate *treatment outcome;* hexagons indicate *treatment modality;* diamonds indicate *diagnostic tests;* and rounded rectangles indicate that you should *refer to original or another algorithm.*

The pentothal pain examination is useful in patients with suspected psychogenic origin of pain, or for patients with a true organic pain generator who have hysteric personality types. The patient's pain response also may be altered when remuneration is expected. Krempen et al.[119] described the pentothal technique well, videotaping and analyzing the procedure as part of the medical record.

## NONINVASIVE PROCEDURES

***Magnetic Resonance Imaging (MRI).*** MRI is indicated four to six weeks after the onset of back pain and is useful in the diagnosis of spinal tumors, hemorrhage, spinal infection, and stenosis. Enhanced MRI with gadolinium contrast is indicated in patients with repeat surgery to differentiate between scar tissue and recurrent disk herniation.[4,171,187]

***Computerized Axial Tomography.*** Computerized axial tomography (CT) is a generally well-accepted and widely used diagnostic procedure especially for assessing bony structures. It is useful when MRI is contraindicated. Intravenous enhanced CT, according to the Oklahoma guidelines,[171] was shown to be equal to MRI for different diagnoses, such as scarring, disk herniation, or spinal cord tumors. However, gadolinium-enhanced MRI is a superior diagnostic modality. This procedure is contraindicated in patients with known allergy to contrast medium or metallic (surgical stainless steel) implants.

***Myelography.*** Myelography is still a widely practiced and well-accepted procedure for low back pain disorders as presurgical information for characteristics, location, and spatial relationships of structures. Combining myelography with CT provides more detailed information.

***Electrodiagnostics.*** Electrodiagnostic tests are useful to differentiate peripheral neuropathy from radicular lesions, spinal cord myelopathy, and myopathy. These procedures are only complementary to the clinical examination in the presence of subjective lower extremity radiculopathy that cannot be pinpointed because of the lack of a clinically objective sign (reflex changes, muscle atrophy, etc.). They have no practical benefit for the acute phase of back pain. Electromyography (EMG) and somatosensory evoked potential (SSEP) are not sensitive for diagnosis of lumbar radiculopathy. Czyrny and Lawrence,[42] showed the sensitivity of EMG to be 59.1% for cervical radiculopathy and 20.4% for lumbar radiculopathy. Although the authors stated that the addition of paraspinal EMG improved detection of more nerve lesions, it must be noted that paraspinal EMG is not feasible in a great number of patients due to discomfort, inability to relax, time constraints, etc. Leblhuber et al[124] compared EMG and SSEP studies and demonstrated that SSEP was more sensitive (85%) in detecting abnormalities than EMG (67%). However, Braune and Wunderlich[27] found the sensitivity of the tests varied depending on the location of the abnormality, i.e., for L4 nerve root lesions the sensitivity of SSEP was 67% and for EMG it was 89%; for L5 lesions the sensitivity of SSEP and EMG were 67% and 87%, respectively; whereas for S1 nerve root lesions, the sensitivity of SSEP was found to be 64% and for EMG it was 53%.

Nerve conduction studies are used in evaluating patients for nerve disease, in assessing disease progression, and in the results of therapeutic intervention. These tests have shown a high degree of variability associated with different examiners but a high degree of intra-examiner reliability.[35,36] This result suggests that if nerve root conduction studies are to be used longitudinally they should be performed by the same examiner to minimize variation.

***Thermography.*** Infrared thermography may help to evaluate radiculopathy. The thermogram examines the sympathetic autonomic component of nerve compression. One study found thermography to be 91% accurate in diagnosing radiculopathy in a surgically treated patient compared to 86% accuracy for myelography.[181] Perhaps the best use of thermography is in detecting suspected reflex sympathetic dystrophy (RSD), a diagnosis difficult to make and even more difficult to manage. Thermography is an adjunct in the diagnosis of radiculopathy and RSD.[213]

### INVASIVE PROCEDURES

While conventional imaging exams such as MRI, CT, and CT myelography remain the standards for spinal pathology diagnosis, they cannot identify the "pain generator" due to their passive nature. Therefore, the source of pain in many spinal syndromes continues to be misunderstood. Direct pressure on spinal nerves or dorsal root ganglions can cause pain, and when associated with radiculopathy, blocking procedures are unnecessary. When imaging procedures do not confirm expected abnormalities or the patient's description of pain is unclear, blocking techniques and provocative diskography may be helpful in identifying the pain source. These percutaneous procedures have become increasingly important in treating disorders of the spine.

Diagnostic blocking techniques are generally performed with short-acting anesthetic and corticosteroids. If a large component of the pain is due to inflammation, steroids may provide a more prolonged relief. Blocking techniques are useful for evaluation of fusion hardware, pars defects (spondylolysis), facet joints, and selective nerves. The technique is also useful as an adjunct to diskography where pain will generally be exacerbated on injection followed by relief for the approximate duration of the anesthetic.

***Trigger Point Blocks.*** Muscles, which are a frequent component of acute back pain (muscle strain), can be a culprit in chronic mechanical low back pain and as such generally warrant blocking procedures. This can be accomplished by injecting several trigger points, usually along the fascia insertion, into the iliac crest or spinous processes.

***Nerve Root Blocks.*** Lumbar nerve root blocks are performed with a posterolateral approach, placing a 22-gauge needle just below the pedicle in the 6 o'clock position as viewed from an anteroposterior (AP) image. Contrast should be injected to identify the target and assure safe positioning of the needle. Once confirmed, 1 cc of mixed lidocaine steroid solution is injected. If multiple nerves are to be injected on the same day, sequential injections can be made by starting with the lower site to decrease the likelihood of contamination of results.

***Facet Injections.*** Lumbar facet areas are approached from the posterior or posterolateral position. Entry can generally be accomplished with either fluoroscopy or CT guidance, or as an alternative an extra-articular facet block can be performed. The latter approach is useful if subsequent rhizotomy is expected. Figure 17-2 illustrates facet joint innervation and blocking procedures.

***Diskography.*** Lumbar diskography is performed using a posterolateral approach. Coaxial needles are preferred with an 18-gauge needle and an inner 22-gauge needle, which can be curved as needed to approach the center of the nucleus pulposus. Once proper positioning of the needle is confirmed in both AP and lateral images, contrast injection should proceed slowly with pressure monitoring. Lumbar volume should be roughly 3 cc. Use of sedation is kept at a minimum to avoid confusing the results. Close monitoring and charting of patient response to pain provocation is crucial. Diskogram reports document approach, contrast volume, pressure, imaging pattern (including x-ray and CT), and pain provocation. Complications from diskography can include discitis, nerve damage, chemical meningitis, and anaphylaxis.

According to Adams et al[3] there are five stages of disk degeneration as identified by plain radiographic diskography (Fig. 17-3). Although diskography was originally introduced for the study of disk herniation, it is no longer used this way, except in the case of lateral disk herniation. The combination of diskography with CT scanning, based on morphology, was the most accurate test for diagnosis of intraforaminal herniation (91%) when comparing CT, myelography, and diskography.[102]

The Dallas CT diskography describes three grades of radial fissure as illustrated in Figure 17-4. Grade 1 fissures reach the inner third of the annulus; grade 2 fissures reach the middle third; and grade 3 fissures reach the outer third. Grade 1 disruptions are rarely painful, but 75% of grade 3 disruptions are associated with exact or similar pain reproduction.[200]

## CLINICAL ORIGINS OF LOW BACK PAIN

### Failed Back Surgery Syndrome—How It Can Be Avoided and Treated

Figure 17-5 represents failed back surgery syndrome. There are numerous causes for failure of lumbar spine surgery with or without fusion, either instrumented or uninstrumented. The failures are multifactorial, forming specific groups that can be di-

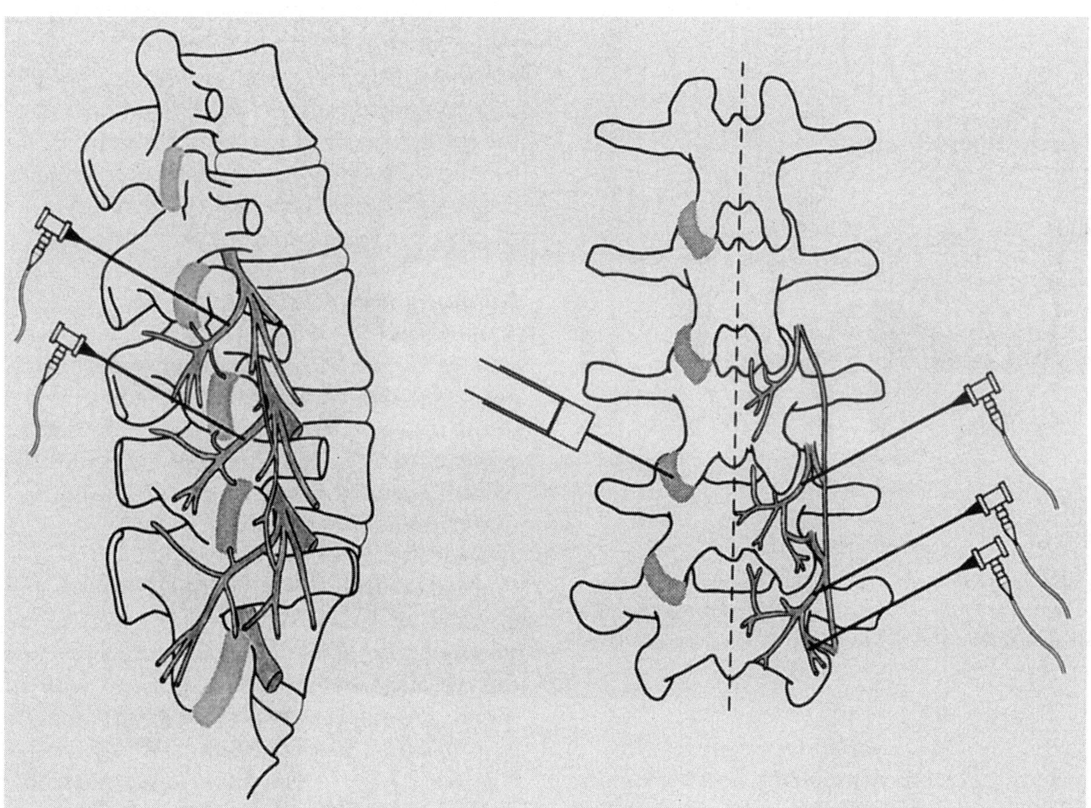

**Figure 17-2**

Lateral and posterior views of the spine illustrating innervation of the facet joints as suggested by Bogduk, with correct probe positioning for intra-articular facet block and radiofrequency rhizolysis. The posterior view also demonstrates a left intra-articular injection of the facet joint.

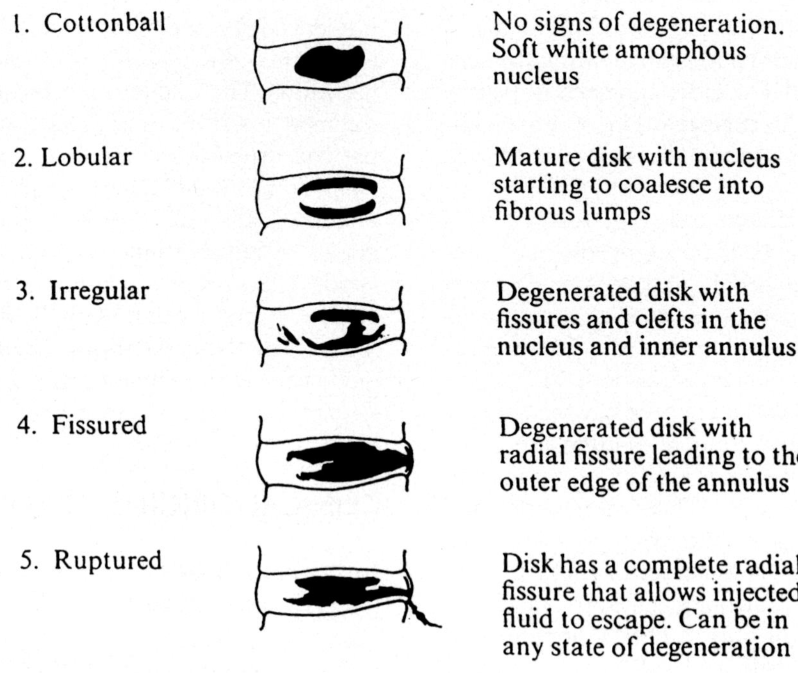


**FIGURE 17-3**

Radiographic patterns of disk degeneration. *From Adams M, Dolan P, Hutton W: The stages of disk degeneration as revealed by discograms,* J Bone Joint Surg *68B:36-41, 1986.*

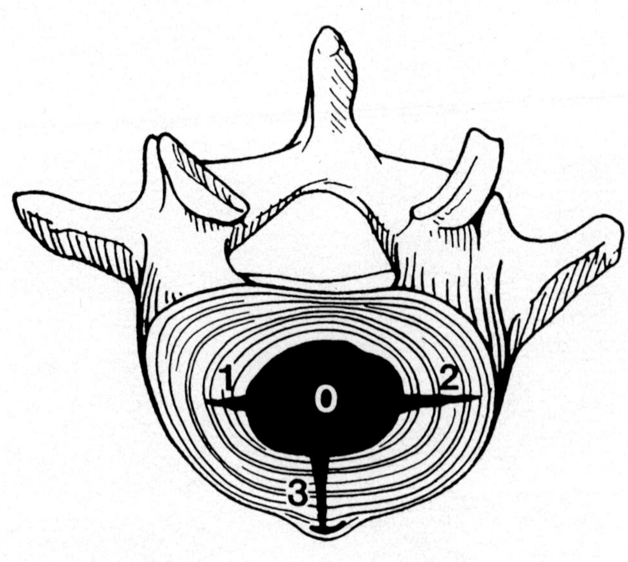


**FIGURE 17-4**

CT diskographic patterns according to Dallas Classification. *From Sachs BL, Vanharanta H, Spivei MA, et al: Dallas discogram description: A new classification of CT/discography in low back disorders,* Spine *12:287-294, 1987.*

vided into surgical technical problems, host biological reaction to injury, selection of patients (abnormal psychology, excessive fibrosis, etc.), and instrumentation-induced complications. Pseudarthrosis, fibrosis, inadequate decompression, nerve root injury, flat back syndrome, and abnormal psychology are major causes of failures. In comparing primary to revisional spine surgeries, we can see immediately that revision surgery has a less favorable outcome.[31,56,58,67,85,230] Despite the literature supporting this finding,[59,125,142] it is not uncommon to repeat a surgery in hopes of alleviating the symptoms from nerve root fibrosis. Failures commonly are influenced by inadequate preoperative location of the pain generator or identification of a correctable pathologic lesion.[12,125,185]

***Noninstrumented Failures.***

RECURRENT DISK HERNIATION. Usually the results of surgery for recurrent disk herniation are encouraging. Microdiskectomy or conventional diskectomy is the treatment of choice for first or second occurrence. Repeat diskectomy for a third recurrence of disk herniation should include fusion in order to improve surgical results.[230]

RESIDUAL SPINAL STENOSIS.

*Residual Bony Spinal Stenosis.* Inadequate decompression of lateral spinal stenosis was reported as a leading cause of lumbar spine surgery failure.[31,89] In this situation, revision laminectomy with fusion responds favorably with good results ranging from 67% to 84% (67% Hadjipavlou,[83] 74% Lehmann and La Rocca,[125] 81% Greenwood,[76] 84% Macnab[143]).

*Stenosis Caused by Fibrosis and Adhesions (Pseudostenosis).* Good revision surgery results are precluded when extensive fibrosis is the predominant cause of previous surgical failure. The reported success rate ranged from 0% to 47%. Spinal fusion in conjunction

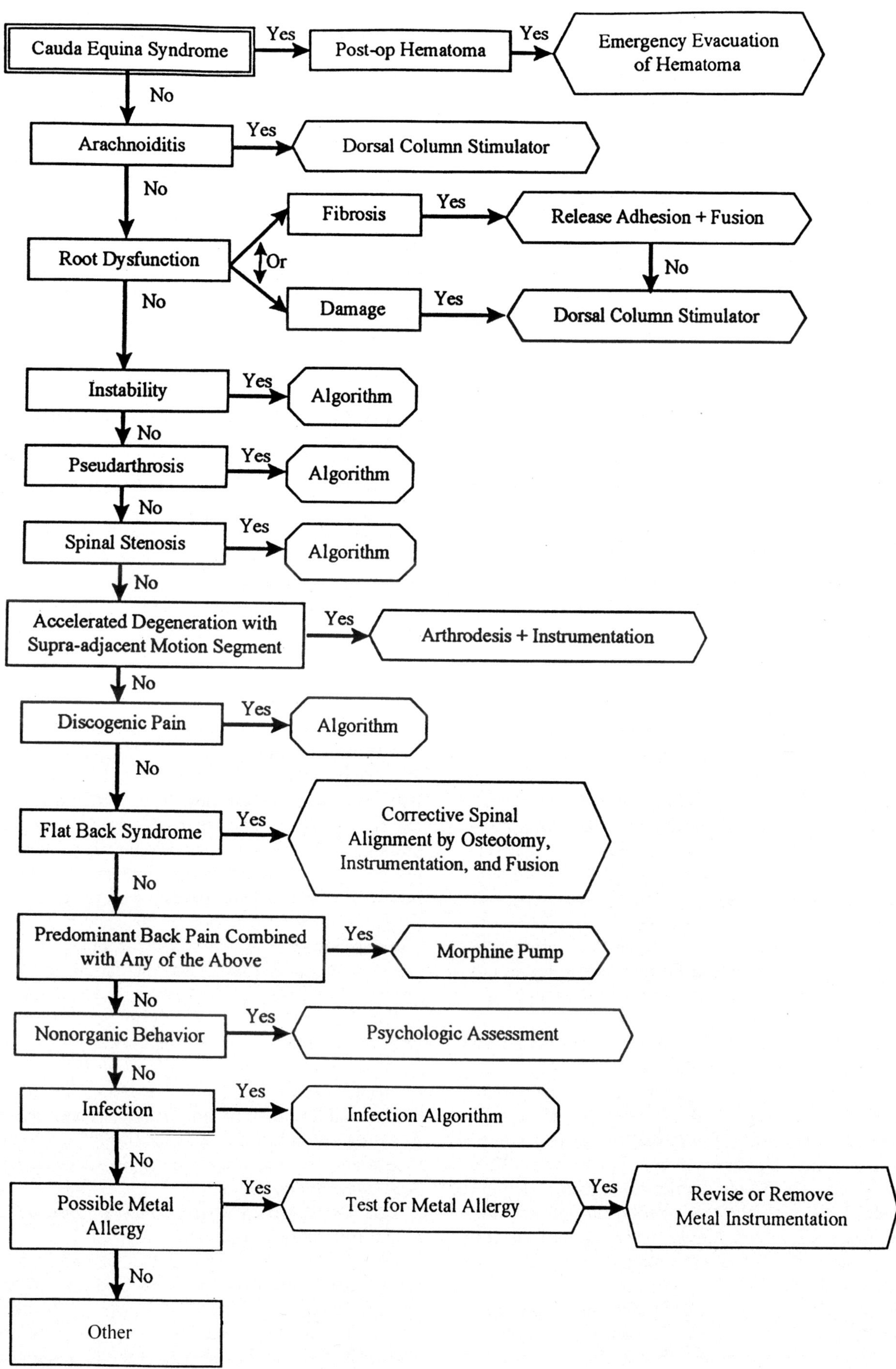


**FIGURE 17-5**

Failed back surgery syndrome.

with laminectomy and lysis of adhesions has yielded results superior to those of revision laminectomy and excision of adhesion alone.[12,59,68,80,110,224,230] The combination of residual bony spinal stenosis and pseudostenosis is also possible.

Other forms of treatment include neuraugmentation, using the dorsal column stimulator or the morphine pump.

Dorsal column stimulation is indicated for intractable leg pain caused by arachnoiditis or adhesive radiculopathy after failed back surgery. It has also been used for ischemic limb pain, phantom limb pain, and peripheral causalgia. This procedure should be tried only if all conservative and surgical modalities have failed previously, and the patient has psychiatric clearance that the pain originates from identifiable pathology. The protocol is indicated as an aid in the management of chronic intractable limb pain, with or without some component of back pain. For trunk pain, this procedure has not fared well. It is contraindicated for patients with cardiac demand pacemakers, for patients who are anticipated to require MRI in the foreseeable future, and for patients in whom the major component is psychiatric or psychological problems. The stimulator should not be permanently implanted unless the patient has had a successful trial of a temporary stimulator.[167]

Intraspinal drug delivery (morphine pump) is indicated for mainly axial or intractable back pain following a failed back surgery, in which all other reconstructive or decompressive surgical options have been exhausted, or for patients with pathology too extensive to be managed surgically in a safe and cost-effective manner. Although the majority of the literature refers to this procedure as a palliative treatment for malignant pain,[172] there are reports indicating that patients with intractable back pain, with appropriate selection and screening, can have an 80% satisfactory outcome.[13,88,118] Morphine pump therapy should not be initiated before a patient has had one or two successful trials of intrathecal morphine injection.

PSEUDARTHROSIS. In general, pseudarthrosis (Fig. 17-6) contributes to unsatisfactory outcomes[38,59,84,125,135,231] as opposed to those who achieve solid fusion.[221] In an experimental canine model, McAfee et al[147] found that the success rate of fusion is much higher with instrumentation (92%) than without (56%). Instrumentation has a definite beneficial effect on the rate of solid fusion; however, solid fusion does not always equal clinical success and the incidence of asymptomatic pseudarthrosis is unknown (Table 17-1).

Repair of pseudarthrosis generally yields unsatisfactory outcomes.[17] Waddell et al[230] reported a success of 17%, while Lehmann et al[125] had a 37% success rate. In the Lauerman et al[123] series for repairing pseudarthrosis, solid fusion was achieved in 49% of cases and correlated well with relief of pain.

However, failure of surgical repair of pseudarthrosis to achieve solid fusion does not necessarily equal an unsatisfactory outcome. Kim and Michelson[111] reported that 81% of patients who underwent surgery for repair of pseudarthrosis and achieved solid fusion demonstrated satisfactory outcomes, while 23% who failed to develop solid fusion also had equally good relief of pain. In another study Frymoyer et al[68,69] showed that patients with a history of repeat fusion surgery had only a 60% satisfaction rate for repair of pseudarthrosis. The results of one- and two-level fusions were superior to fusions of three or more levels.

In our series, the 20% overall pseudarthrosis rate is attributed in part to the use of allograft bone in a substantial number of patients and in part to lengthy fusions (11 of the 20 patients receiving allograft bone developed pseudarthrosis).[85] Therefore, we do not recommend the use of allograft alone in posterolateral spinal fusions, and we conclude that transpeduncular spinal instrumentation does not enhance the rate of fusion in allograft bone recipients. These findings are consistent with prior reports and support the recommendation that lengthy fusions should be avoided[38,59,67,231] or enhanced by other means such as electrical stimulation.[156]

The rate of pseudarthrosis for one-level fusion is 3.5% to 10%; for two-level it is 15% to 20%; and for three-level it is 25% to 40%.[85,103,139]

Methods for diagnosing pseudarthrosis include nonsurgical techniques (plain radiography with flexion/extension views, tomography, CT scan) and invasive blocking techniques (local infiltration with anesthesia agent and diskography).[144] Repair of pseudarthrosis has a poorer response if surgery is repeated to the same bed using the same technique. La Rocca[121] advocated alternate options for pseudarthrosis repair instead of grafting in the same bed. For posterior pseudarthrosis, he advised supplementing the posterolateral graft with instrumentation and a bone growth stimulator or performing anterior interbody fusion. For anterior pseudarthrosis, posterior fusion with instrumentation is recommended.

As reported by others,[238] we observed a tendency for bone graft to resorb between the tranverse processes. This phenomenon is likely caused by stress-shielding secondary to rigid fixation.[236] Oblique tomographic examination was useful in assessing the bone mass under the plates.

POSTLAMINECTOMY INSTABILITY. (See Clinical Spinal Instability section.)

DISK DISRUPTION WITH DISCOGENIC PAIN. The success rate of fusion for discogenic pain is 58% in the revision group and 62% in the primary group, suggesting that discogenic pain may respond to fusion satisfactorily.[85] (Refer to full text in the Discogenic Pain section.)

PSYCHOLOGICAL FACTORS. Patient selection is an important factor in improving surgical out-

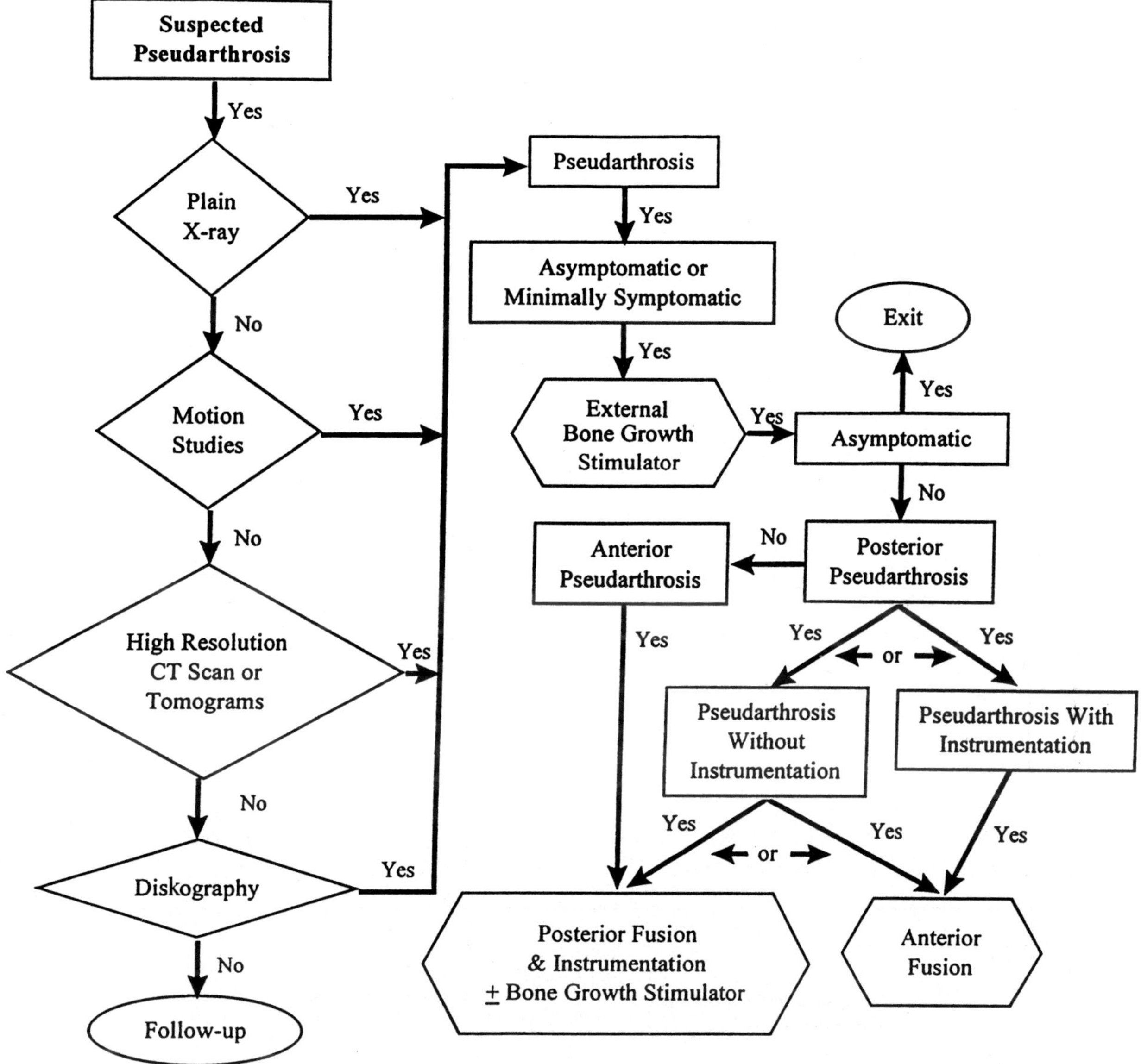


**FIGURE 17-6**

Pseudarthrosis diagnoses.

come.[59,125,230,243] Proper selection of patients with identifiable and correctable lesions, as suggested by Waddell, will provide the most favorable outcomes. The amount of organic pain contributing to a person's perception of pain may be negligible when the pain is magnified by psychological problems. In such cases, surgical removal of the pain generator often does not yield a successful result. We therefore conclude that surgery should be avoided in the presence of abnormal psychology, even if back pain is clearly attributable to an identifiable organic lesion. Only after the patient has undergone appropriate, successful psychological therapy should surgery be considered (Fig. 17-7).

CAUDA EQUINA SYNDROME. (Refer to full text in the Cauda Equina Syndrome section.)

***Instrumentation-Related Failures.***

ACCELERATED DEGENERATION OF AN ADJACENT MOTION SEGMENT. Usually, accelerated degeneration of the adjacent motion segment results in instability. This can be prevented by avoiding damage to the adjacent nonfused facet during instrumentation. If the facet joint becomes damaged, it can be treated by extending the instrumented fusion to the involved segment. Another reason for this complication may be precipitous progression of an already mildly degenerative disk adjacent to the fusion mass. For this reason some argue that the revised fusion mass should also include the adjacent level in the presence of disk degeneration.

PEDICLE SCREW FAILURE. The reported rate of pedicle screw failure in the literature ranges from 2% to 22% (2% Louis,[136] 4% Hadjipavlou et al,[85] 6.6%

**Table 17-1. Comparison of the Pseudarthrosis Rate versus Clinical Success Rate of Instrumented and Noninstrumented Grafts**

| Study | No. of Patients | Type of Instrumentation | Fusion Rate | Clinical Success Rate | Complication Rate |
|---|---|---|---|---|---|
| Zindrick et al[247] | 39 | Pedicle screw | 100% | 80% | 0% |
| | | Noninstrumented | 79% | 59% | |
| Yuan[246] | 2,684 | Pedicle screw | 89% | 89% | 12% |
| | | Noninstrumented | 79% | 90% | 6% |
| Yashiro[245] | 58 | VSP | 91% PLIF, 60% postero-lateral | | 14% 10% |
| West[236] | 62 | VSP | 84% | 71% | 24% |
| Dickman et al[48] | 104 | Cotrel-Dubousset & TSRH | 96% | 80% | 15% |
| Simmons et al[217] | 443 | Simmons Plate System | 98% | | 21.9% (3% device-related) |
| Hadjipavlou et al[83] | 101 | VSP & Cotrel-Dubousset | 77% | 67% primary, 46% revision | 6% |
| Grubb et al[80] | 49 | Instrumented | 94% | 74% | 20% |
| | 52 | Noninstrumented | 65% | 61% | |
| Lorenz et al[135] | | Instrumented | 0% | | |
| | | Noninstrumented | 58.6% | | |
| Zdeblick[248] | 37 | Noninstrumented | 65% | 71% | 7% |
| | 35 | Semirigid pedicle/plate | 77% | 89% | |
| | 52 | Rigid pedicle screw/rod | 95% | 94% | |
| Darden et al[43] | 132 | Pedicle screw | 100% | | |

VSP, Variable Screw Plating; TSRH, Texas Scottish Rite Hospital.

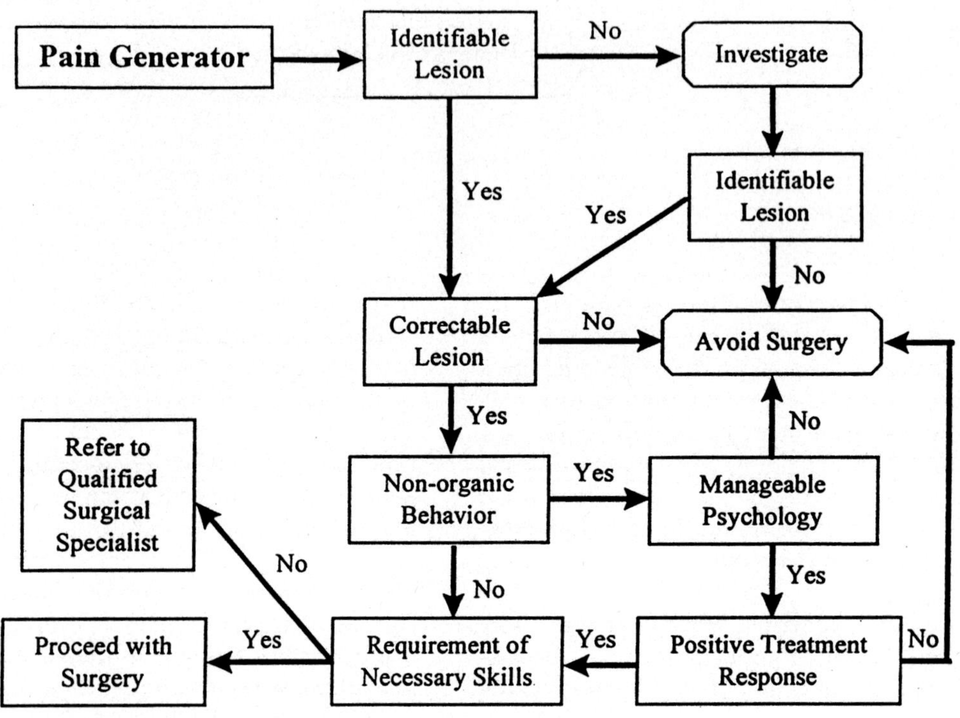


FIGURE 17-7

Psychologic aspects of decision making in instrumented spinal surgery.

Steffee and Brantigan,[225] 10% McAfee et al,[15] 14% West et al,[236] 17% Dickman et al,[48] 17.5% Whitecloud et al,[238] 22% Roy-Camille et al[197]) and can occur independently of solid fusion. Screw failure does not usually contribute to neurological deficits or excessive pain.[48,85,96,136,147,198,225,236,238] If broken screws remain asymptomatic, their removal may not be necessary.[98]

NERVE ROOT INJURY. The overall rate of nerve root injury caused by transpeduncular screws is reported to range between 2% and 5% (2% Dickman et al,[48] 4% Hadjipavlou et al,[85] 3.2% Scoliosis Research Society,[209] 5% West et al,[236] 5% Whitecloud et al[238]). This is lower overall than the reported neurological complication rate of 1.4% to 17% caused by sublaminar wires (1.4% Dove,[49] 10% Herring and Wenger,[91] 11% Schrader et al,[206] 16% Thompson,[227] 17% Wilber[240]). Screw removal may improve nerve root symptomatology caused by misdirected screws.[83,85,238] Usually injury occurs as a result of screw missing the pedicle during surgical instrumentation; however, not all instances are associated with injury. The reported rates are 10% to 28.8% (10% Hadjipavlou,[83] 10% Saillant,[201] 13.5% Roy-Camille,[196] 21% Weinstein et al,[235] 28.8% Robbins and Gertzbein[195]).

Another cause of nerve root injury is instrumentation-induced foraminal stenosis at the adjacent motion segment. This complication can be caused when distraction of one motion segment is performed in order to widen the corresponding intervertebral foramen. At the L4-L5 level distraction may subsequently result in narrowing of the adjacent L5-S1 level and secondary front-back or up-down foraminal stenosis affecting the exiting L5 nerve root.[191]

The complication of nerve root injury can be largely avoided by using appropriate techniques in screw placement, as suggested by Krag,[117] and by avoiding instrumentation-induced foraminal stenosis as suggested by Hsu et al[98] and Hadjipavlou et al.[83] When distracting the peduncular screws, it is essential to begin at the sacrum and progress sequentially to the next level, locking the instrumented vertebrae before distracting the level above. Foraminal distraction of more than 0.5 cm is not necessary; conceptually further distraction may stretch the nerve root and result in traction radiculopathy.

FLAT BACK SYNDROME. Flat back syndrome can occur when fusion is accomplished without previous correction to restore sagittal balance. The symptoms are consistent with backache, fatigue, and pain. Hasday[87] found that loss of lumbar lordosis caused the patient to walk with the hips and knees bent. In this situation surgery is recommended to achieve correction of the sagittal balance by means of an anterior and posterior osteotomy and fusion with instrumentation to support the realigned spine so fusion can occur with the spine in the corrected position.

METAL ALLERGY. Occasionally, patients show signs of an allergic reaction to metal instruments surgically inserted to correct a spinal abnormality. This severe situation requires removal of the instrumentation.

In summary of the failed back surgery syndrome, predictive factors for unsuccessful surgery include excessive fibrosis as the main corrective lesion, abnormal psychology, failure to decompress lateral spinal stenosis, and wrong instrumentation techniques. Figure 17-7 illustrates decision making in spinal surgery requiring instrumentation and is based on a concept proposed by Waddell et al and promoted by La Rocca.[121,231]

## CAUDA EQUINA SYNDROME

Cauda equina syndrome is a rare entity in which there is a sudden onset of pain and weakness of both lower extremities with involvement of the urinary and anal sphincters. It may occur following strenuous physical activity, a cough, sudden body movement, spinal manipulation, or it may occur during sleep.

Postlaminectomy cauda equina is a relatively rare complex and usually is caused by hematoma, especially in patients who have been on aspirin or nonsteroidal anti-inflammatory medication prior to surgery. In this situation immediate surgery is indicated because the prognosis is not good, even with prompt surgery.[107]

The signs and symptoms of cauda equina syndrome include impaired motor function in both lower extremities, as well as widespread hypesthesia and bowel and bladder sphincter impairment. An interesting paradoxical improvement, which may mask the symptoms of cauda equina, is possible in patients with severe unilateral sciatica. In this case, increased intraspinal pressure may lead to complete anesthesia of the nerve root, causing pain to decrease after the onset of motor weakness in the lower extremities, and may mistakenly delay diagnostic imaging tests and surgery.

An expeditious MRI or myelography should be performed to confirm the diagnosis of cauda equina syndrome. This may show a complete cut-off of the dye secondary to the large central disk herniation. The EMG can confirm the extent of radicular involvement. Prompt decompressive laminectomy and diskectomy are necessary. Although the surgery should be performed as soon as the diagnosis is made, there is no predictable recovery of the neurologic function as this is probably determined at the time of the initial injury.[60]

## SPINAL STENOSIS

Figure 17-8 illustrates the diagnosis of spinal stenosis. Degenerative spondylotic changes superimposed on a developmentally narrowed spinal canal produce the symptoms of spinal stenosis in a majority of cases.[53] People with spinal stenosis symptoms (neurogenic claudication and/or back pain) usually have had a narrow

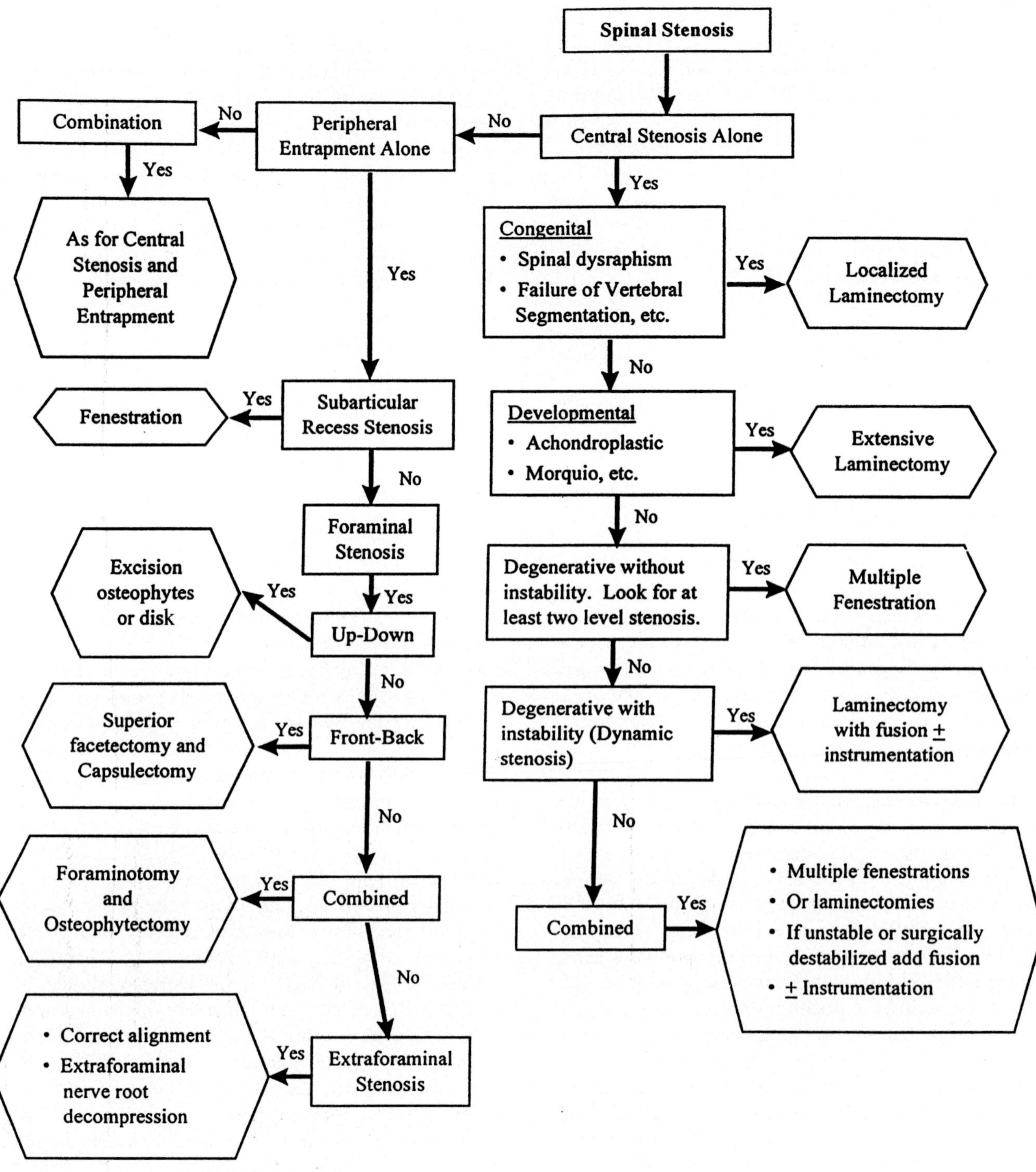


**FIGURE 17-8**

Diagnosis of spinal stenosis.

canal for many years before clinical manifestation of the disease.[40] For this reason a combination of etiological and anatomical classifications is an appropriate, practical guide for the diagnosis and treatment of spinal stenosis.

The classification of spinal stenosis, from an anatomical standpoint, incorporates central stenosis and lateral entrapment syndrome (Table 17-2). Subclassifications for lateral entrapment syndrome include subarticular (lateral recess stenosis), lateral or foraminal stenosis, and extraforaminal or far-out (extracanalicular) stenosis. Ray[191] classified foraminal stenosis as front-back (anteroposterior) caused by facet hypertrophy, up-down (cephalocaudal) stenosis caused by osteophyte formation of the endplate or upward migration of foraminal disk herniation, or combined stenosis (pinhole).

Wiltse[242] first described the phenomenon variously

**Table 17-2. Etiological and Anatomical Classification of Spinal Stenosis**

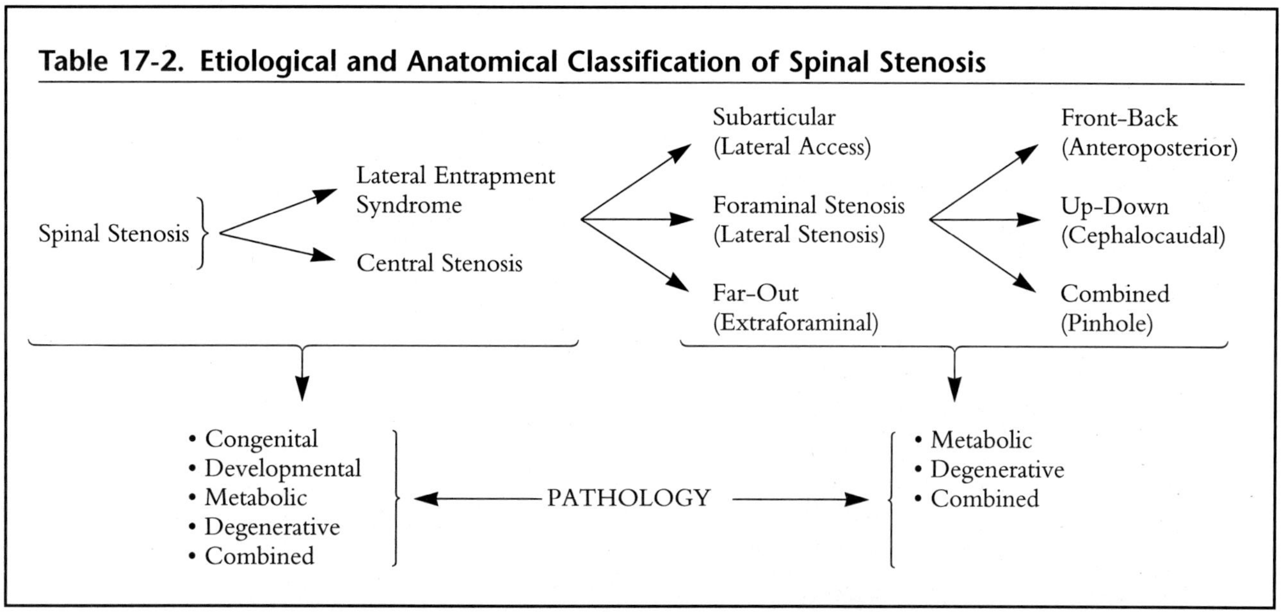


known as extracanalicular, or far-out, or extraforaminal stenosis. This is not a true stenosis under the definition of narrowing of a lumen or canal. It results instead when osteophyte projection from the lateral margin of the caudal vertebral body endplates of L5 and S1 impinges the L5 nerve root in the lateral paravertebral gutter. Apposition of the base of the transverse process of L5 to the adjacent sacral ala can also cause this type of impingement.

Clinical observations support the theory that for spinal stenosis to become symptomatic with neurogenic claudication, there must be more than one level of pathology, such as two-level or multilevel stenosis, or one-level foraminal stenosis and one-level central stenosis, or foraminal stenosis in conjunction with scoliosis. One-level severe spinal stenosis—such as that resulting from spinal tumors, fracture, single central degenerative process, or disk herniation—usually produces low back pain but does not cause neurogenic claudication.[183] This observation correlates well with laboratory experiments. In animals, two-level compression is necessary to bring about radicular vein congestion. In the uncompressed segment between the two levels of compression this congestion results in blood pooling, reduced blood flow with decreased oxygen and nutrition contents, and increased metabolites. The diameter of the spinal canal at the interdiscal level is further compromised by the engorgement of transverse epidural veins as a response to vascular obstruction by the segmental central canal stenosis. This venous "entrapment" can occur in one or more levels.[105,109] It is thus important to make the diagnosis of at least two-level compression, such as the clinical example in Figure 17-9. In the clinical setting these dilatations of conus medullaris and cauda equina draining veins can be demonstrated by intravenous

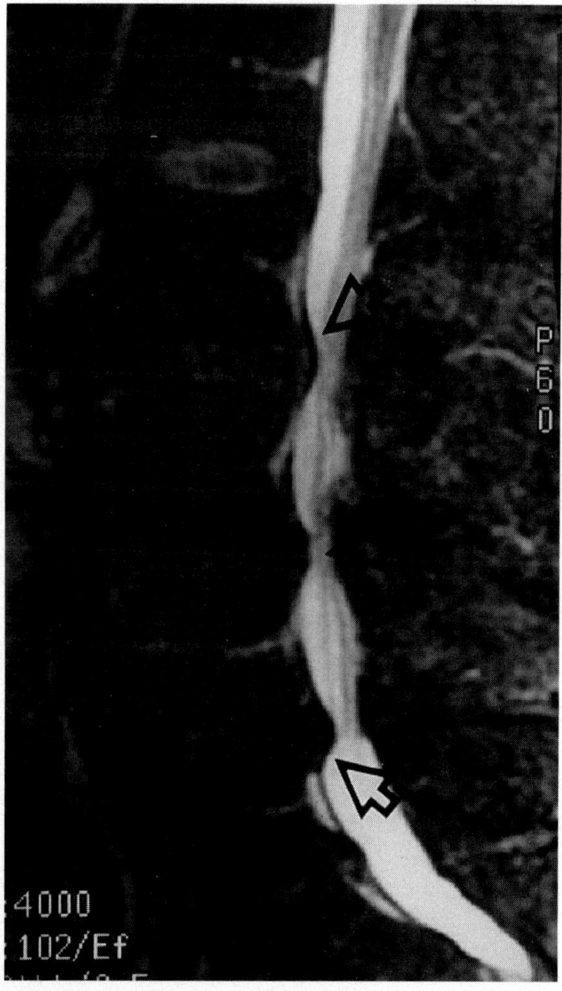


FIGURE 17-9

The MRI of a patient with claudication of spinal stenosis with 3-level spinal canal narrowing. After 3-level bilateral fenestration the patient demonstrated remarkable improvement.

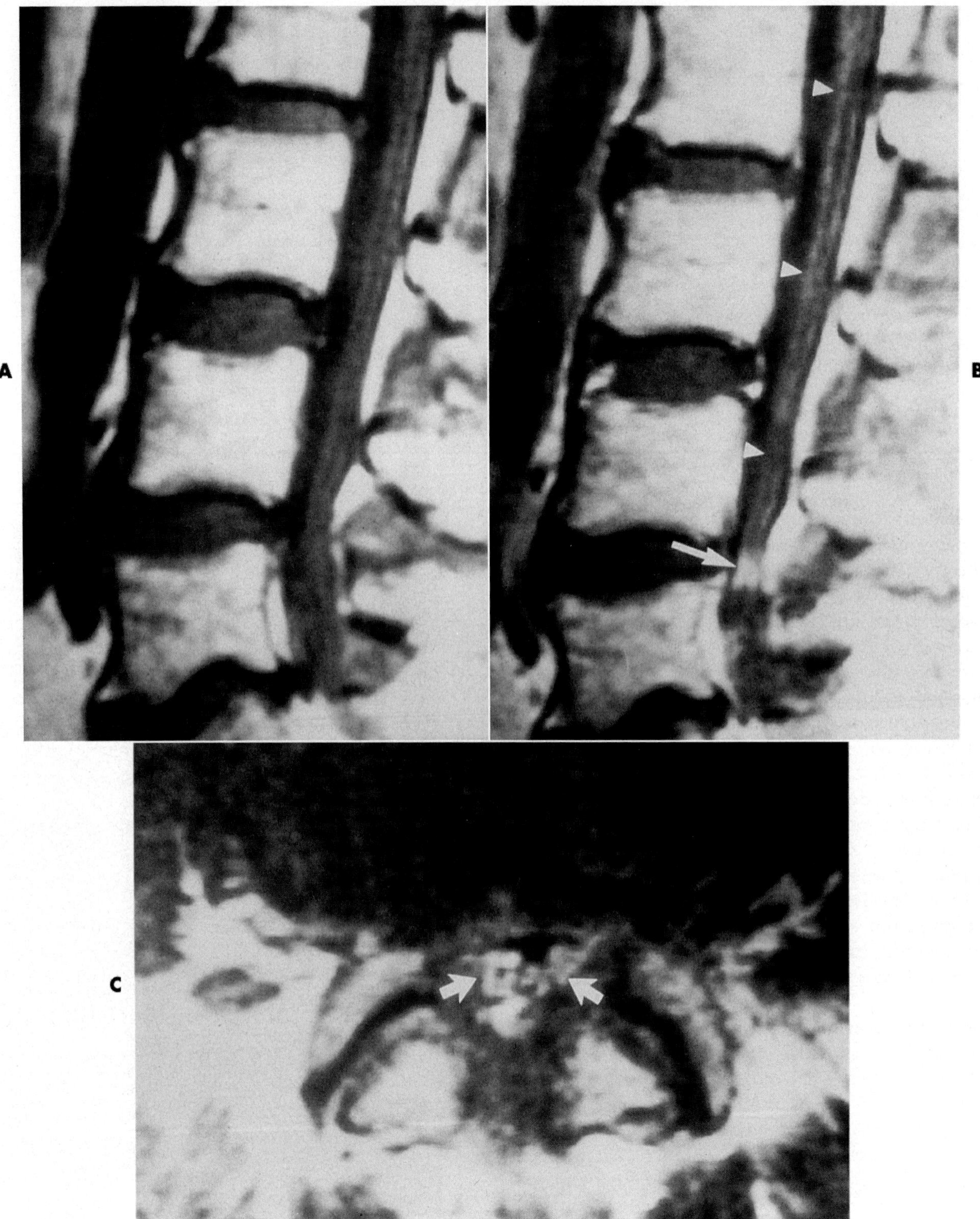


**FIGURE 17-10**

**A,** A T1-weighted conventional spine echo sagittal MRI showing lumbar central canal stenosis with L4-L5 and L5-S1 most severely effected. **B,** Enhanced gadolinium T1-weighted MRI image demonstrating intrathecal enhancement (*long arrow*) and diffuse enhancement of the cauda equina above the stenosis (*short arrows*), which was not depicted in the conventional MRI. **C,** Axial gadolinium-enhanced MRI demonstrating central spinal stenosis of L4-L5 with intrathecal enhancement (arrows) suggesting diffuse breakdown in the blood-nerve barrier.

gadolinium-enhanced MRI (Fig. 17-10). These enhancements may have a linear, curvilinear, or punctate configuration craniad to level(s) of severe lumbar central canal stenosis. Gadolinium-enhanced MRI also has the advantage of demonstrating vein engorgement within the spinal canal that further deteriorates the spinal canal capacity.[105]

According to La Rocca,[121] approximately 80% of patients with spinal stenosis complain of back pain. Spinal stenosis pain may originate either from the resultant neurocompression of the narrow spinal canal or inflammatory process of the various spinal structural elements. Jinkins[105] believes that this somatic/skeletal origin of back pain is caused by an arachnoidal/dural/epidural fibrotic/inflammatory reaction. This reaction occurs in response to the chronic, repetitive trauma to the thecal sac caused by continued spinal motion in the face of marked constrictive stenosis.[54]

When the presentation is highly suggestive of spinal stenosis (neurogenic claudicant symptoms; worsening of back pain and radicular leg pain by ambulation; relieved by bending forward, flexing the low back when sitting, etc.), the next step is to obtain imaging studies to confirm and localize the lesion. Myelography is the least specific imaging. MRI delineates osteophytes as hyperintense, hypointense, or isointense and cannot distinguish very well between soft tissue and osseous elements. CT with or without myelography can distinguish bone from soft tissue degenerative changes.

CT scan is well-suited to assess the osseous dimensions of the spinal canal and can either be combined with MRI or myelography (79% specificity). A true midline osseous sagittal diameter of 10 to 12 mm is suggestive of relative stenosis, with less than 10 mm indicating absolute stenosis. The measurements should determine the distance between the middle of the posterior vertebral bony surface and the junction of the spinous process and lamina.[229] When comparing MRI to CT myelography in the diagnosis of spinal stenosis, Schnebel found 96.6% agreement between the tests.[204] In another clinical study, surgical findings agreed 77% with MRI, 79% with CT, and 54% with myelography.[153] Myelographic studies with sagittal flexion-extension are helpful in demonstrating the instability responsible for dynamic spinal stenosis. In cases involving failed back surgery syndrome, the physician should suspect foraminal stenosis.[31,77,83] Sagittal T1- and proton density-weighted MRI images are recommended to assess this situation (77% specificity).

Jinkins[105] demonstrated significant intrathecal enhancement in patients with central canal lumbar spinal stenosis and neurogenic claudication with intravenous gadolinium-enhanced MRI. He observed that patients who did not have nerve root enhancement on gadolinium fair better with conservative treatment. However, no conclusive proof should be drawn from this observation because of the paucity of clinical findings. On the other hand, he suggested that patients with nerve root enhancement have a greater neural insult and perhaps would be suggestive of a poorer prognosis. From a practical standpoint, in cases of clinical claudication of ambiguous etiology, the presence of intrathecal enhancement unequivocally signifies an underlying neural pathology associated with spinal stenosis.[105]

## DIAGNOSIS AND MANAGEMENT OF SPONDYLOLISTHESIS, DEGENERATIVE SCOLIOSIS, AND OTHER DEFORMITIES

Causes of pain in this situation are investigated according to the algorithms for spondylolisthesis (Fig. 17-11) and degenerative scoliosis and other deformities (Fig. 17-12).

## MECHANICAL LOW BACK PAIN

Clinical mechanical low back pain (Fig. 17-13) is described by exaggeration of pain with motion (effecting the lumbar spine) or by sustaining a position (sitting, standing) for a certain period of time, and is characteristically relieved by rest. The pain may originate in the disk itself (discogenic pain), the facets (facetogenic pain), the spondylolytic defect, or in the myofascial structures (myofascial syndrome). Clinical instability also is characterized by mechanical pain that may originate in any of the above mentioned structures alone or in combination or stretching of the nerve elements.

While there is no question that low back pain is caused most frequently by mechanical structural failure of the lumbosacral spine, there is no consensus of how pain occurs or what structures cause the pain.

***Myofascial Syndrome.*** Careful examination often elicits one or more myofascial trigger points in the paravertebral musculature or occasionally over the interspinous ligaments and insertion of the lumbar fascia along the iliac crests. Patients may relate what appear to be radicular signs emanating from these areas. Infiltration with 5 to 10 cc of lidocaine with steroids often leads to complete, or near complete, resolution of the symptoms. It is occasionally necessary to repeat the injection. There is controversy as to the mechanism and etiology of these trigger points but their existence cannot be ignored.

***Clinical Spinal Instability.*** The spine as a structure is a slender column. Biomechanicians generally concen-

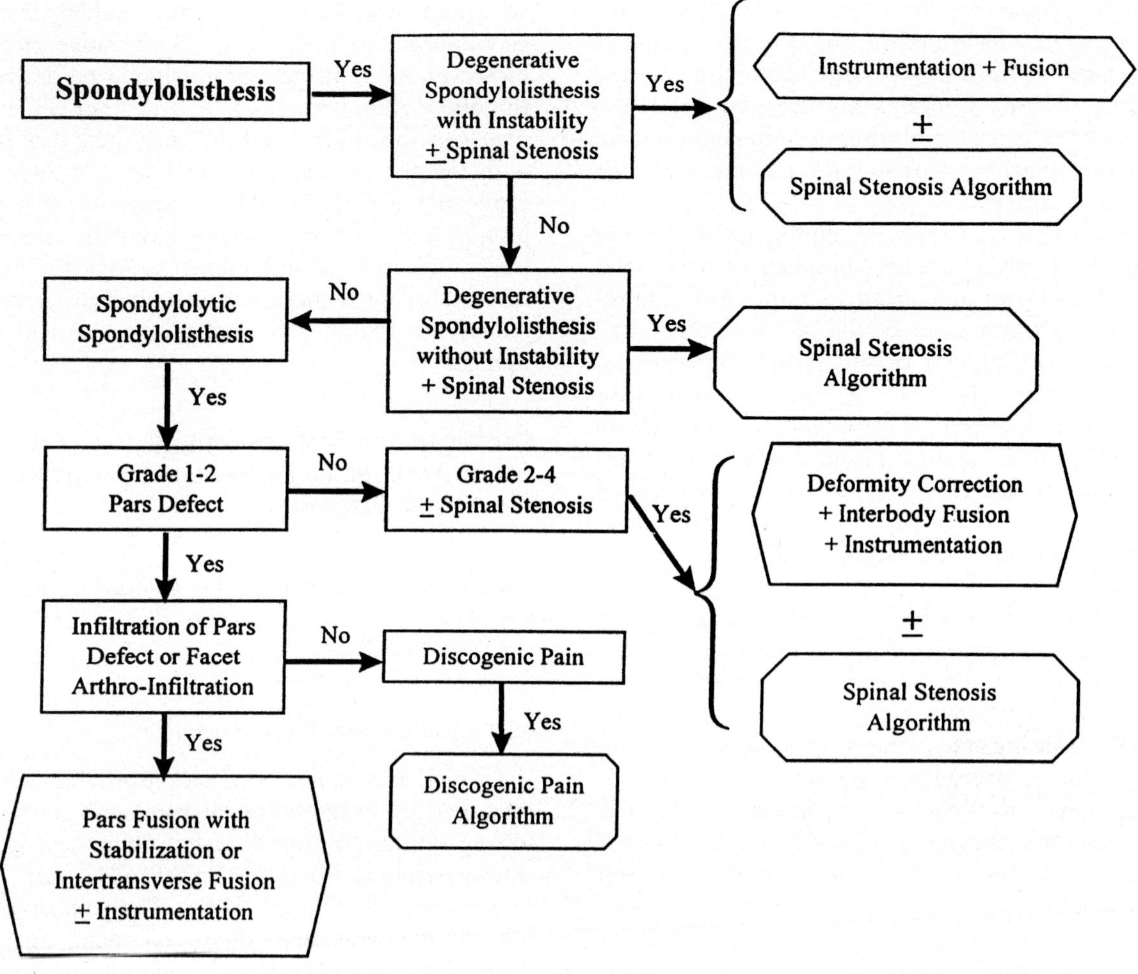


FIGURE 17-11

Causes of pain in cases of spondylolisthesis.

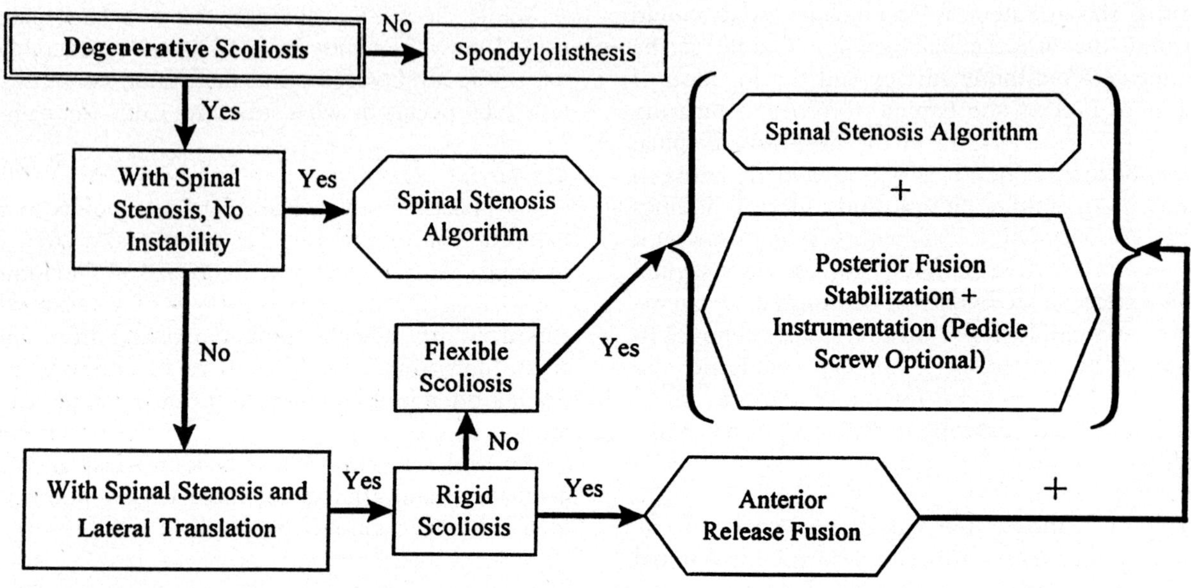


FIGURE 17-12

Causes of pain in cases of degenerative scoliosis and other deformities.

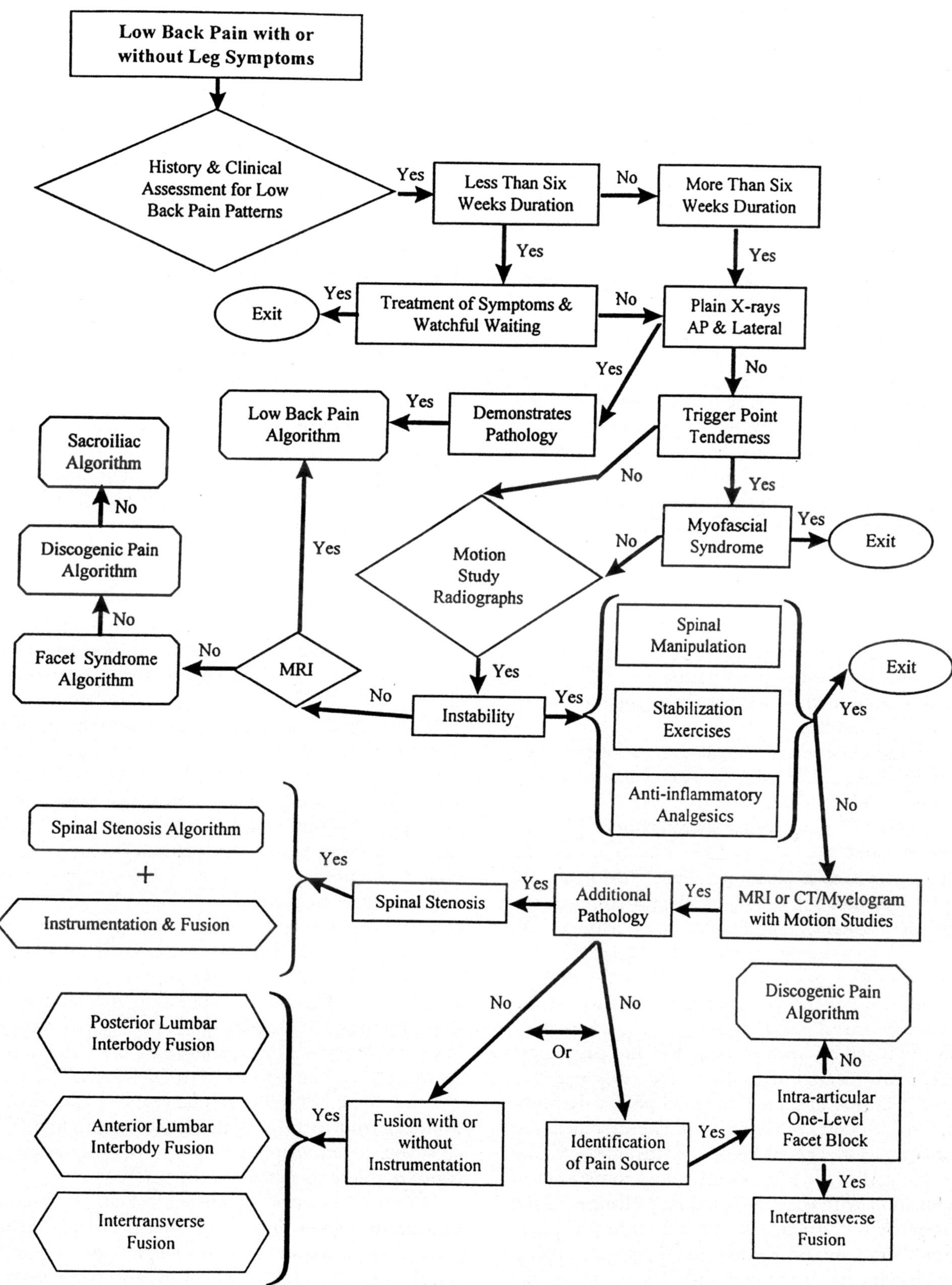


**FIGURE 17-13**

Description of mechanical low back pain.

trate their efforts on the passive (but viscoelastic) structures termed the functional spinal unit (FSU) . This is comprised of the superior and inferior vertebrae, the disk, and the ligaments. The FSU is inherently a stable structure, whereas the spine as a whole is an unstable structure when there are no restraining muscles. An intact spine stripped of its muscles can withstand axial loads of only about 4 kg before buckling occurs.[137] These findings have relevance to the clinical diagnosis and treatment of many conditions affecting the adult lumbar spine in that it gives a fundamental biomechanical importance to the role of muscles especially in rehabilitation. The most important issue has been to qualitatively and quantitatively describe what constitutes instability in the FSU and to apply this knowledge to clinical diagnosis and treatment.

Many biomechanical and clinical definitions have been developed to describe spinal instability. Pope and Panjabi[182] define instability as a lack of stability, which in mechanical terms means decreased stiffness of the FSU, increased mobility, or abnormal motions. These descriptors are implicit in the definition given by the American Academy of Orthopaedic Surgeons, which states that "segmental instability is an abnormal response to applied loads, characterized by motion in motion segments beyond normal constraints."[6] Decreased stiffness and the risk to neurologic structures have been combined in the clinical checklist for spinal stability developed by Posner et al.[184] Their clinical scoring method has particular applicability to lumbar spine trauma.

Knuttson observed that degeneration of the lumbar intervertebral disk led to increased translations of the affected FSU, as measured by flexion/extension radiographs.[5,115] Later, other investigators replicated his experiments and added other directions for the applied stress such as lateral bending.[126] Morgan and King[158] concluded that 25% of all back pain was the result of segmental instability. After Mixter and Barr's[152] description of herniation, that surgical removal of a disk weakened or "destabilized" a motion segment, this general conceptualization formed the rationale for spinal fusion in those patients. Kirkaldy-Willis,[112] based on detailed anatomic and pathologic experiments, concluded that the degenerative process occurred in three sequential phases: dysfunction, instability, and restabilization. The dysfunctional phase was least well-defined, and includes annular tears and earlier nuclear degeneration, sometimes in combination with early osteoarthritic changes in the cartilage of the articular facets. The unstable phase includes reduction of the disk height, gross morphologic changes consistent with disk degeneration, laxity of the spinal ligaments and facet joints, and results in "increased and abnormal range of movement." The later physiologic changes in the disk (such as increased collagen, decreased water content, and spinal osteophytes) tend to reverse this process and result in increased spinal stiffness, i.e., restabilization. In this last stage, spinal stenosis is a possible clinical sequela. Biomechanical studies in vivo and in vitro have provided some confirmation of Kirkaldy-Willis' overall description. Loss of stiffness, accompanied by annular tears, or even nuclear disruption, have been produced in the laboratory by repetitive loading cycles that simulate normal human exposures.[2,30,132] Load applications to degenerative segments have revealed loss of stiffness that in some specimens is quite dramatic.[241] The clinical problem has been to translate these elegant observations into clinical, radiographic, or biomechanical descriptions that could serve as a basis for rational treatment. This problem is detailed by Dupuis et al,[52] who reported that little is known about the true clinical presentation of motion segment laxity.

Clinical signs of instability have included deformities such as intermittent rotoscoliosis, disruptions in the normal smooth arc of lumbar flexion and extension (the "instability" catch),[160] and the intermittent presence of objective neurologic signs such as depressed reflexes. Some observers have noted the presence of a step deformity or the palpation of abnormal motions during flexion and extension, and hypertrophied bands of muscle at the affected level(s).[175] Attempts to establish intra- and interobserver reliability for such observations have not proven successful in clinical studies.[164]

Radiological observations and measurements have been the most consistently reported methods to establish instability, but again there is considerable controversy. These findings include disk space narrowing (sign of significant degeneration). Asymmetric disk space narrowing is an additional observation of questionable significance. However, neither of these findings have proven particularly reliable, because of the common age-related finding of disk space narrowing in asymptomatic individuals.[70] A second radiographic observation has been the presence of traction spurs, as described by Macnab.[142] Based on the analysis of spinal anatomy, he suggested the traction spur resulted from tensile stresses being applied by the outer annular fibers that attach to the vertebral body. The claw spur was hypothesized to be the result of compressive overloads and to be a relatively benign finding. The claw spur is an adaptive and mechanically advantageous response to spinal overloads.[163]

However, the most significant radiologic observation has been the presence of spinal malalignments, particularly when these were observed to progress in spinal sequential radiographs of patients with increasing symptoms. For example, Junghann's[108] original anatomic descriptions and Macnab's[141] subsequent clinical and radiographic analysis strongly implied that degenerative spondylolisthesis was a progressive deformity. Newman and Stone[166] measured these changes, which averaged 2 mm every four years. Spondylolisthesis, once symptomatic, can be thought of as an unstable motion segment.

TRAUMATIC OR DEGENERATIVE INSTABILITY. The most common cause of instability is degenerative and usually results in degenerative spondylolisthesis (pseudospondylolisthesis). Fusion usually yields excellent results; however, in the presence of segmental spinal stenosis, a concomitant laminectomy is indicated.

SPONDYLOLYTIC SPONDYLOLISTHESIS. Pain may be caused by excessive motion if the segment is unstable, by neurocompression in the foramen (protruding disk or osteophytes), or by the fibrocartilage (pseudocallus) of the spondylolytic defect. Fusion usually is the recommended treatment of choice. When spinal stenosis causes neurocompression, decompressive laminectomy or foraminotomy are also indicated.

SPINAL STENOSIS REQUIRING EXTENSIVE DECOMPRESSION. After wide laminectomy and facetectomy for neural decompression caused by spinal stenosis, transpedicular lumbar instrumentation and fusion can be safely used to treat surgically induced instability.[83]

The more common and well accepted assessment of instability has been based on the radiographic observations of Knutsson,[115] who defined instability as 3 mm or more of anterior translation measured between flexion and extension radiographs. Many methods have been developed to more accurately quantify these displacements including Frymoyer et al.[11,52,69,126] It was Woody et al[244] who determined the intra- and interobserver errors for measurements and concluded that a minimum of 4 mm of forward displacement was necessary at the L3-L4 and L4-L5 levels to define instability, whereas at the L5-S1 level, displacements of greater than 5 mm were required for accurate measurement. Others have noted greater accuracy may be possible and that only normal subjects had displacements of 3 mm.[23] For instability the translatory motion should exceed 15% of the endplate width (usually 6 to 7 mm) in order to be outside of the measuring error. Sato and Kikuchi[202] reassessed 50 patients who were diagnosed with radiographic instability 10 years previously and found 20% of cases resolved spontaneously especially when the instability was due to isolated posterior opening. However, combined posterior opening and forward translation inflexion was associated with chronic instability and debilitating symptoms.

A positive Knutsson's sign is the first radiographic evidence of instability, and translational instability can also be represented by degenerative spondylolisthesis. In addition, disk space narrowing and traction spurs have been observed preceding or accompanying the actual deformity.[142] Other signs may include segmentation abnormality or elongation of the L5 transverse process, which effectively stabilizes the L5-S1 level and exposes the L4-L5 level to greater stresses.[140,194]

***Facet Syndrome.*** According to Mooney,[157] facet joints can be the source of pain in a wide array of clinical settings (Fig. 17-14). There seems to be no specific, clear pain pattern that can identify the facet joint as the only source of pain over other potential sources. Some clinical characteristics may, however, be attributed to facet problems. Pain perceived to be in the buttocks, posterior or lateral thigh, or even the calf could originate from the facet joints. Diminished straight leg raising ability could result from a hamstring spasm secondary to facet irritation. Even minor neurologic abnormalities such as reflex changes may be due to pathologic disorders of the facet joints.[157]

In 1938, Oppenheimer first noted that abnormal facet motion may result from disk degeneration.[173] Biomechanical studies by Dunlop et al[51] showed that pressure between the facets increased significantly with narrowing of the disk space and with increasing angles of extension. The higher contact pressure with disk narrowing and extension possibly could damage the facet joints. Therefore, increased pressure or impingement of the facet joints may be a source of pain in patients with reduced disk height. Dunlop's biomechanical study was corroborated with an anatomical observation by Butler et al[32] using CT scan and MRI imaging. They found that patients with facet arthritis almost always had associated disk degeneration whereas only about one-third of the patients with disk degeneration had facet arthritis. This suggests that disk degeneration does not immediately cause facet arthritis, and in fact may even be present without occurrence of the arthritis.

In 1911, Goldthwait first expressed that the facet joints were responsible for low back pain, a concept shared and reinforced by Putti in 1927.[75,186] The term "facet syndrome" was introduced by Ghormley.[72] Later Badgley, Hirsch, and Mooney injected the facet joints with noxious agents and reproduced a clinical pattern of low back pain with referred somatic pain in the lower limbs.[14,93,157] Mooney also observed the presence of tension sciatic signs, EMG, and reflex changes. Hence, the clinical diagnosis of facet syndrome was established.

Several investigators adopted this concept and started reporting various success rates of diagnosing and treating facet syndrome by extra-articular[25] or intra-articular facet joint infiltration[157] with local anesthetic and steroids or facet denervation.[25,192,193,213] Mooney et al noted that intra-articular steroid injection for low back pain with referred somatic pain can achieve long-term relief in 20% and partial relief in 30% of patients.[157] Carrera noted an immediate relief of pain in 65% and long-lasting relief in 30%.[33] Park demonstrated with intra-articular injection a partial to complete long-term relief in 50% of his patients (30% complete relief).[177] Selby and Paris found a long-term positive response to facet

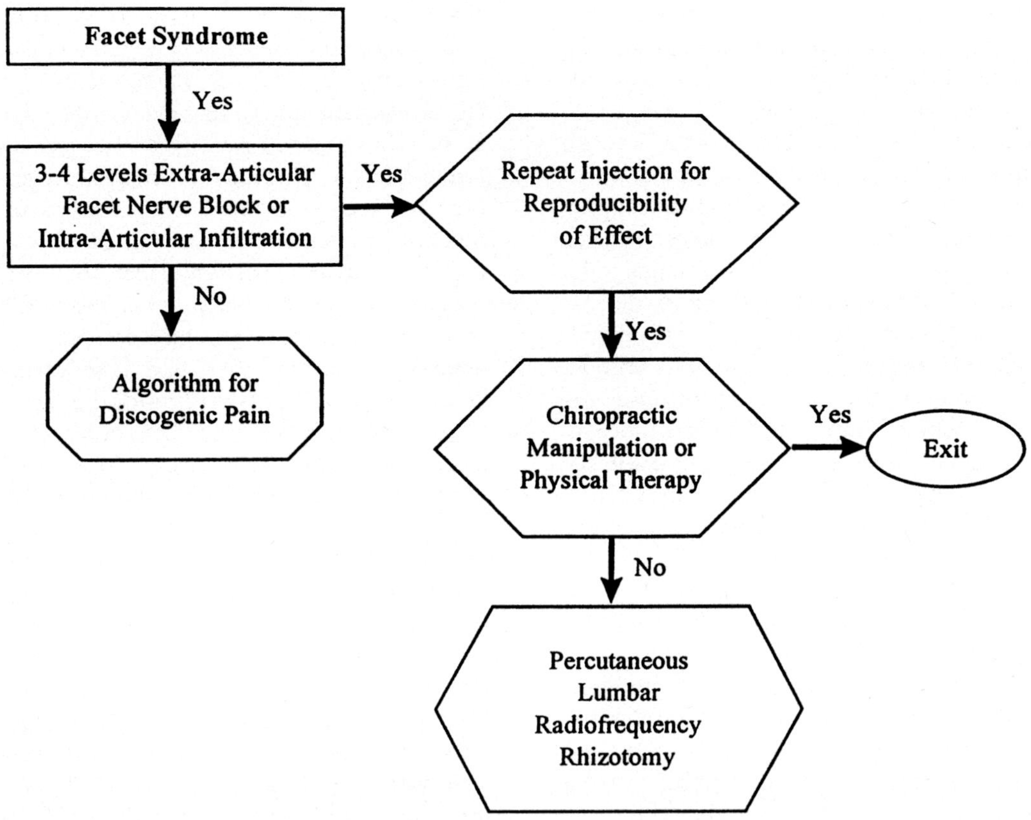


**FIGURE 17-14**

Pain and facet syndrome.

block in 26% of patients with low back pain.[210] In Lippitt's series, the success rate was noted to be 42%.[130] Destouet and Murphy had an overall positive response to facet block in 54% of cases with a long-term relief of pain in 18% of patients.[46] Lynch and Taylor demonstrated that 56% of their patients had partial to complete relief of pain 6 months after injection (complete relief 28%) and that intra-articular injection was far more effective for long-term results than extra-articular injection.[138] Murtagh reported a 94% diagnostic success rate and a steroid long-term therapeutic relief in 54% (greater than 3 months).[159] Helbig and Lee reported an overall prolonged relief of pain in 50% of their series.[90]

The concept of facet syndrome, however, has been challenged. Jackson et al, in a study of 390 patients with low back pain and normal neurological assessment and tension signs, were unable to identify a "clinical facet syndrome" or predict patients who respond better to facet block.[157] They reported an initial relief of pain in 29% of their population. Carrette et al, in a randomized placebo-controlled trial, found that intra-articular facet injection was of little value in the treatment of low back pain.[34] Kuslichs et al, while performing lumbar diskectomies under local anesthesia, tested several spinal and paraspinal tissues for pain sensitivity by mechanical stimulation.[120] He found that the facet synovium generated no pain at all, while the facet capsule generated significant pain in 30% and some pain in 70% of tested tissues.

One must keep in mind that the primary goal of facet joint infiltration is diagnostic rather than therapeutic and that any therapeutic response should be considered as transient and coincidental.[159] According to the Ad Hoc Committee on Diagnostic and Therapeutic Procedures of the North American Spine Society, facet joint injection can be considered a diagnostic analgesic procedure useful for localizing the source of pain.[81] The interpretation of the test result is primarily based on pain response. Until recently the facet joint has been widely considered as a common region of low back pain generator.

TREATMENT. Minimally invasive therapeutic modalities for facetogenic pain are only neurolytic facet blocks and denervation. The success rate of neurolytic facet block with phenol solution was reported to be as high as 80%.[92] Facet rhizotomy is a more specific therapeutic modality for facetogenic pain. In 1971, Rees first performed a facet rhizotomy for facet syndrome and reported 99% success rate, which seems a bit too good to be true.[193] Several other investigators have subsequently reported the success rates of ra-

**Table 17-3. Percutaneous Radiofrequency Lumbar Rhizolysis (Rhizotomy)**

| Success Rate | | | |
|---|---|---|---|
| **Without Previous Surgery** | **After Previous Surgery** | **Overall** | **Authors** |
| 85% | 21% | | Shealy[212] |
| 61% | 26% | 40% | Lora[134] |
| 60% | 21% | | McCulloch and Organ[149] |
| | | 21% | Ogsbury[170] |
| 33% | 41% | | Schaerer[211] |
| | | 28% | Mehta and Sluijter[150] |
| | | 83% Uncompensated<br>74% Compensated | Oudenhoven[174] |
| | | 41% | Ignelzi and Cummings[101] |
| 32% | 54% | | Demirel[143] |
| | | 58% | Fassio and Ginestie[58] |
| | | 70% | Rashbaum[188] |
| | | 62% | Staudte[223] |
| | | 38% | Schulitz[207] |
| | | 32% | Andersen et al[7] |
| 60% | 40% | 58% | Sluijter[219] |
| | | 69% | Silvers[213] |
| | | 54% Uncompensated F<br>48% Uncompensated M<br>32% Compensated F<br>33% Compensated M | Ray[192] |

F, female; M, male.

diofrequency denervation ranging from 21% to 83% (Table 17-3) with less favorable results occurring after previous surgery.

According to Bogduk, the facet joints have bisegmental innervation.[25] The medial division of the posterior primary ramus of the segmental nerve supplies the corresponding facet joint and sends a descending branch to contribute to the innervation of the lower level facet. Paris believes that there is also an ascending branch that innervates the upper level facet joint, which would mean that each facet joint actually has a trisegmental innervation.[176] Consequently, for each intended facet joint denervation, the facet joints above and below should also be denervated.

We may speculate that recurrence of back pain after facet rhizotomy may be due to reinnervation of the facet joints or to pain originating in other anatomical lumbar structures that historically have been asymptomatic. Because the protective warning effects from pain in the facet joints are abolished, torsion injuries may precipitate discogenic pain, which may not have been present before the facet denervation.[57]

Sluijter and Ray both designed radiofrequency probes for use in facet denervation.[190,218] Sluijter designed a thin, flexible radiofrequency probe to be introduced into the core of a 22-gauge disposable insulated needle, while Ray developed a larger solid, insulated 14-gauge probe claiming more precise control of the probe tip. In our series of 217 patients who were chosen for lumbar facet blocks, 74 underwent percutaneous radiofrequency electrocoagulation of the posterior primary ramus, 28 of whom had coagulation using the Sluijter needle and 46 using the Ray needle.[122] At 6 months the success rates in these patients were 21% with the Sluijter probe and 40% with the Ray probe. At 12 months the success rates fell to 11% for Sluijter and 33% for Ray.

Facet radiofrequency denervation should not be considered as a definitive procedure for curing low back pain. It is instead a useful adjunct in controlling pain to allow for better rehabilitation. The successful control of pain by facet block and rhizotomy support the theory of facetogenic origin of pain; however, this represents only a part of the spectrum of low back pain syndrome.

***Discogenic Pain.*** The term "discogenic pain" suggests mechanical pain that originates in the disk substance alone and is not related to lumbar radiculopathy or other spinal pathologies (Fig. 17-15). We are becoming increasingly aware of the contribution of neurogenic and non-neurogenic mediators of pain and their

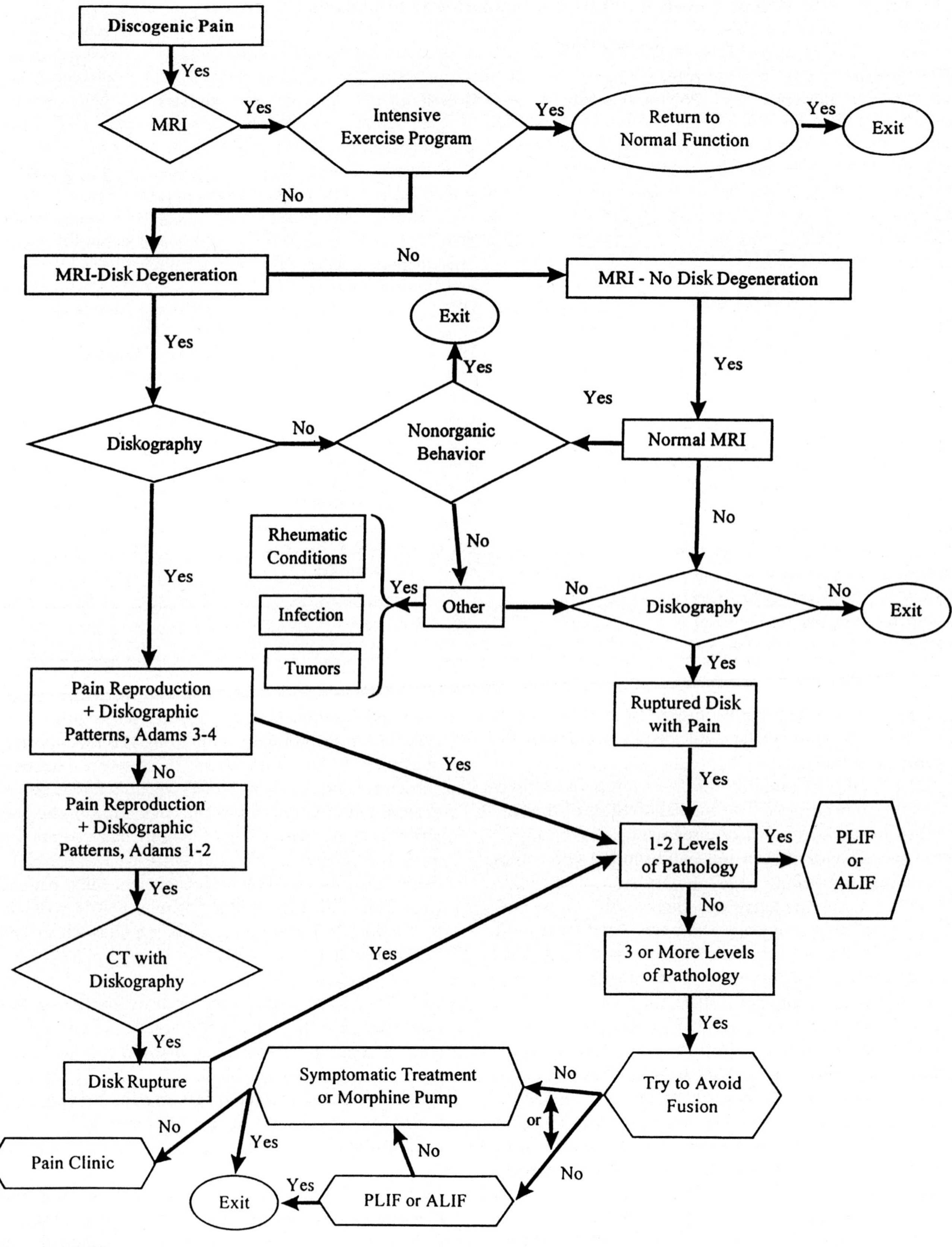


**FIGURE 17-15**

Discogenic pain.

relationship to the development of discogenic pain. Small C-fibers located within the outer 50% of the annulus fibrosus have been identified; these may well be the receptors for pain mediation. They seem to be responsive to chemical irritation and mechanical injuries.[24,106] Recently Freemont et al demonstrated isolated nerve fibers that express substance P deep within diseased intervertebral disks.[65] He concluded that their association with pain suggests an important role for nerve growth into the intervertebral disk in the pathogenesis of low back pain. Franson et al and Saal found increased phospholipase A2 activity within the intervertebral disk.[63,199] Phospholipase A2 is a rate-limiting step in the synthesis of prostaglandins and therefore is considered to be the responsible stimuli in the production of inflammation.[199] Pateromichelakis showed prostaglandin E2 to be capable of increasing mechanically evoked potentials in the peripheral nerve.[179]

The diagnosis of discogenic pain remains problematic. When discogenic pain is clinically suspected, diskography is the only diagnostic modality that can provide two different types of information: descriptive morphology (diskopathy) and clinical data (discogenic symptoms). After excluding spinal stenosis, facet arthropathy, myofascial syndrome, and instability in patients with predominant back pain with or without associated nonradicular leg pain, one is justified in investigating for discogenic pain. Discogenic referred somatic pain is sometimes felt in the region of the greater trochanter or lateral aspect of the thigh and is characteristically described as a dull, deep-seated ache unassociated with the paresthesia or numbness that are hallmarks of radiculopathy. It typically has a mechanical low back pain pattern.

Clinically, discogenic pain is suspected when low back pain, with or without referred somatic pain, is provoked or worsened by maneuvers or positions that increase intradiscal pressure or stresses on the disk. Examples of this are leaning forward, especially when holding a weight at arm's length; sitting also increases intradiscal pressure, especially when vibration is imposed such as in driving; or bending forward while sitting. Discogenic pain is often improved by lying down, walking, or swimming. Clinically, discogenic pain is associated with intervertebral disk resorption,[104] and caused by alteration of the internal disk structure and its metabolic activities.[41] Other situations thought to cause discogenic pain are endplate disruption,[99] acute traumatic interosseous herniation,[148] and posterior annulus fissure.[178] The Farfan compression test seems to be the only clinical test that can clearly identify discogenic pain.[84]

DISKOGRAPHY. The role of lumbar diskography has remained controversial ever since its inception by Lindblom.[127] This controversy stems from several facts. Initially, diskography was compared to myelography as a descriptive radiographic test for neurocompression. Myelography is a diagnostic study for evaluation of anatomy of the spinal canal meant to assess neural elements, and in this context myelography is superior to diskography. However, CT-descriptive diskography has the advantage of clarifying certain false-positive and false-negative findings seen on routine myelography, especially in the case of far lateral disk herniation.[8,180] The incidence of far lateral disk herniation ranges from 1%[168] to 4.6%[86] and 11.7%.[1] Friedman and Goldner and Brodsky and Binder showed that lumbar diskography can produce important information about clinical symptoms even when the myelography is negative.[29,66] Later on, diskography was emphasized as an investigation for determining discogenic pain.

The usefulness of diskography has been reiterated in numerous reports.[3,9,18,20,39,79,81,97,100,104,151,200,214,232,234,249] However, diskography became a controversial test because of the high rate of false positive results reported by Massie (34%) and Holt (37%).[94,146] Essess et al disputed the value of diskography as a predictor of therapeutic response.[55] In a 1988 editorial comment, Nachemson raised great doubts about the use of diskography; however, this opinion has not been shared.[161] Sachs et al reported what they called "Holt false positive results" in 13.5% of cases.[201] Millette et al had 2.1% false positive findings.[151]

In a very detailed prospective study Walsh et al found 0% false positive results when both descriptive (imaging) and provocative (pain pattern) results were considered together as critical for a positive test. Walsh concluded that the specificity of the test can be improved by incorporating a detailed pain assessment into the definition of a positive diskogram, and he emphasized proper placement of the intradiscal needle as a critical factor in test specificity. Walsh and his group found flaws in the Holt study, concluding that Holt's false positive rate would have been substantially better had he interpreted the patient's pain more accurately and correlated his findings with modern imaging techniques. Walsh commented that a radiographic finding suggestive of herniated nucleus pulposus must be correlated with clinical tests such as tension signs and electrodiagnosis; so diskography must be interpreted as a corroboration to discogenic pain only when compared to the patient's exact typical pattern of pain.[232] Colhoun et al suggested that diskography can be used to predict surgical outcomes with an 88% success rate.[39] In 1994, Wetzel et al reported that diskographic studies were able to identify discogenic pain patterns and that solid arthrodesis correlated strongly with symptomatic relief of discogenic pain in 95.6% of patients (22 out of 23).[237]

Gibson et al reported that MRI was more accurate than diskography; however, this study was conducted in a small population of only 22 patients.[73]

Schneiderman et al found a 49% correlation between diskography and MRI and concluded that diskography is not indicated in the face of a normal MRI.[205] This approach was challenged by others who expressed concerns that it could result in a significant number of undiagnosed painful or abnormal disks. In a large study population, Simmons found that 79% of diskographies were abnormal in the face of normal MRI, 5% reproduced exact symptoms, and 2% caused no pain.[216] Bernard demonstrated that CT diskography is more sensitive than MRI in the early stages of disk degeneration.[18] In Bernard's series, 18 out of 177 (10%) disks with normal T2-weighted image exhibited annular tears (radial fissures) with diskography. Brightbill et al shared the opinion that with abnormal diskography, lumbar disk disruption can be present in MRI.[28] Aprill and Bogduk described an 86% incidence of concordantly painful diskography in lumbar disks exhibiting a posterior high-intensity zone on T2-weighted MRI studies of back pain sufferers.[10] They concluded that the high intensity zone is a reliable marker of discogenic pain in symptomatic subjects. This finding was reproduced by Schellhas et al who found that all 87 painful and concordant disks examined exhibited abnormal morphology with annular tears extending into or through the outer third of the annulus fibrosus.[203]

**Box 17-1. Diskography Is a Useful Tool for Evaluating the "Surgical Spine"**

- Pseudarthrosis
- Recurrent disk herniation
- Persistent pain despite apparent adequate fusion
- Annular tear
- Internal disk disruption
- Number of lumbar spine levels to fuse
- Differentiation of organic and psychogenic factors

Smith et al reported 68% of unoperated patients with positive diskogram improved, while 8% remained unchanged and 24% worsened.[220] The patients who improved had a tendency to be older at the onset of back pain (45 versus 33 years) with shorter duration of pain. Psychiatric disease was proven in 66.7% of patients whose condition worsened. Block et al cautioned that even concordant diskographic pain reports are related not only to anatomic abnormalities but also are influenced by personality as assessed by the Minnesota Multiphasic Personality Inventory.[21]

**Table 17-4. Lumbar Fusion**

| Satisfactory Outcome | Poor or Worse | Type of Fusion | Fusion Rate | Remarks | No. of Patients | Authors |
|---|---|---|---|---|---|---|
| 85% | | Global | | | 150 | O'Brien et al[169] |
| 80% | | Global | 91% | | 69 | Kozak and O'Brien[116] |
| 80% | | Global | 72% | Disk disruption & failed surgery | 51 | Linson and Williams[129] |
| 60% | | Posterior | | | 177 | Stauffer and Coventry[224] |
| 68% (16–95%) | | All inclusive | | Review of 47 studies | | Turner[228] |
| 89% | 11% | Anterior | Nonunion excluded | Diskogram-confirmed back pain | | Colhoun et al[39] |
| 36% | 44% | Anterior | | | 83 | Stauffer and Coventry[224] |
| 78% | | Anterior | | | 100 | Goldner[74] |
| 35% | 47% | Anterior | | | 22 | Knox and Chapman[114] |
| 56–100% | | Anterior | | Review of 22 reports | | Watkins[233] |
| 95.6% | | Anterior | | Patients with solid fusion | | Wetzel et al[237] |
| 46% | 54% | | | Overall results | | |
| 74% | | Anterior | 73% | | 34 | Blumenthal et al[22] |
| 86% | | Anterior | 89% | Complication rate 11% | 36 | Newman and Grinstead[165] |
| 60% | | Anterior | 63% | Overall result | | Chow et al[37] |
| | | | 85% | 1 level fused | | |
| | | | 48% | 2 levels fused | | |
| 82% | 7% | Anterior | 81.6% | 1–2 levels, spondylolisthesis or disk degeneration | 45 | Raugstad et al[189] |

Patients with elevated hypochondriasis, hysteria, or depression scales may tend to over-report pain during diskographic injection.

According to the Ad Hoc Committee of Diagnostic and Therapeutic Procedures of the North American Spine Society,[81] diskography may be indicated when the patient has a history of unremitting low back pain, with or without leg pain, which has been unresponsive to all conservative means. The patient should have undergone other diagnostic modalities that have been unable to define the etiology of the patient's complaint. These modalities, though, should not be limited to myelography, CT, and MRI. Diskography may prove useful in evaluation of the spine for prospective surgery.

Interpretation of the procedure should be based on quantification of pain response, volume injected, the pattern of contrast (plain radiography and scan), and the amount of pressure of injecting the contrast medium. Pain response is perhaps the most important part of the procedure (onset, concordant/discordant, nature, character, and distribution). Diskography is an invasive diagnostic procedure and has complications including discitis, nerve damage, chemical meningitis, and anaphylaxis. CT diskography provides further detailed information about morphological abnormality of the disk (Box 17-1)

Diskography is not useful in previously operated disks and it is contraindicated in cases of known allergic reactions.

TREATMENT. The recommended treatment for discogenic pain is anterior interbody fusion.[39,61,165,224] Others found that intertransverse fusion also gave good results for discogenic pain (Table 17-4). When instrumentation was used the fusion rate improved dramatically.

Weatherley et al challenged the indication for intertransverse fusion for discogenic pain, reporting that a series of patients who remained symptomatic after solid intertransverse fusion became asymptomatic only after anterior instrumentation was added. This is exemplified by the case described in Figure 17-16.[234]

## SPINAL INFECTION

Figure 17-17 is a modification of a diagnostic algorithmic approach for investigation of pyogenic infection of the spine.[26] MRI is as sensitive as the gallium-67 bone scan[82,131] in detecting spondylodiscitis but is more specific.[153] Refer to Figure 17-18 for the treatment of infection.

## POSTOPERATIVE INFECTIONS

The use of biomaterial makes the adjacent tissues susceptible to both immediate and delayed infection.[78] Postoperative discitis following standard delayed diskectomy is reported to be between 0.7% to 2.8% with higher incidence following microsurgery (use of operative microscope). When fusion is added, the infection rate increases (0.9% to 6%); with instrumentation, the reported rate of infection is even higher, up to 20%.[64,71,128,133]

Prophylactic antibiotics have been shown to have a beneficial effect.[95] The treatment of choice for infected spinal instrumentation is to open the entire length of the wound. After debridement of necrotic tissues and pus, the wound is irrigated thoroughly with several liters of Ringer's lactate solution. The instrumentation and the autogenous bone grafts are not removed. The wound is either closed over a suction-irrigation system for 5 days[133] or packed open. The wound is redressed in the operating room as necessary three to five days later. If the wound looks good and the infection is brought under control, the wound is closed as if it were primary closure or with the use of muscle flaps providing a good vascularized tissue for closure to promote wound healing. This facilitates antibiotic transport, obliterates dead space and possibly improves leukocyte function, thus inhibiting and eliminating bacterial growth.[113]

Our experience with instrumented infections treated over the past three years[26] consisted of 19 cases of infected instrumentation, treated by exploration of the entire wound, and copious irrigation of instrumentation with a solution of Bacitracin and saline. In addition, 3 to 4 open wound redressings were performed under general anesthesia every 2 to 3 days. The patients were then discharged home and continued to alternate changes of dressing with Dakin's solution or saline 3 to 4 times daily. The wound readily granulated. After the third or fourth week, the skin was approximated, or when the gap was felt to be extensive, muscle flap was transferred to fill the defect. The wounds all healed and there were no complications. Figure 17-19 illustrates the results of serial debridement of infected instrumentation.

## SACROILIAC JOINT DYSFUNCTION

Sacroiliac joint dysfunction as a source of chronic low back pain has remained an enigma to the physician (Fig. 17-20). There is a great controversy between physicians on the one hand and chiropractors and osteopaths on the other. According to the osteopathic literature, one third of low back pain may be directly related to sacroiliac joint dysfunction.[47] Schwarzer et al[208] demonstrated the prevalence of sacroiliac joint dysfunction ranges between 13 and 30%, whereas Bernard and Kirkaldy-Willis[19] stated it to be 22.5%. There is no doubt that pyogenic infection, perinatal or prenatal diastasis of the sacroiliac joints, crystal arthropathy, ankylosing spondylitis, trauma, and damage due to pelvic bone graft can produce sacroiliac joint pain.[50]

*Text continued on p. 244*

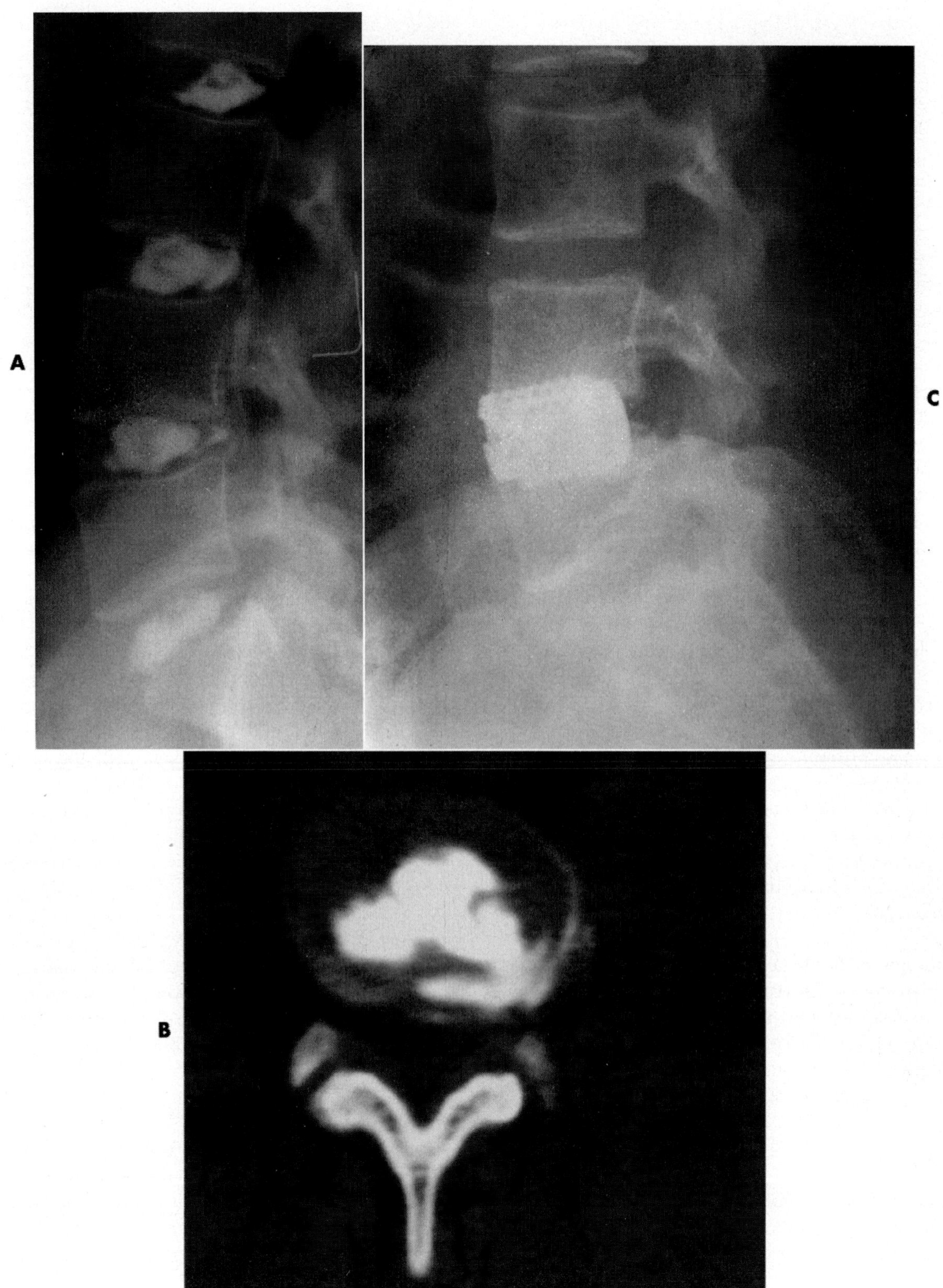


**FIGURE 17-16**

**A,** The lateral radiographic diskography view of a 27-year-old female who complained of three years of intractable back pain and who was unable to work for more than a year. Intensive conservative therapy, consisting of anti-inflammatory medication, analgesics, and physical therapy, failed to provide relief. The diskography demonstrated an Adams Type 5 disk rupture with exact pain reproduction, whereas other diskographic regions, although abnormal, did not reproduce her pain. **B,** CT diskography shows Dallas grade 3 changes. **C,** The patient underwent anterior lumbar fusion with a threaded interbody fusion device and three months later returned to work pain-free.

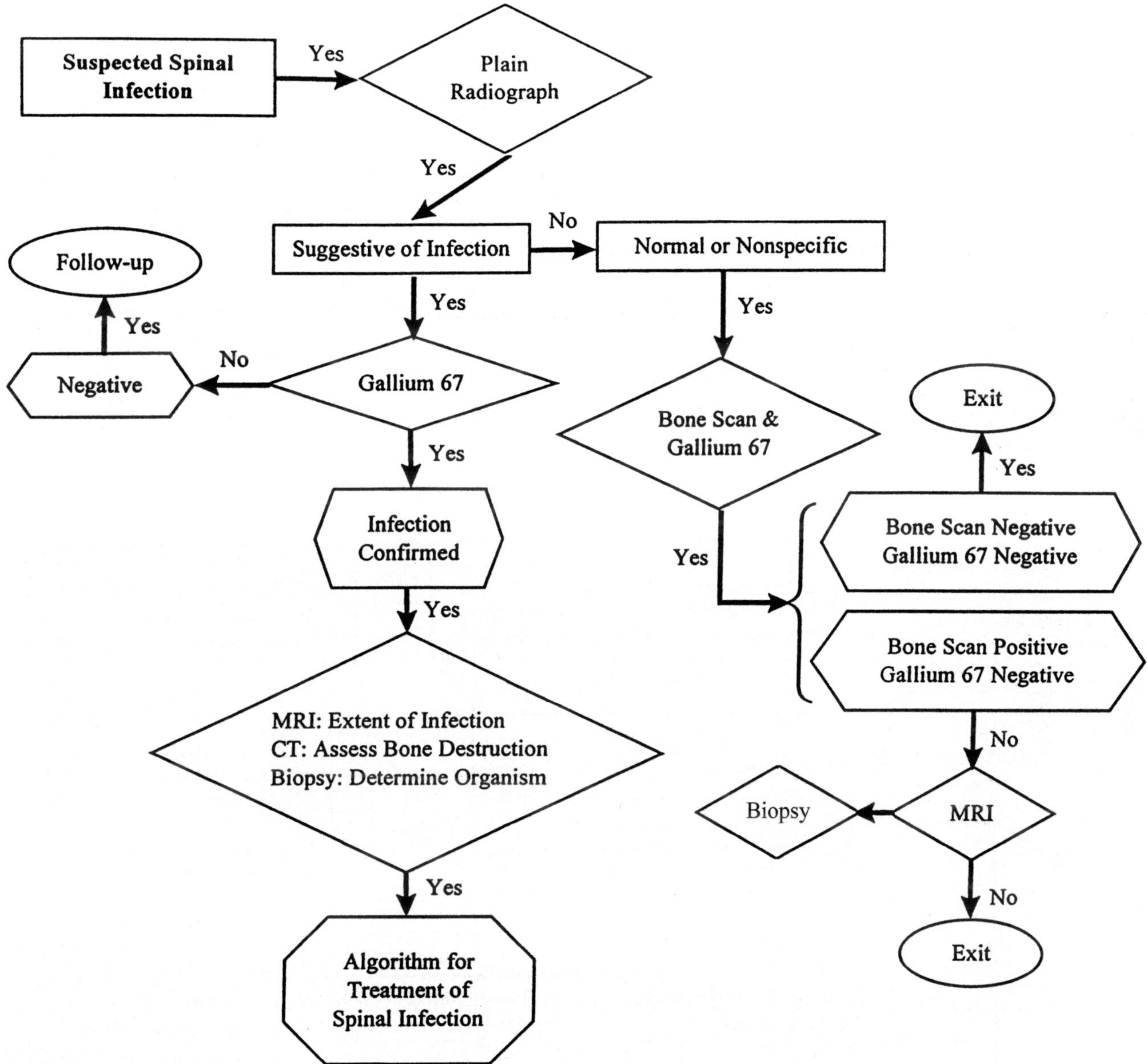


FIGURE 17-17

Diagnosing suspected spinal infection.

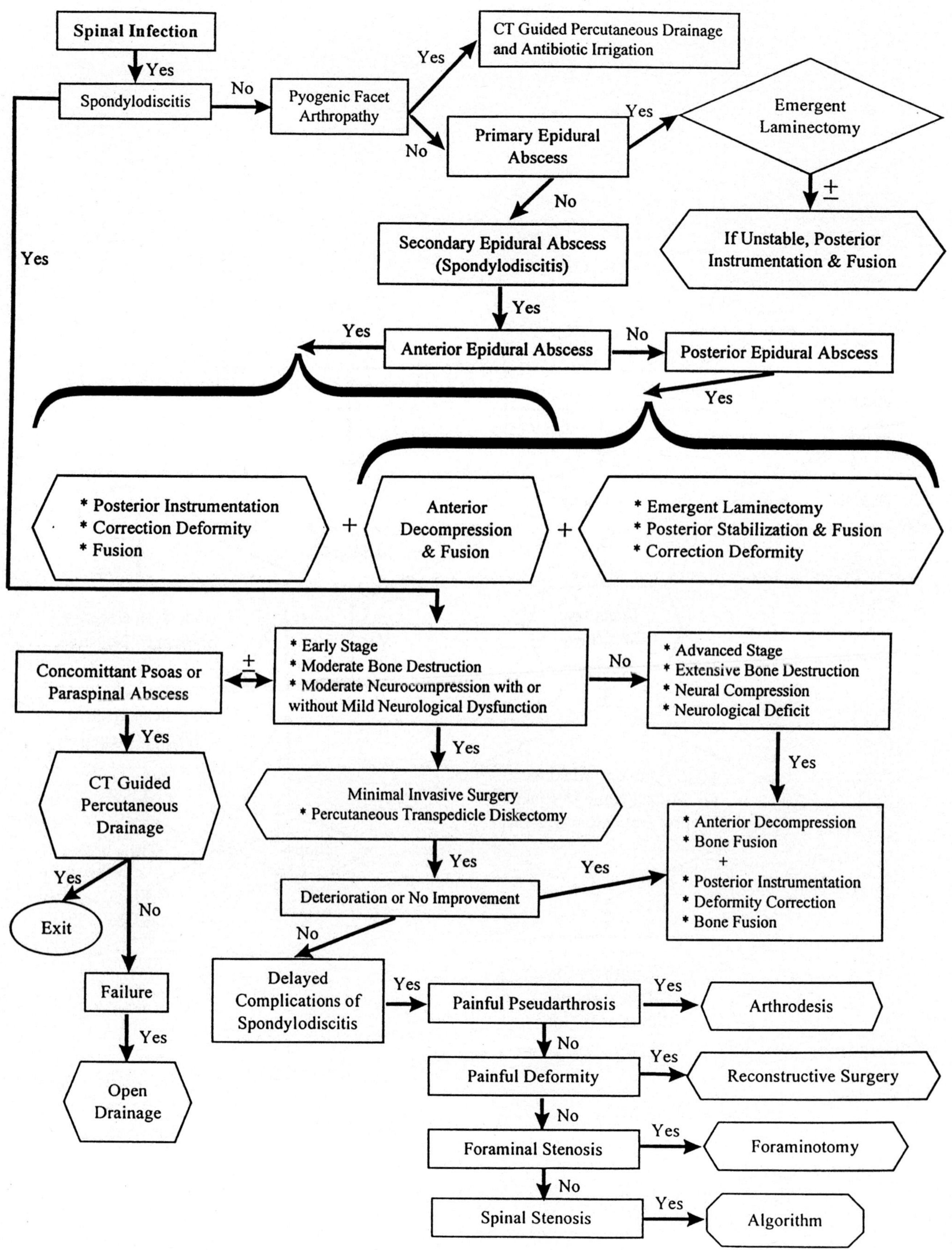


FIGURE 17-18

Therapeutic treatment of spinal infection.

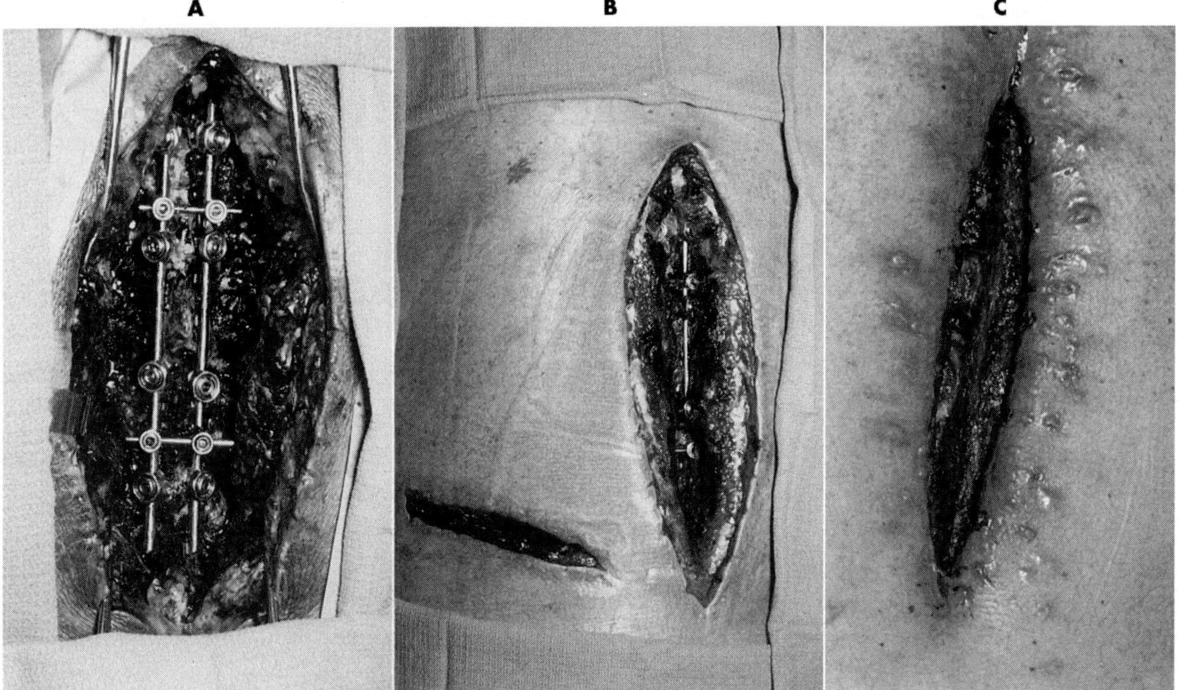


FIGURE 17-19

**A,** The instrumentation was left in situ, the wound was thoroughly irrigated with a solution of saline and Bacitracin, and was redressed every second or third day under general anesthesia. Dressing was continued by the patient at home, alternating saline soaks with Dakin's solution three times daily. **B,** Successful secondary healing took place without surgical intervention within three months, demonstrating progression of spontaneous healing. **C,** Successful progression of wound healing occurred without surgical intervention. Instrumentation was salvaged and the spine consolidated with solid fusion.

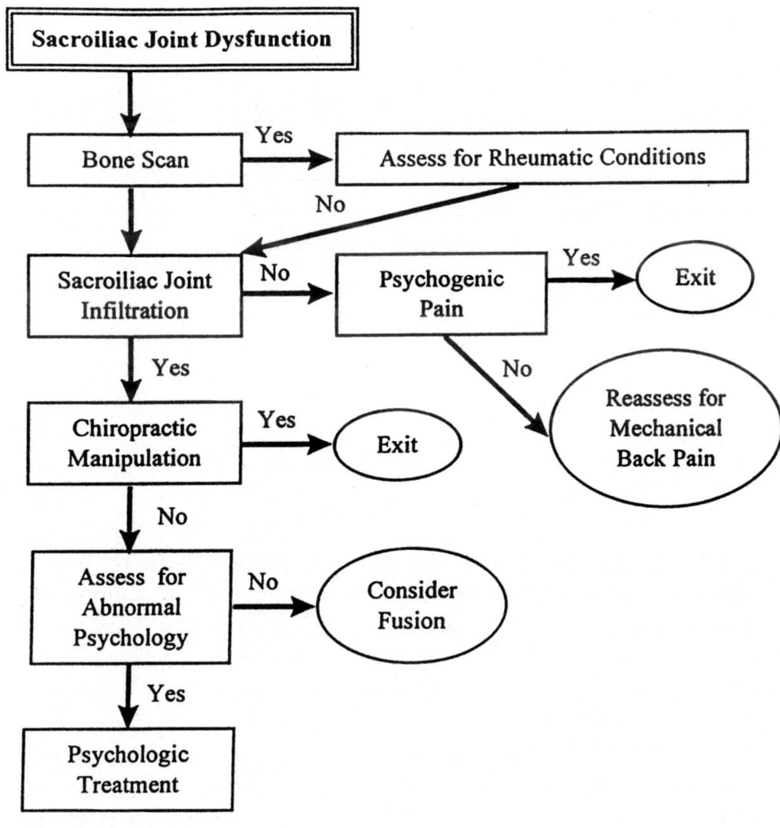


FIGURE 17-20

Sacroiliac joint dysfunction as a source of chronic pain.

**Table 17-5. Relationship Between Clinical Features and the Results of Double Diagnostic Blocks of the Sacroiliac Joint**

| Pain Provocation Test | *P* Value |
|---|---|
| Pain increased by lumbar forward extension | 0.48 |
| Pain increased by lumbar extension | 0.43 |
| Pain increased by lumbar ipsilateral flexion | 0.26 |
| Pain increased by lumbar contralateral flexion | 0.15 |
| Pain increased by distraction test | 0.35 |
| Pain increased by compression test | 0.52 |
| Pain increased by sacral pressure test | 0.23 |
| Pain increased by Gaenslen test | 0.43 |
| Pain increased by Patrick test | 0.09 |
| Pain increased by resisted external rotation of the hip | 0.67 |
| Pressure on the pubic symphysis | 0.34 |
| Pain provocation during arthrography | 0.51 |

Maigne JY, Aivaliklis A, Pfefer F: Results of sacroiliac joint double block and value of sacroiliac pain provocation tests in 54 patients with low back pain. *Spine* 21(16):1889–1892, 1996.

Fortin et al demonstrated in healthy volunteers that intra-articular injection of contrast medium produces pain in the sacroiliac joints that could also be felt in the buttocks and posterior thigh region.[62] This pain has been shown to get substantial relief after injection with local anesthetic.[15,16] There are several clinical tests for assessing sacroiliac joint dysfunction. According to Maigne the dysfunction is an uncommon but real source of low back pain, and the accuracy of some tests was questioned as shown in Table 17-5.[145]

The treatment for sacroiliac joint dysfunction is sacroiliac manipulation with local anesthesia, steroids, and prolotherapy; and in well-established diagnosis refractory to conservative therapy, fusion can be rewarding.[44]

## CONCLUSION

As cited previously, the overall clinical picture of facet syndrome, discogenic pain, and sacroiliac joint dysfunction remains confusing and unclear despite meticulous assessment. One can easily gather from the literature review that there is only circumstantial evidence suggesting pain originates in the lumbar facet joints (facetogenic pain), intervertebral disks (discogenic pain), sacroiliac joints, and that spinal instability can be a source of pain. Conclusive evidence can only be obtained through randomized clinical trials. Sensitivity, accuracy and specificity of facet block, sacroiliac joint infiltration and diskography are not yet established. If the diagnosis cannot be made with a good degree of certainty, surgery should not be undertaken (Fig. 17-7).

The use of an algorithmic approach—combining imaging resources, clinical observation and treatment outcomes—will allow data accumulation for epidemiological studies and provide useful information for potential structural origin and classification of low back pain.

## ACKNOWLEDGMENT

The authors greatly appreciate the contribution of Pamela Necessary, technical writer, to the preparation of this chapter.

## REFERENCES


1. Abdullah AF, Ditto EW 3d, Byrd EB, Williams R, Extreme-lateral lumbar disc herniations. Clinical syndrome and special problems of diagnosis, *J Neurosurg* 41(2):229-234, 1974.
2. Adams M, Hutton WX: Prolapsed intervertebral disc: a hyperflexion injury, *Spine* 7:184-191, 1982.
3. Adams M, Dolan P, Hutton W: The stages of disc degeneration as revealed by discograms, *J Bone Joint Surg* 68B:36-41, 1986.
4. Agency for Health Care Policy and Research (AHCPR): Acute low back problems in adults: assessment and treatment. Publication 95-0643. Rockville, MD: U.S. Department of Health and Human Services, 1994.
5. Allbrook D: Movements of the lumbar spinal column. *J Bone Joint Surg* 39B:339-345, 1957.
6. American Academy of Orthopaedic Surgeons: A glossary on spinal terminology. *Chicago American Academy of Orthopaedic Surgeons,* p. 34.
7. Andersen KH, Mosdal C, Vaernet K: Percutaneous radiofrequency facet denervation in low- back and extremity pain, *Acta Neurochirurgia* 87:48-51, 1987.
8. Angtuaco EJ, Holder J, Boop WC, Binet EF: Computed tomographic discography in the evalua-

tion of extreme lateral disc herniation, *Neurosurg* 14: 350-351, 1984.
9. Antti-Poika I, Soini J, Tallroth K, Yrjonen T, Konttinen Y: Clinical relevance of discography combined with CT scanning, *J Bone Joint Surg* 72B:480-485, 1990.
10. Aprill C, Bogduk N: High-intensity zone: A diagnostic sign of painful lumbar disc on magnetic resonance imaging, *Br J Radiol* 65:1361-1368, 1992.
11. Arkin AM: The mechanism of rotation in combination with lateral deviation in the normal spine, *J Bone Joint Surg* 32A:180-188, 1950.
12. Armstrong JR: The causes of unsatisfactory results from the operative treatment of lumbar disc lesions, *J Bone Joint Surg* 33B:31-35, 1951.
13. Auld A, Maki-Jokela A, Murdoch D: Intraspinal narcotic analgesia in the treatment of chronic pain, *Spine* 10:777-781, 1985.
14. Badgely CE: The articular facets in relation to low back pain and sciatic radiation, *J Bone Joint Surg* 23:481-496, 1941.
15. Barnsley L, Lord S, Bogduk N: Comparative anesthetic blocks in the diagnosis of cervical zygopophysial joints pain, *Pain* 55:99-106, 1993.
16. Barnsley L, Lord SM, Wallis BJ, Bogduk N: The prevalence of chronic cervical zygopophysial joint pain after whiplash, *Spine* 20:20-26, 1995.
17. Barr JS, Riseborough EJ, Freedman PA: Failed surgery for low back pain and sciatica, *J Bone Joint Surg* 45A:1553, 1963.
18. Bernard T: Lumbar discography followed by computed tomography: refining the diagnosis of low back pain, *Pain* 15:640-707, 1990.
19. Bernard TN, Kirkaldy-Willis WH: Recognizing specific characteristics of nonspecific low back pain, *Clinical Orthop* 217:266-280, 1987.
20. Birney TJ, White JJ Jr, Berens D, Kuhn G: Comparison of MRI and discography in the diagnosis of lumbar degenerative disc disease, *J Spine Disord* 5:417-423, 1992.
21. Block AR, Vanharanta H, Ohnmeiss DD, Guyer RD: Discographic pain report. Influence of psychological factors, *Spine* 21:334-338, 1996.
22. Blumenthal SL, Baker J, Dossett A, Selby DK: The role of anterior lumbar fusion for internal disc disruption, *Spine* 1988; 13:566-569, 1988.
23. Boden SD, Wiesel WS: Lumbosacral segmental motion in normal individuals. Presented at the meeting of the International Society for the Study of the Lumbar Spine. Kyoto, Japan, 1989.
24. Bogduk N: The nerves to the intervertebral discs, *J Anat* 132:39-56, 1981.
25. Bogduk N, Long DM: The anatomy of the so-called articular nerves and their relationship to facet denervation in the treatment of low back pain, *J Neurosurg* 51:172-177, 1979.
26. Borowksi A, Crow, WN, Hadjipavlou, AG, Chajub G, Mader JT, Cesani F; vanSonnenberg E: Percutaneous management of pyogenic spondylodiscitis, *Am J Roentgenolog.* In Press 1997.
27. Braune HJ, Wunderlich MT: Diagnostic value of different neurophysiological methods in the assessment of lumbar nerve root lesions, *Arch Phys Med Rehabil* 78:518-520, 1997.
28. Brightbill TC, Pile N, Eichelberger RP, Whitman M Jr: Normal magnetic resonance imaging and abnormal discography in lumbar disc disruption, *Spine* 19: 1075-1077, 1994.
29. Brodsky AE, Binder WF: Lumbar discography. Its value in diagnosis and treatment of lumbar disc lesions, *Spine* 4:110-120, 1983.
30. Brown T. Hansen RH, Yorra AJ: Some mechanical tests on the lumbosacral spine with particular reference to the intervertebral discs. A preliminary report, *J Bone Joint Surg* 39A:1135-1164, 1957.
31. Burton CV, Kirkaldy-Willis WH, Yong-Hing K, Heithoff KB: Causes of failure of surgery on the lumbar spine, *Clin Orthop* 157:191-199, 1981.
32. Butler D, Traimow JH, Andersson GB, McNeill TW, Huckman MS: Disks degenerate before facets, *Spine* 15:111-113, 1990.
33. Carrera GF: Lumbar facet joint injection in low back pain and sciatica: description of technique, *Radiology* 137:661-664, 1980.
34. Carrette S, Marcoux S, Truchau R, Grondin C, Gognon J, Albert Y, Latulippe M: A controlled trial of corticosteroid injection into facet joints for chronic low back pain, *N Engl J Med* 325:1002-1006, 1991.
35. Chaudhry V, Cornblath DR, Mellits ED, Avila O, Freimer ML, et al: Inter- and intra-examiner reliability of nerve conduction measurements in normal subjects, *Ann Neurol* 30:841-843, 1991.
36. Chaudhry V, Corse AM, Freimer ML, Glass JD, Kuncl RW, et al: Inter- and intra-examiner reliability of nerve conduction measurements in patients with diabetic neuropathy, *Neurology* 44:1459-1462, 1994.
37. Chow SP, Long JC, Ma A, Yau AC: Anterior spinal fusion or deranged lumbar intervertebral disc, *Spine* 5:452-458, 1980.
38. Cleveland M, Bosworth DM, Thompson FR: Pseudoarthrosis in the lumbosacral spine, *J Bone Joint Surg* 30A:302-312, 1948.
39. Colhoun E, McCall IW, Williams L, Cassar Pullicino VN: Provocation discography as a guide to planning operations on the spine, *J Bone Joint Surg* 70B:267-271, 1988.
40. Critchley EM: Lumbar spinal stenosis [editorial]. *B Med J Clin Res Ed* 284(6329):1588-1589, 1982.
41. Crock HV: A reappraisal of intervertebral disc lesions, *Jed J Australia* 1:983-989, 1970.
42. Czyrny JJ. Lawrence J: The importance of paraspinal muscle EMG in cervical and lumbosacral radiculopathy: Review of 100 cases, *Electromyog Clin Neurophys* 36:503-508, 1996.

43. Darden BV, Wood KE, Hatley MK: Evaluation of pedicle screw insertion monitored by intraoperative evoked electromyography, *J Spinal Disord* 9:8-16, 1996.
44. Daum WJ: The sacrioliac joint: an unappreciated pain generator, *Am J Orthop* 24:475-478, 1995.
45. Demirel T: [Experience with percutaneous facet-neurectomy]. [German] Medizinische Welt. 31(29-30):1096-1098, 1980.
46. Destouet JM, Murphy W: Lumbar facet block. Indications and technique, *Orthop Rev* 14:280-288, 1985.
47. DeJung B: Iliosacralgelenksblockierungen. Ein Verlauf-studie. Manuelle Medizin 23:109-115, 1994.
48. Dickman CA, Fessler RG, Mac Millan M, Haid RW: Transpedicular screw-rod fixation of the lumbar spine: Operative technique and outcome in 104 cases, *J Neurosurg* 77:860-870, 1992.
49. Dove J: Segmental wiring for spinal deformity: A morbidity report, *Spine* 14:229-231, 1989.
50. Dreyfuss P, Michaelsen M, Pauza K, McLarty J, Bogduk N: The value of medical history and physical examination in diagnosing sacroiliac joint pain, *Spine* 21:2594-2602, 1996.
51. Dunlop RB, Adams MA, Hutton WC: Disco space narrowing and the lumbar facet joints, *J Bone Joint Surg* 66B:706-710, 1984.
52. Dupuis PR, Young-Hing K, Cassidy JD, Kirkaldy-Willis WH: Radiologic diagnosis of degenerative lumbar spinal instability, *Spine* 10:262-276, 1985.
53. Edwards WC, La Rocca H: The developmental segmental sagittal diameter of the cervical spinal canal in patients with cervical spondylosis, *Spine* 8:20-27, 1983.
54. Epstein JA, Epstein BS, Lavine LS, Rosenthal AD, Decker RE, Carras R: Obliterative arachnoiditis complicating lumbar spinal stenosis, *J Neurosurg* 48:252-258, 1978.
55. Esses SI, Botsford J, Kostuik JP: The role of external spinal skeletal fixation in the assessment of low-back disorders, *Spine* 14:594-601, 1988.
56. Fager CA, Freidberg SR: Analysis of failures and poor results of lumbar spine surgery, *Spine* 5:87-94, 1980.
57. Farfan HF, Cossette JW, Robertson GH, et al: The effects of torsion on the lumbar intervertebral joints: the role of torsion in the production of disc degeneration, *J Bone Joint Surg* 52A:468-497, 1970.
58. Fassio B, Ginestie JF: [Intersomatic lumbar arthrodesis by posterior approach (Cloward) in the treatment of lumbago]. [French], *Acta Orthop Belgica* 47(4-5): 667-671, 1981.
59. Finnegan WJ, Fenlin JM, Marvel JP, Nardini RJ, Rothman RH: Results of surgical intervention in the symptomatic multiply-operated back patient, *J Bone Joint Surg* 61A:1077-1082, 1979.
60. Finneson B: *Low back pain*. Philadelphia, 1980, JB Lippincott, pp 199-327.
61. Fischgrund JS, Montgomery DM: Diagnosis and treatment of discogenic low back pain, *Orthop Rev* 22:311-318, 1993.
62. Fortin JD, Dwyer AP, West S, Pier J: Sacroiliac joint: pain referral maps upon applying a new injection/arthrography technique Part I: Asymptomatic volunteers, *Spine* 19:1475-1482, 1994.
63. Franson RC, Saal JS, Saal JA: Human disc phospholipase A2 is inflammatory, *Spine* 17(suppl 6):S219-S231, 1992.
64. Fraser RD, Osti OL, Vernon-Roberts B: Discitis after discography, *J Bone Joint Surg* 69B(1):26-35, 1987.
65. Freemont AJ, Peacock TE, Goupille P, Howland JA, O'Brien J, Jayson MIV: Nerve ingrowth into diseased intervertebral disc in chronic back pain, *The Lancet* 350:178-181, 1997.
66. Friedman J, Goldner MZ: Discography in evaluation of lumbar disc lesions, *Radiology* 65:653-661, 1955.
67. Frymoyer JW, Hanley EN, Howe J, et al: Disc excision and spine fusion in the management of lumbar disc disease: a minimum ten-year follow-up, *Spine* 3:1-6, 1978.
68. Frymoyer JW, Matteri RE, Hanley EN, Kuhlman D, Howe J: Failed lumbar disc surgery requiring second operation, *Spine* 3:7-11, 1978.
69. Frymoyer JW, Hanley EN Jr, Howe J, Kuhlmann D, Matteri RE: A comparison of radiographic findings in fusion and non-fusion patients, ten or more years following lumbar disc surgery, *Spine* 4:435-440, 1979.
70. Frymoyer JW, Newberg A, Pope MH, Wilder DG, Clements J, MacPherson G: Spine radiographies in patients with low-back pain, *J Bone Joint Surg* 66A: 1048-1055, 1984.
71. Gepstein R, Eismont FI: *Post-operative spine infections.* In Weinstein JN and Wiesel SW, editors: *The Lumbar Spine*. Philadelphia, 1990, WB Saunders.
72. Ghormley RK: Low back pain with specific reference to the articulation facets with presentation of an operative procedure, *JAMA* 101:1773-1777, 1933.
73. Gibson M, Buckley J, Mawhinney R, Mulholland RC, Worthington BS: Magnetic resonance imaging and discography in the diagnosis of disc degeneration, *J Bone Joint Surg* 68B:369-373, 1986.
74. Goldner JL, Urbaniak JR, McCollum DE: Anterior disc excision and interbody spinal fusion for chronic low back pain, *Orthop Clin North Am* 2:543-568, 1971.
75. Goldthwait JE: The lumbosacral articulation. An explanation of many cases of lumbago, sciatica and paraplegia, *Boston Med Surg* 164:365-372, 1911.
76. Greenwood J, McGuire T-H, Kimbell F: A study of the cause of failure in the herniated intervertebral disc operation, *J Neurosurg* 9:15-20, 1952.
77. Grenier N, Kressel HY, Schiebler ML, Grossman RI, Dalink MK: Normal and degenerative posterior spinal structures: MR imaging, *Radiology* 165:517-525, 1987.
78. Gristina AG, Costerton JW: Bacterial adherence and

the glycocalyx and their role in musculoskeletal infection, *Orth J Clin North Am* 15:517-535, 1984.

79. Grubb SA, Lipscomb HJ, Guilford WB: A relative value of lumbar roentgenograms, metrizamide myelography, and discography in the assessment of patients with chronic low back syndrome, *Spine* 12:282-286, 1987.
80. Grubb SA, Lipscomb HJ: Results of lumbosacral fusion for degenerative disc disease with and without instrumentation: two to five year follow-up, *Spine* 17:349-355, 1992.
81. Guyer RD, Ohnmeiss DD: Contemporary concepts in spine care: Lumbar discography. Position statement from the North American Spine Society Diagnostic and Therapeutic Committee, *Spine* 20:2048-59, 1995.
82. Hadjipavlou AG, Cesani-Vazquez F, Villanueva-Meyer J, Mader JT, Necessary JT, Crow W, Jensen RE, Chaljub G: The effectiveness of Gallium citrate[67] radionuclide imaging in vertebral osteomyelitis revisited, *Am J Orthop* 17:179-183, 1998.
83. Hadjipavlou AG, Enker, P, Dupuis P, Katzman S, Silver J: The causes of failure of lumbar transpedicular spinal instrumentation and fusion: a prospective study, *Int Orthop (SICOT)* 20:35-42, 1996.
84. Hadjipavlou AG, Farfan HF, Simmons JW: *The clinical signs of lumbago and sciatica.* In Hadjipavlou AG, Farfan HF, Simmons JW, editors: *The sciatic syndrome,* Thorofare, New Jersey, 1996, Slack, Inc., Chapter 7:141-164.HHa
85. Hadjipavlou AG, Katzman S, Dupuis P, Silver J: Failures of lumbar transpeduncular instrumentation and fusion. A prospective study presented at the North Amer Spine Soc, San Diego, October 1993.
86. Hadjipavlou AG, Lander PH, Antoniou J: The effect of chymopapain on low back pain with a correlation of clinical results to disc to disc space height and CT resolution, *Orthop Rev* 21:733-738, 1992.
87. Hasday CA, Passof TL, Perry J: Gate abnormalities arising for iatrogenic loss of lumbar lordosis: Secondary Harrington instrumentation in lumbar fracture, *Spine* 8:501-511, 1983.
88. Hassenbusch SJ, et al: Constant infusion of morphine for intractable cancer pain using an implanted pump, *J Neurosurg* 73:405-409, 1990.
89. Heithoff KB: Computed tomography and plain film diagnosis of the lumbar spine. In Weinstein J, Wiesel SW, editors: *The lumbar spine.* Int Soc Study Lumbar Spine, Saunders Co, 1990.
90. Helbig T, Lee CK: The lumbar facet syndrome, *Spine* 13:61-64, 1988.
91. Herring JA, Wenger DR: Early complications of segmental spinal instrumentation, *Orthop Trans* 6:22, 1982.
92. Hickey RF, Tregonning GC: Denervation of the spinal facet joints for the treatment of chronic low back pain, *N Engl J Med* 85:96-99, 1977.
93. Hirsch C, Inglemark B, Miller M: The anatomical basis for low back pain, *Acta Orthop Scand* 33:1, 1963.
94. Holt E: The question of lumbar discography, *J Bone Joint Surg* 50A:720-726, 1968.
95. Horowitz NH, Curtin JA: Prophylactic antibiotics and wound infections following laminectomy for lumbar disc herniation, *J Neurosurg* 43:727-31, 1975.
96. Holmes HE, Rothman RH: The Pennsylvania Plan: an algorithm for the management of lumbar degenerative disc disease, *Spine* 4:156-162, 1979.
97. Horton WC, Daftari TK: Which disc as visualized by magnetic resonance imaging is actually a source of pain? *Spine* 1992;17:S164-S171, 1992.
98. Hsu K, Zucherman JF, White AH, Wynne G: *Internal fixation with pedicle screws.* In White AH, Rothman RH, Ray CD, editors: *Lumbar spine surgery.* St. Louis, 1987, Mosby, pp 322-327.
99. Hsu KY, Zucherman JF, Derby R, et al: Painful lumbar end plate disruption: a significant discogenic finding, *Spine* 13:76, 1988.
100. Hudgins WR: The predictive value of myelography in the diagnosis of ruptured lumbar discs, *J Neurosurg* 32:152-162, 1970.
101. Ignelzi RJ, Cummings TW: A statistical analysis of percutaneous radiofrequency lesions in the treatment of chronic low back pain and sciatica, *Pain* 8:181-7, 1980.
102. Jackson RP, Cain JE Jr, Jacobs RR, Cooper BR, McManus BE: The neuroradiographic diagnosis of lumbar herniated nucleus pulposus: I. A comparison of computed tomography (CT), myelography, CT/myelography, discography, and CT/discography, *Spine* 14:1362-1367, 1989.
103. Jackson RP, Jacobs JJ, Montesano PX: 1988 Volvo award in clinical sciences. Facet joint injection in low back pain. A prospective statistical study, *Spine* 13:966-971, 1988.
104. Jaffray D, Hoyle M, O'Brien JP: Isolated intervertebral disc resorption. A source of mechanical and inflammatory back pain? *Spine* 10:397-401, 1986.
105. Jinkins JR: Gd-DTPA Enhanced MR of the lumbar spinal canal in patients with claudication, *J Computer Assisted Tomography* 17:555-562, 1993.
106. Jinkins JR, Whitmore AR, Bradley WG: The anatomical basis of vertebrogenic pain and the autonomic syndrome associated with lumbar disc extrusion, *AJR Am J Roentgenol* 152:1277-1289, 1989.
107. Jönsson BO, Strömquist B, Vist MG: Lumbar spine surgery in elderly: complications and surgical results, *Spine* 21:982-994, 1996.
108. Junghanns H: Spondylolisthesen ohne Spalt in Zwischengelenkstueck, *Archiv fuer Orthopadische Unfalichirurgie* 29:118-127, 1930.
109. Kaiser MC, Capesius P, Roilgen A, Sandt G, Poos D, Gratia G: Epidural venous stasis in spinal stenosis: CT appearance, *Neuroradiology* 26:435-438, 1984.
110. Kelley JH, Voris DC, Svien JH, Ghormley RL:

Multiple operations for protruded intervertebral discs, *Proc Staff Meet Mayo Clin* 29:546-550, 1954.
111. Kim SS, Michelsen CB: Revision surgery for failed back surgery syndrome, *Spine* 17:957-960, 1992.
112. Kirkaldy-Willis WH, Farfan HF: Instability of the lumbar spine, *Clin Orthop* 165:110-123, 1982.
113. Klink BK, Thurman T, Wittpenn GP, Lauerman WC, Cain JE: Muscle flap closure for salvage of complex back wound, *Spine* 19:1467-1470, 1994.
114. Knox BD, Chapman TM: Anterior interbody fusion for discogram concordant pain, *J Spinal Disord* 6:242-244, 1993.
115. Knutsson F: The instability associated with disc degeneration in the lumbar spine, *Adult Radiol* 25:593-609, 1944.
116. Kozak JA, O'Brien JP: Simultaneous combined anterior and posterior fusion: an independent analysis of a treatment for the disabled low-back pain patient, *Spine* 15(4):322-328, 1990.
117. Krag MH: Biomechanics of thoracolumbar spinal fixation: A review, *Spine* 16(3S): S84-S89, 1991.
118. Krames ES, Lanning RM: Intrathecal infusion analgesia for nonmalignant pain. American Pain Society, November 1991.
119. Krempen JR. Silver RS, Hudley J: An analysis of differential epidural spinal anesthesia and pentothal pain study in the differential diagnosis of back pain, *Spine* 4:452-259, 1979.
120. Kuslichs SD, Ulstrom CL, Michael CJ: The tissue origin of low back pain and sciatica, *Orthop Clin North Am* 22:181-187, 1991.
121. La Rocca HS: *Failed lumbar surgery: Principles of management.* In Weinstein J and Weisel S, editors: *The lumbar spine.* International Society for the Study of the Lumbar Spine, Saunders Co, 1990, pp 872-881.
122. Lander PH, Hadjipavlou AG: Radio-frequency electrocoagulation of the lumbar dorsal ramus in the treatment of facet syndrome: preliminary results. 74th Scientific Assembly and Annual Meeting, The Radiological Society of North America. Chicago, Illinois. December, 1988.
123. Lauerman WC, Bradford DS, Ogilvie JW, Transfeldt EE: Results of lumbar pseudarthrosis repair, *J Spinal Disord* 5:149-157, 1992.
124. Leblhuber F, Resisecker F, Boehm-Jurkovic H, Witzmann A, Deisenhammer E: Diagnostic value of different electrophysiological tests in cervical disk prolapse, *Neurology* 38:1879-1881, 1988.
125. Lehmann TR, La Rocca HS: Repeat lumbar surgery. A review of patients with failure from previous lumbar surgery treated with spinal canal exploration and lumbar spine fusion, *Spine* 6:615-619, 1981.
126. Lindahl O: Determination of the sagittal mobility of the lumbar spine. *Acta Orthop Scand* 37:241-254, 1966.
127. Lindblom K: Diagnostic puncture of intervertebral disk in sciatica, *Acta Orthop Scand* 17:231-239, 1948.
128. Lindholm TS, Pylkkanen P: Discitis following removal of intervertebral disc, *Spine* 7(6):618-622, 1982.
129. Linson MA, Williams H: Anterior and combined anteroposterior fusion for lumbar disc pain. A preliminary study, *Spine* 16(2):143-145, 1991.
130. Lippit AB: The facet joint and its role in spine pain, *Spine* 9:746-750, 1984.
131. Lisbona R, Derbekyan F, Novales-Diaz J, Veksler A: Gallium-67 scintigraphy in tuberculous and nontuberculous infectious spondylitis, *J Nucl Med* 34:853-859, 1993
132. Liu YK, Goel VK, DeJong A, Njus GO, Wu HC: Torsional fatigue of the lumbar intervertebral joints. In: Proceedings of the International Society for the Study of the Lumber Spine, Cambridge England, 1983.
133. Lonstein J, Winter R, Moe J, Gaines D: Wound infection with Harrington instrumentation and spine fusion for scoliosis, *Clin Orthop* 96:222-233, 1973.
134. Lora J: So-called facet denervation. *Spine* 1:121-126, 1976.
135. Lorenz M, Zindrick M, Schwaegler P et al: A comparison of single level fusion with and without hardware. *Spine* 16[Suppl 8]:S455-458, 1991.
136. Louis R: Fusion of the lumbar and sacral spine by internal fixation with screw plates. *Clin Orthop* 203:18-35, 1986.
137. Lucas D, Bresler B: Stability of ligamentous spine. In: Biomechanics Laboratory Report 40. San Francisco: University of California, 1961.
138. Lynch MC, Taylor JF: Facet joint injection for low back pain, *J Bone Joint Surg* 68B:138-141, 1986.
139. MacDonald G, Dennel G: Lumbar spine fusion. Presented at workmen's compensation course, Toronto, Canada, June, 1966.
140. MacGibbon B, Farfan HF: A radiologic survey of various configurations of the lumbar spine, *Spine* 4:258-266, 1979.
141. Macnab I: Spondylolisthesis with an intact neural arch-the so-called pseudo-spondylolisthesis, *J Bone Joint Surg* 32B:325-333, 1950.
142. Macnab I: The traction spur. An indicator of segmental instability, *J Bone Joint Surg* 53A:663-670, 1971.
143. Macnab I: Negative disc exploration, *J Bone Joint Surg* 53A:891-903, 1971.
144. Macnab I, Johnson RG: Localization of symptomatic lumbar pseudarthroses by use of discography, *Clin Orthop* 197:170-194, 1985.
145. Maigne JY, Aivaliklis A, Pfefer F: Results of sacroiliac joint double block and value of sacroiliac pain provocation tests in 54 patients with low back pain, *Spine* 21(16):1889-1892, 1996.
146. Massie WK, Stevens DB: A critical evaluation of discography. Scientific Exhibit. In: Proceedings of the American Academy of Orthopedic Surgeons, *J Bone Joint Surg* 49A:1243-1244, 1967.

147. McAfee PC, Weiland DJ, Corlov JJ: Survivorship. Analysis of pedicle spine instrumentation, *Spine* 16:S422-427, 1991.
148. McCall IW, Park WM, O'Brien JP, Seal V: Acute traumatic intraosseous disc herniations, *Spine* 10:134, 1985.
149. McCulloch JA, Organ LW: Percutaneous radiofrequency lumbar rhizolysis (rhyzotomy), *CMA Journal* 116:30-32, 1976.
150. Mehta M, Sluijter ME: The treatment of chronic back pain. A preliminary survey of the effect of radiofrequency denervation of the posterior vertebral joints, *Anaesthesia* 34(8):768-775, 1979.
151. Millette PC, McLanson D: A reappraisal of lumbar discography, *J Can Assoc Radiologists* 176:182, 1982.
152. Mixter WJ, Barr JS: Rupture of the intervertebral disc with involvement of the spinal canal, *N Engl J Med* 211:210-215, 1934.
153. Modic MT, Pavlicek W, Weinstein MA, et al: Magnetic resonance imaging of intervertebral disc disease, *Radiology* 152:103-111, 1984.
154. Mooney V: Surgery and post-surgical management of the patient with low back pain, *Phys Ther* 59:1000, 1979.
155. Mooney V: Where is the pain coming from: Presidential address to the International Society for the Study of the Lumbar Spine, Dallas, 1986, *Spine* 12(8):754-759, 1987.
156. Mooney V: A randomized double-blind prospective study of the efficacy of pulsed electromagnetic field for interbody lumbar fusions, *Spine* 15:708-712, 1990.
157. Mooney V, Robertson J: The facet syndrome, *Clin Orthop* 115:149-156, 1976.
158. Morgan FP, King T: Primary instability of lumbar vertebrae as a common cause of low-back pain, *J Bone Joint Surg* 39B:6-22, 1957.
159. Murtagh FR: Computed tomography and fluoroscopy guides. Anesthesia and steroid injection in facet syndrome. *Spine* 13:686-689, 1988.
160. Nachemson A: Lumbar spin instability. A critical update and symposium summary, *Spine* 10:290-291, 1985.
161. Nachemson A: Lumbar discography-Where are we today? *Spine* 13:1343, 1988.
162. Nachemson A: The lumbar spine: an orthopaedic challenge, *Spine* 1(1):59-71, 1976.
163. Nathan H: Osteophytes of the vertebral column. An anatomical study of their development according to age, race, and sex with considerations as to their etiology and significance, *J Bone Joint Surg* 44A:243-268, 1962.
164. Nelson RM: Low back atlas of standardized tests/measures, NTIS Publication PB 89-165-096, 1989.
165. Newman MH, Grinstead GL: Anterior lumbar interbody fusion for internal disc disruption, *Spine* 17(7):831-833, 1992.
166. Newman PH, Stone KH: The etiology of spondylolisthesis, *J Bone Joint Surg* 45B:39-59, 1963.
167. North R, et al: Failed back surgery syndrome: five-year follow-up after spinal cord stimulator implantation, *Neurosurgery* 28(5):692-699, 1991.
168. Novetsky GJ, Berlin L, Epstein AJ, Lobo N, Miller SH: The extraforaminal herniated disk: Detection by computed tomography, *AJNR* 3(6):653-655, 1982.
169. O'Brien JP, Dawson MH, Heard CW, Momberger G, Speck G, Weatherly CR: Simultaneous combined anterior and poterior fusion. A surgical solution for failed spinal surgery with a brief review of the first 150 patients, *Clin Orthop* 203:191-195, 1986.
170. Ogsbury JS 3d, Simon RH, Lehmann RA: Facet "denervation" in the treatment of low back syndrome, *Pain* 3(3):257-63, 1977.
171. Oklahoma Physician Advisory Committee: Low back pain treatment guidelines. Oklahoma City: Oklahoma Worker's Compensation Court, 1996.
172. Onofrio B, Yaksh T: Long term relief produced by intrathecal morphine infusion in 53 patients, *J Neurosurg* 72:200-209, 1990.
173. Oppenheimer A: Diseases of the epiphyseal (intervertebral) articulation, *J Bone Joint Surg* 20:285-313, 1938.
174. Oudenhoven RC: The role of laminectomy, facet rhizotomy, and epidural steroids, *Spine* 4(2):145-7, 1979.
175. Paris SV: Physical signs of instability. *Spine* 10:277-279, 1985.
176. Paris SV, Nyberg R, Mooney V: Three level innervations of the lumbar facet joints. Presented at the 7th annual meeting of the International Society for the study of the Lumbar Spine, New Orleans, Louisiana, 1980.
177. Park WM: The place of radiology in the investigation of low back pain, *Clin Rheum Dis* 61:93-132, 1980.
178. Park WM, McCall IW, O'Brien JP, Webb JK: Fissuring of the posterior annulus fibrosis in the lumbar spine, *Br J Radiology* 52(617):382-387, 1979.
179. Pateromichelakis S, Rood JP: Prostaglandin E2 increases mechanically evoked potentials in the peripheral nerve, *Experientia* 37(3):282-284, 1981.
180. Patrick BS: Extra-lateral rupture of lumbar intervertebral disc, *Surg Neurol* 3:301-304, 1975.
181. Pochaczevsky R: The value of liquid crystal thermography in diagnosis of spinal root compression syndrome, *Ortho Clin North Am* 14(1):271-288, 1983.
182. Pope MH, Panjabi M: Biomechanical definitions of spinal instability, *Spine* 1:235-256, 1985.
183. Porter RW, Ward D: Cauda equina dysfunction. The significance of two-level pathology, *Spine* 17:9-15, 1992.
184. Posner I, White AA, Edwards WT, et al: A biomechanical analysis of the clinical stability of the lumbar and lumbosacral spine, *Spine* 7:374-389, 1982.
185. Prothero ST, Parker JC, Stinchfield FE: Complications after low back fusion in 1000 patients: A com-

parison of two series one decade apart, *J Bone Joint Surg* 48A:57-65, 1966.

186. Putti V: Lady Jares lecture on new concepts in pathogenesis of sciatic pain, *Lancet* 2:53-60, 1927.
187. Quebec Task Force on Spinal Disorders: Scientific approach to the assessment and management of activity-related spinal disorders. A monography for clinicians. *Spine* 12(7):S1-S59, 1987.
188. Rashbaum RF: Radiofrequency facet denervation. A treatment alternative in refractory low back pain with or without leg pain, *Orthop Clin North Am* 14(3):569-575, 1983.
189. Raugstad TS, Harbo K, Oogberg A, et al: Anterior interbody fusion of the lumbar spine, *Acta Orthop Scand* 53:561-565, 1982.
190. Ray CD: Percutaneous radiofrequency facet nerve blocks. Treatment of the mechanical low-back syndrome. Monograph published by Radionics Inc., Burlington, Massachusetts, 1982: pp 1-28.
191. Ray CD: Excessive lumbar decompression. Autostabilization and other variations. In: White AH, Rothman RH, Ray CD, editors: *Lumbar spine surgery*. St. Louis, 1987, Mosby, pp 217-229.
192. Ray CD: Facet syndrome: pathophysiology, clinical picture & treatment, *Giorn Int Ant* 1:80-94, 1991.
193. Rees WES: Multiple bilateral subcutaneous rhizolysis of segmental nerves in the treatment of the intervertebral disc syndrome, *Ann Gen Proc* 16:126-127, 1971.
194. Rosenberg NJ: Degenerative spondylolisthesis. Predisposing factors, *J Bone Joint Surg* 57A:467-474, 1975.
195. Robbins and Gertzbein: Proc Ortho Trauma Assoc Meeting, Dallas, Texas, 1988.
196. Roy-Camille R: Experience with Roy-Camille fixation for the thoracolumbar and lumbar spine: Acute spinal injuries. Current Management Techniques, U of Mass CME Course, Sturbridge, Mass, October, 1987.
197. Roy-Camille R, Saillent G, Berteaux D, Marie-Anne S: Vertebral osseosynthesis using metal plate: Its different uses, *Chirurgie* 105(7):597, 1979.
198. Roy-Camille R, Saillent G, Mazel C: Plating of thoracic, thoracolumbar and lumbar injuries with pedicle screw plates, *Orthop Clin North Am* 17:147-159, 1986.
199. Saal JS: High levels of inflammatory phospholipase A2 activity in lumbar disc herniation, *Spine* 15:674-678, 1989.
200. Sachs BL, Vanharanta H, Spivei MA, et al: Dallas discogram description. A new classification of CT/discography in low back disorders, *Spine* 12:287-294, 1987.
201. Saillant G: [Anatomical study of the vertebral pedicles. Surgical application]. Rev Chir Orthop 62(2):151-160, 1976.
202. Sato H, Kikuchi S: The natural history of radiographic instability of the lumbar spine, *Spine* 18(14):2075-2079, 1993.
203. Schellhas KP, Pollei SR, Gundry CR, Heithoff KB: Lumbar disc high-intensity zone. Correlation of magnetic resonance imaging and discography, *Spine* 21(1):79-86, 1996.
204. Schnebel B, Kingston S, Watkins R, Dillin W: Comparison of MRI to contrast CT in the diagnosis of spinal stenosis, *Spine* 14:332-337, 1989.
205. Schneiderman G, Flannigan B, Kingston S, et al: Magnetic resonance imaging in the diagnosis of disc degeneration: Correlation with discography, *Spine* 12:276-281, 1987.
206. Schrader WC, Bethem D, Scebin V: The chronic local effect of sublaminar wires; an animal model, *Spine* 13:499-502, 1988.
207. Schulitz KP, Lenz G: Das facetten syndrom-klinik und terapie. In Hohman D, Kügelgen B, Liebig K, Schirmer M, editors: *Neuroorthopädie 2,* Berlin, 1984, Springer.
208. Schwarzer AC, Aprill CN, Bogduk N: The sacroiliac join in chronic low back pain, *Spine* 20:31-37, 1995.
209. Scoliosis Research Committee: Morbidity and Mortality Committee, 1987.
210. Selby DK, Paris SV: Anatomy of facet joints and its correlation with low back pain, *Contemp Orthop* 312:1097-1103, 1981.
211. Shaerer JP: Radiofrequency facet rhyzotomy in the treatment of chronic neck and low back pain, Int Surg 63:53-59, 1978.
212. Shealy CN: Percutaneous radiofrequency denervation of spinal facets. Treatment for chronic back pain and sciatica, *J Neurosurg* 43(4):448-451, 1975.
213. Silvers HR: Lumbar percutaneous facet rhizotomy, *Spine* 15(1):36-40, 1990.
214. Simmons EH, Segil CM: An evaluation of discography in the localization of symptomatic levels in discogenic disease of the spine, *Clin Orthop* 108:57-69, 1975.
215. Simmons JW: An algorithmic approach to treatment of low back pain, *Orthop Rev* XI: 81-84, Jan 1982.
216. Simmons JW: Awake Discography. A comparison study with magnetic resonance imaging, *Spine* 16(6):S216-S221, 1990.
217. Simmons JW, Andersson GB, Hadjipavlou AG, Russell GS: A prospective study of three hundred-forty-two patients using transpedicular fixation instrumentation for lumbosacral spine arthrodesis, *J Spinal Disord* (In Press), 1998.
218. Sluijter ME: Percutaneous thermal lesions in the treatment of back and neck pain. Radionic Procedure Technique Series, Radionics, Burlington, Mass., 1981.
219. Sluijter ME: The use of radiofrequency lesions for pain relief in failed back patients, *Intl Disab Studies* 10(1):37-43, 1988.
220. Smith SE, Darden BV, Rhyne AL, Wood KE:

Outcome of unoperated discogram-positive low back pain, *Spine* 28(18):1997-2000, 1995.

221. Soini J: Lumbar disc space height after external fixation and anterior intervertebral fusion: A prospective two year followup of clinical and radiographic results, *J Spine Disord* 7:487-494, 1994.
222. Spengler DM: Chronic low back pain: The team approach, *Clin Orthop* 179:71, 1983.
223. Staudte HW, Hild A, Niehaus P: Kinische Ergebnisse nit der facetten-Koagulation des ramus articularis der unteran ledenwirbelsaüle. In Hohman D, Kügelgen B, Liebig K, Schirmer M, editors: *Neuroorthopädie* 2, Berlin, 1984, Springer.
224. Stauffer, RN, Coventry MB: Posterolateral lumbar spine fusion, *J Bone Joint Surg* 54A:1195-1204, 1972.
225. Steffee A, Brantigan JW: The variable screw placement spinal fixation system: Report of a prospective study of 250 patients enrolled in Food and Drug Administration clinical trials, *Spine* 18:1160-1171, 1993.
226. Strömquist B: Posterolateral noninvasive fusion, *Acta Orthop Scand* 26:97-99, 1993.
227. Thompson GH, Wilber RG, Shaffer JW, Scoles PV, Nash CL: Segmental spinal instrumentation in idiopathis scoliosis. A preliminary report, *Spine* 10(7): 623-30, 1985.
228. Turner JA, Ersek M, Herron L, Deyo R: Surgery for lumbar spinal stenosis. Attempted meta-analysis of the literature, *Spine* 17:1-8, 1992.
229. Verbiest H: The significance and principles of computerized axial tomography in idiopathic developmental stenosis of the bony lumbar vertebral canal, *Spine* 4:379-390, 1979.
230. Waddell G, Kimmel EG, Lotto WN, Graham JD, Hall H, McCulloch JA: Failed lumbar disc surgery and repeat surgery following industrial injuries, *J Bone Joint Surg* 61A:201-207, 1979.
231. Waddell G, Main CS, Morris EW, Dipaola M, Gray IC: Chronic low back pain. Psychologic distress and illness behavior, *Spine* 9:204-213, 1984.
232. Walsh TR, Weinstein JN, Spratt KF, Lehmann TR, Aprill C, Sayre H: Lumbar discography in normal subjects. A controlled, prospective study, *J Bone Joint Surg* 72A(7):1081-1088, 1990.
233. Watkins RM: Assessment of results and complications of anterior lumbar fusion. In: Lumbar Interbody Fusion. Lin K (ed.), Aspen Publishers Inc., Rockville, MD, pp. 153-169, 1989.
234. Weatherley CR, Brickett CF, O'Brien JP: Discogenic pain persisting despite solid posterior fusion, *J Bone Joint Surg* 68B:142-143, 1986.
235. Weinstein JN, Spratt KF, Spengler D, Brick C, Reid S: Spinal pedicle fixation: reliability and validity of roentgenogram-based assessment and surgical factors on successful screw placement, *Spine* 13:1012-18, 1988.
236. West JL 3d, Bradford DS, Ogilvie JW: Results of spinal arthrodesis with pedicle screw plate fixation, *J Bone Joint Surg* 73A:1179, 1991.
237. Wetzel FT, LaRocca SH, Lowery GL, Aprill CN: The treatment of lumbar spinal pain syndromes diagnosed by discography. Lumbar arthrodesis, *Spine* 19(7):792-800, 1994.
238. Whitecloud TS 3d, Butler J, Cohen J, Candelora P: Complications with the variable spinal plating system, *Spine* 1989; 14:472-476.
239. Wiesel SW, Feffter LH, Rothman RH: *A lumbar spine algorithm: The lumbar spine.* The International Society for the Study of the Lumbar Spine, Weinstein JN, Wiesel SW, editors, WB Saunders Co., 1990.
240. Wilber RG: Postoperative neurological deficits in segmental spinal instrumentation, *J Bone Joint Surg* 1984;66A:1178-1187.
241. Wilder DG, Pope MH, Frymoyer JW: The biomechanics of lumbar disc herniation and the effect of overload and instability, *J Spinal Disord* 1:16-35, 1988.
242. Wiltse K, Kirkaldy-Willis W, McIvor GWD: Treatment of spinal stenosis, *Clin Orthop* 1987;115(6): 83-91.
243. Wiltse LL, Roccio PD: Preoperative psychological tests as predictors of success of chemonucleolysis in the treatment of low back syndrome, *J Bone Joint Surg* 1975; 57A:578-482.
244. Woody J, Lehmann T, Weinstein J, et al: Excessive translation on flexion-extension radiographs in asymptomatic populations. Presented at the meeting of the International Society for the Study of the Lumbar Spine. Miami, Florida, 1988.
245. Yashiro K, Homme T, Hokari Y, et al: The Steffee variable screw placement system using different methods of bone grafting, *Spine* 16:1329, 1991.
246. Yuan HA, Garfin SR, Dickman CA: A historical cohort study of pedicle screw fixation in thoracic, lumbar, and sacral spinal fusions, *Spine* 19(suppl 20): 2279S-2296S, 1994.
247. Zindrick M, Schwaegler P, Lorenz M, Collatz M, Vrbox L, Behal R, Cram R: A comparison of single level fusion with & without hardware. Annual meeting of the North American Spine Society, Monterey, California, 1990.
248. Zdeblick TA: A prospective randomized study of lumbar fusion: Preliminary results, *Spine* 1993; 18:983-991.
249. Zucherman J, Derby R, Hsu K, et al: Normal magnetic resonance imaging with abnormal discography, *Spine* 13:1355-1359, 1988.

# 18

# REVISION CERVICAL SPINE SURGERY: ANTERIOR, POSTERIOR, OR BOTH?

**Gary L. Lowery, M.D., Ph.D.**
**Richard F. McDonough, B.S.**



The decision process in revision of failed cervical fusions cannot be written as a simple algorithm. Correct analysis of the factors that led to the unsuccessful outcome is of paramount importance. Similar pitfalls must be avoided to ensure a successful revision. The type of failure (i.e., pseudarthrosis, kyphotic deformity, or failed hardware) also determines whether the corrective surgery is best achieved through anterior, posterior, or combined approaches. This chapter will illustrate our solutions to many of the difficult problems encountered in revision cervical spine surgery. Our philosophy will hopefully serve as a blueprint to be considered when surgical revision is necessary. A general list of references is included to provide a historical framework for better understanding of this topic. Surgical case examples illustrate the important concepts of our philosophy.

## GENERAL PHILOSOPHY

### Anterior Revisions

A common complication of anterior surgery is pseudarthrosis. To avoid a repeat occurrence, it is important to identify the factors contributing to the nonunion. Possible contributing factors include the number of levels attempted in the fusion, the type of bone graft, and the use or absence of anterior instrumentation. Constitutional factors such as osteoporosis, smoking, diabetes, and chronic steroid use also need consideration.

Autograft is the gold standard and should be employed whenever possible, especially when revising a failed allograft fusion. In many instances, a single-level revision can be accomplished by meticulously preparing vertebral body receptor sites and using a wedge-shaped autologous tricortical iliac crest graft. If foraminal or central stenosis is present (secondary to osteophytes or fibrous pseudarthrosis), this can be addressed via an anterior microsurgical technique using high-speed burr and kerrisons. In certain cases to ensure complete decompression, the posterior longitudinal ligament should be resected for better visualization of the underlying roots and the uncinate processes.

We emphasize the importance of lordotic positioning of each individual level (C3 to C7) in primary or revision surgery. Lordotic positioning places the anterior grafts in an optimal biomechanical and biological environment. Revision surgeries performed in a similar manner will ensure a normal lordotic posture of the cervical spine from C3 to C7.

We advocate anterior cervical plates in revision surgery. Anterior instrumentation aids in stabilizing the local reconstruction, especially when the posterior longitudinal ligament has been sacrificed. Torsional forces and shear forces (flexion and extension) are reduced, and anterior fusion is promoted. We feel anterior instrumentation prevents excessive graft compression, which can lead to fragmentation and collapse, resultant nonunion, and potential kyphosis. Lordotic position of the spinal reconstruction can be maintained when a constrained plate is applied in neutralization (Fig. 18-1). Even in the presence of con-

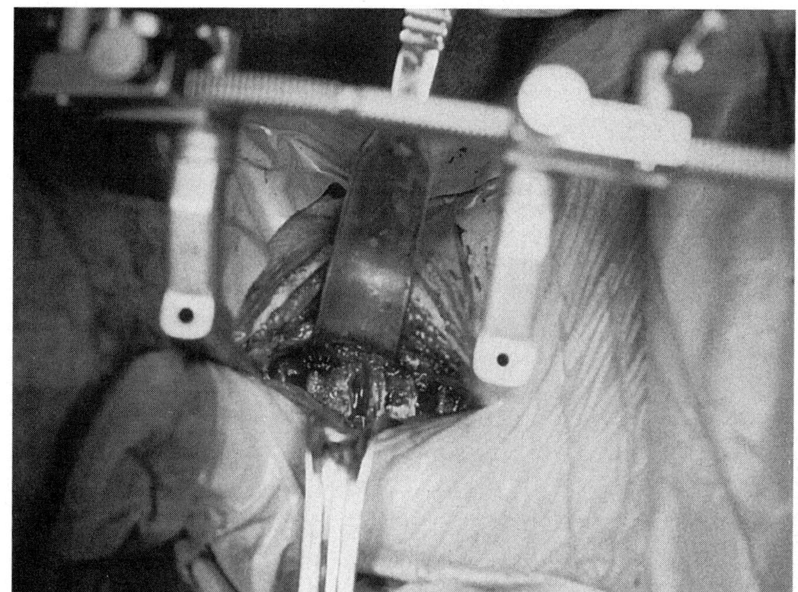

**FIGURE 18-1**

Intraoperative image of a unique lordotic distractor.

strained plating, the grafting techniques are most important, because rigid or constrained plates may stress-shield the grafts. We advocate critical attention to the "fit and fill" of the graft with flush cancellous contact surfaces at the vertebral receptor sites (Fig. 18-2).

In constructs in which screws are not locked into the anterior plate, the screws may toggle as the grafts settle into compression. Theoretically, compression may increase the likelihood of fusion. In our experience, however, this vertebral settling in the midcervical spine leads to localized kyphosis, an unnatural biomechanical and physiological state (Fig. 18-3, *A,B,* and *C*).

All reconstructive surgeons struggle with how much of the vertebral body can be safely resected while still preserving structural support for the anterior grafts. When the subchondral endplates are violated, substantial support is lost, and grafts inevitably subside.[5] Fusion theoretically is enhanced, but kyphosis is the usual end result. Excessive forces are transmitted to the anterior plate, predisposing it to failure usually in the form of screw fracture or loosening (Fig. 18-4, *A* and *B*).

Careful preservation of the supportive endplates is not always possible in revision surgery. When an extensive portion of the vertebral body (>30%) needs to be resected, we advocate performing a diskectomy of the adjacent level and removing the remainder of the affected vertebral body. This provides good biomechanical support for the graft by preparing a fresh subchondral endplate receptor surface. In addition, the endplate aids in obtaining and supporting the reconstructed lordotic position (Fig. 18-5). Inclusion of another level will further reduce cervical motion, but studies demonstrate that each lower cervical level makes a minimal contribution to the overall rotation (2° or 6%) and flexion-extension (6 to 10° or 10% to 15%).[8] This additional loss of motion may be necessary in order to achieve a successful fusion in a more anatomic position and elimination of pain via a solid fusion.

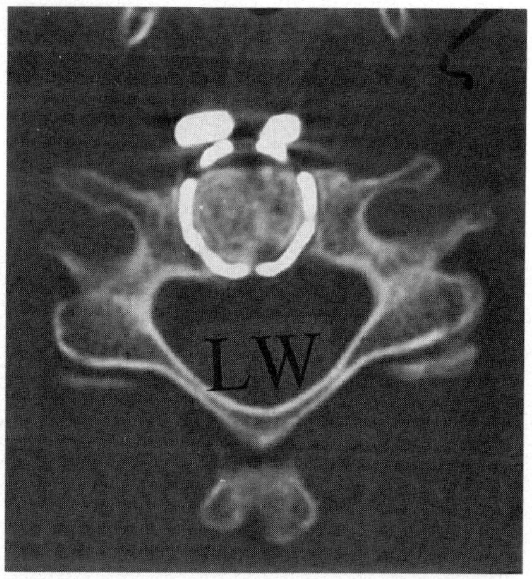


**FIGURE 18-2**

Axial computed tomography demonstrating the "fit and fill" of the composite graft and side-to-side healing of the construct.

Corpectomy has additional advantages for the treatment of failed anterior cervical fusion.[7,10,18] A thorough decompression can be completed more safely and quickly via this "macroscopic" approach. A pedicle-to-pedicle decompression can be performed, usually while maintaining the integrity of the posterior longitudinal ligament. The extracted bone can be saved for autologous graft reconstruction. We prefer a

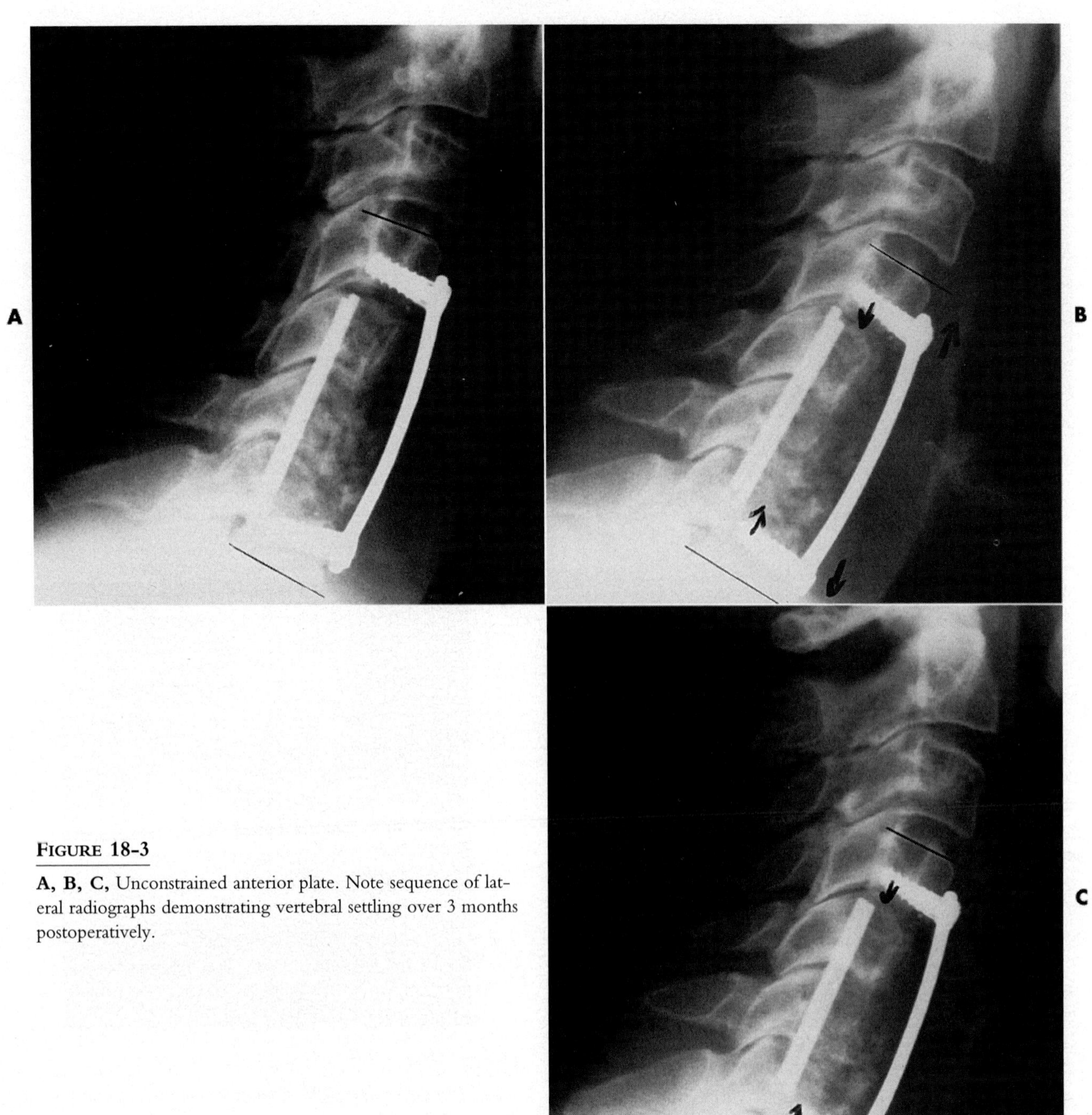


**FIGURE 18-3**

**A, B, C,** Unconstrained anterior plate. Note sequence of lateral radiographs demonstrating vertebral settling over 3 months postoperatively.

composite graft technique combining structural support (titanium surgical mesh or carbon fiber conduits) with autologous grafting (locally harvested autograft). These composites have biomechanical and biological properties similar to autologous iliac crest struts, and our clinical results bear out this premise (Fig. 18-6, *A* and *B*).[15,21]

Certain principles need to be strictly followed for a successful revision. Prepare punctate bleeding surfaces while maintaining the integrity of the subchondral endplate. Smooth flush cancellous surfaces should be prepared for maximum contact area to promote fusion and provide adequate anterior column support. Strong structural contact areas are necessary to withstand forces transmitted through lordotically fashioned struts (autograft, allograft, or composite grafts).

To achieve a more natural anatomic position intraoperatively, we use a special method of lordotic distraction (Fig. 18-7). Maximum neuroforaminal distraction is possible while maintaining lordosis. When traditional linear distraction is used, the relative position of the involved vertebrae is kyphotic, and the facets become un-

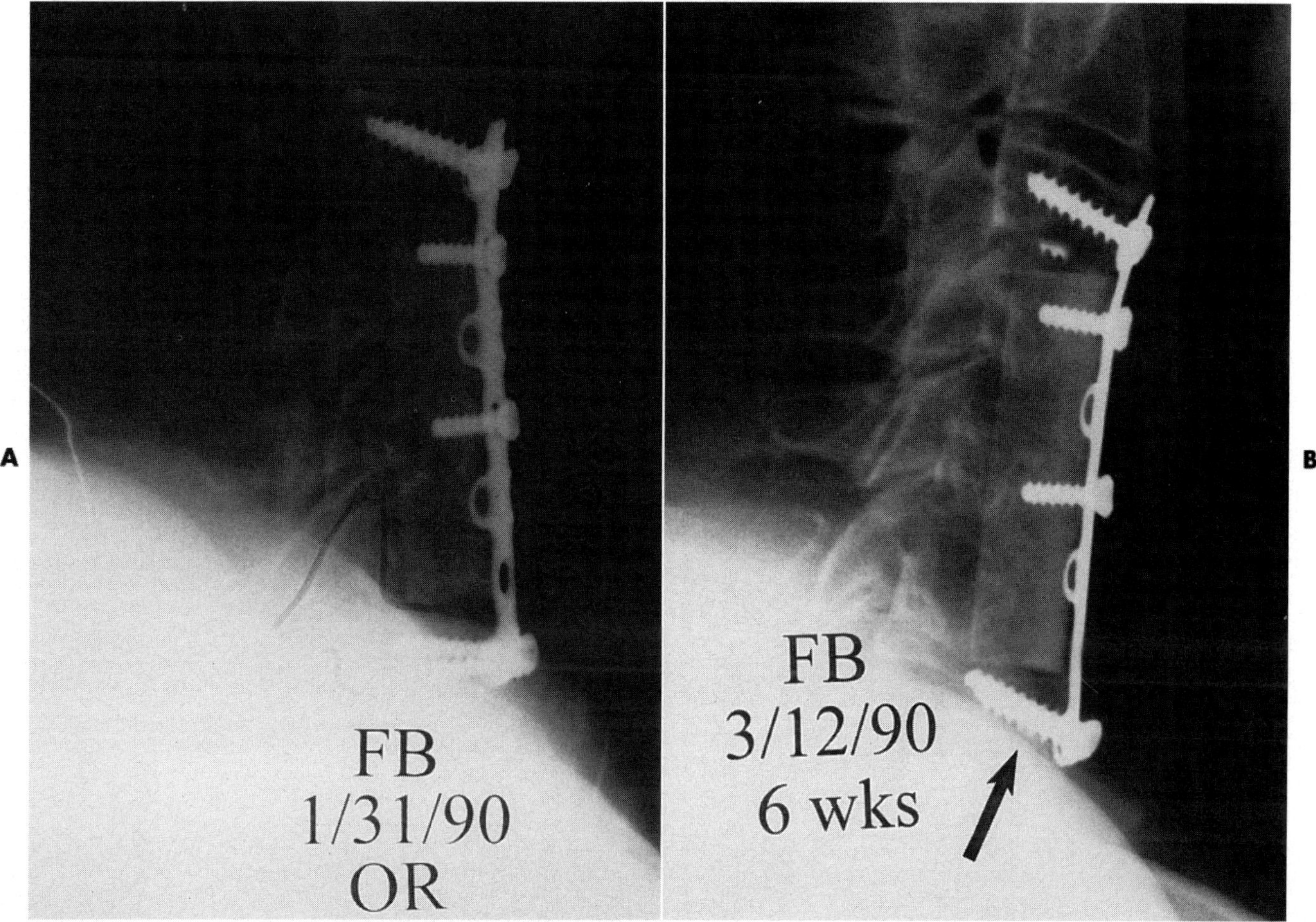


FIGURE 18-4

**A,** Intraoperative lateral radiograph showing intact anterior plate and strut graft with inferior screws placed into partially resected vertebral body. **B,** After six weeks, the strut graft has settled into the cancellous bone of the partially resected inferior vertebrae. As a result, the anterior plate has subsided into the disk space below.

locked. When the facets remain overlapped (locked) in a more favorable biomechanical position, the facet joints help control rotational and shearing forces (Fig. 18-8). This reduces stress on the anterior implants, which work best in the mode of neutralization (no excessive compression or distraction).[12]

Another principle for revision reconstruction is the "fit and fill" of the strut graft. Typically, we perform a wide pedicle-to-pedicle decompression of 16 to 18 mm. Adequate reconstruction entails filling this space completely. Side-to-side contact between the strut graft and the side walls of the corpectomy defect increases the biomechanical stability of the reconstruction. This allows large tricortical grafts and fenestrated composite grafts (Fig. 18-2) to heal side-to-side as well as end-to-end. Immediate biomechanical stability is achieved, and, as healing progresses, there is "biological enhancement of biomechanics." As bone grows into the strut or composite graft, a segmental interlock occurs, and the reconstruction becomes stronger as the ingrowth matures. Large corpectomy voids filled only partially with a fibular strut are at a disadvantage since healing occurs only end-to-end (Fig. 18-9). In such constructs, torsional and shear forces are only controlled through endplate-graft contacts and the stability of the cephalad and caudal plate-screw mechanism.

## POSTERIOR REVISIONS

An alternative approach to anterior revision is to perform an instrumented posterior cervical fusion spanning the levels of the pseudarthrosis. In our results and those in the literature, the rate of successful fusion is between 95% and 100%.[4,5,16,20] In many cases, the anterior nonunion will consolidate and heal as the posterior fusion progresses (Fig. 18-10, *A* and *B*). There are many posterior cervical techniques.[3,9,11,19] For a single-level fusion, we often use facet wiring and interspinous wiring to stabilize the posterior fusion (Fig. 18-11). This traditional method allows bone grafting of the facets and wiring of bicortical iliac crest to the interspinous area. If a laminectomy has been

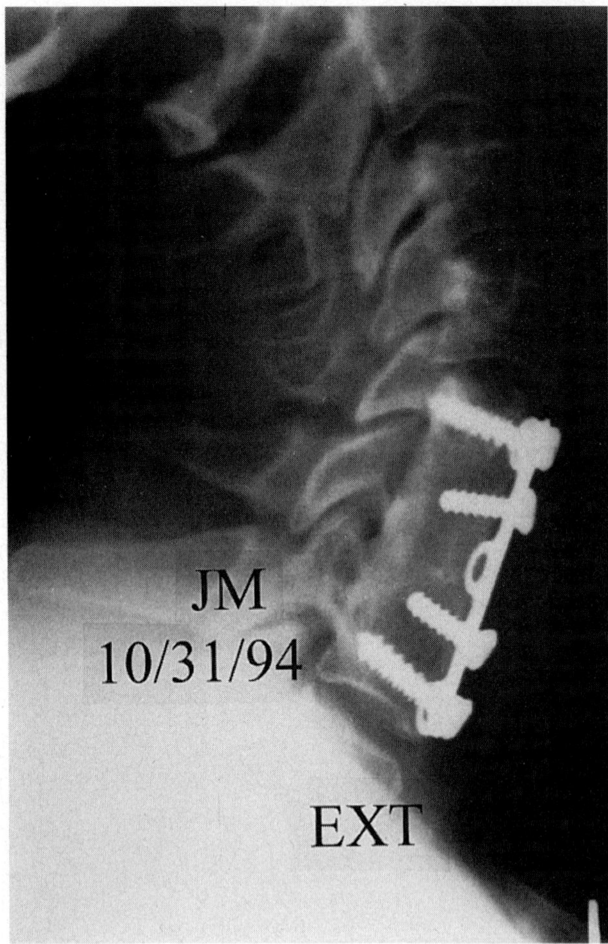


**FIGURE 18-5**

Multilevel interbody fusion with excellent lordotic position of the cervical spine.

performed or multiple levels need to be addressed, additional stability can be achieved via articular pillar plates and screws. This segmental reconstruction is more stable, reducing the need for external immobilization.

For longer reconstructions, especially those spanning the C6 to T1 area, we prefer to apply a posterior cervical plate with cephalad articular pillar screws and caudal pedicle screws. We classify this as posterior cervical hybrid reconstruction.[13] Although more technically demanding, this is a stronger biomechanical construct. In the lower cervical spine, pedicle screws are easier to apply than articular pillar screws.[1,2,22] Improperly placed articular pillar screws provide little support if they cut out or loosen. In addition, the superior and inferior facet joints are not violated in hybrid reconstruction (Fig. 18-12).

## THE DECISION PROCESS

We prefer to solve an anterior pseudarthrosis with a repeat anterior procedure; in many cases, a partial or near-total corpectomy with excision of the fibrous

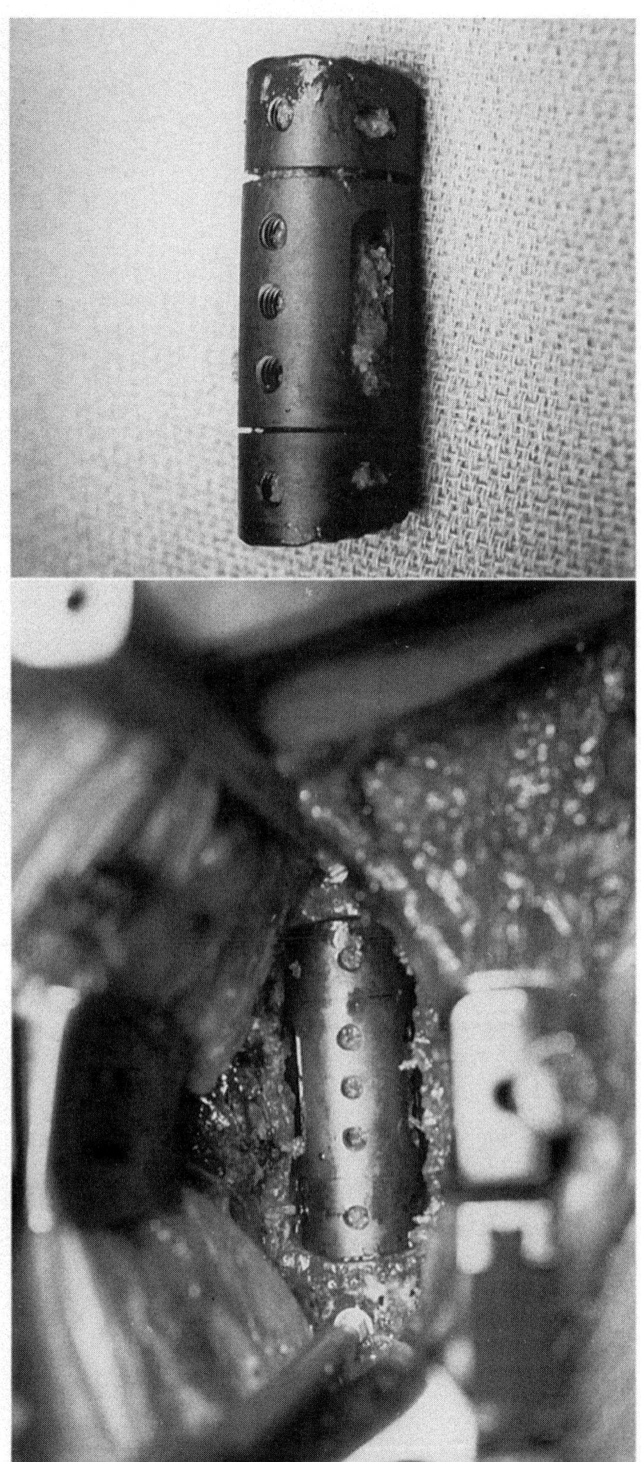


**FIGURE 18-6**

**A,** Close-up of a custom carbon fiber strut packed with local bone graft prior to implantation. **B,** Intraoperative view of the carbon fiber strut implanted to fill a corpectomy defect.

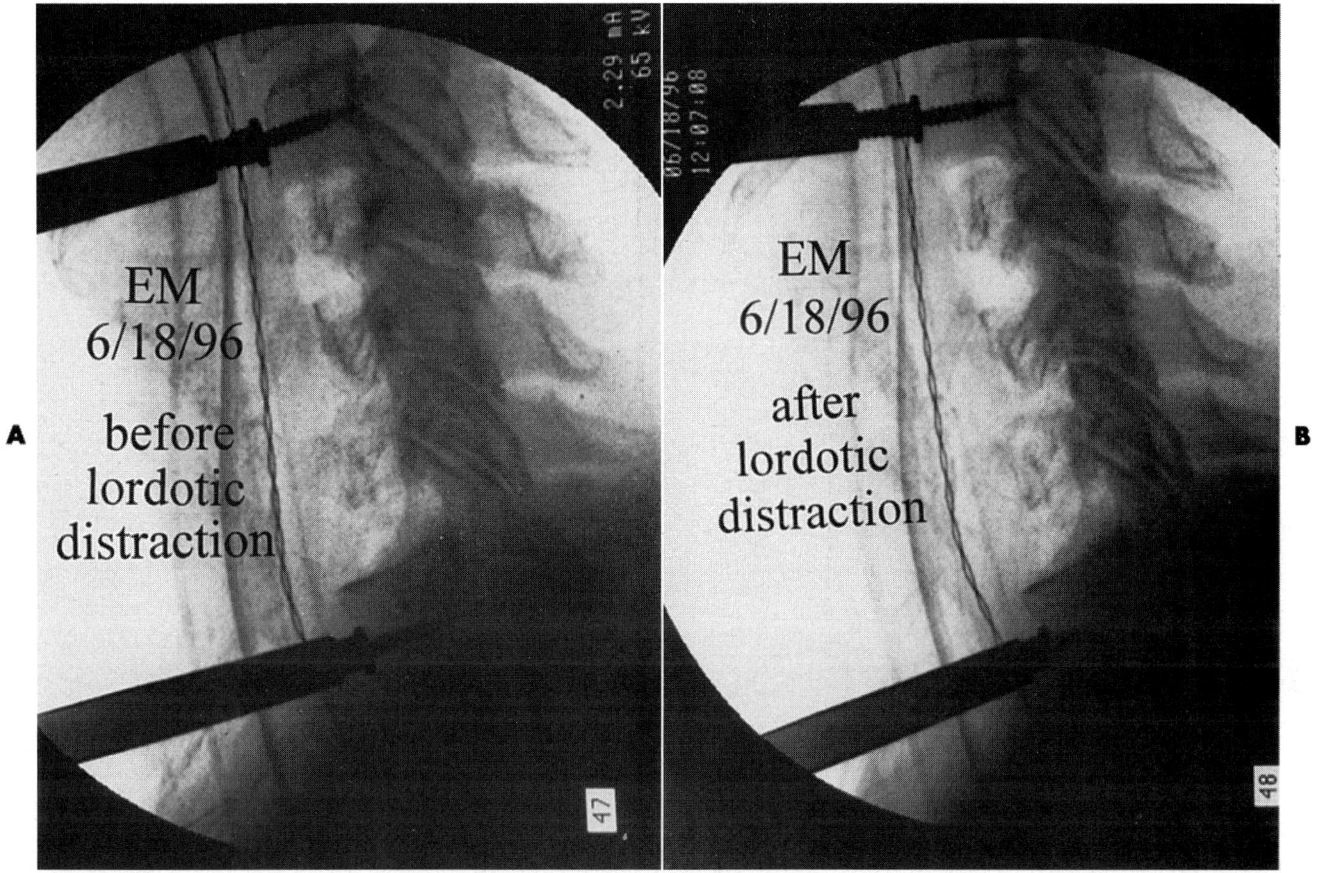


FIGURE 18-7

**A,** Intraoperative view of a unique distractor that allows lordotic distraction instead of the traditional linear distraction used in the cervical spine; **B,** View following distraction.

pseudarthrosis tissue provides a more favorable biological environment. The addition of a constrained anterior cervical plate in neutralization to a properly reconstructed anterior column is all that is needed. Our results with composite graft struts (titanium surgical mesh or carbon fiber) compare favorably with autologous iliac crest struts, both in terms of fusion rate and clinical result. The repeat anterior approach has the theoretical increased risk to neurovascular structures, but we have not experienced these complications. Even in revision surgery, the anterior approach results in less soft tissue morbidity than stripping fascia and posterior musculature from the spine. We find that patients who have a wide posterior exposure continue to experience muscle fatigue and chronic symptoms.

An anterior approach is necessary when there are residual osteophytes that were not fully decompressed. To solve the resultant deformity and incomplete decompression, we operate from a single approach whenever possible. If anterior hardware from the primary surgery has failed, this is accessible from an anterior approach. Whether the original surgery used an anterior or posterior approach, often an additional level must be included in the reconstruction.

Revision surgery may be necessary when hardware has failed. Asymptomatic broken plates are not routinely removed. Hardware failure can be addressed during nonunion repair or kyphosis correction. If screws loosen early (more frequently with nonconstrained plates), careful radiographic follow-up is mandated. If screw loosening progresses over 6 weeks, the plate and screws should be revised. Later screw loosening (>6 months) is highly suggestive of a nonunion. In a recent review of our patients with minimum one-year follow-up (range, 1 to 7 years), we noted that only 5% of patients had the potential for tracheoesophageal problems from failed hardware. However, upon exploration, all implants were fully enveloped in soft tissue and presented no problems to neighboring structures.[14]

Kyphotic deformities can result from postlaminectomy instability, collapse of uninstrumented anterior fusions, or anterior pseudarthrosis. We prefer to address these from an anterior or combined anteroposterior approach. An anterior release can involve an opening wedge osteotomy or diskectomies and insertion of wedged grafts. Opening-wedge osteotomy can be performed extending through the foramen. A wedged-shaped graft (autologous, allograft, or composite) is used, and the correction is stabilized. If sufficient lor-

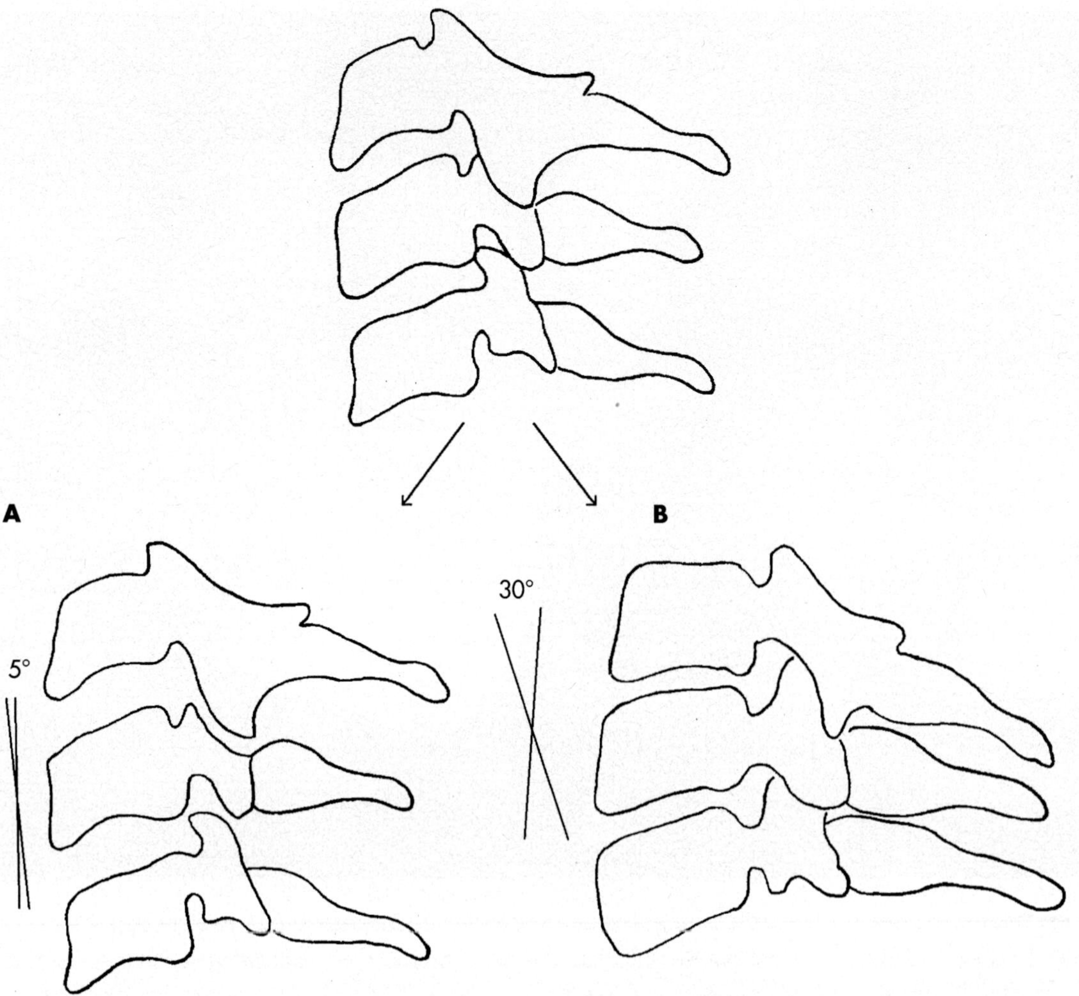


FIGURE 18-8

**A,** Linear distraction unloads the facets and decreases contact area. **B,** Lordotic distraction improves biomechanics with load sharing by posterior elements. Flexion, shear, and torsional forces are minimized.

FIGURE 18-9

Fibula graft that does not entirely fill the corpectomy defect. In these cases, only end-to-end healing is possible.

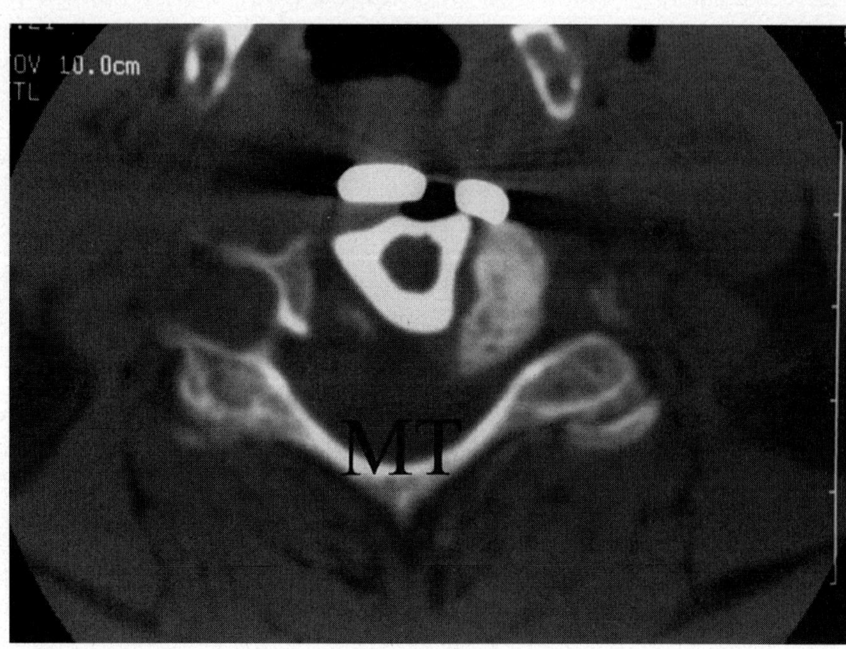

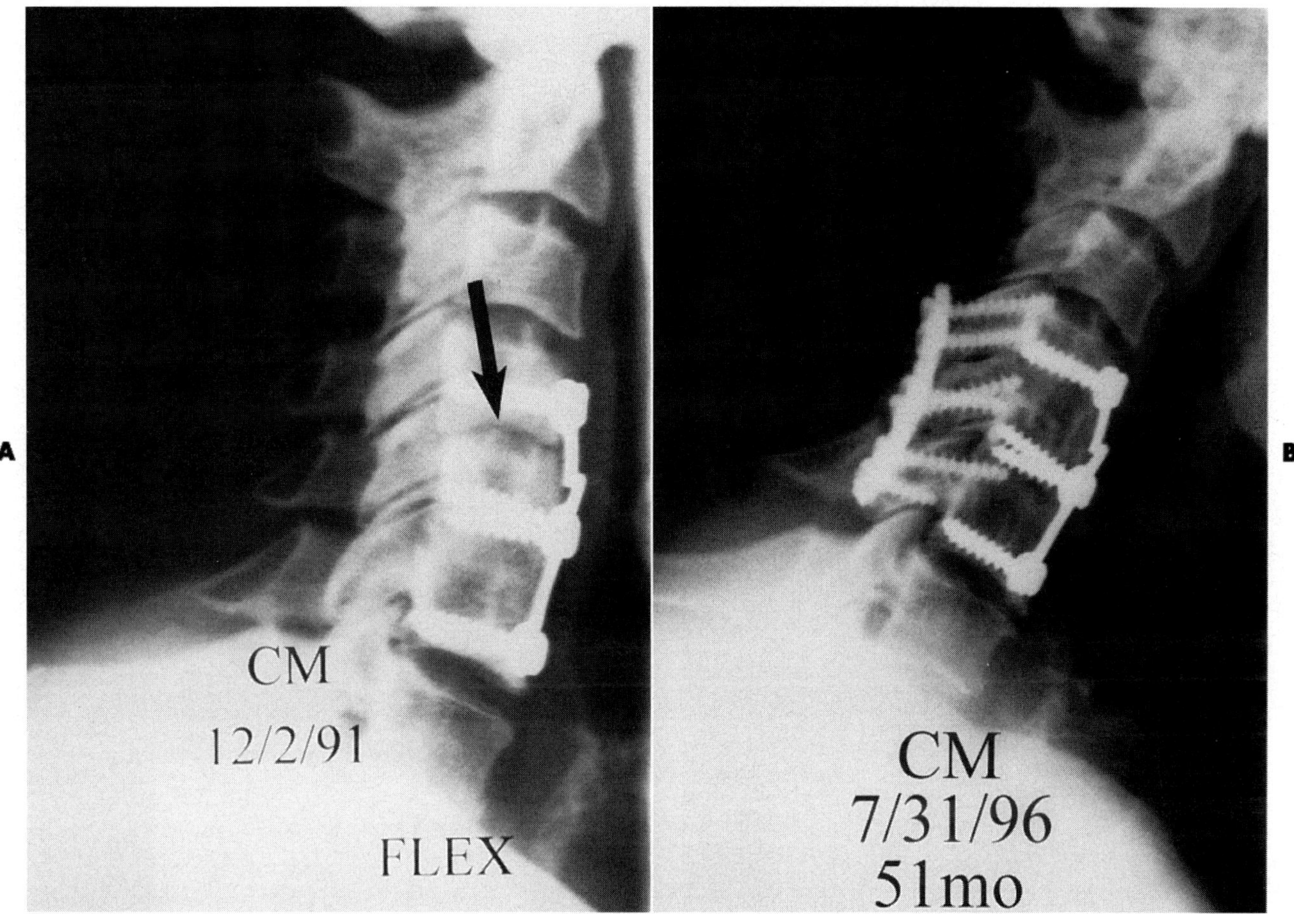


**FIGURE 18-10**

**A,** Anterior nonunion and hardware failure. **B,** Postoperative radiograph demonstrating consolidation of an anterior nonunion after a posterior revision.

dosis is obtained, we prefer to span the osteotomy reconstruction with a constrained anterior cervical plate. When further correction is necessary via posterior release (i.e., foraminotomy and partial laminectomy), an anterior buttress plate can be used to stabilize the graft(s) while turning the patient (Fig. 18-13). After the posterior release, the position of the head and neck is altered via preoperatively placed Mayfield tongs. The final steps are posterior cervical hybrid reconstruction as previously described[13] and posterior cervical fusion.

When cascading spinal deformities are present due to postlaminectomy kyphosis, we feel most patients can be revised through an anterior approach. When fixed deformities are noted, the options are varied. Multiple anterior releases or multiple posterior releases can be performed without grafting. If posterior releases are the first procedure, we close the posterior wound and turn the patient in tongs. Anteriorly, we perform multilevel wedged interbody grafts and instrumentation if appropriate lordosis has been obtained via head and neck positioning. We feel anterior and posterior instrumentation and fusion is needed in these difficult cases.

Finally, when should the patient be treated both anteriorly and posteriorly? In our experience, revisions over 3 vertebral levels (4 disks) have a high nonunion rate (>50%) unless posterior instrumentation is added. We also advocate anterior grafting at C7-T1 and posterior instrumentation to T2 or T3 when the need arises to cross the cervicothoracic junction.

## CORPECTOMY TECHNIQUE

General endotracheal intubation is performed after placement of intravenous lines, intraarterial lines, and a Foley catheter. A roll under the neck and between the shoulder blades is often helpful to maintain a lordotic posture of the cervical spine. Slight distraction with head halter traction may prevent abnormal cervical positioning, such as rotation, during cervical instrumentation. The neck is then sterilely prepared and draped in the usual fashion.

A standard left-sided approach is then performed. A transverse incision can be readily used for one- and two-level corpectomies, whereas more extensive soft tissue dissection is routinely required for corpectomies

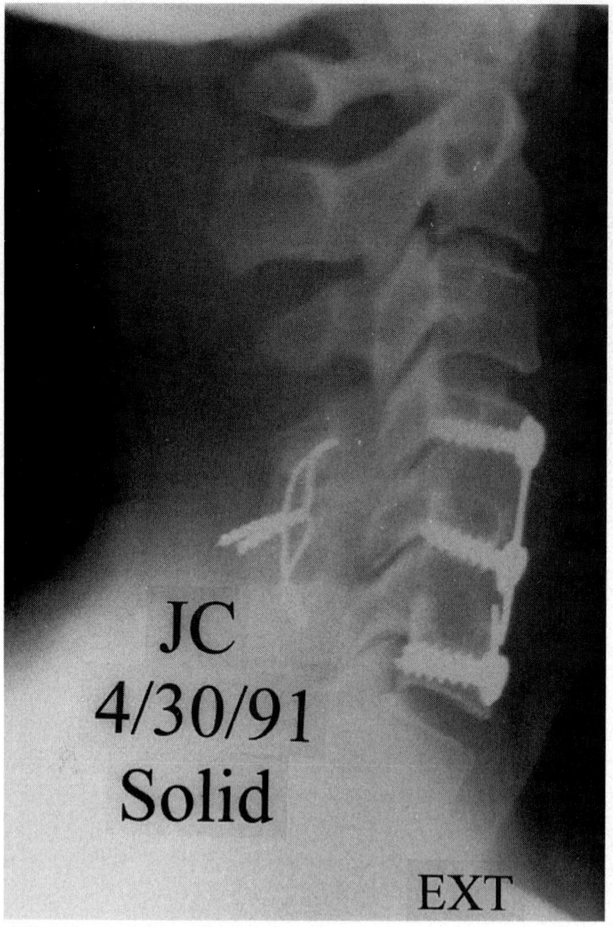


FIGURE 18-11

Postoperative radiograph of posterior cervical fusion and wiring to correct an anterior nonunion.

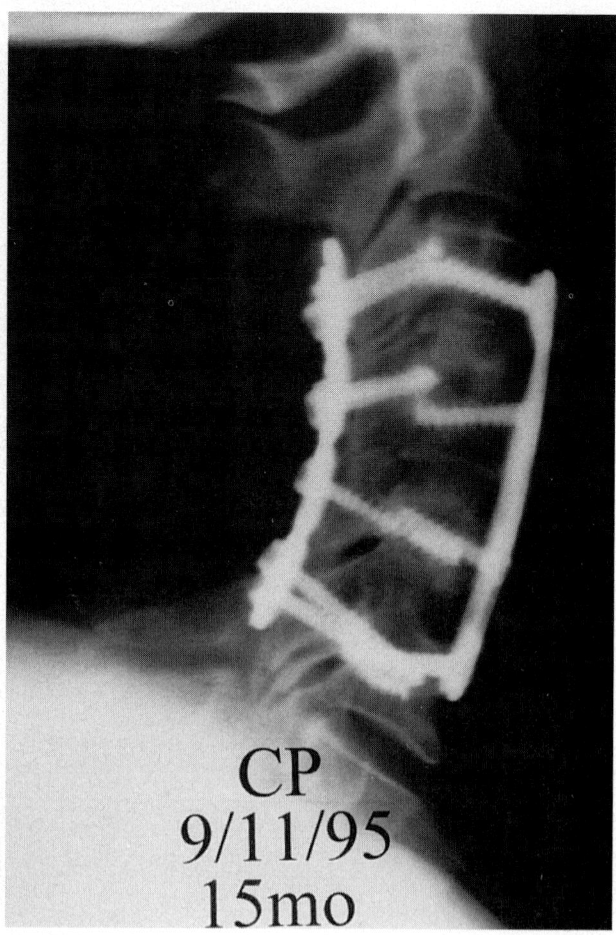


FIGURE 18-12

Postoperative radiograph demonstrating solid anterior and posterior fusions after a circumferential procedure.

spanning three or four levels. A carotid incision minimizes the soft tissue retraction when the procedure requires decompression of three or more levels. Anterior cervical instrumentation and composite graft construct insertion are more safely performed through a carotid incision.

The appropriate disk levels to be excised are confirmed on x-ray or fluoroscopy. The disk spaces are excised with a #15 blade, and discal material is removed with pituitary rongeurs and curettes (Fig. 18-14). Care is taken to preserve the bony subchondral plate upon which the supportive reconstructive strut construct will rest. It is important to clearly identify the uncinate processes, because these serve as the anatomical landmarks for adequate central decompression and for nerve root decompression via anterior foraminotomies. Proper strut construct insertion and positioning of an anterior cervical plate also depend on identifying this anatomy.

Next, a sagittal saw blade is used to make three vertical cuts in the vertebral body. One cut is in the midline, and one cut is made on either side of the midline while remaining within the confines of the uncinate processes (Fig. 18-15). The vertebral cuts should not be made to penetrate more than 14 mm. A Lexel rongeur is then used to remove this bone, which is saved for the cancellous graft (Fig. 18-16). This process is repeated for each level. Cancellous bone bleeding from the side walls can be controlled with bone wax (removed prior to reconstruction/grafting).

After harvesting of the local autograft is completed, a high-speed burr is used to widen the subtotal corpectomy site further. The uncinate processes again serve as the limit for subtotal decompression. The width of the decompression should be a minimum of 15 to 16 mm in order to accommodate the reconstructive strut construct. Although not mandatory, keyhole foraminotomies and pedicle-to-pedicle decompression are easily performed after resection of the posterior longitudinal ligament.

An appropriate autograft or allograft strut is selected (Fig. 18-17). Alternatively, either a titanium surgical mesh conduit (16-mm diameter) is trimmed for trial implantation (Fig. 18-18, *A*) or a stackable carbon fiber

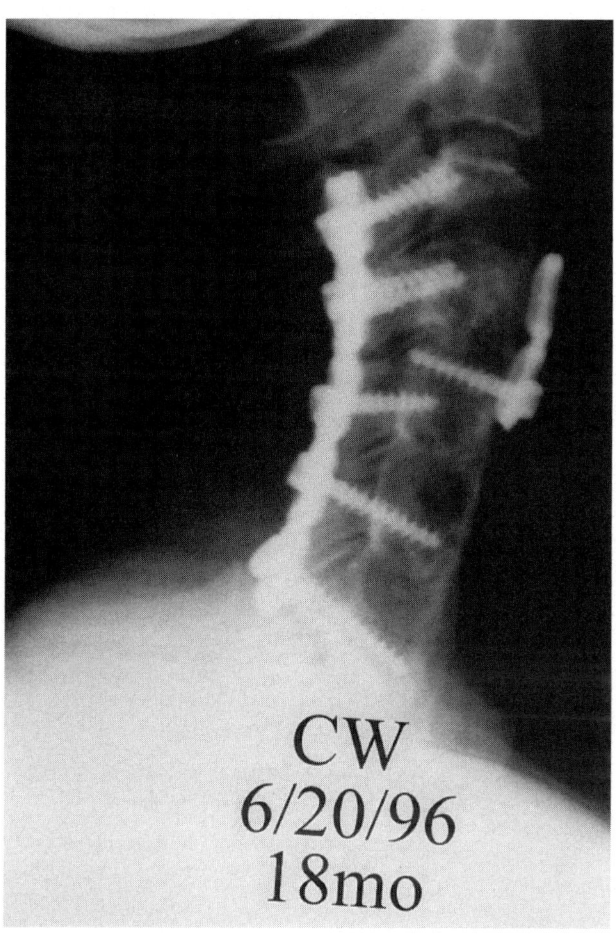


**FIGURE 18-13**

Note the anterior buttress plate used to prevent anterior graft dislodgment.

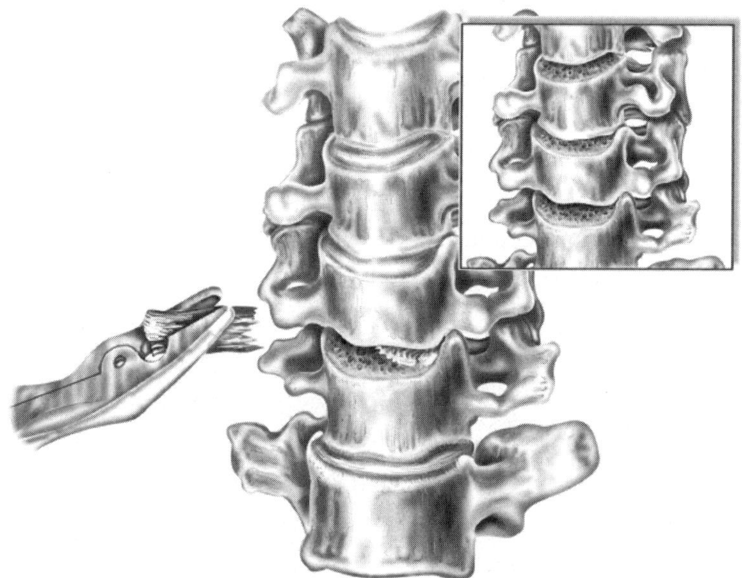

**FIGURE 18-14**

Three-level diskectomy performed visualizing the uncinate processes with a blow up of the disk spaces after diskectomy. © Neil BioMedical Art Co.

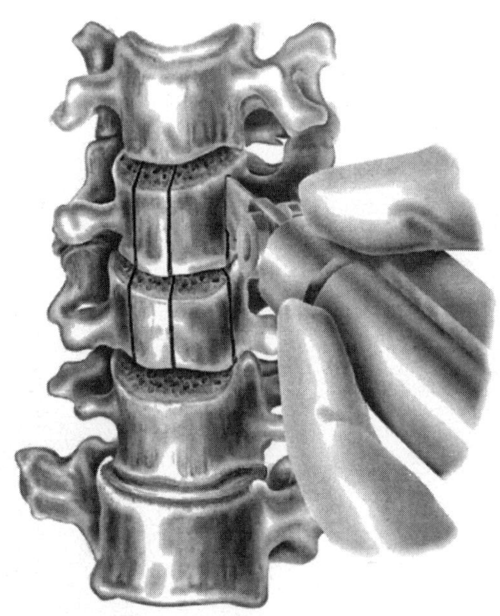

**FIGURE 18-15**

Use of a sagittal saw to prepare local vertebral bone for extraction. © Neil BioMedical Art Co.

spacer is assembled (Fig. 18-18, *B*). Bioceramics are also becoming popular in reconstructing thoracolumbar corpectomy defects in tumor surgery, and their use is being expanded to include spondylotic disease processes.[17,23]

The subtotal corpectomy defect is measured, and the reconstructive strut is fashioned with wedge-shaped ends to help ensure a lordotic cervical posture. A trial implantation is performed with slight distraction (10 to 15 pounds traction). It is imperative not to overdistract the facets linearly. Although the compression on the construct is favored with increased distraction, this may impart excessive loads on the strut with subsequent settling. Either anterior cervical plating in neutralization or posterior cervical hybrid plating with articular pillar screws and pedicle screws is considered mandatory for optimal stability of the reconstruction. Excessive settling of the construct predisposes the anterior cervical plate and screws to failure (see Fig. 18-4, *B*). The implant then undergoes increased cyclical loading when compared to the initial loads in neutralization. In addition, linear distraction unloads the facets and causes a kyphotic cervical posture. A combination of slight distraction with preservation of lordosis ("lordotic distraction" or "locking the facets") helps to maintain a normal cervical posture and minimizes the loads on the anterior construct (Fig. 18-18, *A* and *B*).

The composite graft construct is fashioned appropriately and packed with the autologous cancellous bone saved from the corpectomy procedure. Again with minimal cervical distraction, the construct is gently impacted into the subtotal corpectomy defect. The construct is impacted just past the anterior vertebral edge, and the distraction is released. The stability of the construct is tested prior to anterior cervical plate stabilization.

Prior to anterior cervical plate stabilization, radiographic confirmation of appropriate construct position is required for optimal stabilization of the reconstruction. Whether or not to add posterior stabilization depends on the type of pathology, the number of levels reconstructed, and any preexisting dynamic instability. The wound is then irrigated and closed over a drain in a routine fashion.

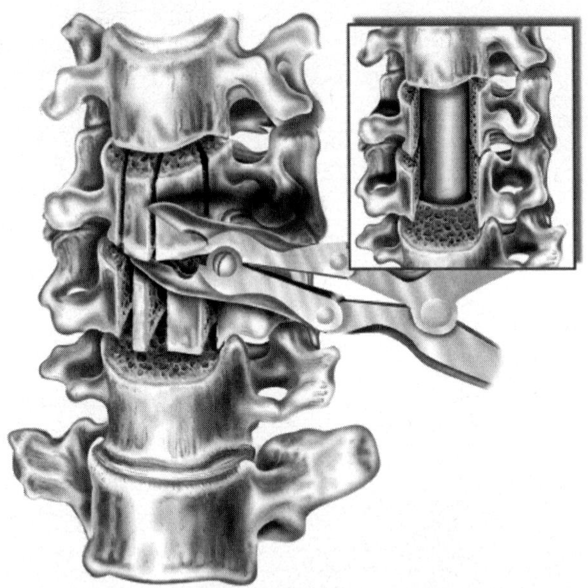

**FIGURE 18-16**

Rongeurs are used to extract cancellous bone and perform two-level corpectomy. © Neil BioMedical Art Co.

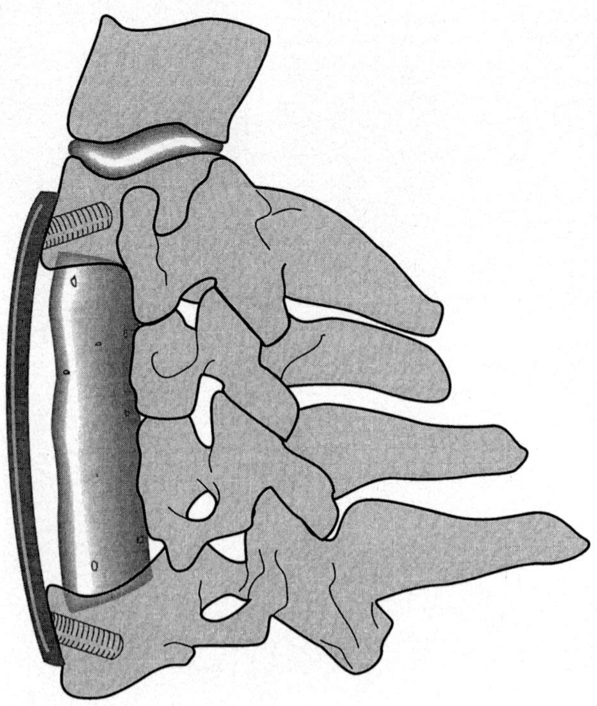

**FIGURE 18-17**

Lateral view of autologous tricortical iliac crest strut reconstruction with ventral cervical plate.

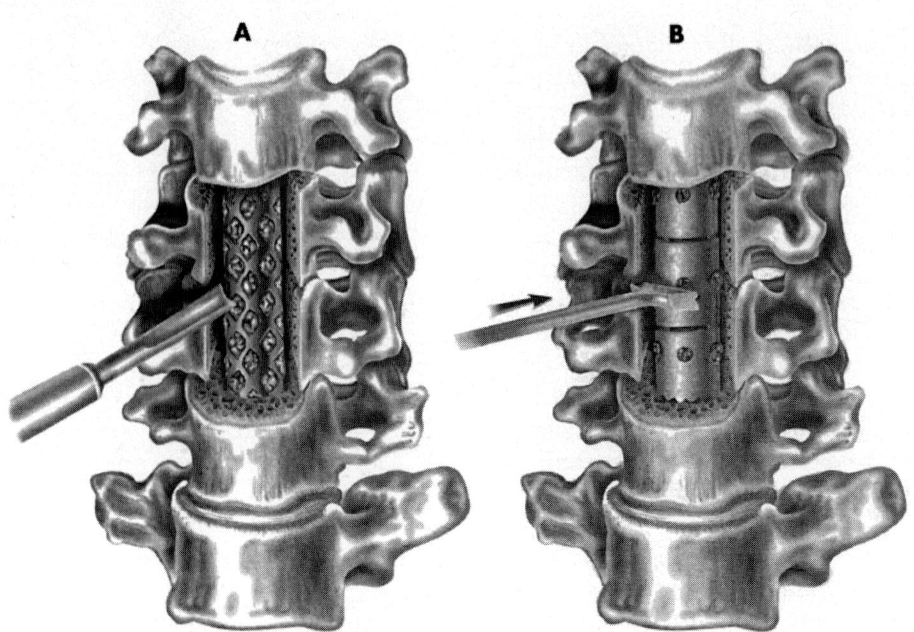


**FIGURE 18-18**

**A,** Insertion and impaction of titanium surgical mesh/cancellous bone construct. **B,** Insertion and impaction of assembled carbon fiber strut/cancellous bone construct. © Neil BioMedical Art Co.

## CASE STUDIES

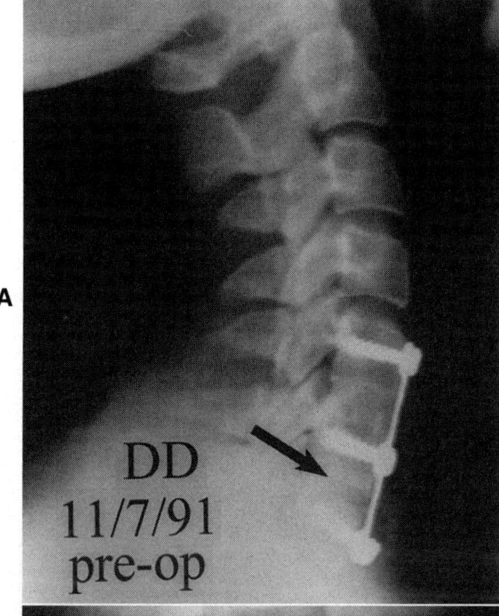


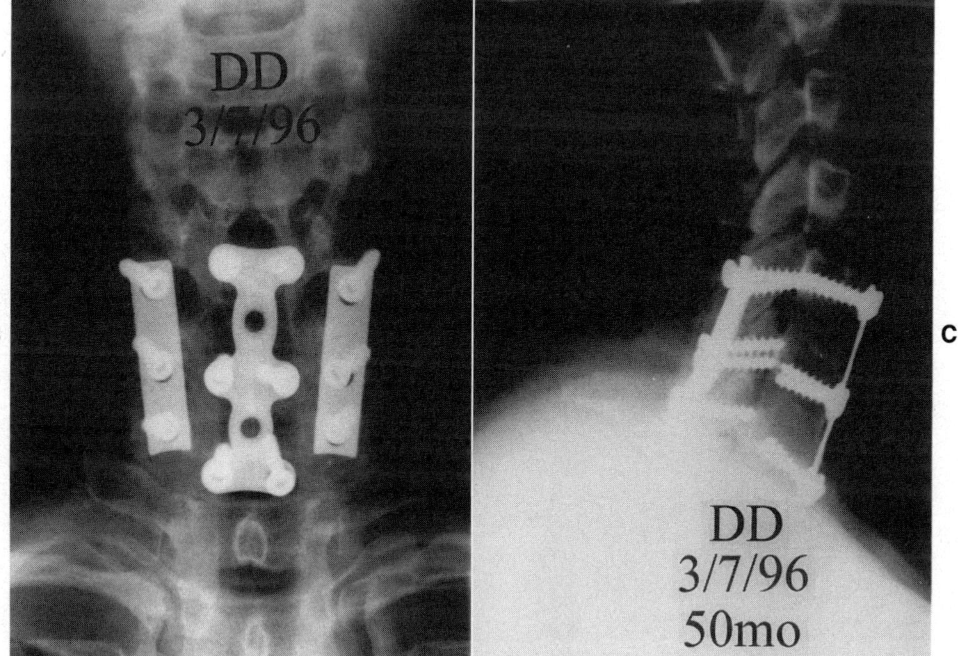


**FIGURE 18-19**

**A,** Lateral radiograph demonstrating an anterior nonunion at the C6-C7 grafting site. **B,** Postoperative anteroposterior radiograph showing placement of posterior cervical plates and articular pillar screws. **C,** Postoperative lateral radiograph demonstrating consolidation of the anterior nonunion.

### CASE 1

This 25-year-old woman initially underwent an anterior procedure for cervical spondylosis and intractable neck pain. Her surgery included a two-level anterior cervical diskectomy, tricortical iliac crest allograft interbody grafting, and Orozco anterior plating. Her symptoms completely resolved after surgery, and she resumed her daily activities. Two years after surgery, her symptoms had returned, and radiographic studies revealed a nonunion at C6-C7 (Fig. 18-19, *A*). A posterior procedure was determined to be the best solution to her recurrent pain and nonunion. A posterior cervical fusion with posterior plating and articular pillar screws was performed (Fig. 18-19, *B* and *C*). The patient's own cancellous iliac bone was used to achieve a solid posterior fusion. Her pain resolved after this procedure, and she has remained symptom-free for more than four years. Both anterior and posterior grafting sites healed within three months of her revision procedure.

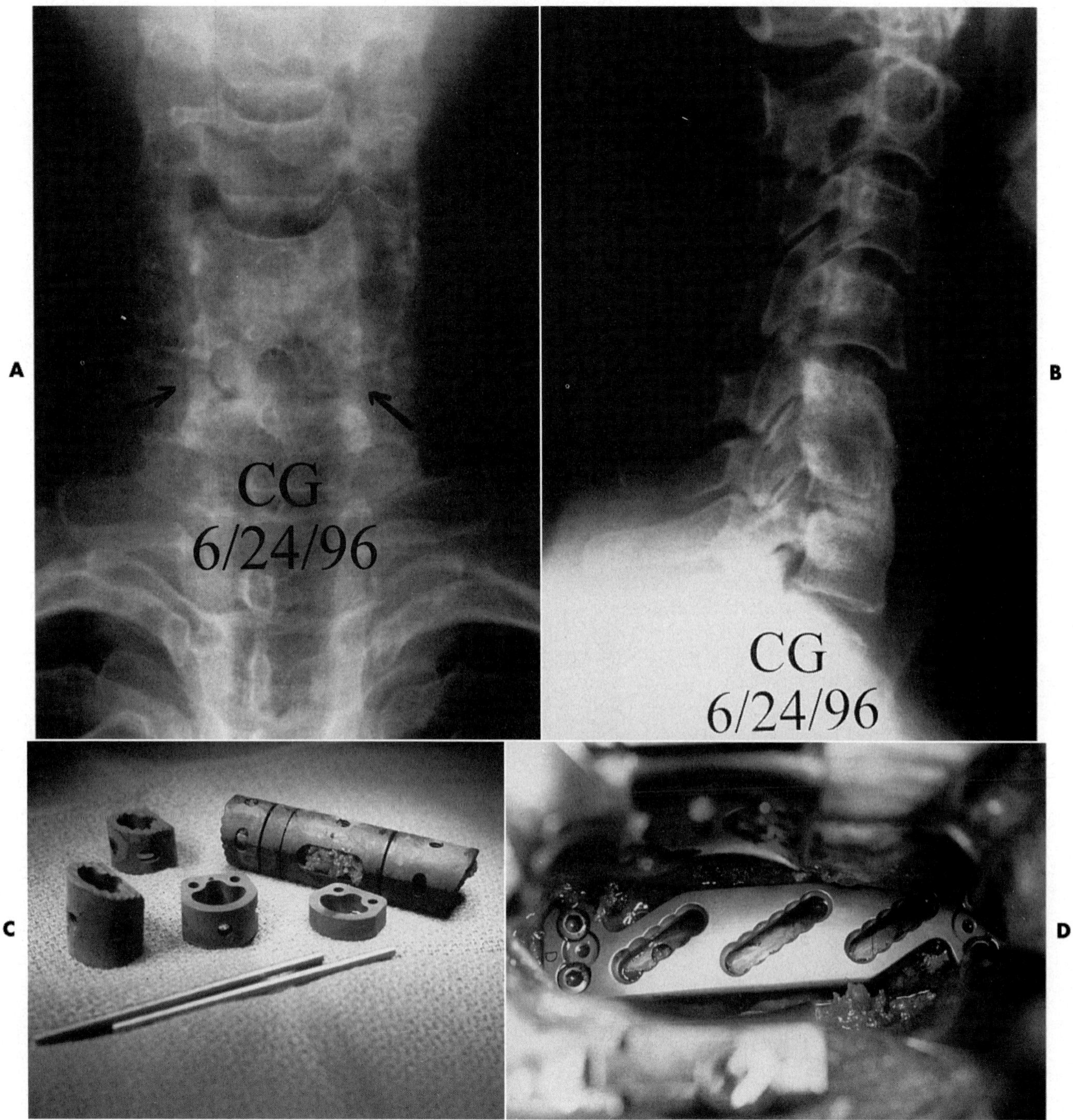


**FIGURE 18-20**

**A,** Anteroposterior view of an anterior nonunion with a clear radiolucent line through the disk space. **B,** Lateral radiograph of the attempted fusion sites. **C,** Intraoperative image of carbon filter implants. **D,** Intraoperative image with anterior cervical plate in place.

*Continued*

## CASE 2

This 48-year-old woman initially had neck pain in 1992 and underwent anterior cervical grafting at C5-C6 and C6-C7. She was pain-free for two years, but she began to have increased neck pain and left shoulder pain that radiated into the arm and hand. She was referred to the first author for a second opinion. In addition to a C6-C7 nonunion, she had signs and symptoms consistent with advanced degeneration of the levels above and below the operated levels (Fig. 18-20,

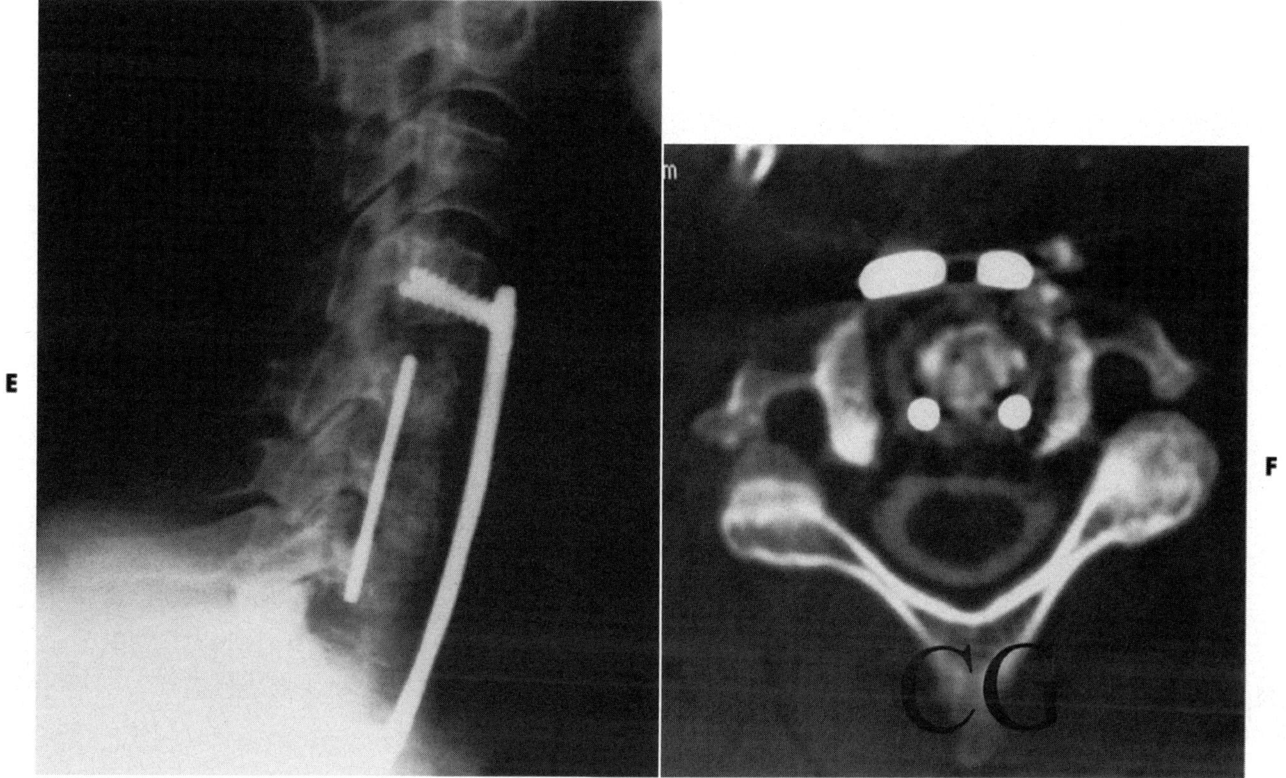

FIGURE 18-20 CONT'D

**E,** Postoperative lateral radiograph of proper plate and composite graft alignment. **F,** Axial computed tomography showing pedicle-to-pedicle decompression and proper "fit and fill" of the composite strut.

*A* and *B*). To achieve adequate decompression of the multilevel pathology and prepare fresh grafting sites, a three-level corpectomy was performed. A custom carbon fiber spacer packed with local bone filled the corpectomy defect, and an anterior plate was placed to stabilize the reconstruction (Fig. 18-20, *C* through *F*). She has significantly improved with regard to numbness and has only minimal pain. Her fusion became solid over 6 months, and all implants are intact after 18 months postoperatively.

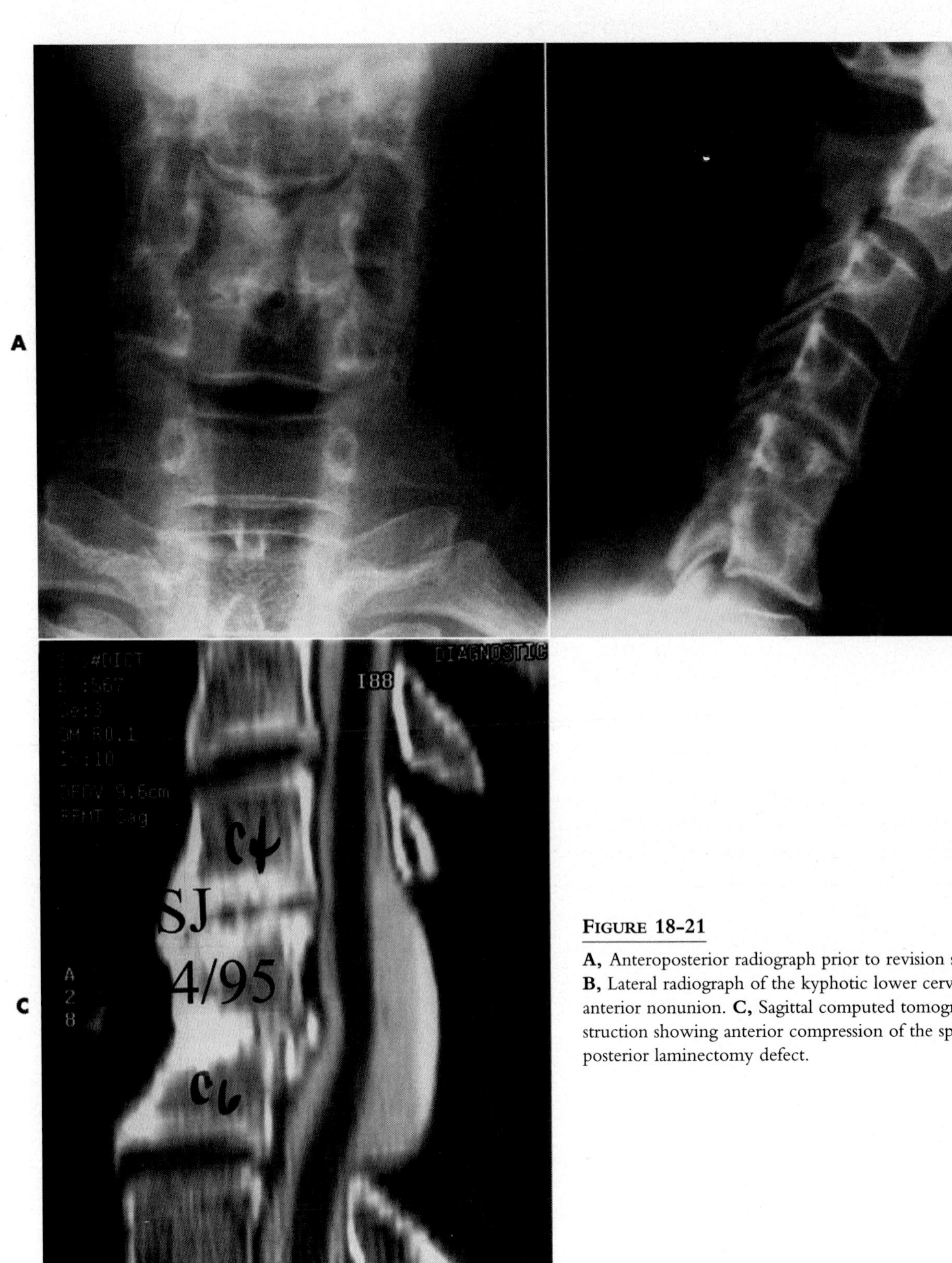


**FIGURE 18-21**

**A,** Anteroposterior radiograph prior to revision surgery. **B,** Lateral radiograph of the kyphotic lower cervical spine and anterior nonunion. **C,** Sagittal computed tomography reconstruction showing anterior compression of the spinal cord and posterior laminectomy defect. *Continued*

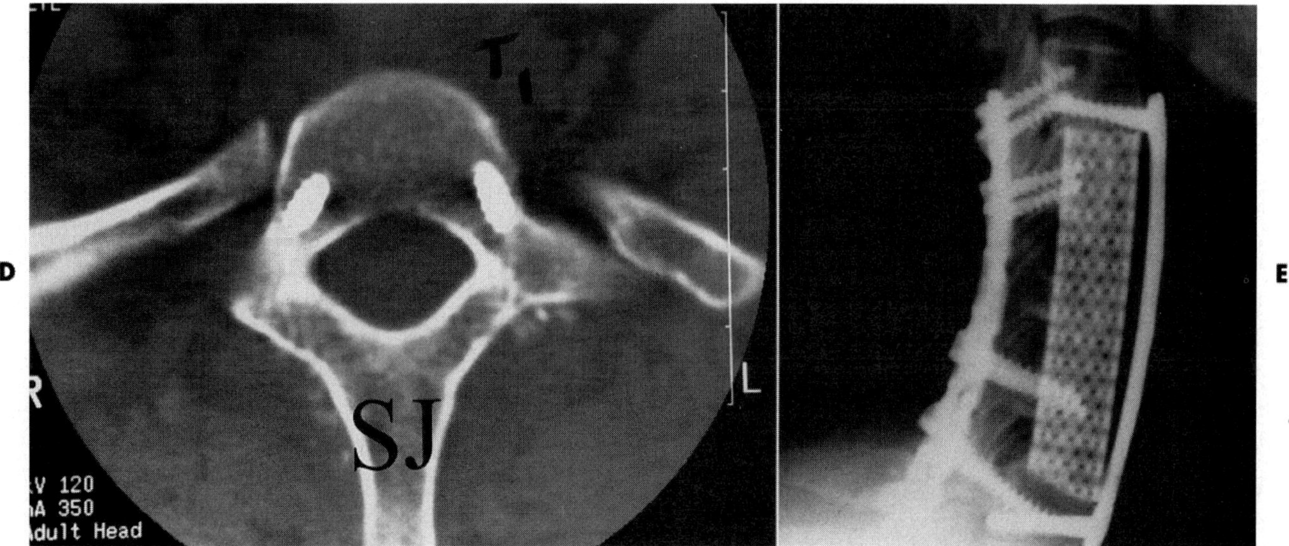


**FIGURE 18-21 CONT'D**

**D,** Postoperative computed tomography of T1 pedicle screws placed safely within each pedicle. **E,** Lateral postoperative radiograph 15 months after surgery demonstrating excellent alignment of the circumferential reconstruction.

## CASE 3

This 43-year-old man had an anterior procedure in March 1989 and multiple laminectomies in October 1990. In 1995, he presented with radicular and myelopathic symptoms. Radiographic studies demonstrated anterior pseudarthrosis and postlaminectomy kyphosis with anterior pathology that impinged on the thecal sac (Fig. 18-21, *A* through *C*). An anteroposterior procedure was performed to address this complicated multilevel problem. A three-level corpectomy was performed to address the significant anterior neural compression. Titanium surgical mesh (TSM) packed with local bone filled the defect, and this was stabilized with an anterior cervical plate. To ensure adequate fixation and further decompression, a posterior procedure also was performed. This included posterior cervical fusion and posterior cervical hybrid plate-screw reconstruction using cephalad articular pillar screws and caudal pedicle screws (Fig. 18-21, *D* and *E*). All myelopathic and radicular symptoms resolved, and his neck pain is minimal. The anterior and posterior fusions have progressed well, and all implants are in place.

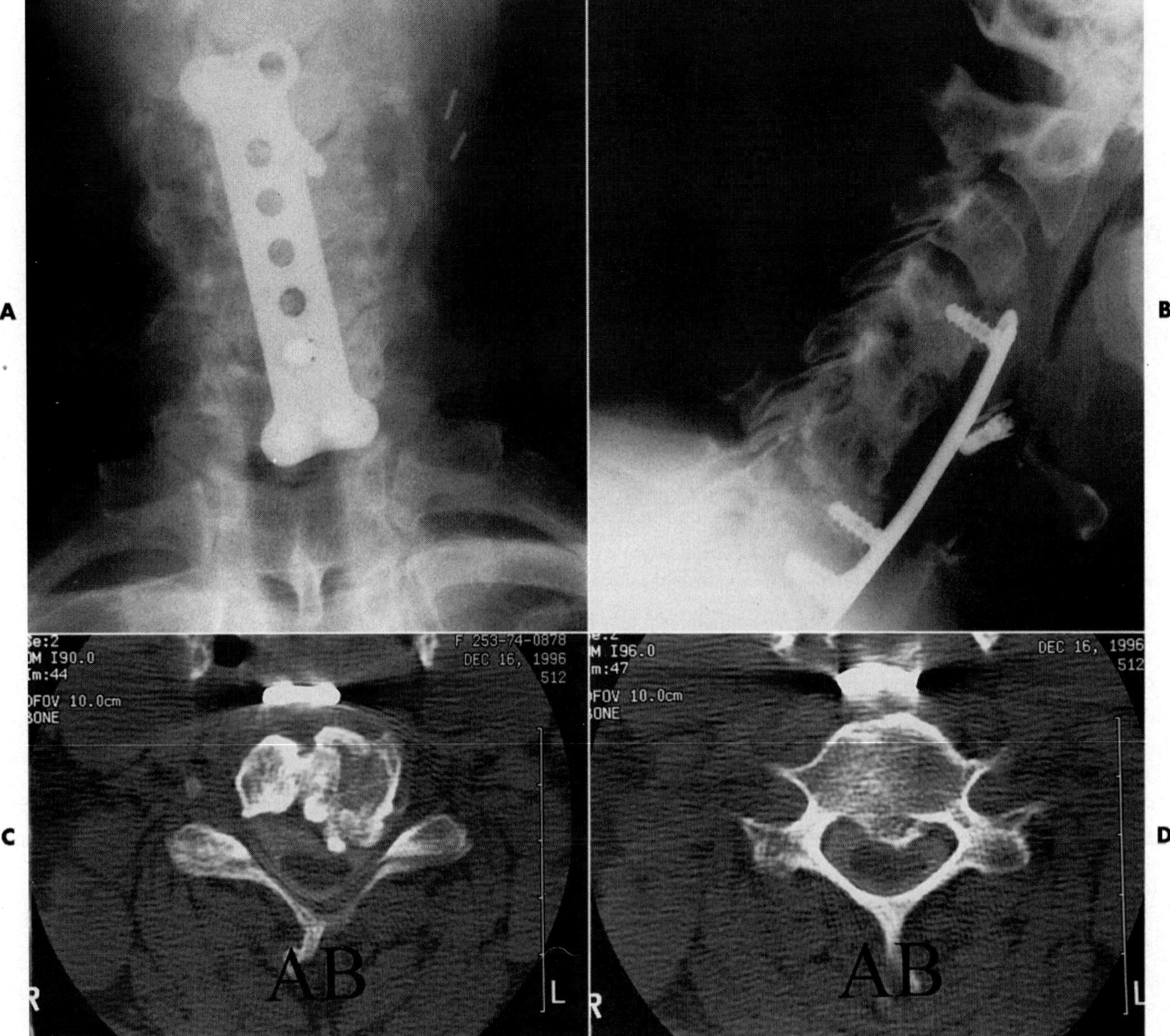


**Figure 18-22**

**A,** Anteroposterior radiograph. One of the superior screws has disengaged from the plate, and the plate is tilted. **B,** Lateral radiograph. The screw is visible in the anterior soft tissues. A kyphotic deformity is present, and osteophytes have formed at the superior end of the plate. **C,** Computed tomography of C5-C6. An inadequate decompression was performed previously. **D,** Computed tomography of C6. A central osteophyte impinges on the spinal cord, and the loosened plate is also evident.

*Continued*

## CASE 4

This 55-year-old woman had an anterior surgery with grafting and anterior plating in June 1994 for neck and shoulder pain. After surgery, her pain intensified, and she was unable to return to work. She presented to our office with persistent severe axial and appendicular pain, and radiographic studies demonstrated hardware failure, nonunion, inadequate decompression, and degeneration across the cervicothoracic junction (Fig. 18-22, *A* through *D*). An anteroposterior procedure was performed to correct her multilevel problem. A four-level corpectomy was performed, and the defect was reconstructed with a custom carbon fiber spacer (packed with local bone) and stabilized with an anterior plate. A posterior fusion was performed, and a custom rod-plate with midcervical articular pillar screws and thoracic pedicle screws was used to stabilize the cervicothoracic junction (Fig. 18-22, *E* and *F*). Her progress in the first four weeks is slow due to the chronic nature of the condition, but pain and weakness have improved (Fig. 18-22, *G* and *H*).

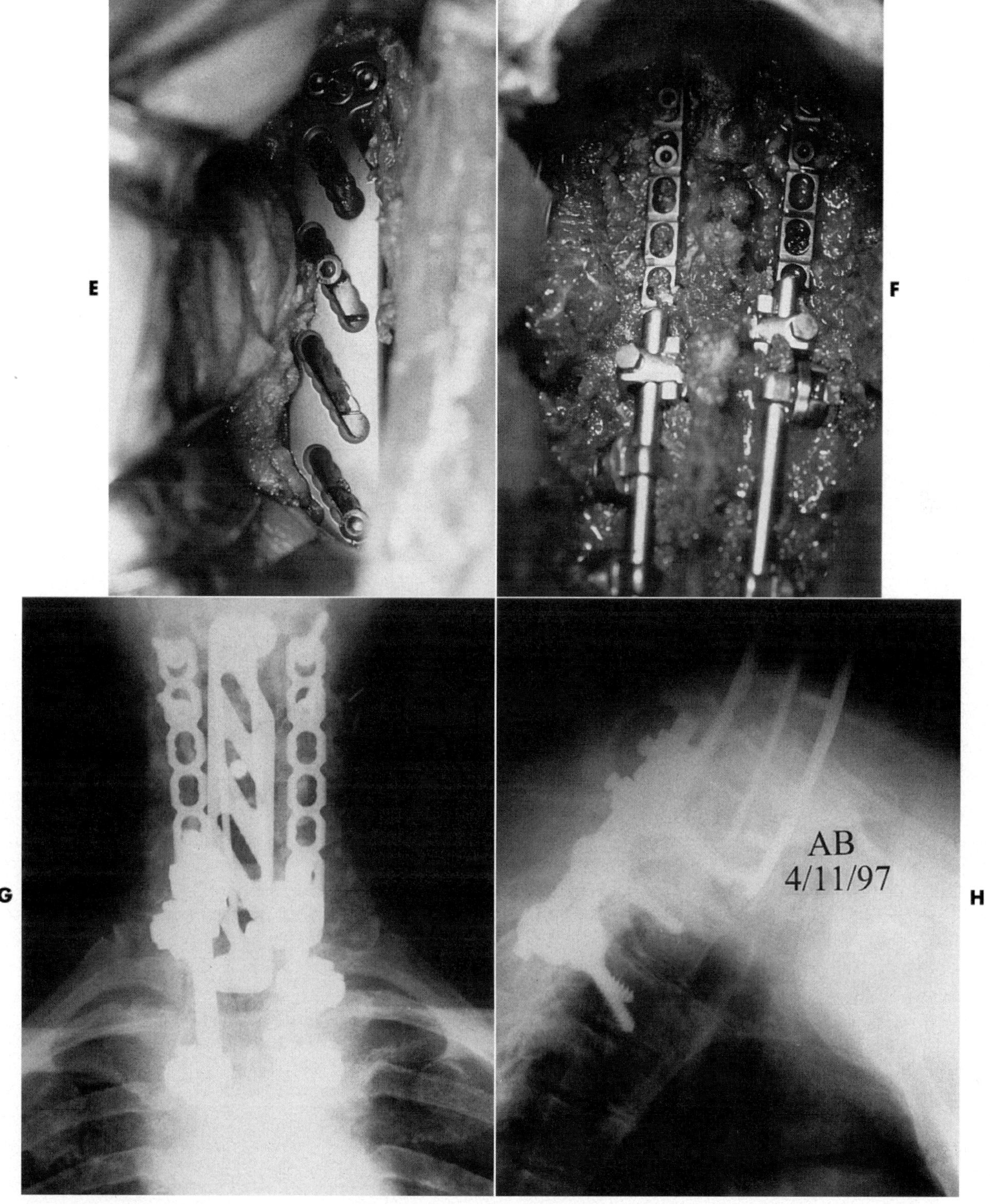


**FIGURE 18-22 CONT'D**

**E,** Intraoperative image with anterior cervical plate in place. **F,** Intraoperative image of custom cervicothoracic rod-plate construct. **G,** Anteroposterior radiograph of the cervical and upper thoracic spine. The anterior plate and custom rod-plates are in place with bone graft surrounding the posterior implants. **H,** Lateral view of the circumferential reconstruction.

## REFERENCES

1. Abumi K, Itoh H, Taneichi H, Kaneda K: Transpedicular screw fixation for traumatic lesions of the middle and lower cervical spine: description of the techniques and preliminary report, *J Spinal Disord* 7:19-28, 1994.
2. An HS, Gordin R, Renner K: Anatomic considerations for plate-screw fixation of the cervical spine, *Spine* 16:S548-S551, 1991.
3. Anderson PA, Henley MB, Grady MS, Montesano PX, Winn HR. Posterior cervical arthrodesis with AO reconstruction plates and bone graft, *Spine* 16:S72-S79, 1991.
4. Brodsky AE, Khalil MA, Sassard WR, Newman BP: Repair of symptomatic pseudarthrosis of anterior cervical fusion: posterior versus anterior repair, *Spine* 17:1137-1143, 1992.
5. Emery SE, Bolesta MJ, Banks MA, Jones PK: Robinson anterior fusion: comparison of the standard and modified techniques, *Spine* 19:660-663, 1994.
6. Farey ID, McAfee PC, Davis RF, Long DM: Pseudarthrosis of the cervical spine after anterior arthrodesis, *J Bone Joint Surg* 72-A:1171-1177, 1990.
7. Fernyhough JC, White JI, LaRocca H: Fusion rates in multilevel cervical spondylosis comparing allograft fibula with autograft fibula in 126 patients, *Spine* 16:S561-S564, 1991.
8. Goel VK, Clark CR, McGowan D, Goyal S: An in vitro study of the kinematics of the normal, injured, and stabilized cervical spine, *J Biomech* 17:373-376, 1984.
9. Graham AW, Swank ML, Kinard RE, Lowery GL, Dials BE: Posterior cervical arthrodesis and stabilization with a lateral mass plate: clinical and computed tomographic evaluation of lateral mass screw placement and associated complications, *Spine* 21:323-329, 1996.
10. Hanai K, Fujiyoshi F, Kamei K: Subtotal vertebrectomy and spinal fusion for cervical spondylotic myelopathy, *Spine* 11:310-315, 1996.
11. Jónsson H, Rauschning W: Anatomical and morphometric studies in posterior cervical spinal screw-plate systems, *J Spinal Disord* 7:429-438, 1994.
12. Lowery G: *Three-dimensional screw divergence and sagittal balance: a personal philosophy relative to cervical biomechanics*. In Merola A, editor: *SPINE: State of the art reviews*, vol. 10, no.2, Philadelphia, 1996, Hanley and Belfus, pp 343-356.
13. Lowery G, Carmody C, McDonough R, Allen A: Posterior cervical hybrid plate reconstruction: articular pillar screws and pedicle screws. Presented at the American Association of Neurological Surgeons 1997 Annual Meeting, Denver, Colorado, April 12-17, 1997.
14. Lowery G, McDonough R: The significance of hardware failure in anterior cervical plate fixation: patients with 2- to 7-year follow-up, *Spine* 23:181-187, 1998.
15. Lowery G, Swank M, Bhat A, McDonough R, Allen A. Titanium surgical mesh in cervical spine reconstruction: North American experience. Presented at the 64th Annual Meeting of the American Academy of Orthopaedic Surgeons, San Francisco, California, February 13-17, 1997.
16. Lowery G, Swank M, McDonough R. Salvage reconstruction for failed anterior cervical fusions: articular pillar plating or anterior revision, *Spine* 20:2436-2441, 1995.
17. Matsui H, Tatezaki S, Tsuji H: Ceramic vertebral body replacement for metastatic spine tumors, *J Spinal Disord* 7:248-254, 1994.
18. Meding JB, Stambough JL: Critical analysis of strut grafts in anterior spinal fusions, *J Spinal Disord* 6:166-174. 1993.
19. Montesano PX, Jauch E, Jonsson H: Anatomic and biomechanical study of posterior cervical plate arthrodesis: an evaluation of two different techniques of screw placement, *J Spinal Disord* 5:301-305, 1992.
20. Riley LH, Robinson RA, Johnson KA, Walker E: The results of anterior interbody fusion of the cervical spine, *J Neurosurg* 30:127-133, 1969.
21. Swank M, Lowery G, Bhat A, McDonough R: Anterior cervical allograft arthrodesis and instrumentation: multilevel interbody grafting and strut graft reconstruction, *Eur Spine J* 6(2), 1997.
22. Xu R, Ebraheim NA, Yeasting R, Wong F, Jackson T: Anatomy of C7 lateral mass and projection of pedicle axis on its posterior aspect, *J Spinal Disord* 8:116-120, 1995.
23. Yamamuro T: AW glass-ceramic in spinal repair. In Wilson J, Hench L, Greenspan D, editors: *Bioceramics* 8:123-127, 1995.

# 19

# NEUROLOGIC DEFICITS FOLLOWING SURGERY

Jens R. Chapman, M.D.
Robert Goodkin, M.D.
Sohail K. Mirza, M.D.



Spine surgery is undertaken with the goal of enhancing a patient's quality of life. Neurologic deterioration in a patient undergoing spine surgery can potentially negate all of these efforts and cause further anguish. Avoidance of such an incident is of obvious fundamental importance. Despite best efforts, any surgical procedure involving dissection or manipulation of or about neural tissue carries a theoretical risk of injury to neural tissue and possible deterioration of its accompanying functional capacities.[26]

Neurologic deficit following spine surgery may present in multiple manifestations and in any location of the central nervous system, directly or indirectly, as a result of even the best intended and performed intervention. As much as possible, the treating clinician should have knowledge of a patient's preoperative neurologic status in order to avoid confusion with possible postoperative findings. Pertinent to spine surgery, neurologic function can be assessed by evaluation of mental status, vision and cranial nerve function, extremity motor strength, various components of sensory function, deep tendon reflexes and pathologic reflexes, bowel and bladder control, anal sphincter function, sexual function by history and pain in a radicular distribution. The completeness of evaluation has to be individualized to match a patient's specific needs. Pertinent findings are preferably documented to allow for meaningful comparison later on.[5]

Particularly in elective procedures, preoperative patient education and discussion of risks including neurologic deterioration and its implications to the patient should be undertaken. Individualized preoperative planning can enhance the success of the intended surgical procedure by minimizing the influence of avoidable events surrounding the actual surgical procedure. Preoperative consults to address patient comorbidity, selection of appropriate anesthetic technique, patient positioning and assessment for transfusion and electrophysiologic monitoring needs are as important as the decision of surgical approach and decompression as well as reconstruction strategies. From the standpoint of minimizing neurologic deterioration in association with spinal surgery, the potential benefits of intraoperative electrophysiologic monitoring in patients undergoing instrumentation with or without deformity correction should be considered. This chapter deals with the occurrence, detection, and management of neurologic injuries to the spine following surgical intervention. Implications of intradural surgery exceed the scope of this chapter and are therefore not addressed. Due to differences in etiology and treatment, the time of identification of neurologic compromise relative to the surgical intervention was used to structure the various subsections.

## PRESURGICAL FACTORS

It is desirable that a surgeon performing spine surgery be actively involved in preoperative patient preparation. Intubation techniques should take the stability of the cervical spine into account as manual in-line traction or nasal intubation techniques may cause undue spinal canal encroachment or distraction.[20,47] Awake fiberoptic intubation can minimize cervical spine excursion during endotracheal intubation in cases with significant instability or deformity.

Any spine procedure starts with proper patient positioning. Proper patient positioning is important in avoiding incidental neurologic deficits such as loss of vision or peripheral nerve compression.

Awake patient positioning can be used to monitor neurologic changes in patients with unstable spinal column. Alternatively, prepositioning baseline electrodiagnostic function or a postpositioning wake-up test can be performed. For patients with unstable cervical spine pathology fluoroscopy enhances the ability of the treating surgeon to monitor spinal alignment for final positioning.

Should deterioration of neurologic function be noted with any of these tests, prompt return of the patient into the prepositioning status, hopefully, will reverse all or most neurologic deficits. In case of electrodiagnostic deterioration of signals, a Stagnara wake-up test can be used to corroborate these findings.[59] Factors such as changes of anesthetic levels and hemodynamic changes should be taken into account. If there is concern about a spinal cord injury, early administration of intravenous methylprednisolone according to the North American Spinal Cord Injury part II and III (NASCIS II and NASCIS III) protocols can be considered. From an anesthetic aspect, any hypotension, hypoxia, and relevant anemia should be corrected promptly. Aside from concerns for spinal cord perfusion, the differential diagnosis of positioning-induced neurologic deterioration centers around spinal cord impingement from changes in alignment or mass effect upon the cord from other sources. Correction of any malalignment with repositioning should be a first step in counteracting the neurologic deterioration. Intraoperative imaging tools such as fluoroscopy and plain radiographs are useful for this purpose. Should clinically concerning neurologic deterioration be identified, the treating surgeon is faced with the option of delaying or discontinuing the procedure or proceeding with it. Discontinuation of the surgical procedure can be used to further study the patient's condition. Emergent reimaging with plain radiographs, magnetic resonance imaging (MRI), or computed tomography (CT) scan can help in the understanding of the causative event and can be useful in addressing the underlying problem. The patient subsequently can be monitored for any further neurologic changes and the type and timing of definitive treatment can be reevaluated. However, for patients with significant instability or deformity, delay of surgery may lead to progressive cord damage or risk to general well-being in the case of prolonged recumbency. In such a situation, the patient may be better served by proceeding with an appropriate decompression and reconstruction procedure with best possible realignment of the spinal canal followed by reimaging of the spine postoperatively.

When positioning a patient for spine surgery, head, neck, and extremities have to be protected and padded adequately to minimize the risk of pressure palsies. Eyes should not be exposed to direct pressure and a prolonged dependent head position is preferably avoided.

## INTRAOPERATIVE LOSS OF NEUROLOGIC FUNCTION

There are two basic methods of identifying intraoperative neurologic injury: observation of direct physical injury to neural tissue or indirect signs seen on electrodiagnostic monitoring devices or pertinent changes in vital signs.

Obvious injury to neurologic structures may occur during surgical dissection around neural tissue by contusion, laceration, or excessive traction of neural tissue. Incidental tears or lacerations of neural tissue have been reported in incidences of 0.3% to 13% and may be caused by virtually any cutting or grasping tools, curettes, drills, or high-speed burrs.[35] In the case of an iatrogenic dural laceration, efforts should be undertaken to visually identify all potentially injured structures and to repair torn dura with the goal of achieving containment of neural tissue and cerebrospinal fluid.[27,35] Patients who sustained incidental durotomies that have been repaired are expected to have no compromise of their final result.[35] Attempts at repair of traumatically separated neural elements such as spinal cord, roots, and rootlets are currently not supported by prevalent publications. Recovery of reanastomosed nerve roots is currently not known to enhance chances for any neurologic recovery. Technical difficulties in achieving a surgical reanastomosis of neural tissue, which is frequently avulsed, within reasonable exposure, are further challenges to accomplishing a potentially successful neurologic repair.

Intraoperative spinal cord or cauda equina contusion may be incurred during exposure or as result of impaction. Such an event may be accompanied by sudden waking up of the patient or jerky sudden motion of involved extremities. Inspection of the involved neural tissue should be performed to rule out lacerated dural membranes. A Valsalva maneuver can be used to rule out an occult dural tear. Presence or absence of spinal cord pulsation may be a relevant finding but lacks scientific background for prognostication purposes.

Indirect neural tissue injury can also be caused by high temperatures created by use of high-speed burrs during extended bone dissection. Use of cooling irrigants, sharp cutting devices, or alternate bone dissection techniques should be considered to avoid thermal damage to adjacent neural tissue.

More indirect signs of neurologic deterioration can be found in unexplained changes of vital signs during surgery at the spinal cord level. Such changes could consist of bradycardia in presence of hypotension in absence of pharmacologic or volume status changes. Utilization of an intraoperative wake-up test or correlation with electrophysiologic tests can be considered. As in all patients with possibly impaired spinal cord function, normotension, a hematocrit near or above 30, and full oxygenation are believed important for optimal cord perfusion.[41]

Spinal cord monitoring is a useful method to identify intraoperative neurologic impairment in patients undergoing manipulation of the spinal column. The two basic methods for intraoperative spinal cord monitoring are wake-up test or continuous electrophysiologic monitoring. The wake-up test as described by Vauzelle and Stagnara[59,65] is conceptually simple and has been described as effective for deformity surgery. Although the concept of a wake-up test appears straightforward, the routine clinical application is quite cumbersome and test results may be difficult to interpret. Winter describes major drawbacks of this technique as lacking continuous monitoring capability and requiring an experienced anesthesiologist with a compliant, interactive patient.[69]

Most commonly, somatosensory evoked potentials (SSEP) are utilized for spine surgery involving manipulation or realignment of the spinal cord. This monitoring technique assesses electrical posterior column function only by means of stimulating major nerves in the upper and lower extremities and identifying responses at cervical, subcortical, and cortical sites. Intraoperative signal changes are of concern with an amplitude drop of 50% or more and delay of response of 10% or more. Decreasing signal changes probably reflect evolving spinal cord ischemia rather than direct neural trauma and occur with a delay of about 15 minutes.[52,55] Following the introduction of routine intraoperative spinal cord monitoring, a considerable drop in the incidence of severe neurologic events has been noted.[44,52] This observation, however, does not reflect upon the introduction of more sophisticated spine instrumentation systems and improved decision-making and patient management skills. Despite its popularity in most major spine centers, concerns arise out of the possibility for false-negative results in cases of preponderant anterior column dysfunction, and absent real-time display due to its sampling and averaging technology.[8,15] False-positive readings of SSEPs have been reported to range from 1.7% to 17%,[28,57] with false-negative results being between 0% and 0.2%.[55] Winter has suggested that this limitation may be caused by the "sensory-side" monitoring capacity of SSEP.[57,69] Faulty or poorly performed monitoring techniques may contribute significantly to the reported false-negative rates. In our experience of more than 3000 monitored instrumentation cases, the false-negative rate remains zero.

Motor evoked potentials (MEP) have been described by several authors as a technique to intraoperatively monitor the functionally perhaps more relevant anterior spinal column.[28,37] MEP is an evolving technique that requires further development due to its considerable implications on stimulation and anesthetic technique.[42] The routine clinical application of MEP has not been duplicated by a majority of spine centers to date because of cost and technical issues. In areas of surgery at or below the level of the conus, intraoperative electromyography has been described as real-time feedback to avoid excessive stretching or impingement to nerve roots or undue physical impingement of nerve roots through objects such as hardware.[31] We have found this technique to be very valuable for assessment of root function during posterior cervical and lumbar instrumentation and use it to supplement our SSEP monitoring. Although the technique allows for identification of neurotonic discharge during manipulation of nerve roots, actual nerve root transsection is not recorded by this technique.

If electrophysiologic monitoring identifies signal changes, technical malfunction should be ruled out promptly and the type, location, and consistency of signal changes interpreted. Correlation with anesthetic technique and changes in vital signs should be performed. In the case of persistent signal changes, the differential diagnosis includes aberrant hardware placement, manipulation of the spinal cord in excess of its tolerance for such excursions, and undue impingement of neurologic structures. Other considerations are changes in anesthetic levels, spinal cord perfusion, changes in vital signs, and duration of surgery. If signal changes occurred following instrumentation, especially with distraction, prompt hardware removal has been advocated in some circumstances.[15,44,69] If it is felt to be clinically important, correlation with an intraoperative wake-up test can be performed. In our experience, such tests are helpful early feedback techniques but can be cumbersome to execute and rely on an experienced anesthesiologist.

Impairment of spinal cord perfusion is a feared complication of spine surgery due to its usually severe and commonly irreversible resultant neurologic deficit. Intraoperative hypotension, prolonged hypoxia, or a hematocrit below 30 can adversely affect spinal cord perfusion.[9,40] In particular, hypotension has repeatedly been implicated in intraoperative loss of spinal cord function. Controlled hypotension is popular for patients receiving correction of spinal deformities in order to minimize blood loss and to optimize visualization.[46] Maintenance of a mean arterial blood pressure of around 60 mm Hg is suggested. Elective hypotensive anesthesia may, however, be undesirable in patients in need of extensive spinal column or cord manipulation.[41] Correction of intraoperative blood loss is important to minimize decrease of spinal cord perfusion. Ligation of multiple segmental arteries during anterior thoracolumbar approaches or combined anterior and posterior spine surgeries have been implicated in possible disruption of spinal cord perfusion. In a series of 1197 consecutive neurologically intact scoliosis patients with over 6000 vessel ligations, Winter et al found no patients with paralysis secondary to ligation of up to 8 segmental vessels.[68] Our experience in trauma patients with incomplete spinal cord injury undergoing anterior surgery to date has shown no neurologic deterioration secondary to segmental vessel ligation. Bridwell found a statistically significant increase of neurologic deficits with same day anterior and posterior corrective deformity surgery (2% incidence) compared with staged anterior and posterior surgery (0.5% incidence).[15] Extensive same-day anterior and posterior spinal surgery with deformity correction and circumferential disruption of spinal cord blood supply may contribute to neurologic deterioration in some patients. Overdistraction of the spinal cord, distraction over an anterior mechanical obstacle, shortening of the spinal canal, and cord swelling are possible causes of indirect disruption of spinal cord perfusion and should be taken into account when analyzing possible causes of impaired neurologic function. Correction of hyperkyphosis was associated with a 1% risk of deterioration in Bridwell's series.[15] In patients receiving surgery to the cervical spine, disruption of normal blood flow to the carotid or vertebral arteries may cause strokelike symptoms. Postoperative flow studies of noninvasive or invasive type can be utilized to work up such clinical presentations.

The overall risk of neurologic deterioration associated with spine surgery was reported at 5.95% in a review of 2855 patients operated for a wide variety of conditions at one institution.[9] Permanent spinal cord damage was encountered in 1.43% of patients. Severe cervical stenosis and dedifferentiated malignant tumors were identified as major risk factors for neurologic deterioration.[9,70] Spinal implants have become essential components of many components of spine surgery. Spinal fixation devices have evolved from hardware aimed at correcting deformities to implants capable of stabilizing all areas of the spine for a wide variety of indications. During the years 1974 to 1979, thoracolumbar deformity surgery was reported to carry a risk of neurologic impairment ranging from 0.72% to 17%. More recently, the risk of complete neurologic impairment for these indications was reported as 0.3%.[44,69] In anterior cervical diskectomies and fusion, a 0.1% incidence of severe myelopathic deterioration has been reported.[17,25] For segmental posterior cervical instrumentation, neurologic complications of 0.6% rate of root injuries with no myelopathic deterioration were found.[29] In the thoracolumbar spine all presently used posterior fixation techniques such as sublaminar wires, hooks, and screws have been associated with rare instances of neurologic injury.

Hardware removal remains an option in patients with intraoperative neurologic deterioration in association with instrumentation. Initially, rods or plates can be removed with the goal of allowing the spine to resume its preinstrumentation alignment.[51] If signal recovery is accomplished with this measure, consideration should be given to instrument the spine in situ with no attempts at deformity correction. While evaluating the effect of rod removal, hooks or screws should be evaluated for proper placement. Spinal cord abnormalities, such as a diastematomyelia, may lead to cord compromise in the presence of posterior spine fixation devices that invade the spinal canal, such as sublaminar wires or hooks.[69] Preoperative visualization of the spinal cord in patients with the possibility of having a spinal cord abnormality can help in preoperative planning.

Intraoperative imaging is helpful in the evaluation of neurologic deterioration of spine patients. Unanticipated alignment changes, displacement of structural grafts, and hardware position can be checked with plain radiographs or fluoroscopy.[54] Identification of any of these occurrences with these radiographic techniques in the operating room (OR) allows the surgeon to correct the possible problem. Use of a fully radiolucent OR table enhances the surgeon's ability to visualize the spinal column for possible cord impingement. Intraoperative myelography allows for limited visualization of the epidural space to rule out gross mechanical impingement. This technique is of marginal value due to technical difficulties in achieving adequate contrast visualization in an operating room setting. High-resolution ultrasound, intraoperative CT, and MRI scan are evolving technologies that could be of some benefit for intraoperative cord visualization.

In a patient with an intraoperative event leading to suspected or likely neurologic deterioration, postoperative imaging immediately following completion of the surgical procedure has been recommended.[15] Visualization of the spinal cord in the area of neurologic deterioration is the goal. If titanium alloy implants have been used, an MRI scan has some advantages over myelography/CT myelography. An MRI scan with gadolinium contrast is noninvasive, can be performed rapidly, and can visualize the spinal cord structure itself. Hardware interference and expected postsurgical changes, however, can distort images, thus requiring cautious interpretation.[56] Myelography with postmyelography CT over the entire length of an instrumentation system is preferable in patients with stainless steel implants. For circumstances in which hardware and bone graft visualization is of interest a noncontrast CT scan may suffice.

In the event of a suspected acute intraoperative spinal cord injury prompt administration of intravenous methylprednisolone in doses as recommended by the NASCIS II study can be considered.[12,13] Although there is no study supporting this suggestion, the potentially beneficial therapeutic effects of membrane stabilization and minimization of necrosis propagation follow the same mechanism as in acute spinal cord injury patients.

## POSTOPERATIVE NEUROLOGIC DEFICIT

There are multiple possible causes for postoperative neurologic deterioration. The most common causes of neurologic deterioration with spine surgery are intraoperative spinal cord injury, changes in alignment, graft displacement, and epidural hematoma.[9,70] Any of these etiologies may not be identified intraoperatively, even in the presence of electrophysiologic monitoring, and may become manifest postoperatively or may evolve secondarily.

Because the timing of onset of neurologic deterioration is a helpful parameter in investigating potential causes, postoperative assessment of a patient's neurologic status is an important part of completion of the surgical procedure. *Immediate* onset of postoperative neurologic deficit can be defined as identifying a persistent deterioration of neurologic function on the first postoperative examination within one hour from completion of surgery. *Delayed* onset of neurologic deficit can be defined as manifestation of neurologic deterioration in reference to the initial postoperative neurologic examination until early soft tissue healing is completed by about three weeks postoperatively. *Late* neurologic deterioration can be defined as onset ranging from the completion of early soft tissue healing at three weeks to years or decades following a surgical intervention. Discussion of postoperative neurologic compromise therefore is best divided by the time of deficit occurrence.

### IMMEDIATE POSTOPERATIVE NEUROLOGIC DEFICIT

It is desirable to assess the neurologic function of a patient with completed spine procedure at the earliest feasible postoperative time. A neurologic evaluation in a postoperative patient can be difficult and confusing in light of postanesthetic changes affecting the central and peripheral nervous systems.[62] Upon achieving postoperative compliance with simple commands, basic neurologic abilities including visual and cognitive functions can be assessed. Although detailed motor, sensory, and reflex function assessment may be premature, compliance with simple functional commands should be possible. In patients with preoperatively altered mental status, such as in mental retardation, unconsciousness and presence of large doses of narcotic drugs, particular vigilance in the postoperative phase is important.[21] Certain anesthetic agents such as midazolam and fentanyl have been associated with the temporary enhancement of preoperative motor deficits.[62] Basic sensory function tests assessing light touch or pin prick may be helpful in defining neurologic levels of dermatomal distribution of deficits and looking for sensory sparing. The assessment of deep tendon reflexes and clinical tests for long tract signs may be unreliable, usually for up to one hour after completion of an anesthetic because of residual effects of depolarizing or muscle relaxant agents. Repeat neurologic assessment of a patient with completed spine surgery is desirable and can be timed to match the patient's individual circumstances.[16]

In the presence of unexplainable persistent profound neurologic deficits, early postoperative imaging tests are helpful. The type of imaging test can range from simple plain radiographs in two plains to MRI or CT scans with or without contrast. Their use should match the suspected etiology of neurologic deficit and should be compatible with any hardware used.[56] Primary concerns in this immediate postoperative phase are directed at hardware placement, graft position, attenuation, or tethering of the spinal cord or a mass effect, such as a postoperative hematoma.[1,36]

Correct hardware and structural graft placement can most commonly be identified by well-centered radiographs.[54] If radiographic visualization of the spine segments involved in the presumed neurologic incident is not possible, the surgeon is confronted with the decision to perform an emergent surgical reintervention or obtain further imaging studies to gain improved understanding of the process involved. Should immediate CT or MRI scanning facilities be available such tests may be helpful prior to considering surgical reintervention. Noncontrast CT scans can be useful in more questionable cases of invasion of the spinal canal or neuroforamina. This is particularly relevant in complex cervical spine or sacral fixation cases and in presence of abnormal or unusual bony anatomy. Computed tomography with reformatted views can be used to assess the spinal canal alignment for possible cord tethering or impingement. A mass effect can be created by a displaced structural bone graft, a retained foreign body, a herniated nucleus pulposus, infolded ligamentum flavum, displaced bony fragments, or an expanding hematoma. An indirect mass effect can be created by swelling of neural tissue with subsequent encroachment by surrounding structures. Identification of the cause of a mass effect can be possible by noncontrast CT scan, however, it may require an MRI scan or myelography/CT myelogram if soft tissue visualization is limited on the CT scan alone.[16]

The choice of therapeutic countermeasures to attempt reversal of any neurologic deficit is difficult and can vary from observation and reassurance to emergent surgical reintervention. Multiple variables enter the decision making process and make simple decision making algorithms nearly useless. If an obvious mass effect upon or displacement of the spinal cord is identified, early surgical reintervention may aid neurologic recovery, provided the patient's condition allows for such further surgery. The merits of such a decompressive surgery have to be weighed with possible complicating circumstances of additional surgery, such as additional blood loss and coagulopathies. Supplemental pharmacologic treatment with intravenous methylprednisolone may be helpful and has been discussed above. In patients with incomplete and perceived minor neurologic deterioration a more elective approach can be taken. Swelling and neuropraxic etiologies may be causative factors of such deficits and should lead to a progressive improvement over time. Appropriate electrodiagnostic or imaging studies can be obtained as the further patient status warrants.

Examples of peripheral neurologic impairment can be found following anterior spinal procedures. Anterior surgery to the cervical spine can be associated with recurrent laryngeal nerve palsy, Horner's syndrome as a result of an injury to the sympathetic chain, and esophageal dysphagia as a result of segmental denervation during exposure.[17,25] Transthoracic approaches can be associated with intercostal radiculopathy, with similar complication rates described for open and thoracoscopic procedures.[45] Lumbosacral approaches can be associated with unilateral sympathectomy symptoms, retrograde ejaculation in males and dysfunction of ilioinguinal, iliofemoral, and lateral femoral cutaneous nerves.[24] In absence of surgical transsection of any of these structures, the majority of these neurologic deficits are expected to recover spontaneously.

Visual loss following spine surgery in a prone position is a troublesome neurologic occurrence.[49] Currently, it is not standard practice to use intraoperative monitoring techniques for visual integrity, making timely postoperative assessment of visual function following lengthy spine procedures important. Prone positioning, head placement, low hematocrit with intraoperative blood loss, and hypotension have been associated with visual impairment following spine surgery. Delayed onset up to three weeks after surgery has been reported.[61]

## EARLY POSTOPERATIVE NEUROLOGIC DEFICITS

Neurologic deficits that develop after the immediate postoperative observation period to approximately three weeks postoperatively may have a variety of causes specific for this time period. Presence of neural tissue swelling is a possible and usually a spontaneously reversible condition. An epidural hematoma or an early wound infection are examples of evolving soft tissue masses that can adversely affect neural function and warrant timely workup and therapeutic intervention. While animal experiments and studies on preoperative patients support delays of surgical decompression between 8 and 24 hours no such studies exist for postsurgical patients. Therefore it is recommended that spinal cord compression in association with an evolving postoperative neurologic deficit preferably be treated as an emergency with attempt at early decompression.[30]

Postoperative epidural hematomas may be caused by persistent wound hemorrhage, reopening of coagulated or clotted vessels, or emerge secondary to anticoagulants or comorbid coagulopathies. Recently, the use of low molecular weight heparin as routine postoperative deep venous thrombosis prophylaxis has been associated with an increased incidence of postoperative epidural hematoma formation.[23] Persistent wound hemorrhage may be caused by isolated nonoccluded larger vessels or a coagulopathy (Fig. 19-1). Certain comorbid conditions such as prostate carcinoma and other metastatic neoplastic diseases may predispose patients for coagulopathies. Retained foreign bodies such as cottonoid sponges, bone wax, or Gelfoam, if left next to the spinal cord in a confined space, may lead to neural tissue compression. Quadriparesis has been described in anterior cervical diskectomies as a result of Gelfoam sponges left posterior to the bone plug.[1]

Early postoperative wound infection can lead to neurologic deterioration. Septic events, urinary tract or respiratory infections, and persistent wound drainage in a postoperative patient are common infectious foci.[60] In patients with delayed onset of neurologic deterioration following anterior neck surgery, esophageal perforation should be considered.[38,64] Epidural abscess or empyema formation can be a diagnostic challenge, especially in immunocompromised patients.[58] Insidious occurrence of soft tissue swelling in the general operative area and temperature spikes for unknown reasons can be possible diagnostic clues, but most frequently clinical signs are vague. Patients treated with immunosuppressant medications such as steroids and cytostatic medications pose particular diagnostic challenges due to absence of obvious sepsis signs. Unexplained neurologic symptoms in such patients may be best worked up with an MRI screen rather than relying on a traditional sepsis workup alone. Following identification of a possible source, surgical resection of all abscess material and necrotic debris is recommended. In addition to potentially causing worsening neurologic deficit, delay of surgical debridement can lead to more widespread soft tissue and bony involvement and may require more extensive surgical reconstructive efforts (Fig. 19-2).[63]

Postoperative mental status changes are worrisome for multiple possible etiologies. Embolic causes or meningitis may be possible causes. Cerebellar herniation may be caused by continuous loss of cerebrospinal fluid from a dural leak in presence of a pleural fistula or wound drain.[3]

In patients with diskectomy, a recurrent disk herniation should be considered in case of return or worsening of preoperatively present radicular symptoms. The incidence of such an event has been suggested to reach as high as 15%.[18] Repeat diagnostic imaging with an MRI scan and contrast can be difficult to interpret due to postsurgical changes but remains a preferred imaging test for early decision making in this scenario. The indication for surgical reintervention is a treatment choice that depends upon recovery potential of the patient and size and location of an offending disk fragment.

In patients with hardware, early loss of reduction or hardware displacement should be considered as possibilities. Plain radiographs and comparison with initial postoperative studies should suffice to make this diagnosis. In such situations early reintervention may be technically easier than hoping for possible further

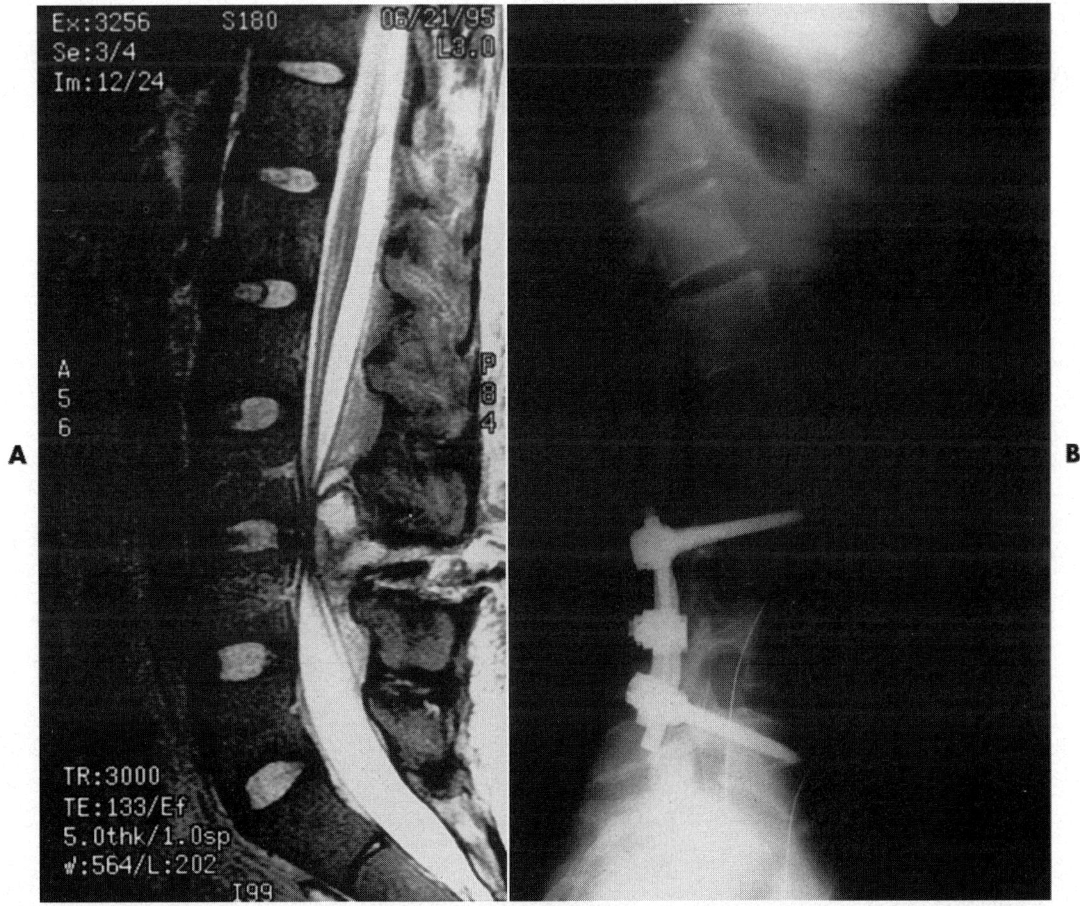


**FIGURE 19-1**

**A,** Sagittal lumbar MRI scan of an 18-year-old patient one week after being placed in a hyperextension cast for an L3-L4 Chance-type injury. The patient had initially been neurologically intact but developed an acute cauda equina syndrome due to an epidural hematoma on post injury day seven. **B,** Lateral lumbar radiograph demonstrates posterior segmental instrumentation bridging L3 to L5 placed following emergently performed posterior decompression. The patient fortunately recovered neurologic function. The epidural hematoma was believed to have resulted from routine postoperative thromboembolism prophylaxis with heparin.

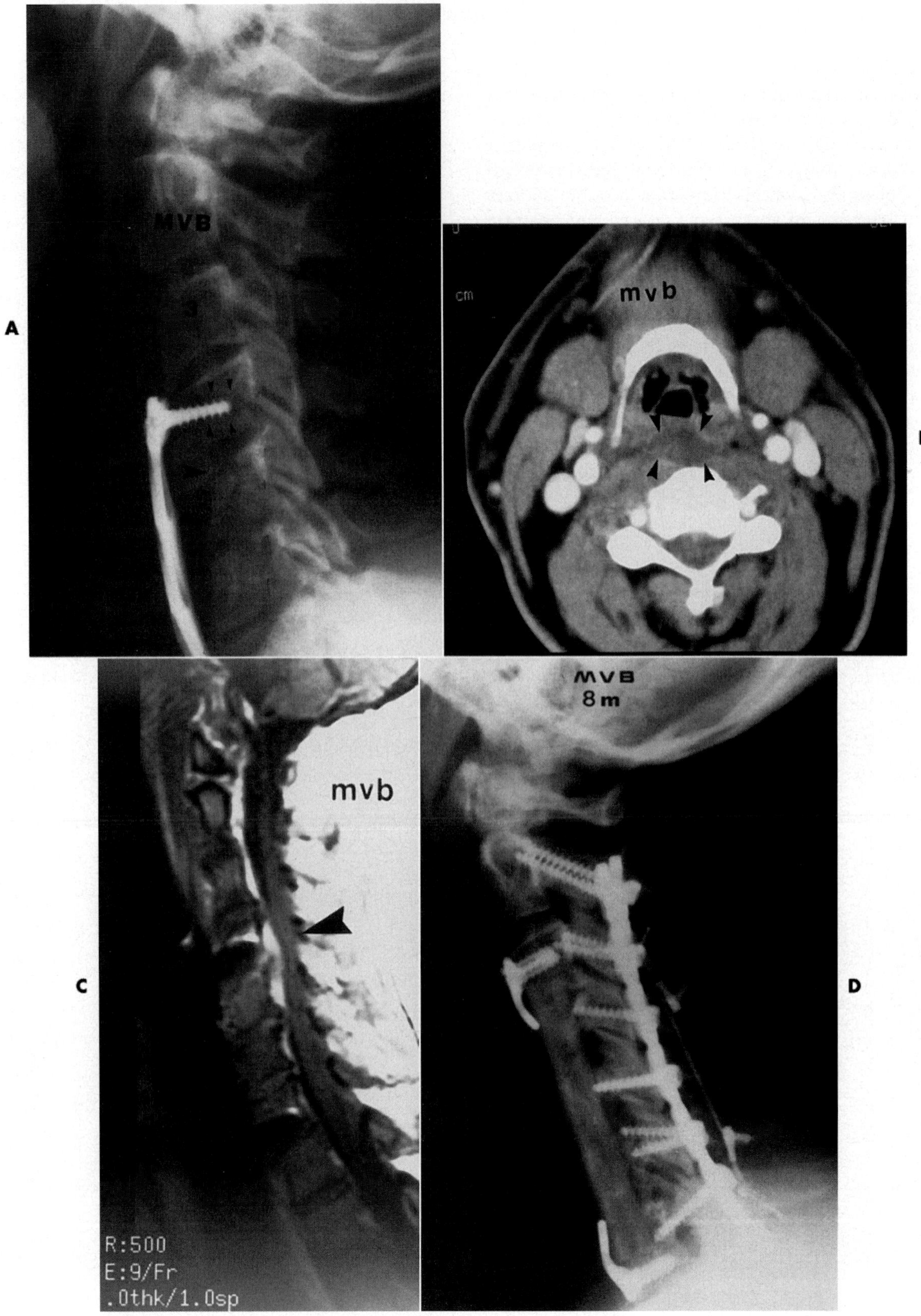


**FIGURE 19-2**

**A,** This 56-year-old male presented with myelopathic deterioration 3 weeks after C5 and C6 corpectomy and strut grafting. He was mildly febrile and complained of sudden-onset hoarseness and difficulty swallowing. This lateral cervical radiograph shows loosening of the rostral screws (*small arrows*) and displacement of the strut graft. **B,** A postoperative CT scan reveals a retropharyngeal fluid collection (*four arrows*). A gastrografin swallowing test showed no esophageal perforation. **C,** This MRI scan demonstrates an epidural mass effect on the ventral spinal cord (*large arrow*). An emergent decompression was performed with staged anterior and posterior reconstruction. **D,** At his 8-month follow-up the patient had recovered a normal neurologic function. Satisfactory bony healing could be verified on postoperative radiographs.

consolidation to take place. Delayed postoperative ascending paraparesis has been reported up to 30 hours upon completion of a scoliosis surgery in absence of any hardware displacement.[48] Urgent decompression of the spinal cord upon completion of spinal cord imaging is recommended.

An unusual cause for neurologic deterioration can be the development of a postoperative extremity compartment syndrome. This may be associated with positioning, such as knee-chest position, prolonged surgical time, and large-scale intravascular volume changes resulting in breakdown of the blood membrane barrier. In trauma patients reevaluation for possibly missed extremity injuries should be considered. Use of thromboembolism prevention devices such as TED hoses and sequential compression devices may obscure physical evaluation of extremities. Awareness of the possibility of this condition and complete physical examination in the presence of concerning neurologic findings are helpful in such situations.

## LATE NEUROLOGIC DETERIORATION

Following completion of initial soft tissue healing at approximately two to three weeks, a variety of other developments may adversely affect spinal cord function. Loss of spine reduction and malunion or nonunion of spine fusions may cause late onset of neurologic deficit through mechanical cord compression.[21] Understanding the causes and counteracting with corrective surgical reconstruction should carry a favorable prognosis for recovery of deficits.[2,11] Similarly, a late infection may cause a deteriorating neurologic status of a patient. Late infection can occur in a variety of manifestations from a wide spectrum of causes. Vertebral osteomyelitis or soft tissue infections with epidural or paraspinal extension should be considered in patients with late-onset neurologic deterioration and worked up with serologic and imaging studies.[60,63,66] Identification of a source and eradication of it are important components of the overall treatment.

From approximately three weeks postoperatively and on, neurologic compromise frequently manifested by pain or return of a radiculopathy may be caused by a pseudomeningocele.[50] With continued expansion of such a cyst in a space confined by bony margins, progressive compression of neural tissue is possible. In the cervical spine herniation of the spinal cord into a pseudomeningocele has been described as a cause for gait disturbance.[32] MRI with and without gadolinium contrast can demonstrate a pseudomeningocele. Avoidance of a pseudomeningocele by best possible repair or closure of a dural leak is preferred. Lumbar drainage or surgical reexploration with the goal of dural closure are treatment options (Fig. 19-3).[27]

The most common cause of late deterioration of neurologic function in a posttraumatic setting is the development of syringomyelia.[71] The etiology of a posttraumatic syrinx is still incompletely understood but involves development of myelomalacia with cord atrophy and evolution of cerebrospinal fluid (CSF)-filled cysts. Time of symptomatic clinical onset ranges from 3 weeks post injury to decades. The mechanism of expansion from a simple cyst to an expansile dissecting structure remains subject of speculation but is probably related to pressure changes within the CSF space during coughing and straining with resultant propagation of syrinx fluid into the spinal cord.[67] Its incidence has been estimated to be 20% as incidental findings on MRI scans, with approximately 3.2% being clinical symptomatic.[4] The most common presenting symptom is pain but symptoms can include worsening pain and numbness, increase in spasticity and, at a later stage, ascending motor deficits. Diagnostic workup preferably consists of an MRI scan with gadolinium contrast. Further confirmation or delineation of the lesion can be achieved with a myelogram/CT myelography and delayed repeat CT scan to better assess syrinx expansion. Tube drainage of a syrinx can be associated with complications such as infection, blockage, displacement, or overdrainage of cerebrospinal fluid leading to an acquired Arnold-Chiari syndrome.[10] Treatment of a syrinx is case-dependent and includes observation and repeat scans, surgical drainage with a shunt or an expansion duraplasty.[43] Although lasting recovery of neurologic function in patients with this condition is unlikely, deterioration can, hopefully, be stabilized or delayed (Fig. 19-4).

Other conditions that can adversely affect spinal cord function are cord tethering, or advancing mechanical compression by events caused by non- or malunions of the spine. Postoperative kyphosis can lead to progressive cord impingement in the area of the kyphotic apex and lead to subsequent neurologic deterioration. Iatrogenic destabilization of the spine or nonunion of a fusion construct are common causes for postoperative kyphosis and should be considered for surgical correction and stabilization.[14,34] Similar to kyphosis, other deformities such as postoperative scoliosis or hyperlordosis may occur and lead to neurologic symptoms.[36] The efficacy of the concept of surgical decompression, arthrodesis and stabilization of the spinal column has been demonstrated up to 12 months following spinal cord trauma.[2,11] Surgical treatment strategies for such conditions are described in previous chapters.

In patients with fusion, breakdown of levels above or below in the form of a transfer lesion may lead to neurologic entrapment by spinal stenosis, olisthesis, disk herniation, or a combination of these findings. Radiographic degenerative changes in disks adjacent to fusion levels were found in 9% of patients on aver-

**FIGURE 19-3**

**A,** This sagittal cervical MRI scan was obtained in a 45-year-old male who presented with progressive cervical myelopathy in association with postlaminectomy kyphosis. Cord signal changes can be seen between C4 and C6. **B,** The patient received a three-level corpectomy and posterior instrumentation as demonstrated on this postoperative lateral radiograph. A small dural leak during the C3-C4 diskectomy was not repairable but was sealed with fibrin glue. Aside from this, the procedure was carried out without complications. The patient's initial postoperative examination was unchanged from his preoperative status. **C,** The patient's motor status in both upper extremities suddenly deteriorated 36 hours postoperatively. The emergently obtained MRI scan revealed a circumferential fluid pocket encroaching the spinal cord (*arrows*). Upon emergent surgical decompression a postsurgical pseudomeningocele was encountered and decompressed. A lumbar drain and bed rest prevented recurrence. The patient experienced full neurologic recovery.

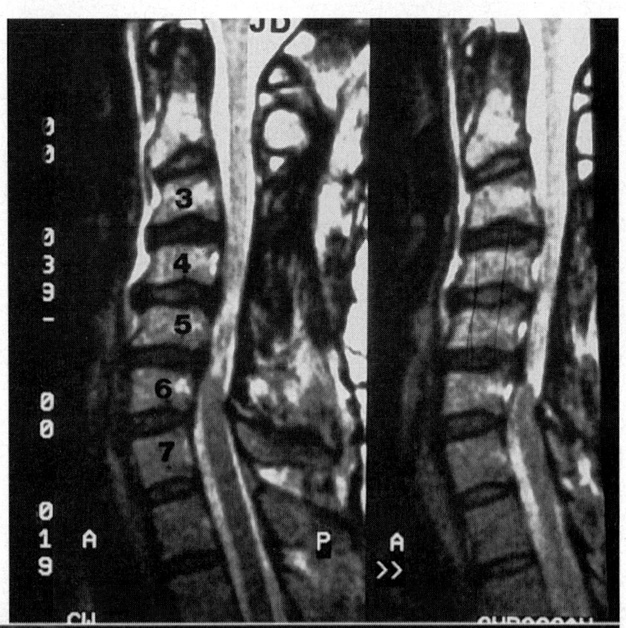


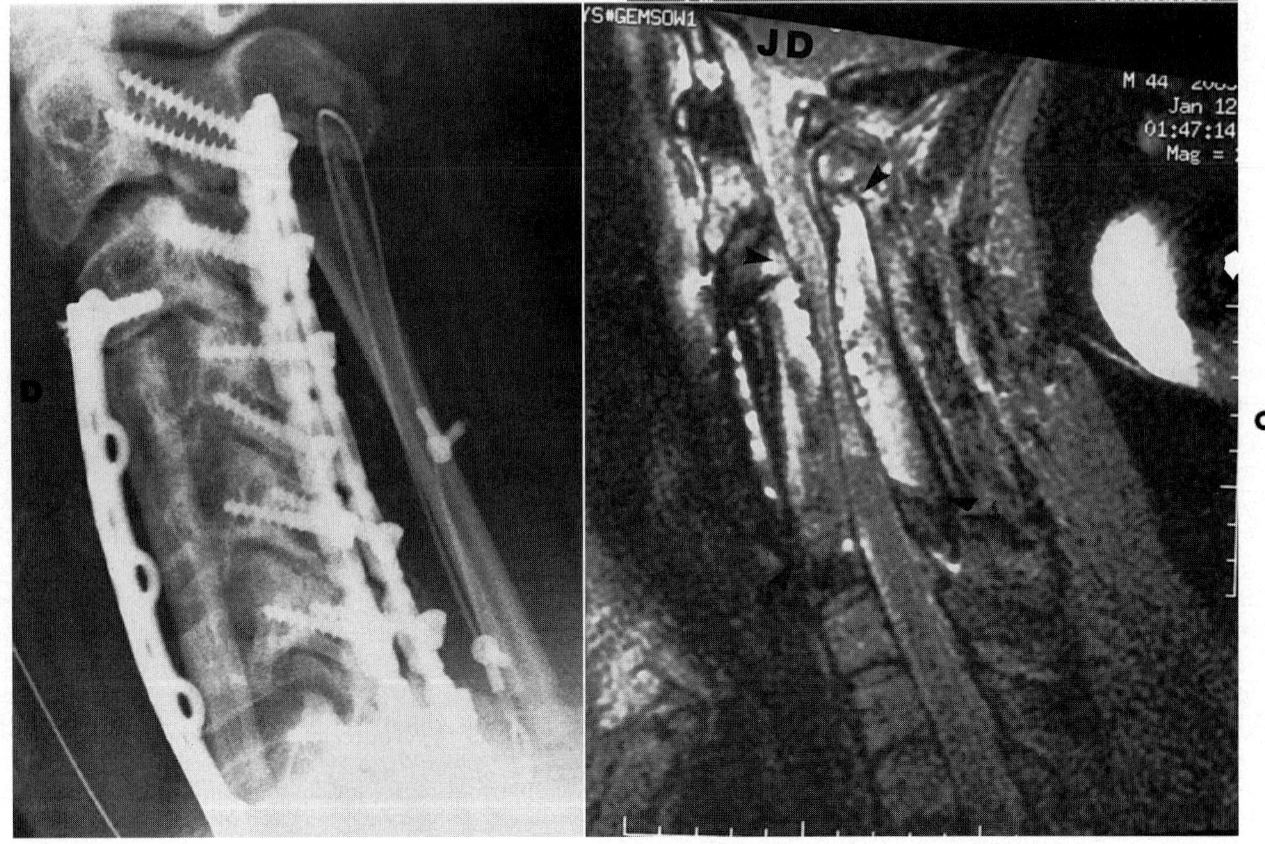

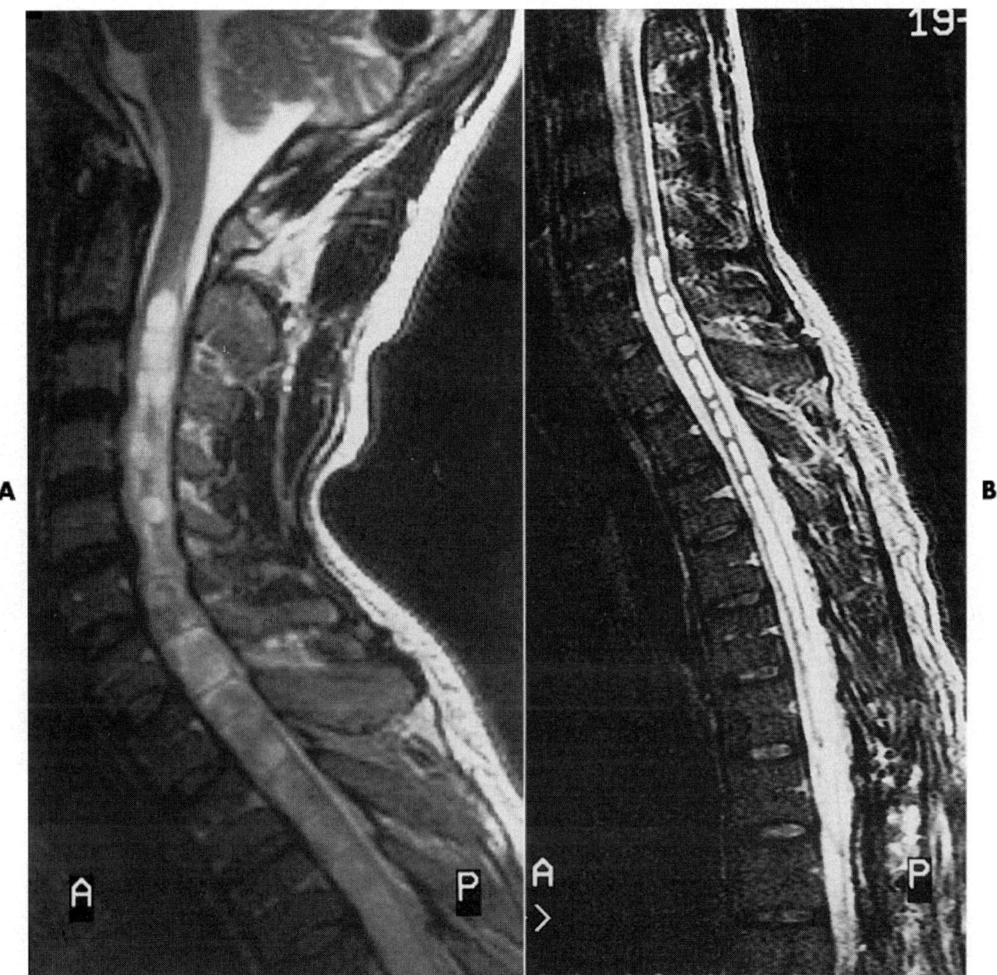


FIGURE 19-4

**A,** This MRI scan shows the cervical spine of a 57-year-old male 9 years after sustaining a gunshot wound to T8 with resulting complete spinal cord injury. He presented with progressive loss of upper extremity function and inability to breathe. The MRI scan confirmed presence of an extensive post-traumatic syrinx extending to the C2 segment. **B,** Following placement of a syringopleural shunt this MRI demonstrates collapse of the syrinx to the C7 segment. The patient was successfully weaned off the respirator and regained use of his hand function. He requires regular follow-up examinations and MRI scans to assure continued decompression of the syrinx.

age 8 years after cervical spine fusions for trauma.[33] Awareness of this risk on the part of the treating physician is important in the diagnosis of such conditions. Availability of comparison radiographs and other imaging studies from earlier treatments are helpful in assessing the rate of progression of such transfer lesions. There are currently no statistics that allow for an estimation of neurologic deficits arising from transfer lesions.

Epidural fibrosis and arachnoiditis have been associated with chronic radicular pain syndromes, although a clear etiology has not definitely been shown.[19] Treatment options are limited although antiscar formation devices may help in the future.[22,53]

Intrathecal granuloma formation has been identified as a cause of neurologic deterioration years after implantation of intrathecal morphine pumps and in presence of retained other foreign bodies such as bullets. Reimaging and intradural reexploration is recommended in such circumstances.[6,39]

In patients with complete spinal cord injuries longstanding evolving conditions may cause worsening neurologic symptoms. Presence of an epidural abscess or vertebral osteomyelitis should be ruled out. Similarly, a nonunion of a fusion may have gone unnoticed for longer than usual. Finally, a Charcot arthropathy may cause worsening neurologic symptoms if perineural cysts cause cord compression. A technetium-99 bone scan is a suitable screening tool for these conditions. Treatment of a Charcot arthropa-

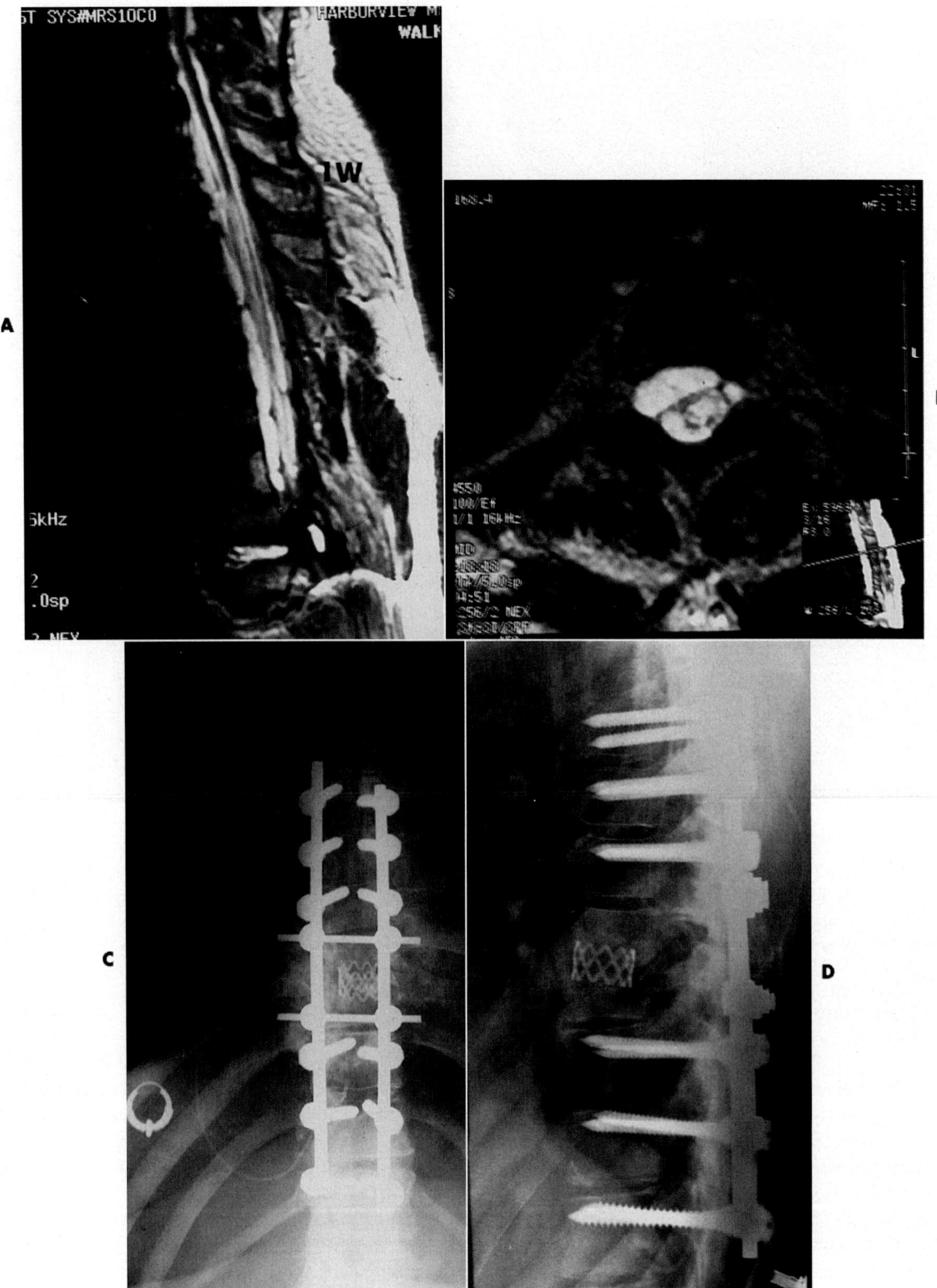


**FIGURE 19-5**

**A,** This 44-year-old man presented with loss of lower cervical strength 17 years after suffering a midthoracic spinal cord injury. The thoracic MRI scan reveals a high signal intensity at the T8-T9 disk space communication with the epidural space. **B,** Axial MRI cuts show large perineural cysts displacing the spinal cord circumferentially. **C, D,** Postoperative anteroposterior and lateral views demonstrate segmental instrumentation and cage placement into the T8-T9 disk space. An unstable Charcot arthropathy was found to have developed at T8-T9, which then decompressed a pseudarthrosis capsule into the spinal canal. The patient has regained the same neurologic level of function that he had after his initial injury.

thy is directed at resection of the destructive process and stabilization of anterior and posterior spinal columns (Fig. 19-5).

## CONCLUSIONS

Neurologic deterioration of patients undergoing spine procedures is an undesirable but to a certain degree unavoidable side effect. Timely diagnosis and intervention may reverse or ameliorate some of these events. Ignoring neurologic deterioration, however, may be associated with irreversible loss of function. The past two decades have brought a tremendous improvement of spinal instrumentation and reconstruction techniques. As surgical technologies in spine care continue to evolve rapidly, surgeons should remain aware of their patients' physiologic responses and possible associated complications. For patients with permanent neurologic deficits the hope remains that the next two decades will bring improvements in the capabilities to repair neural tissue similar to the scale of development that spinal implant technologies have experienced.

## REFERENCES

1. Alander DH, Stauffer ES: Gelfoam induced acute quadriparesis after cervical decompression and fusion, *Spine* 29(8):970-971, 1995.
2. Anderson PA, Bohlmann HH: Anterior decompression and arthrodesis of the cervical spine: long term motor involvement: II. Improvement in complete traumatic quadriplegia, *J Bone Joint Surg* 74-A:671-682, 1992.
3. Andrews RT, Koci TM: Cerebellar herniation and infarction as a complication of an occult postoperative lumbar dural defect, *Am J Neuradiol* 16(6):1312-1315, 1995.
4. Anton HA, Schweigel JF: Posttraumatic syringomyelia: the British Columbia experience, *Spine* 11(9):865-868, 1986.
5. American Spinal Injury Association: "Standards for neurological and functional classification of spinal cord injury," revised, 1992.
6. Bejjani GK, Karim NO, Tzortzidis F: Intrathecal granuloma after implantation of a morphine pump: a case report and review of the literature, *Surg Neurol* 48(3):288-291, 1997.
7. Ben David B, Haller G, Taylor P: Anterior spinal fusion complicated by paraplegia. A case report of a false-negative somatosensory evoked potential, *Spine* 12(6):536-539, 1987.
8. Ben David B: Spinal cord monitoring, *Orthop Clin North Am* 19(2):427-448, 1988.
9. Benazet JP, Thoreux P, Saillant G, Roy-Camille R: Neurologic complications of surgery of the spine in adults, *Chirurgie* 120(11):39-42, 1994.
10. Biyani A, El Masry WS. Post-traumatic syringomyelia: a review of the literature, *Paraplegia* 32:723-731, 1994.
11. Bohlmann HH, Anderson PA: Anterior decompression and arthrodesis in the cervical spine: long-term motor improvement: I. Improvement in incomplete traumatic quadriparesis. *J Bone Joint Surg* 74-A:659-670, 1992.
12. Bracken MB,Shepard MJ, Collins WF, Holford TR, Young W, Baskin DS, Eisenberg HM, Flamm E, Leo-Summers L, Maroon J, Marshall LF, Perot PL, Piepmeier J, Sonntag VKH, Wagner FC, Wilberger JE, Winn HR: A randomized, controlled trial of methylprednisolone or Naloxone in the treatment of acute spinal cord injury, *N Engl J Med* 322:1405-1411, 1990.
13. Bracken MB, Shepard MJ, Collins WF Jr, Holford TR, Baskin DS, Eisenberg HM: Methylprednisolone or naloxone treatment after acute spinal cord injury: 1-year follow-up data. Results of the Second National Spinal Cord Injury study, *J Neurosurg* 76:23-31, 1992.
14. Bradford DS, McBride GG: Surgical management of thoracolumbar spine fractures with incomplete neurologic deficits, *Clin Orthop* 218:201-216, 1987.
15. Bridwell KH, Lenke LG, Baldus C, Blanke K: Major intraoperative neurologic deficits in pediatric and spinal deformity patients: incidence and etiology at one institution, *Spine* 23 (3):324-332, 1998.
16. Chapman JR, Anderson PA: *Cervical spine trauma.* In Frymoyer JR, editor in chief: *The Adult Spine: Principles and Practice,* 2nd ed, Philadelphia, 1997, Lippincott-Raven.
17. Cloward RB: Complications of anterior cervical disc operation and their treatment, *Surgery* 69(2):175-182, 1971.
18. Davis RA: A long term outcome analysis of 984 surgically treated herniated lumbar discs, *J Neurosurg* 69: 415-421, 1994.
19. De La Porte, Siegfried J : Lumbosacral fibrosis, *Spine* 8:593-603, 1983.
20. Donaldson WF, Heil BV, Donaldson VP, Silvaggio VJ: The effect of airway maneuvers on the unstable C1-C2 segment: a cadaver study, *Spine* 22(11):1215-1218, 1997.
21. Doyle JS, Lauerman WC, Wood KB, Krause DR: Complications and outcome of upper cervical spine arthrodesis in patients with Down syndrome, *Spine* 21(10):1223-1231, 1997.
22. Einhaus SL, Robertson JT, Dohan FC, Wujek JR,

Ahmad S. Reduction of peridural fibrosis after lumbar laminectomy and discectomy in dogs by a resorbable gel (Adcon-L), *Spine* 22(13):1440-1447, 1997.

23. Federal Drug Administration: Bulletin 1/98: Complications in the use of Lovenox following spine surgery. February 1998.
24. Ford L: Local complications following spine surgery, *J Bone Joint Surg* 50-A:418-428, 1968.
25. Flynn TB: Neurologic complications of anterior cervical interbody fusion, *Spine* 7(6):536-539, 1982.
26. Goodkin R, Laska LL: *Medicolegal implications of complications of lumbar spine surgery*. In Hardy RW Jr, editor: *Lumbar disc disease,* 2nd edition. New York, 1993, Raven Press.
27. Goodkin R, Laska LL: Unintended "incidental" durotomy during surgery of the lumbar spine: Medicolegal implications, *Surg Neurol* 43:4-14, 1995.
28. Haghigi SS, York DH, Gaines RW, Oro JJ. Monitoring of motor tracts with spinal cord stimulation, *Spine* 19:1518-1524, 1994.
29. Heller JG, Viroslav S, Hudson T: Complications of posterior cervical plating, *Spine* 20:2442-2448, 1995.
30. Hoi Sang U, Wilson CB: Postoperative epidural hematoma as a complication of anterior cervical discectomy, *J Neurosurg* 49:288-291, 1978.
31. Holland NR, Kostuik JP: Continuous electromyographic monitoring to detect nerve root injury during thoracolumbar scoliosis surgery, *Spine* 22(21):2547-2550, 1997.
32. Hosono N, Yonenobu K, Ono K: Postoperative cervical pseudomeningocele with herniation of the spinal cord, *Spine* 20(19):2147-2150, 1995.
33. Jenkins LA,Capen DA, Zigler JE, Nelson RW, Nagelberg S. Cervical spine fusions for trauma. A long-term radiographic and clinical evaluation, *Orthop Rev* Suppl:13-19, 1994
34. Jodoin A, Gillet P, Dupuis PR, Maurais G: Surgical treatment of post-traumatic kyphosis: a report of 16 cases, *Can J Surg* 32(1):36-42, 1989.
35. Jones AA, Stambough JL, Balderston RA, Rothman RH, Booth RE Jr: Long term results of lumbar spine surgery complicated by unintended incidental durotomy, *Spine* 14(4):443-446, 1989.
36. Kimura S, Homma T, Uchiyama S, Yamazaki A, Imura K: Posterior migration of cervical spinal cord between split laminae as a complication of laminoplasty, *Spine* 20(11):1284-1288, 1995.
37. Kitawaga H, Itoh T, Takano H, Takakuwa K, Yamamoto N, Yamada, Tsuji H: Motor evoked potential monitoring during upper cervical spine surgery, *Spine* 14(10):1078-1083, 1989.
38. Krespi YP, Grossman BG, Berktold RE, Sisson GA: Mediastinitis and neck abscess following cervical spine fracture, *Am J Otolaryngol* 6:29-31, 1985.
39. Kuijlen JM, Herpers MJ, Beuls EA: Neurogenic claudication, a delayed complication of a retained bullet, *Spine* 22(8):910-914, 1997.
40. Lam AM: Spinal cord injury and management, *Curr Op Anesth* 5:632-639, 1992.
41. Lam AM : Acute spinal cord ischemia: implications for anesthetic management, *Adv Anesth* 10:247-273, 1993.
42. Lang EW, Beutler AS, Chesnut RM, Patel PM, Kennelly NA, Kalman CJ, Drummond JC, Garfin SR: Myogenic motor-evoked potential monitoring using partial neuromuscular blockade in surgery of the spine, *Spine* 21(14):1676-1686, 1996.
43. Levi ADO, Sonntag VKH: Management of posttraumatic syringomyelia using an expansile duraplasty. A case report, *Spine* 23(1):128-132, 1998.
44. MacEwen GD, Bunnell WP, Sriram K. Acute neurologic complications in the treatment of scoliosis, *J Bone Joint Surg* 57-A:404-408, 1975.
45. McAfee PC, Regan JR, Zdeblick T, Zuckerman J, Picetti GD 3rd, Heim S, Geis WP, Fedder IL: The incidence of complications in endoscopic anterior thoracolumbar spinal reconstructive surgery. A prospective multi center study comprising the first 100 consecutive cases, *Spine* 20(14):642-1632, 1995.
46. McNeill JW, DeWald RL, Kuo KN, Bennett EJ, Salem MR. Controlled hypotensive anesthesia in scoliosis surgery, *J Bone Joint Surg* 56-A:1167-1172, 1974.
47. Meschino A, Devitt JH, Szalai JP, Koch JP, Schwartz M. The safety of awake tracheal intubation in cervical spine injury, *Can J Anaesth* 39:114-117, 1992.
48. Mineiro J, Weinstein SL: Delayed postoperative paraparesis in scoliosis surgery. A case report, *Spine* 22(14):1668-1672, 1977.
49. Myers MA, Hamilton SR, Bogosian AJ, Smith CH, Wagner TA: Visual loss as a complication of spine surgery: a review of 37 cases, *Spine* 22(12):1325-1329, 1997.
50. Nairus JG, Richman JD, Douglas RA: Retroperitoneal pseudomeningocele complicated by meningitis following a lumbar burst fracture, *Spine* 21(9):1090-1093, 1996.
51. Naito M, Owen JH, Bridwell KH, Sugioka Y: Effects of distraction on physiologic integrity of the spinal cord, spinal cord blood flow, and clinical status, *Spine* 17:1154-1158, 1992.
52. Nash CL, Brown RH: Spinal cord monitoring. Current Concepts Review, *J Bone Joint Surg* 71-A(4): 627-630, 1989.
53. Nygaard OP, Kloster R, Dullerud R, Jacobsen EH, Wellgren SI: No association between peridural scar and outcome after lumbar microdiscectomy, *Acta Neurochir* 139:1095-1100, 1997.
54. Odgers CJ 4th, Vaccaro AR, Pollack ME, Cotler JM: Accuracy of pedicle screw placement with the assistance of lateral plain radiography, *J Spinal Disord* 9(4):334-338, 1996.
55. Robinson LR, Slimp JC, Anderson PA, Stolov WC: The efficacy of femoral nerve intraoperative somatosensory evoked potentials during surgical treatment of thoracolumbar fractures, *Spine* 18(13):1793-1797, 1993.

56. Rudisch A, Kremser C, Peer S, Kathrein A, Judmaier W, Daniaux H: Metallic artifacts in magnetic resonance imaging of patients with spinal fusion. A comparison of implant materials and imaging sequences, *Spine* 23(6):692-699, 1998.
57. Shufflebarger HL, Papazian O, Morrison G, Corredor C: SSEP changes during cordotomy. Scoliosis Research Society, 1984.
58. Spiegelmann R, Findler G, Faibel M, Ram Z, Shacked I, Sahar A: Postoperative spinal epidural empyema. Clinical and computed tomography features, *Spine* 16(10):1146-1149, 1991.
59. Stagnara P. Experience with the wake-up test in 623 cases (1970-1977). Presented to the Italian Society for Spinal Deformity, Rome, Italy, 1977
60. Stahl RS, Burstein FD, Lieponis JV, Murphy MJ, Piepmeier JM: Extensive wounds of the spine: a comprehensive approach to debridement and reconstruction, *Plast Reconstr Surg* 85(5):747-753, 1991.
61. Stevens WR, Glazer PA, Kelley SD, Lietman TM, Bradford DS. Ophthalmic complications after spinal surgery, *Spine* 22(15):1319-1324, 1977.
62. Thal GD, Szabo MD, Lopez-Breshnahan M, Crosby G: Exacerbation or unmasking of focal neurologic deficits by sedatives, *Anesthesiology* 85(1):21-25, 1996.
63. Thalgott JS, Cotler Hb, Sasso RC, La Rocca H, Gardner V. Postoperative infections in spinal implants. Classification and analysis—a multicenter study, *Spine* 16(8):981-984, 1991.
64. Tomaszek DE, Rosner MJ: Occult esophageal perforation associated with cervical spine fracture, *Neurosurgery* 14:492-494, 1984.
65. Vauzelle C, Stagnara P, Jovinroux P: Functional monitoring of spinal cord activity during spinal surgery, *Clin Orthop* 93;173-178, 1973.
66. Viola RW, King H, Adler SM, Wilson CB: Delayed infection after elective spinal instrumentation and fusion: a retrospective analysis of eight cases, *Spine* 22(20):2444-2451, 1997.
67. Williams B: Posttraumatic syringomyelia, an update, *Paraplegia* 8:296-313, 1990.
68. Winter RB, Lonstein JE, Denis F, Leonard A, Garamella J. The risk of paraplegia secondary to segmental vessel ligation: an analysis of 1197 consecutive anterior procedures, *Spine* 21:1232-1234, 1996.
69. Winter RB: Neurologic safety in spinal deformity surgery, *Spine* 22(13)1527-1533, 1977.
70. Yonenobu K, Hosono N, Iwasaki M, Asano M, Ono K: Neurologic complications of surgery for cervical compression myelopathy, *Spine* 16(11):1277-1282, 1991.
71. Zdeblick TA, Ducker TB: *Posttraumatic syringomyelia.* In Frymoyer JW, editor: *The adult spine: principles and practice,* 2nd ed, Philadelphia, 1997, Lippincott-Raven.

# 20

# WHEN NOT TO OPERATE

**Yizhar Floman, M.D.**
**Nahshon Rand, M.D.**



Spinal surgery consists of decompression of the neural elements (cord, cauda equina, and nerve roots), reconstruction of the load-bearing capacity of the vertebral column (bone grafting and internal fixation) and correction of spinal deformities. Many of these procedures are performed in concert, including spinal fusion. Failure of spinal surgery to relieve pain, improve neurologic deficit, to correct deformity, or to achieve a solid fusion may necessitate revision surgery. In some instances the index or latest surgery was successful in achieving its goals, but resulted, in due time, in adjacent-segment instability or deformity. Revision surgery may be attempted to achieve the goals of the primary surgery (i.e., decompress, fuse, correct deformity, relieve pain, and enhance neural recovery). In many instances, reoperation may be indeed successful. There are certain instances, however, in which expectations of revision surgery may be unrealistic in achieving these goals. Factors such as the general condition of the patient, ongoing pathology not amenable to surgery, severe osteopenia precluding firm internal fixation, loss of soft tissue coverage, and severe infection that can not be eradicated may preclude the possibility of safely performing revision spine surgery.

Taylor et al[41] reported that the rate of surgery for degenerative lumbar disk disease has increased by over 50% during the decade of 1980–1990. It is therefore not surprising that the rate of performance of revision surgery has also significantly increased. In major spine centers revision spine surgery accounts for more than 40% of all surgical interventions. In our own spine center 41% of all surgical interventions done for degenerative disk disease, during 1996, were revision procedures.

Because revision surgery is fraught with many complications there are certain questions to be asked before embarking on additional surgery. Is revision surgery going to achieve pain relief, promote neurological recovery, will it correct existing deformity or achieve spinal fusion and if so, can these goals be achieved with reasonable risk to the patient? If the answers to these questions are positive then revision surgery is indeed indicated. On the other hand, if these questions can not be answered positively, then revision spine surgery should not be performed.

Because of the complexity of revision spine surgery and the lack of adequate data bank in many types of revisions, it would seem logical to obtain a mandatory "second opinion" consultation prior to almost any attempt of revision.

For reasons of convenience, the discussion on when not to reoperate will be separated into several categories: failure of decompression surgery, failure to achieve fusion, failed deformity correction, failed surgery of spinal trauma, and failed tumor surgery. Although it is realized that many of the patients in need of repeat spine surgery have undergone a combination of some of the above-mentioned procedures, for the sake of simplicity these are artificially separated to different categories.

## THE SURGEON

Revision spine surgery is a complex and difficult surgery with many inherent complications including a higher possibility for infliction of neurological deficit. Therefore, this kind of surgery should be performed by a well-trained and experienced spine surgeon (with formal training in a spine fellowship program). Surgeons who perform spinal operations occasionally, rather than on a routine basis, should refrain from undertaking the highly demanding tasks of revision spine surgery.

## FAILURE OF FUSION

Modern spine surgery coincides with the first in situ posterior spine fusion as a surgical "remedy" for tuberculous spondylitis performed at the beginning of the twentieth century by Hibbs and by Ablee. Gradually spinal fusion was applied to other types of spinal pathology such as deformity correction, fracture fixation, and degenerative disk disease. The recent proliferation of modern segmental spinal instrumentation systems and in particular pedicle screw fixation, resulted in ever increasing numbers of spinal arthrodesis. Today, spinal fusion has become the most common type of spinal surgery performed.

Nevertheless, spondylodesis remains a controversial procedure, especially in the management of degenerative disorders of the spine. Although theoretically it is performed because of so-called instability, fusion does not necessarily restore segmental stability and may even result in an accelerated process of degeneration and instability, mostly in the adjacent motion segments.

Failure to achieve solid arthrodesis in the index surgery remains the leading cause for revision spine surgery.[23,33] Although pseudarthrosis may be occasionally asymptomatic[10] a better clinical outcome is usually encountered in patients in whom a solid spondylodesis was obtained.[18]

There are many factors that affect the rate of spinal fusion, such as the biomechanical environment of the fusion area (the arthrodesis area is under loading, compression, distraction, or under continuous segmental instability), local biological factors (blood supply, scarring), systemic factors (hormones, drugs, nutritional status, smoking), and bone graft factors (autograft, allograft, graft bed preparation, various growth factors). For example, osteoporosis and malnutrition, both being common conditions in the elderly, may adversely affect the ability to form a solid spine arthrodesis.[3,14] The presence of severe osteopenia may preclude the application of firm internal fixation. With severe osteopenia it is sometimes better to use laminar hooks rather than pedicle screws[8] but even this combination may eventually fail (Fig.20-1). Nonsteroidal anti-inflammatory drugs (NSAIDs), which are commonly used to control spinal pain including in the postoperative period, have been shown to interfere with bone formation and spine fusion.[26] Smoking has been shown to inhibit bone formation and the rate of spine fusion after surgery for degenerative disk disease.[34] Smokers have been found to have significantly lower fusion rates compared to nonsmokers.[5,47] Thus, before reoperation the nutritional status of the patient should be corrected, ingestion of NSAIDs should be stopped, and the patient should quit cigarette smoking. Inability of the patient to quit smoking should be considered a major drawback to revision surgery.

A careful analysis of the biological and mechanical milieu of the failed fusion (coronal and sagittal alignment as well as the type of instrumentation and the mode of application) is also mandatory when considering revision surgery.

Biological factors are also important in the success of obtaining a solid spondylodesis. Bone morphogenetic proteins (BMP) and other local growth factors are important for the bony fusion process.[45] Several of these factors are already available through recombinant protein technology. Biological manipulation of the fusion process may be possible in the very near future, obviating the need for revision surgery due to pseudarthrosis.

Recent research and limited clinical trials have focused on the role of BMP in attaining spinal arthrodesis. These preliminary reports are promising and point out that in the future spinal fusion will be obtained almost universally with minimum need for bone graft (and its associated morbidity) just by local application of BMP.

Boden and collaborators demonstrated that bovine BMP extract increased the fusion rate from 62% using autogenous iliac crest bone graft to 100% using BMP.[2] Schimandale et al showed that a fusion rate of 100% was achieved by using recombinant human BMP-2 delivered in a collagen carrier.[33] The use of osteoinductive BMPs may result in a more rapid and stronger fusion. Pseudarthrosis may then be eliminated altogether. Thus, revision surgery for failed fusion may soon become a thing of the past.

Other alternatives to refusion: direct constant current electrical stimulation and pulsating electromagnetic field coils have been used to enhance the rate of spine fusion. The use of these devices has been shown to enhance the rate of fusion in experimental animals and in human clinical trials.[25,28,35] Simmons reported on the use of pulsed electromagnetic fields in the management of failed posterior lumbar interbody fusion. Solid arthrodesis occurred in 77% of the patients within 4 months of treatment.[35] Similar results were reported by Mooney.[28] One should therefore consider the use of electric stimulation of the attempted fusion

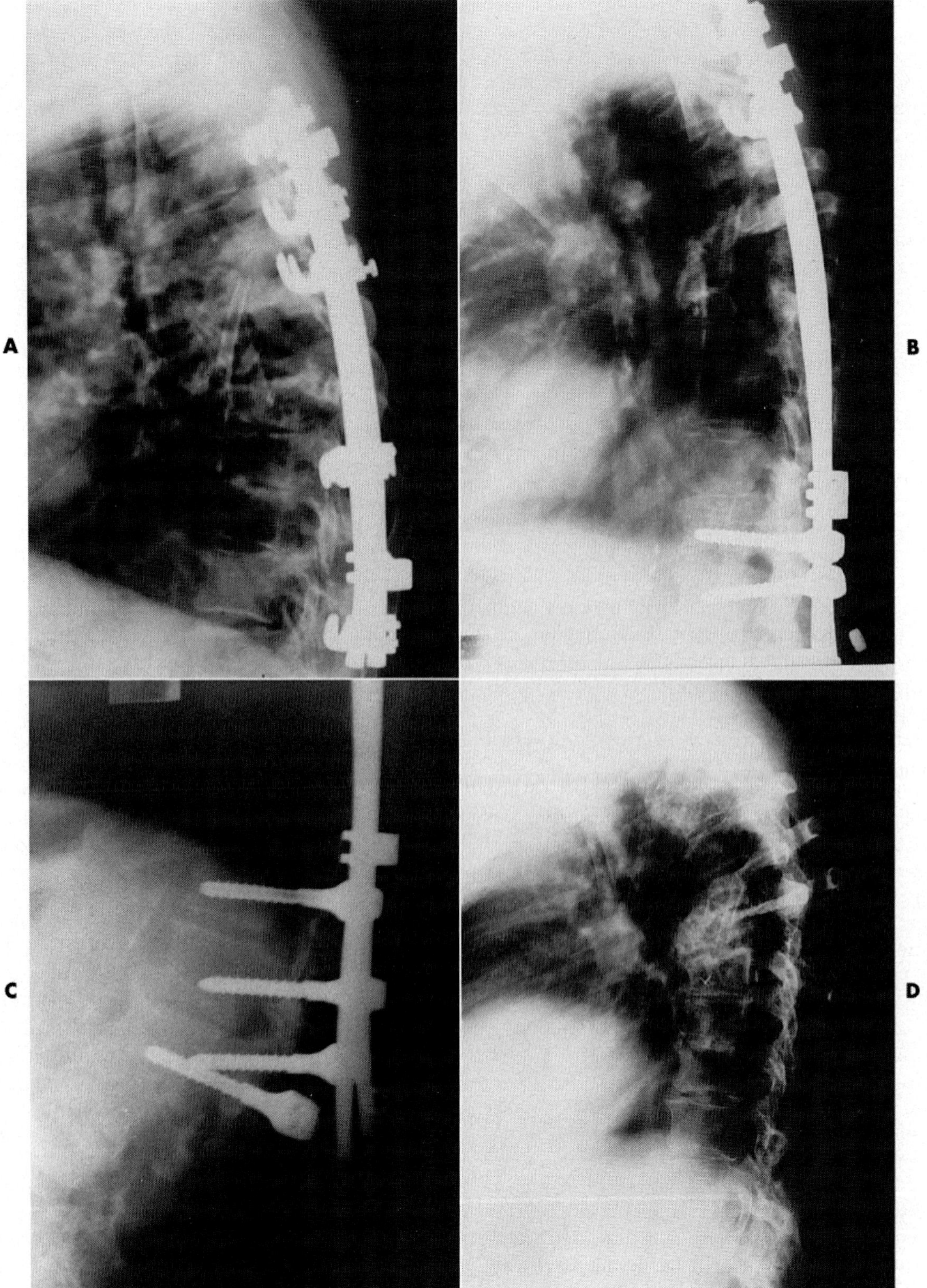


**FIGURE 20-1**

**A,** A 75-year-old woman with vertebral osteomyelitis (T6-T7) and marked paraparesis underwent anterior decompression and strut grafting as well as posterior spine fusion with instrumentation under a single anesthesia. A significant neurological recovery was observed, however pull-out of the instrumentation due to severe osteopenia was observed. Revision with proximal claw at T2-T4 and distal fixation with pedicle screws at T12, L1, and L2 **(B)** failed as well because of the marked osteopenia **(C)**. **D,** The patent was therefore managed with external support, and subsequent removal of the hardware. Although the spine has fused in marked and somewhat painful kyphosis, the infection has been eradicated and the patient has regained ambulation.

area before submitting the patient to more surgery. This is certainly true for a patient who has had several previous attempts at spinal arthrodesis, including posterior and anterior approaches.

Degenerative changes adjacent to a fusion (usually above the fusion) occur with time in up to 50% of the operated patients.[27] Most of these changes are not associated with symptoms. Careful evaluation of the patient by the managing clinician should be exercised, to ascribe these changes to the patient's persistent symptoms before embarking on more surgery. Cast immobilization test and provocative injection procedures may indicate whether these imaging abnormalities account for the patient's symptoms. Even with the use of pain-aggravating injection tests, the decision whether to reoperate and at what level may be difficult because these tests have a rather low sensitivity and specificity.

## FAILURE OF DECOMPRESSIVE SURGERY IN DEGENERATIVE DISK DISEASE

Nowhere in clinical medicine is the risk:benefit ratio closer to parity as in patients with failed surgery due to degenerative disk disease undergoing revision surgery. The final outcome of multiply operated back patients may often result in chronic back and leg pain with or without neural deficit. Repeat surgery in such a case has a high likelihood of resulting in repeat failure. In many of these cases salvage surgery may be therefore a fallacy or mirage. Success is unrealistic and impossible. At best, the patient's symptoms will remain the same, more often, however, the patient will be left worse than before the last surgical intervention.

There are many reasons for failure in degenerative spine surgery. Certain etiologies leading to failure are correctable with additional surgery, however, many etiologies are not.[16,29] It is imperative for the surgeon to be as objective as possible in evaluating the patient who is a candidate for reoperation. The surgeon who performed the index or the last operation on a patient who is now a candidate for revision, is often in the worst position to make an objective decision about the efficacy and necessity of a repeat operation.[19]

The most common causes of failure of the primary surgery can be described as the "3 Ws": wrong diagnosis, wrong patient, and wrong surgery. If the original surgery was performed on the wrong patient or because of a wrong diagnosis, or both, revision surgery is contraindicated. The wrong patient category consists of either a situation in which, by surgically addressing the demonstrated pathology, symptomatic relief can not be expected or that the patient's psychosocial background precludes favorable outcome of the surgery. It is only in the category of wrong or inadequate surgery that revision may result in some improvement. For example, if the previous surgery was performed at the wrong level, reoperation at the appropriate level will result in pain relief and improved function. Likewise, gratifying results may be obtained in cases of new (different level) or recurrent disk herniation (Fig. 20-2).[16]

Because many changes and findings on imaging studies are nonspecific and are common in nonsymptomatic individuals, one must heavily rely on correlation of symptoms with these imaging abnormalities as well as on pain provocation procedures. One should not decide on revision surgery if the diagnostic tests do not reveal the cause of persistent pain or failure. By the same token, exploration has almost no place in either primary or revision surgery (the only exception being exploration of the fusion mass). If the primary procedure was performed without validation that the pathology addressed by it was related to the patient's symptoms, then performing revision surgery to correct any abnormalities or symptoms that persisted following the primary surgery is bound to fail. The initial decision concerning the primary surgical intervention is thus the most crucial one.[38] Moreover, if the index operation is overprescribed for nonspecific nonmechanical back pain, it too is bound to fail. Therefore if there was a faulty decision to perform the original surgery, further surgery will lead to further disability and suffering. In these circumstances the decision not to reoperate may be in the best of the patient's interests no matter how "miserable" and incapacitated he or she is.

People with psychological disorders, social disarray, or both, are also poor candidates for revision surgery or the index surgery.[24,37,44] Likewise, patients involved with workman's compensation or litigation are also non-ideal candidates for this type of surgery.[42]

The availability of modern spinal fixation has enabled the revision surgeon to perform a wider, more thorough decompression without the fear of creating postoperative segmental instability. However, hopes to improve the success rate of revision surgery using modern segmental fixation have not been met yet. Although the use of modern segmental fixation is widespread and is probably associated with increased fusion rates,[47] it is technically demanding and fraught with complications and failures. A complication rate of up to 45% was reported in multiply operated backs when pedicle screw fixation was used.[15]

Early or mid-term failure, following disk or decompression surgery, may indicate that epidural fibrosis is at fault, and revision surgery should not be considered. Endoneural or perineural fibrosis, a serious sequela of lumbar decompressive surgery, results in an incurable painful radiculopathy.[43] Chronic intrinsic radiculopathy,[32] which develops after persistent nerve root compression with resultant ischemia of the nerve root, will also not respond to decompressive surgery. Likewise, symptoms arising from arachnoiditis, not to be confused with peridural fibrosis, will not be relieved by re-

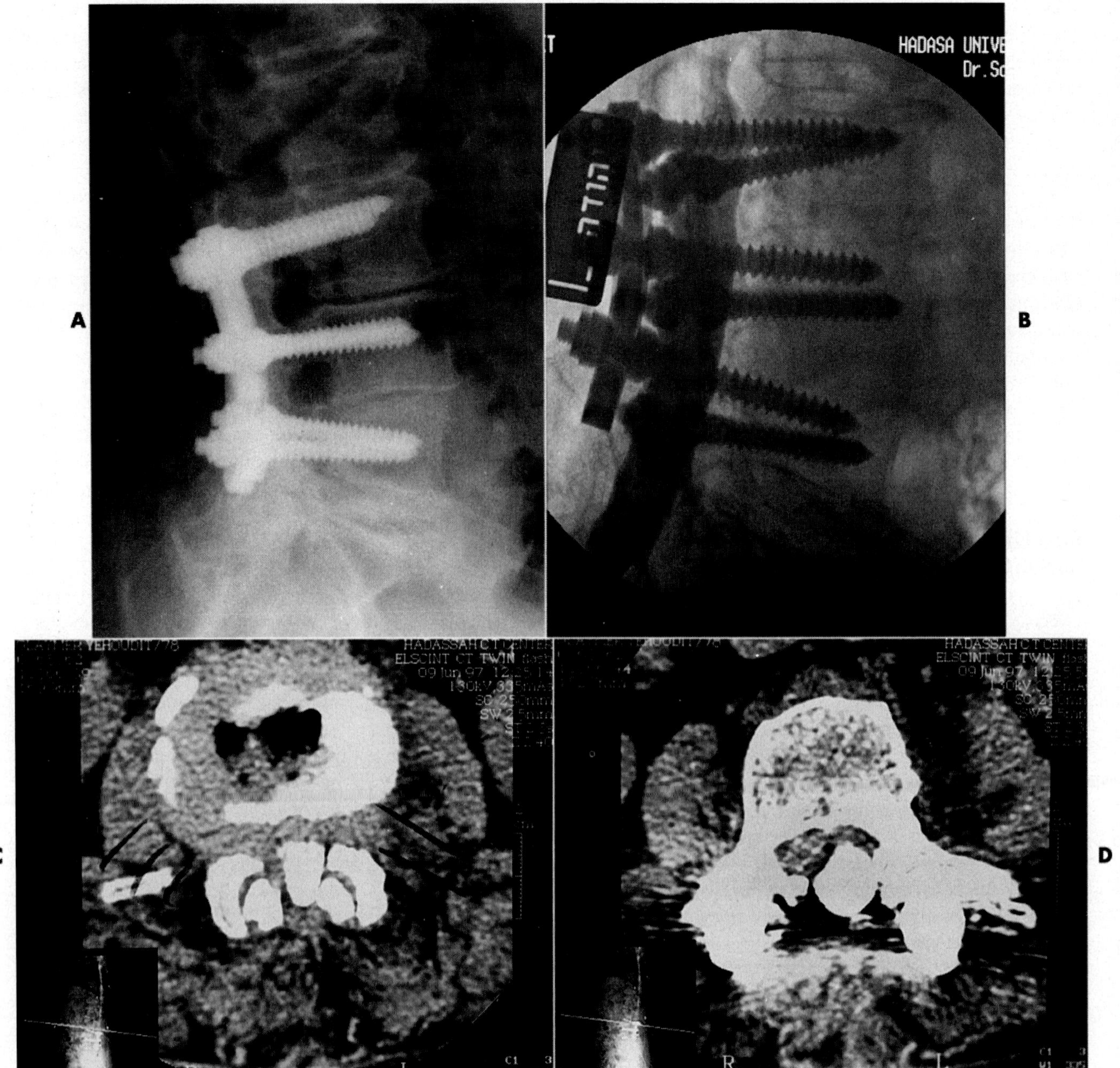

**FIGURE 20-2**

**A,** A 78-year-old woman has had three previous decompression and fusion procedures (L3-L5 with Dynalock). She presented with severe bilateral leg pain accompanied by marked proximal muscle weakness. Myelography **(B)** followed by CT revealed a massive disk herniation proximal to the instrumentation as well as a free fragment at the level of the right L3 pedicle level **(C, D).** At revision surgery multiple free disk fragments were removed.

vision surgery of any kind. According to Burton,[6] 16% of the patients with failed lumbar surgery suffer from arachnoiditis. Surgery in such circumstances is unrewarding. It is unrealistic to expect that intrinsic neural pathology will be improved by a repeat surgical intervention. In such circumstances, participation in a pain control program or implantation of spinal cord stimulation[30] should be considered as an alternative to repeat surgery. North et al[31] conducted a randomized controlled trial of spinal cord stimulation and reoperation in patients with persistent radicular pain after lumbosacral spine surgery. The primary outcome measure was the frequency of cross-over to the alternative procedure at 6-month follow up. Six months after surgery, spinal cord stimulation showed a statistically significant advantage over reoperation.[31]

## FAILURE OF SPINAL DEFORMITY CORRECTION

Failure of previous deformity correction may be due to pseudarthrosis, adding on, crankshaft phenomena, or surgeon's miscalculation. More importantly, failure to achieve coronal and sagittal balance may result in awkward posture and incapacitating back pain. The flat back syndrome and residual thoracolumbar kyphosis are well-known examples of failed attempts of deformity correction. Although idiopathic scoliosis patients with flat back syndromes are ideal candidates for revision surgery, revision of deformities secondary to congenital scoliosis, cerebral palsy, progressive muscular dystrophy, or paralytic scoliosis associated with amyotonia may be problematic.[46]

One of the major reasons for revision surgery in spinal deformities is the persistence of an unsightly and unbalanced torso deformity. It is not uncommon for the patient to have unrealistic expectations that the deformity will vanish with an additional surgical intervention. The surgeon must be sure that he or she can improve the cosmesis of the patient with minimal risk. This may be unrealistic in some patients and embarking on complicated, multistage revision surgery would be unwise. Sometimes, simple and effective thoracoplasty may be all that is needed. Resection of the prominent ribs of the hump (usually the fifth through the eleventh ribs) results in improved cosmesis, without significant risks. Most patients tolerate the procedure, and the likelihood of adversely affecting the mechanical efficiency of breathing is remote. Likewise, the surgeon must be sure that he or she can effectively rebalance the spine with minimal risk to the patient. An analysis of the causes for the lack of spinal fusion should precede the attempt at pseudarthrosis repair.

It is not rare that a fracture of a rod or screw is noted on follow-up x-rays of patients who have had deformity corrective surgery. If such a fracture is not associated with pain and the spinal deformity is stable, further surgery should not be considered. Although a pseudarthrosis was probably the cause of hardware fracture, it may have healed in the meantime, or the pseudarthrosis does not endanger the patient and, because the spinal deformity is stable, revision surgery should not be performed (Fig. 20-3). One of the most challenging types of deformity surgery is to obtain a long fusion down to the sacropelvis. Galveston-type instrumentation is the most efficient way to achieve such a fusion, especially in neuromuscular scoliosis. Nevertheless, a "windshield wiper" effect can be noted on follow-up x-rays around the iliac posts (Fig. 20-4). Although this may indicate a pseudarthrosis, the lack of symptoms in many of these cases is a contraindication for revision surgery.

The main problems leading to revision surgery are persistent pseudarthrosis, curve progression, too short fusion, adding on, and decompensation in the frontal plane or sagittal plane.[17] In addition, degenerative disk disease in the adjacent segments mainly caudal to the instrumented spine may also occur. Symptoms due to these problems are usually a combination of pain, increasing deformity, and, occasionally, progressive shortness of breath.

Patients with congenital scoliosis,[9] infantile scoliosis, or early-onset juvenile idiopathic scoliosis may have severe restrictive lung disease precluding the possibility to perform extensive reconstructive spinal surgery. Cor pulmonale is a contraindication for surgery.[4] Vital capacity of less than 25% and minute ventilation volume of less than 30% of the expected should be considered as an unacceptable high risk for revision surgery.

In adult patients with scoliosis surgical reintervention for pain reduction and improved cosmesis and function may be disappointing.[39] In view of the high risk involved and the limited benefit to patients even following the primary surgery, revision in adult patients should be considered only if a major gain is anticipated.[39]

If revision surgery for flat back syndrome is technically not feasible within the spinal column itself, pelvic osteotomy should be considered.[13]

## FAILURE OF SPINAL TRAUMA SURGERY

Revision of previously failed surgery for thoracolumbar fractures is usually the result of failure to adequately decompress the spinal canal, because of the development of posttraumatic kyphosis and as a result of failed short segment posterior fixation in bursting injuries (due to loss of anterior load sharing capacity). Less often, a simple pseudarthrosis has developed following an attempt at spinal arthrodesis. There are almost no circumstances in which the performance of revision surgery in such cases is contraindicated.[20] There are however two exceptions. In cases of incomplete decompression of a burst fracture in a neurologically intact patient, there is no need for further decompression. In elderly patients with severe osteopenia and posttraumatic kyphosis, internal fixation, including pedicle screw fixation, may fail because of the extremely poor bone purchase. The use of bone cement may enable one to perform such reconstruction.

## FAILURE OF BONE TUMOR SURGERY

There are numerous classifications that have been proposed to predict the usefulness of surgery in metastatic spine disease.[1] The variables that appear to be most consistently significant for neural recovery

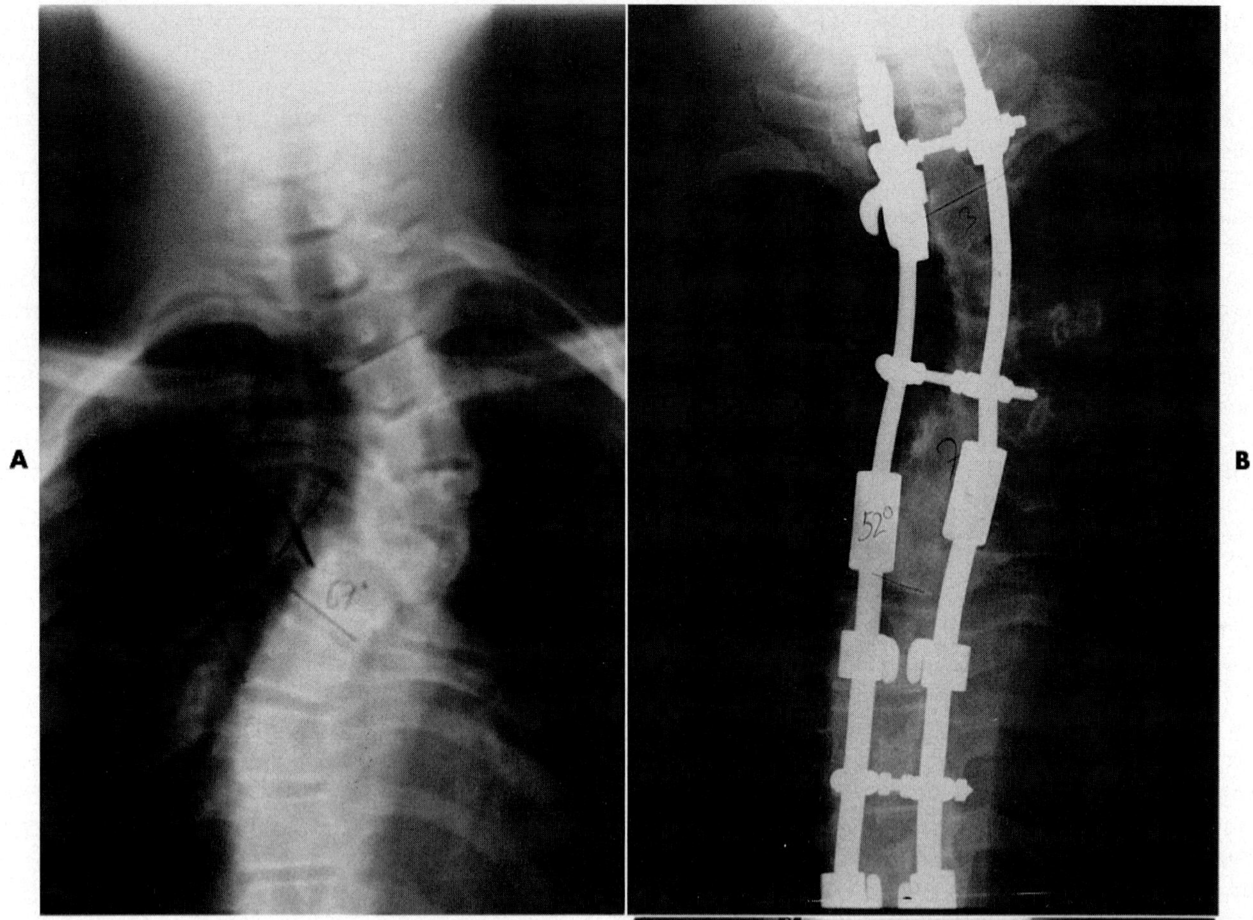

A

B

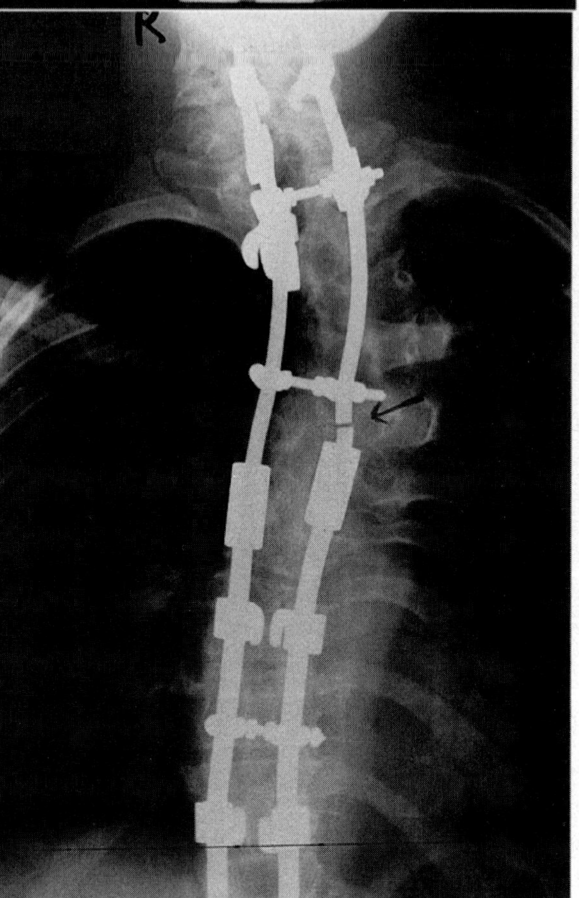

C

**FIGURE 20-3**

A 17-year-old man with dystrophic scoliosis (67 degrees) secondary to neurofibromatosis **(A),** underwent spinal fusion with instrumentation from C7 to T1 1 (a combination of pediatric and adult CD) **(B).** At 5 years following surgery, one of the pediatric 5-mm rods is broken, although the patient remains pain-free and the deformity is stable **(C).**

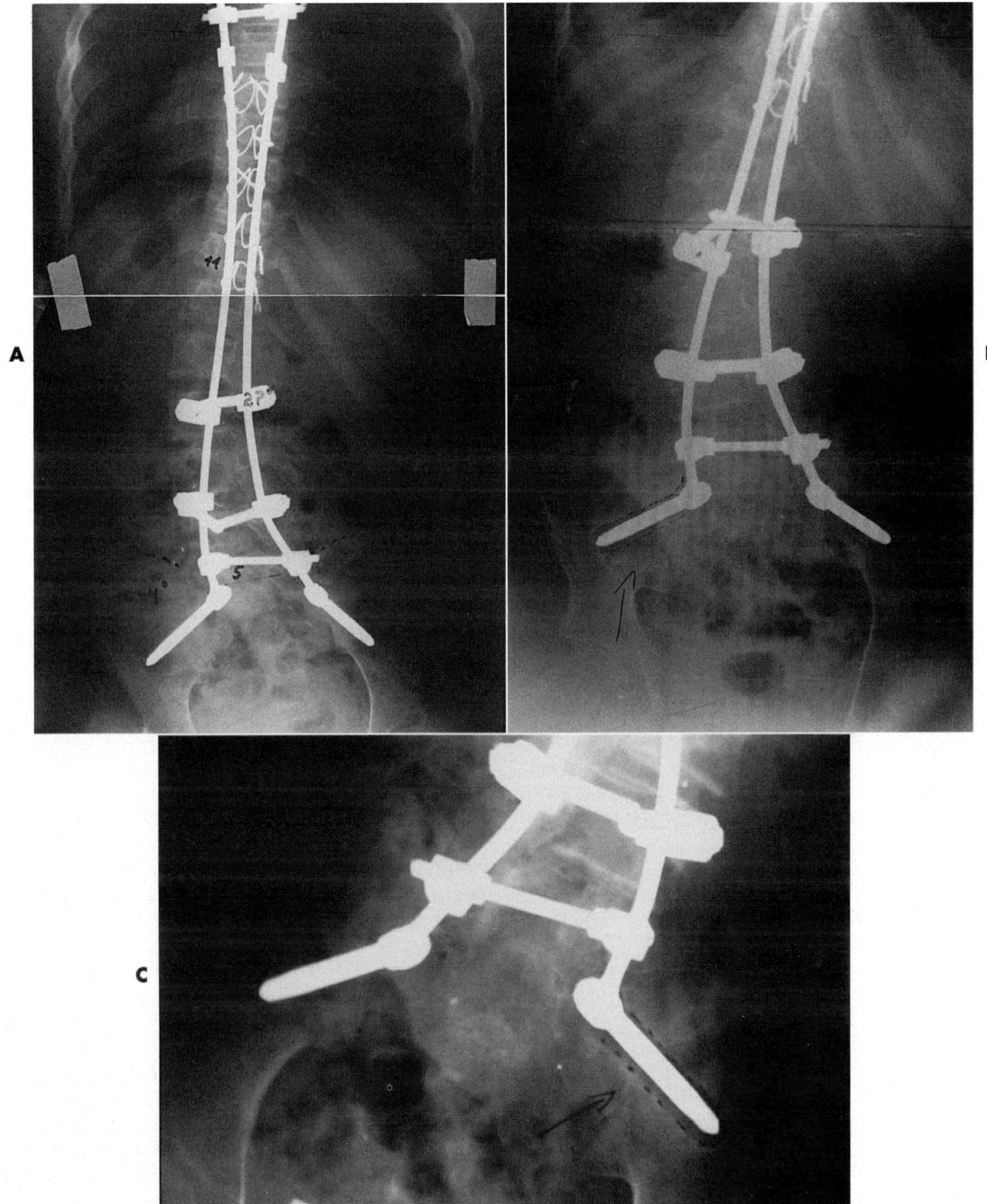

**Figure 20-4**

**A,** An 18-year-old man with scoliosis secondary to poliomyelitis, underwent anterior and posterior fusion to the sacropelvis utilizing Galveston-type iliac posts (Isola). **B, C,** Although a "windshield wiper" effect is noticed around one of the iliac screws, the patient is asymptomatic and the deformity stable.

are: pretreatment ambulatory status of the patient, rate of neurologic deterioration (the slower the better, while rapid deterioration carries the worst prognosis), the presence of normal autonomic function and the biological characteristics of the tumor.[1] The decision whether to reintervene because of tumor recurrence should be made on the basis of tumor biology, life expectancy of the patient, as well as the nutritional and immunological status of the patient.[11]

For the sake of establishing a logical and useful treatment and to estimate prognosis for patients with metastatic spine disease, DeWald et al[11] devised a classification system based on five general scenarios or classes. These classes are: (1) moderate pain with vertebral body collapse but without deformity, (2) immunocompetent patients with moderate deformity and collapse, (3) immunodeficient patients with collapse and moderate deformity, (4) immunocompetent patients with marked collapse deformity and paralysis, and (5) immunodepressed patients with marked deformity and paralysis. The latter patients (with marked deformity and collapse, paralysis, and immune depression) should probably be considered very high-risk patients for revision surgery with a dubious outcome. A decision about nonoperative treatment in such cases should be made as a joint decision by the spine surgeon and the oncologist.

Other circumstances in which revision surgery is not advocated are presence of multiple myelographic blocks, widespread metastatic disease, and prognosis for shorter than 3 months' survival.[21] One must also remember that the biological behavior of all metastases is not alike. Patients with recurrent spinal cord compression due to renal and lung carcinoma have the worst prognosis and probably are the worst candidates for revision surgery.

## GENERAL CONSIDERATIONS

In the aging population, osteopenia, associated medical comorbidities, and diminished response to attempted fusion may preclude additional corrective surgery. For example, patients with long-standing diabetes do poorly when operated on for degenerative disk disease and spinal stenosis.[36] It is also difficult to distinguish between true radicular pain and neuropathic pain due to diabetes in these patients.[29] Patients with combined neural and vascular claudication may also do poorly even after an adequate spinal canal decompression.[12,40] Patients with degenerative pathology in the cervical, thoracic, and lumbar spine may also do poorly after revision because their pathology is widespread and is beyond surgical remedy. On the other hand, advanced age per se is not a contraindication for revision spine surgery.

## REHABILITATION

Constant pain and an inability to function normally lead to inactivity and to physiological and structural changes. Although most patients expect to return to near normal functioning following decompression and/or fusion surgery, many patients may continue to suffer from the same symptoms as before surgery. These symptoms will lead to impaired lower extremity and trunk mobility, impaired muscle strength, and impaired cardiovascular fitness. These alterations may be further compounded by the patient's fear of injuring themselves, thus leading to even poorer functional outcome.

With some patients, a rehabilitation program may be mandatory before any consideration is given for revision surgery. Impairment in trunk function can be improved in the presence of chronic pain and should not result in increased pain or disability.[22] Likewise, cardiovascular conditioning is vital in patients with failed back surgery. Cardiovascular rehabilitation will increase the pain threshold, decrease secondary depression, and enable the patient to exercise with more will and less pain and fatigue.[7]

## CONCLUSIONS

Revision spine surgery is a complex surgery with many, sometimes serious, complications. The decision to reoperate should be made only after serious consideration of the alternatives and the efficacy of such an endeavor. Factors such as ongoing pathology that will not be influenced by additional surgery, serious medical comorbidity, epidural fibrosis and/or arachnoiditis, psychological overlay, and severe osteopenia usually signify that revision surgery should not be contemplated.

If reoperation results in a "better looking" x-ray, but fails to relieve pain or enhance functional restoration, then revision surgery should not be undertaken. Likewise, if the risk:benefit ratio of the procedure is such that more complications are likely to occur than successes that bring patient satisfaction, surgery should be avoided.

## REFERENCES


1. Asoudrian PL: *Metastatic disease of the spine.* In Bridwell KH, DeWald RL, editors: *Textbook of spinal surgery,* ed 2, Philadelphia, 1997, Lippincott-Raven, pp 2007-2051.
2. Boden SD, Schimandale JH, Hutton WC: Lumbar intertransverse-process spinal arthrodesis with use of a bovine bone-derived osteoinductive protein. A preliminary report, *J Bone Joint Surg* 77A:1404-1417, 1995.
3. Boden SD and Schimandale JH: *Biology of lumbar fusion and bone graft materials.* In *The lumbar spine,* ed 2, International Society for the Study of the Lumbar Spine, Philadelphia, 1996, Saunders, p 1289.
4. Bowen RM: *Respiratory management in scoliosis.* In Lonstein JE, Bradford DS, Winter RB, Oglievi JW, editors: *Moe's textbook of scoliosis and other spinal deformities,* ed 3, Philadelphia, 1995, Saunders, pp 576.
5. Brown CW, Orme TJ, Richardson D: The rate of pseudoarthrosis in patients who are smokers and patients who are non smokers: a comparison study, *Spine* 11:942-943, 1986.
6. Burton CV: Lumbosacral arachnoiditis, *Spine* 3:24-27, 1978.
7. Chocron S, Etievent JP, Viel JF: Prospective study of quality of life before and after open heart operations, *Ann Thorac Surg* 61:153-157, 1996.
8. Coe JD, Warden KE, Herzig MA, McAfee PC: Influence of bone mineral density on the fixation of thoracolumbar implants: a comparative study of transpedicular screws, laminar hooks, and spinous process wires, *Spine* 15:902-907, 1990.
9. Day GA, Upadhyay SS, Ho EKW, Leong JCY, Ip M: Pulmonary functions in congenital scoliosis, *Spine* 19:1027-1031, 1994.
10. DePalma AF, Rothman RH: The nature of pseudoarthrosis, *Clin Orthop* 59:113-118, 1968.
11. DeWald RL, Bridwell KH, Prodromas C, Rodts MF: Reconstructive spinal surgery as palliation for metastatic malignancies of the spine, *Spine* 10:21-26, 1985.
12. Dodge LD, Bohlmann HH, Rhodes RS: Concurrent lumbar spinal stenosis and peripheral vascular disease: a report of 9 patients, *Clin Orthop* 230:141-148, 1988.
13. Doherty JH: Complications of fusion in lumbar scoliosis, *J Bone Joint Surg* 55A:438 (abstract), 1973.
14. Einhorn TA, Bonnarens F, Burstein HA: The contribution of dietary protein and minerals to the healing of experimental fractures. A biomechanical study, *J Bone Joint Surg* 68A:1389-1395, 1986.
15. Esses SI, Sachs BL, Dreyzin V: Complications associated with the technique of pedicle screw fixation. A selected survey of ABS members, *Spine* 18:2231-2238, 1993.
16. Finnigan WJ, Fenlin JM, Marvel JP, Nardini RJ, Rothman RH: Results of surgery in the symptomatic multiply operated back patient: analysis of 67 cases followed 3-7 years, *J Bone Joint Surg* 61A:1077-1082, 1979.
17. Floman Y, Penny JN, Micheli LJ, Riseborough EJ, Hall JE: Osteotomy of the fusion mass in scoliosis, *J Bone Joint Surg* 64A:1307-1316, 1982.
18. Frymoyer JW, Hanley EN, Howe J, Kuhlmann D, Matteri RE: A comparison of radiographic findings in fusion and non fusion ten years or more after lumbar disc surgery, *Spine* 4:435-440, 1979.
19. Gill K, Frymoyer JW: *Management of treatment failures after decompressive surgery.* In Frymoyer JW, editor: *The adult spine: principles and practice,* ed 2, Philadelphia, 1997, Lippincott-Raven, p 2112.
20. Glassman SD, Farcy JPC: *Late deformities.* In Floman Y, Farcy JPC, Argenson C, editors: *Thoracolumbar spine fractures,* Philadelphia, 1993, Raven Press, pp 449-462.
21. Hammemberg KW: Surgical treatment of metastatic spine disease, *Spine* 17:1148-1153, 1992.
22. Hazard RG, Fenwick JW, Kalisch SM, Redmond J, Reeves V, Reid S, Frymoyer JW: Functional restoration with behavioral support. a one year prospective study of patients with chronic low back pain, *Spine* 14: 157-161, 1989.
23. Heggeness MH, Esses SI: Classification of pseudoarthroses of the lumbar spine, *Spine* 16:S249-S254, 1991.
24. Hurme M, Alaranta H: Factors predicting the results of surgery for lumbar intervertebral disc herniation, *Spine* 12:933-938, 1987.
25. Kahanovitz N, Arnoczky SP, Nemzek J, Shores A: The effect of electromagnetic pulsing on posterior lumbar spinal fusions in dogs, *Spine* 19:705-709, 1994.
26. Lebwohl NH, Starr JK, Milne EL, Latta LL, Malinin TI: Inhibitory effect of ibuprofen on spinal fusion in rabbits. American Academy of Orthopedic Surgeons Annual Meeting, New Orleans 1994, p. 278.
27. Lehmann TR, Spratt KF, Tozzi J: Long term follow-up of lower lumbar fusion patients, *Spine* 12:97-104, 1987.
28. Mooney V: A randomized double-blind prospective study of the efficacy of pulsed electromagnetic fields for interbody lumbar fusions, *Spine* 15:708-712, 1990.
29. Naftulin S, Fast A, Thomas M: Diabetic lumbar radiculopathy: sciatica without disc herniation, *Spine* 18:2419-2422, 1993.
30. North RB, Ewend MG, Lawton MT, Kidd DH, Piantadosi S: Failed back surgery syndrome: 5 year follow up after spinal cord stimulation implantation, *Neurosurgery* 28:692-699, 1991.
31. North RB, Kidd DH, Piantadosi S: Spinal cord stimulation versus reoperation for failed back surgery syndrome: a prospective, randomized study design, *Acta Neurochir.* Suppl64:106-108, 1995.
32. Rydevik B, Brown MD, Lundborg G: Pathoanatomy and pathophysiology of nerve root compression, *Spine* 9:7-15, 1984.
33. Schimandale JH, Boden SD, Hutton WC: Experi-

mental spinal fusion with recombinant human bone morphogenetic protein-2, *Spine* 20:1326-1337, 1995.

34. Silcox DH, Daftari T, Boden SD, Schimandale JW, Hutton W, Whitesides TE: The effect of nicotine on spine fusion, *Spine* 20:1549-1553, 1995.
35. Simmons JW: Treatment of failed posterior lumbar interbody fusion of the spine with pulsed electromagnetic fields, *Clin Orthop* 193:127-132, 1985.
36. Simpson JM, Silveri CP, Balderstone RA, Simeone FA, An HS: The results of operations on the lumbar spine in patients who have diabetes mellitus, *J Bone Joint Surg* 75A:1823-1829, 1993.
37. Spengler D, Freeman CW: Patient selection for lumbar discectomy: an objective approach, *Spine* 4:129-134, 1979.
38. Spengler DM, Freeman C, Westbrook R, Millar JW: Low back pain following multiple lumbar spine procedures. Failure of initial selection, *Spine* 3:356-360, 1980.
39. Sponseller PD, Cohen MS, Nachemson AL, Hall JE, Wohl ME: Results of surgery for adults with idiopathic scoliosis, *J Bone Joint Surg* 69:667-675, 1987.
40. Stansby G, Evans G, Shieff C, Hamilton G: Intermittent claudication due to spinal stenosis in a vascular surgical practice, *J Royal Coll Surg Edinb* 39:83-85, 1994.
41. Taylor VM, Deyo RA, Cherkin DC, Kreuter W: Low back pain hospitalization: recent United States trends and regional variations, *Spine* 19:1207-1213, 1994.
42. Waddell G, Kummel EG, Lotto WN, et al: Failure of lumbar disc surgery and repeat surgery following industrial injuries, *J Bone Joint Surg* 61A:201-207, 1979
43. Wetzel FT, LaRocca H: The failed posterior lumbar interbody fusion, *Spine* 16:839, 1991.
44. Wiltse LL, Rocchio HL, Borenstein DG: Preoperative psychological tests as predictors of successes of chemonucleolysis in the treatment of low back syndrome, *J Bone Joint Surg* 57A:478, 1975.
45. Wozney JM: Bone morphogenetic proteins, *Prog Growth Factor Res* 1:267-280, 1989.
46. Wright M, DeWald RL: *Flat back syndrome*. In Margulies JY, Floman Y, Farcy JCP, Neuwirth MG, editors: *Lumbosacral and spinopelvic fixation*, Philadelphia, 1996, Lippincott-Raven, p 698.
47. Zdeblick TA: A prospective, randomized study of lumbar fusion. Preliminary results, *Spine* 18:983-991, 1993.

# 21

# DECISION MAKING AND PERIOPERATIVE CARE OF THE PATIENT

**Vincent J. Devlin, M.D.**
**Denise A. Williams, R.N.**



The outlook for patients requiring revision spinal surgery is better today as a result of advances in spinal instrumentation, anesthesia, and perioperative care. Delivery of complex spine care is challenging within our current health care system. Comprehensive preoperative assessment, adequate personnel and institutional support, and a coordinated multidisciplinary team approach are essential for achieving a successful outcome in revision spinal procedures. The perioperative care of the patient undergoing revision spinal surgery will be evaluated with respect to preoperative evaluation, intraoperative care, and postoperative management. Our goal is to examine possible methods to minimize complications and improve outcome for patients requiring revision surgery.

## PREOPERATIVE PHASE

### Patient Assessment

Patient selection is the most important variable in spinal surgery that is under control of the spinal surgeon. Patient assessment involves a thorough and comprehensive evaluation of the factors that resulted in a less than optimal outcome following the initial procedure. It is helpful to assess whether the presenting problem can be attributed to decision-making errors or technical difficulties[15] relating to the initial surgical procedure (Box 21-1). If a poor surgical outcome can be attributed to initial errors in surgical strategy or surgical technique with respect to the index procedure, revision surgery may provide a reasonable chance of improved outcome. However, surgical failures attributed to errors in diagnosis or inappropriate patient selection for surgical treatment may not have an improved outcome if further surgery is performed. Accurate diagnosis and definition of the patient's problem is the goal of the initial patient assessment.

> **Box 21-1. Decision-Making Versus Technical Errors in Spinal Reconstructive Surgery[15]**
>
> **Decision-Making Errors**
> Wrong patient
> Wrong diagnosis
> Wrong procedure
> - Procedure inadequate to address all aspects of patient's spinal pathology
> - Improper fusion level selection
> - Failure to provide anterior column support when necessary
>
> **Technical Errors**
> Inadequate decompression
> Decompression at wrong level
> Neural impingement by fixation devices
> Failure to maintain or restore lumbar lordosis
> Failure to provide anterior column support when necessary
> Unstable instrumentation construct
> Facet joint impingement or soft tissue disruption at end of instrumentation construct leading to transitional syndrome

## History

Evaluation begins with a detailed history including the nature and duration of symptoms prior to the index procedure. The patient's response to prior surgical procedures both in the immediate postoperative period as well as over time is assessed. Are the patient's symptoms the same, better, or worse following surgery? Are the current symptoms similar or different from those present before surgery? The health care provider must be sensitive and knowledgeable regarding the wide range of spinal pathology that may present in various age groups and appropriately focus evaluation on pertinent issues. The assessment of the pediatric patient with a less-than-optimal result following spinal deformity surgery will differ markedly from evaluation of the senior citizen with persistent axial and radicular pain following surgery for spinal stenosis. It is important to define the patient's chief complaint and tailor subsequent evaluation to determine whether this problem is amenable to surgical treatment or best treated by other means. Spinal deformity, neurologic dysfunction, axial, and/or radicular pain as well as cosmetic concerns may present singularly or in combination. The severity of the patient's symptoms can be estimated by their effect on activities of daily living including work and recreational pursuits. Factors that aggravate and relieve patient symptoms should be determined. It is important to have a realistic assessment of a patient's function preoperatively and consider this in surgical decision making. Prior treatment including medication, orthoses, physical therapy, and injection treatments should be documented. Details of prior surgical procedures including operative reports and prior imaging studies should be obtained and reviewed. A thorough medical history is mandatory. Tobacco is a contributing factor to failure of fusion and has been linked to progressive disk degeneration. It is desirable that smoking be discontinued prior to revision surgery. Assessment of the patient's psychosocial circumstances and expectations regarding future treatment are important. The patient's present work situation and the status of possible compensation claims and litigation merit consideration.

## Physical Examination

The patient's overall medical condition requires assessment. Patients with a history of significant medical problems or patients over age 40 should be evaluated by an internist prior to surgical scheduling. The patient's overall spinal alignment is assessed in both the coronal and sagittal plane. Spinal range of motion is evaluated. A general neurologic assessment is routinely performed. Physical examination is tailored to the particular spinal pathology under evaluation. When cervical spine disorders are evaluated, shoulder pathology, brachial plexus disorders, and conditions involving the peripheral nerves should not be overlooked as a potential source of symptoms. When evaluating lumbar spine problems, the hip joints, sacroiliac joints, and prior bone graft sites should be evaluated. Examination of peripheral pulses is routinely performed to rule out vascular insufficiency.

## Diagnostic Imaging

Prior imaging studies are reviewed and correlated with the patient's present clinical symptoms. Erect plain radiographs provide assessment of the extent, level, and type of prior surgery. Important information may be obtained regarding prior laminectomy defects, fusion masses, spinal fixation devices, spinal deformities, and degenerative changes adjacent to previously operated spinal levels. Assessment of spinal deformities is best accomplished with standing 36-inch posteroanterior (PA) and lateral radiographs. Recumbent anteroposterior (AP) side-bending films or push-prone films are useful for assessing flexibility of coronal plane spinal deformities. Hypertension lateral radiographs are utilized to assess flexibility of sagittal plane spinal deformities. Lateral flexion-extension views may be useful in demonstrating postoperative lumbar spinal instability or pseudarthrosis. Magnetic resonance imaging (MRI) or computed tomography (CT) myelography may be indicated depending upon the patient's symptoms, the presence or absence of spinal implants, and the specific spinal problem requiring evaluation. MRI provides optimal visualization of the neural elements and associated bony and soft tissue structures. However, MRI quality is subject to degradation by metal artifact that may arise from microscopic metal debris remaining at the initial surgical site or from spinal implants especially if the latter are non-titanium implants. CT myelography is of great utility in evaluating the previously operated spine, especially in the presence of spinal deformity or extensive metallic spinal implants. Other imaging studies that are occasionally utilized are bone scans, diskography, and selective nerve root blocks. Bone mineral density studies may be used to document osteopenia and guide preoperative treatment for patients with coexistent metabolic bone disease.

## DECISION MAKING AND SURGICAL INDICATIONS

The physician must form an opinion as to the etiology of the patient's problem and decide whether further surgery should be considered. Commonly encountered reasons for poor outcomes following initial spinal procedures include: (1) poor patient selection for initial surgery, (2) failure to make the correct initial diagnosis, (3) inappropriate surgical indications, and (4) technical problems related to the index procedure. Alternatively, it may be apparent that a poor outcome was due to an unavoidable complication of appropriately performed surgery or that the problem arose due to progression of an underlying disease process. Fusion procedures (Table 21-1) and decompression procedures (Box 21-2) each have their own specific complications and modes of failure. Kostuik[15,16] has stressed the importance of the time of presentation of the patient's symptoms relative to the index surgical procedure. Did the patient report a

### BOX 21-2. CLASSIFICATION OF FAILURES AFTER SPINAL DECOMPRESSION PROCEDURES[15]

**1. Lack of improvement immediately after surgery with persistent or unchanged radicular symptoms**

*A Wrong preoperative diagnosis*
- Tumor
- Infection
- Metabolic disease
- Psychosocial causes
- Discogenic pain syndrome
- Decompression performed too late

*B Technical error*
- Surgery performed at wrong level(s)
- Inadequate decompression performed
- Missed disk fragment
- Failure to treat both spinal stenosis and disk protrusion when necessary
- Conjoined nerve root

**2. Temporary relief with recurrence of pain**

*A Early recurrence of symptoms (within 6 weeks)*
- Hematoma
- Infection
- Meningeal cyst

*B Midterm failure (6 weeks to 6 months)*
- Recurrent disk herniation
- Stress fracture of pars interarticularis
- Battered root syndrome
- Arachnoiditis
- Unrealistic patient expectation regarding surgical outcome

*C Long-term failure (greater than 6 months)*
- Recurrent stenosis
- Adjacent level stenosis
- Instability

**Table 21-1. Classification of Failures After Spinal Fusion Procedures[16]**

| Time of Appearance | Back Pain Predominant | Leg Symptoms Predominant |
|---|---|---|
| **Early (weeks)** | Infection<br>Wrong level fused<br>Insufficient levels fused<br>Psychosocial distress | Neural impingement by fixation devices<br>Foraminal stenosis due to change in spinal alignment (e.g., after spinal osteotomy) |
| **Midterm (months)** | Pseudarthrosis<br>Adjacent level degeneration<br>Sagittal imbalance<br>Graft donor site pain<br>Inadequate reconditioning<br>Fixation loose, displaced or broken | Neural compression due to pseudarthrosis<br>Adjacent level degeneration<br>Graft donor site pain |
| **Long-term (years)** | Pseudarthrosis<br>Adjacent level instability<br>Acquired spondylolysis<br>Abutment syndrome<br>Compression fracture adjacent to fusion<br>Adjacent level degeneration | Adjacent level stenosis<br>Adjacent level disk herniation |

pain-free interval following surgery? What time period elapsed between surgery and the recurrence of symptoms? For example, if a patient reports no immediate improvement in symptoms following a decompression procedure, one must consider whether the wrong diagnosis has been made or the wrong procedure has been performed. In the patient who describes immediate relief of symptoms followed by recurrent symptoms within weeks to months after surgery, new pathology or a complication of the index procedure must be considered. In the patient who reports good relief of symptoms for months to years following the index procedure and subsequently presents with recurrent symptomatology, a pseudarthrosis, new pathology, or a problem arising due to a degenerative process occurring adjacent to the previously operated levels should be considered.

In certain circumstances the need for additional surgery is obvious whereas in other cases the indications are less certain. Surgical decision making should proceed only after all attempts have been made to diagnose the problem as precisely as possible. A clear diagnosis-symptom relationship should be established. Decision making should consider the natural history of the specific spinal pathology requiring treatment. The risk-benefit ratio should favor the decision for surgery. The patient should be able to safely undergo a procedure of the magnitude that is proposed. The condition requiring surgery should be responsible for significant functional limitation, pain, or deformity. Failure to perform surgery should have adverse consequences for the patient in the present or future. The proposed surgical procedure should have a reasonable chance of improving patient function, decreasing pain, and/or improving spinal deformity.

Following comprehensive assessment, revision surgery may be a reasonable and desirable consideration. The indications for surgical intervention will generally fall into one or more of the following categories:

1) Decompression may be required to relieve encroachment upon the spinal cord and/or nerve roots that has persisted following prior procedures or has developed subsequent to prior spinal procedures.
2) Spinal realignment may be indicated if a spinal deformity is present that requires correction and/or stabilization. Indications for surgery include unacceptable kyphotic deformities, progressive deformities, and deformities associated with neurologic deficit or chronic pain.
3) Spinal stabilization may be required if pain, deformity progression, or neurologic compromise is attributed to compromise of the load-carrying capacity of the spinal column.
4) Adjunctive procedures may be required for a variety of miscellaneous problems. For example, surgery may be needed to remove broken or loose spinal instrumentation. Cosmetic concerns may be addressed through a variety of procedures such as thoracoplasty for persistent thoracic deformity or scar revision for a cosmetically unacceptable surgical incision. Occasionally soft tissue coverage procedures may be indicated for soft tissue defects arising as a result of wound infection or following radiation therapy.

**BOX 21-3. BASIC PRINCIPLES OF REVISION SPINE SURGERY**

1. Adequate preoperative assessment
2. Optimization for fusion including smoking cessation
3. Perform definitive surgical procedures (combined anterior and posterior procedures often required)
4. Complete neural decompression
5. Restoration or maintenance of sagittal alignment
6. Adequate internal fixation
7. Autogenous bone graft used somewhere within the construct
8. Appropriate postoperative immobilization
9. Postoperative rehabilitation

Careful preoperative planning is essential before arriving at a specific surgical treatment plan (Box 21-3). The proposed surgical procedure should be comprehensive in nature and attempt to address the patient's problem in such a manner that, in most cases, the need for further surgery is unlikely. Revision surgery for spinal deformity problems is extremely challenging and decision making requires considerable experience and expertise in complex reconstructive spinal surgery (see Table 21-2 and Figs. 21-3 through 21-5).

## SCHEDULING PROCESS FOR REVISION SPINAL SURGERY

Once the decision has been made to pursue surgical treatment, the patient enters the next phase of evaluation. Depending on the protocols of the specific institution, the nurse coordinator, spine surgeon, physician assistant, and other office health care providers work together to coordinate future care.[2] It is beneficial to have a designated health care provider other than the spinal surgeon who can function as the patient's primary contact person and surgery coordinator during this process. Issues that require attention during the scheduling process include: (1) facilitation of appropriate interdisciplinary evaluation to confirm that the patient is a reasonable medical candidate for surgery; (2) coordination of the technical requirements for surgical procedures (e.g., special instrumen-

**Table 21-2. Salvage and Reconstructive Surgery for Spinal Deformities[3,6,8,9,13,17–20,27,32,35,36,41]**

| Presenting Problem | Surgical Solutions |
|---|---|
| Simple pseudarthrosis | Posterior fusion with compression instrumentation |
| Complex pseudarthrosis (Charcot arthropathy, kyphosis, lumbosacral junction) | Anterior and posterior fusion with posterior instrumentation ± anterior instrumentation |
| Proximal fusion extension required | Posterior spinal instrumentation with proximal fusion extension |
| Distal fusion extension required | Posterior spinal instrumentation and distal fusion extension. Anterior fusion required if pseudarthrosis present or fusion requires extension to sacrum |
| Patient fused out of balance in sagittal plane (postsurgical flat back) | Posterior spinal osteotomy ± anterior fusion/osteotomy (Smith-Peterson vs. decancellation type) |
| Patient fused out of balance in coronal and sagittal planes | Multiple anterior and posterior osteotomies vs. vertebral column resection procedure |
| Crankshaft phenomenon | Anterior fusion vs. anterior and posterior spinal osteotomies |
| Residual rib prominence | Thoracoplasty |

tation, spinal monitoring, allograft); and (3) patient education regarding diagnosis, treatment, and eventual recovery.

The patient's overall medical status requires assessment prior to surgery. A detailed medical history and current medication history is obtained. The use of aspirin and/or nonsteroidal anti-inflammatory medication should be discontinued within 2 weeks prior to surgery to avoid potential bleeding problems due to these agents. Patients who use tobacco are advised of the need to stop smoking due to the adverse effects of nicotine on healing of spinal fusion as well as the increased rate of pulmonary complications in smokers following surgery.[4] Preoperative testing may include complete blood count (CBC), electrolytes, coagulation profile, electrocardiogram (ECG), chest radiographs, and pulmonary function tests as indicated. A preoperative nutritional assessment is obtained and further treatment based upon the magnitude of the planned surgical procedures and the patient's general health status. Preoperative risk assessment by a pediatrician or internist is generally obtained prior to surgery. Patients who are anticipated to require postoperative intensive care unit or ventilatory support are generally assessed by a pulmonary or intensive care specialist. These patients include those with impaired pulmonary function prior to surgery, patients undergoing same-day multilevel anteroposterior spinal procedures, and patients undergoing extensive anterior cervical procedures due to the risk of postoperative neck edema with resultant airway obstruction. Evaluation by the anesthesiologist prior to the day of surgery can avoid delay or cancellation of procedures due to incomplete medical workup. Preoperative anesthesia assessment can facilitate activities on the day of surgery by providing the opportunity to prepare for special patient needs such as awake fiberoptic intubation or Swan-Ganz line placement.

The technical and equipment requirements for revision spinal surgery vary depending upon the specific spinal problem. Standard protocols ensure that all necessary areas are considered in the preoperative period and that the operating suite is prepared for the day of surgery. Specific patient information (Fig. 21-1) should be readily available during the scheduling process. Detailed information (Fig. 21-2) must be provided to the operating room staff prior to the day of surgery in order to ensure that arrangements can be made to accommodate all equipment and necessary resources for the procedure.

Patients are frequently overwhelmed upon learning that further surgery is recommended for their spinal problem. The typical patient is only able to partially assimilate details regarding future surgical treatment presented by the spinal surgeon during a standard office encounter. The interval between first learning that additional surgery is indicated and the day of hospital admission is a critical period for the patient. Patient education is an important part of the scheduling process and requires time, compassion, and a health care provider knowledgeable in details regarding spinal reconstructive surgery. A comprehensive patient conference (Box 21-4, p. 312) is an important element of the preoperative scheduling process. This provides the patient a final opportunity to review questions or concerns which persist or which have arisen follow-

*Text continued on p. 309*

KAISER PERMANENTE
Fontana, California

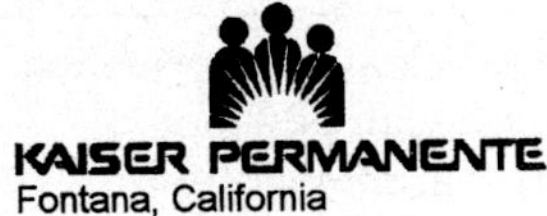

Patient Imprint Area

Date Of Surgery: ____________ Date Scheduled: ____________
Pre-Op. # 1: ____________ Pre-Op # 2: ____________
Estimated Time: ____________ Patient's Age: ____________

Diagnosis:

Procedure:

Surgeon: ____________ Critical Care MD: ____________
Assistant Surgeon ____________ Internist : ____________
P.A. Assistant: ____________

Medical History:

Medications: ____________ Known Allergies: ____________
____________ Latex Sensitive: Yes No
____________

Cardiac Problems: ____________ Respiratory Problems: ____________

Other Medical Problems: ____________

Blood: Yes No # Units ____________ Auto Direct Bank

Date Form Faxed: ____________

Fibrin Glue: Yes No

Prior Blood Transfusions: Yes No Hepatitis: Yes No

**FIGURE 21-1**

Reconstructive Spine Surgery Preoperative Worksheet. Use of a detailed form by the scheduling staff keeps important patient information readily available during the scheduling process.

*Continued*

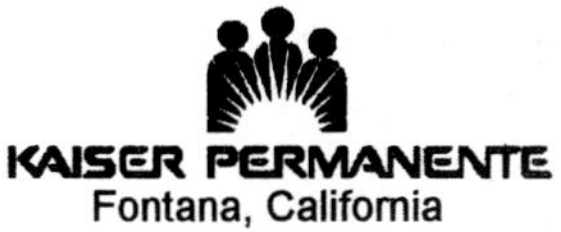


Patient Imprint Area

Pre-Op Brace Appointment: Yes No Contact:________________ Date:______________________

Spinal Monitoring: Yes No Contact: ________________ Date: ______________________

Industrial: Yes No Contact: ________________ Date: ______________________

Post-Op Bed: **ICU** **Step Down** **Pediatric Unit** **Adult Unit**

Aspirin - NSAID Use Yes No Smoking Yes No

Pre-Operative Evaluation:

Radiology Studies:

Pre-Operative X-rays Taken: ______________________________

Bending Films:________________________________________

CT Scan: ____________________________________________

Myelogram: __________________________________________

MRI: _______________________________________________

CXR/EKG PFT's CBC UA LFT HIV BS LYTES BUN CR

Handouts Given: ______________________________ Admit:__________________________

Spinal Surgery Booklet: __________________________ Surgery Booklet: __________________

Other:

FIGURE 21-1 CONT'D

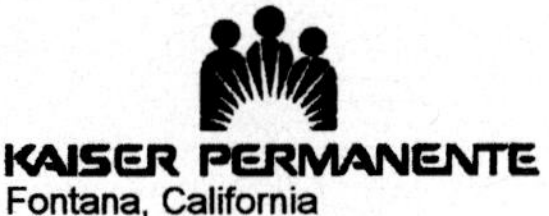


Patient Imprint Area

Date Of Surgery: ____________________ Date Scheduled: ____________________
Pre-Op. # 1: ____________________ Pre-Op # 2: ____________________
Estimated Time: ____________________ Patient's Age: ____________________

Diagnosis:

Procedure:

Surgeon: ____________________ Critical Care MD: ____________________

Assistant Surgeon ____________________ Internist : ____________________

P.A. Assistant: ____________________

Blood: Yes No # Units ____________ Auto Direct Bank Form
Faxed: ____________

Fibrin Glue: Yes No

Pre-Op Brace Appointment: Yes No Contact: ____________________
Date: ____________________

Spinal Monitoring: Yes No Contact: ____________________
Date: ____________________

Industrial: Yes No Contact: ____________________
Date: ____________________

Post-Op Bed: ICU Step Down Pediatric Unit Adult Unit

**FIGURE 21-2**

Reconstructive Spinal OR Worksheet. Use of a specific form can establish a protocol and assist the surgeon in working together with the operating room staff to ensure that all necessary equipment and services are available on the day of surgery.

*Continued*

KAISER PERMANENTE
Fontana, California

Patient Imprint Area

| | | | | | |
|---|---|---|---|---|---|
| **Position:** | Supine Prone | Rt. Lateral | Lt. Lateral | Sitting | |
| **Head Holders:** | Mayfield | Horseshoe | Donut | Halo | |
| **Neck Support:** | Halter | Garner Wells | Cervical Collar | soft-hard | |
| **Table:** | Jackson | Skytron | Andrews | Other | |
| **Frame/Support:** | 4 -Poster | Rolls | Bean Bag | Wilson | Other |
| **Radiology:** | C-Arm | Intra-operative x-ray | | | |
| **Cell Saver:** | Yes No | | | | |
| **Power Equipment:** | Midas | Hall Drill | | | |

**Spinal Instrumentation:**

Type: ____________________
Type: ____________________
Contact: __________ Phone #: __________
Date: __________

**Bone Graft Site:** ____________________

Bank Bone Yes No Allograft Type: __________

Antibiotics: Ancef Vancomycin Other: __________

Intraop Hypotension: Yes No CVP A-Line

Foley: Thigh Ted Hose Sequential Stockings

FIGURE 21-2 CONT'D

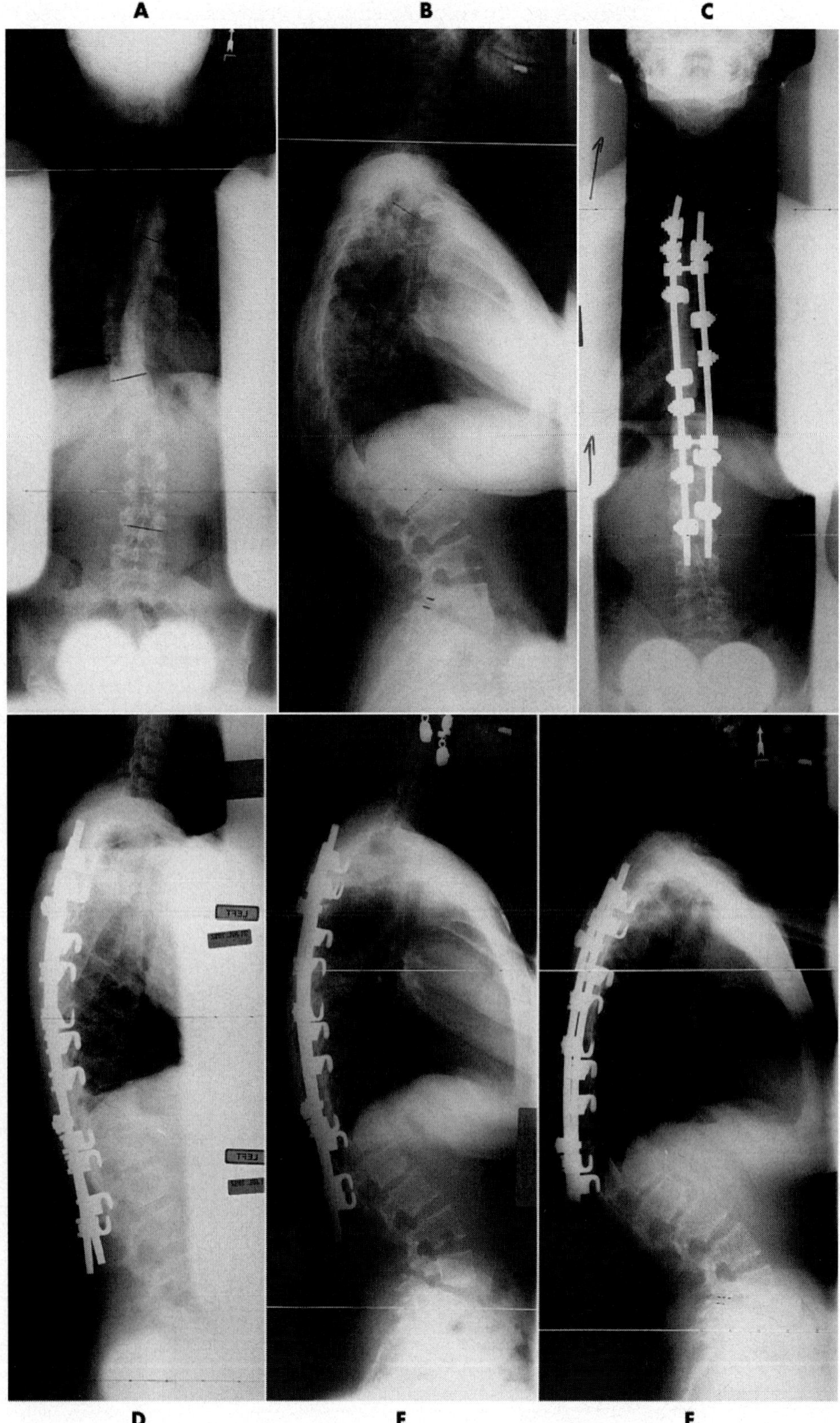


## FIGURE 21-3

PA **(A)** and lateral **(B)** radiographs of a 17-year-old woman with mild scoliosis with hyperkyphosis and grade 1 isthmic L5 spondylolisthesis. Prior to referral, the patient's deformity was treated with a posterior multisegmental hook-rod system and posterior spinal fusion **(C,D)**. Distal fixation failure occurred **(E)** and a deep infection developed at the distal extent of the instrumentation. The initial surgeon treated the problem by irrigation and debridement with removal of the distal rod prominence. The patient was referred for chronic thoracolumbar pain, progressive kyphotic deformity, and radiographic evidence of multiple posterior pseudarthroses **(F)**.

*Continued*

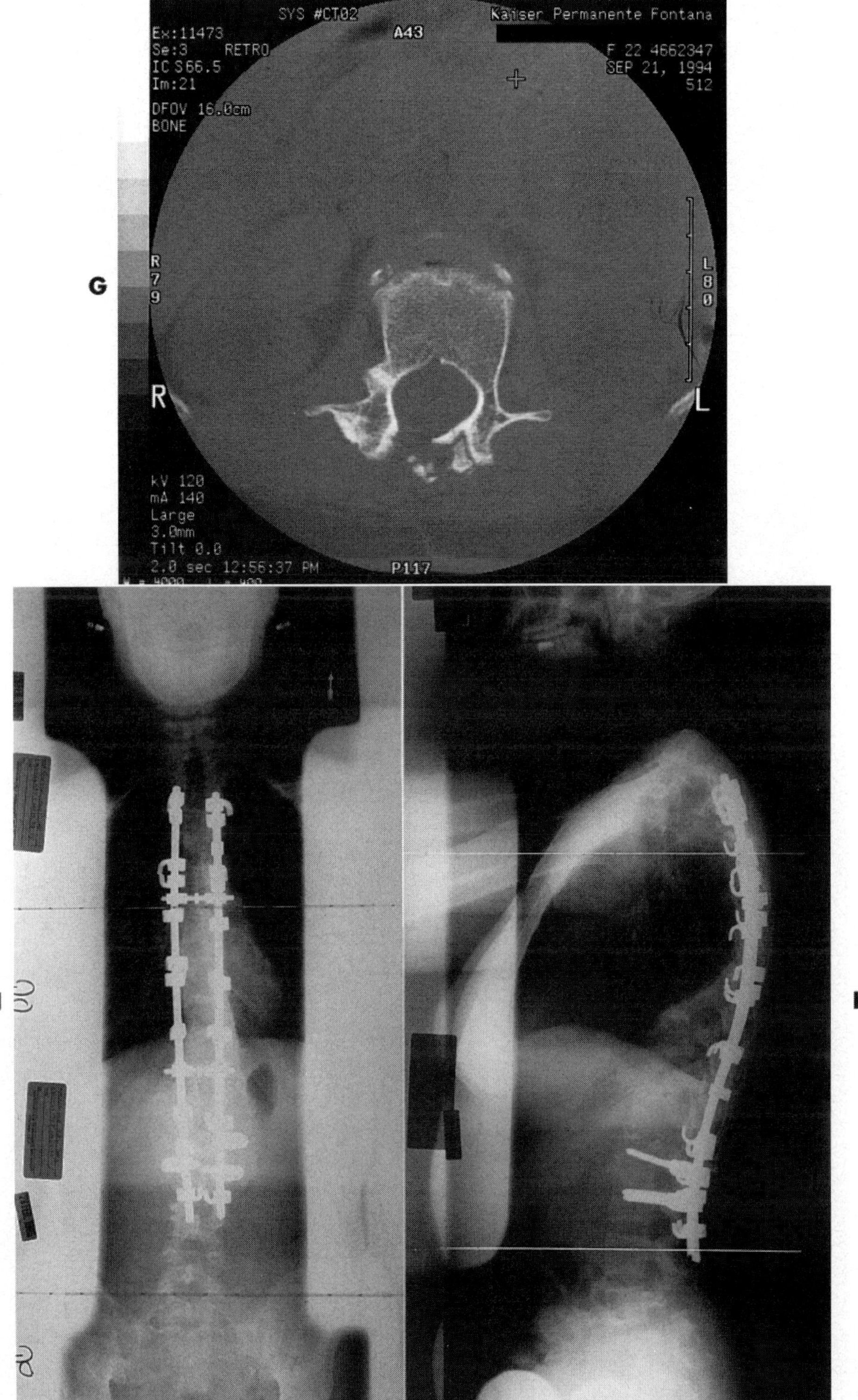


**FIGURE 21-3 CONT'D**

Note that a unilateral pedicle fracture is present at the L2 level **(G).** Treatment consisted of multilevel anterior diskectomies and interbody fusions, posterior repair of multilevel pseudarthroses, posterior compression instrumentation, and iliac crest autograft with successful restoration of coronal and sagittal alignment **(H,I).**

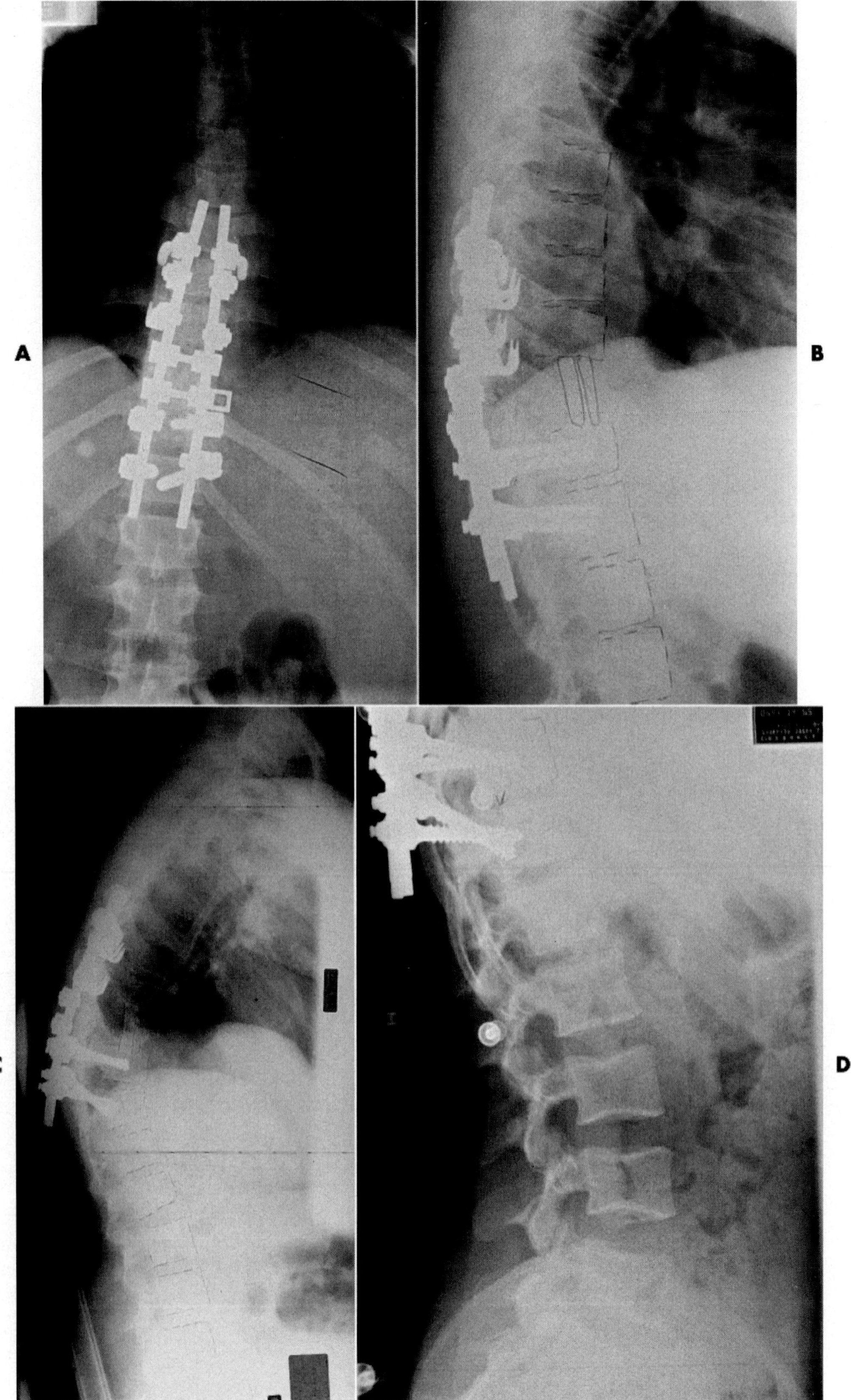

**FIGURE 21-4**

A 28-year-old man sustained a complete paraplegia secondary to a T10 burst fracture that was treated elsewhere by posterolateral spinal canal decompression with rib strut grafting and posterior segmental spinal fixation **(A,B).** The patient remained a complete paraplegic following surgery. Consultation was obtained two months postoperatively due to a thoracolumbar prominence that was exacerbated by sitting erect in a wheelchair. Lateral radiographs **(C,D)** show distal screw pull-out at the T11 and T12 levels with resultant vertebral body and pedicle fracture at the T12 level. The distal screw diameters were quite large (7.5 mm) and may have predisposed to this mode of failure.

*Continued*

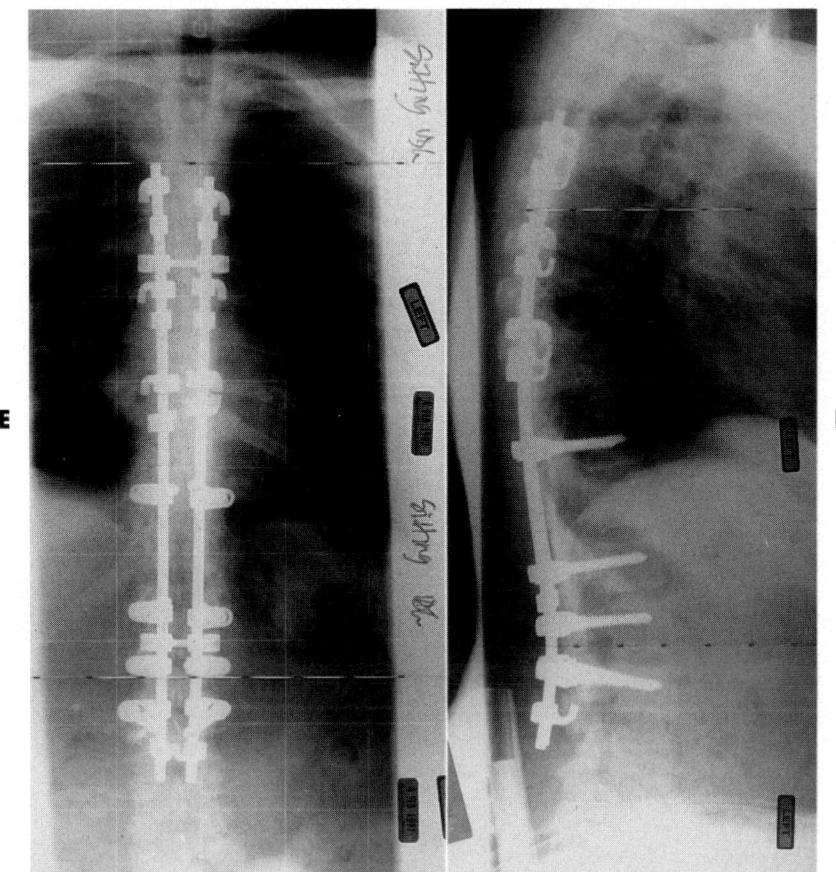

**FIGURE 21-4 CONT'D**

Revision surgery was performed posteriorly consisting of instrumentation revision achieving six points of fixation distal to the level of fracture **(E,F)** thereby permitting brace-free mobilization of this patient following surgery.

ing the preoperative scheduling and education process. It is generally recommended that family members or significant others who will participate in the care of the patient following surgery attend this conference with the surgeon.

## INTRAOPERATIVE CONSIDERATIONS

Intraoperative care of the patient is the mutual responsibility of the surgeon, anesthesiologist, and nursing staff. A coordinated team approach can maximize the opportunity for a good outcome. Members of the spine surgical team should be knowledgeable in all aspects of operative care, including patient positioning, blood salvage, neurologic monitoring, fundamentals of spinal instrumentation, intraoperative imaging requirements, and potential intraoperative problems and their management.

### NURSING CONSIDERATIONS

The time period from arrival of the patient in the presurgical holding area until the patient is brought to the operating suite is an opportunity to facilitate the upcoming surgical procedure. The nurse has the opportunity to decrease patient anxiety and apprehension regarding surgery. Potential problems such as medication or tape allergies can be identified. The availability of preoperatively donated blood, completed imaging studies, and necessary equipment can be confirmed. If a sequential procedure is planned that requires changing patient position between procedures (e.g., anterior and posterior procedures), availability of the appropriate positioning aids and the exact sequence of surgery can be confirmed.

### ANESTHESIA CONSIDERATIONS

Revision spinal procedures are routinely performed under general anesthesia. Overall anesthetic-induced morbidity and mortality are extremely low. Accurate knowledge of preexisting medical conditions is crucial to modify anesthetic risk. Capnography and pulse oximetry are routinely utilized. Intraoperative hemodynamic monitoring is performed when indicated using an arterial line, central line, and, occasionally, a Swan-Ganz catheter. A Foley catheter is routinely used

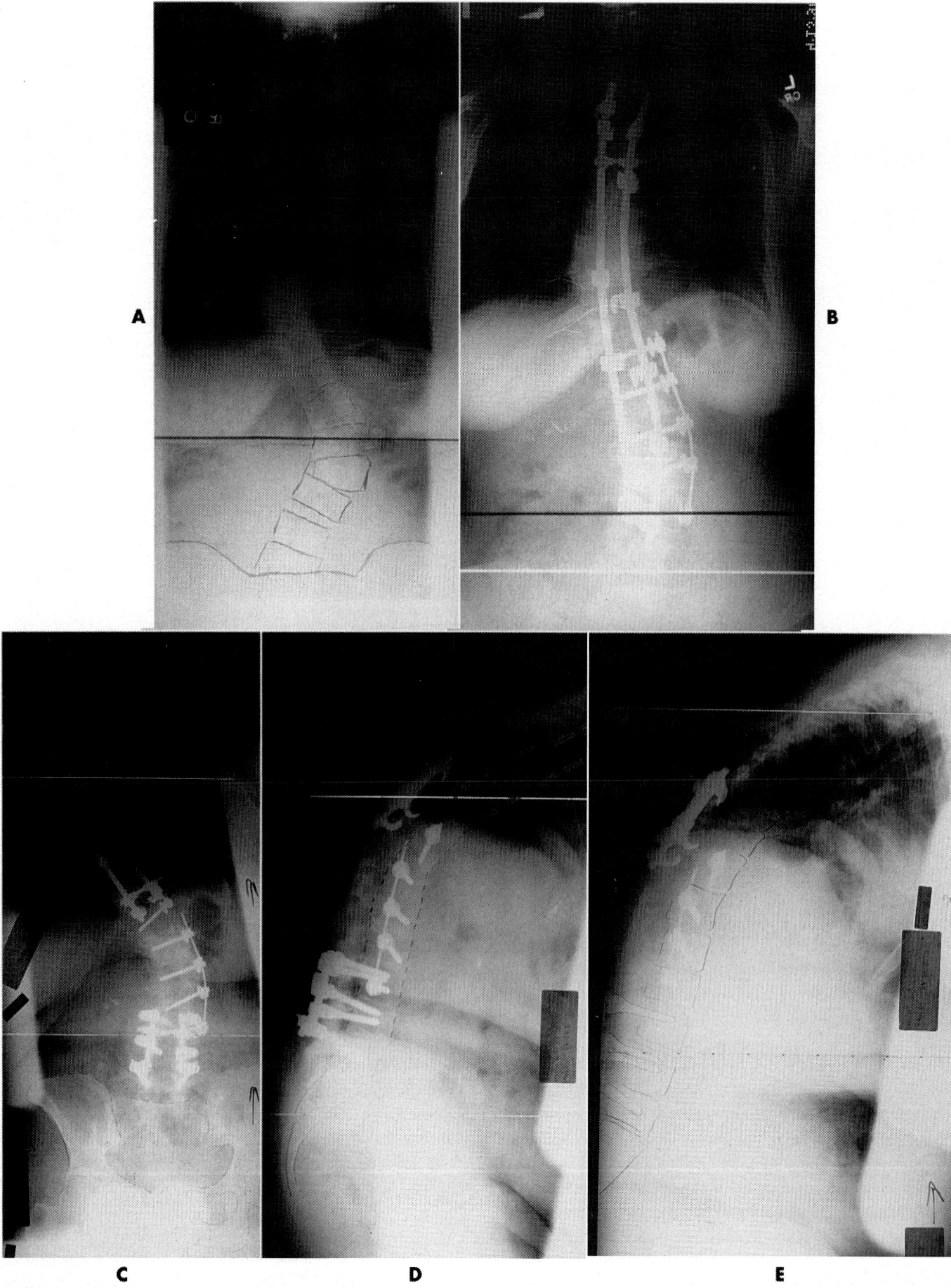

**FIGURE 21-5**

A 25-year-old female presented with thoracolumbar scoliosis **(A)** and was treated elsewhere with combined anterior and posterior surgery **(B).** The patient developed increasing lumbar pain and subsequently underwent further treatment by the initial surgeon consisting of distal fusion extension to L5, removal of the proximal instrumentation, and repair of a pseudarthrosis in the thoracic region. A significant coronal and sagittal plane deformity **(C,D,E)** developed following this procedure.

*Continued*

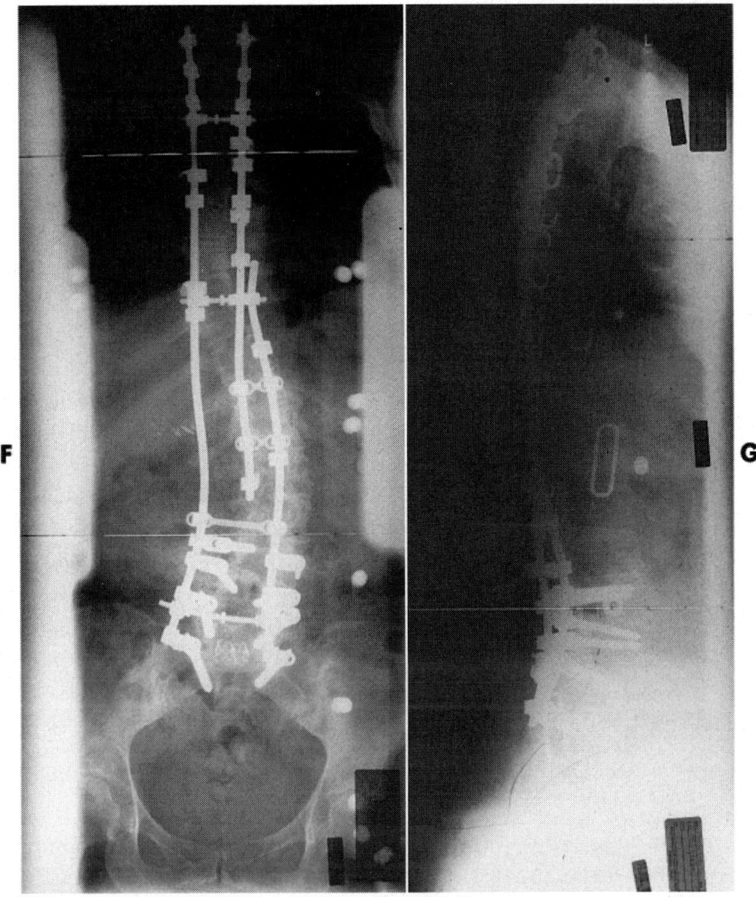


**FIGURE 21-5 CONT'D**

Extensive revision surgery was required **(F,G).** First-stage surgery consisted of anterior grafting of the thoracolumbar spine with removal of the broken anterior spinal instrumentation. Second-stage surgery included posterior realignment and extension of fusion to the sacrum. A posterior interbody fusion of L5-S1 was performed to provide structural anterior column support because extensive scarring encountered during the anterior procedure did not permit safe exposure of the lumbosacral junction anteriorly. Acceptable coronal and sagittal alignment were achieved with this approach.

to assess urine output. The anesthetic technique may be varied according to the type of procedure, the type of spinal monitoring utilized, the need to perform a wake-up test, and the requirement for a hypotensive effect to reduce intraoperative blood loss. Certain surgeons prefer to perform anterior thoracic procedures with the assistance of one lung ventilation as a means of improving surgical access. This can be achieved with placement of a double-lumen endotracheal tube. Use of a forced air warming system has proven beneficial in maintaining normal core body temperature during extensive spinal procedures.[24]

## PATIENT POSITIONING

Attention to detail is essential when positioning the patient for complex spinal procedures. The patient should be positioned in the manner that provides the best operative exposure, facilitates required intraoperative imaging, and maintains appropriate body alignment. Care must be taken to protect bony prominences from pressure irritation and minimize pressure problems in the axillary, breast, and genital areas. Specific attention must be given to ensuring that the eyes and face are protected. Blindness has been reported as a complication following spinal procedures. The position of the neck should be specifically assessed prior to surgery. A position of mild cervical flexion without significant rotation is preferred. Prolonged unphysiologic cervical extension may have disastrous consequences during a thoracolumbar procedure in a patient with coexistent cervical stenosis.

Many equipment options exist for use in positioning the patient undergoing spine surgery. Although a standard operating room table may be used, specific

**BOX 21-4. ISSUES FOR THE PRESURGERY PATIENT/FAMILY CONFERENCE**

- Review patient's specific spinal problem and treatment alternatives
- Review pertinent diagnostic studies with patient/family
- Explain specific surgical procedure using spinal models
  - Incisions
  - Bone graft
  - Spinal instrumentation
  - FDA status of spinal devices
- Discuss realistic expectations and goals of surgical treatment
  - Pain relief
  - Deformity correction
  - Neurologic improvement
  - Likely outcome of procedure
- Discuss possible surgical complications and obtain informed consent
- Confirm arrangements for
  - Blood donation
  - Cessation of aspirin and anti-inflammatory medication
  - Cessation of smoking
  - Orthosis (if needed)
  - Wake-up test, spinal monitoring
  - Hospital tour and familiarization
- Order any additional imaging studies required for preoperative planning
- Review final recommendations and evaluations by consultants (anesthesiologist, internist, intensivist)
- Review events on the day of surgery for patient and family
  - Check-in procedure and surgical waiting area
  - Duration of surgery
  - Patient's postoperative location (ICU vs. step-down unit vs. standard nursing floor)
- Discuss anticipated hospital course and discharge arrangements
  - Anticipated length of stay
  - Discharge planning concerns
  - Work-related issues
- Discuss need for psychologic support during postoperative period
- Discuss chemical dependency issues relating to preoperative use of narcotic medication

spine surgery tables (e.g., Jackson table, Andrews table) offer advantages over conventional tables. Specialized positioning frames such as a Wilson frame or Relton-Hall frame may be used with any of the surgery tables. Additional supportive devices such as the Mayfield head holder, cervical tongs, halo, and lateral stabilizers may be required. If sequential procedures are performed under a single anesthetic, the operating room staff must have the specific equipment ready to facilitate changing position of the patient (e.g., supine to prone position) after completion of the first procedure. Simultaneous anterior and posterior procedures have been popularized and require customization of existing positioning equipment to permit two surgical teams to simultaneously operate on both the anterior and posterior spine.[39]

General principles apply to patient positioning for posterior surgical procedures regardless of the specific table or frame utilized. Pressure should be distributed evenly over the chest and anterior thighs. The abdomen should be positioned so that it is free of pressure in order to permit venous drainage of the lower extremities and decrease shunting of blood through Batson's plexus. The brachial plexus and upper extremities should be protected from traction or compression injury. The shoulders should not be abducted past 90° and the elbows should be kept flexed with the ulnar nerve areas well padded. When fusion procedures are performed in the lumbar region, the patient should generally be positioned with the hips in full extension at the beginning of the procedure. This will position the lumbar spine in lordosis and help prevent inadvertent creation of a flat back syndrome.[11,34] Often positioning alone is not sufficient to create appropriate lordosis and adjunctive procedures such as osteotomies and interbody fusions are required. Following an osteotomy, the surgeon generally achieves osteotomy closure using segmental spinal instrumentation. The operating table may be used as an adjunct to achieve closure of a lumbar osteotomy. This is accomplished by positioning the patient on a four-poster frame with the bottom of the frame located above the hinge of the operating table. Extension of the distal portion of the table will rotate the hips, pelvis, and lower lumbar spine, thereby shortening the posterior spinal column and providing for closure of the osteotomy. A unique situation arises in the patient presenting with severe hyperlordosis (e.g., neuromuscular scoliosis) requiring fusion to the pelvis. In this situation, it is helpful to position the patient's hips in flexion to facilitate placement of intrailiac fixation and enhance correction of hyperlordosis.

Positioning of the patient for anterior spinal surgery depends on the specific spinal problem requiring treatment, the specific region of the spine requiring exposure, and whether spinal instrumentation is utilized in the course of the procedure. Exposure of the thoracic region and thoracolumbar junction is generally performed with the patient in the lateral position. Use of an axillary roll is important to prevent compression of vital neurovascular structures. The patient may be tilted 30 degrees from the true lateral position to facilitate visualization when multilevel diskectomy and fusion procedures are performed to create flexibility in the presence of a rigid spinal deformity. However, when anterior instrumentation is utilized, patient positioning in the true lateral position is preferred. This facilitates radiographic evaluation of the operative site and prevents creation of a secondary deformity due to intraoperative positioning. Patient positioning for anterior lumbar procedures is variable and both the supine and lateral positions can be utilized. Considerations in decision-making include the spinal levels requiring exposure, preference for a retroperitoneal or transperitoneal approach, requirement of a specific laparoscopic or open approach, and whether spinal instrumentation is utilized.

## BLOOD LOSS AND BLOOD CONSERVATION

Blood loss during spinal surgery depends on patient factors, the extent of surgery, type of surgical procedure, and surgical technique. Patients frequently donate autologous blood a short time prior to surgery and a baseline CBC immediately prior to surgery is helpful to provide an accurate baseline measure of hemoglobin and hematocrit. Anesthesia staff should confirm that the patient has ceased routine use of aspirin and anti-inflammatory medication prior to surgery. Desmopressin (DDAVP) has been shown to decrease blood loss in extensive posterior spinal fusion procedures. Multilevel posterior spinal fusion procedures are often accompanied by significant blood loss and cell-saver devices for intraoperative autotransfusion are routinely used. These systems wash collected red cells to eliminate debris and in the process also remove platelets and clotting factors. In cases in which significant volumes of salvaged blood are transfused, replacement with fresh frozen plasma and platelets may be required to restore adequate hemostasis. Hypotensive anesthesia can reduce blood loss in spinal fusion procedures. Caution must be used in elderly patients, patients with compromised spinal cord function, and patients with cerebrovascular disease or diminished cardiac output. Careful calculation of administered fluids and estimates of blood loss should be communicated to the surgical team on an hourly basis and should be used to guide intraoperative fluid and blood replacement. Surgically controllable factors for reducing blood loss include use of a subperiosteal dissection technique, meticulous control of bleeding, use of thrombostatic and hemostatic agents (Gelfoam, thrombin, Avitene, bone wax) and delay of complete decortication of the fusion bed to as late in the procedure as possible.

## NEUROLOGIC MONITORING AND PREVENTION OF NEUROLOGIC COMPLICATIONS

Neurologic injury during spinal surgery is a dreaded complication. Neurologic injury may involve the spinal cord or individual nerve roots. Spinal cord injury during surgery is reported to occur in less than 1% of cases.[25] Spinal cord injury may occur secondary to ischemia or mechanical damage. Current techniques permit monitoring of both sensory and motor pathways within the spinal cord.

Initially, spinal cord monitoring was performed by recording mixed nerve somatosensory evoked potentials (SEPs). SEPs are sensitive to the functional integrity of the dorsal medial tracts within the spinal cord. Because the SEPs are sensory based, they provide only indirect information regarding the functional integrity of the spinal cord motor tracts. Damage to the spinal cord can occur without a concomitant change in SEPs. Recording of only SEPs will detect approximately 70% of surgically induced insults to the spinal cord.[26] Various factors have been shown to have an adverse affect on SEP recordings including operating room power equipment, halogenated anesthetic agents, hypothermia, and hypotension. The surgeon must be notified when SEPs show a 50% to 60% reduction from baseline amplitude or a 10% increase from baseline latency to allow assessment of these changes. It has been shown that the best time to collect baseline data is following completion of the surgical exposure because this eliminates the variables of anesthetic level and patient core temperature. If SEP deterioration occurs during surgery, a standard protocol should be followed.[23] This includes checking that electrodes have not become displaced, increasing the concentration of inspired oxygen, elevating the mean blood pressure, ceasing further anesthetic inhalation agents, discontinuing instrumentation including release of any distraction forces, and irrigating the wound with warm saline. An arterial blood gas analysis should be obtained to assess for an unrecognized metabolic abnormality or unrecognized low hemoglobin level. If SEPs fail to return, a wake-up test should be performed. Depending upon the patient's response, the instrumentation may require removal and the use of steroids (spinal injury protocol) may be considered.

In many institutions, motor evoked potentials (MEPs) are used in combination with SEPs to provide a direct measure of spinal cord motor tract function thereby increasing the efficacy of spinal monitoring. The most common method of recording MEPs is by electrical stimulation of the spinal cord using percutaneous-percutaneous electrodes, nasopharyngeal-percutaneous electrodes, or translaminar electrodes. MEPs can be recorded either from a peripheral mixed nerve (NMEP) or recorded directly from muscle (MEP-EMG).

Lumbosacral nerve root injury with subsequent postoperative radiculopathy occurs much more commonly than spinal cord injury following spinal reconstructive surgery. The reported incidence of nerve root injury following adult thoracolumbar scoliosis surgery is in the range of 10%. Monitoring of mixed nerve

SEPs, the most common monitoring modality used to monitor spinal cord function, is not a sensitive technique for detecting nerve root injury. EMG monitoring is required to detect and prevent injury to individual nerve roots.[7] EMG procedures are classified into two categories based on their method of elicitation: mechanical and electrical. Mechanically elicited EMGs should be used during the dynamic phases of surgery (pedicle screw preparation and insertion, nerve root manipulation) and electrically elicited EMGs should be used during the static phases of surgery (immediately before or after pedicle screw placement). Dermatomal SEPs (DSEPs) are not sufficiently sensitive to be used as a method of protecting nerve roots during placement of transpedicular instrumentation. However, DSEPs have been recommended for determining the level of nerve root involvement prior to surgery and for determining the adequacy of nerve root decompression during surgery.

Intraoperative monitoring using SEPs may also be useful in the prevention of peripheral neuropathies due to patient positioning on the operating room table. During posterior spinal procedures, ulnar nerve SEPs are monitored to assess for possible brachial plexopathy. During anterior procedures, peroneal and femoral SEPs are monitored. Monitoring of the integrity of the peroneal nerve can alert the team to the onset of an impending peroneal nerve palsy secondary to pressure of the leg against the operating room table. A permanent injury can be averted by moving the patient's leg or adjusting the padding. Monitoring of femoral nerve function can alert the surgeon to excessive traction on the iliopsoas muscle and the adjacent nerve roots during an anterior procedure, thereby avoiding a potential femoral nerve palsy.

Neurologic monitoring is not routinely utilized for revision lumbar decompression procedures unaccompanied by spinal instrumentation. The incidence of neural injury in this setting is estimated to range from 0.2% to 2.5%. An injury may result from excessive neural retraction, contusion, laceration, or electrocauterization.[33] The key to avoiding neural injury is meticulous surgical technique and adequate exposure of neural structures. Initial exposure must respect the absent posterior bony elements and proceed from known bony landmarks toward the area of previous surgery. An operative plane should be developed by elevating scar and dura away from the margins of the prior decompression using curettes and dural elevators. Scar tissue covering the dura in the midline does not require removal. Sufficient bone should be removed laterally to visualize the lateral edge of the nerve root. Each nerve root is then identified and decompressed. It is safest to work from proximal to distal when performing lateral nerve root decompressions, thereby remaining parallel to the root and minimizing the risk of inadvertent transection of a nerve root. Decompression should continue until the nerve root is adequately decompressed as judged by visualization, palpation, and nerve root mobility. If a significant portion of the facet joints requires removal or the extent of decompression violates the integrity of the pars interarticularis, then a fusion should accompany the decompression procedure. Dural tears may occur during revision lumbar decompression procedures. These should be handled with standard suture repair techniques to achieve a water-tight closure. Fibrin glue is a useful adjunct to supplement dural repair and facilitates early patient mobilization following surgery.

## INSTRUMENTATION CONSIDERATIONS

The ultimate goal in revision spinal procedures utilizing spinal instrumentation is to achieve a balanced spine in the coronal and sagittal planes that will progress to a solid arthrodesis over the instrumented levels without significant complications. Decisions regarding spinal instrumentation can be made only after careful analysis of the presenting spinal problem with respect to alignment in the sagittal, coronal, and axial planes. Appropriate levels for spinal instrumentation and fusion as well as the operation or sequence of operations most likely to address the patient's spinal problem must be determined in advance of the surgery date. Revision procedures present many unique challenges to the spinal reconstructive surgeon. Deficient posterior spinal elements, deficient sacral and pelvic bone stock, osteopenia, broken spinal instrumentation, pseudarthroses, and coronal and/or sagittal imbalance make subsequent spinal instrumentation and fusion procedures challenging.[38] The surgeon must have available in the operating room a variety of anterior and posterior spinal instrumentation options that can be adapted to these unique problems. Various modular instrumentation systems are currently available and provide versatile options for achieving segmental fixation of the thoracolumbosacral spine utilizing hooks, screws, wires, and iliac posts. Fixation spanning the lumbosacral junction remains problematic, especially when long fusions are required. The spine team should have a detailed working knowledge of the spinal instrumentation systems available in their hospital in order to expedite these complex procedures.

Risk factors for instrumentation failure after revision surgery have been reviewed.[22] Factors under the control of the surgeon include (1) appropriate placement of hook, screw, and wire implants, (2) appropriate rod contouring, (3) appropriate application of corrective forces, (4) selection of an adequate number of fixation points to achieve a stable construct, and (5) achievement of postoperative coronal and sagittal balance. Patient factors that cannot readily be controlled by the surgeon include osteoporosis and compliance with postoperative activity restrictions. The surgeon must consider both patient biology and biomechanics in determining an appropriate procedure. Circumferential surgery should be performed when indicated. Anterior and posterior procedures are most commonly indicated for kyphotic deformities, rigid deformities, revision surgery for failed posterior fusions, long fusions to the sacrum, and for patients who smoke or have significant osteoporosis.

### INTRAOPERATIVE IMAGING

The operating room should have the capacity for excellent quality spinal imaging. AP and lateral radiographs are useful for spinal level localization and documenting placement of spinal implants. Fluoroscopy may be used to monitor implant placement and spinal realignment procedures. Capability for PA 36-inch radiographs is required when long fusions are performed to the sacrum. It is critical to clearly visualize the alignment of C7 and the head over the sacrum before concluding such procedures in order to ensure that iatrogenic spinal imbalance has not been created. New techniques such as computer-assisted image guidance may play a future role in intraoperative imaging as new minimally invasive spinal procedures are developed.

## POSTOPERATIVE CARE

Following extensive spinal reconstructive procedures, the patient is initially best managed in a critical care unit or postsurgical step-down unit. In this setting the patient can be monitored continually by nursing staff experienced in the care of spine patients and critical care specialists are readily available to participate in patient care.[28] In this manner, postsurgical complications can be recognized early and appropriate intervention can be implemented. Postsurgical complications most commonly encountered involve the pulmonary, cardiovascular, and gastrointestinal systems.[31] Although neurologic complications following surgery are rare, neurologic status should be carefully monitored because early recognition of neurologic problems may prevent permanent neurologic deficits if urgent treatment is instituted. Consideration must also be given to nutritional and pain control issues in the postsurgical spine patient.

### RESPIRATORY SYSTEM CONCERNS

Pulmonary problems are common following extensive spinal procedures and can arise due to a variety of factors. In general, it is desirable to extubate most patients following spinal procedures. Exceptions include patients who undergo extensive anterior cervical procedures due to concerns about airway obstruction secondary to postoperative edema. Patients with compromised preoperative respiratory status may require postoperative ventilator support, especially if extensive anteroposterior reconstructive procedures are performed. Following extubation, most patients develop some degree of atelectasis secondary to impaired coughing and breathing secondary to pain or hypoventilation due to residual narcotics or muscle relaxants. Routine treatment with an incentive spirometer is generally effective. Nebulizers and chest physical therapy may help prevent significant atelectasis and subsequent pneumonia. All patients should be monitored for shortness of breath or chest discomfort and a chest radiograph should be obtained if symptoms persist. Patients with chest tubes in place following anterior thoracic spinal procedures are managed according to standard general surgical protocols. Hemothorax and pneumothorax may develop even when a posterior surgical approach has been utilized due to inadvertent entry into the chest cavity. This may occur during preoperative central line placement, during exposure of the spine, or following rib resections performed during posterior spinal deformity procedures. Treatment for hemothorax or pneumothorax is placement of a chest tube.

Less common problems occurring after spinal procedures include chylothorax and acute respiratory distress syndrome (ARDS). Chylothorax may develop following anterior spinal procedures during which an injury to the lymphatic system occurs. Chylothorax may present as a persistent pleural effusion following chest tube removal. Treatment includes chest tube drainage, a low fat diet, and, occasionally, total parenteral nutrition (TPN). ARDS may develop after extensive spinal procedures and is associated with an increase in pulmonary compliance, decrease in lung volume, and progressively increased shunting with resultant decreased PaO2. Bilateral infiltrates are noted on chest radiographs. ARDS is commonly associated with fluid overload but may develop secondary to shock, sepsis, or fibrin and platelet microemboli introduced following massive transfusions.

### CARDIOVASCULAR SYSTEM CONCERNS

Persistent blood loss and cardiovascular instability are concerns following extensive spinal procedures. Careful monitoring of blood pressure, central venous pressure, urine output, and wound drainage is essential following surgery. Postoperative cardiovascular problems may present as hypotension or hypertension. Hypotension is most often the result of hypovolemia due to blood loss or third spacing. The treatment is generally fluid resuscitation. If low blood pressure persists despite adequate volume replacement, the problem may be due to either cardiac dysfunction or decreased systemic vascular resistance. Central pressure monitoring and critical care consultation are essential in sorting out these problems. The possibility of acute myocardial infarction or myocardial ischemia must be assessed. Hypertension may occur following surgery as a result of vasoconstriction secondary to pain, hypoxemia, hypercarbia, or hypothermia. Prompt treatment of pain and maintenance of normal body temperature using a forced air warming system are generally effective initial measures for treatment of this problem.

The reported incidence rate for deep vein thrombosis following major reconstructive spinal surgery ranges from 0.9% to 14%.[40] However, when mechanical prophylaxis consisting of combined graduated compression stockings and pneumatic compression stockings is utilized, the incidence of deep vein thrombosis following major spinal procedures (including anterior lumbar procedures) is 0.3%.[29] In most situations, the risk-benefit ratio does not favor prophylaxis with Coumadin due to concerns regarding bleeding complications, especially epidural hematoma and possible cauda equina syndrome.

## Gastrointestinal and Nutritional Issues

Patients are generally maintained on NPO status except for ice chips immediately following surgery. When bowel sounds have returned on the first or second day following surgery, a clear liquid diet is initiated and advanced to a regular diet as tolerated by the patient. Postoperative ileus may develop following correction of severe scoliosis or kyphosis, after anterior lumbar fusion or secondary to postoperative analgesics. Decompression with a nasogastric tube for 24 to 48 hours usually leads to resolution of this problem.

Patients undergoing major spinal procedures are at risk of postoperative protein malnutrition with resultant increase in likelihood of wound infection.[14] This appears especially problematic for patients undergoing staged anterior and posterior reconstructive procedures due to the catabolic state induced by the initial surgical procedure.[5] The use of intravenous hyperalimentation is recommended for these patients. It has been shown that normalization to preoperative nutritional status in such patients occurs generally within six weeks after surgery. Risk factors for prolonged return to baseline preoperative nutritional status include increased number of fusion levels (>10), patients undergoing anterior and posterior procedures whether performed on the same day or in a staged manner, and patients older than 40 especially if multiple level fusion procedures are performed.[21]

A variety of common gastrointestinal problems may require management following surgery. Patients at risk for stress gastritis or ulcer are treated with ranitidine or cimetidine in the postoperative period. Constipation frequently develops as a result of postoperative analgesic use and is treated effectively with stool softeners and suppositories. Occasionally, diarrhea may develop due to a variety of factors. Antibiotic-associated colitis may result in diarrhea and is initially treated by hydration and cessation of antibiotics. If symptoms persist and cultures show that symptoms are secondary to toxin production by *Clostridium difficile,* treatment with vancomycin is required. Occasionally, a superior mesenteric artery syndrome may develop following deformity correction secondary to compression of the third part of the duodenum in the angle between the superior mesenteric artery and the aorta. Such patients present with nausea, vomiting, and high-pitched bowel sounds. Initial treatment is restriction of oral intake, decompression with a nasogastric tube, intravenous hydration, maintenance of fluid and electrolyte balance, and occasionally hyperalimentation.[37]

## Neurologic Evaluation

Following surgery a detailed neurologic assessment of upper and lower extremity function should be performed upon arrival in the postsurgical unit. Neurologic deficits may occur at the level of spinal surgery or at remote sites due to traction or compression injuries secondary to patient positioning during surgery. If the initial assessment is normal, serial examinations based on the location of the spinal procedure are carried out every 2 hours during the first 24 hours and every 4 hours over the next 48 hours and then once every shift until the patient is discharged. Neurologic evaluation should include assessment of extremity motor strength, sensation, and reflexes. Bladder function and rectal tone should be monitored carefully because impaired function may be the first sign of neurologic deterioration.

Patients who are neurologically intact immediately following surgery may develop neurologic problems later in the postoperative period. Delayed onset paraplegia may develop 24 to 96 hours following spinal deformity procedures. The onset of symptoms may be insidious with complaints limited to paresthesias or a feeling of heaviness in the extremities. A rapid response to any change in neurologic status is essential and the nursing staff should notify the surgeon promptly. Depending on the specific situation, the operating room should be alerted of the potential for emergent surgery, radiographs and neural imaging studies should be obtained, and a spinal cord injury steroid protocol should be initiated. Delayed-onset paraplegia is attributed to a vascular etiology in many cases and surgical intervention may be of little benefit in this setting. However, Hall[12] has reported recovery in 4 patients following emergent decompression in this setting and attributed the neurologic deterioration to edema that developed during the postoperative period. Another cause of postoperative neurologic deterioration is cauda equina syndrome. This may develop secondary to a variety of etiologies including hematoma, disk herniation, tumor, infection, fracture, or spinal stenosis. Symptoms are variable and may include severe low back pain, urinary retention, sciatica, bowel dysfunction, and widespread numbness of buttocks and perineum. Neurodiagnostic imaging studies are required to determine the etiology of cauda equina syndrome and to determine the spinal levels responsible for the problem. Treatment is complete decompression of the involved neural elements.

## WOUND INFECTION

The reported rate of infection following spinal fusion with instrumentation ranges from 0% to 35%.[1] This wide range of infection rates is partially the result of use of spinal instrumentation in high-risk patient groups such as the elderly, neuromuscular scoliosis and myelodysplasia in whom effective treatment could not be provided prior to the development of modern segmental spinal fixation techniques. When these high-risk groups are excluded from consideration, reported rates for infection associated with spinal instrumentation approach an average of 7% with a reported range from 0% to 13%.[30] Prior spine surgery increases the risk of infection by a factor of two when an instrumented fusion is performed. A history of prior spine infection increases the risk of subsequent infection by a factor of five if an instrumented spinal fusion is performed. Other patient-related factors associated with postoperative infection risk include malnutrition, obesity, smoking, steroid use, concurrent illness or infection, prolonged preoperative hospitalization, and prolonged postoperative immobilization. Use of prophylactic antibiotics have been shown to decrease the incidence of postoperative wound infection and should be continued for 24 to 48 hours following surgery. Generally, prophylaxis is administered for gram-positive organisms but the changing spectrum of spinal infections in some areas has led to routine prophylaxis against both gram-positive and gram-negative organisms.

The diagnosis of acute postoperative spinal infection is difficult since the clinical findings are often subtle and the incision may appear unremarkable. The most common presentation is persistent temperature elevation or atypical pain that is out of proportion for the time elapsed since surgery. The patient may report that pain initially decreased in the first few days following surgery but then pain recurred and intensified. If a superficial infection is present, the wound edges may be edematous or erythematous and a small amount of drainage may present from the incision. If a deep wound infection is present, the incision may appear normal. Laboratory tests such as erythrocyte sedimentation rate (ESR) and C-reactive protein are nonspecific and are generally elevated after any surgical procedure. Elevation of white blood cell (WBC) count is not a constant finding and may be normal in infections with low virulence organisms. Radiographic studies such as radionuclide scans and MRI are generally not helpful because of their inability to discriminate normal postoperative changes from infection. If drainage is noted from the incision beyond 3 to 4 days following surgery, Gram stain and cultures should be obtained and the patient should undergo exploration of the wound in the operating room prior to discharge or transfer from the hospital. Expectant management of a draining incision is not recommended. If no drainage is noted and a postoperative wound infection is suspected, a wound aspiration at the superficial and deep layers of the wound is performed under sterile conditions and any fluid obtained is sent for Gram stain and culture.

## PAIN MANAGEMENT

Adequate postoperative pain management is an important component of patient management following reconstructive spinal surgery. Adequate analgesia can facilitate respiratory care and enable early patient mobilization and ambulation. Preoperative education can decrease anxiety following surgery and facilitate pain management. The mainstay for postoperative pain relief immediately following spinal procedures are systemic opioids. Patient-controlled analgesia (PCA) using morphine provides acceptable pain relief in the majority of cases. The PCA device can be programmed to deliver a set dose of narcotic at a defined time interval when triggered by the patient. A lockout period (usually 6 to 10 minutes) prevents excessive drug administration. In some cases, a continuous background infusion is used in addition to the patient-triggered dosages. Such basal rate infusions should be used cautiously in the elderly or in patients with an increased risk of respiratory depression (e.g., chronic obstructive pulmonary disease, sleep apnea). Use of an apnea monitor and pulse oximeter is recommended in such patients. Naloxone (Narcan) should be kept readily available in case of overmedication or respiratory depression. Morphine is a preferred narcotic due to its predictable side effects and lack of accumulated metabolites. Hydromorphone (Dilaudid) is also an effective drug with an acceptable safety profile for use in this setting. Meperidine (Demerol) should be used with caution due to potential for accumulation of a toxic metabolite, normeperidine, which may lead to agitation, delirium, or seizures. Side effects of opioids include nausea and pruritus. Recently, Ketorolac (Toradol), an injectable nonsteroidal anti-inflammatory drug (NSAID), has been utilized as an analgesic in a variety of postoperative settings. Presently this agent cannot be recommended for use in the patient undergoing spinal fusion because a recent study[10] documented that patients treated with Ketorolac were five times more likely than controls to develop a pseudarthrosis. Intravenous narcotics are generally utilized during the first 48 to 72 hours following surgery or until the patient is able to tolerate fluids and oral medication. At this time the patient may be shifted to oral narcotics such as hydrocodone. Muscle spasm may be problematic, especially following posterior procedures, and agents such as lorazepam may be utilized for treatment of these symptoms. Physical modalities such as heat, cooling massage, or transcutaneous electrical nerve stimulation may be used to supplement drug therapy. Assistance with proper turning technique, instruction in body mechanics and bed exercises may reduce discomfort after spinal surgery.

## SUMMARY AND CONCLUSIONS

Management of the patient requiring revision spinal surgery is a challenge. A coordinated multidisciplinary team approach can minimize complications and improve patient outcome in these challenging cases. The best treatment for complex spinal problems requiring surgical intervention is appropriate initial surgical treatment in order to minimize the need for subsequent revision surgery.

## REFERENCES


1. An HS, Glover JM: *Complications and revision surgery in adult spinal deformity.* In Bridwell KH, DeWald RL, editors: *The textbook of spinal surgery,* ed 2, Philadelphia, 1997, Lippincott-Raven, pp 797-820.
2. Baldus C, Blanke K: *Preoperative nursing care.* In Bridwell KH, DeWald RL, editors: *The textbook of spinal surgery,* ed 2, Philadelphia, 1997, Lippincott-Raven, pp 3-10.
3. Bradford DS, Tribus CB: Current concepts and management of patients with fixed decompensated spinal deformity, *Clin Orthop* 306:64-72, 1994.
4. Brown CW, Orme TJ, Richardson JD: The rate of pseudarthrosis in patients who are smokers and patients who are non-smokers. A comparison study, *Spine* 11:942-943, 1986.
5. Boachie-Adjei O: *Implications of malnutrition in the surgical patient.* In Bridwell KH, DeWald RL, editors: *The textbook of spinal surgery,* ed 2, Philadelphia, 1997, Lippincott-Raven, pp 101-112.
6. Boachie-Adjei O, Bradford DS: Vertebral column resection and arthrodesis for complex spinal deformities, *J Spinal Disord* 4:193-202,1991.
7. Clements DH, Morledge DE, Martin WH, et al: Evoked and spontaneous electromyography to evaluate lumbosacral pedicle screw placement, *Spine* 21:600-604, 1996.
8. Dewald RL: Revision surgery for spinal deformity. Instructional Course Lectures. Vol XLI. Ed Eilert RL. American Academy of Orthopaedic Surgeons, 1992, pp 235-250.
9. Gertzbein SD, Harris MB: Wedge osteotomy for the correction of post-traumatic kyphosis, *Spine* 17:374-379, 1992.
10. Glassman SD, Rose SM, Dimar JR, et al: The effect of postoperative nonsteroidal antiinflammatory administration on spinal fusion. North American Spine Society 12th Annual Meeting, October 22-25, 1997, New York, New York.
11. Guanciale AF, Dinsay JM, Watkins RG: Lumbar lordosis in spinal fusion—a comparison of intraoperative results of patient positioning on two different operative table frame types, *Spine* 21:964-969, 1996.
12. Hall JE: Management of intraoperative or early postoperative neurologic deficits. Scoliosis Research Society—The surgical treatment of complex spinal deformities, September 25, 1996, Ottawa, Canada.
13. Heinig CF: *Eggshell procedure.* In Luque ER, editor: *Segmental spinal instrumentation,* Thorofare, NJ, 1984, Slack Inc, pp 221-234.
14. Klein JD, Hey LA, Yo CS, et al: Perioperative nutrition and postoperative complications in patients undergoing spinal surgery, *Spine* 21:2676-2682, 1992.
15. Kostuik JP: *The surgical treatment of failures of laminectomy and spinal fusion.* In Andersson GB, McNeil TW, editors: *Lumbar spinal stenosis,* St. Louis, 1992, Mosby Yearbook, pp 425-470.
16. Kostuik JP: *Failures after spinal fusion.* In Frymoyer JW, editor: *The adult spine—principles and practice,* edition 2, Philadelphia,1997, Lippincott-Raven, pp 2277-2328.
17. Kostuik J, Maurais GR, Richardson WJ, et al: Combined single anterior and posterior osteotomy for correction of iatrogenic lumbar kyphosis, *Spine* 13:257-266, 1988.
18. LaGrone M, Bradford DS, Moe JH, et al: Treatment of symptomatic flatback after spinal fusion, *J Bone Joint Surg* 70:569-580, 1988.
19. Lauerman WC, Bradford DS, Transfeldt EE, et al: Management of pseudarthrosis after arthrodesis of the spine for idiopathic scoliosis, *J Bone Joint Surg* 73:222-236, 1991.
20. Lehmer SM, Keppler L, Biscup RS, et al: Posterior transvertebral osteotomy for adult thoracolumbar kyphosis, *Spine* 19:2060-2067, 1994.

21. Lenke LG, Bridwell KH, Blanke K, et al: Prospective analysis of nutritional status normalization after spinal reconstructive surgery, *Spine* 20:1359-1367, 1995.
22. Lenke LG: Complications of adult spinal deformity surgery: kyphosis and revision surgery. AAOS Instructional Course Lectures. Course No. 238, San Francisco, 1996.
23. Meyer PR, Cotler HB, Gireesan GT: Operative neurological complications resulting from thoracic and lumbar spine internal fixation, *Clin Orthop* 237:125-131, 1988.
24. Nielsen CH: *Preoperative and postoperative anesthetic considerations for the spinal surgery patient.* In Bridwell KH, DeWald RL, editors: *The textbook of spinal surgery,* edition 2, Philadelphia, 1997, Lippincott-Raven, pp 31-38.
25. Owen JH: *Monitoring during surgery for spinal deformities.* In Bridwell KH, DeWald RL, editors: *The textbook of spinal surgery,* edition 2, Philadelphia, 1997, Lippincott-Raven, pp 39-60.
26. Owen JH, Tolekis JR: *Nerve root monitoring.* In Bridwell KH, DeWald RL, editors: *The textbook of spinal surgery,* edition 2, Philadelphia, 1997, Lippincott-Raven, pp 61-76.
27. Rawlins BA, Boachie-Adjei O: Revision adult spinal deformity surgery, *Semin Spine Surg* 9:169-180, 1997.
28. Rodts MF: *Perioperative and postoperative nursing care for the spinal surgery patient.* In Bridwell KH, DeWald RL, editors: *The textbook of spinal surgery,* edition 2, Philadelphia, 1997, Lippincott-Raven, pp 11-30.
29. Rokito SE, Schwartz MC, Neuwirth MG: Deep vein thrombosis after major reconstructive spinal surgery, *Spine* 21: 853-859, 1996.
30. Slucky AV, Eismont FJ: *Spinal infection.* In Bridwell KH, DeWald RL, editors: *The textbook of spinal surgery,* edition 2, Philadelphia, 1997, Lippincott-Raven, pp 2141-2184.
31. Smith GF: *Perioperative care of the spine patient.* In White AH, editor: *Spine care—operative treatment.* St. Louis, 1995, Mosby, pp 964-983.
32. Smith-Petersen MN, Larson CB, Aufranc OE: Osteotomy of the spine for correction of flexion deformity in rheumatoid arthritis, *J Bone Joint Surg* 27:1-11, 1945.
33. Stambough JL, Simeone FA: *Neurogenic complications in spine surgery.* In Rothman RH, Simeone FA, editors: *The spine,* edition 3, Philadelphia, 1992, WB Saunders, pp 1885-1891.
34. Stephens GC, Yoo JJ, Wilbur G: Comparison of lumbar sagittal alignment produced by different operative positions, *Spine* 21:1802-1807, 1996.
35. Thiranont N, Netrawichen P: Transpedicle decancellation closed wedge osteotomy for treatment of fixed flexion deformity of the spine in ankylosing spondylitis, *Spine* 18:2517-2522, 1993.
36. Thomasen E: Vertebral osteotomy for correction of kyphosis and ankylosing spondylitis, *Clin Orthop* 194:142-152, 1985.
37. Transfeldt EE: *Complications of treatment.* In Lonstein JF, Winter RB, Bradford DS, Ogilvie JW, editors: *Moe's textbook of scoliosis and other spinal deformities,* edition 3, Philadelphia,1995, WB Saunders, pp 451-481.
38. Vaccaro AR, Mirkovic S, Bauer RD, Garfin SR: *Revision lumbar and cervical degenerative spine surgery-indications and techniques.* In Bridwell KH, DeWald RL, editors: *The textbook of spinal surgery,* edition 2, Philadelphia, 1997, Lippincott-Raven, pp 1457-1494.
39. Weidenbaum M, Farcy JP: *Surgical management of thoracic and lumbar burst fractures.* In Bridwell KH, DeWald RL, editors: *The textbook of spinal surgery,* edition 2, Philadelphia, 1997, Lippincott-Raven, pp 1839-1880.
40. West JL III: *Deep vein thrombosis in the adult spinal deformity patient.* In Bridwell KH, DeWald RL, editors: *The textbook of spinal surgery,* edition 2, Philadelphia, 1997, Lippincott-Raven, pp 93-100.
41. Winter RB, Denis F, Lonstein JE, Dezen E: Salvage and reconstructive surgery for spinal deformity using Cotrel-Dubousset instrumentation, *Spine* 16:S412-S417, 1991.

# VI

# SPECIFIC CONSIDERATIONS RELATED TO PATHOLOGICAL ENTITIES

# 22

# MANAGEMENT OF LATE KYPHOTIC DEFORMITY OF FRACTURES

**Stanley D. Gertzbein, M.D., F.R.C.S. (C)**



Failure to recognize the extent of bony and soft tissue trauma in spine injuries may result in inadequate stabilization of an unstable lesion. Despite better methods of spine fracture evaluation and treatment, late deformities are not uncommon, often resulting in pain and occasional neurological compromise.[9,15,16,18,20,21] Kyphotic deformity greater than 30 degrees is generally accepted as a significant deformity often associated with pain.[4,16,22] Pain may derive from the site of the deformity itself (the injured disk or a pseudarthrosis) or from the lordotic compensation above and below the deformity site when added stresses are placed on the respective facet joints. Injuries associated with distraction of the soft tissue posterior elements are particularly prone to this deformity and not uncommonly result in a progressive chronic pain syndrome (Fig. 22-1). As a late consequence, over a period of months or years, a neurological deficit may develop or progress, particularly when associated with intraspinal bony fragments (Fig. 22-2).[1]

Posttraumatic kyphosis usually results from failure of the initial treatment method. If recognized early it can be corrected; however, if discovered late, the deformity represents a therapeutic challenge.[2,13] Iatrogenic kyphosis secondary to laminectomy to decompress the spinal canal following a spine fracture is mentioned only to be avoided as this procedure often leads to further kyphosis, especially if the anterior column has been injured.

A thorough understanding of the extent of instability associated with any given spine injury is crucial to avoid under-diagnosing significant injuries. The following classification provides an improved understanding of the extent of instability of spine injuries.

## CLASSIFICATION OF THORACIC AND LUMBAR FRACTURES IN SPINE INSTABILITY

The Comprehensive Classification advocated by Magerl and coworkers identifies progressive instability as one moves through the classification (Fig. 22-3).[11,14] *Type A injuries* include those associated with compressive lesions with relative intactness to the posterior elements. *Type B injuries,* for the most part are distraction injuries; that is, a transverse disruption of the posterior elements along with disruption anteriorly either through the disk or through the vertebral body. The third category, *Type C injuries,* are disruptions with associated rotation, whereby multiple vectors produce forces, which result in the most unstable of all spine injuries. Instability increases as one progresses through the classification from Type A to Type C.

If significant instability has been recognized, then surgical measures must be undertaken to stabilize the injury and prevent posttraumatic kyphosis. If these more serious injuries go unrecognized and are treated nonoperatively, in many cases they progress to further kyphotic deformity and late pain.

## EVALUATION OF KYPHOTIC DEFORMITY

The extent of kyphotic deformity must be evaluated. This is determined on lateral radiographs by the

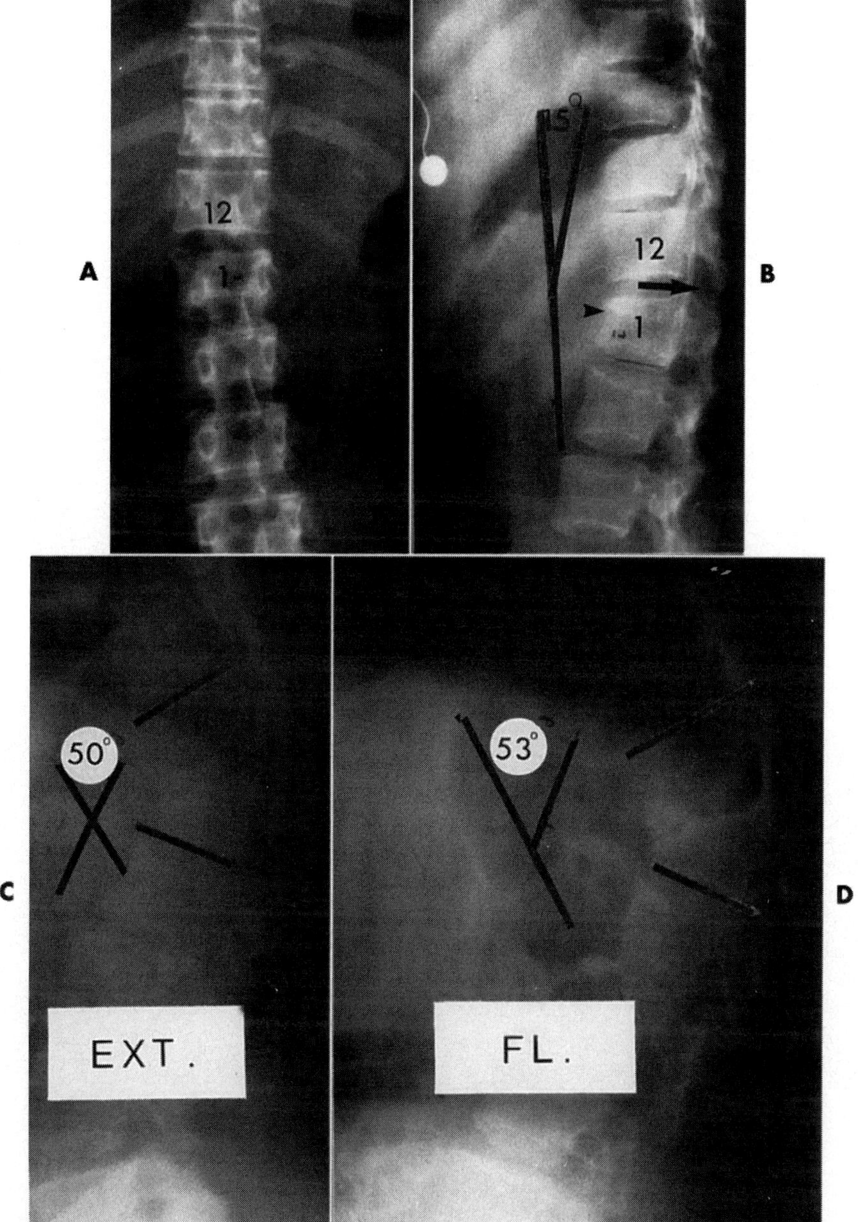


**FIGURE 22-1**

Type B injury with soft tissue disruption posteriorly and loss of vertebral height anteriorly. **A, B,** This seemingly innocuous fracture of the vertebral body (*arrowhead*) is combined with posterior disruption of the soft tissues (*arrow*). The kyphosis initially measured 15 degrees. **C,D,** Extension and flexion radiographs two years later demonstrate a marked kyphotic deformity of 50 and 53 degrees, respectively, due to the lack of posterior tensile and anterior compressive support. Marked pain was a sequelae of this deformity. *(With permission Gertzbien SD: Fractures of the thoracic and lumbar spine, Baltimore, 1992, Williams & Wilkins.)*

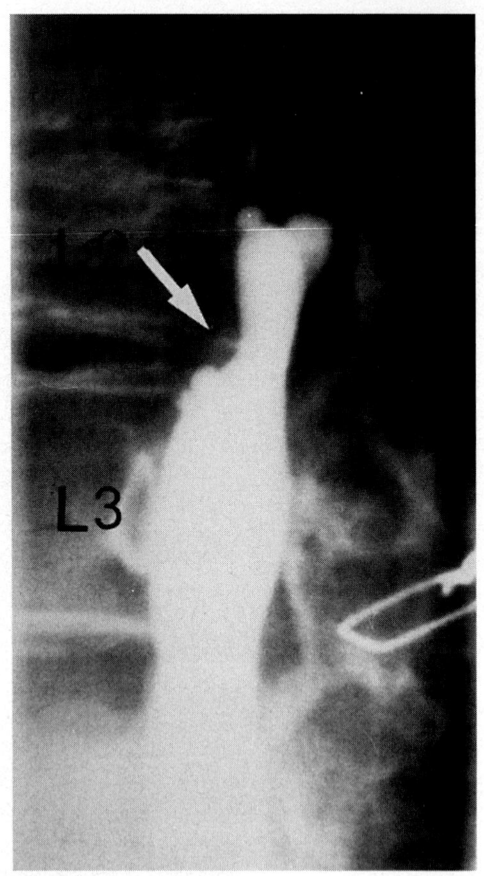


**FIGURE 22-2**

Spinal stenosis with neurological signs. This 45-year-old woman treated with laminectomy for a burst fracture of L2 17 years earlier, developed progressive weakness in the lower limbs secondary to the deformity and the intraspinal fragment (*white arrow*) and a kyphotic deformity. *(With permission Gertzbien SD: Fractures of the thoracic and lumbar spine, Baltimore, 1992, Williams & Wilkins.)*

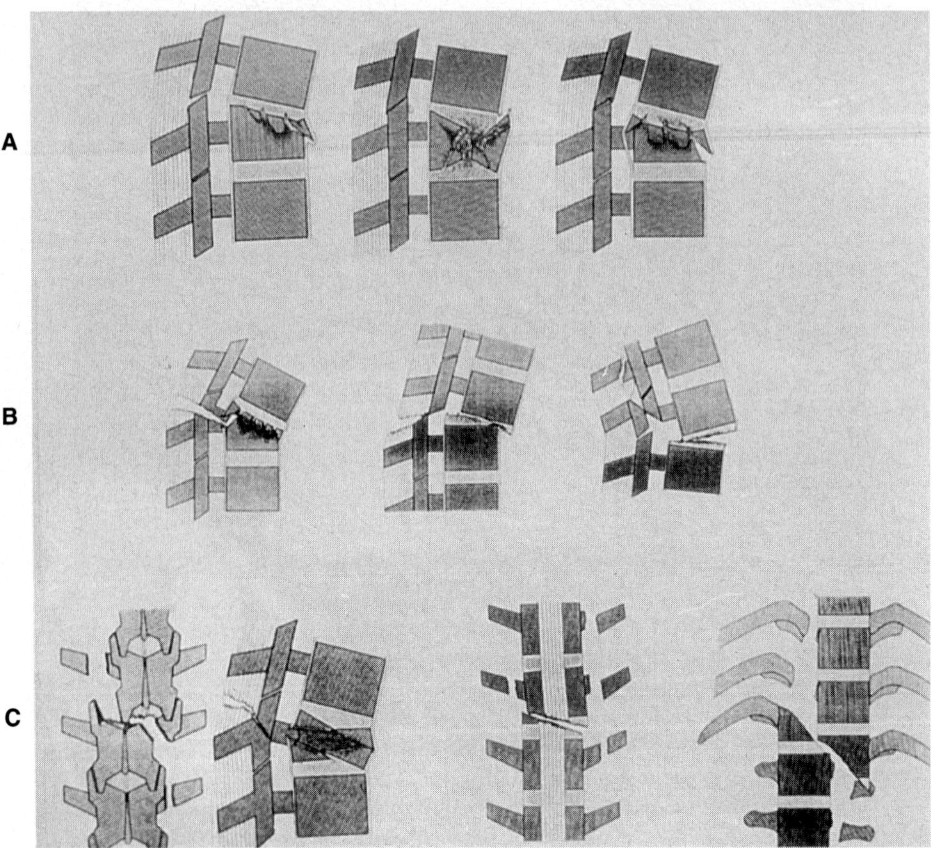


**FIGURE 22-3**

Comprehensive classification of thoracic and lumbar fractures. Type A injuries include wedge fractures, coronal split fractures (pincer), and burst fractures. Type B injuries involve distraction, usually posteriorly with disruption anteriorly through the vertebral body or disk, and occasionally distraction anteriorly with fracture of the posterior element. Type C injuries are those associated with rotation and may include additional injuries associated with distraction and/or shear.

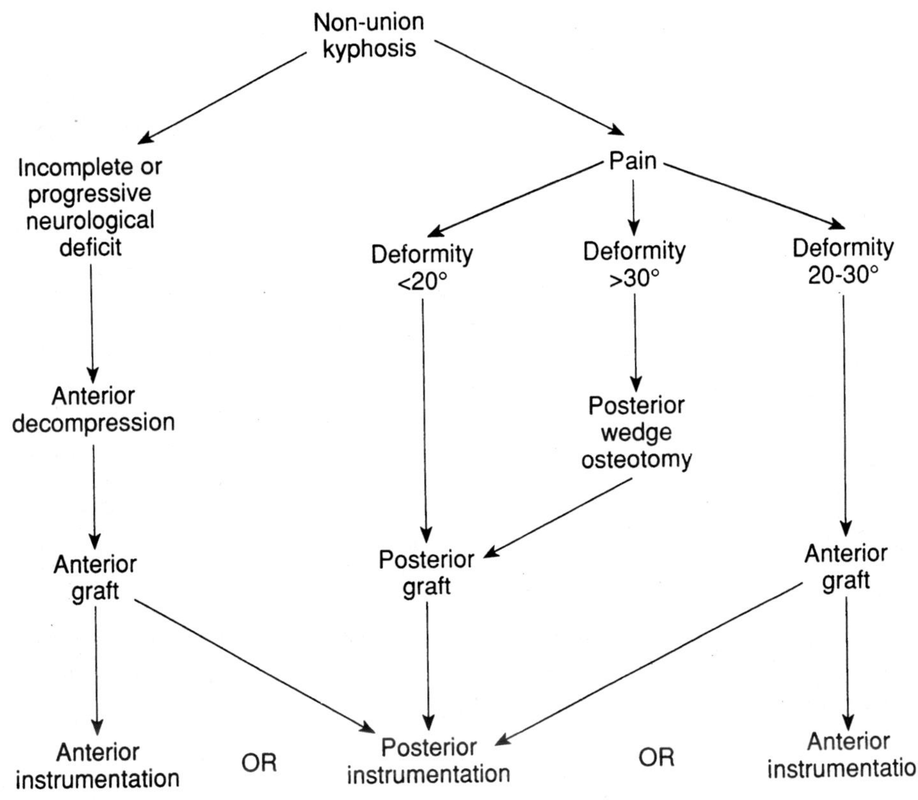


**FIGURE 22-4**

Algorithmn for the management of posttraumatic kyphosis. *(With permission Gertzbien SD: Fractures of the thoracic and lumbar spine, Baltimore, 1992, Williams & Wilkins.)*

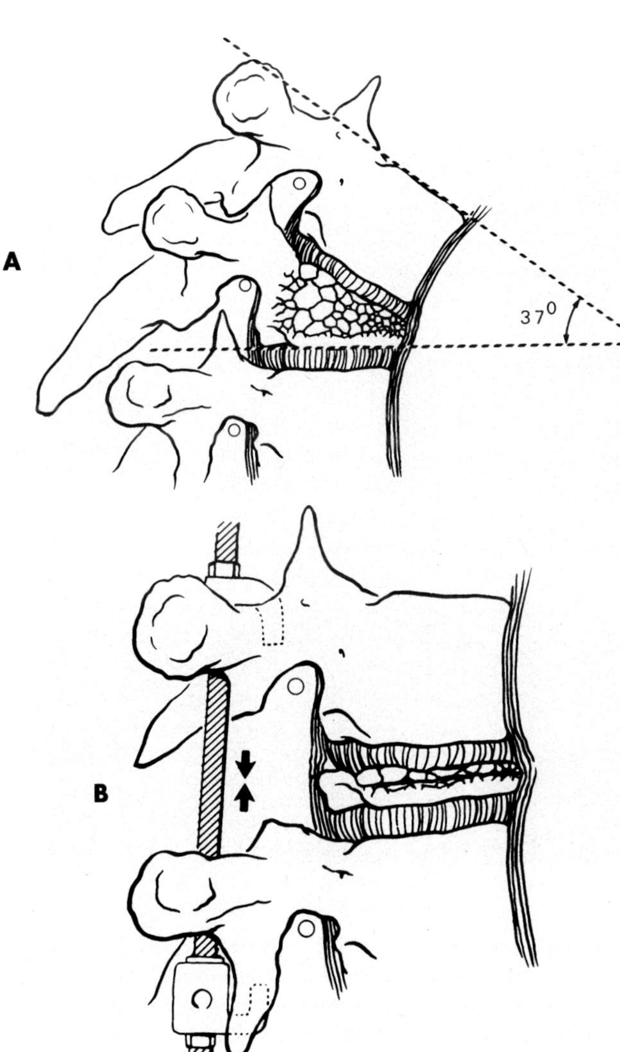


**FIGURE 22-5**

Posttraumatic kyphosis correction. Dorsal wedge osteotomy. **A,** Diagrammatic representation of a Type A complete burst fracture with a 37-degree kyphotic deformity. **B,** After wedge resection and compression posteriorly using a compressive device, the deformity is reduced to a normal anatomical alignment. *(With permission Gertzbien SD: Fractures of the thoracic and lumbar spine, Baltimore, 1992, Williams & Wilkins.)*

Cobb technique measuring the inferior endplate of the involved vertebrae and the superior endplate of the vertebra above. Careful assessment of pain is also essential. Facet blocks above or below the lesion and diskogram pain studies at the level of the lesion may be helpful. Flexion/extension views may be useful in identifying motion at a pseudarthrosis site and tomograms may confirm the nonunion.

## ALGORITHM FOR MANAGEMENT OF POSTTRAUMATIC KYPHOSIS

The degree of deformity is variable and dictates the approach to management. Lesser kyphotic angles require a different approach than the more severe deformities (Fig. 22-4).[3] In cases in which there is incomplete or progressive neurological deficit, an anterior approach should be taken to decompress the neural elements. Anterior correction, strut graft, and anterior instrumentation are recommended as the treatment of choice under these circumstances. If anterior instrumentation techniques are not familiar to the treating surgeon, the anterior strut graft should be supplemented with posterior instrumentation, because there is a significant progression of the deformity after the anterior grafting without instrumentation.[5]

If mechanical back pain is the primary indication for surgery, and the patient is neurologically intact, consideration should be given to whether the deformity is less than 20 degrees, between 20 and 30 degrees, or greater than 30 degrees. In most cases in which there is less than a 20-degree deformity, and the deformity is mobile, as proven by flexion/extension views, then posterior fusion with a compressive device (such as pedicle screw fixation or other compressive instrumentation) should be undertaken. If the deformity is rigid, however, posterior fusion and splinting with instrumentation is recommended without an attempt at correction. In cases where there is a 20- to

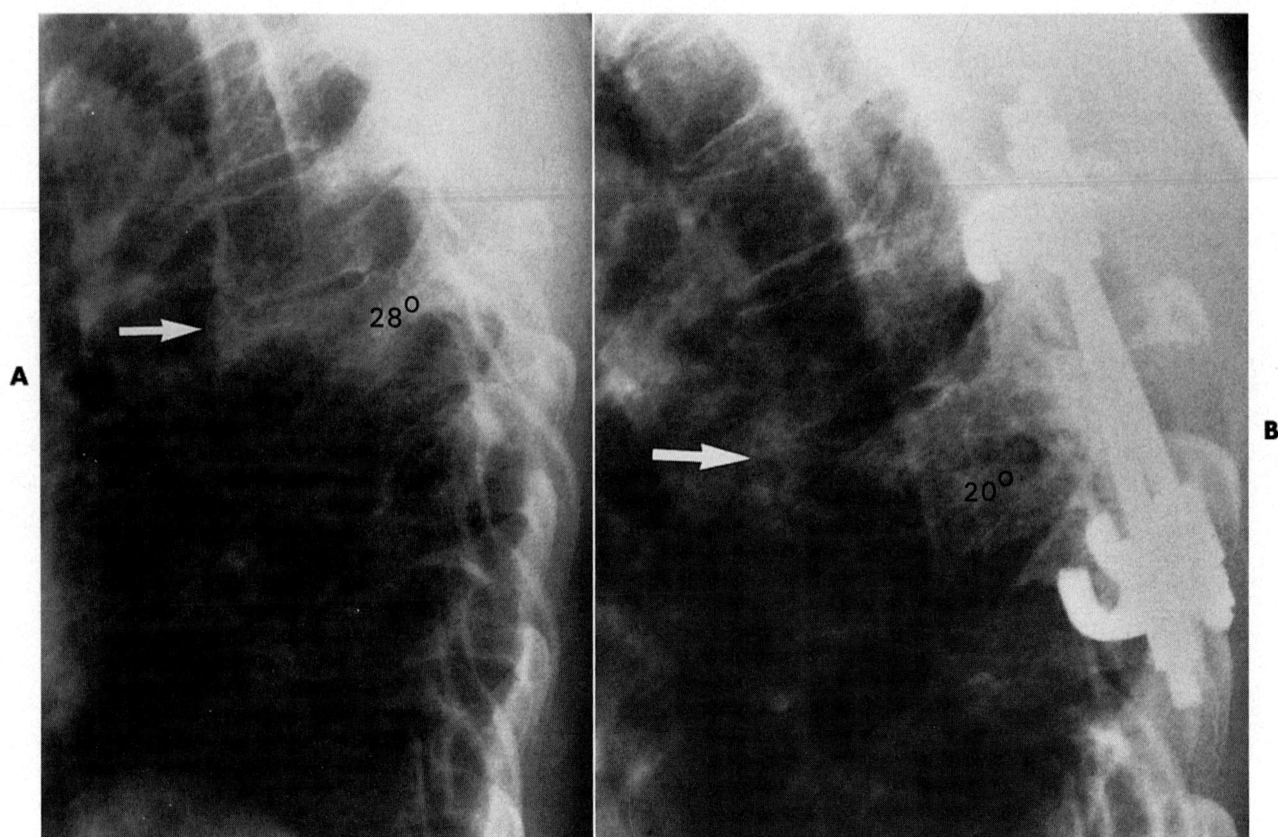


**FIGURE 22-6**

Posttraumatic kyphosis. **A,** This patient had a Type A complete burst fracture (*white arrow*) presented one year later with a 28-degree kyphotic deformity and local pain. Facet blocks alleviated most of the pain. **B,** Following compression rod instrumentation one level above and below, coupled with an in situ bone graft, a modest correction of the deformity was obtained and the symptoms alleviated. *(With permission Gertzbien SD: Fractures of the thoracic and lumbar spine, Baltimore, 1992, Williams & Wilkins.)*

30-degree deformity, anterior strut grafting and instrumentation can be considered, particularly if there is significant spinal stenosis.

Where the deformity is greater than 30 degrees, anterior grafting and posterior instrumentation are the standard treatment; however, recently, a full-wedge osteotomy has been described involving both the anterior and posterior elements with the use of a bone graft and posterior compression instrumentation (Fig. 22-5).[6,14]

## SURGICAL TECHNIQUES

A number of surgical techniques have been reported to correct kyphotic deformity of the spine[7-12,15-21,23-25] and should be reviewed before embarking on correction of the deformity. These include anterior corpectomy, correction of deformity and stabilization with a strut graft, or cage devices with graft. Anterior or posterior internal fixation are added for additional stabilization. The recent description of full posterior wedge osteotomy is an effective technique for correction for the appropriate indications (Figs. 22-6, 22-7, and 22-8).[6,14]

In summary, unstable fractures of the thoracic and lumbar spine may result in development of posttraumatic kyphosis if inadequately treated. The surgical approach may be anterior, posterior, or both, depending on the severity of the deformity.

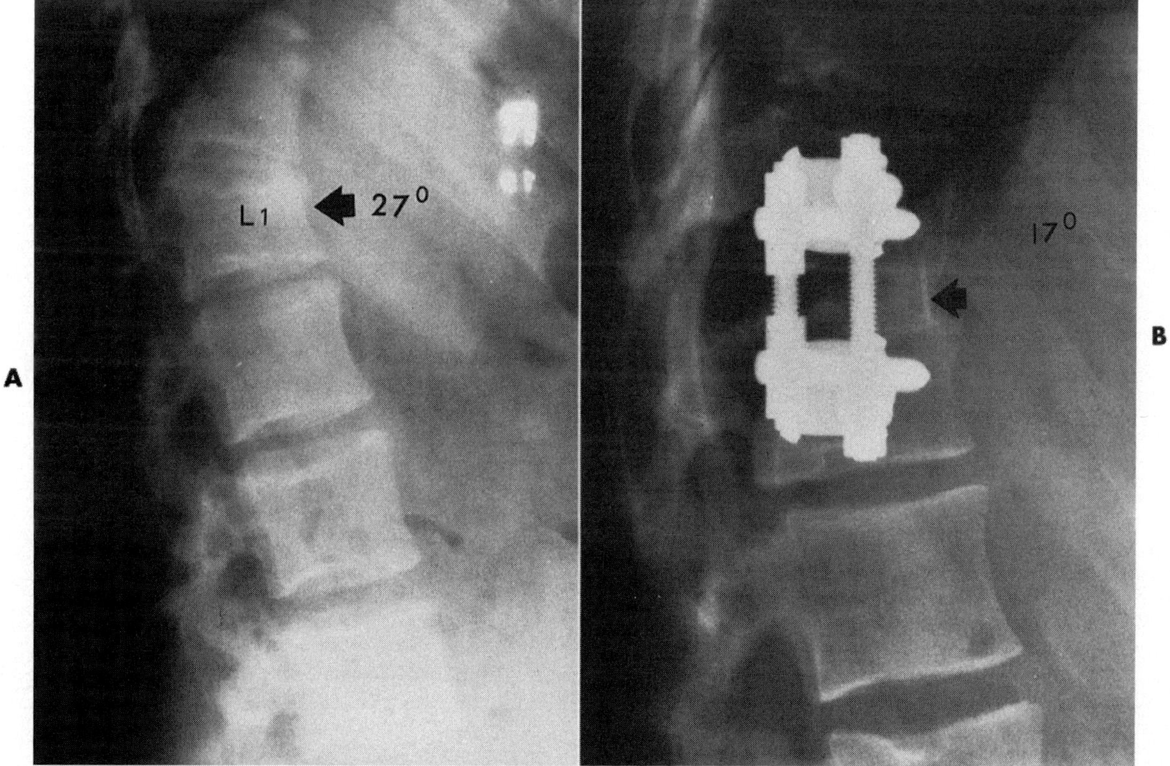


**FIGURE 22-7**

Posttraumatic kyphosis. **A,** This Type A wedge injury of 27 degrees is associated with significant local back pain two and a half years following the fracture. A diskogram pain study was positive at T12-L1. **B,** Anterior excision of the disk, insertion of the tricortical graft (*arrow*), and anterior instrumentation resulted in correction of the deformity with complete relief of symptoms. *(With permission Gertzbien SD: Fractures of the thoracic and lumbar spine, Baltimore, 1992, Williams & Wilkins.)*

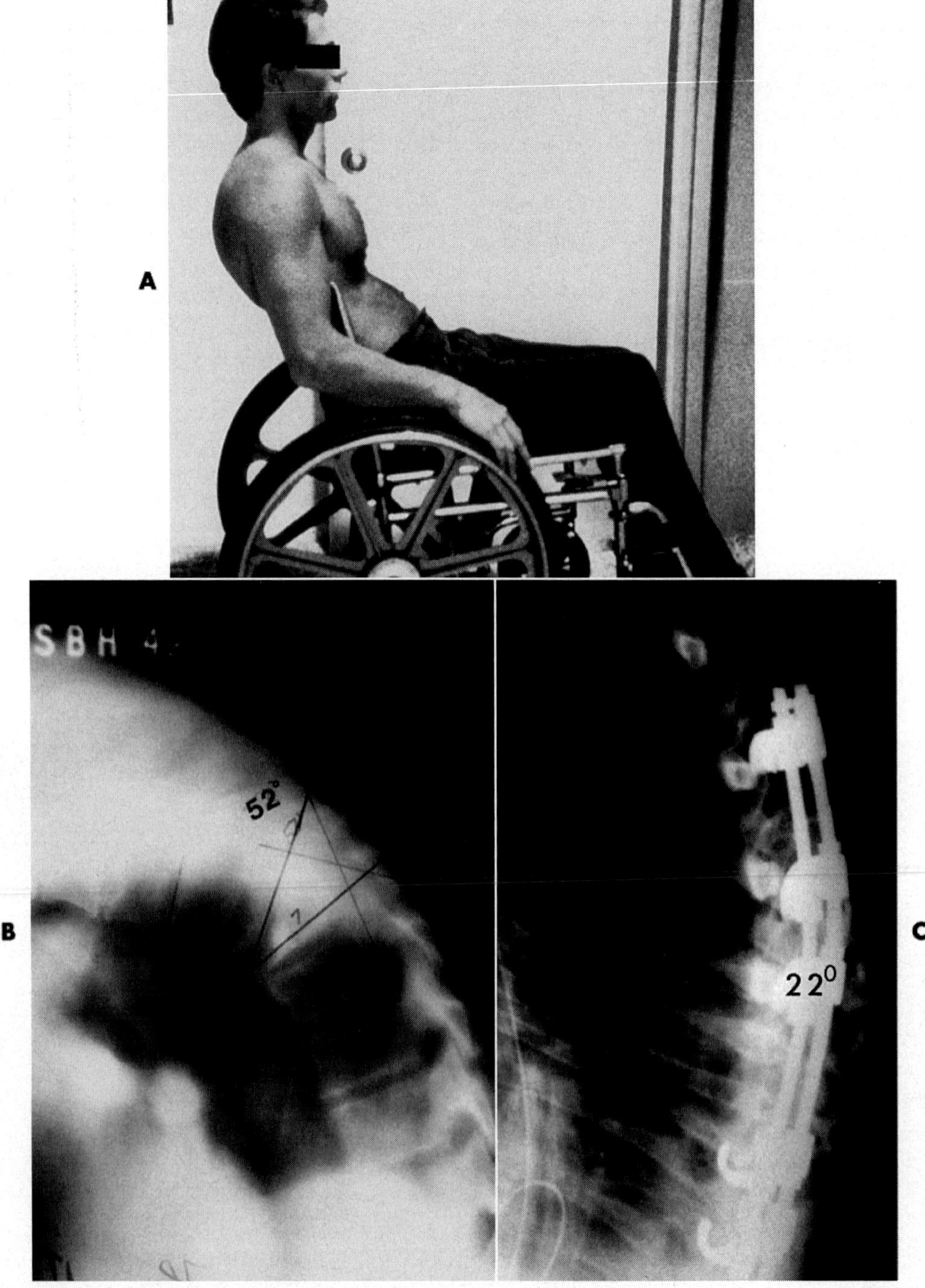


**FIGURE 22-8**

Posttraumatic kyphosis. Dorsal wedge osteotomy. **A,** This patient with a moderate kyphosis in the midthoracic spine, had to sit slouched in his wheelchair to comfortably see straight ahead. **B,** The kyphotic deformity, secondary to a Type C injury, measured 52 degrees. **C,** Following dorsal wedge osteotomy, alignment was restored with a residual kyphosis of 22 degrees, improving the sitting posture.

## REFERENCES

1. Bohlmann HH, Anderson P: Anterior decompression and arthrodesis of the cervical spine: long term motor improvement. Part I: Improvement in incomplete traumatic quadriparesis, *J Bone Joint Surg* 74A(5):671-682, 1992.
2. Bradford DS, Ganjavian S, Antonious D, et al: Anterior strut grafting for the treatment of kyphosis: review of experience with forty-eight patients, *J Bone Joint Surg* 64A:680-690, 1982.
3. Gertzbein SD: Fractures of the thoracic and lumbar spine. Baltimore, 1992, Williams and Wilkins.

4. Gertzbein SD: Multicenter spine fracture study, *Spine* 17(5) 528-540, 1992.
5. Gertzbein SD, Court-Brown CM, Jacobs RR, et al: Decompression and circumferential stabilization of unstable spinal fractures, *Spine* 13(8):892-895, 1988.
6. Gertzbein SD, Harris MB: Wedge osteotomy for the correction of post-traumatic kyphosis, *Spine* 17(3):374-379, 1992.
7. Goel MK: Vertebral osteotomy for correction of fixed flexion deformity of the spine, *J Bone Joint Surg* 50A:287-294, 1968.
8. Heinig CF, Boyd BM Jr: One-stage vertebrectomy or eggshell procedure. Personal communication.
9. Jodoin A, Gillet P, Dupuis PR, Maurais G: Surgical treatment of post-traumatic kyphosis: a report of 16 cases, *Can J Surg* 32:36-42, 1989.
10. Johnson JTH, Robinson RA: Anterior strut grafts for severe kyphosis: results of 3 cases with a preceding progressive paraplegia, *Clin Orthop* 56:25-36, 1968.
11. Kaneda K, Abumi K, Fujiya M: Burst fractures with neurologic deficits of the thoracolumbar-lumbar spine: Results of anterior decompression and stabilization with anterior instrumentation, *Spine* 9:788-795, 1988.
12. Kaneda K, Durakami C, Minami A: Free vascularized fibular strut graft in the treatment of kyphosis, *Spine* 13:1273-1277, 1988.
13. Kostuik JP, Matsusaki H: Anterior stabilization instrumentation, and decompression for post-traumatic kyphosis, *Spine* 14:379-386, 1989.
14. Lehmer SM, Keppler L, Biscut RS, et al: Posterior transvertebral osteotomy for adult thoracolumbar kyphosis, *Spine* 19(18):2060-2067, 1994.
15. Magerl F, Aebi M, Gertzbein SD, Harms J, Nazarian S: *Eur Spine J* 3:184-201, 1994.
16. Malcolm BW, Bradford DS, Winter RB, Chou SN: Post-traumatic kyphosis: a review of forty-eight surgically treated patients, *J Bone Joint Surg* 63A:891-900, 1981.
17. McAfee PC, Bohlmann HH, Yuan HA: Anterior decompression of traumatic thoracolumbar fractures with incomplete neurological deficit using a retroperitoneal approach, *J Bone Joint Surg* 67A:89-104, 1985.
18. McBride GG, Bradford DS: Vertebral body replacement with femoral neck allograft and vascularized rib strut graft: a technique for treating post-traumatic kyphosis with neurologic deficit, *Spine* 8:406-415, 1983.
19. McMaster PE: Osteotomy of the spine for fixed flexion deformity, *J Bone Joint Surg* 44A:1207-1216, 1962.
20. Roberson JR, Whitesides TE Jr: Surgical reconstruction of late post-traumatic thoracolumbar kyphosis, *Spine* 10:307-312, 1985.
21. Roy-Camile R, Saillant G, Mazel CH, et al: The surgical treatment of post-traumatic vertebral deformities, *Ital J Orthop Traumatol* 12:419-426, 1986.
22. Soreff J: Assessment of the late results of traumatic compression fractures of the thoracolumbar vertebral bodies: a clinical radiological and medical/social computer conducted survey, Thesis, Gotenburg, Sweden, 1977.
23. Smith-Peterson MN, Larson CB, Aufranc OE: Osteotomy of the spine for correction of flexion deformity in rheumatoid arthritis, *J Bone Joint Surg* 27:1-11, 1945.
24. Streitz W, Brown JC, Bonnet CA: Anterior fibular strut grafting in the treatment of kyphosis, *Clin Orthop* 128:140-148, 1977.
25. Yuan HA, Mann KA, Found EM, et al: Early clinical experience with the Syracuse I-plate: an anterior spinal fixation device, *Spine* 13:278-285, 1988.

# 23

# REVISION OF THORACOLUMBAR FRACTURES TREATED SURGICALLY: POSTTRAUMATIC KYPHOSIS

**John R. Klein, M.D.**
**Frank J. Schwab, M.D.**
**Jean-Pierre C. Farcy, M.D.**



Posttraumatic kyphotic deformities of the spine remain a significant challenge to the spine surgeon. Significant evolution in surgical technique and instrumentation has occurred over the past decades and yet progressive kyphosis after acute surgical stabilization continues to plague specialists. Crucial to understanding this issue is a comprehension of spinal stability after injury. Numerous classification systems have been developed to create a common language in defining spine fractures. Their ability in guiding treatment and avoiding long-term problems such as kyphosis is not absolute. Much agreement now exists in the treatment of mild injury patterns such as minimal compression fractures, or very unstable patterns such as fracture-dislocations. Guidelines on burst fractures in the thoracolumbar region remain a topic of great debate. Although there are many problems related to nonoperatively treated burst fractures, there are also surgically treated burst fractures that lead to long-term complications related to progression of deformity. It is these surgically treated injuries and their progression into kyphotic deformity that will be addressed in this text.

## INSTABILITY AND PROGRESSION OF DEFORMITY

Posttraumatic kyphosis is a common complication of untreated or inadequately treated thoracolumbar burst fractures. The development of kyphosis and its progression is due to the presence of instability. The definition of what constitutes spinal instability has evolved over time and continues to this day to be a controversial and much debated subject.

Nicoll is credited with the first attempt at classifying fractures into stable and unstable categories.[56] Nicoll recognized that unstable fractures were likely to undergo progression of deformity and required treatment with plaster immobilization. Holdsworth is recognized for coining the term "burst fracture."[34,35] He described the burst fracture as a stable entity because he believed that this fracture did not disrupt the posterior ligament complex, which he considered critical to maintaining spinal stability.

The concept of the two-column spine was introduced by Kelly and Whitesides in 1968.[39] In this model, the anterior column consists of the vertebral bodies, whereas the posterior column is made up of the neural arches. Using the two-column model as his guide, Whitesides pointed out that anteriorly the spine is subjected to compressive forces and posteriorly the spine is placed under tensile forces. According to Whitesides, the inability of the spine to withstand either of these forces leads to kyphosis and its progression.[73] In their review of the biomechanics of kyphosis, White et al[72] note that the initial anterior wedging of the vertebrae creates an increased moment arm. This moment arm increases the amount of eccentric loading that is placed on the vertebrae. Thus, the greater the initial amount of anterior angulation of the vertebrae, the greater the degree of loading that is placed on the vertebrae, thereby increasing the risk of further progression of the kyphotic deformity.

In 1983, Denis introduced the concept of the three-column spine.[15,16] Using the three-column spine as his model, Denis defined the burst fracture as a failure of the anterior and middle columns, secondary to an axial compressive load. McAfee et al further added to the concept of instability by classifying burst fractures into stable and unstable categories.[47] A stable burst fracture is defined as a disruption of the anterior and middle columns, whereas the unstable burst fracture is defined as a disruption of all 3 columns. More recently, Farcy proposed a detailed scoring system for thoracolumbar fractures that considers anterior column collapse as well as ligamentous support from all three columns. This scoring system is applied in a useful treatment algorithm.[23,24,29]

## SURGICAL TREATMENT OF THORACOLUMBAR FRACTURES—EVOLUTION OF TECHNIQUES AND LATE COMPLICATIONS

The indications for the acute surgical treatment of thoracolumbar burst fractures are controversial. Most clinicians agree that patients with incomplete neurologic injury or progressive neurologic involvement require early surgical intervention. Many other clinicians believe that unstable burst fractures require early surgical stabilization in order to prevent progressive kyphotic deformity and neurologic injury. The goals of internal fixation of thoracolumbar burst fractures are reduction of deformity, stabilization, and decompression of the neural canal. Proponents argue that acute surgical fixation allows for earlier patient mobilization and facilitates patient rehabilitation. This, in turn, leads to fewer complications associated with prolonged bed rest and decreases hospital length of stay.

## HARRINGTON INSTRUMENTATION

Harrington instrumentation was one of the earliest and most widely used treatment modalities for thoracolumbar burst fractures. Despite its widespread use and initial acceptance, Harrington instrumentation has been associated with a high complication rate.[3,14,17,25,27,48,55,59,76]

One of the goals of Harrington instrumentation is the correction of deformity and maintenance of reduction. Several studies have revealed that Harrington instrumentation has been associated with a high incidence of inadequate correction and loss of reduction.[27,48,59,76] In their review of the literature, Riebel et al determined that the overall average loss of correction associated with the use of Harrington instrumentation in the treatment of thoracolumbar fractures was 5.5 degrees.[59] McAfee and Bohlman in their series on the complications associated with Harrington instrumentation noted inadequate reduction of deformity in 9 out of 40 patients.[48] Gertzbein et al similarly reviewed their use of Harrington instrumentation in the treatment of thoracolumbar fractures.[27] In this series, 19 of 36 patients had unsatisfactory correction of deformity. In 4 of these patients no correction was achieved. Moreover, 12 of 21 (57%) burst fractures were noted to have significant loss of reduction on follow-up (= 5 degrees). The authors postulated that the association of Harrington instrumentation with the loss of reduction in burst fractures is due to the lack of anterior bone stock seen in many burst fractures. Due to this lack of anterior support, the Harrington rods, unable to withstand the bending and tension forces, fail, leading to a loss of correction. Consequently, Gertzbein et al recommend that, in fractures in which anterior column support is deficient, Harrington instrumentation should be augmented with anterior grafting.

Postoperative removal of Harrington rods used for the treatment of thoracolumbar fractures has been advocated by many clinicians. These clinicians argue that the early removal of Harrington rods preserves the unfused motion segments spanned by the rods (the rod-long, fuse-short technique). Several studies have demonstrated, however, that early removal of the Harrington rods leads to a significant loss of reduction.[3,14,55,59] In essence, this uninstrumented posterior fusion mass fails to withstand the tensile forces and progresses into kyphosis. Akbarnia et al reported on their results of 13 patients suffering from thoracolumbar fractures treated with Harrington instrumentation.[3] After removal of the Harrington rods, average loss of correction was 9 degrees with 9 patients losing more than 7 degrees of correction. Riebel et al note that the literature reflects an overall average loss of correction of 11 degrees in a series in which patients have had their Harrington rods removed.[59]

One of the basic principles of Harrington instrumentation is that it achieves decompression of the spine through ligamentotaxis. It is thought that distraction of the posterior longitudinal ligament (PLL) with its attachment to the posteriorly displaced bone fragments allows for the indirect decompression of the spine.[17,48,59,70] Nevertheless, studies have demonstrated that inadequate decompression of the neural canal is one of the major complications associated with Harrington instrumentation.[5,14,48,60] McAfee and Bohlman in their review of Harrington rod complications reported that 16 patients with burst fractures required an additional anterior decompression for persistent neural compression after posterior Harrington instrumentation.[48]

Overdistraction of the spine by Harrington instrumentation is thought to be prevented by the intact PLL.[17,48] However, the PLL can be disrupted in burst fractures. McAfee and Bohlman noted that in their series there were 4 cases of overdistraction, resulting in increased neurologic injury in 3 patients and the eventual death of 1 patient due to ascending paralysis.[48] On exploration the PLL was found to be lax in each case.

Instrument-related failure is another highly reported complication associated with the use of Harrington instrumentation.[17,21,25,48,59] In one of the first reports on the use of Harrington rods in the treatment of thoracolumbar fractures, Flesch et al noted 2 broken rods and 2 dislodged rods.[25] Dickson et al reported 6 instances of broken rods and 6 cases of hook dislodgement.[17] McAfee and Bohlman reported 16 cases of rod dislodgment or disengagement with resultant loss of fixation.[48] Overall, Riebel et al state that the average rod-related complication rate is 15.5 percent.[59]

Recently, attention has been focused on the flat back syndrome and its association with Harrington instrumentation. It is believed that when Harrington rods extend into the lumbosacral spine, the distraction of the rods leads to a loss of lordosis in the lumbar spine.[18,40,42,59] This loss of sagittal spine contour eventually leads to the flat back syndrome, in which patients develop the sensation of falling forwards. In order to maintain an erect posture, patients keep their hips and knees flexed. The strain associated with this hip and knee flexion leads to fatigue, back pain, and lower extremity pain. Progressive pain and disability often require surgical intervention to alleviate these symptoms.

## SEGMENTAL SPINAL INSTRUMENTATION—SUBLAMINAR WIRING

Clinicians have investigated the use of segmental spinal instrumentation, popularized by Luque,[43,44,45] in the treatment of thoracolumbar fractures.[2,7,11,26,69] Initially used in the treatment of scoliosis, segmental instrumentation involves the passage of sublaminar wires at each noninjured instrumented level. These wires are then attached to two individual L-shaped rods. In comparison to Harrington instrumentation, segmental instrumentation is a more rigid and stable fixation system due to its multiple sites of fixation, which distribute the load over a wider area.[4,6,11,30,71,77] Accordingly, Luque and others believe that one of the advantages of segmental instrumentation is that, due to this increased stability, patient immobilization with casting or bracing is unnecessary.[2,4,7,26,43,45]

Because segmentally instrumented L-rods do not have distraction hooks, one of the perceived deficiencies of Luque segmental fixation is that no distractive force can be generated in the treatment of thoracolumbar fractures. In order to overcome this deficiency, Luque et al described the use of a Harrington outrigger, prior to application of Luque instrumentation, to distract and reduce thoracolumbar fractures.[45] Many clinicians, however, do not use the Luque rods in the treatment of thoracolumbar fractures. Instead, spine surgeons have often used Harrington distraction rods with sublaminar wiring in order to combine the benefits of both systems.

Biomechanical testing has confirmed that the combination of sublaminar wiring with Harrington rods provides increased rigidity and stability compared to Harrington rods alone.[49,54,71] McAfee et al demonstrated that segmentally wired Harrington rods, in comparison to Luque segmental instrumentation and Harrington rods alone, provided greater axial stability for unstable burst fractures.[49]

The increased risk of passing wires through the epidural space has prompted several investigators to use interspinous wiring as a means of segmental fixation.[19,57,58] Phillips et al examined the use of Harrington rods supplemented with interspinous wiring in the treatment of unstable thoracolumbar fractures.[58] This group of patients was compared retrospectively to patients who had been treated with Harrington rods alone. The Harrington rod group revealed a significant average loss of correction postoperatively (10.4 degrees). In contrast, the segmentally wired group had an average loss of reduction of 3.4 degrees. There was also a statistically significant greater number of instrument-related failures and reoperations in the Harrington rod group. The investigators concluded that the increased rigidity and stability of the segmentally wired Harrington rods contributed to the decreased incidence of instrument-related failure and improved maintenance of postoperative correction.

One of the disadvantages of segmental instrumentation is that it is a more technically demanding operation. In spite of its ability to improve stability, segmental instrumentation has also been associated with wire breakage and subsequent loss of reduction.[6] Of note, the greatest disadvantage of segmental instrumentation is the potential risk of neurologic injury. Passage of the wires through the posterior epidural space or breakage of the wires postoperatively can lead to injury of the spinal cord, dura, or nerve roots.[4,6,11,13,30,37,43,74,77] Wilber et al in their review documented a 17% incidence of neurologic complications associated with segmental instrumentation.[74] Although most of these cases involved temporary sensory changes, 3 patients suffered a significant spinal cord injury. Accordingly, these potential neurologic complications associated with segmental instrumentation have diminished its popularity in the treatment in thoracolumbar fractures.

## COTREL-DUBOUSSET INSTRUMENTATION

Cotrel-Dubousset (CD) instrumentation and other pedicle screw fixation systems have recently taken the forefront in treatment of thoracolumbar spine fractures. Initially developed for the treatment of scoliosis, CD instrumentation has evolved to a versatile instrumentation system providing rigid and stable fixation through the use of multiple hooks, pedicle screws, and transverse cross-links. Unlike Harrington instrumentation, the CD rods can be segmentally attached and contoured to optimize the sagittal contour of the spine.

Several biomechanical studies have investigated the rigidity and stability provided by CD instrumentation. Gurr et al demonstrated that under axial loading, flexion, and rotational testing, CD instrumentation provided greater stability than the Harrington and Luque instrumentation systems.[32] Farcy et al also compared the stiffness and stability of CD instrumentation to segmentally wired Harrington rods and Luque instrumentation.[22] Biomechanical testing revealed that one-level CD instrumentation provided the greatest rotational stability, whereas two-level CD instrumentation gave superior axial stability.

Despite clear advantages of the CD instrumentation in the treatment of thoracolumbar fractures, long-term complications do occur. In a clinical series, Moreland et al reported an average postoperative loss of correction of 3.6 degrees.[53] One hardware failure (a broken pedicle screw) did not require reinstrumentation. McBride retrospectively reported on 45 patients suffering from unstable thoracolumbar fractures.[51] Three patients underwent additional anterior procedures. A minimum of 3 vertebral levels above and below the injured vertebrae were instrumented. Three different types of CD constructs were used depending on the type of injury. Postoperative loss of reduction averaged 3.8 degrees. There were 2 cases of instrument failure with concomitant loss of correction, which required reinstrumentation. No case of iatrogenic neurologic injury was noted postoperatively. Graziano reported similar results (n = 14).[31] Loss of correction averaged 0.5 degrees postoperatively. There was 1 case of screw failure that did not require reinstrumentation.

In spite of the many reports documenting the efficacy and low complication rate associated with CD instrumentation in the treatment of thoracolumbar fractures, some have documented a significant complication rate associated with short-segment fixation using pedicle screw fixation systems.[8,12,20,52,67] Carl et al reviewed the results of 38 patients treated with short-segment CD instrumentation.[12] Thirty-two patients had instrumentation and fusion of one vertebra cephalad and caudad to the injured vertebrae. Postoperative loss of correction was significant, averaging 6.5 degrees. Ten cases of hardware failure were documented. McLain et al also reported a high complication rate associated with CD instrumentation.[52] The majority of patients in this study were instrumented 1 level above and below the disrupted vertebrae. Ten out of 19 patients were noted to have a loss of reduction greater than 5 degrees. Two of these patients required additional surgery for stabilization. This significant incidence of loss of correction was attributed to the high rate of hardware failure. Twenty-nine percent of the pedicle screws placed cephalad to the injured vertebrae were bent, while 36 percent of the screws immediately caudad to the damaged vertebrae were either bent or broken. The authors also noted that in all patients with residual anterior column instability, there was significant loss of reduction. The authors concluded that in patients who have anterior column instability the screws in short-segment fixation are subject to increased bending moments which can lead to an increased rate of hardware failure.

Loss of reduction and hardware failure is not only seen with short-segment CD instrumentation.[8,20] Ebelke et al reported their experience with Variable Screw Placement (VSP) instrumentation in the treatment of thoracolumbar burst fractures.[20] Short-segment fixation was used in which plates spanned one vertebra above and below the burst fracture. Eight out of 21 patients received additional anterior bone grafting. Only 1 patient in the bone grafting group experienced hardware failure. However, in the nonaugmented group, 54% of the patients suffered from instrument failure. Loss of correction was not addressed. The authors concluded that the use ofVSP instrumentation, without anterior bone grafting, in the treatment of thoracolumbar burst fractures can lead to a high rate of failure.

Several biomechanical studies have investigated the use of short-segment instrumentation in the treatment of thoracolumbar burst fractures.[33,63,64] Gurwitz et al documented that axial stiffness of short-segment posterior instrumentation is significantly less than posterior instrumentation augmented with an anterior strut graft or anterior instrumentation with anterior strut grafting.[33] The authors state that the use of posterior instrumentation alone in the treatment of burst fractures does not provide adequate rigidity and stiffness to the spine. Slosar et al also investigated the biomechanical stability of three different short-segment transpedicular systems.[64] The investigators also revealed that short-segment fixation fails to adequately restore the axial stability of the spine. The authors state that transpedicular systems may need to be augmented especially if there is a three-column injury.

Farcy and Weidenbaum retrospectively reviewed their experience with CD instrumentation in the treatment of 27 patients with unstable spine fractures.[23] The majority of cases had 2 levels above and below the injured vertebrae instrumented. All 11 burst fractures were treated with additional anterior strut grafting and fusion. In all cases there were no instances of instrument failure or loss of correction. It is the senior author's belief that all burst fractures with significant loss of anterior bone stock and ligamentous injury require additional anterior strut grafting and fusion to provide adequate stability.

## EVALUATION OF POSTTRAUMATIC KYPHOSIS

Kyphotic deformity after spinal trauma can be a significantly disabling condition. Kyphosis and its progression may lead to chronic back pain, new-onset or progressive neurologic involvement, fatigue, and failure of patient rehabilitation. New-onset or progressive neurologic involvement is usually secondary to anterior cord compression in which the cord becomes tented over the apex of the deformity. Patients may also suffer from symptoms of spinal stenosis. Findings on physical examination can range from back pain (usually concentrated over the apex of the kyphosis), to paresthesias and radiculopathy of the lower extremity, lower extremity weakness, and bladder, bowel, or sexual dysfunction. Skin breakdown may also be noted over the apex of the deformity.

Radiographic analysis preoperatively includes anteroposterior, lateral, and flexion-extension radiographs. The degree of kyphosis is measured by the Cobb technique. Plumb line measurements are taken to assess the degree of sagittal malalignment. A myelogram with delayed computed tomography (CT) imaging should be obtained in order to evaluate the degree of canal compromise and to identify areas of dural and nerve root impingement. Magnetic resonance imaging (MRI) scans are also important in the preoperative assessment. The MRI, with its unrivaled ability to image the soft tissues, provides important information on the posterior ligamentous structures, spinal cord, and disks.

## TREATMENT OPTIONS FOR SURGICALLY TREATED POSTTRAUMATIC KYPHOSIS

The literature on the surgical treatment of posttraumatic kyphosis is surprisingly sparse with little consensus on the preferred technique for its treatment.[1,9,10,28,36,41,46,50,61,62,75] The goals of surgical treatment include: (1) correction of kyphosis, (2) the adequate decompression of neural structures, and (3) spinal stabilization. Clinically, the improvement or elimination of back pain and resolution of neurologic symptoms is sought.

Anterior decompression in combination with anterior strut grafting (rib, iliac, fibula) is one of the potential treatment modalities for traumatic kyphosis. Bradford et al reviewed their use of anterior rib or fibular strut grafting for kyphosis in 48 patients.[10] To augment fixation, posterior arthrodesis and instrumentation were employed in more than half of the patients. The average postoperative immobilization was 9 months. Average length of follow-up was 41 months.

The authors reported that 16 out of 17 patients with preexisting back pain reported complete relief of their pain postoperatively. Eight patients underwent anterior decompression for preexisting neurologic involvement. Fifty percent of these patients demonstrated neurologic improvement by one Fränkel class. Postoperative correction of kyphosis averaged 59 degrees. However, there was a significant overall loss of correction, with 10 patients losing an average of 19 degrees of correction. Interestingly, 7 of these patients had undergone an additional posterior arthrodesis with instrumentation. The complication rate in this series was quite high, with 4 fractures of the strut graft, 4 pseudarthroses, and 2 cases of graft dislodgment. Three patients required a repeat anterior procedure secondary to excessive loss of reduction. As a consequence of these complications, Bradford et al recommended a second-stage posterior procedure for all cases in which a reduction of kyphotic deformity is attempted.

One of the earliest series on the treatment of posttraumatic kyphosis was done by Malcolm et al.[46] A total of 48 patients were treated with either an anterior or posterior procedure or a combination of both procedures. Postoperative immobilization averaged 9.3 months. Average time of follow-up was 33 months. Twenty-four of these patients had undergone previous surgical treatment. Two patients had been treated with posterior instrumentation and laminectomy and 22 patients with laminectomy alone.

Postoperatively, back pain was completely relieved in 67% of the patients. An additional 31% of patients reported a significant improvement in their back pain. Fourteen patients underwent an anterior decompression for preexisting neurologic involvement. Five patients were noted to be improved neurologically and 4 patients demonstrated no change in their neurologic status postoperatively. Significant complications in this series were noted. Four patients experienced postoperative neurologic deterioration. None of these 4 patients regained their preoperative neurologic status. One of these patients required a posterolateral decompression for progressive neurologic deterioration. There were 2 pseudarthroses and 4 reoperations for significant loss of correction (5 to 10 degrees) and/or pain. Overall loss of correction in this series was not discussed, however, the data show an average loss of correction of 6 to10 degrees for patients with thoracic or thoracolumbar deformity. All told, 50 percent of the solitary anterior procedures went on to failure and 40 percent of the patients experienced a postoperative complication. Recognizing this high complication rate in their series, the authors recommend an additional posterior arthrodesis to augment anterior fixation.

As seen in this series, anterior strut grafting, even when used in combination with a second-stage posterior procedure, is associated with a high complication rate. The need for long-term immobilization of these patients is deemed important in order to allow for incorporation and consolidation of the strut graft. Structurally the graft is weakest at 6 months and it can take as long as 2 years before bony union of the strut graft is achieved.[10,38,41] Even with long-term patient immobilization, graft fracture, graft dislodgment, and pseudarthrosis are common complications.[10,68] As a consequence, significant loss of correction is common. In addition, long-term immobilization of patients can lead to a high incidence of other complications such as deep vein thrombosis, pulmonary embolism, and decubitus ulcers.[10,46,68]

Kostuik and Matsusaki were one of the first to report on a series of 37 patients treated for posttraumatic kyphosis using one treatment method.[41] Sixteen of these patients had undergone acute surgical treatment. Ten patients had been treated with posterior Harrington instrumentation, 4 with laminectomy, and two with anterior decompression and anterior strut grafting. In this series, patients were treated with an anterior arthrodesis and anterior instrumentation (Kostuik-Harrington). Bi- or tricortical iliac crest graft was used to augment anterior arthrodesis. Patients were ambulated several days postoperatively with the use of an orthosis or cast brace. Follow-up ranged from 3 to 10 years. All patients suffered from back pain preoperatively. Postoperatively, eighteen (49%) patients reported complete or almost complete relief of pain. There was 1 case of nonunion. The degree of correction was not discussed. On follow-up, 4 patients were noted to have significant loss of correction, averaging 11 degrees. Three out of 8 patients who had preexisting neurologic involvement showed significant functional improvement postoperatively after anterior decompression. No patient experienced postoperative neurologic deterioration.

Kostuik and Matsusaki advocate an anterior approach for the treatment of posttraumatic kyphosis. They note that because the anterior cortex heals rapidly into a kyphotic position after injury, an anterior release is essential for adequate reduction. Thus, they believe that a solitary posterior arthrodesis with instrumentation cannot adequately reduce the kyphotic deformity. In their review, 36 out of 37 patients went on to union. Kostuik and Matsusaki attribute this success to the added stability provided by the anterior Kostuik-Harrington instrumentation.

Wu et al reported on the use of a solitary posterior arthrodesis and transpedicular instrumentation of 13 patients suffering from posttraumatic kyphosis.[75] All patients were placed in a brace for 3 to 4 months until bony union was achieved. Follow-up was at least 2 years in all patients. Posterior correction of the kyphotic deformity was accomplished through a transpedicular removal of the vertebral body, known also as the "eggshell" procedure. After transpedicular decancellation of the vertebral body a partial wedge osteotomy is performed. Through compression of transpedicular Schanz screws placed above and below the deformity, distraction and fracture of the anterior cortex and the anterior soft tissues is achieved. With additional manipulation of the operating room table final reduction of the deformity is accomplished.

In the series reported by Wu et al, the average kyphosis preoperatively averaged 40 degrees. Postoperative kyphosis averaged 1.5 degrees. At final follow-up the average kyphosis was 3.8 degrees. No patient demonstrated a preoperative neurologic deficit and no patients exhibited a neurologic deficit postoperatively. All patients went on to successful union and the issue of pain was not addressed. Wu et al, although advocating this technique in the treatment of posttraumatic kyphosis, do concede that there is a potential neurologic risk with this technique and careful attention to detail and technique are essential to minimizing this risk. The senior author of this chapter notes that this procedure is technically demanding and because it does not allow for release of the soft tissues anteriorly, it is often necessary to perform a large posterior osteotomy. This, in turn, increases the risk of potential neurologic damage to the conus or cauda equina because during the reduction maneuver the dura may become impinged.[1]

Böhm et al presented one of the first papers advocating the use of combined anterior and posterior procedures for the treatment of posttraumatic kyphosis.[9] Forty patients were treated in this series with segmental transpedicular fixation, anterior arthrodesis, and anterior instrumentation. The majority of these procedures were performed sequentially under one sitting. Correction achieved postoperatively was on average 22.5 degrees. On follow-up, loss of correction averaged 1 degree. Thirty percent of patients with preexisting neurologic involvement were noted to have improvement. There were no cases of postoperative neurologic deterioration. Although all cases went on to successful union, one patient was noted to have a broken rod with delayed union of the fibula strut graft.

**Table 23-1. Summary of Thoracolumbar Spine Fractures**

| Mechanical Instability | |
|---|---|
| *SI* <15 | Instability 1–2 → Bed rest + brace |
| 15< *SI* <25 | Instability 1–3 → Cast 3 months |
| 25< *SI* <35 | Instability 4–6 → Posterior approach |
| 35< *SI* | Instability 4–6 → Ant/Post simultaneous |

- Based on 3 columns, score 1–6.
- SI-Sagittal index.

## PREFERRED TREATMENT

With the advent of the MRI and its superior ability to image the soft tissues of the spine, Farcy et al have modified the concept of the three-column spine in an effort to further define spinal instability.[23,29] In this revised model each column principally consists of 1 bony element and 1 major ligament. All told, the spine has a total of 6 elements. Thus, each ligament and bony structure represent separate units of stability. When 3 or more of these elements are disrupted, the spine is suspected of being potentially unstable.

Farcy et al have also devised the sagittal index as a means of predicting the late progression of kyphotic deformity in thoracolumbar burst fractures.[24] The sagittal index is the difference between the measured segmental kyphosis at the affected vertebrae and the baseline sagittal curve at that level. The baseline sagittal curves are estimated to be the following: thoracic, 5 degrees; thoracolumbar junction, 0 degrees; lumbar, −10 degrees. These estimates are based on the patterns seen in Stagnara's studies.[65,66] Farcy et al believe that a sagittal index of 25 degrees or greater represents an injury of sufficient magnitude where bony healing will not occur. Thus, the authors believe that an instability score of 3 or greater in combination with a sagittal index of 25 degrees or greater are good predictors of which patients are at risk for late progression of kyphotic deformity. Treatment guidelines have thus been proposed based upon the sagittal index and the instability score (Table 23-1).

Although the proposed sagittal index and instability score was designed to assess initial stability and guide treatment, identical concepts should be applied in approaching the posttraumatic kyphosis. When planning revision surgery it is essential to provide for adequate anterior column support as well as posterior tension band forces to stabilize a corrected deformity. A major factor in the late complication of kyphosis is that a rigid deformity with instrumentation and fusion is frequently in place. To properly address this situation all columns of the spine must thus be treated for an optimal result.

It is our impression that a solitary posterior procedure is inadequate treatment for posttraumatic kyphosis. Such an approach does not allow for adequate anterior release of deformity or decompression of the neural structures. An isolated posterior approach will not permit adequate reduction of deformity and thus the fusion will be placed under excessive tension, which can lead to subsequent implant failure, pseudarthrosis, and again progressive loss of reduction. A solitary anterior procedure is also often insufficient because the posterior structures can impede an adequate reduction of deformity. In addition, a solitary anterior fusion often fails because it is subjected to excessive loading from a large moment arm and the tension band posteriorly is not reconstructed. Accordingly, it is our belief that only with a combined anterior and posterior procedure will adequate decompression, reduction, and stability be achieved.

## CLINICAL EXPERIENCE

In our retrospective series, we treated 31 patients suffering from posttraumatic kyphosis with simultaneous anterior and posterior surgery.[1] All patients had an instability score of 3 or greater at the time of initial injury and the initial sagittal index ranged from 18 to 52 degrees. The time interval between the initial injury and surgery for late complications associated with posttraumatic kyphosis averaged 4 years. Twenty-two of these patients had been treated acutely with surgical stabilization. Two patients had been treated with anterior instrumentation, 7 with Harrington instrumentation and laminectomies, and 13 with posterior segmental instrumentation. Follow-up averaged 29 months.

Postoperatively, the sagittal index improved to an average of +4 degrees (range of +10 degrees to −2 degrees). Three of 4 patients who presented with preexisting neurologic involvement demonstrated complete neurologic recovery postoperatively. Pain was graded on a scale of 1 to 10. Preoperatively, pain scores averaged 6.2 and decreased postoperatively to an average of 2.4. There were no cases of pseudarthrosis. One patient required a reoperation secondary to the anterior strut graft impinging posteriorly on the dura and neural elements. Patients were immediately mobilized out of bed postoperatively. A brace was used only during physical therapy.

Although technically demanding, simultaneous spine surgery offers several advantages to staged anterior and posterior procedures. With experienced teams, the simultaneous procedures can offer decreased operating time, blood loss, and hospital length of stay compared to sequential or staged procedures. Simultaneous surgery also offers several clear technical advantages. It avoids multiple patient positionings, which can lead to acute instability of the spine and anterior graft dislodgment. Simultaneous anterior and posterior visual control also allows for the safe, gradual, and direct correction and reduction of the kyphosis, thereby decreasing the risk of injury to the neural structures.

## CONCLUSION

Untreated or inadequately treated thoracolumbar burst fractures can lead to posttraumatic kyphosis. The acute treatment of burst fractures has evolved significantly over time. New techniques and instrumentation systems have led to shorter fusions and perhaps improved clinical results. Essential to the treatment of these injuries has been the understanding of what defines instability. A variety of classification systems and treatment guidelines have been developed to address this issue. Although opinions still differ on what constitutes instability, it appears that burst fractures with significant risk for progressive deformity should be surgically treated from the outset. In those injuries with significant posterior ligamentous disruption and anterior loss of support, a posterior instrumentation should be augmented with anterior structural stabilization in order to prevent loss of reduction and long-term complications.

The treatment of patients who have developed posttraumatic kyphosis after acute surgical stabilization has similarly evolved with our improved understanding of spinal instability. The use of anterior strut grafting without posterior instrumentation has demonstrated a high complication rate. Excessive loading of the graft from the large moment arm without posterior tension band support leads to a large incidence of graft failure and loss of correction. Solitary posterior approaches inadequately release the anterior column limiting correction of deformity and decompression of the spinal canal in cases of neurologic compromise.

In the management of posttraumatic kyphosis, anterior, middle, and posterior column pathology must frequently be addressed in one surgical procedure. The need for combined anterior and posterior procedures has thus become recognized. It is our belief that the ideal treatment of posttraumatic kyphosis is through the use of simultaneous anterior and posterior approaches. Simultaneous surgery may decrease the risk of neurologic injury through the direct visual monitoring of controlled reduction of the deformity. A simultaneous technique also obviates the need for multiple patient positionings, which can be risky in a destabilized spine. Finally, this technique, when compared to a sequential or staged procedure, may lead to decreased operative time, decreased blood loss, and shorter hospital length of stay.

## CASE STUDY

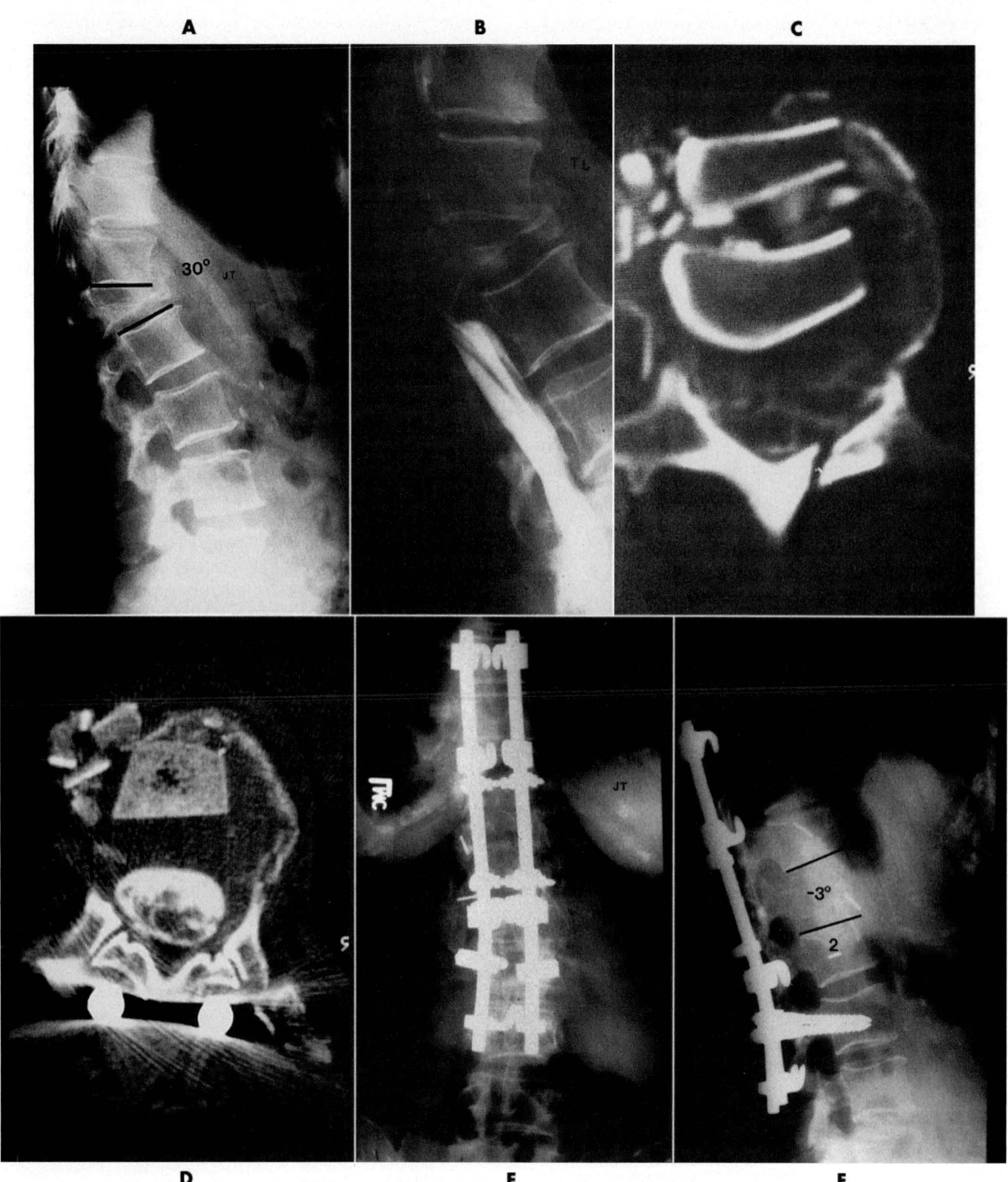


FIGURE 23-1

**A,** Preoperative lateral radiograph demonstrating an L1 burst fracture with a measured kyphosis of 30 degrees. Retropulsed bone into the canal is evident. **B,** Preoperative lateral myelogram revealing complete blockage of dye at the level of the burst fracture. **C,** CT myelogram after the first surgical decompression and bone grafting. The scan demonstrates significant obstruction of the spinal canal. Decompression is inadequate with obvious impaction of the posterior wall of L1 with structural grafts into the spinal canal. **D,** CT my-elogram of spine after repeat anterior decompression and fusion with simultaneous posterior instrumentation. Complete canal decompression is evident with free flow of contrast. **E,** Postoperative anteroposterior radiograph, note the use of the two-rod technique. **F,** Lateral radiograph demonstrating the use of the two-rod technique. A hook claw configuration is present above the injury site, double-threaded screws reinforced with hooks placed caudally. Postoperative kyphosis is measured to be −3 degrees.

## CASE 1

The patient is a 56-year-old female who suffered a fall in Mexico and sustained a burst fracture of L1. She was taken to a local hospital where she was found to have an incomplete paraplegia and thus underwent an anterior decompression and fusion. No neurologic recovery was noted postoperatively. She was subsequently transferred back to the United States.

On physical examination the patient was noted to have diffuse weakness of the right lower extremity. Sensation was diminished in the right lower extremity with numbness and anesthesia to pin prick in the region of L4-L5 dermatome. CT myelogram revealed significant compression of the cord at the level of the conus. This obstruction of the canal was due to impacted portions of the posterior vertebral body and the surgically placed anterior graft.

The patient thus underwent a proper anterior decompression and fusion with simultaneous posterior application of the two-rod technique using pedicle screw instrumentation. The patient had an uneventful postoperative course and gradually regained full neurologic function (Fig. 23-1,*A-F*).

## REFERENCES


1. Acaroglu, ER, Schwab FJ, Farcy J: Simultaneous anterior and posterior approaches for correction of late deformity due to thoracolumbar fractures, *Eur Spine J* 5:56-62, 1996.
2. Akbarnia BA, Fogarty JP, Tayob A: Contoured Harrington instrumentation in the treatment of unstable spinal fractures: the effect of supplementary sublaminar wires, *Clin Orthop* 189:186-194, 1984.
3. Akbarnia BA, Crandall DG, Burkus K, Matthews T: Use of long rods and a short arthrodesis for burst fractures of the thoracolumbar spine: a long-term follow-up study, *J Bone Joint Surg* 76A:1629-1635, 1994.
4. Allen BL Jr: Segmental spinal instrumentation with L-rods, *Instr Cours Lect* 32:202-208, 1983.
5. Benson DR: Unstable thoracolumbar fractures, with emphasis on the burst fracture, *Clin Orthop* 230:14-29, 1988.
6. Bernard TN, Jr, Johnston CE, II, Roberts JM, Burke SW: Late complications due to wire breakage in segmental spinal instrumentation: Report of two cases, *J Bone Joint Surg* 65A:1339-1345, 1983.
7. Bernard TN, Jr, Whitecloud TS, III, Rodriguez RP, Haddad RJ, Jr: Segmental spinal instrumentation in the management of fractures of the thoracic and lumbar spine, *South Med J* 76:1232-1236, 1983.
8. Bernucci C, Maiello M, Silvestro C, Francaviglia N, Bragazzi R, Pau A, Viale GL: Delayed worsening of the surgical correction of angular and axial deformity consequent to burst fractures of the thoracolumbar or lumbar spine, *Surg Neurol* 42:23-25, 1994.
9. Böhm H, Harms J, Donk R, Zielke K: Correction and stabilization of angular kyphosis, *Clin Orthop* 258:56-61, 1990.
10. Bradford DS, Ganjavian S, Antonious D, Winter RB, Lonstein JE, Moe JH: Anterior strut-grafting for the treatment of kyphosis: Review of experience with forty-eight patients, *J Bone Joint Surg* 64A:680-690, 1982.
11. Bryant CE, Sullivan JA: Management of thoracic and lumbar spine fractures with Harrington distraction rods supplemented with segmental wiring, *Spine* 8:532-537, 1983.
12. Carl AL, Tromanhauser SG, Roger DJ: Pedicle screw instrumentation for thoracolumbar burst fractures and fracture-dislocations, *Spine* 17:S317-S324, 1992.
13. Cervellati S, Bettini N, Bianco T, Parisini P: Neurological complications in segmental instrumentation: Analysis of 750 patients, *Eur Spine J* 5:161-166, 1996.
14. Dekutoski MB, Conlan ES, Salciccioli GG: Spinal mobility and deformity after Harrington rod stabilization and limited arthrodesis of thoracolumbar fractures, *J Bone Joint Surg* 75A:168-176,1993.
15. Denis F: The three-column spine and its significance in the classification of acute thoracolumbar spinal injuries, *Spine* 8:817-831, 1983.
16. Denis F: Spinal instability as defined by the three-column spine concept in acute spinal trauma, *Clin Orthop* 189:65-76, 1984.
17. Dickson JH, Harrington PR, Erwin WD: Results of reduction and stabilization of the severely fractured thoracic and lumbar spine, *J Bone Joint Surg* 60A:799-805, 1978.
18. Doherty JH: Complications of fusion in lumbar scoliosis, *J Bone Joint Surg* 55A:438, 1973.
19. Drummond D, Guadagni J, Keene JS, Breed A, Narechania R: Interspinous process segmental spinal instrumentation, *J Pediatr Orthop* 4:397-404, 1984.
20. Ebelke DK, Asher MA, Neff JR, Kraker DP: Survivorship analysis of VSP spine instrumentation in the treatment of thoracolumbar and lumbar burst fractures, *Spine* 16:S428-S432, 1991.
21. Erwin WD, Dickson JH, Harrington PR: Clinical review of patients with broken Harrington rods, *J Bone Joint Surg* 62A:1302-1307, 1980.
22. Farcy J, Weidenbaum M, Michelsen CB, Hoeltzel DA, Athanasiou KA: A comparative biomechanical study of spinal fixation using Cotrel-Dubousset instrumentation, *Spine* 12:877-881, 1987.

23. Farcy J, Weidenbaum M: A preliminary review of the use of Cotrel-Dubousset instrumentation for spinal injuries, *Bull Hosp Jt Dis Orthop Inst* 48:44-51, 1988.
24. Farcy JC, Weidenbaum M, Glassman SD: Sagittal index in management of thoracolumbar burst fractures, *Spine* 15:958-965, 1990.
25. Flesch JR, Leider LL, Erickson DL, Chou SN, Bradford DS: Harrington instrumentation and spine fusion for unstable fractures and fracture-dislocations of the thoracic and lumbar spine, *J Bone Joint Surg* 59A:143-153, 1977.
26. Gaines RW, Breedlove RF, Munson G: Stabilization of thoracic and thoracolumbar fracture-dislocations with Harrington rods and sublaminar wires, *Clin Orthop* 189:195-203, 1984.
27. Gertzbein SD, Macmichael D, Tile M: Harrington instrumentation as a method of fixation in fractures of the spine: a critical analysis of deficiencies, *J Bone Joint Surg* 64B:526-529, 1982.
28. Gertzbein SD, Harris MB: Wedge osteotomy for the correction of post-traumatic kyphosis: a new technique and a report of three cases, *Spine* 17:374-379, 1992.
29. Glassman SD, Farcy JC: *Late deformities*. In Floman Y, Farcy JC, Argenson C, editors: *Thoracolumbar spine fractures,* New York, NY, 1993, Raven Press, pp 449-462.
30. Goll SR, Balderston RA, Stambough JL, Booth RE, Cohn JC, Pickens GT: Depth of intraspinal wire penetration during passage of sublaminar wires, *Spine* 13:503-509, 1988.
31. Graziano GP: Cotrel-Dubousset hook and screw combination for spine fractures, *J Spinal Disord* 6:380-385, 1993.
32. Gurr KR, McAfee PC, Shih C: Biomechanical analysis of anterior and posterior instrumentation systems after corpectomy: a calf-spine model, *J Bone Joint Surg* 70A:1182-1191, 1988.
33. Gurwitz GS, Dawson JM, McNamara MJ, Federspiel CF, Spengler DM: Biomechanical analysis of three surgical approaches for lumbar burst fractures using short-segment instrumentation, *Spine* 18:977-982, 1993.
34. Holdsworth FW: Fractures, dislocations, and fracture-dislocations of the spine, *J Bone Joint Surg* 45B:6-20, 1963.
35. Holdsworth F: Fractures, dislocations, and fracture-dislocations of the spine, *J Bone Joint Surg* 52A:1534-1550, 1970.
36. Jodoin A, Gillet P, Dupuis PR, Maurais G: Surgical treatment of post-traumatic kyphosis: a report of 16 cases, *Can J Surg* 32:36-42, 1989.
37. Johnston CE, II, Happel LT, Jr, Norris R, Burke SW, King AG, Roberts JM: Delayed paraplegia complicating sublaminar segmental spinal instrumentation, *J Bone Joint Surg* 68A:556-563, 1986.
38. Kaneda K, Kurakami C, Minami A: Free vascularized fibular strut graft in the treatment of kyphosis, *Spine* 13:1273-1277, 1988.
39. Kelly RP, Whitesides TE, Jr: Treatment of lumbodoral fracture-dislocations, *Ann Surg* 167:705-717, 1968.
40. Kostuik JP, Maurais GR, Richardson WJ, Okajima Y: Combined single stage anterior and posterior osteotomy for correction of iatrogenic lumbar kyphosis, *Spine* 13:257-266, 1988.
41. Kostuik JP, Matsusaki H: Anterior stabilization, instrumentation, and decompression for post-traumatic kyphosis, *Spine* 14:379-386, 1989.
42. Lagrone MO, Bradford DS, Moe JH, Lonstein JE, Winter RB, Ogilvie JW: Treatment of symptomatic flatback after spinal fusion, *J Bone Joint Surg* 70A:569-580, 1988.
43. Luque ER: Segmental spinal instrumentation for correction of scoliosis, *Clin Orthop* 163:192-198, 1982.
44. Luque ER: The anatomic basis and development of segmental spinal instrumentation, *Spine* 7:256-259, 1982.
45. Luque ER, Cassis N, Ramirez-Wiella G: Segmental spinal instrumentation in the treatment of fractures of the thoracolumbar spine, *Spine* 7:312-317, 1982.
46. Malcolm BW, Bradford DS, Winter RB, Chou SN: Post-traumatic kyphosis: A review of forty-eight treated patients, *J Bone Joint Surg* 63A:891-899, 1981.
47. McAfee PC, Yuan HA, Fredrickson BE, Lubicky JP: The value of computed tomography in thoracolumbar fractures: An analysis of one-hundred consecutive cases and a new classification, *J Bone Joint Surg* 65A:461-473, 1983.
48. McAfee PC, Bohlman HH: Complications following Harrington instrumentation for fractures of the thoracolumbar spine, *J Bone Joint Surg* 67A:672-686, 1985.
49. McAfee PC, Werner FW, Glisson RR: A biomechanical analysis of spinal instrumentation systems in thoracolumbar fractures: Comparison of traditional Harrington distraction instrumentation with segmental spinal instrumentation, *Spine* 10:204-217, 1985.
50. McBride GG, Bradford DS: Vertebral body replacement with femoral neck allograft and vascularized rib strut graft: A technique for treating post-traumatic kyphosis with neurologic deficit, *Spine* 8:406-415, 1983.
51. McBride GG: Cotrel-Dubousset rods in surgical stabilization of spinal fractures, *Spine* 18:466-473, 1993.
52. McLain RF, Sparling E, Benson DR: Early failure of short-segment pedicle instrumentation for thoracolumbar fractures: A preliminary report, *J Bone Joint Surg* 75A:162-167, 1993.
53. Moreland DB, Egnatchik JG, Bennett GJ: Cotrel-Dubousset instrumentation for the treatment of thoracolumbar fractures, *Neurosurgery* 27:69-73, 1990.
54. Munson G, Satterlee C, Hammond S, Betten R, Gaines RW: Experimental evaluation of Harrington rod fixation supplemented with sublaminar wires in stabilizing thoracolumbar fracture-dislocations, *Clin Orthop* 189:97-102, 1984.
55. Myllynen P, Böstman O, Riska E: Recurrence of deformity after removal of Harrington's fixation of spine

fracture: Seventy-six cases followed for 2 years, *Acta Orthop Scand* 59:497-502, 1988.

56. Nicoll EA: Fractures of the dorso-lumbar spine, *J Bone Joint Surg* 31B:376-394, 1949.
57. Noel SH, Keene JS, Rice WL: Improved postoperative course after spinous process segmental instrumentation of thoracolumbar fractures, *Spine* 16:132-136, 1991.
58. Phillips DL, Brick GW, Spengler DM: A comparison of Harrington rod fixation with and without segmental wires for unstable thoracolumbar injuries, *J Spinal Disord* 1:151-161, 1988.
59. Riebel GD, Yoo JU, Fredrickson BE, Yuan HA: Review of Harrington rod treatment of spinal trauma, *Spine* 18:479-491, 1993.
60. Riska EB, Myllynen P, Bostman O: Anterolateral decompression for neural involvement in thoracolumbar fractures. A review of 78 cases, *J Bone Joint Surg* 69B:704-708, 1987.
61. Roberson JR, Whitesides TE, Jr,: Surgical reconstruction of late post-traumatic thoracolumbar kyphosis, *Spine* 10:307-312, 1985.
62. Roy-Camille R, Saillant G, Mazel CH, Gagna G, Caubel P, Ciniglio M: The surgical treatment of post-traumatic vertebral deformities, *Ital J Orthop Traumatol* 12:419-426, 1986.
63. Shono Y, McAfee PC, Cunningham BW: Experimental study of thoracolumbar burst fractures: A radiographic and biomechanical analysis of anterior and posterior instrumentation systems, *Spine* 19:1711-1722, 1994.
64. Slosar PJ, Jr, Patwardhan AG, Lorenz M, Havey R, Sartori M: Instability of the lumbar burst fracture and limitations of transpedicular instrumentation, *Spine* 20:1452-1461, 1995.
65. Stagnara P: *Spinal deformity,* Sumerset, England, 1988, Butterworth & Co.
66. Stagnara P, DeMauroy JC, Dran G, Gonon GP, Costanzo G, Dimnet J, Pasquet A: Reciprocal angulation of vertebral bodies in sagittal plane: approach to the references for the evaluation of kyphosis and lordosis, *Spine* 7:335-342, 1982.
67. Stephens GC, Devito DP, McNamara MJ: Segmental fixation of lumbar burst fractures with Cotrel-Dubousset instrumentation, *J Spinal Disord* 5:344-348, 1992.
68. Streitz W, Brown JC, Bonnett CA: Anterior fibular strut grafting in the treatment of kyphosis, *Clin Orthop* 128:140-148, 1977.
69. Sullivan JA: Sublaminar wiring of Harrington distraction rods for unstable thoracolumbar spine fractures, *Clin Orthop* 189:178-184, 1984.
70. Vornanen MJ, Böstman OM, Myllynen PJ: Reduction of bone retropulsed into the spinal canal in thoracolumbar vertebral body compression burst fractures: a prospective randomized comparative study between Harrington rods and two transpedicular devices, *Spine* 20:1699-1703, 1995.
71. Wenger DR, Carollo JJ, Wilkerson JA, Jr, Wauters K, Herring JA: Laboratory testing of segmental spinal instrumentation versus traditional Harrington instrumentation for scoliosis treatment, *Spine* 7:265-269, 1982.
72. White AA, III, Panjabi MM, Thomas CL: The clinical biomechanics of kyphotic deformities, *Clin Orthop* 128:8-17, 1977.
73. Whitesides TE, Jr: Traumatic kyphosis of the thoracolumbar spine, *Clin Orthop* 128:78-92, 1977.
74. Wilber RG, Thompson GH, Shaffer JW, Brown RH, Nash CL, Jr: Postoperative neurological deficits in segmental spinal instrumentation: a study using spinal cord monitoring, *J Bone Joint Surg* 66A:1178-1187, 1984.
75. Wu S, Hwa S, Lin L, Pai W, Chen P, Au M: Management of rigid post-traumatic kyphosis, *Spine* 21:2260-2267, 1996.
76. Yosipovitch Z, Robin GC, Makin M: Open reduction of unstable thoracolumbar spinal injuries and fixation with Harrington rods, *J Bone Joint Surg* 59A:1003-1015, 1977.
77. Zindrick MR, Knight GW, Bunch WH, Miller MC, Butler DM, Lorenz M, Behal R: Factors influencing the penetration of wires into the neural canal during segmental wiring, *J Bone Joint Surg* 71A:742-750, 1989.

# 24

# PRINCIPLES OF REVISION SURGERY FOLLOWING FAILED CERVICAL SPINAL INJURY

**Alexander R. Vaccaro, M.D.**
**William P. H. Charlton, M.D.**
**Jerome M. Cotler, M.D.**



Cervical spine trauma is a devastating reality in our modern society of sophisticated high-speed travel, the potential excessives of alcohol and drug use, the popularity of dangerous recreational activities, as well as the aging of our population with its attendant metabolic consequences (i.e., osteoporosis). Appropriate recognition and management of a cervical spine injury, whether nonoperative or operative, are critical to the neurological and therefore functional well-being of this patient population. In patients requiring surgical decompression and/or stabilization, an unfavorable outcome may be the result of a poor understanding of the mechanism of injury and the degree of bony and ligamentous instability, the choice of an incorrect surgical approach or procedure, or a lack of understanding of the biomechanics of the chosen instrumentation. Unfortunately, failure of the initial cervical spine procedure may result in spinal instability with the potential for neurological deterioration.

A revision operation following failed surgical treatment of a cervical spine injury serves four purposes: (1) restore or preserve neurologic function; (2) create a stable construct that immobilizes a minimum number of spinal segments while maximizing the potential for a successful spinal fusion; (3) restore rapid, pain-free functional recovery; and (4) prevent late instability and the potential for late neurological embarrassment.

Essential in the majority of revision surgical procedures of the cervical spine is the appropriate choice and application of various fixation devices. Various kinds of instrumentation, including wires, cables, plates, screws, and hooks are used in the cervical spine. Each has its own biomechanical properties, anatomical benefits, and limitations. This understanding is essential for planning a successful surgical revision of a failed cervical fusion. This chapter briefly reviews the common surgical mistakes made in the initial surgical management of cervical spine trauma as well as the biomechanical principles underlying sound reconstruction techniques in the revision of these surgical failures.

## INADEQUATE NEURAL DECOMPRESSION

Inadequate neural decompression following a cervical spinal cord injury with anterior or posterior thecal sac compression may result in persistent neurological compromise and possible acute or late neurological deterioration. Various studies have documented the potential for neural recovery after decompression following spinal injury.[10,44] Appropriate postsurgical imaging evaluation for potential cord compression includes a plain radiographic survey followed by myelography, myelography with computerized tomography (CT), or magnetic resonance imaging (MRI) (Fig. 24-1). Myelography supplemented with CT scanning may be more useful than MRI in situations

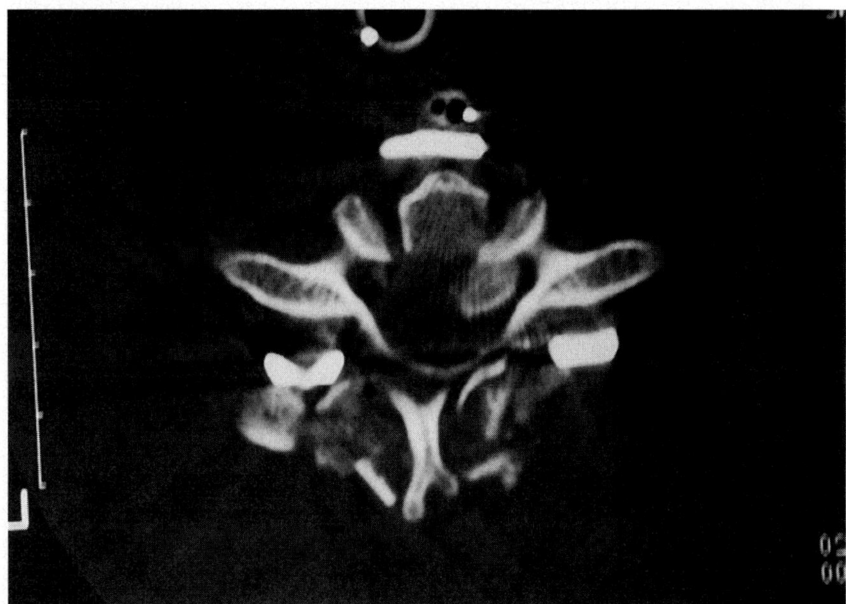

**FIGURE 24-1**

Transaxial CT scan following an anterior cervical corpectomy and fusion revealing evidence of an inadequate decompression of the spinal canal.

in which cervical internal fixation has been used, especially stainless steel, in order to avoid scatter artifact within the epidural space. A common mistake made, resulting in an inadequate anterior cervical decompression, is not recognizing the midline of the cervical vertebral body and therefore performing an eccentric bony decompression. This is seen more frequently when anatomic landmarks are obscured such as in advanced spondylosis or in metabolic spinal disease such as ankylosing spondylitis or diffuse idiopathic skeletal hyperostosis. Suggestions to avoid this potential complication include obtaining a localizing anteroposterior (AP) radiograph prior to surgical decompression as well as a postdecompression AP radio-graph with dilute water-soluble radiographic dye to document the extent of the cervical decompression. The surgeon should determine the transverse width of the anticipated decompression by measurements obtained on preoperative axial MRI or CT images.

## SURGICAL APPROACH

The method of fixation chosen for the surgical management of cervical spine trauma is a complex decision requiring a thorough knowledge of the anatomy and biomechanics of the cervical spine and a working knowledge of the biomechanics of spinal instrumentation techniques. Preoperative recognition of the mechanism of injury as well as the associated resulting bony and ligamentous injury is imperative for determining the appropriate treatment. Constructs used for cervical stabilization will fail if the true extent of bony and ligamentous instability is not recognized preoperatively. The decision to use an anterior or a

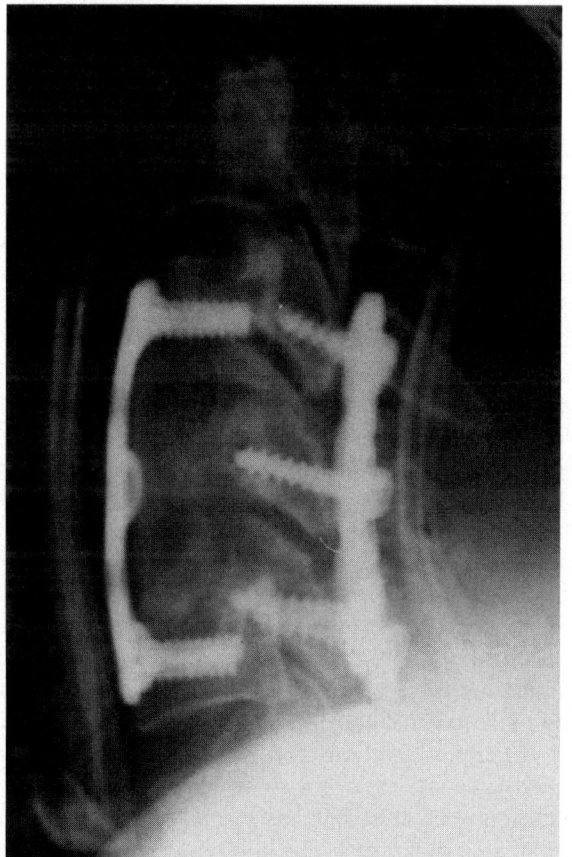

**FIGURE 24-2**

Lateral radiograph revealing a postoperative anterior and posterior cervical decompression and fusion for an advanced stage flexion compression injury with significant anterior and posterior circumferential instability.

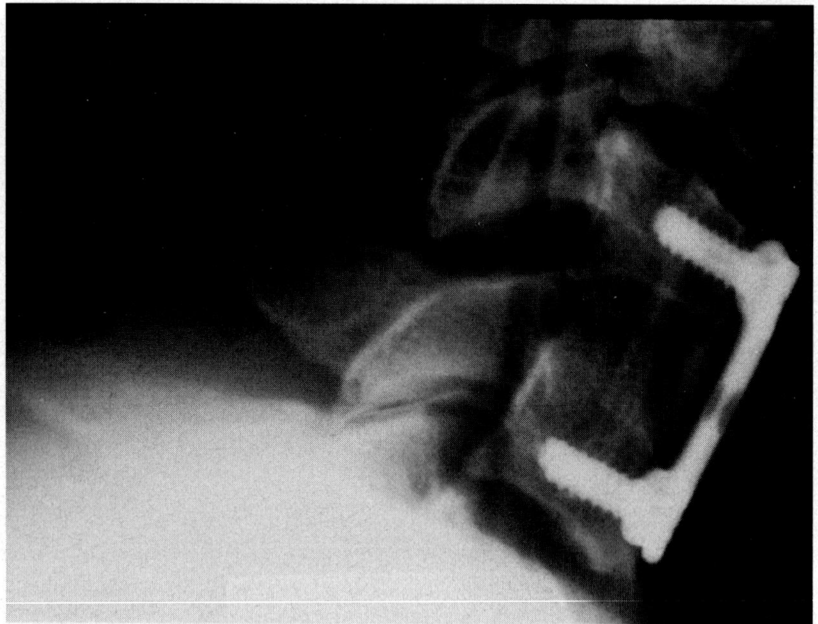

**Figure 24-3**

Lateral plain radiograph revealing excessive distraction of the posterior facets following anterior graft placement and instrumentation.

posterior or a combined anteroposterior surgical approach depends on the location and degree of ligamentous instability and the presence or absence of neural compression. A posterior or anterior cervical fusion alone often may be unable to achieve a stable spine in the presence of a severe three column injury (Fig. 24-2).[21] An anterior bone grafting and stabilization procedure alone in the presence of circumferential instability that occurs with advanced-stage flexion compression injuries has been shown to be biomechanically inadequate in animal and cadaveric spines,[18,71,74,78,80,81] although clinical articles have reported successful outcomes.[47] An anterior interbody or strut graft fusion with or without instrumentation, without posterior stabilization may result in excessive facet subluxation and possible dislocation in the presence of posterior element compromise if excessive distraction is applied to the vertebral elements with an oversized bone graft (Fig. 24-3). Facet subluxation should be noted on an intraoperative plain lateral radiograph necessitating graft revision, and in most cases a supplemental posterior stabilization procedure. The choice between posterior wiring or lateral mass plating with optional pedicle screw placement depends on the quality of the bony reconstruction anteriorly and the degree of instability posteriorly. The absence of stable spinous processes and lamina posteriorly makes the choice of lateral mass plating obligatory.

## OCCIPITOCERVICAL INSTABILITY

An occipitocervical fusion is required rarely for acute traumatic instability of the occipitocervical junction because of the exceedingly high mortality rate associated with this injury.[66] This injury is usually fatal, hence the true incidence of this type of injury is probably much higher than presently believed. Multiple techniques for occipitocervical arthrodesis have been advocated,[29,34,47] but the technique described by Wertheim and Bohlman is the most widely accepted.[77] This latter procedure involves the use of three wires through the external occipital protuberance, around the posterior arch of C1, and around the spinous process of C2. These wires are then secured to two contoured corticocancellous iliac grafts. The stability of the construct depends upon the integrity of bone graft. Fracture of one of the corticocancellous bone grafts destabilizes the construct and is an important mechanism of failure using this technique. Wire breakage is another reason for failure, but is rare in posterior cervical fusions occurring in 1% to 2% of cases.[15] Several other types of fixation devices can be used for occipitocervical arthrodesis including metallic loops with wire or cable attachments, a hook-rod construct, or plates and screws.[40,57,64,70]

Contoured plating of the occipitocervical junction, originally described by Roy-Camille,[64] requires screws in the skull and lateral masses. The contoured plate provides rigid internal fixation and is independent upon the lamina and spinous processes. Because of the plates' biomechanical strength and position lateral to the midline posterior elements, occipitocervical plating is an ideal choice for patients with a failed occipitocervical arthrodesis. The screws placed in the skull can be unicortical or bicortical. Biomechanical studies have demonstrated no significant differences between these screw depths. Screws placed into the inion can be longer in length and potentially have a higher pull-out strength.

Newer designs for contoured plate constructs and techniques for cervical pedicle identification allow the

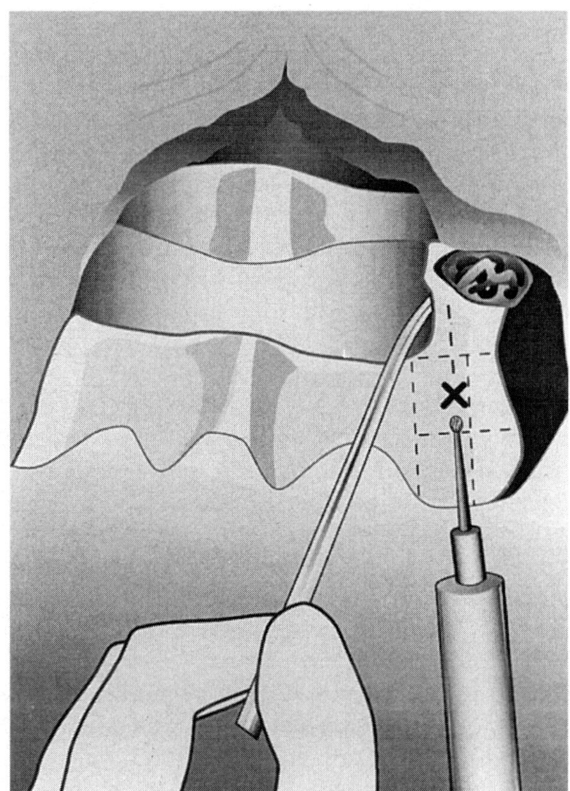

FIGURE 24-4

Illustration of the surgical technique describing placement of a C2 pedicle or isthmus screw.

additional placement of cervical pedicle screws at C2 and C7, thus providing a rigid construct that can improve the chances of fusion and require less postoperative external immobilization. Prior to C2 pedicle (isthmus) screw placement, a transaxial CT scan of the C2 vertebral body should be obtained to determine the width and angulation of the C2 pedicle as well as to identify the vertebral artery anatomy. A routine posterior midline surgical approach is used to expose the second cervical vertebrae. During exposure of the C2 pedicle, dissection is carried laterally along the superior border of the C2 lamina to its junction with the C2 pedicle. A Penfield #4 is then used to gently palpate the inner or medial wall of the C2 pedicle or isthmus to determine appropriate screw direction (Fig. 24-4). The starting point for screw insertion should be the upper medial quadrant of the C2 lateral mass to avoid the vertebral artery, which courses from inferomedially to superolaterally within the C2 foramen. The direction of screw passage is approximately 15 to 20 degrees medially and 15 to 20 degrees superiorly allowing passage of the screw into the dense subchondral bone of the C2 superior articular facet. A 3.5-mm cancellous screw measuring 14 to 20 mm is used most frequently within the C2 pedicle.

## ATLANTOAXIAL INSTABILITY

A time-honored method of atlantoaxial stabilization involves wiring together the posterior elements of C1 and C2.[32,33] The Gallie or Brooks techniques are two wiring methods that have been utilized frequently to achieve an atlantoaxial arthrodesis.[11,24,25,30,39] These techniques differ in specific wire placement and grafting methods and depend upon intact lamina and spinous processes for sublaminar and spinous processing wiring. The Gallie technique uses a sublaminar wire passage at C1 and a spinous process wire passage at C2 with the placement of bone graft extending from the dorsal lamina of C1 to the spinous process of C2.

The Brooks technique uses two sets of sublaminar wires passed at C1 and C2 and two bone graft blocks wedged between the lamina at this level.[73] The Gallie technique is considered safer because it utilizes the spinous process of C2 and minimizes sublaminar wire placement to the C1 level.[47,52] Although safer, the Gallie construct lacks stability in extension and rotation as well as suboptimal resistance to subluxation, all of which are important mechanisms of failure of this technique. The Brooks technique provides greater stability in extension and rotation than other atlantoaxial fusion techniques, and prevents overcompression of adjacent segments.[47,49,63] Because of its biomechanical superiority, the Brooks fusion technique is often applicable for patients with a failed fusion following the Gallie technique or interlaminar clamp fixation, unless a narrow spinal canal precludes the use of sublaminar wires. Extreme caution must be employed when passing sublaminar wires particularly in a reoperated field. Neurological complications associated with C1-C2 fusions are most frequently the result of passing sublaminar wires. Nordt and Stauffer reported two patients with quadriplegia following the passage of sublaminar wires in the presence of anterior C1 subluxation.[53] Careful complete subperiosteal dissection of the sublaminar surfaces of both C1 and C2 must be carried out from the midline for approximately at least 15 mm laterally prior to any attempted wire passage.

Interlaminar clamps including the Halifax and Apofix devices may also be used to stabilize the atlantoaxial joint.[2,3,22,35] These devices consist of sublaminar hooks connected by a threaded screw or rod. For C1-C2 stabilization, the Halifax clamp is frequently placed from C1 to C3 to lower the risk of dislodgment that can occur with clamps bridging C1 to C2,[1,35] even though this fuses a stable motion segment unnecessarily. The hook design carries the adherent risk associated with all sublaminar instrumentation and can not be used with deficient or destabilized posterior elements.[19] The clamp mechanism in addition provides little biomechanical stability in extension and rotation. The Halifax clamp was used originally without bone grafting and its size limited the surface area available for grafting. Although some reports have documented good results despite the absence of bone grafting,[35] this latter construct is currently not recommended. The Halifax clamp can dislodge in extension or rotation with resulting destabilization of the construct.

Posterior C1-C2 transarticular screw fixation[43,75] involves placing a screw through the posterior lateral mass of C2, across the C1-C2 articulation and into the lateral mass of C1. This technique can be used in patients with deficient or unstable posterior elements at these levels and provides rigid fixation of the C1-C2 articulation, which is equal to or biomechanically superior to that of the Brooks and interlaminar hook techniques.[50] In this method a 3.5-mm cortical screw is placed obliquely in the sagittal plane beginning at the posterior inferior C2 facet and traversing superiorly through the C2 superior articular process into the inferior C1 articular process ending within the C1 lateral mass. A preoperative CT with sagittal reconstruction is necessary for identification of the pertinent surrounding anatomy including the proximity of the vertebral artery. A Mayfield pin holder is secured to the patient's skull to allow optimum patient positioning and fluoroscopic visualization. The C2-C1 facet joints are exposed with careful attention to avoid the lesser occipital nerve (C2), which exits between the C1 and C2 lamina. The surgical exposure is limited to the C1-C2 level. The appropriate entry level to allow percutaneous placement of the 3.5-mm cortical screw is confirmed by lateral fluoroscopy and is at approximately the C6 to T1 level. Drilling using a 2.5-mm drill through a cannulated system is performed under lateral fluoroscopy as well as visual inspection of the medial aspect of the C2 pedicle to avoid canal breach. After drilling, a 3.5-mm cortical tap is used followed by screw placement. The starting point of screw fixation is a point approximately 2 mm lateral to the lamina/lateral mass junction of C2 at the posteroinferior border of the C2 inferior facet. The path of the drill in the coronal plane is parallel to the canal to avoid canal penetration. The sagittal plane direction is determined by fluoroscopy and is usually 50 to 60 degrees from the horizontal. A Gallie or Brooks fusion is routinely added at the completion of the procedure in order to augment fusion of the C2-C1 articulation. Prior to tightening both screws, cancellous bone graft is placed within the C2-C1 decorticated facet joints. The Magerl procedure is a technically demanding procedure that places at risk the vertebral artery both laterally and inferiorly and the spinal cord medially. This is a viable salvage procedure following a failed sublaminar wire atlantoaxial arthrodesis (Fig. 24-5) in the setting of compromised posterior laminas or when spinal canal compromise prohibits the passage of sublaminar wires. An occipitocervical fusion with plating and C2 pedicle screw fixation may occasionally be chosen following a failed C1-C2 fusion but with the unfortunate sacrifice of motion at the occipitocervical articulation.

The anterior approach may occasionally be utilized in revision of a failed posterior atlantoaxial arthrodesis. The earliest anterior surgical approaches to this region, such as the transoral and tongue splitting approaches, had associated infection rates in some reports of up to 50%.[46,48,69A] Later surgical exposures exploiting the retropharyngeal passageway to the upper cervical spine negating the need to traverse the oral cavity, drastically decreased the incidence of infection associated with fusion procedures at this level.[63] Anterior arthrodesis using C1-C2 articular facet screws[6,67] was described by Barbour in 1971.[8] Exposure for this procedure is through the standard Smith-Robinson surgical approach[69] usually centered over C5 to allow for the appropriate superolateral trajectory for screw placement. The dissection is carried cephalad to the inferior-anterior edge of the C2 vertebra. Prior to screw placement the facet joints are debrided of articular cartilage and packed with cancellous bone graft. Under biplanar fluoroscopic visualization, two 4.0-mm cancellous lag screws are directed superolaterally from the mid anterior lateral surface of the C2 body into the lateral mass of the C1 body. Various authors have described the placement of a T-type plate across the C1-C2 articulation with short screw fixation into the C1 lateral mass and the C2 body. This technique is not adequately described in the literature and is without significant patient follow-up.

An alternative means of fusing the C2-C1 joint in instances in which a posterior approach is not feasible is the lateral approach to the upper cervical spine, as described by Whitesides.[82] This approach exposes the lateral aspect of the upper cervical vertebrae through dissection posterior rather than anterior to the carotid sheath.[83] At the completion of the exposure, the anterior articular facet of C2-C1 is exposed. The intertransverse membrane between the C1 and C2 transverse processes is preserved and the articular cartilage is subsequently denuded within the C2-C1 joint surface in preparation for autologous bone grafting. Once completed, a 2 mm guide wire is placed at the anterior base of the C1 transverse process and directed 25 degrees inferiorly in the coronal plane and 10 degrees posteriorly in the sagittal plane. This is done bilaterally and confirmed with intraoperative fluoroscopy. A cannulated drill is then placed over the guide wire followed by an appropriate length 3.5-mm cortical lag screw (Fig. 24-6). The C1 lateral mass can be over drilled with a 3.5 mm cannulated drill in order to compress the facet joint at screw insertion. This technique is rarely useful, but should be considered when

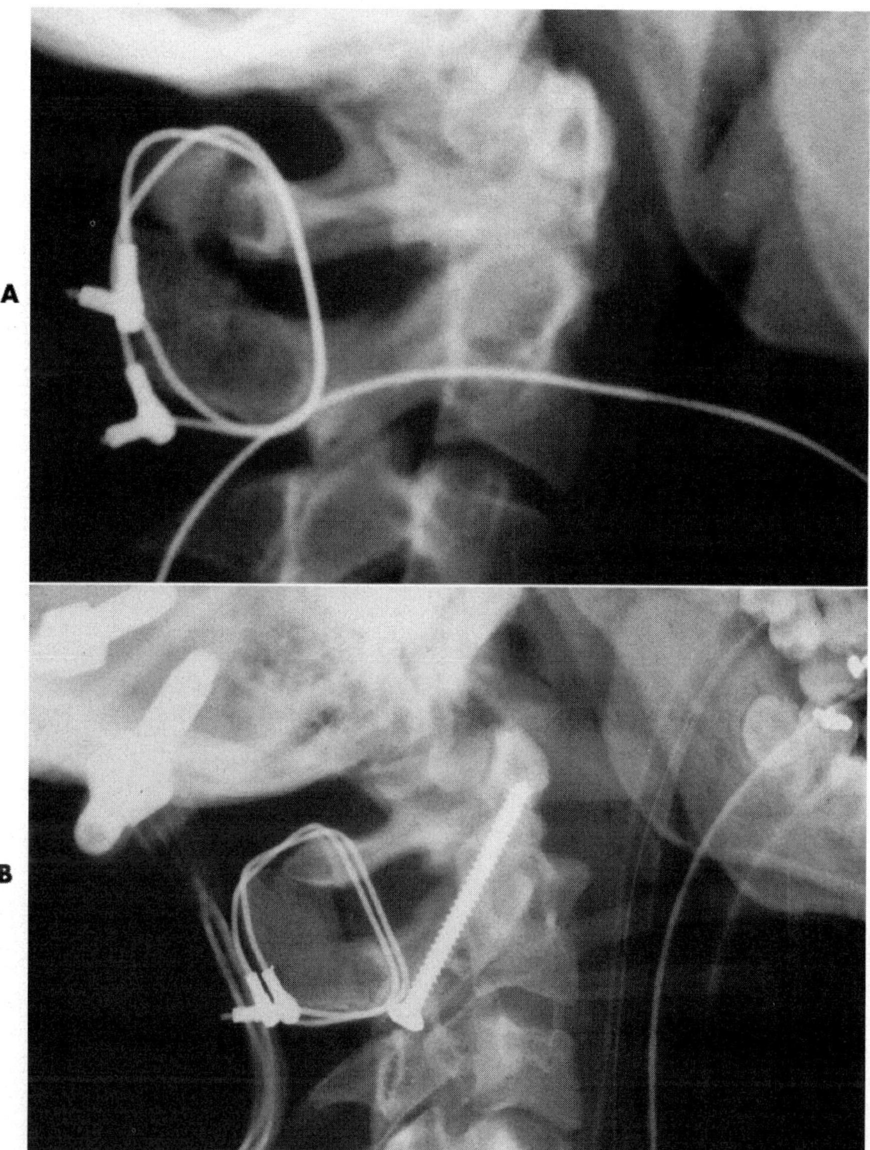


**FIGURE 24-5**

**A,** Lateral plain radiograph revealing evidence of a nonunion between the graft and the C1 posterior lamina following a Brooks fusion. **B,** The patient subsequently underwent a revision posterior C2-C1 facet screw fixation with a supplemental fusion.

other approaches may not be technically feasible in cases of failed atlantoaxial fusion.

## SUBAXIAL SPINE

### POSTERIOR STABILIZATION TECHNIQUES

Posterior spinous process wiring, originally described by Rogers,[61,62] provides good stability in flexion but little stability to extension and rotational loading.[4] As a result of the increased cord-to-canal ratio in the subaxial spine as compared to the upper cervical region, sublaminar wire placement is discouraged, because the potential for neurological compromise is significant. Spinous process wiring requires intact and stable posterior elements. Several modifications of the traditional wiring technique have been described.[9,13,14,23,47,54,65,76] The Bohlman triple-wire technique combines interspinous wiring with corticocancellous bone graft compression. This triple-wire technique has been shown to be safe and effective and biomechanically superior to other wiring constructs.[9,18,45,71] Complications of these wiring techniques include wire breakage and cutout. Cahill reported recurrent dislocation in four patients with interspinous wiring for facet dislocations,[13] and Edwards et al[23] noted that spinous process wiring for facet subluxation may allow partial recurrence of rotation because of the axial pull of the wire that is 65 degrees off from the obliquely oriented facet. The oblique wiring technique,[13,23,84] originally described by Robinson and Southwick,[60] involves wiring the inferior facet of the superior vertebrae to the spinous process of the inferior vertebrae. This construct acts as a diagonal tension band from the dislocated facets to the spinous process below.[1]

Facet wiring is another technique utilized in poste-

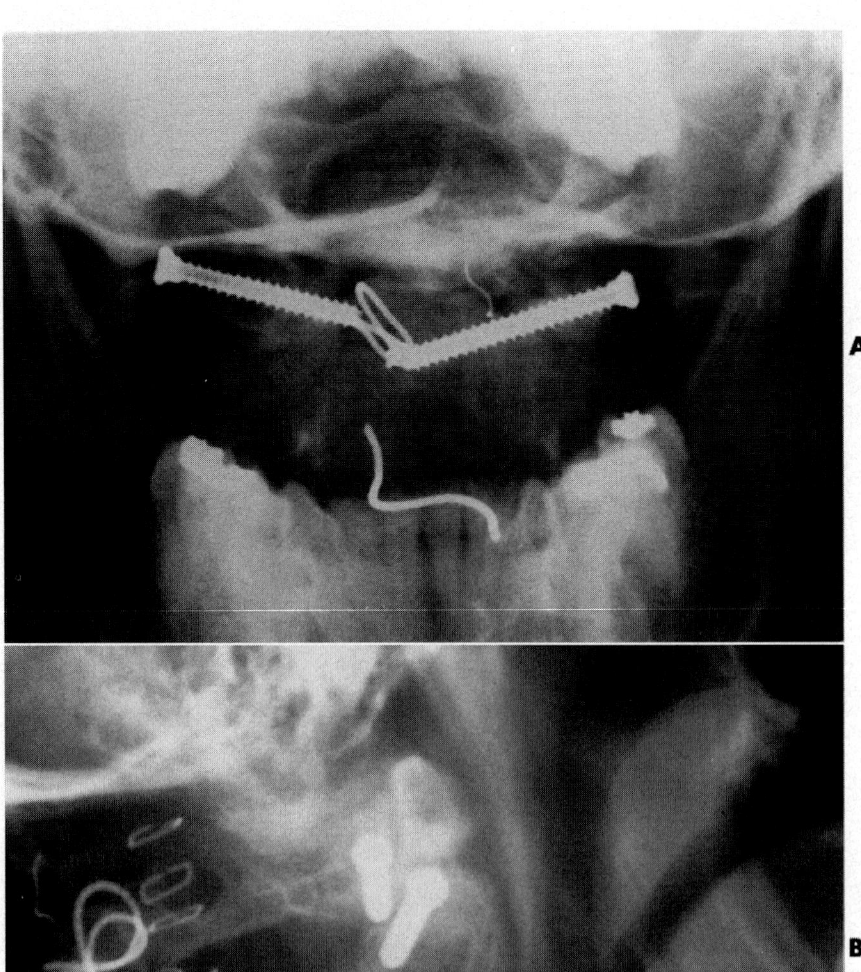


**FIGURE 24-6**

**(A)** An anterior posterior and **(B)** lateral plain radiograph illustrating C2-C1 facet screw fixation through the lateral approach of Whiteside.

rior cervical fusions. Originally described by Robinson and Southwick,[60] this technique is useful for patients with deficient or unstable lamina and spinous processes. Graft breakage destabilizes the construct and has been associated with nonunion.[14] Facet wiring has been shown to provide excellent stability against flexion and lateral bending moments in biomechanical testing but was found to offer little stability with either extension or axial rotational forces.[56]

The Hook plate,[31,36,42,43] developed by Magerl, uses superior screw fixation with inferior sublaminar hooks. The strength of this construct has been confirmed by in vitro biomechanical testing. However, these tests have also shown the Hook plate to have insufficient biomechanical advantage over conventional posterior wiring techniques to warrant the neurological risks associated with cervical sublaminar hook placement.[18,71]

The development of lateral mass plating with optional C2 and/or C7 pedicle screw placement is an important advance in revision surgery for failed cervical spine reconstruction. Lateral mass plates, initially developed and popularized by Roy-Camille,[64] provide rigid fixation that is not dependent upon the posterior elements. The construct relies upon screw fixation into the lateral masses, but is contraindicated in the presence of osteoporotic bone or other conditions associated with suboptimal bone quality. The plates are placed bilaterally in the lateral masses. By maximizing their distance from the instantaneous axis of rotation, they provide greater rotational stability than conventional midline fixation devices. This technique, although technically more demanding than traditional wiring methods, provides superior biomechanical stability over spinous process wiring in rotational and extension loads. Preoperative CT visu-

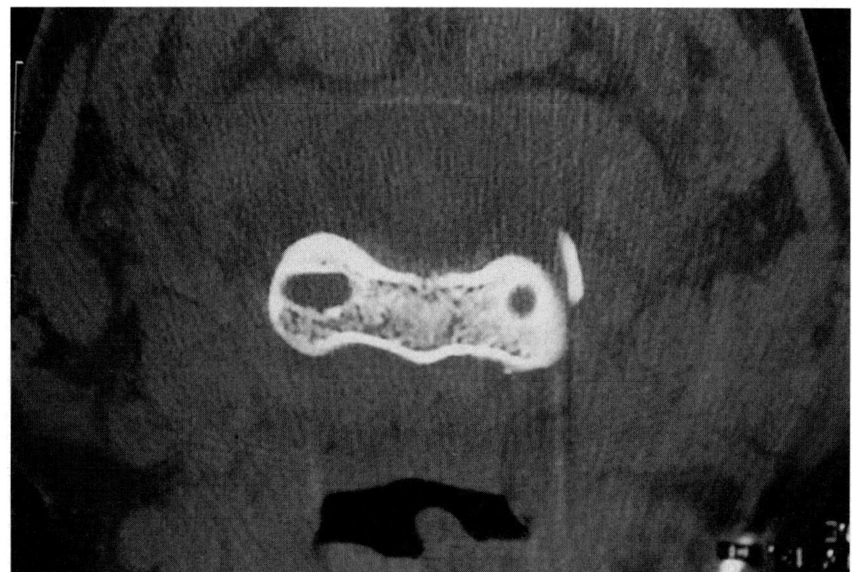

FIGURE 24-7

Transaxial CT scan revealing a tortuous C2 foramen transversarium potentially placing the vertebral artery at risk during C2 pedicle screw placement.

alization of the anatomy of the lateral mass and its relationship to the neural foramen and vertebral artery are critical to the success of this technique. There are several techniques for lateral mass screw placement including the Roy-Camille,[63] the Magerl,[36] the Anderson,[7] and the An[4] methods. The method used most frequently by the senior authors is the technique by An. In this method, following bilateral exposure of the lateral masses, the articular pillars are identified and the cortex is entered 1 mm medial to the center of each pillar with a small burr. A 2.5-mm drill bit is used and directed laterally 25 to 30 degrees and cephalad approximately 15 degrees for the C3 to C6 levels. Following penetration of the opposite cortex, the drill hole is tapped with a 3.5-mm tap. A 3.5-mm diameter and appropriate length cortical screw is then inserted to secure a contoured posterior cervical plate. A cadaveric study by An has demonstrated this screw direction to be the safest.[5]

The latest advances in spinal imaging using frameless stereotactic CT techniques have allowed a more reliable and accurate identification of cervical spine anatomy for cervical lateral mass, pedicle, and transarticular screw placement. The placement of cervical pedicle screws within the correct anatomic zone by the use of topographical landmarks has been shown to be most reliable at the C2 and C7 pedicle although palpation of the medial pedicle or isthmus border is recommended at the time of screw placement. Placement of pedicle screws at other levels has been shown to be associated with a significant risk of penetration of the spinal canal or foramen transversarium, causing a potential injury to the spinal cord or vertebral artery.[38] Preoperative CT and MRI are essential to visualize the pedicle dimension as well as vertebral artery location (Fig. 24-7). It has been noted that long posterior lateral mass fusions from C3 to C7 frequently result in inferior screw loosening with possible loss of sagittal alignment. Revision plating with the addition of C2 and C7 cervical pedicle screw fixation improves significantly the rigidity of the long fusion constructs and allows for early postoperative mobilization.

## ANTERIOR CERVICAL RECONSTRUCTION

The complication of anterior cervical graft extrusion following reconstruction of cervical spine trauma is related to the degree of initial instability, the use or nonuse of instrumentation, the type of immobilization, and the length and type of bone graft (Fig. 24-8).[20] Anterior instrumentation was originally designed to provide immediate stability to the reconstructed cervical spine. It maintains appropriate cervical alignment, provides a buttress support to the bone graft to prevent extrusion, and functions in a load-sharing capacity due to its limited flexibility, thereby adding to the stability of the construct.[12,16,27] Bicortical screw purchase for plate fixation was initially utilized for earlier designs.[16,17,28,55] This technique was more demanding[27,75] and had a complication rate as high as 40%.[68,79] Fluoroscopic guidance was required to prevent overpenetration into the spinal canal. The use of a locking unicortical screw for the fixation of anterior plates proposed by Lesoin,[41] and later by Morscher,[51] improved the neurological safety of this procedure. In fact, biomechanical studies have demonstrated no particular advantage to the use of bicortical screws for anterior plate fixation.[37] The most frequent causes for failure of anterior fusion, namely graft collapse and extrusion, have been signif-

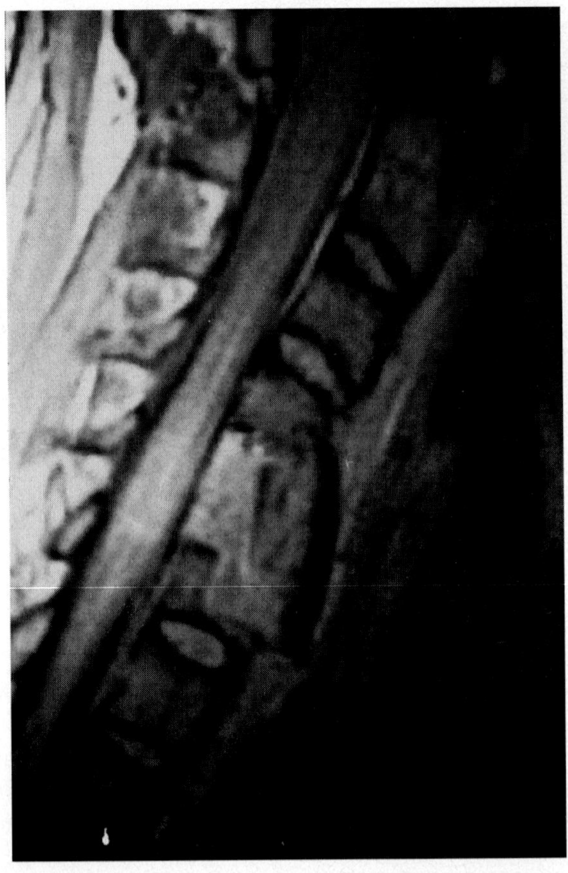

FIGURE 24-8

A sagittal MRI revealing an anterior strut graft dislodgment following an anterior cervical corpectomy and graft fusion for an advanced stage flexion compression injury.

icantly reduced by using anterior instrumentation. However, it must be remembered that an anterior plate is no substitute for sound grafting and fusion techniques. The quality of bone present as a substrate and the type of interbody bone graft chosen determine the overall stability of the construct, with tricortical iliac crest bone graft being the strongest.[58] Anterior cervical spine instrumentation has become a more popular technique in recent years.[26,59] The anterior plate biomechanically functions as a tension band,[68] being most effective in extension and least effective in flexion. In vitro biomechanical comparison between anterior and posterior cervical instrumentation has demonstrated anterior plates to be significantly weaker than posterior fixation devices for compression and flexion induced strain[18,71,72] although they provide good stability in extension. Anterior instrumentation may fail as a result of screw pull-out or breakage and at times due to plate fatigue in the setting of a failed fusion. Long anterior plate stabilization has been shown in clinical studies to have a propensity for early plate fixation failure due to inferior screw/bone failure. In such situations, the addition of a posterior cervical stabilization procedure is recommended.

## CONCLUSION

Many good and acceptable techniques exist to assist in obtaining cervical spine fusion in patients with cervical spine instability following trauma. These techniques are not successful without strict adherence to the sound principles and details of an adequate decompression of compromised neural elements and a stable spinal fusion. Additionally, the potential for a failed surgical procedure may be minimized by a thorough knowledge of the biomechanical principles and anatomical limitations of techniques of cervical spine instrumentation.

## REFERENCES


1. Abdu WA, Bohlman HH: Techniques of subaxial posterior cervical spine fusions: an overview, *Orthopedics* 15:287-295, 1992.
2. Aldrich EF, Crow WN, Weber PB, Spagnolia TN: Use of MR imaging-compatible Halifax interlaminar clamps for posterior cervical fusion, *J Neurosurg* 74: 185-189, 1991.
3. Aldrich EF: Halifax interlaminar clamps: indication and operative technique, *Contemp Neurosurg* 15:1-6, 1993.
4. An HS: *Posterior instrumentation of the cervical spine.* In An HS, Cotler JM, editors: *Spinal instrumentation,* Baltimore, 1992, Williams & Wilkins.
5. An HS, Gordin R, Renner K: Anatomic consideration for plate-screw fixation of the cervical spine, Presented at Cervical Spine Research Society, San Antonio, November 1990.
6. Anderson LD, Clark CR: *Fractures of the odontoid process of the axis.* In Sherk HH and the Cervical Spine Research Society, editors: *The cervical spine,* Philadelphia, 1989, JB Lippincott.
7. Anderson PA, Henley MB, Grady MS, Montesano PX, Winn GR: Posterior cervical arthrodesis with AO reconstruction plates and bone graft, *Spine* 16: 72-79, 1991.
8. Barbour JR: Screw fixation and fractures of the odontoid process, *S Australian Clin* 5:20-24, 1971.
9. Bohlman HH: Acute fractures and dislocations of the cervical spine: an analysis of 300 hospitalized patients

and review of the literature, *J Bone Joint Surg* 61A:1119-1142, 1979.

10. Bolesta MJ, Bohlman HH: *Late complication of cervical fractures and dislocations and their management.* In Frymoyer JW, editor: *The adult spine,* New York, 1991, Raven Press.
11. Brooks AL, Jenkins EB: Atlanto-axial arthrodesis by the wedge compression method, *J Bone Joint Surg* 60A:279-284, 1978.
12. Brown JA, Havel P, Ebraheim N, Greenblatt SH, Jackson WT: Cervical stabilization by plate and bone fusion, *Spine* 13:236-240, 1988.
13. Cahill DW, Bellegarrigue R, Ducker TB: Bilateral facet to spinous process fusion: a new technique for posterior spinal fusion after trauma, *Neurosurgery* 13:1-4, 1983.
14. Callahan RA, Johnson RM, Margolis RN, Keggi KJ, Albright JA, Southwick WO: Cervical facet fusion for control of instability following laminectomy, *J Bone Joint Surg* 59A:991-1002, 1977.
15. Capen DA, Garland GE, Waters RL: Surgical stabilization of the cervical spine, *Clin Orthop* 196:229-237, 1985.
16. Casper W, Barbier DD, Klara PM: Anterior cervical and Casper plate stabilization for cervical trauma, *Neurosurgery* 25:491-502, 1989.
17. Casper W: *Anterior stabilization with trapezoid osteosynthetic technique in cervical spine injuries.* In Kehr P, Weidner A, editors: *Cervical spine* , New York, 1987, Springer-Verlag.
18. Coe JD, Warden KE, Sutterlin CE III, McAfee PC: Biomechanical evaluation of cervical spine stabilization methods in a human cadaveric model, *Spine* 14:1122-1131, 1989.
19. Cooper PR: Posterior stabilization of the cervical spine, *Clin Neurosurg* 16:286-320, 1992.
20. Cotler JM, Star AM: *Complications of spinal fusions.* In Cotler JM, Cotler HB, editors: *Spinal fusions: science and technique,* New York, 1990, Springer-Verlag.
21. Cybulski GR, Douglas RA, Meyer PA, Rovin RA: Complications in three column cervical spine injuries requiring anterior-posterior stabilization, *Spine* 16:253-256, 1991.
22. Cybulski GR, Stone JL, Crowell RM, Rifai MH, Gandhi Y, Glick R: Use of Halifax interlaminar clamps for posterior C1-2 arthrodesis, *Neurosurgery* 22:429-431, 1988.
23. Edwards CC, Matz SO, Levine AM: The oblique wiring technique for rotational injuries of the cervical spine, *Orthop Trans* 10(3):455, 1986.
24. Gallie WE: Skeletal traction in the treatment of fractures and dislocations of the cervical spine, *Ann Surg* 106:770-776, 1937.
25. Gallie WE: Fractures and dislocations of the cervical spine, *Am J Surg* 46:495-499, 1939.
26. Garvey RA, Eismont FJ, Roberti LJ: Anterior decompression, strut bone grafting, and Casper plate stabilization for unstable cervical spine fracture and or dislocation, *Spine* 17:S431-S435, 1992.
27. Gassman J, Seligson D: The anterior cervical plate, *Spine* 8:700-707, 1983.
28. Goffin J, Plets C, Van den Bergh R: Anterior cervical fusion and osteosynthetic stabilization according to Casper: a prospective study of 41 patients with fracture and/or dislocations of the cervical spine, *Neurosurgery* 25:865-871, 1989.
29. Grantham SA, Dick HM, Thompson RC, Stinchfield FE: Occipitocervical arthrodesis, *Clin Orthop* 65:118-129, 1969.
30. Griswold DM, Albright JA, Schiffman E, Johnson R, Southwick WO: Atlanto-axial fusion for instability, *J Bone Joint Surg* 60A:285-292, 1978.
31. Grob D, Magerl F: Dorsal spondylosis of the cervical spine using a hooked plate, *Orthopaedics* 16:66-61, 1987.
32. Hadra BE: The classic wiring of the vertebrae as a means of immobilization in fractures and Potts' disease, *Clin Orthop* 112:4-8, 1975.
33. Hadra BE: Wiring of the spinous process in injury and Potts disease, *Orthopaedics Assoc* 4:206, 1981.
34. Hamblen DL: Occipito-cervical fusion, *J Bone Joint Surg* 49B:33-45, 1967.
35. Holness RO, Huestis WS, Howes WJ, Langille RA: Posterior stabilization with an interlaminar clamp in cervical injuries: technical note and review of the long-term experience with the method, *Neurosurgery* 14:318-322, 1984.
36. Jeanneret B, Magerl F, Halterward E, Ward EH, Ward JC. Posterior stabilization of the cervical spine with hook plates, *Spine* 16:S56-S63, 1991.
37. Krag MH: *Biomechanics of the cervical spine, including bracing, surgical constructs, and orthoses.* In Frymoyer JW, editor: *The adult spine: principles and practice,* New York, 1991, Raven Press.
38. Kramer D, Ludwig S, Vaccaro A, Albert T, Foley K, Balderston R: Placement of pedicle screws in the cervical spine: comparative accuracy of cervical pedicle screw placement using three techniques, Presented at Cervical Spine Research Society, Palm Beach, FL, December 5-7, 1996.
39. Larsson S, Toolanen G: Posterior fusion for atlanto-axial subluxation for rheumatoid arthritis, *Spine* 11:525-530, 1986.
40. Lesoin F, Autricque A, Jomin M: Use of C-D instrumentation for cranio-cervical junction osteosynthesis, 6th Proc Internat Cong on Cotrel-Dubousset instrumentation, Montpellier, France, Sauramps Medical, 249, 1989.
41. Lesoin F, Cama A, Lozes G, Servato R, Kabbag K, Jomin M: Anterior approach and plates in lower cervical posttraumatic lesions, *Surg Neurol* 21:581-587, 1984.
42. Magerl F, Grob D, Seemann P: *Stable dorsal fusion of the cervical spine (C2-T1) using hook plates.* In Kehr P,

Weidner A, editors: *Cervical spine,* ed 1, New York, 1987, Springer-Verlag.

43. Magerl F, Seemann PS. *Stable posterior fusion of the atlas and axis by transarticular screw fixation.* In Kehr P, Weidner A, editors: *Cervical spine,* ed 1 New York, 1987, Springer-Verlag.
44. McAfee PC: *Cervical spine trauma.* In Frymoyer JW, editor: *The adult spine: principles and practice,* New York, 1991, Raven Press.
45. McAfee PC, Bohlman HH, Wilson WL: The triple wire fixation technique for stabilization of acute cervical fracture-dislocations: a biomechanical analysis, *Trans Orthop* 9:142, 1985.
46. McAfee PC, Bohlman HH, Riley LH, Robinson RA, Southwick WO, Nachlas NE: The anterior retropharyngeal approach to the upper part of the cervical spine, *J Bone Joint Surg* 69A:1371-1383, 1987.
47. Meyer PR, Heim S: *Surgical stabilization of the cervical spine.* In Meyer PR, editor: *Surgery of spine trauma,* New York, 1989, Churchill Livingstone, pp 397-523.
48. Meyer PR, Rusin JJ, Haak MH: *Anterior instrumentation of the cervical spine.* In An HS, Cotler JM, editors: *Spinal instrumentation,* Baltimore, 1992, Williams & Wilkins.
49. Miz G: *Cervical spine instability and biomechanics of treatment.* In Errico TJ, Bauer RD, Waugh T, editors: *Spinal trauma,* ed 2, Philadelphia, 1991, JB Lippincott.
50. Montesano PX, Juach EC, Anderson PA, Benson DR, Hansen PB: Biomechanics of cervical spine internal fixation, *Spine* 16:10-16, 1991.
51. Morscher E, Sutter F, Jenny H, Olerud S: Anterior plating of the cervical spine with the hollow screw-plate system of titanium, *Chirurg* 57:702-707, 1986.
52. Murphy MJ, Southwick WO: *Surgical approaches and techniques.* In Sherk HH, Dunn EJ, Eismont FJ et al, editors: *The cervical spine,* ed 2, Philadelphia, 1989, JB Lippincott.
53. Nordt JC, Stauffer ES: Sequelae of atlantoaxial subluxation in two patients with Down syndrome, *Spine* 6:437-440, 1981.
54. Oro JJ, Watts C: Sublaminar and epilaminar wire fusion: a new technique for posterior subluxation injuries of lower cervical spine, *Trans Orthop* 9:142, 1985.
55. Papadopoulas SM: Anterior cervical instrumentation, *Clin Neurosurg* 15:273-285, 1992.
56. Pelker RR, Duranceau JS, Panjabi MM: Cervical spine stabilization-a three dimensional, biomechanical evaluation of rotational stability, strength, and failure mechanism, *Spine* 16:117-122, 1991.
57. Ransford AO, Crockard HA, Pozo JL, Thomas NP, Nelson IW: Craniocervical instability treated by contoured loop fixation, *J Bone Joint Surg* 68B:173-177, 1986.
58. Reinsel T, Krag M: *Cervical spine biomechanics.* In An HS, Simpson MJ, editors: *Surgery of the cervical spine,* London, 1994, Martin Dunitz.
59. Ripa DR, Kowall MG, Meyer PR: Series of ninety-two traumatic cervical spine injuries stabilized with anterior ASIF plate fusion technique, *Spine* 16:S46-S55, 1991.
60. Robinson RA, Southwick WO: Indication and techniques for early stabilization of the neck in some fracture dislocations of the cervical spine, *South Med J* 53:565-579, 1960.
61. Rogers WA: Treatment of fracture-dislocation of the cervical spine, *J Bone Joint Surg* 24:245-258, 1942.
62. Rogers WA: Fractures and dislocation of the cervical spine: an end result study, *J Bone Joint Surg* 39A:341, 1957.
63. Roy-Camille R, Saillant G, Berteaux D, Serge MA: *Early management of spinal injuries.* In McKibbon B, editor: *Recent advances in orthopaedics,* Edinburgh, 1987, Churchill Livingstone.
64. Roy-Camille R, Saillant G, Mazel C: *Internal fixation of the unstable cervical spine by a posterior osteosynthesis with plates and screws.* In Bailey RW, Sherk HH, et al, editors: *The cervical spine,* ed 2, Philadelphia, 1989, JB Lippincott.
65. Schlicke LH, Schulak DJ: Wiring of the cervical spinous process, *Clin Orthop* 154:319-320, 1981.
66. Scott EH, Haid RW, Peace D: Type I fractures of the odontoid process: implications for atlanto-occipital instability, *J Neurosurg* 72:488-492, 1990.
67. Simmons EH, Du Toit G: Lateral atlantoaxial arthrodesis, *Orthop Clin North Am* 9:1101-1114, 1978.
68. Simpson MJ, Sutton D, Rizzolo SJ, Cotler JM: *Traumatic injuries of the lower cervical spine.* In An HS, Simpson MJ, editors: *Surgery of the cervical spine,* London, 1994, Martin Dunitz.
69. Smith GW, Robinson RA: The treatment of certain cervical spine disorder by anterior removal of the intervertebral disc and interbody fusion, *J Bone Joint Surg* 40A:607-624, 1958.

69A. Stauffer ES: *Direct transoral anterior approaches to the upper cervical spine.* In Sherk HH, Dunn EJ, Eismont FJ et al, editors: *The cervical spine,* ed 2, Philadelphia, 1989, JB Lippincott, pp 805-822.

70. Steib JP, Kehr P, Mitteau M: C1-C2 instrumentation with C-D pediatric material, 6th Proc Internat Cong on Cotrel-Dubousset instrumentation, Montepellier, France, Sauramps Medical, 245, 1989.
71. Sutterlin CE III, McAfee PC, Warden KE, Rey RM Jr, Farey ID: A biomechanical evaluation of cervical spine stabilization methods in a bovine model: static and cyclical loading, *Spine* 13:795-802 1988.
72. Ulrich C, Worsdorfer O, Claes L, Magerl F: Comparative study of the stability of anterior and posterior cervical spine fixation procedures, *Arch Orthop Trauma Surg* 106:226-231, 1987.

73. Vaccaro AR, Cotler JC: *Traumatic injuries of the adult upper cervical spine.* In An HS, Simpson MJ, editors: *Surgery of the cervical spine,* London, 1994, Martin Dunitz.
74. Van Peterghem PK, Scheweifel JF: The fractured cervical spine rendered unstable by anterior cervical fusion, *J Trauma* 19:110-114, 1979.
75. Weidner A: *Internal fixation with metal plates and screws.* In The Cervical Spine Research Society, editors: *The cervical spine,* ed 2, Philadelphia, 1989, JB Lippincott.
76. Weiland DJ, McAfee PC: Posterior cervical fusion with triple-wire strut graft technique: one hundred consecutive patients, *J Spine Dis* 4:15-21, 1991.
77. Wertheim SB, Bohlman HH: Occipitocervical fusion. *J Bone Joint Surg* 69A:833-836, 1987.
78. White AA, Panjabi MM: *Clinical biomechanics of the spine,* Philadelphia, 1978, JB Lippincott.
79. White AA: Clinical biomechanics of cervical spine implants, *Spine* 14:1040-1045, 1989.
80. White AA, Southwick WO, Panjabi MM: Clinical instability in the cervical spine, *Spine* 1:15-27, 1976.
81. Whitehill R, Barry JC: The evolution of stability in cervical spinal constructs using either autogenous bone graft or methylmethacrylate cement. A follow up report on a canine in vivo model, *Spine* 10:32-41, 1985.
82. Whitesides TE, Kelly RP: Lateral approach to the upper cervical spine for anterior fusion, *South Med J* 59:879, 1966.
83. Whitesides TE, McDonald AP: Lateral retropharyngeal approach to the upper cervical spine, *Orthop Clin North Am* 9:1115-1127, 1978.
84. Wilber RG, Peters JG, Likavec MJ: *Surgical techniques in cervical spine surgery.* In Errico TJ, Bauer RD, Waugh T, editors: *Spinal trauma,* Philadelphia, 1991, JB Lippincott.

# 25

# LOAD-SHARING CLASSIFICATION: PREVENTING IMPLANT FAILURE FOLLOWING SURGICAL TREATMENT

**Eldin E. Karaikovic, M.D.**
**Robert W. Gaines, Jr., M. Sci**



There are three fundamental questions that every spine surgeon has to answer when facing a patient with a spine fracture. These are: first, how should a patient be treated—nonoperatively or operatively; second, how many segments should one instrument and fuse—short- versus long—segment fusion; and third, which approach should one use—anterior or posterior.

Our clinical success with short-segment instrumentation (one level above to one level below the injury), from the anterior or posterior approach, has been so rewarding since adoption of the Load-Sharing Classification (Fig. 25-1),[28] that we only rarely use long-segment fixation (virtually always in patients who are *unreliable* in brace-wear) based on their premorbid personality, their injuries, or both, or in high thoracic injuries in which preservation of motion segments is less important than lower in the spine.

We quantify fracture comminution by our Load-Sharing Classification and do anterior vertebrectomy and strut grafting with the Kaneda device[24] for more highly comminuted injuries, or use posterior pedicle screw-based short segment spinal instrumentation[22] for minimally comminuted injuries.

Fracture-dislocations (injuries with translational displacement) (Fig. 25-2) are initially stabilized posteriorly to realign the translational displacement, because realignment of the translation is easier to achieve, particularly if grotesque, from a posterior than from an anterior approach. If vertebral body comminution is minimal or modest, posterior short-seg-

# Comminution/Involvement

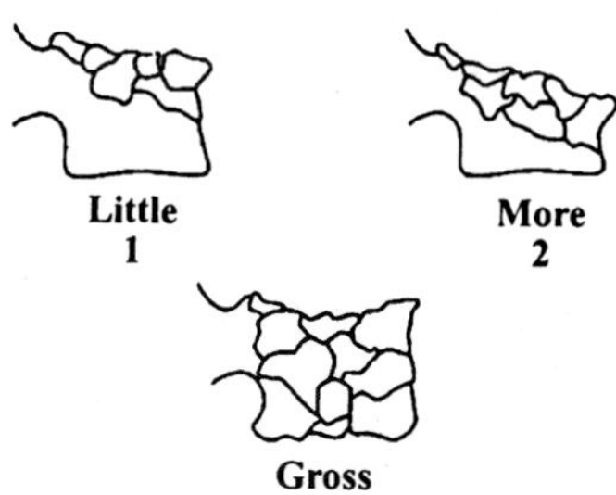


1 Little = < 30% Comminution on sagittal plane section CT

2 More = 30% - 60% Comminution

3 Gross = > 60% Comminution

# Apposition of Fragments

1 Minimal = Minimal displacement on axial CT cut.

2 Spread = At least 2mm displacement of < 50% cross section of body.

3 Wide = At least 2mm displacement of > 50% cross section of body.

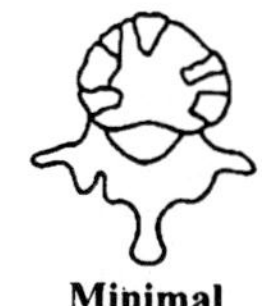


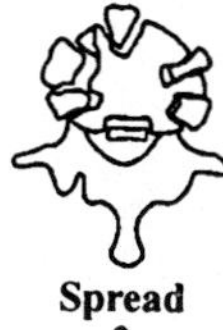


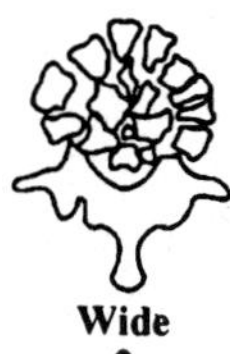


# Deformity Correction

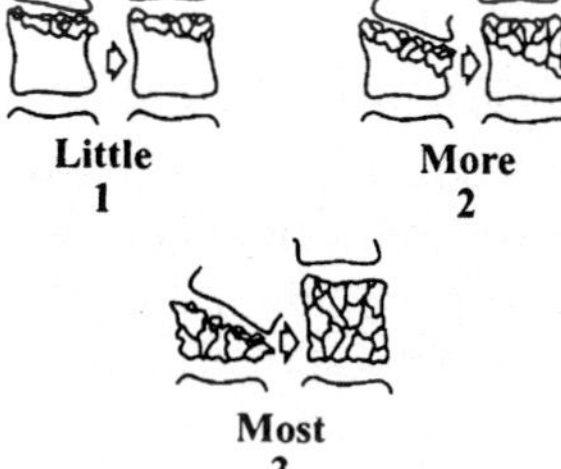


1 Little = Kyphotic correction ≤ 3° on lateral plain films.

2 More = Kyphotic correction 4° - 9°.

3 Most = Kyphotic correction ≥ 10°.

FIGURE 25-1

The Load-Sharing Classification of thoracolumbar fractures.

ment instrumentation and fusion is sufficient, even for fracture-dislocations. If the comminution assessment rates seven points or more on our Load-Sharing Classification scale, short-segment instrumentation and fusion is performed first, then an anterior strut graft without anterior implants is performed, usually in a staged manner.

## SHORT-SEGMENT INSTRUMENTATION AND FUSION—CLINICAL ADVANTAGES

The introduction of pedicle screw-related implants, anterior spinal implants, and improvements in understanding of fracture biomechanics have led to the ability to perform short-segment instrumentation and fusion from either the anterior or posterior approach to preserve motion segments. Early reports encouraged the use of these systems but offered no guidelines for the selection of patients, postoperative care, or technical application.[7,16,21]

A canine study showed that lumbosacral motion and facet loading were significantly increased after long-segment immobilization of proximal segments, and that the amount of the increase was dependent on the number of immobilized segments. This indicated that immobilization of long segments of the spine influences the remaining mobile segments by increasing the load and motion not only at the immediately adjacent segment but also at the distal segments.[36] This data provides basic science support for short-segment instrumentation and fusion compared with long-segment instrumentation, along with the obvious clinical advantages for active patients.

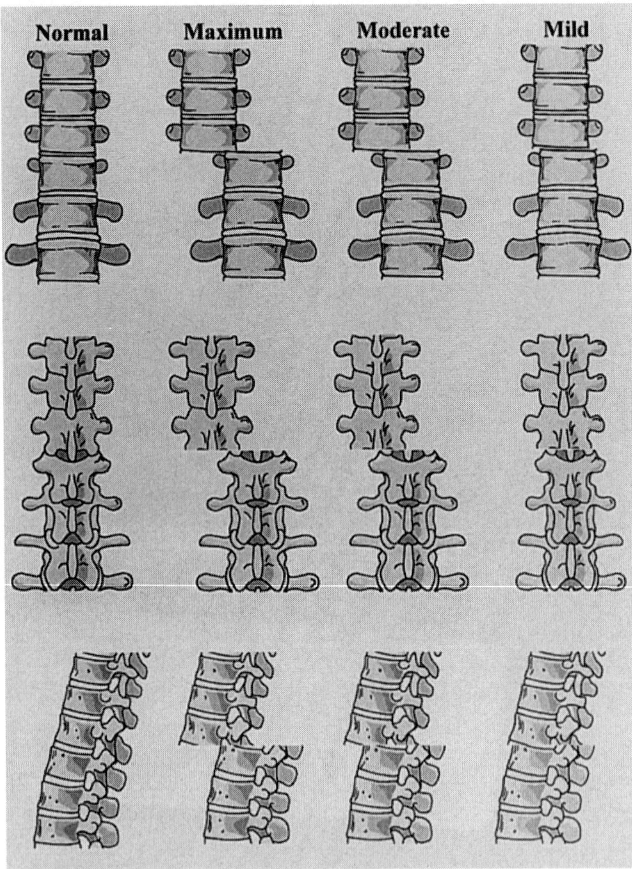


FIGURE 25-2

Anteroposterior, posteroanterior, and lateral views of translational displacement in a thoracolumbar fracture. The drawing on the left represents an intact spine, and is followed by drawings of different degrees of translation from gross to subtle.

## LOAD SHARING

The emphasis on load sharing (the ability of the fracture site itself to transfer a part of an externally applied load along with an applied implant)[3] came from our laboratory investigations regarding the biomechanics of spinal fracture repair. Our work with spine fracture constructs with seven different implants showed that the load transfer *through the fracture site itself* was far more important in clinically successful spine reconstruction than the type of implant used to repair the fracture.[12] This is especially important when short-segment instrumentation is used for spine fracture treatment. The absence of load sharing (i.e., extensive comminution, overcorrection, or fracture gaps) regularly leads to implant failure, loss of reduction, deformity, and nonunion (Fig. 25-3).[9,29,30,44]

We have come to realize that a preoperative analysis of bony fracture comminution is much more useful in guiding successful spinal fracture treatment than previously used mechanistic or column-based classifications. Because comminution and initial fracture displacement have been proven to control the amount of shortening and deformity in patients with long bone fractures treated nonoperatively,[40] an understanding of comminution also helps predict the structural and also the likely functional outcome of nonoperatively treated spinal fracture patients. If surgical treatment is chosen, particularly short-segment instrumentation, then the Load-Sharing Classification can guide the surgeon to the anterior or posterior approach.

## IMPLANT SURVIVORSHIP AND LOSS OF REDUCTION AFTER POSTERIOR PEDICLE SCREW-BASED SHORT-SEGMENT INSTRUMENTATION AND FUSION

Survivorship is a term borrowed from oncology that spinal surgeons now use to identify implant failure, or "death" of an implant. This was defined as breakage, loosening, significant change in position (Cobb angle change of more than 8°), or implant removal/revision for any implant-related problem.[9]

Loss of correction and failure of implants are more common in spine fractures that had short-segment fixation with pedicle screws. A literature review suggested an incidence of around 20% within 6 months.[1,2,4,9,10,25,30,31,42,44,46,47] A series that used anterior strut graft and anterior instrumentation had an incidence rate of 6%.[21] The mean loss of correction of kyphosis ranged from 3 to 12 degrees in the reported pedicle screw studies, whereas the mean loss of correction in the Kaneda series was only 1 degree. Nevertheless, most mentioned pedicle screw studies report high fusion rates and good clinical results despite the high implant failure rate (Fig. 25-3).

Failure of short-segment pedicle screw-based instrumentation seems to regularly occur regardless of the type of instrumentation used. The angle-stable plate,[4] the AO Fixateur Interne,[1,10] the AO dynamic compression (DC) plate,[41,42] Cotrel-Dubousset instrumentation,[2,29,30,46] the Dick internal fixator,[25,44] Olerud posterior segmental fixator,[47] and the variable screw placement (VSP) plates[9,20,47] have all shown fractured screws. None of the patients who had good load sharing through fractured vertebral bodies had measurable progression, whereas, regardless of the length of follow-up, patients who had poor load sharing had an average of 10 degrees of progression resulting in more symptoms and/or functional disability that required reoperation in some cases.[30]

Lack of anterior column support after posterior correction and instrumentation is an obvious source of the failure of posterior short-segment spinal instrumentation.[4,7,9,28,29,30,45] Some surgeons have tried to supplement the anterior column by a posterior approach and transpedicular grafting and one suc-

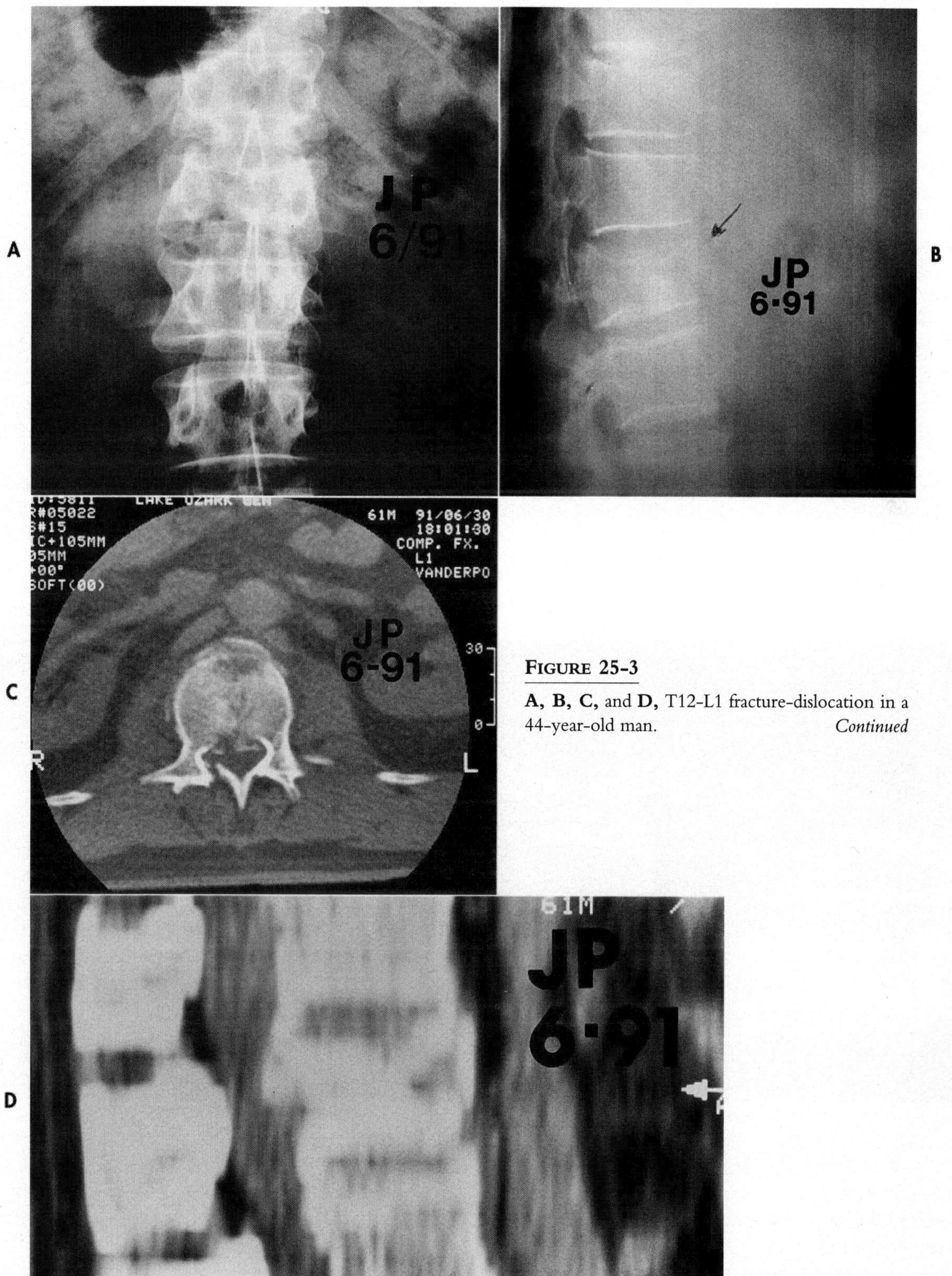


**FIGURE 25-3**

**A, B, C,** and **D,** T12-L1 fracture-dislocation in a 44-year-old man. *Continued*

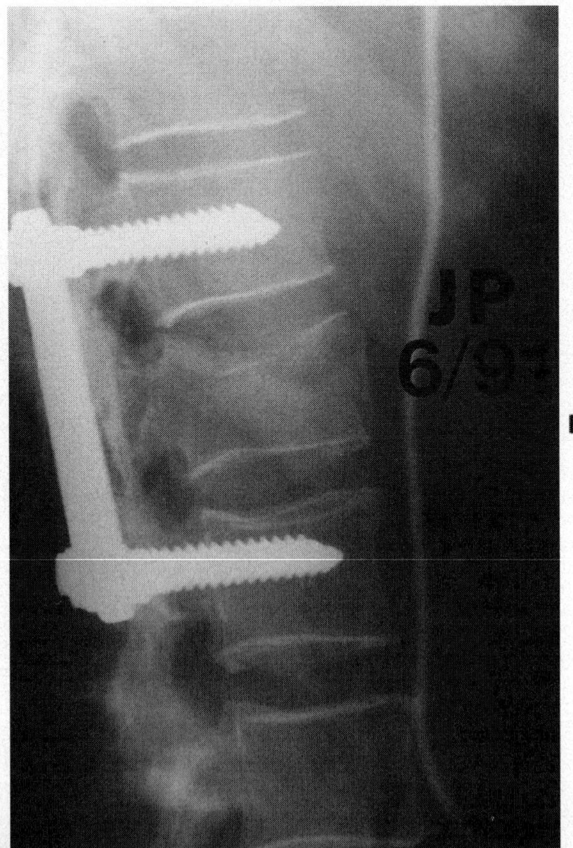


FIGURE 25-3, CONT'D

**E,** Excellent postoperative reduction and **F,** progressive collapse at the fracture site without an implant fracture were seen within a few months. This indicates the value of the Load-Sharing Classification in predicting the fate of short-segment constructs that neglect "load sharing." Full bony union was achieved and the patient is clinically fine. See the text for details.

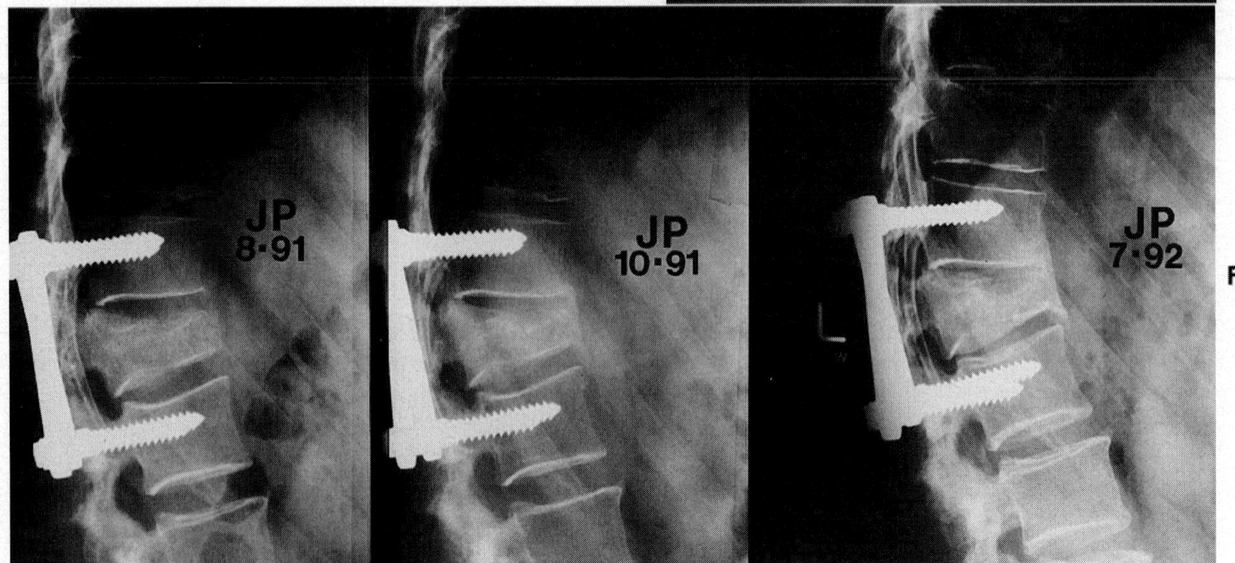


ceeded.[9] However, the largest series of this technique with the longest follow-up seriously failed.[44] The anterior strut graft has been clearly shown to be the most reliable technique to achieve and maintain adequate vertebral height with the least statistical complications in the largest series with the longest follow-up.[21,23,39]

## BASIC BIOMECHANICS

When using wooden blocks as vertebral models with total lack of load sharing (a corpectomy model), Carson showed that untransfixed, 0-degree pedicle-to-pedicle angle bilevel constructs are unstable 4R-4bar linkages that will collapse until impingement of fragments in the fracture site resist the applied load. The same untransfixed, but non-0-degree pedicle-to-pedicle angle constructs are stable structures. However, as the pedicle-to-pedicle angle approaches 0 degrees, these constructs become increasingly flexible (unstable) to lateral loads and, when displaced from the rectangular configuration, to axial loads. Rapid increase in flexibility (instability) began at a pedicle-to-pedicle angle of approximately 30 degrees. This can cause premature implant failure unless load sharing takes place and/or the facets sufficiently constrain the unstable lateral linkage motion. Transfixating bilevel constructs stabilizes them to all modes of loading, and reduces excessive linkage instability, even in the absence of load sharing and/or facets.[3]

## CLINICAL BIOMECHANICS

When a patient who has had a spinal fracture internally fixed with a posterior implant system and fusion stands erect, the loaded intervertebral disks under the fusion mass lose water and height and produce strain in the posterior spinal fusion mass and implant system. This strain causes fatigue loading in the posterior fixation device. Under these conditions stiff implants can break or bend or lose fixation at the bone-implant interface,[37] if the load sharing through the spine itself is too low.[28]

When the load applied to Harrington rods used in tests was measured postoperatively, rapid and dramatic decreases were noted after six weeks.[37] Loads sustained by Harrington rods used for patients with idiopathic scoliosis also showed a rapid decrease in axial load transmission over the 10 days following their application.[34] This loss occurs due to the adaptation of the disks separating the vertebral bodies anteriorly[37] and loosening of the hook sites due to toggling of Harrington hooks and/or bone resorption at the hook sites. The spinal implants briefly decreased the loads on the disks and limited the motion of the underlying vertebrae, but did not eliminate load or motion completely.[35]

In spinal fracture patients, although intraoperative distraction helps achieve radiographically pleasing anatomical reconstruction of vertebral bodies,[1,7,10,25] the absence of load sharing (i.e., extensive comminution) overcorrection, or fracture gaps[8] regularly leads to failure of posteriorly placed implants, loss of reduction, deformity, and nonunion.[7,10,25,30] We agree with other authors[30] that prestressing of the screws, through forced compression, distraction, or in situ bending, should be avoided. The amount of load transmitted through the distracted segment is a function of the rigidity of the internal fixation device and the load-transmitting characteristics of the tissue in the fracture site, such as an interbody bone graft or damaged vertebral body or disk.[17] Posterior fixation devices lead to stress-shielding of vertebral bodies under the implants, leading to stress relief-induced osteopenia. This osteopenia subsides in months due to implant loosening.[43] A decrease in stress-shielding through the vertebral body promotes healing and explains why the moderate loss of correction that may occur after an implant fracture after short-segment posterior spinal fusion is accompanied by prompt fusion. Therefore, collapsed vertebral bodies should be left axially shortened with a surgically decompressed spinal canal if posterior fusion is used, or, if distraction is performed and full height of comminuted injuries restored, the construct must be supplemented with anterior strut grafting.[9,21,27,29,31,44]

Our early experience with short-segment pedicle screw-based plating for spine fractures indicated that the occurrence of screw fracture was based solely on fracture selection criteria.[20] To recognize this fact, and to help the surgeon face a patient with a thoracolumbar spine fracture, we published a new approach to fracture assessment, the Load-Sharing Classification of thoracolumbar spine fractures (Fig. 25-1).[28] After 5 years' experience (1986-1991) with short-segment spinal fracture instrumentation with VSP screws and plates and treating several cases with screw fracture, we reviewed a consecutive series of cases to determine the causes of pedicle screw fracture with or without loss of correction. Our review demonstrated an impelling relationship between the *amount of comminution* in the most injured vertebra and the success of posterior short segment instrumentation with VSP plates and screws.[28]

## LOAD-SHARING CLASSIFICATION IN TREATMENT DECISION MAKING

Our classification was developed after we recognized that by preoperatively quantifying the comminution of the most injured vertebral body (regardless of the mechanism of injury, and without being column-specific regarding the comminution), we could predict, with great accuracy, the occurrence of postoperative pedicle screw fracture for spine fractures treated with pedicle screws one level above to one level below the injury.

All currently used classifications,[5,6,11,14,15,18,19,26,33] including ours,[28] accept the fact that imaging techniques provide only a static view of spinal displacement. Unidentified ligamentous ruptures, spontaneously reduced thoracolumbar subluxations, and even dislocations, and inability to demonstrate the maximal displacement of any given injury by available imaging techniques are liabilities of any and all classifications. However, clinically our classification was evaluated and found to be reliable and easy to use.[32]

Three fundamental principles underlie the Load-Sharing Classification. First, fracture anatomy can *never* be used *alone* to determine fracture treatment and/or surgical indications because *any fracture,* regardless of comminution or displacement, can be treated either operatively or nonoperatively. Details regarding the patient's general age and health, neurologic injury, other system injuries, activity level and the expertise of the medical system available are as essential a component of treatment decision making as the anatomy of the fracture itself.[13] The second principle is the concept of load sharing, and, the third, short-segment instrumentation and fusion.

We must emphasize that the assessment of comminution provided by the Load-Sharing Classification, does not, by itself, recommend a decision for operative or nonoperative treatment of a certain spine fracture. However, it does help the surgeon to understand the likely amount of kyphosis that will develop through the fracture if it is treated nonoperatively and/or the pattern of stresses transferred through a spinal implant construct after surgical fixation if it is operated, particularly if short-segment instrumentation is used.

## CLASSIFICATION COMPONENTS (RATING A FRACTURE)

The Load-Sharing Classification of thoracolumbar fractures[28] is generated by the review of preoperative plain radiographs and sagittal and axial CT scans that provide data regarding three separate characteristics of the fracture site. All three factors used in our system quantify the comminution of the vertebral body that may have occurred during the injury. Each of these factors is subdivided into three degrees of severity and awarded 1 point for mild, 2 points for moderate, and 3 points for most severe (see Fig. 25-1).

### AMOUNT OF INVOLVEMENT/COMMINUTION

The first factor used in our system is the amount of involvement/comminution as best seen on sagittal CT reconstructions of the fracture site. This factor describes the amount and extent of comminution of the most injured vertebra. Comminution controls collapse if nonoperative treatment is selected and influences load sharing if operative treatment is selected.

After this parameter is assessed, 1 point is given for damage to 30% of the body or less; 2 points for 30% to 60% comminution of the body; and 3 points for comminution greater than 60% of the vertebral body.

### APPOSITION/DISPLACEMENT OF FRAGMENTS

The second factor in our classification system is apposition/displacement of fragments as best seen on axial CT. This component of the classification assesses the ability of fracture fragments to transmit axial load through the fracture site and heal if they are in apposition. The wider the displacement of fracture fragments, the more poorly they transmit load; if displacement is wide enough, as seen in some particularly grotesque injuries, they may never heal.

After this parameter is assessed, 1 point is given for 0 to 1 mm displacement of fragments from the intact rim of the fractured vertebra as viewed on axial CT; 2 points for at least 2 mm of displacement in less than 50% of the cross-sectional area of vertebral body; and 3 points for 2 mm or greater displacement in over 50% of the cross-sectional area.

### CORRECTION OF KYPHOTIC DEFORMITY (ANGULAR DEFORMITY)

The third factor in our classification system includes the amount of correction of kyphotic deformity, which is necessary to restore physiologic sagittal plane alignment at the involved motion segment, as best measured on lateral radiographs. Obviously, the desired amount of correction of kyphosis differs on different levels. This component quantitates the gap in the vertebral body that occurs when the traumatic kyphosis associated with severe fractures is corrected. This fracture site gap has been well-described by DeWald and others.[8] When severe traumatic kyphosis due to vertebral body crushing is well corrected by a posterior rod or plate technique, this gap is unavoidable. The creation of such a gap totally eliminates anterior column load sharing and exposes pedicle screw based spinal implants to the highest possible cantilever bending loads.

After the amount of necessary correction of kyphotic deformity is assessed, 1 point is given to a fracture for which correction of three degrees or less is necessary to achieve preinjury sagittal plane contour of the vertebra: 2 points for four to nine degrees correction; and 3 points to a fracture that requires correction of ten degrees or greater to restore normal sagittal plane alignment.

Using this classification means that *every* fracture (regardless of mechanism) can be graded from a minimum total of three points to a maximum total of nine points.

## TRANSLATIONAL DISPLACEMENT

To complete the assessment of any fracture, the only remaining task is to identify the presence or absence of translational displacement (see Fig. 25-2). If present, translation indicates serious multiple spinal ligament disruption, which we use in our classification to define a fracture-dislocation. Sometimes the amount of displacement is grotesque and easy to recognize. However, in many cases the displacement is subtle. Careful clinical evaluation (local swelling, a palpable defect in posterior interspinal ligaments), and evaluation of a pedicle position and/or spinous process malalignment (rotatory displacement) on anteroposterior radiographs can indicate this type of injury. Translational displacement commonly exists without rotational displacement. Of course, the radiographic appearance may be influenced by spontaneous reduction of a fracture on a backboard or x-ray table. Therefore, attention to subtle translation is extremely important. Axial computed tomography scans may show various degrees of subluxation of facet joints. The existence of translational displacement (indicating multiple spinal ligament and/or capsular ligament injuries) creates a much more impelling tendency toward operative treatment, than a fracture without translation. However, even in fracture-dislocations with severe comminution of the vertebral body (point total of 7 and more) we use staged short-segment posterior pedicle screw fixation and then an anterior strut graft for our reliable (brace wear for 3 months) patients (see Fig. 25-8).

## INJURIES OF THE INTERVERTEBRAL DISK IN THORACOLUMBAR FRACTURES

Disk injuries accompanying thoracolumbar fractures are important but, until recently, were poorly defined factors in acute and chronic spinal instability. Oner et al[38] discussed a classification of traumatic disk injuries (Utrecht Classification) and reviewed their influence on clinical outcome on fractures treated operatively and nonoperatively. Based on midsagittal sections of T2-weighted magnetic resonance images, they classified disk injuries in six types: a normal or near-normal disk, a black disk, an isolated Schmorl impression, collapse and/or herniation of predominantly the anterior one-third of the disk, massive herniation of the nucleus pulposus through the endplate with the nucleus still discernible as a bright space, and total collapse of the disk space with irregularity of the endplate.[38]

In nonoperatively treated fractures, the type and extent of disk injury and the degree of intervertebral disk degeneration seemed to be the cause of late pain. Analyzing the data of 35 patients with thoracolumbar spine fractures (13 treated nonoperatively and 22 operatively), Oner et al proposed that two disk types (types 4 and 6) were associated with high pain scores in nonoperatively treated patients (Fig. 25-4). The same type disk injuries were also the types associated with recurrence of kyphosis in surgically treated patients.[38]

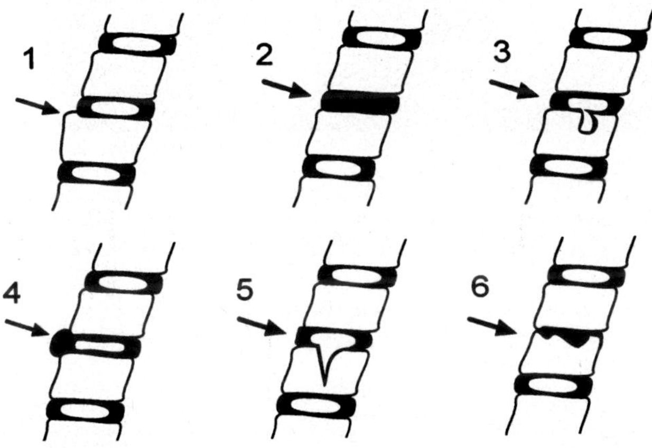


**FIGURE 25-4**

Schematic representation of disk types based on midsagittal sections of T2-weighted MRI (the arrows point to the anterior side of the spine): **1,** Normal or near-normal disk; except for some change of the shape of endplates there are no abnormalities of the disk. **2,** Black disk. The normal shape and size with only diffuse loss of signal. **3,** Isolated Schmorl impression. **4,** Collapse and/or herniation of predominantly the anterior one third of the disk. **5,** Massive herniation of the nucleus pulposus through the endplate. The nucleus is still discernible as a bright space. **6,** Total collapse of the disk space with irregularity of the endplate. (*Courtesy of FC Oner et al*[38])

## APPLICATION OF THE LOAD-SHARING CLASSIFICATION

To decide on operative versus nonoperative treatment, a clinician merely needs to assess first, the severity and location of spinal ligament injury (by physical examination, assessment of translational displacement on plain x-ray, or MRI); second, the patient's general preinjury health, activity level, neurologic injury, and other injuries; and third, quantify the fracture comminution with the Load-Sharing Classification. Following this, a good judgement regarding the risk-benefit ratio of operative versus nonoperative treatment can be done.

If the judgment leans toward nonoperative treatment, appropriate braces are chosen. If operative treatment is chosen, short-segment instrumentation and fusion are used for most surgery patients. Posterior fixation only is used for low point total injuries (Fig. 25-5), anterior fixation only for point totals of 7 and over (Fig. 25-6), posterior fixation only for fracture-dislocations with point totals less than 7 (Fig. 25-7), and posterior fixation and staged anterior strut grafting for fracture-dislocations with point totals 7 or more (Fig. 25-8). Due to the position of the iliac vein anterior to the L4 and L5 levels, which prevents the use of an anterior fixation device, we treat high total point nonfracture-dislocation burst fractures (point totals 7 and more) at these levels with posterior short-segment instrumentation, and staged anterior strut grafting. If the anterior procedure cannot be performed, posterior short-segment instrumentation and fusion and 4 to 6 weeks of bed rest with subsequent careful gradual ambulation can be successfully used.

Our only indications for long segment instrumentation are: first, unreliable or elderly patients (unable to

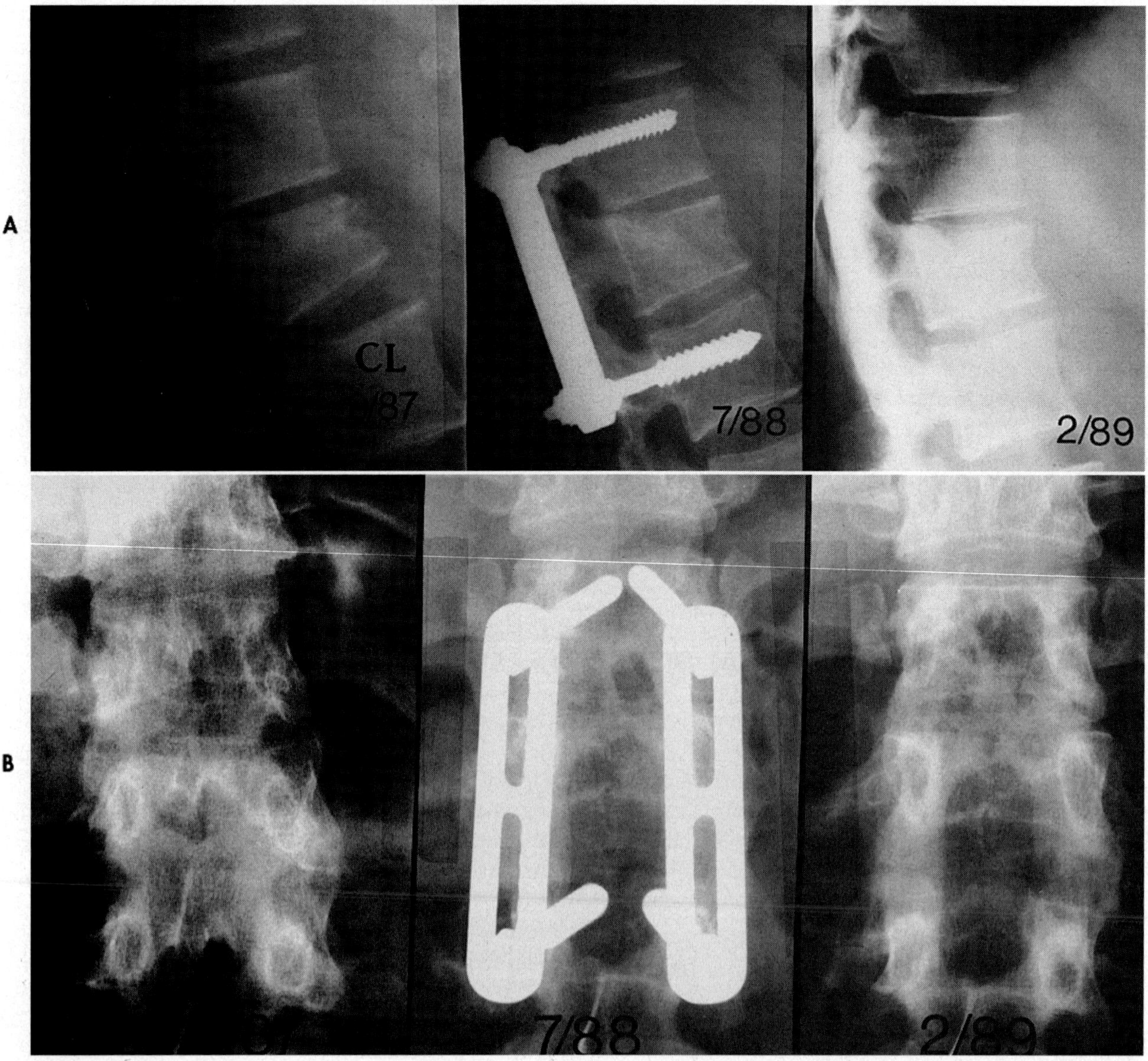


FIGURE 25-5

**A,** Mild burst fracture involves only the top third of the body (1 point), only mild (<2 mm) fragment displacement over <50% of the body (2 points), and correction of 4 to 9 degrees for restoration of normal alignment (2 points). Thus, the point total is 5 points and the fracture is successfully handled by posterior pedicle screw-based short-segment instrumentation and fusion. Follow-up films at 11 months and 18 months (after implant removal) document the fusion mass and proper healing. **B,** Anteroposterior preoperative, postoperative, and follow-up radiographs after implant removal in the same patient. Posterolateral decompression was used to relieve canal encroachment.

use bracing for 3 to 4 months) or, second, high thoracic injuries (in which maintenance of motion segments is less important than in the lumbar or thoracolumbar spine).

## DOCUMENTATION OF CLINICAL SUCCESS

A clinical review of a consecutive $4\frac{1}{2}$-year series of 46 consecutive operated fractures using short-segment instrumentation and fusion documented the reliability of our classification to eliminate failure of pedicle screw-based implants from our practice. All nonfracture dislocations with low point totals (<6) treated with VSP instrumentation[22] (23 patients) healed with no implant failures. The average preoperative kyphotic deformity was 11 degrees, the mean intraoperative correction was 12 degrees, and loss of correction on the last follow-up was 4 degrees (well within measurement error).

All but one of 16 patients of more comminuted injuries (point total of 7, 8, or 9) treated with the Kaneda device and strut grafting[24] healed, again with

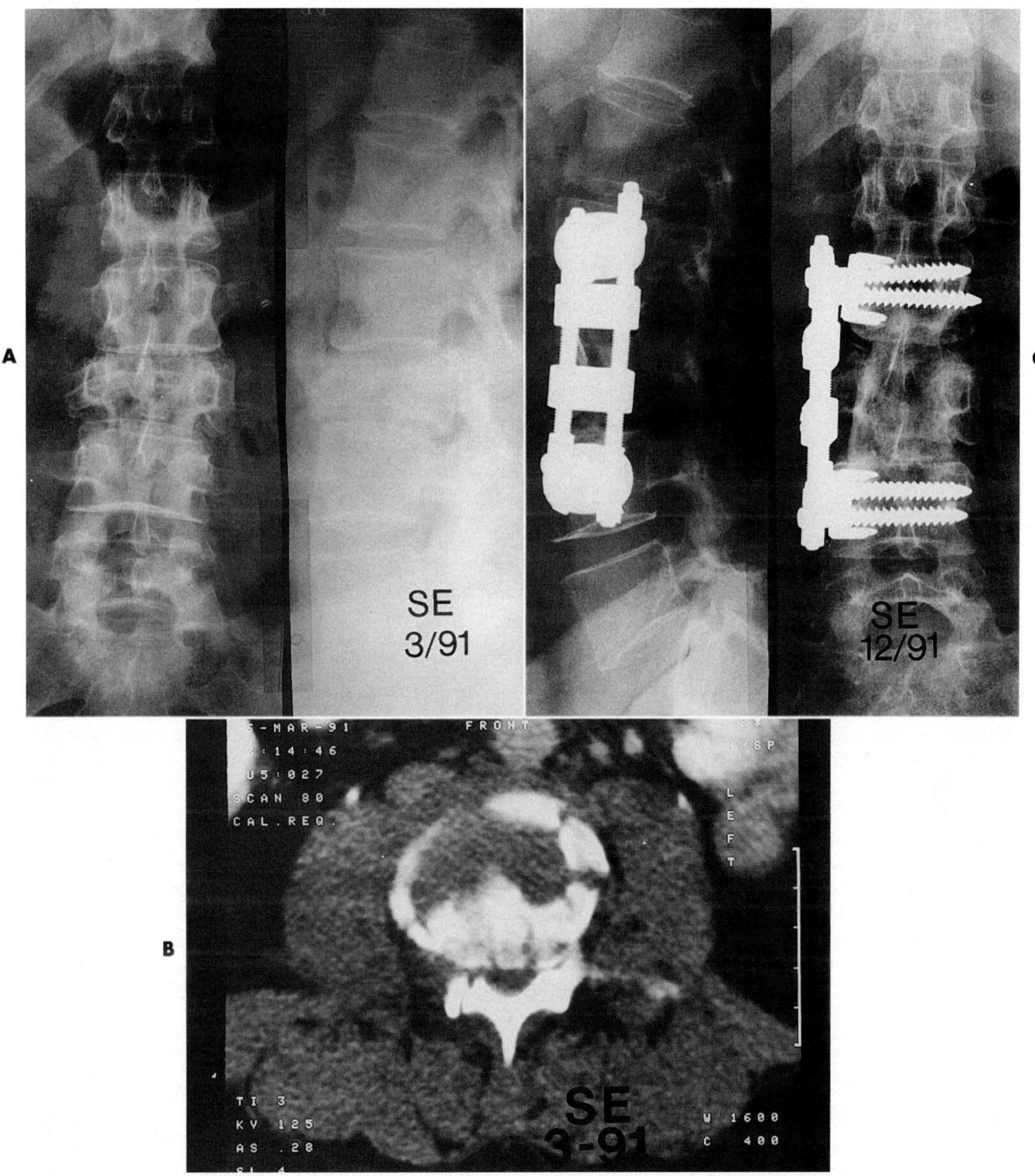


FIGURE 25-6

**A,** 21-year-old woman with total body involvement (3 points), with **B,** widespread fragments on CT (3 points), that needs greater than 10-degree sagittal plane correction because the injury is at L3 (3 points); point total is 9. Thus, the patient is operated from the anterior approach with the Kaneda device and strut graft. **C,** Proper healing with no loss of reduction was illustrated at the 9 month.

*Continued*

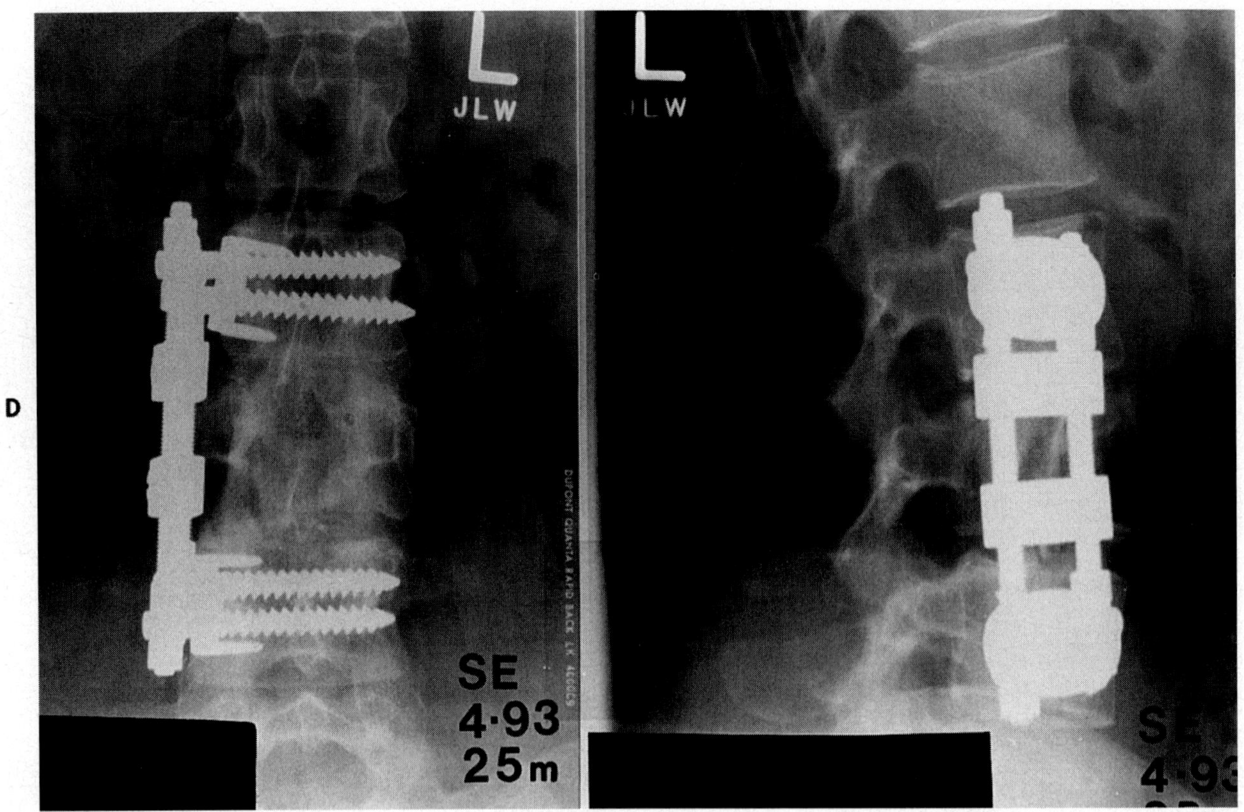


**FIGURE 25-6, CONT'D**

**D,** Proper healing with no loss of reduction was illustrated at the 25-month follow-up radiographs.

loss of correction within the range of measurement error. The average preoperative kyphotic deformity was 23 degrees, the mean intraoperative correction was 16 degrees, and loss of correction on the last follow-up was 4 degrees.

One Kaneda patient showed implant fracture and loss of correction of 32 degrees. However, tomograms show union of the iliac crest strut graft and his implants have not been revised. This patient had a history of sociopathic personality disorder preoperatively, did not comply with postoperative bracing, and should have not been chosen for short-segment instrumentation.[39]

## FRACTURE ANALYSIS

Analysis of the fracture in Figure 25-3 (*A, B,* and *C*), using our Load-Sharing Classification, shows the involvement of the entire vertebral body (more than two-thirds) 3 points; the fracture fragments are displaced over 2 mm anteriorly and posteriorly (more than 50% endplate surface) 3 points; but the necessity for sagittal plane correction to restore normal sagittal plane is very low (less than 3 degrees) 1 point. Thus, the 7-point total indicates the need for an anterior strut graft if short-segment instrumentation is used. Because the patient's pulmonary condition was poor, his strut graft was not performed (Fig. 25-3, D). Progressive collapse at the fracture site without implant failure developed (Fig. 25-3, E). This indicates the value of the classification in predicting the fate of short-segment constructs that neglect load sharing. The patient is clinically fine.

## SPINAL CANAL DECOMPRESSION

In a patient with no neurologic injury, decompression of the spinal canal should not be routinely performed. In a patient with neurologic injury, neural decompression is accomplished by the approach used to instrument the fracture. If posterior short-segment instrumentation with pedicle screws is used for fracture repair, decompression of the spinal canal can be successfully achieved by transpedicular decompression, avoiding ligamentotaxis as a reduction tool. Ligamentotaxis inevitably creates a gap in the vertebral body. It is better to leave a fractured body with some axial collapse to provide adequate load sharing, so long as the spinal cord and nerve roots are decompressed and the sagittal plane alignment is normal.

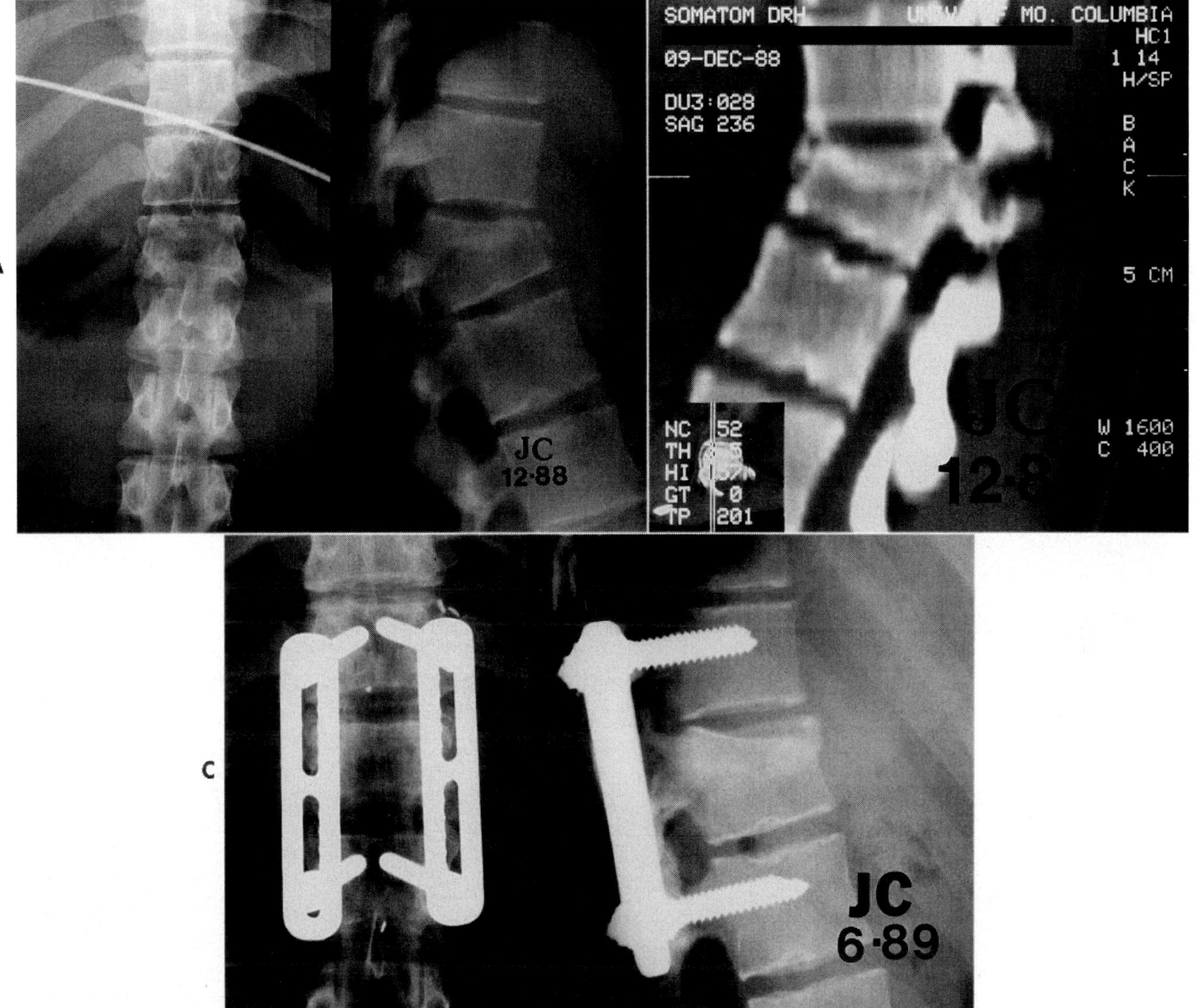


FIGURE 25-7

**A,** Typical flexion-distraction injury involves only top half of the vertebral body (2 points), minimal fragment displacement on the CT scan (1 point), and greater than 10-degree correction of kyphosis to restore normal sagittal plane alignment at T12 (3 points). Thus, the point total is 6 points. **B,** Sagittal reconstruction of the CT scan is helpful in assessing point totals. **C,** The 7-month postoperative radiographs showing short-segment reconstruction and healing in normal alignment.

## CLASSIFYING MULTIPLE FRACTURES

Although we have not done a formal review of the Load-Sharing Classification in these patients, we suggest *adding* together the point totals of the separate fractures. The total for most injuries will be over 7, suggesting that most of these patients with adjacent level fractures need to be treated anteriorly by strut graft. If fractures are multiple, but independent, they can each be described and treated independently.

## CONCLUSIONS

In our hands, the Load-Sharing Classification helps the treating physician determine the results of nonoperative treatment (by quantifying comminution and the fracture's potential for collapse); assist in making the operative/nonoperative treatment decision; and decide on the anterior versus the posterior approach if short segment surgical treatment is selected.

The classification is easy to learn and remember

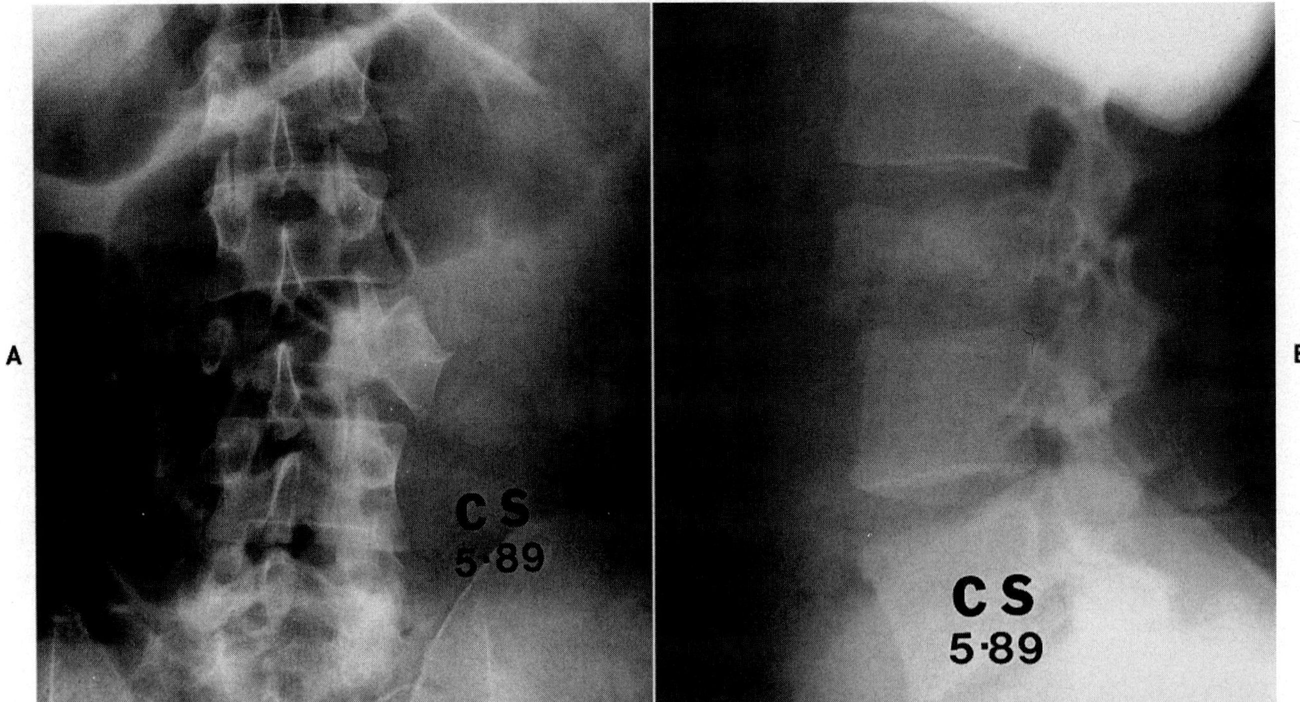


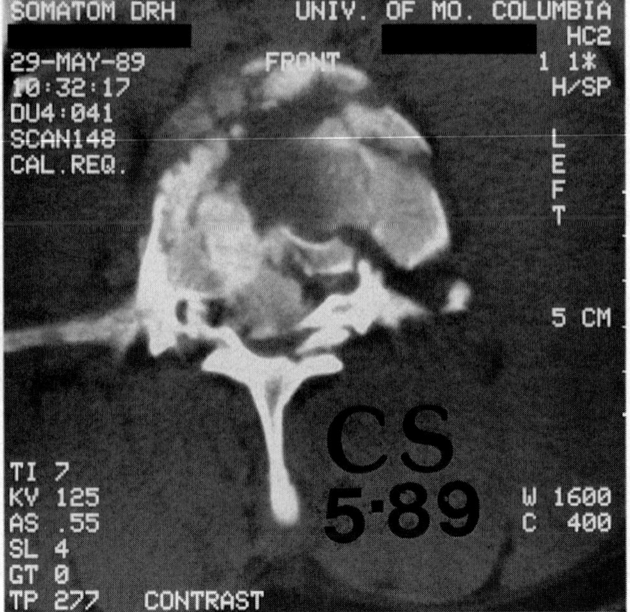


**Figure 25-8**

**A, B, C,** Highly comminuted L3 fracture-dislocation (with obvious but subtle translational displacement) involves entire body (3 points), has wider than 2-mm displacement of fragments over entire body (3 points), but requires only 4 to 9 degrees of correction to restore the normal sagittal plane (2 points). Translational displacement defines this injury as a fracture-dislocation though the displacement is only moderate.

*Continued*

and it can predict the outcome of either operative or nonoperative treatment. The use of our Load-Sharing Classification has made short-segment instrumentation and fusion our preferred treatment method and eliminated pedicle screw fractures from our clinical spine fracture practice. Our experience validates the successful clinical application of the classification and secondarily establishes short-segment instrumentation as a high quality, low morbidity, injury-specific treatment technique for isolated fractures in patients cooperative with 3 to 4 months of postoperative bracing.

## ACKNOWLEDGMENT

The fundamental contributions made by William L. Carson, Ph.D., Professor of Mechanical and Aerospace Engineering, University of Missouri-Columbia, to the understanding of spinal fracture fixation are very gratefully acknowledged.

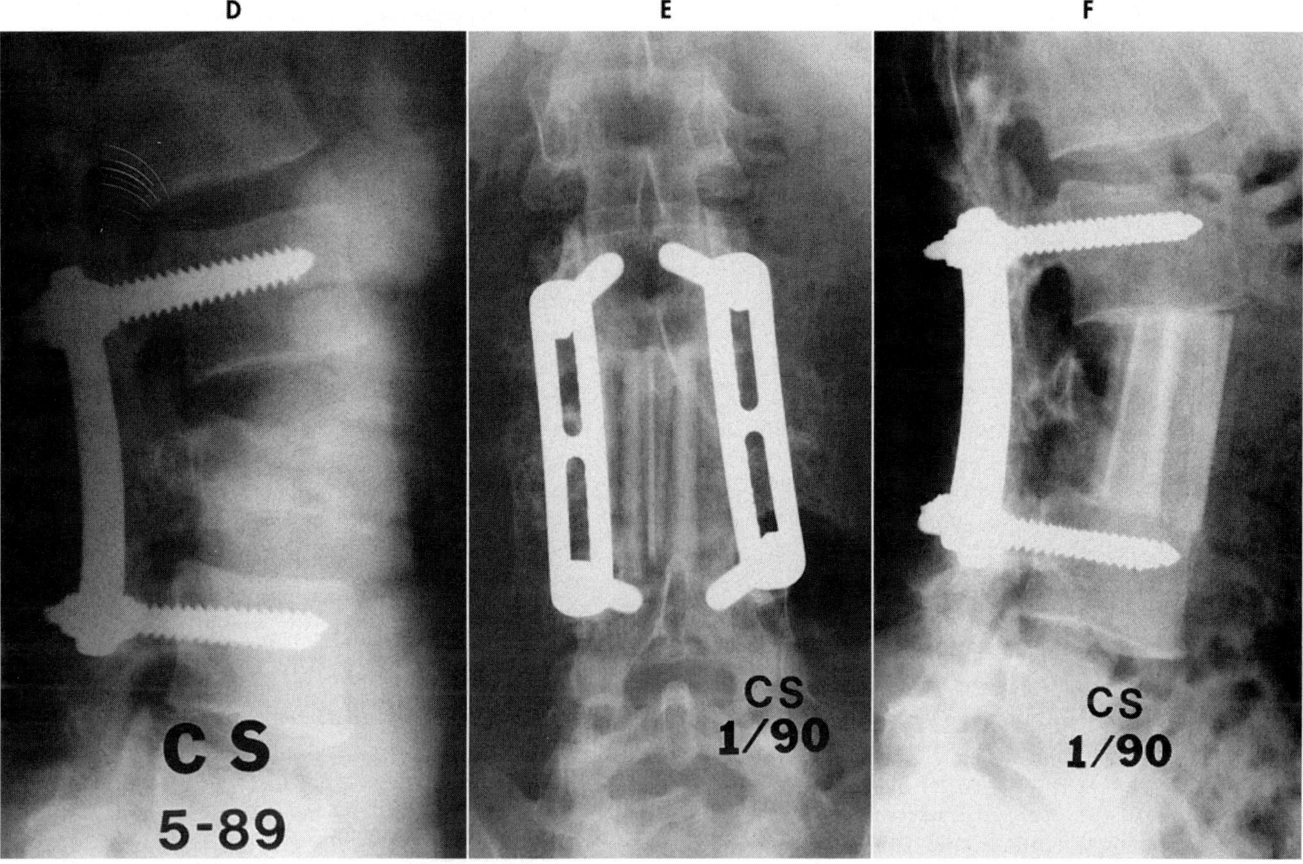


FIGURE 25-8, CONT'D

**D,** Initial treatment involved posterior instrumentation, posterolateral decompression with suture of dural laceration and containment of displaced roots, and posterolateral fusion with autograft. **E, F,** Second-stage fibular strut autograft was carried out one week later to mechanically support the posterior construct. Healing and neurologic recovery is obvious at 8 months postoperatively.

## REFERENCES

1. Benson DR, Burkus JK, Montesano PX, Sutherland TB, McLain RF: Unstable thoracolumbar and lumbar burst fractures treated with the AO fixateur interne, *J Spinal Disord* 5:335-343, 1992.
2. Carl AL, Tromanhauser SG, Roger DJ: Pedicle screw instrumentation for thoracolumbar burst fractures and fracture-dislocations, *Spine* 17(8S):S317-S324, 1992.
3. Carson WL: Biomechanical fundamentals for spinal instrumentation construct design. British Scoliosis Society, 22nd Annual Scientific Meeting, Stratford-upon-Avon, March 19-21, 1997.
4. Daniaux H, Seykora P, Genelin A, Lang T, Kathrein A: Application of posterior plating and modifications in thoracolumbar spine injuries. Indication, techniques, and results, *Spine* 16(3S):S125-S133, 1991.
5. Denis F: The three column spine and its significance in the classification of acute thoracolumbar spine injuries, *Spine* 8:817-831, 1983.
6. Denis F: Spinal stability as defined by the three-column spine concept in acute spinal trauma, *Clin Orthop* 189:65-76, 1984.
7. Devito DP, Tsahakis PJ: Cotrel-Dubousset instrumentation in traumatic spine injuries. Proceedings of the Sixth International Congress on Cotrel-Dubousset Instrumentaiton, Montpellier, Sauramps Medical, 1989:41-46.
8. DeWald RL: Burst fractures of the thoracic and lumbar spine, *Clin Orthop* 189:150-161, 1984.
9. Ebelke DK, Asher MA, Neff JR, Kraker DP: Survivorship analysis of VSP spine instrumentation in the treatment of thoracolumbar and lumbar burst fractures, *Spine* 16(8S):428-492, 1991.
10. Esses SI, Botsford DJ, Kostuik JP: Evaluation of surgical treatment for burst fractures, *Spine* 15:667-673, 1990.
11. Ferguson RL, Allen BL Jr: A mechanistic classification of thoracolumbar spine fractures, *Clin Orthop* 189:77-88, 1984.

12. Gaines RW, Carson WL, Satterlee CC, Groh GI: Experimental evaluation of seven different spinal fracture devices using non-failure stability testing—The load-sharing and unstable mechanism concepts, *Spine* 16:902-909, 1991.
13. Gaines RW, Humphreys WG: A plea for judgment in management of thoracolumbar fractures and fracture dislocations, *Clin Orthop* 189:36-42, 1984.
14. Gertzbein SD: Classification of thoracic and lumbar fractures, *Spine* 19(5):626-628, 1994.
15. Gertzbein SD: Neurologic deterioration in patients with thoracic and lumbar fractures after admission to the hospital, *Spine* 19(15):1723-2725, 1994.
16. Gillet P, Meyer R, Fatemi F, Lemaire R: Short segment internal fixation using CD instrumentation with pedicular screws: biomechanical testing. Proceedings of the Sixth International Congress on Cotrel-Dubousset Instrumentation, Montpellier, Sauramps Medical, 1989:19-24.
17. Goel VK, Lim TH, Gwon J, Chen JY, Winterbottom JM, Park JB, Weinstein JN, Ahn JY: Effects of rigidity of an internal fixation device. A comprehensive biomechanical investigation, *Spine* 16(3S):S155-S161, 1991.
18. Harms VJ. Classification of fractures of the thoracic and lumbar vertebrae (Klassifikation der BWS- und LWS-Frakturen), *Fortschr Med* 105 Jg 28:545-548, 1987.
19. Holdsworth F: Fractures, dislocations and fracture-dislocations of the spine, *J Bone Joint Surg Am* 52:1534-1551, 1970.
20. Holt BT, McCormack T, Gaines RW: Short segment fusion-anterior or posterior approach? The load-sharing classification of spine fractures, *Spine State of Art Reviews* 7(2):277-285, 1993.
21. Kaneda K, Taneichi H, Abumi K, Hashimoto T, Satoh S, Fujiya M: Anterior decompression and stabilization with the Kaneda device for thoracolumbar burst fractures associated with neurological deficits, *J Bone Joint Surg Am* 79(1):69-83, 1997.
22. Karaikovic EE, Gaines RW: *Short segment fixation using VSP plates and pedicle screws for trauma.* In *Spinal instrumentation techniques,* Scoliosis Research Society, 1994.
23. Karaikovic EE, Holt B, Gaines RW: Clinical and radiographic follow-up of Kaneda device reconstruction of thoracolumbar burst fractures, *Orthop Trans,* 17(3):885, 1993-1994.
24. Karaikovic EE, Kaneda K, Akbarnia BA, Gaines RW: *Kaneda instrumentation for spinal fractures.* In Bridwell KH, DeWald RL, editors: *The textbook of spinal surgery,* ed 2, Philadelphia, 1997, Lippincott-Raven, pp 1899-1924.
25. Lindsey RW, Dick W: The Fixateur Interne in the reduction and stabilization of thoracolumbar spine fractures in patients with neurologic deficit, *Spine* 16(3S):S140-S145, 1991.
26. Magerl F, Aebi M, Gertzbein SD, Harms JV, Nazarian SM: Comprehensive classification of the thoracic and lumbar injuries, *Eur Spine J* 3(4):184-201, 1994.
27. McAfee PC, Yuan HA, Fredrickson BE, Lubicky JP: The value of computed tomography in thoracolumbar fractures, *J Bone Joint Surg Am* 65(4):461-473, 1983.
28. McCormack T, Karaikovic E, Gaines RW: The Load-Sharing Classification of Spine Fractures, *Spine* 19(15):1741-1744, 1994.
29. McKinley LM, Obenchain TG, Roth KR: Loss of correction: late kyphosis in short segment pedicle fixation in cases of posterior transpeduncular decompression. Proceedings of the Sixth International Congress on Cotrel-Dubousset Instrumentation, Montpellier, Sauramps Medical, 1989:37-39.
30. McLain RF, Sparling E, Benson DR: Early failure of short-segment pedicle instrumentation for thoracolumbar fractures, *J Bone Joint Surg Am* 75:162-167, 1993.
31. McNamara MJ, Stephens GC, Spengler DM: Transpedicular short-segment fusions for treatment of lumbar burst fractures, *J Spinal Disord* 5:183-187, 1992.
32. Moore KD, Gaines RW: Intraobserver reproducibility and interobserver reliability of the Load-Sharing Classification of spine fractures. *Spine* (submitted for publication) 1998.
33. Morsher E. Classification of spinal column injuries (Klassifikation von Wirbelsäulenverletzungen), *Orthopäde* 9:2-6, 1980.
34. Nachemson A, Elfstrom G: Intravital wireless telemetry of axial forces in Harrington distraction rods in patients with idiopathic scoliosis, *J Bone Joint Surg Am* 53:445-465, 1971.
35. Nachemson A, Morris J: "In vivo" measurement of intradiscal pressure, *J Bone Joint Surg Am* 46:1077-1092, 1964.
36. Nagata H, Schendel MJ, Transfeldt EE, Lewis JL: The effects of immobilization of long segments of the spine on the adjacent and distal facet force and lumbosacral motion, *Spine* 18(16):2471-79, 1993.
37. Nagel DA, Edwards WT, Schneider E: Biomechanics of spinal fixation and fusion, *Spine* 16(3S):S151-S154, 1991.
38. Oner FC, v.d. Rijt R, Ramos MPL, Dhert WJA, Verbout AJ: Disc degeneration patterns after compression type fractures of the thoracolumbar spine. A classification based on MRI of 35 patients with minimal 2 year follow-up, *Spine* 1998 (submitted for publication).
39. Parker JW, Lane JR, Karaikovic EE, Gaines 45. RW: Successful short segment instrumentation and fusion for thoracolumbar spine fractures—A consecutive $4\frac{1}{2}$ year series, *Spine,* 1997 (submitted for publication).
40. Sarmiento A, McKellop HA, Llinas A, Park SH, Stetson W, Rao R: Effect of loading and fracture motions on diaphyseal tibial fractures, *J Orthop Res* 14(1):80-84, 1996.
41. Sasso RC, Cotler HB: Posterior instrumentation and fusion for unstable fractures and fracture-dislocations of

the thoracic and lumbar spine. A comparative study of three fixation devices in 70 patients, *Spine* 18(4):450-60, 1993.

42. Sasso RC, Cotler HB, Reuben JD: Posterior fixation of thoracic and lumbar spine fractures using DC plates and pedicle screws, *Spine* 16(3S):S134-S139, 1991.
43. Smith KR, Hunt TR, Asher MA, Anderson HC, Carson WL, Robinson RG: The effect of a stiff spinal implant on the bone mineral content of the lumbar spine in dogs, *J Bone Joint Surg Am* 73:115-123, 1991.
44. Speth MJGM, Oner FC, Kadic MAC, de Klerk LWL, Verbout AJ: Recurrent kyphosis after posterior stabilization of thoracolumbar fractures. 24 cases treated with a Dick internal fixator followed for 1.5-4 years, *Acta Orthop Scand* 66(5):406-410, 1995.
45. Steffee AD, Biscup RS, Sitkowski DJ: Segmental spine plates with pedicle screw fixation. A new internal fixation device for disorders of the lumbar and thoracolumbar spine, *Clin Othop* 203:45-53, 1986.
46. Stephens GC, Devito DP, McNamara MJ: Segmental fixation of lumbar burst fractures with Cotrel-Dubousset instrumentation, *J Spinal Disord* 5:344-348, 1992.
47. Viale GL, Silvestro C, Francaviglia N, Carta F, Bragazzi R, Bernucci C, Maiello M: Transpedicular decompression and stabilization of burst fractures of the lumbar spine, *Surg Neurol* 40:104-111, 1993.

# 26

# POSTSURGICAL INSTABILITY OF THORACOLUMBAR FRACTURES

**Daniele A. Fabris, M.D., Ph.D.**

THE ABSENCE OF FUSION
TREATMENT

The three major objectives when surgically treating thoracolumbar injuries are the reduction of the fracture-dislocation, the decompression of the spinal cord and/or nerve roots, and stabilization of the reduction by internal fixation. The importance of surgical decompression for thoracolumbar injuries was known before the turn of the century. Even though this concept was clear, three case reports found in the literature prior to 1900 all ended with unsuccessful results.

When a thoracolumbar injury occurs, one of the first priorities is to rule out any neurologic injury. Decompression must be performed immediately, because the clinical feature of a complete paraplegia does not always represent the true anatomic lesion of the spinal cord; and further, discriminative elements are available from somatosensory evoked potential (SEP) or magnetic resonance imaging (MRI) studies. The utilization of stabilization techniques following thoracolumbar injury was not routine until Raimond Roy-Camille in 1970 and Paul Harrington in 1976, began proving its success. During the 1970s, each of these surgeons had a different system based on their individual philosophies of reduction and stabilization.

The Roy-Camille plate uses a three-point deflection method for reduction, followed by a multisegmental fixation system. Although being the first surgeon to acknowledge the importance of the pedicle as the key site for spinal stabilization, his instrumentation system had shortcomings. The major drawback to his system was that it did not have the ability to distribute multidirectional forces during reduction. For proper reduction of different vertebral injuries, distraction, extension, and derotation may all be necessary. His system was not capable of doing this. Some other drawbacks of his system were the need for long instrumentation, three levels above and three levels below the injury were needed for fixation, and the poor resistance to pull-out of the screws.

The use of pedicle screws in the thoracic spine often leads to mobilization of the hardware, kyphosis, and late instability. On the contrary, Harrington rods have the capacity to distribute reductive strains. Distraction is, however, this system's only true method of obtaining reduction. With time, Harrington's system began to show inadequacies that included little resistance to torsion of the double-rod assembly, presence of only two constraint points between the rod and the spine, the application of reductive forces far from the injured level, and the system's use of long instrumentation, which increased the risk of degenerative changes especially in the vertebral bodies below the instrumentation.

At the beginning of the 1980s a new instrumentation system was introduced that began a true Copernican revolution in spinal fixation. The theoretical notion that different corrective strains are necessary to reduce various injuries became obsolete. In the mid- to late-1980s, Cotrel-Dubosset (CD) instrumentation was being used in the treatment of thoracolumbar fractures. New innovative options now included different assemblies available for different levels of the spine and different kinds of injuries, and the possibility to use hooks, screws, and claws. These new techniques brought about their own complications. Postsurgical instability is a late sequelae following stabilization. The two major etiologies of postsurgical instability are improper technical use of instrumentation and underestimation of the importance of biologic stabilization.[1]

Technical errors are caused by the use of an instru-

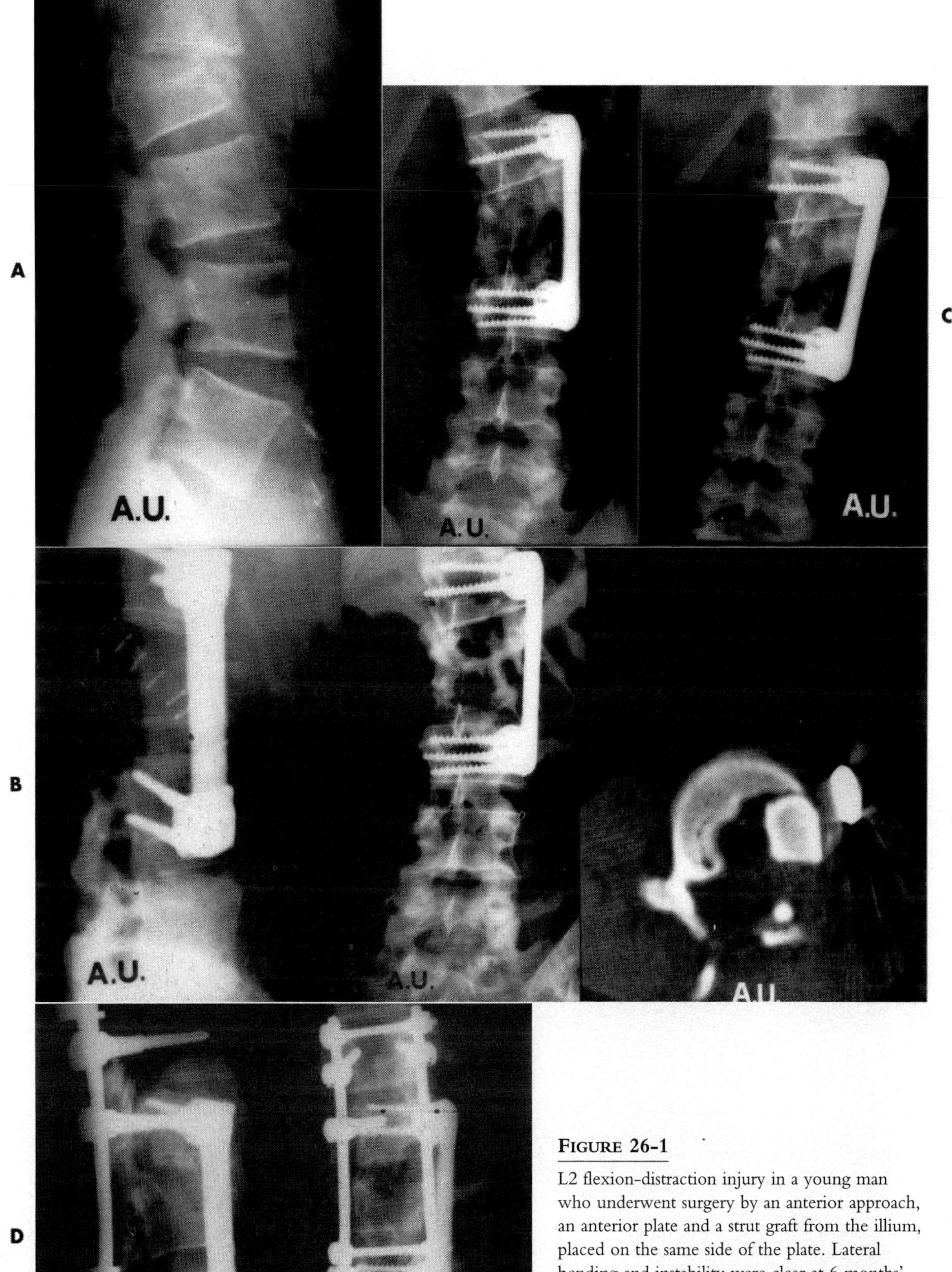


**FIGURE 26-1**

L2 flexion-distraction injury in a young man who underwent surgery by an anterior approach, an anterior plate and a strut graft from the illium, placed on the same side of the plate. Lateral bending and instability were clear at 6 months' follow-up; a posterior approach, a solid instrumentation and a posterior fusion, then were carried out with a fair result.

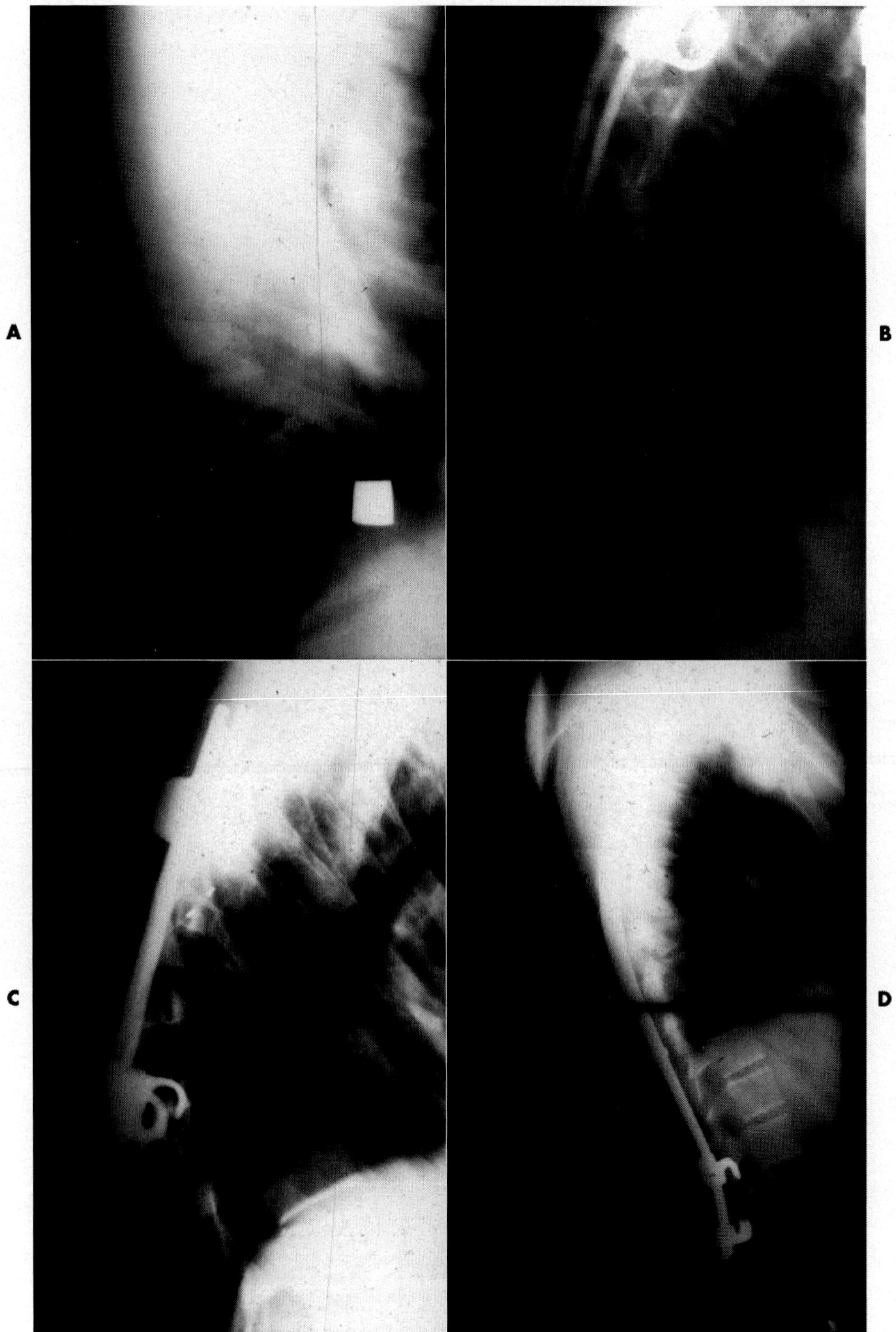


FIGURE 26-2

A 21-year-old man with thoracic injury and complete paraplegia who underwent operation using a new instrumentation device, with hook claws but too short an assembly. Kyphotic instability appeared early, and revision surgery with longer instrumentation and interbody fusion was carried out with restoration of a normal kyphosis stable assembly.

mentation device that does not obtain solid primary stability. This lack of stability leads to mobilization of the hardware, resulting in postsurgical instability. An uncorrected interaction between hardware and an anterior fusion can also lead to instability (Fig. 26-1).

Strategic errors occur when the surgeon makes a wrong choice for the assembly, such as selecting to fuse the wrong level or not using enough instrumentation claws in relation to the level of the pathomechanics of the injury.[3] In other words, strategic errors occur when a stable instrumentation device is applied with an unstable hook-screw pattern (Fig. 26-2).

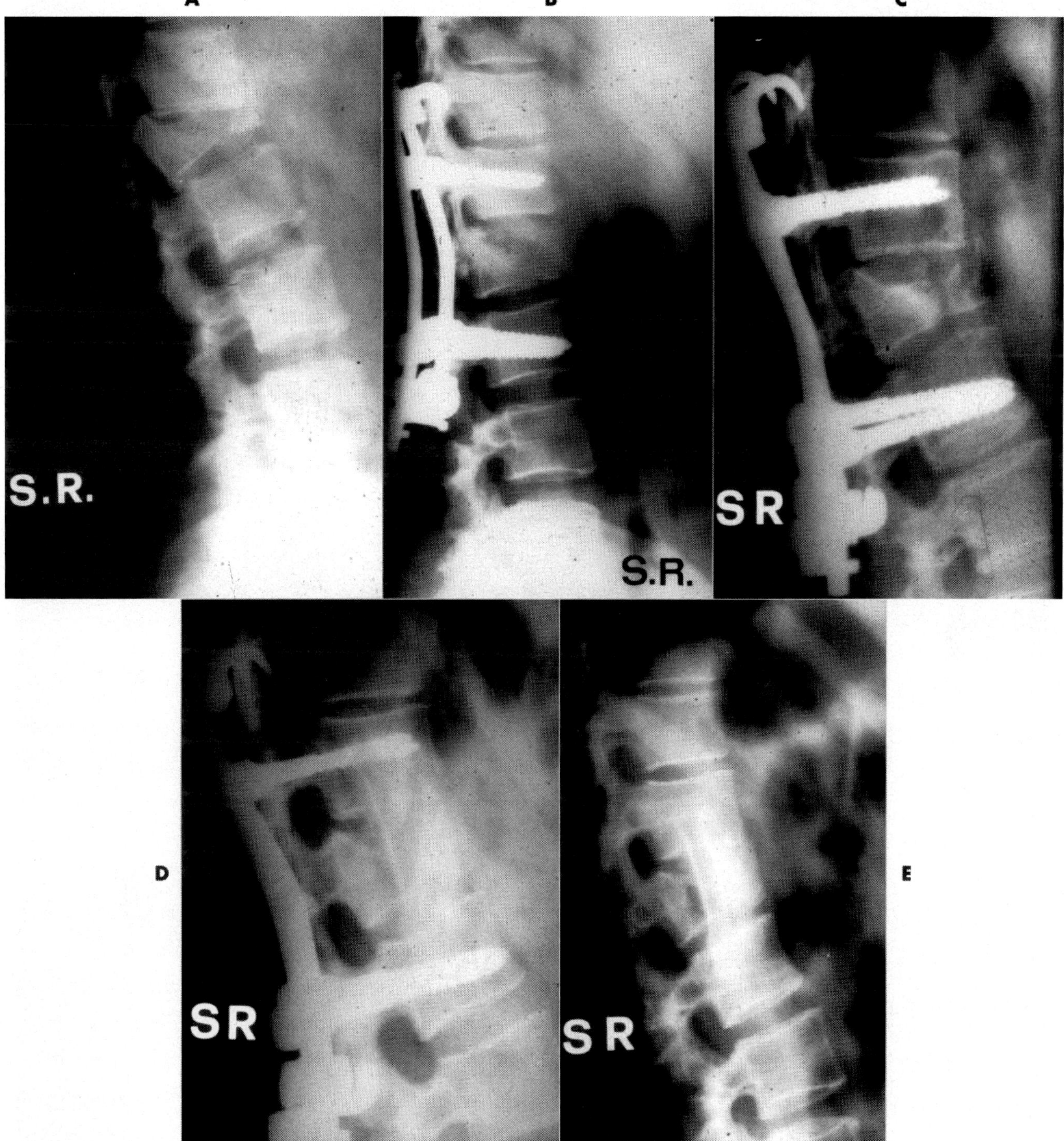


**FIGURE 26-3**

L1 burst fracture and incomplete paraplegia; the patient underwent an emergency surgery with a posterior reduction and stabilization and fair neurological recovery (Frankel B to D); 4 months later an anterior collapse was evident, and an anterior strut graft was performed with acceptable results. Removal of the hardware 6 months later shows the good biological stability of the spine.

Although the first step in the treatment of thoracolumbar injuries is the restoration of spinal stability by means of instrumentation, biologic stabilization must be achieved for successful long-term results. Hardware only acts as a temporary stabilizer while biologic fusion forms. Late-term postsurgical instability can therefore occur when the absence of biologic fusion or complete fusion does not occur. In my opinion, a poor mechanical quality of fusion means that a posterolateral fusion does not result in biologic stabil-

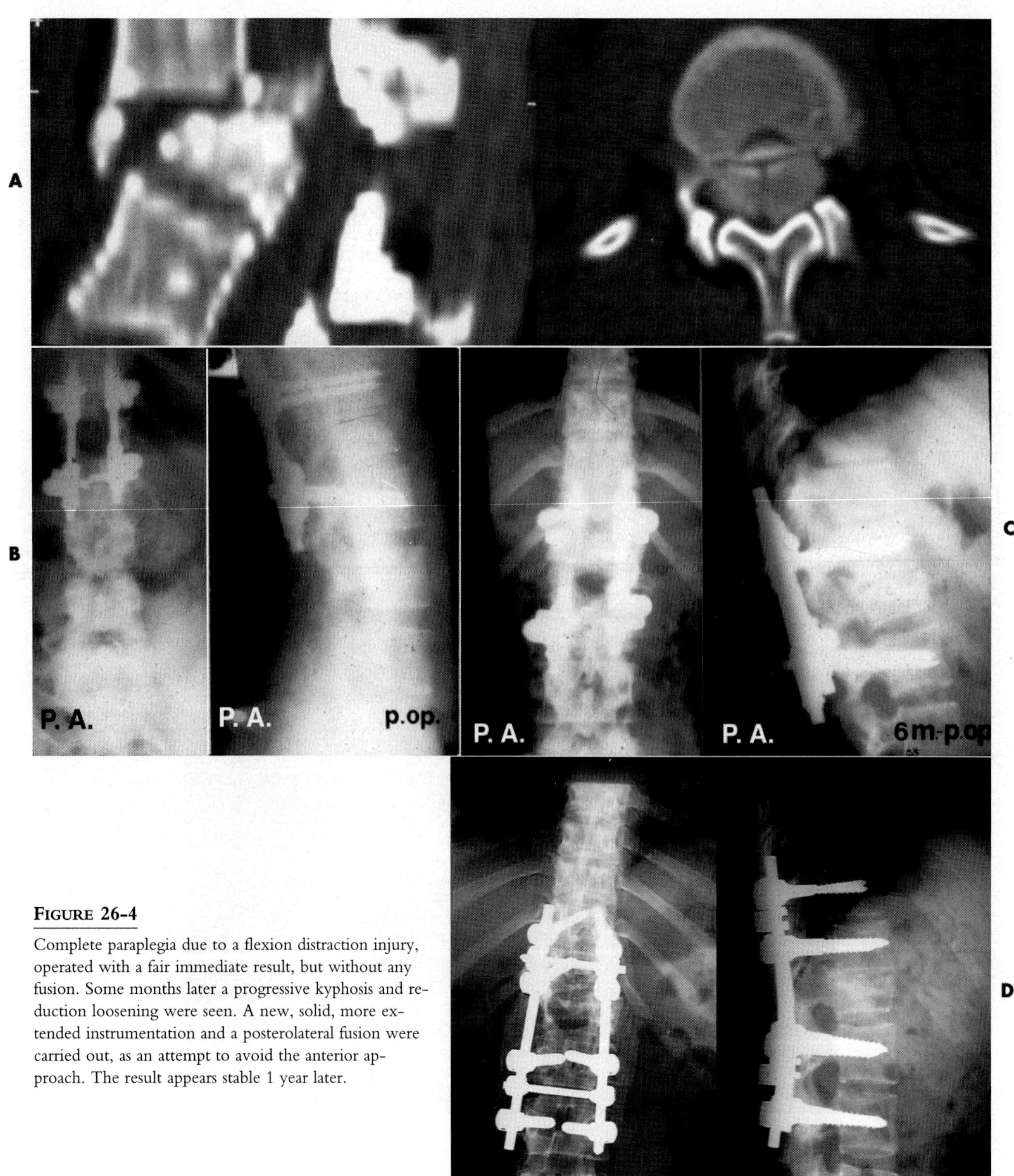


**FIGURE 26-4**

Complete paraplegia due to a flexion distraction injury, operated with a fair immediate result, but without any fusion. Some months later a progressive kyphosis and reduction loosening were seen. A new, solid, more extended instrumentation and a posterolateral fusion were carried out, as an attempt to avoid the anterior approach. The result appears stable 1 year later.

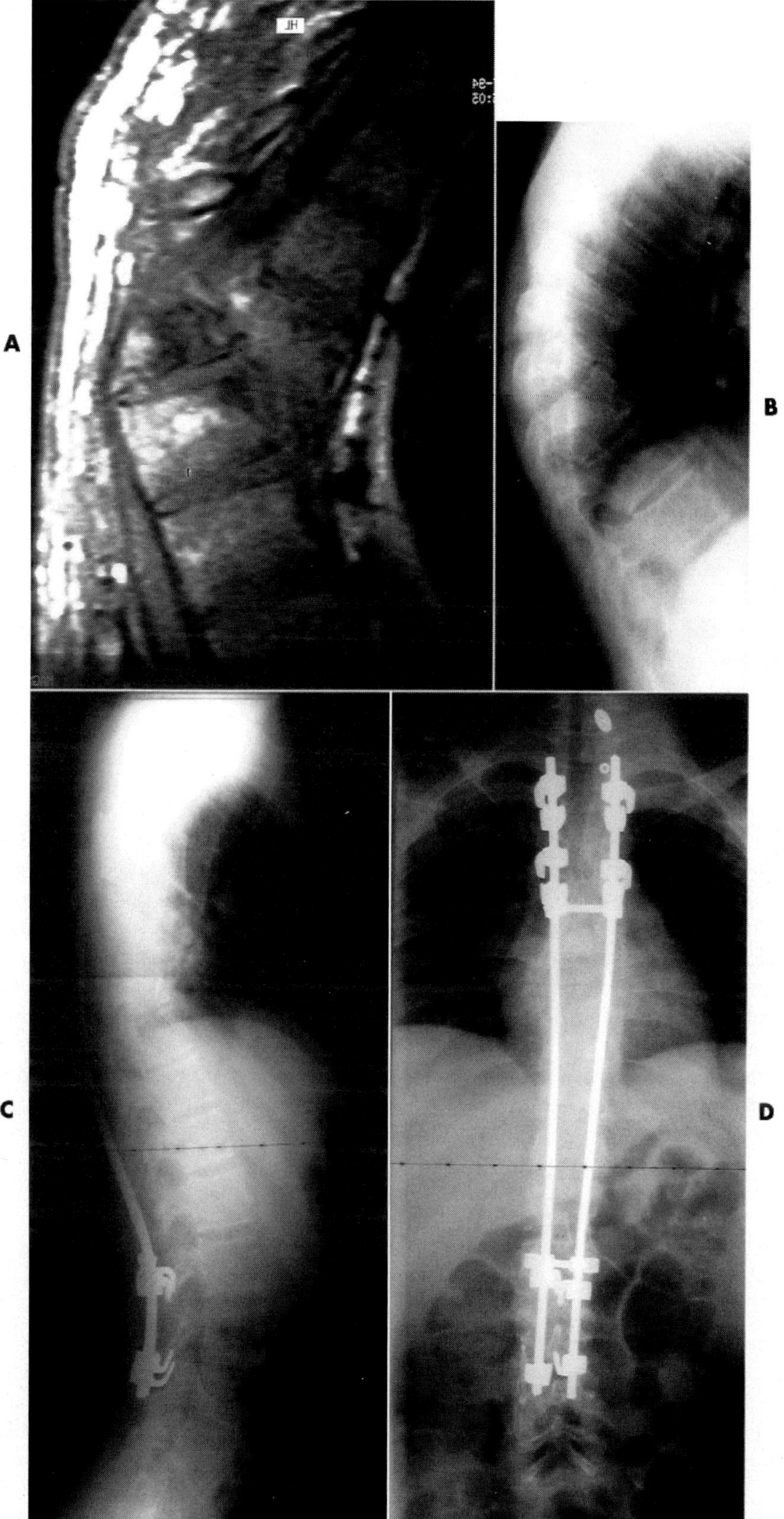

FIGURE 26-5

An 18-year-old man, with complete paraplegia due to thoracic fracture/dislocation and a postsurgical instability due to postoperative infection and hardware removal. A posterior approach, a vertebrectomy and a posterior interbody strut graft with a long instrumentation, were performed with stable results.

ity. This occurs when anterior instability is the true ideology.[2,5,6] Therefore it is important to recognize chronic anterior instabilities that are due to a pseudarthrosis of a somatic fracture. Because these surgical patients were approached posteriorly and treated by a posterior arthrodesis, guarantee against anterior collapse is not possible. It is impossible to predict an anterior somatic pseudarthrosis and its resulting chronic instability. This is why I recommend universal posterolateral fusions on all patients who receive posterior surgery for thoracolumbar injuries. Clinically, instability may not present for 3 to 4 months after the initial procedure. At that time, the presence of pain and the evidence of a loosened reduction may reveal the instability and the need for an anterior strut graft (Fig. 26-3).

## THE ABSENCE OF FUSION

Underestimation of fusion is an increasing problem, frequently occurring when the physician uses hardware as the ultimate and only stabilizer of the spine, without adding bone graft.

## TREATMENT

The main goal when treating thoracolumbar injuries is to restore the stability by using instrumentation thereby buying enough time to guarantee a solid biologic fusion. If fusion does not occur, revision surgery must be performed. Clinically, the patient will complain of pain without any radiographic sign of anterior collapse. Kyphosis frequently occurs several months after the original surgery. If at that time there is clear evidence of complete absence of posterolateral fusion, a revision posterior surgical procedure must be performed with a posterolateral fusion (Fig. 26-4). This revision must be done using a new construct. I believe that replacement of the old hardware with new instrumentation is required to get the best possible successful arthrodesis. Old instrumentation is not acceptable even when good stability was previously obtained, because micromotion secondary to the absence of posterolateral fusion is the cause of the patient's complaint of pain.

The use of an anterior approach in the treatment of thoracolumbar injuries is controversial. When deciding if an anterior approach should be performed, the amount of and type of neurologic injury deficit must be considered.[3] In a patient with complete paraplegia, I perform a posterior interbody fusion by means of a posterolateral approach (Fig. 26-5). This option avoids a thoracotomy and its related morbidity. This is especially important in paraplegic patients because they lack ideal ventilation capabilities. Technically, this procedure allows easy access to the vertebral bodies without having to manipulate the spinal canal. This approach also allows relative ease when placing the interbody strut graft. With partial paraplegic or neurologically intact patients, the anterior approach by thoracotomy or thoracoscopy may be considered. Although technically demanding, thoracoscopic procedures seem promising.

In conclusion, there are two goals when treating the thoracolumbar-injured patient. The first is initial stabilization of the spine followed by biologic fusion. If biologic fusion does not occur, revision surgery must be performed. Today there are many approaches including posterior, posterolateral, anterior, and thoracoscopic. With the understanding of thoracolumbar injuries, new stabilization techniques, and an increasing evolution of possibilities it is important that a skilled spine surgeon perform these surgeries in order to preserve as much neurologic function as possible.

## REFERENCES


1. Bolesta MJ, Bohlman HH: *Late sequelae of thoracolumbar fractures and fracture-dislocations.* In Frymoyer JW, editor: *Surgical treatment in the adult spine: principles and practice,* New York, 1991, Raven Press, p 1331.
2. Bradford DS, Ganjavian S, Antonious D, Winter RB, Lonstein JE, Moe JH: Anterior strut grafting for the treatment of kyphosis. Review of experience with forty-eight patients, *J Bone Joint Surg* 64A:680, 1982.
3. Fabris D: Post-traumatic post-surgical instabilities; principles of instrumentation and fusion. Cons. Conf. Revision Surgery, Cortina, January 1998.
4. Kostuik JP: *Adult kyphosis.* In Frymoyer JW, editor: *The adult spine: principles and practice,* New York 1991, Raven Press, p 1369.
5. Kostuik JP, Maurais GR, Richardson WJ, Okajima Y: Combined single stage anterior and posterior osteotomy for correction of iatrogenic lumbar kyphosis, *Spine* 13: 257, 1988.
6. Roberston JR, Whitesides TE Jr: Surgical reconstruction of late post-traumatic thoracolumbar kyphosis, *Spine* 10:307, 1985.

# 27

# REVISION OF DISK SURGERY

Dieter Grob, Dr. med., M.D., P.D.



Since Mixter and Barr[23] published their paper in 1934 the herniated disk is a well-defined clinical entity. The surgical procedure with removal of the compressive disk is generally the common accepted surgical approach in acute and painful cases with progressive neurologic deficit resistant to conservative management. Controversies remain about the indication in chronic disk disease. Similar long-term results after adequate conservative treatment and nucleotomy are reported in the literature.[25] However, intractable pain and persistent motor deficit that corresponds to radiological findings remain as guidelines for the surgical approach to the problem.

Despite the well-defined pathoanatomy, there is a considerable failure rate of 10% to 60% after disk surgery found in the literature, varying according to the evaluation criteria used.[7,20] Several reasons for disappointing results may be listed. Failure to achieve pain relief after disk surgery may be due to the wrong diagnosis or to technical insufficiency during surgery. Some of the postoperative pain syndromes may also be due to recurrence of the disk herniation or to a new pathology such as segmental instability. The psychosociologic aspects must also be taken into account when dealing with failure after disk surgery.[19]

The following presentation analyzes various causes for revision of disk surgery. According to the postoperative course and the onset of pain, different categories of reasons for failures after disk surgery may be established. Diagnostic problems and therapeutical modalities are addressed.

## CAUSES FOR FAILURES AFTER DISK SURGERY

### POSTOPERATIVE PERSISTING SYMPTOMS

***Missed Disk Fragments.*** Postoperative persistence of preoperative symptoms may be due to failure of localization or identification of the pain-provoking pathology. Multiple fragmented disk herniations can be dislocated and dispersed to the next segment. Overlooked fragments or only partial removal leads to partial pain relief, making revision necessary. Displaced disk fragments beneath nerve root, dura, or the posterior longitudinal ligament need to be carefully excluded by meticulous palpation of the spinal canal. Intraforaminal or lateral disk herniations may cause persisting root irritation if not properly removed. From a diagnostic view, it has to be taken into account that lateral disk herniations may provoke pain and symptoms of the root from the level above, indicating clinically the adjacent level for surgical exploration. In cases of prior spine surgery, epidural scar formations and adhesions may create adverse situations in which the exploration for disk protrusion or herniation may be difficult. The relevant disk fragment may be missed.

Exact preoperative imaging of the pathology and its localization in the spinal canal is mandatory to avoid such failures. Computed tomography (CT) and/or magnetic resonance imaging (MRI) reveal unusual fragmented disks and allow precise surgery. The use of gadolinium helps to differentiate between scar formation and disk material.

***Incorrect Diagnosis.*** The clinical entity of nerve root irritation may be due to other reasons than simple disk pathology. Up to 76% of abnormal disk changes on MRI are not associated with clinical symptoms.[3,4] Therefore, the presence of a degenerated disk does not necessarily implicate it as the source of pain. Narrowing of the lateral spinal canal with encroachment of the nerve root may be primarily due to degenerative facet hypertrophy. The incidentally found concomitant disk bulging is insignificant in provocation of radicular symptoms. If only the disk is removed, radicular symptoms are likely to persist after surgery.

Tumors or infection instead of disk protrusion may be responsible for the radicular pain. Systemic or metabolic diseases may mimic radicular symptoms and lead erroneously to the diagnosis of disk pathology. Affection of the hip or knee or peripheral nerve injuries can be responsible for similar symptoms.

Meticulous diagnostic evaluation with clinical investigation, neurological and neurophysiological examination, and the requirement of correct correlation to the imaging diagnostic tools minimize the failure rate.

***Incorrect Vertebral Level.*** At first glance, various reasons for this unlikely mistake may be listed. The similarity of the different segments by posterior surgical approach may favor a erroneous selection of the level. Prevention can be achieved by using fluoroscopy before or during surgery to identify the correct level. However, an obliquely orientated C-arm may create confusion about the appropriate level. Loosening or incorrect fixation of the metallic marker during the radiologic examination may mislead the surgeon. The incidence of surgery on the wrong level at our institution is about 0.3%.

Surgery of the wrong level can be minimized with a thorough knowledge of the anatomy of the lumbar spine. The lumbosacral level and the adjacent L4-L5 level can easily be identified by the intraoperative palpation of the sacrum. The twelfth rib and the different contours of the facet joints of the thoracolumbar level (T12-L1) allow intraoperative orientation; however, anatomical variations include misjudgment. Therefore, surgery of T12 to L3 requires intraoperative or preoperative radiographic control. Preoperative radiographically controlled injection of methylene blue may be of further help. Finally, if the pathology in the spinal canal is not found or differs considerably from what was to be expected, a wrong level should always be suspected and excluded by radiographic reconfirmation.

## RECURRENCE OF SYMPTOMS

***Recurrent Disk Herniation.*** In this group of patients, only those should be included that experienced successful disk surgery with relief of their initial radicular pain for a certain amount of time. They have to be separated from the patients with successful nucleotomy and subsequent lateral stenosis due to narrowing of the foramen as a consequence of postoperative disk narrowing.

The incidence of recurrent disk herniation has been reported to be approximately 3%.[11] The most common site of recurrent disk herniation is at the same level on the same side (60% to 80%), followed by the contralateral side (10% to 20%). Recurrent herniated nucleus pulposus at a different level is uncommon (5%).[22]

True recurrent disk fragment in the spinal canal may be the source of pain within 3 to 6 months after the primary intervention. The diagnosis is made by gadolinium-enhanced MRI, which allows separation of recurrent disk material from intraspinal scar formation.[14] To prevent recurrent herniation of nucleus pulposus, Ahlgren[2] recommends a simple slit incision of the anulus fibrosus entering the disk space during diskectomy. A small incision leads to a shorter healing phase and a more stable scar situation than a full window excision of the anulus.

***Lateral Stenosis.*** Disk narrowing creates retrolisthesis due to the oblique orientation of the facets. The downward gliding of the inferior articular process of the superior vertebra produces facet protrusion into the foramen with decreased available space for the nerve root in the foramen. As nucleotomy is likely to produce subsequent disk narrowing, secondary lateral stenosis may be responsible for recurrence of symptoms after months or years.

***Segmental Instability and Facet Degeneration.*** Mixter and Barr[23] in their original paper emphasized the fact that, as a consequence of removing disk material, segmental instability may result. Despite the ill-defined term of segmental instability, it might be assumed that removal of disk material alters the segmental motion pattern. As a consequence, accelerated degeneration of the facets is observed. Formation of degenerative space-occupying alterations, such as facet cysts or osteophytes, might create radicular symptoms similar to the preoperative situation.

***Nonsurgical Factors.*** Psychological factors, nonorganic symptoms, sociodemographic factors, and depression may be negative predictors for lumbar disk surgery.[19] These nonsurgical factors may lead to disappointing results and cause both persisting or recurrent pain after nucleotomy. Neurophysiological diagnostic means such as somatosensory and motor evoked potentials may help to identify nonorganic paralysis in these cases.[16] Obviously in these patients reoperation should not be considered.

### New Symptomatology

***Instability.*** A torn disk represents a disturbance of the normal motion pattern of a functional spinal unit. Additional surgical removal of the disk, laminas, and facets may lead to instability of the operated segment.[23] The typical clinical history reveals excellent relief of radicular symptoms but gradually increasing low back pain originating from the operated segment after weeks or several months.

***Infection.*** Wound infection after diskectomy or decompressive procedures may be favored by the hypovascularization of large subcutaneous fat tissue. Swelling, pain, or wound dehiscence are the clinical symptoms. Laboratory data may show infectious parameters, confirming the diagnosis. Subfascial wound infections with low activity in the lumbar spine are sometimes difficult to detect clinically. Discitis or spondylodiscitis after disk surgery may be caused by direct intraoperative or hematogenous contamination. The symptomatology differs considerably from the preoperative pain. Intense low back pain independent of physical activity and often persisting at night appears typically after a pain-free postoperative interval.

Consequent prophylactic antibiotics minimizes the risk of postoperative infections.[9] Diagnostic procedure should include needle aspiration of infected tissue. This invasive procedure allows adequate antibiotic treatment by identification of the types of bacteria and their resistance to antibiotic treatment.

***Arachnoiditis.*** The role of arachnoiditis is unclear, but it is said that it may produce symptoms after disk surgery by adhesions around the cauda equina or nerve roots. Steroids and conservative management are indicated rather than surgical exploration.

***Epidural Scar Formation.*** As a natural consequence of intraspinal surgery, scar formation is observed. It is unclear why only a few patients get symptomatic. Any possible cause for the presented clinical symptoms other than scar formation has to be excluded. The value of revision surgery other than fusion is questionable in these cases.[10]

***Epidural Hematoma.*** Increasing pain in the first 24 to 48 hours postoperatively with rapidly progressive neurological deficit suggests the formation of a compressive epidural hematoma. Continuous hemorrhage after wound closure may build up pressure in the subfascial compartment, which leads to neurological damage. Hemorrhage of the epidural veins may also escape to the adjacent, not decompressed segment. Increasing pressure is created by a valvelike mechanism by the dura and the lamina. Immediate wound revision and evacuation may prevent further neurological damage.

The prevention of epidural hematoma includes a preoperative evaluation of the patient's coagulability. All medication creating hypocoagulability should be stopped one week prior to surgery. During surgery, meticulous coagulation of the paraspinal muscles should be performed. Bleeding epidural veins should be compressed and packed with hemostatic tissue (fibrin) rather than coagulated in order to avoid circulatory disturbances of the nerve roots.[6]

***Pseudomeningocele.*** Dural tear during surgical decompression with leakage of cerebrospinal fluid may create postoperative spinal headache and local swelling. Persistent leakage may lead to the formation of a pseudomeningocele. There is increased risk of infection of the epidural space if the skin is perforated. The incidence of clinically relevant pseudomeningocele formation after disk surgery has to be reported up to 2%.[13] Symptomatic pseudomeningocele require surgical revision and closure of the dural defect (Fig. 27-1).

## DIAGNOSTIC PROBLEMS

Difficulties are frequently encountered when identifying the painful segment in unoperated lumbar spines. The situation gets worse if the symptomatology is compounded by previous surgery. Any of the factors mentioned earlier in this chapter may create nonspecific low back pain with or without radicular symptoms. Overlying disappointment by treatment failure or recurrent symptoms may further complicate the situation. Therefore, indication for additional surgery is difficult to establish and requires meticulous investigation of the situation.

*Imaging:* Disk space narrowing, retrolisthesis, or abnormal motion are visible on conventional or functional radiographs. Partial or complete facetectomies can be detected in oblique views. Soft tissue changes in the spinal canal are an indication for MRI investigation, whereas bony abnormalities are seen on CT scans. Enhancement with gadolinium allows differentiation between disk material and scar formation.

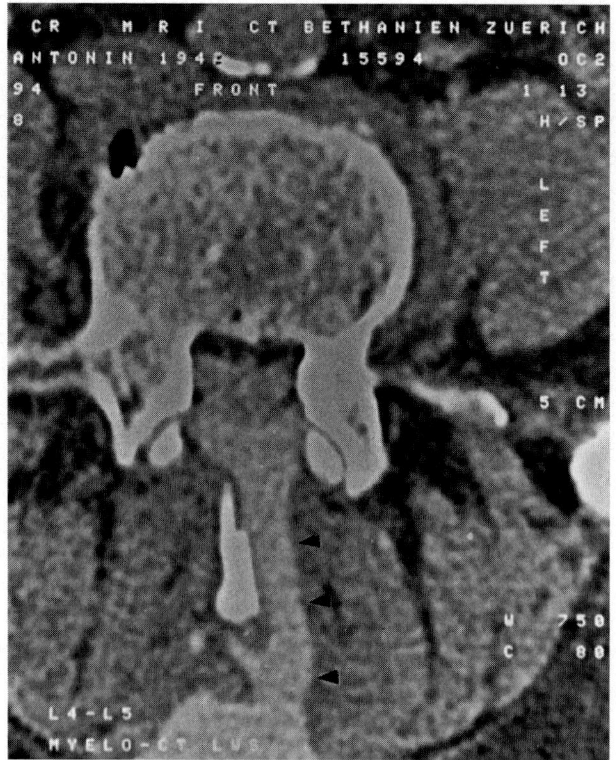


**FIGURE 27-1**

Patient after decompression and nucleotomy. Postoperative painless swelling in the lumbosacral area in the midline. The CT scan reveals a dural leak with liquid connection to the subfascial layer; pseudomeningocele.

*Epidural injections* may be advocated for diagnostic procedures in primary surgery[5] but are of limited value in reinterventions. The distribution of the epidurally injected corticosteroid is limited by epidural scar formation and the interpretation of the result is unreliable.

*Nerve root blocking* (Fig. 27-2) with injection of the sleeve of the spinal nerve extraforaminally is a specific diagnostic tool and may be used to identify the painful level with suspected root irritations.

*Diskography:* Injection of the disk may produce memory pain and indicate the source of pain.

*Temporary external fixation:* This invasive diagnostic procedure has to be carefully indicated in a well-selected patient population. However, it represents the only means to simulate lumbar fusion and therefore predict the result of a permanent spondylodesis.[17]

Schanz screws are inserted percutaneously under fluoroscopy. Alternating external fixation and release allow evaluation of the corresponding changes of pain by a visual analogue pain scale. If there is reproducible pain relief during fixation, the instrumented segment is likely to be the source of pain and accessible to permanent fusion (Fig. 27-3).

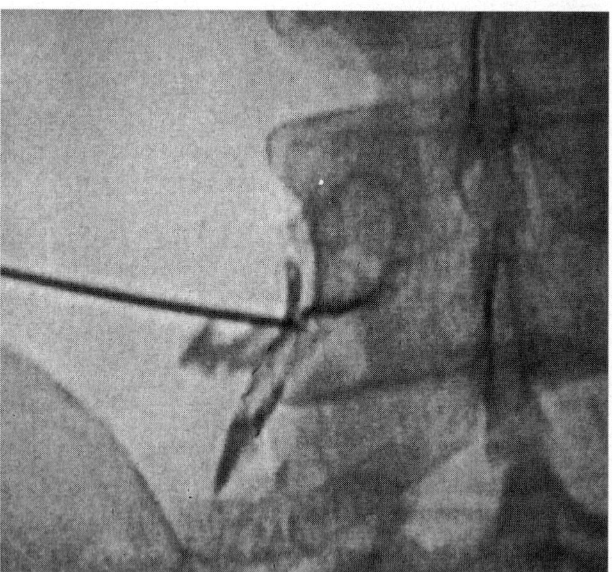

**FIGURE 27-2**

Diagnostic nerve root block by paravertebral injection of the perineural sleeve. This diagnostic procedure allows conclusions about the involved nerve root to be drawn.

## THERAPY

### CONSERVATIVE TREATMENT

The value of conservative treatment in failed disk surgery is limited because of the altered anatomy after surgery. However, epidural scar formation and arachnoiditis represent indications for conservative management with administration of steroids.

Incapacity of identifying the painful level may necessitate conservative treatment modalities. Apart from physical exercises, analgetic treatment with epidural injections or nerve root blocks may be considered.

### SURGICAL TECHNIQUES

The goal of revision surgery is pain relief and restoration of function; it does not, therefore, differ from those of primary surgery. However, due to scar formation, epidural adhesions and altered anatomy reinterventions do not have the same prognosis as primary interventions. These difficulties require special attention and vast experience of the surgeon.

### PATIENT INFORMATION

The patient undergoing revision surgery requires a different approach than a patient facing primary intervention. Disappointment, persistence or recurrence of pain and negative socioeconomic situation after the first intervention make the patient more suspicious

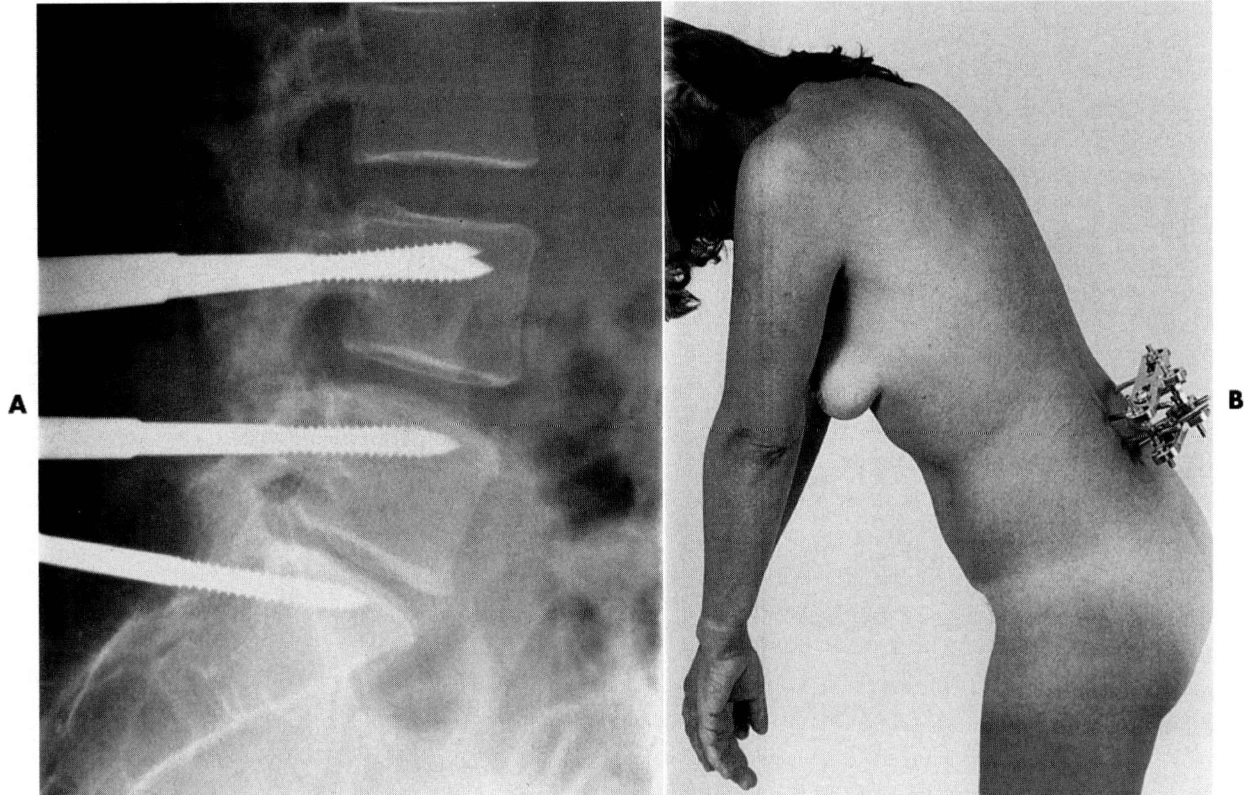


FIGURE 27-3

**A,** Diagnostic external fixator. **B,** The suspected painful segments are instrumented with percutaneously inserted transpedicular Schanz screws. External alternative fixation of each segment and subsequent corresponding pain relief allow identification of the pain source and prognosis of a possible permanent fusion in the future.

and nervous than a patient entering the hospital for primary surgery. This patient deserves careful information about the revision and its associated risks and benefits. Complications such as nerve injury, dural tear, infection, and others need to be discussed. The patient has to be informed that unforeseen procedures such as additional fusion might be necessary.

## DECOMPRESSION

The site of compression has to be identified by clinical symptoms and correlated to preoperative imaging. This determines the choice of surgical approach, which in the case of postlaminectomy syndromes will be mostly posterior.

Extensive scar tissue in the erector spinae might be encountered. Simple subperiosteal dissection and orientation are impossible and may require extension of the skin incision until untouched tissue is seen. From the normal anatomy adjacent to the previously explored area careful dissection may proceed, the bony structures serving as secure landmarks. Radiographs and CT scans have to be studied in order to anticipate defects such as missing spinous processes, facets, or laminas. The scar tissue is removed from solid bone to obtain orientation if solid adhesions to the dura are encountered. The scar tissue might be left in place in order to avoid dural tears.

The extent of epidural scar formation has to be assessed. In order to avoid dural tears, it is recommended to begin dissection and visualization of the dura in a previously untouched area. With an osteotome a small part of the lamina adjacent to the compressive agent may be removed until the dura is visible. From there, the appropriate tissue layer may be identified and the dissection proceeded to the obstruction. In this situation, the use of a microscope is helpful to distinguish dural and scar tissue. Only after complete adhesiolysis, decompression with removal of the compressive agent should be undertaken. Special attention is required by retracting the dura or nerve roots with nerve hooks. Remaining adhesions may create unexpected lever arms and increase pressure and/or tension on the retracted nerve (Figs. 27-4 through 27-7).

With such mobilized nerve root and dura, decompression with widening of the lateral aspects of the spinal canal and foraminotomy may be performed. Resection of the medial aspect of the facet removes

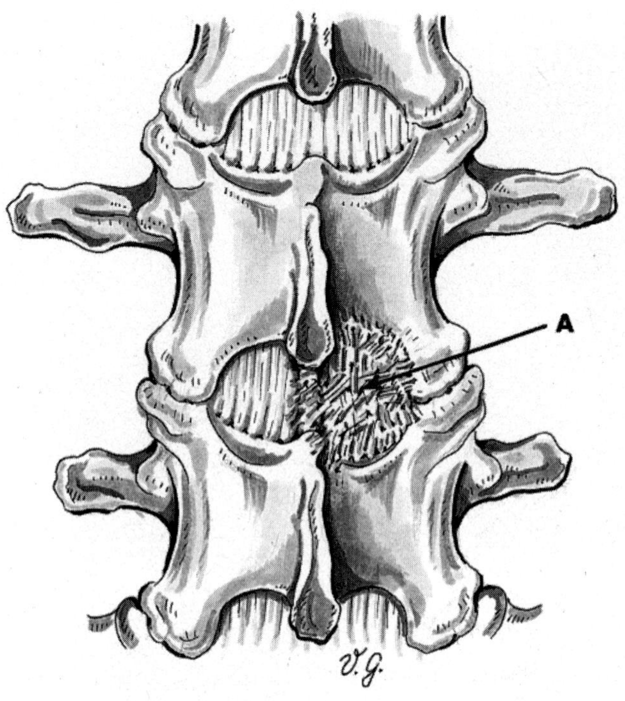


**FIGURE 27-4**

After visualization of the posterior aspects of the spinous process, lamina, and facet joints, the scar tissue overlying the interlaminar space (*A*) and the bony edges of the remaining caudal and cranial lamina are identified. Drawing by Vladomir Golyakhovsky, M.D., Ph.D., New York.

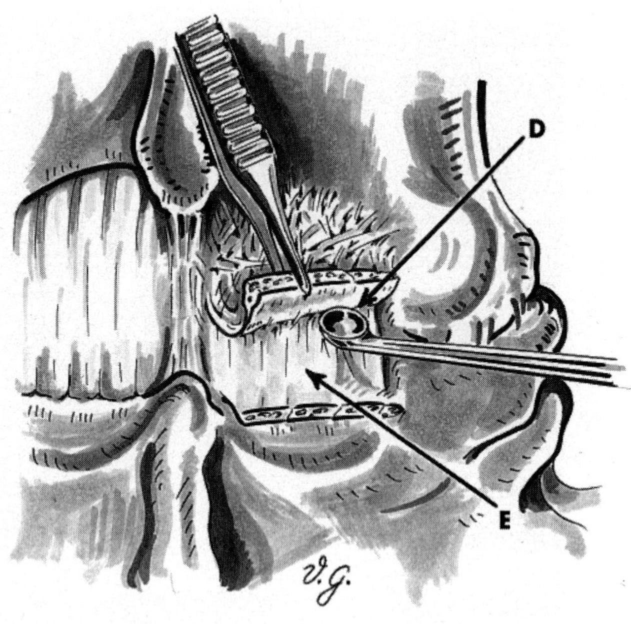


**FIGURE 27-6**

The bone and scar are gently pulled cranially, using gentle dissection with a curette (*D*) to separate the scar from the dura (*E*). Removal of the scar tissue is performed to allow orientation and safe access to the space-occupying lesion. Drawing by Vladomir Golyakhovsky, M.D., Ph.D., New York.

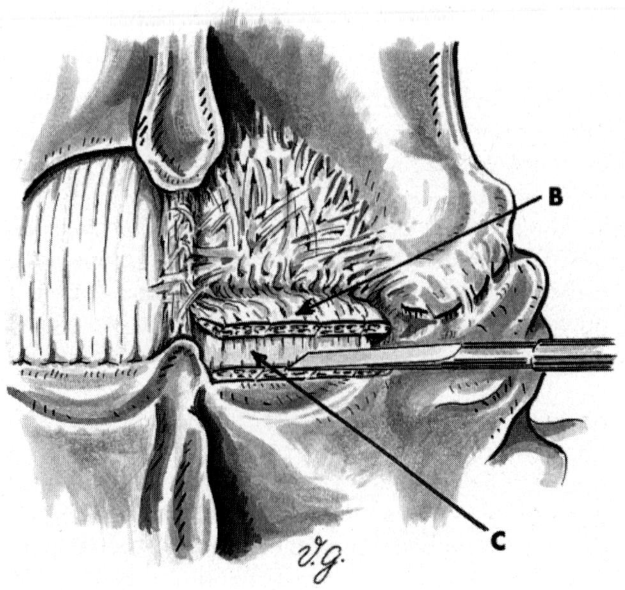


**FIGURE 27-5**

To reach the untouched dura without scar adherence, a rim of the lamina is osteotomized (*B*). A small piece of bone, adherent to the scar tissue (*C*) is elevated and allowed to enter the spinal canal safely. Drawing by Vladomir Golyakhovsky, M.D., Ph.D., New York.

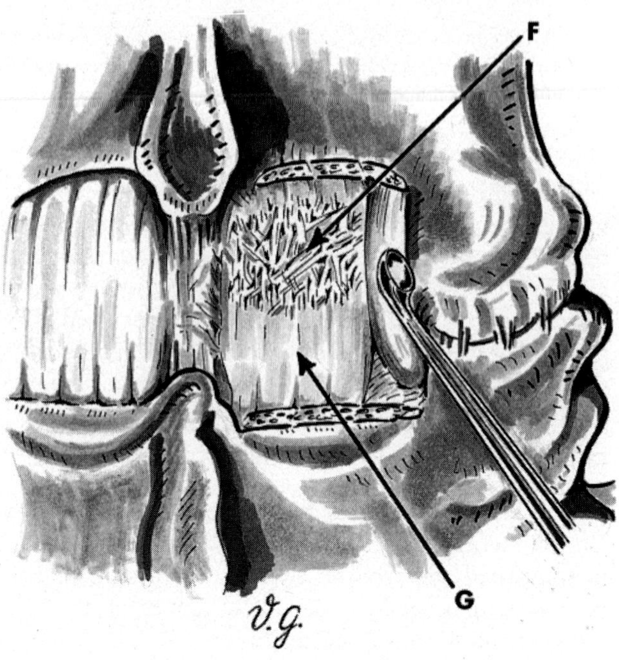


**FIGURE 27-7**

Scar tissue (*F*), which could not be separated from the dural sac (*G*) is left untouched. Access to the disk and anterior part of the spinal canal can be achieved by careful dissection with a curette, which allows for the mobilization of the dura and nerve root. Drawing by Vladomir Golyakhovsky, M.D., Ph.D., New York.

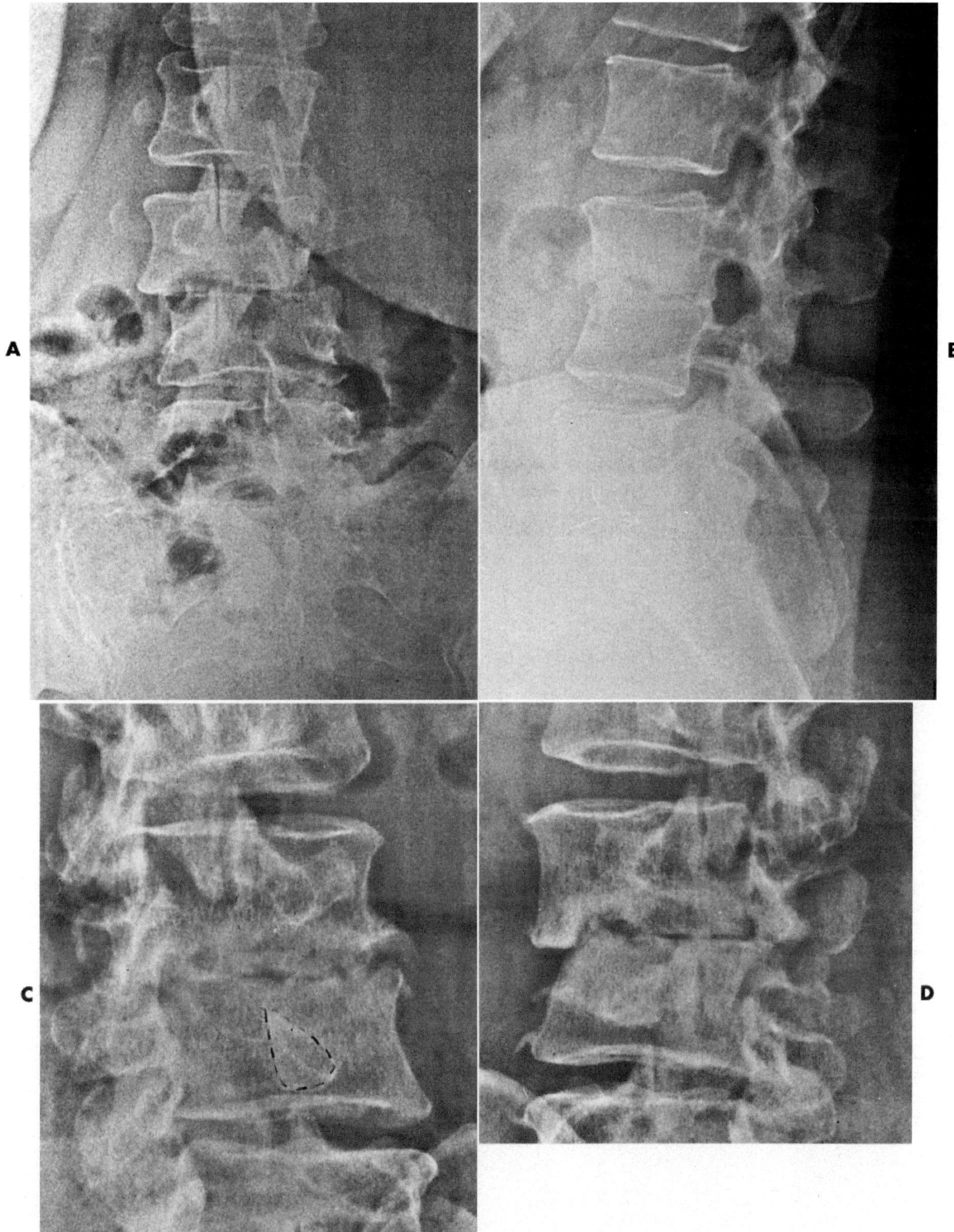


FIGURE 27-8

Lumbar spine after nucleotomy with facetectomy L3/4. The AP and lateral views **(A, B)** show a rotary displacement between L3 and L4 and a kyphotic deformity due to disk resorption. The oblique views **(C, D)** demonstrate the missing partner of the upper articular process of L4 (*dotted line, left*).

pressure of the lateral dura and uncovers the exiting nerve root. The pedicle and its medial face indicate the maximum width of the spinal canal obtainable without aggressive procedures and severe destabilization. Lateral bone resection of the caudal lamina allows decompression of the nerve root and the ganglion. Difficulties may be encountered in reaching recurrent disk herniations by adherent nerve roots to the posterior longitudinal ligament. Careful mobilization should be attempted and both lateral and medial approaches to the nerve root should be considered to remove the disk fragment.

If a dural tear is realized during surgery, immediate closure should be attempted (see Fig. 27-1). A watertight running suture represents the classic procedure. However, this may be time-consuming or technically

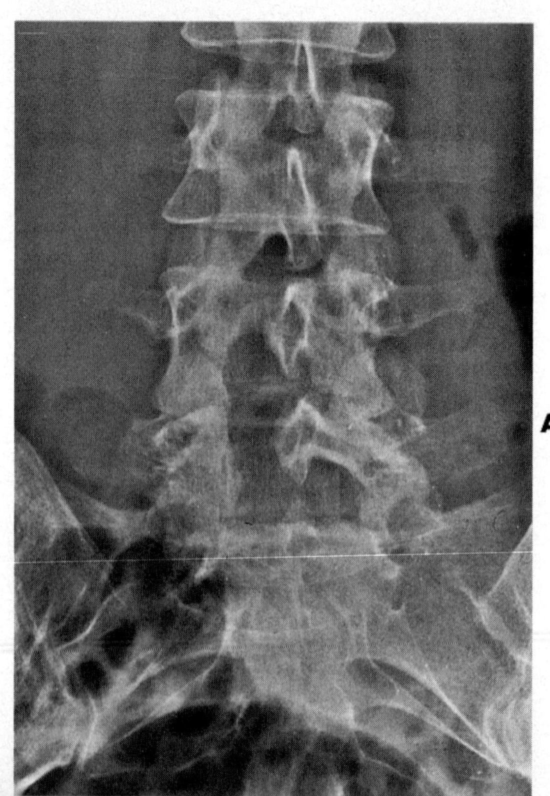

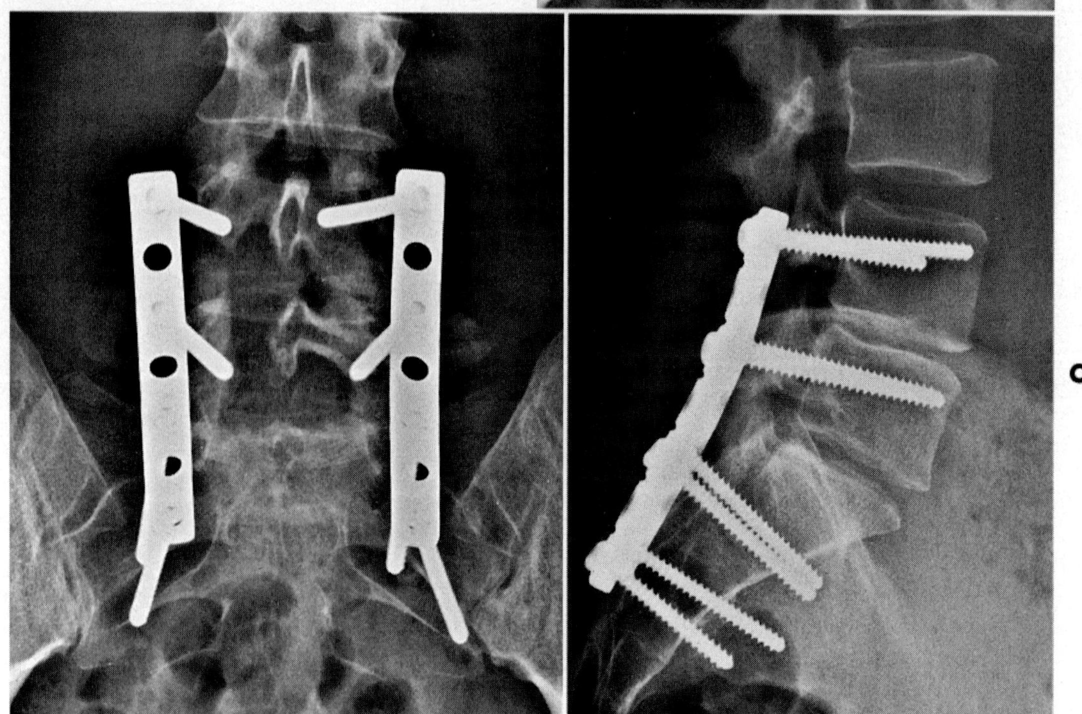

**FIGURE 27-9**

**A, B,** Patient after nucleotomy and extensive bone resection. After initial pain relief, sudden local back pain was felt. Conservative physiotherapy and analgesics were administered. Radiological investigation because of persisting pain revealed a fracture of the weakened right interarticular portion of L4. **C,** Same patient after posterior transpedicular fusion. Immediate pain relief after fusion.

difficult in limited and stability preserving surgical exposures of the dura with intact lamina. Fat pads fixed with fibrin glue may be considered to close the leak in these situations (see Fig. 27-1). In extensive dural tears it is recommended that the bone be removed in order to obtain adequate exposure to perform the suturing. Additional stabilization has to be considered if removal of more than 50% of the facet had to be performed.[1]

### Stabilization

There is no general consensus about fusion at the time of primary nucleotomy. Although Vaughan[24] reports significantly better long-term results after nucleotomy and fusion than after fusion alone, simultaneous fusion has not become generally accepted. There is no consensus about fusion in revision procedures either. The proponents for fusion argue that scar formation and segmental motion may contribute to irritation of the nerve roots and cause pain. After extensive decompression with bone removal, the segmental motion pattern is disturbed (Fig. 27-8) and instability may be prevented by simultaneous immobilization and fusion. Anterior, posterior, or combined approaches are described. From posterior, the transpedicular internal fixations provide reliable stability and fusion rates of 75% to 95% (Fig. 27-9). However, there is a considerable complication rate by misplaced screws.[8,12] In revision cases with extensive scar formation, the intraoperative orientation to recognize the landmark for correct screw placement requires special surgical skill. The translaminar facet screws represent a safe and technically easy method for segmental stabilization.[15,21] Intact anterior column and preserved lamina and facets, however, are requirements for this procedure. Recently, anterior techniques have become more popular by introduction of new implants such as cages and cylinders. The anterior approach is indicated if pain generation is motion-induced and no posterior decompression is required. Multiple posterior procedures increase scar formation and diminish the prognosis of solid fusion by hypovascularization of the surrounding tissue. In this situation an anterior procedure reduces the risk of pseudarthrosis. Circumferential anterior/posterior fusion procedures are rarely indicated but might be considered as a solution in severely affected segmental instability after extensive posterior bone resection.

Discitis or spondylodiscitis should be approached by direct puncture of the focus. Posterior soft tissue infection may be treated by conservative means and administration of antibiotics. However, aggressive treatment with debridement and wound excision usually shortens the time needed for consolidation considerably. An anterior approach is indicated if the spondylodiscitis is associated with loss of stability or in the presence of an abscess, which may be diagnosed by MRI. Evacuation and reconstruction and fusion with autologous bone graft are recommended. In severe cases, anterior debridement and temporary posterior transpedicular external fixation as a first intervention and secondary reconstruction and fusion anteriorly lead to satisfactory results.[18]

## REFERENCES


1. Abumi K, Panjabi M, Kramer K: Biomechanical evaluation of lumbar spinal stability after graded facetectomies, *Spine* 15:1142-1147, 1990.
2. Ahlgren BD, Vasavada A, Brower RS, Lydon BS, Herkowitz HN, Panjabi MM: Anular incision technique on the strength and multidirectional flexibility of the healing intervertebral disc, *Spine* 19:948-954, 1994.
3. Boden S, McCowin P, Davis DO, Dina TS, Mark AS, Wiesel S: Abnormal magnetic resonance scans of the cervical spine in asymptomatic subjects, *J Bone Joint Surg* 72A:1178-1183, 1990.
4. Boos N, Rieder R, Schade V, Spratt K, Semmer N, Aebi M: The diagnostic accuracy of magnetic resonance imaging, work perception and psychological factors identifying symptomatic disc herniations, *Spine* 20:2613-2625, 1995.
5. Bowman SJ, Wedderburn L, Whaley A, Grahame R, Newman S: Outcome assessment after epidural corticosteroid injection for low back pain and sciatica, *Spine* 18:79-83, 1993.
6. Crock H: *A short practice of spinal surgery*. Wien, New York, 1993, Springer Verlag.
7. Deyo RA, Cherkin DC, Loeser JD, Bigos SJ, Ciol MA: Mortality in association with operations on the lumbar spine, *J Bone Joint Surg* 74A:536-544, 1992.
8. Esses S, Botsford D, Kostuik J: The role of external spinal skeletal fixation in the assessment of low-back disorders, *Spine* 14:594-601, 1989.
9. Fraser RD, Vernon Roberts B, Osti OL: *Iatrogenic discitis*. In Wiesel S, Weinstein JN, Herkowitz H, Dvorak J, Bell G, editors: *The lumbar spine,* Philadelphia, 1996, WB Saunders, pp 899-916.
10. Fritsch EW, Heisel J, Rupp S: The failed back surgery syndrome. Reasons intraoperative findings and long term results: a report of 182 operative treatments, *Spine* 21:626-633. 1996.

11. Garfin SR, Glover M, Ooth RE: A review of the Pennsylvania Hospital Experience, *J Spinal Disord* 1:116-133, 1988.
12. Gertzbein S, Robbins S: Accuracy of pedicle screw placement in vivo, *Spine* 15:4-11, 1990.
13. Hadani FG, Knoler N, Tadmor R: Entrappment lumbar nerve root in pseudomeningocele after laminectomy: Report of three cases, *Neurosurgery* 19:405-407, 1986.
14. Hueftle MG et al: Lumbar spine: postoperative MR imaging with Gd-DTPA, *Radiology* 167:817-824, 1988.
15. Humke T, Grob D, Dvorak J, Messikommer A: Translaminar screw fixation of the lumbar and lumbosacral spine: A five year follow-up, *Spine* (In Press) 1997.
16. Janssen BA, Theiler R, Grob D, Dvorak J: The role of motor evoked potentials in psychogenic paralysis, *Spine* 5:608-611, 1995.
17. Jeanneret B, Jovanovic M, Magerl F: Percutaneous diagnostic stabilization for low back pain: correlation with results after fusion operations, *Clin Orthop* 304:130-138, 1994.
18. Jeanneret B, Magerl F: Treatment of osteomyelitis of the spine using percutaneous suction/irrigation and percutaneous spinal fixation, *Spinal Dis* 7:185-205, 1994.
19. Junge A, Dvorak J, Ahrens S: Predictors of bad and good outcomes of lumbar disc surgery, *Spine* 20:460-468, 1995.
20. Korres DS, Loupassis G, Stamos K: Results of lumbar discectomy: a study using 15 different evaluation methods, *Eur Spine J* 1:20-24, 1992.
21. Marchesi DG, Boos N, Zuber K, Aebi M: Translaminar facet joint screws to enhance segmental fusion of the lumbar spine, *Eur Spine J* 1:125-130, 1992.
22. McCulloch JA: *Principles of microsurgery for lumbar disc disease.* New York, 1989, Raven Press, pp 257-264.
23. Mixter WJ, Barr JS: Rupture of the intervertebral disc with involvement of the spinal canal, *N Engl J Med* 2A:210-215, 1934.
24. Vaughhan PA, Malcolm B, Maistrelli GL: Results of L4-L5 disc excision alone versus disc excision and fusion, *Spine* 13:690-695, 1988.
25. Weber H: The lumbar disc herniation. A controlled prospective study with ten years of observation, *Spine* 8:131-140, 1983.

# 28

# FAILED BACK SURGERY: CLINICAL RESULTS OF THE INSTRUMENTED POSTEROLATERAL FUSION

**Carlos Villanueva, M.D., Ph.D.**



The number of spinal surgeries is growing year after year in western countries due to the increasing number of surgeons and also to the global pressure of the industry and the patients; consequently, the spine units are facing an unprecedented number of patients previously operated with a poor result.[2]

Persistence of pain and disability after a well-indicated lumbar procedure has been attributed to a great number of different causes. The most common of them are segmental instability, persistence of the radicular entrapment, and postlaminectomy fibrosis. There is no scientific evidence that pure fibrosis, which is a common finding in magnetic resonance imaging (MRI) exams after every surgical procedure, can be responsible for persistent radicular pain. Cases with an unusual amount of fibrosis that retracts the dural sac and includes the nerve root suggest a possible traumatic previous surgery and consequent nerve root damage (battered root).[1]

## DIAGNOSIS

Clinical diagnosis of segmental instability is characterized by predominant back pain with eventual dynamic sciatica. These patients report inability to stand and progressive irradiated pain. Pain improves or disappears in supine position. Patients with segmental instability also report acute lumbar pain in relation to torsion or flexion-extension of the trunk. Some cases show radiological evidence of disk degeneration and, in the most severe cases, gross instability in flexion-extension and/or spondylolisthesis can be radiologically demonstrated. MRI is less specific, showing only the typical black disk.

Patients with persistent radicular compression have predominant leg pain and neurogenic claudication. Clinical examination may show positive straight leg raising test (SLR) and reflex anomaly, but this finding is very common among operated patients no matter the clinical result. MRI has little value after disk excision because of reported persistent posterior contour abnormalities of the disk causing mass effect on the thecal sac or nerve roots.[3] Tulberg et al found no consistent correlation between 1-year postoperative outcome and the MRI findings.[7] In cases with persistent radiculopathy, myelography is probably the best choice.

Classic indication for failed back surgery syndrome (FBSS) has been decompression, if needed, and posterolateral fusion. However, the clinical results of this technique, using pedicle screw instrumentation, have not been reported. The main question is whether a secondary surgery has a reasonable expectancy of improvement. Previously reported results by Spangfort[6] and Weber[9] in large series of primary disk excisions confirm that complete relief of symptoms occurs only in 60% of the total group. Revision surgery has worse expectancies. Waddell reported only a 50% rate of good results in second surgeries with 20% of the patients considering themselves in worse condition.[8]

In my practice, I perform fusion (without decompression) in those cases with predominant back pain with or without dynamic sciatica after failure of conservative treatment. In cases of predominant sciatica with consistent evidence of radicular compression, I perform decompression as wide as necessary.

## REVIEW OF CASES

My colleagues and I were able to review 118 patients who had surgery from 1986 to 1993. This number represents 77% of the total number of lumbosacral fusions in that time period. All patients were reviewed by an independent orthopedic surgeon with a minimum follow-up of 2 years after surgery. Eighty patients were primary cases and the remaining 38 were failed back surgeries. The purpose of our study was to compare the clinical outcomes of both the FBSS cases and the primary cases.

Both of the groups had similar ages (FBSS, mean age 42.5, range of 2 to 61 years old; primary cases, mean age 46.6, range of 16 to 71 years of age), jobs, marital status, and gender distribution (Fig. 28-1).

Health status was also very similar in both groups; almost the same proportion of patients in each group had systemic diseases (Fig. 28-2).

Isthmic spondylolisthesis and degenerative disk disease were the most common diagnoses among the primary group with a smaller number of degenerative spondylolisthesis and few cases of spinal stenosis. Postdiskectomy instability was, by far, the most common diagnosis among the operated group with a small number of spinal stenosis, spondylolisthesis, and pseudarthrosis of a previous fusion (Fig. 28-3).

The clinical pattern in primary group was predominant low back pain and/or dynamic sciatica in 57% of the cases; the remaining cases had predominant sciatica. In the FBSS group, 83% had predominant sciatica and 17% had predominant low back pain. Low back pain with dynamic sciatica was more frequent in the primary group because of the higher percentage of isthmic spondylolisthesis in this group (Fig. 28-4).

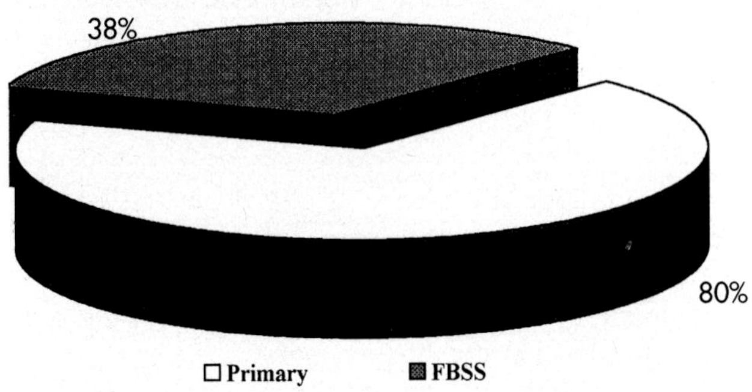


FIGURE 28-1

Clinical outcomes of both primary and FBSS cases.

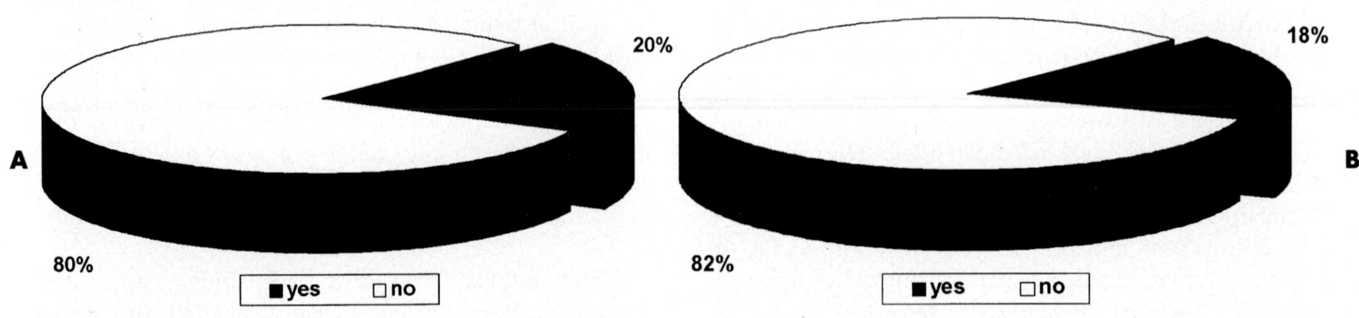


FIGURE 28-2

**A,** Primary cases: systemic diseases. **B,** FBSS: systemic diseases.

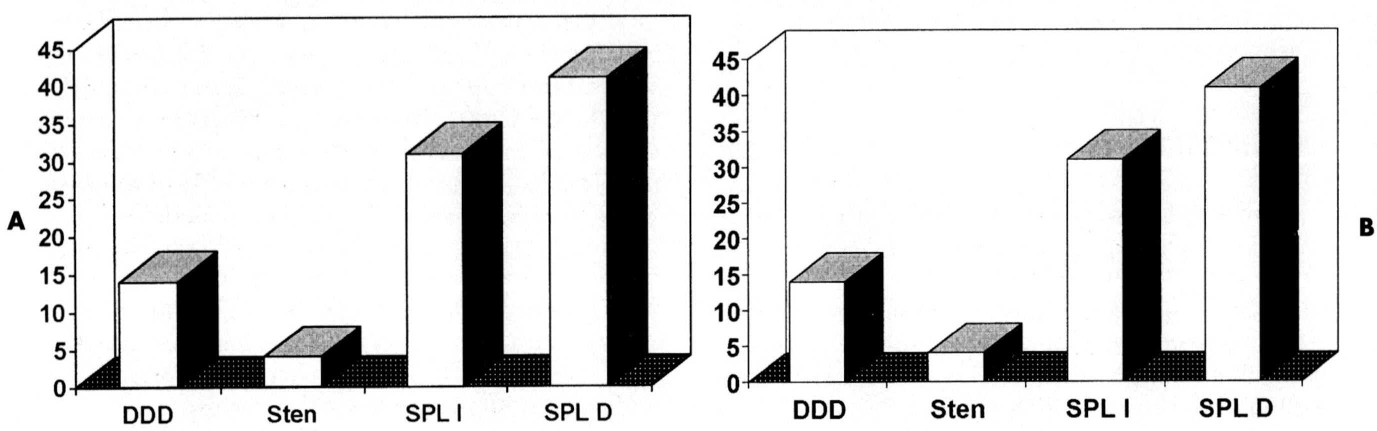


FIGURE 28-3

**A, B,** Primary cases: diagnosis.

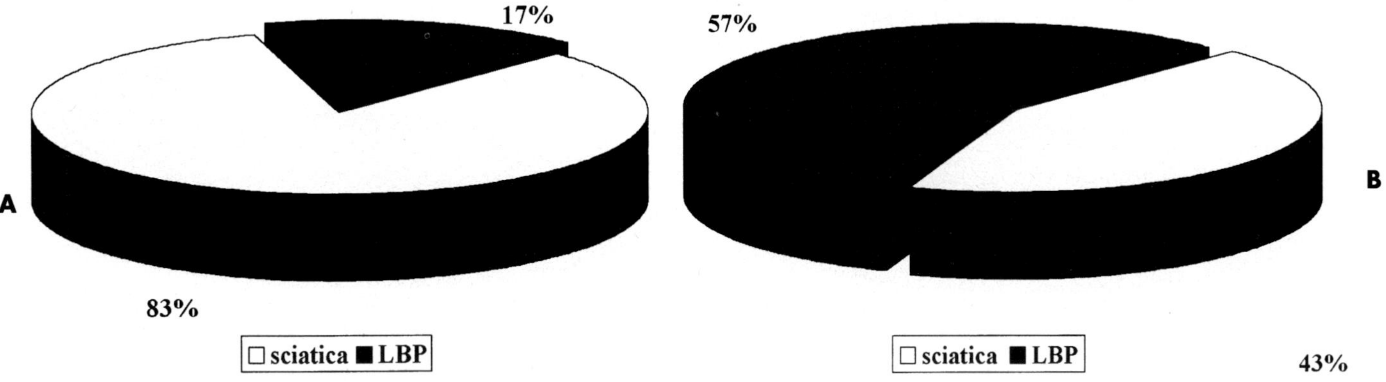


FIGURE 28-4

**A,** Clinical patterns in FBSS. **B,** Clinical pattern in primary cases.

Tobacco consumption was clearly more prevalent in the FBSS group (52.6%) than in the control group (28.5%). Tobacco consumption has been associated with a higher rate of pseudarthrosis but until present no relation with FBSS has been demonstrated (Fig. 28-5).

Among the operated patients, the majority of them had previous diskectomy and/or decompression procedures with only nine attempted fusions. Ten patients had two previous surgeries; in eight patients, this was the second diskectomy-decompression, one patient had a fusion and rhizotomy, and one patient had a fusion. Finally, one patient had a third surgery (wide laminectomy and fusion).

The delay since the first operation varies from 1.8 months to 435 months with a mean value of 66.3 months. This important delay minimizes the importance of a possible spontaneous improvement of the natural history.

Concerning the surgical technique, all patients had at least instrumented bilateral, lateral fusion; patients with diagnoses of compressive radiculopathy also had neural decompression as wide as needed. The number of fused levels was slightly higher in the primary group and the floating fusion percentage was almost identical (Fig. 28-6).

The revision protocol was designed to evaluate the clinical outcome as well as the operative complication rate, psychologic postoperative status, and radiological status.

Perioperative complications were very similar in both groups. Dural laceration was the most common complication, with 8 cases in the primary surgeries and 4 cases in the FBSS patients. There was a single case in each group of a screw in the wrong position and one more case of symptomatic pedicle violation among the primary cases. Neurological postoperative deficits were also almost equal. There was 1 postoperative radicular deficit in a primary case and 2 persistent radicular pains in both of these groups.

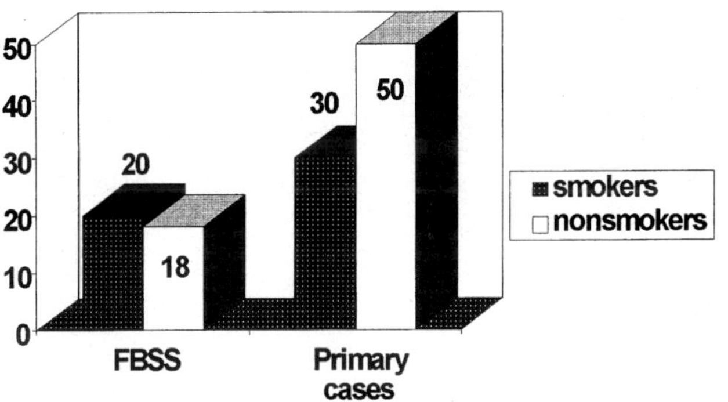


FIGURE 28-5

Tobacco use in FBSS versus primary cases.

All the screws (three) responsible for radicular pain or deficit were removed. No cases of radicular pain or neurological deficit persisted at the time they were evaluated. Other complications, such as postoperative seroma or infection, were very rare, again in the same proportion in both of groups, 70 of the primary case patients and 35 of the FBSS patients had a postoperative course without any complication (Fig. 28-7).

Radiological outcome was assessed by posteroanterior and lateral standing films as well as flexion-extension films. We looked for radiological signs of disk degeneration or segmental instability in the segments adjacent to the fusion area. No case of disk collapse or radiological signs of segmental instability (lysthesis) were found in the FBSS group.[5] Among the primary cases one patient had floating fusion L4-L5, with a L5-S1 black disk on preoperative MRI, and needed a fusion extension to sacrum. Clinical outcome was assessed by Visual Analogue Scale, Prolo index, and Wadell subjective incapacity score. Of the primary cases, 67.8% had good or very good results, but only 58% of the FBSS group had the same results; however,

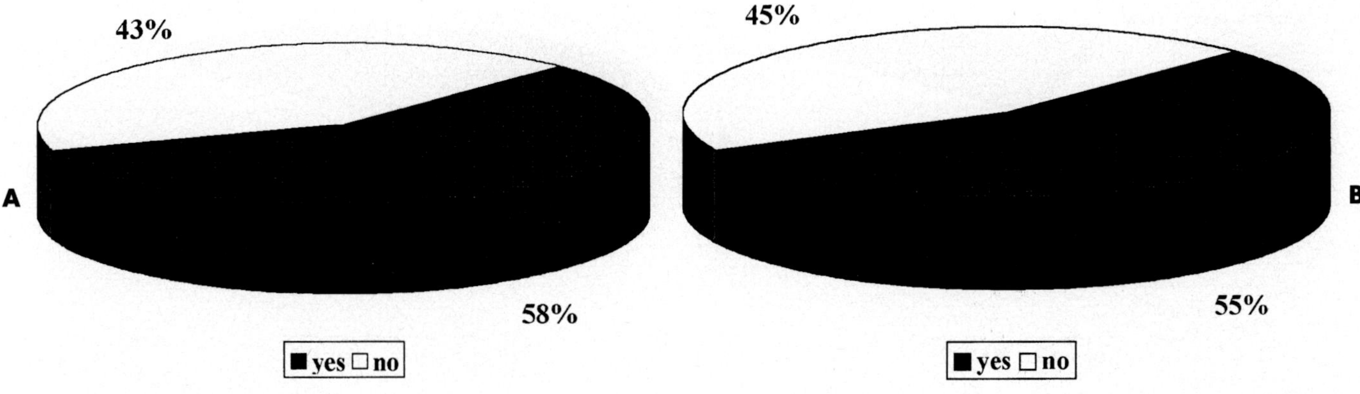


FIGURE 28-6

**A,** FBSS: fusion to sacrum. **B,** Primary cases: fusion to sacrum.

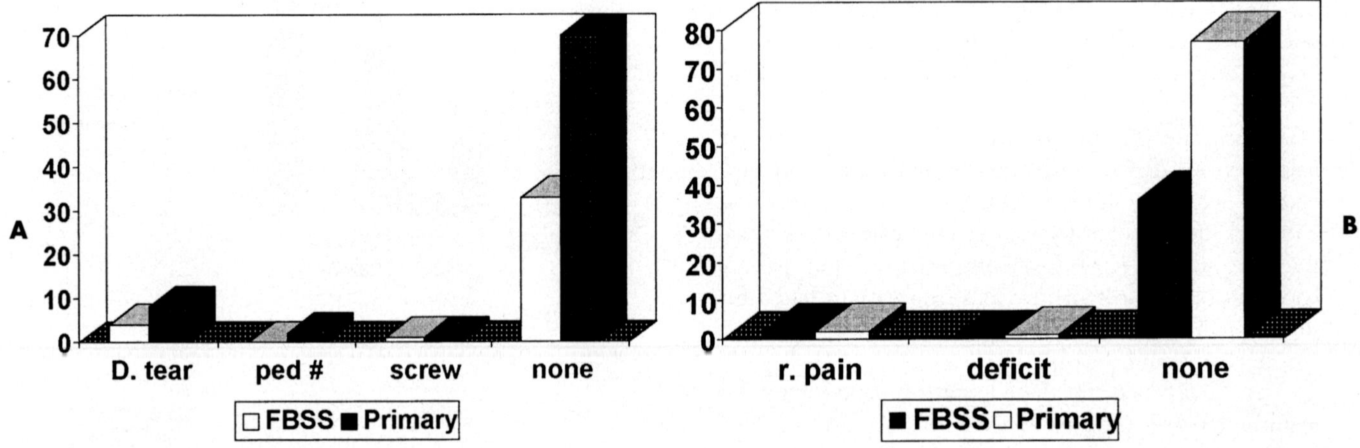


FIGURE 28-7

**A,** Preoperative complications. **B,** Postoperative complications.

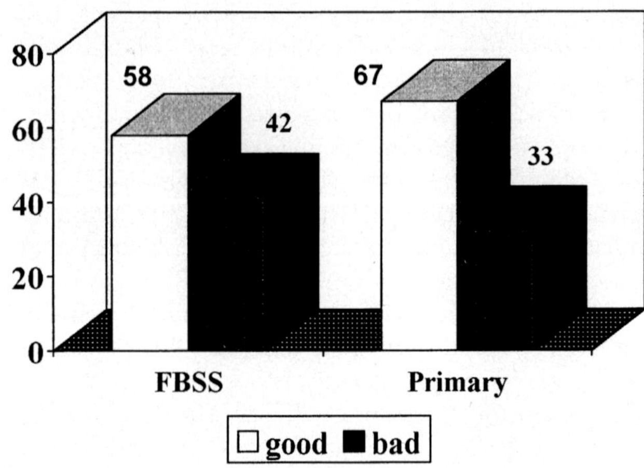


FIGURE 28-8

The results of FBSS versus primary cases.

this difference was not statistically significant (Fig. 28-8).

Psychological outcome was assessed with Minnesota Multiphasic Personality Inventory, STAI anxiety questionnaire, and Beck depression index (BDI). All of the groups had very similar numbers of psychological problems. In a multivariate regression analysis, depression ($p = 0.0086$), hypochondriasis ($p = 0.001$), hysteria ($p = 0.007$), and schizophrenia ($p = 0.02$) were the only factors related to bad results with statistical significance. However, this retrospective study can not conclude if these factors are preoperative predictors of bad results or, on the contrary, if the psychologic disturbances are a consequence of the failed surgery and the persistence of severe pain and disability.

Posterolateral lateral fusion in failed back surgery

patients, with proper patient selection and adequate technique, has a reasonably good result rate compared with those from the primary cases.[4] Results of instrumented fusion seem to be better than previously reported without instrumentation.[8] We strongly believe that increment of fusion technique (360° fusion) can give some improvement beyond the results of these series. However, there is still a significant number of patients discarded for revision surgery who remain without any reasonable solution to their problem.

## REFERENCES


1. Bertrand G: The battered root syndrome, *Orthop Clin North Am* 6(1):305-310, 1975.
2. Biondi J, Greenberg B: Redecompression and fusion in failed back syndrome patients, *J Spinal Disord* 3(4):212-217, 1990.
3. Deustch et al: Lumbar spine following successful surgical discectomy, *Spine* 15(12):1366-1369, 1993.
4. Finnegaan WJ, Fenlin JM, Marvel JP, Nardini RJ, Rothman RH: Results of surgical intervention in the symptomatic multioperated back patient. Analysis of 67 cases followed for three to seven years, *J Bone Joint Surg (Am)* 61:1077-1082, 1979.
5. Pellisé C, García L, Veras J, Bagó C, Villanueva C: Sagittal displacement of the vertebra above a lumbar fusion. Presented at the 8th Annual Meeting of the European Spine Society. Kos (Greece) September 11-13, 1997.
6. Spangfort EV: The lumbar disc herniation, *Acta Orthop Scand* (suppl.):142, 1972.
7. Tullberg T, Grane P, Isaccson J: Gadolinium-enhanced magnetic resonance imaging of 36 patients one year after lumbar disc resection, *Spine* 19(2):176-182, 1994.
8. Wadell G, Kummel EG, Lotto WN: Failed lumbar disc surgery and repeated surgery following industrial injuries, *J Bone Joint Surg* 61A:201-207, 1979.
9. Webber H: A prospective study of prognostic factors including a controlled trial. *J Oslo City Hosp* 28:33-61, 91-113, 1978.

# 29

# REVISIONS IN DEGENERATIVE LUMBAR DISEASES

**Se-Il Suk, M.D.**
**Won-Joong Kim, M.D.**



Degenerative spine disease is a broad spectrum of spinal disorders caused by degenerative changes of the bone, joints, and the connective tissues of the spinal column. It spans from simple, seemingly innocent degenerative arthritis to degenerative spinal deformities such as spondylolisthesis and scoliosis with neurologic compromise.

Today, treatment of degenerative spine disorders comprises a greater portion of all spine surgeries performed throughout the world and will be of a greater percentage in the future. Though improved surgical techniques and instruments will continue to reduce the percentage of patients requiring revision in the future, the absolute number of revisions for degenerative disease is expected to increase considerably with this tremendous increment of surgery. The purpose of this chapter is to delineate the problems commonly encountered in revision surgery for degenerative diseases of the lumbar spine and to offer an appropriate guideline for management of specific problems.

## INCIDENCE AND CAUSES

The incidence of revision for degenerative diseases of the lumbar spine is widely variable, depending on the primary procedure undertaken, skill and training of the surgeon who has performed the primary surgery, and the philosophy of the treating surgeons making the decision for revision.

Reported overall incidence of revision in degenerative lumbar disease ranges from 5% to 18% with slightly higher rates of revision in patients with degenerative deformities, as these deformities mandate an adequate stabilization following a decompressive surgery.[12]

The causes of revision surgery, when rephrased, are the causes of unsatisfactory results of the primary surgery for which surgical treatment is indicated. As in primary surgery, the major complaints arise from a single or one of the combinations of neurologic compromises, instability, deformity, back pain without mechanical instability, psychosocial distress, or a biochemical pathology (as in disk disruption). They may be caused by wrong or misdirected primary surgery, surgical complications, and progression of degenerative changes in operated and/or unoperated levels.

In establishing a probable diagnosis, it is useful to look into both the time interval between the primary surgery and the presentation of the complaints and similarities between the original complaint for the primary surgery and the postoperative complaints. Wrong or misdirected surgery presents with symptoms and signs similar to the previous complaints in the early postoperative period within weeks. Surgical complications often have a set of symptoms quite different from the original complaints and usually present months after the primary surgery. Progression of the degenerative process in operated and other virgin levels presents years after the primary surgery with usual symptoms of degenerative disease that may or may not be similar to the original complaints. Table 29-1 is a classification of cause of failures of primary surgery by the major offending pathology.

## ASSESSMENT

In assessing patients with apparent primary surgery failures, the clinical history is of prime importance in determining a probable cause. As stated before, the nature of the presenting complaint and its similarities with the symptoms prior to the operation and the duration of the initial symptom-free interval following the primary surgery may point to the underlying causes. Other important factors to be sought for in the history are the duration of the illness prior to the surgical treatment, presence of other systemic illness that might adversely affect the outcome of the primary surgery, and psychosocial factors such as worker's compensation, low socioeconomic status, heavy job requirements, cigarette smoking, psychological disturbance, and litigation. These factors are known to have predictive values on the failures of the surgery.[9,35] Though the presenting symptoms of the patients with failed surgery are more often vague, predominant pathology may be determined by the clinical manifestations. When neurologic compromise is the predominant complaint, it is more often related to the pathology affecting the neural structures. When back pain is the predominant complaint, it is usually related to the pathologies affecting the disk, bony architecture, or the stability of the vertebral column. When deformity

**Table 29-1. Classification of Cause of Failure**

| Predominant pathology | Neurologic compromise | Instability | Deformity | Others |
|---|---|---|---|---|
| Wrong or misdirected operation | 1. Wrong diagnosis<br>a. Tumor<br>b. Metabolic diseases and peripheral neuropathy<br>2. Decompression done too late for compressive neuropathy<br>3. Technical errors<br>a. Missed level or levels<br>b. Failure to perform an adequate decompression | 1. Technical errors<br>a. Missed instability<br>b. Insufficient fusion levels | 1. Technical errors<br>a. Missed instability<br>b. Insufficient fusion levels | 1. Wrong diagnosis<br>a. Infection<br>b. Discogenic pain<br>c. Psychosocial distress |
| Surgical complications | 1. Root injury<br>2. Neural impingement by bone graft, cement or fixation devices<br>3. Meningeal cyst<br>4. Perineural scarring<br>5. Arachnoditis | 1. Pseudarthrosis<br>2. Implant failures<br>3. Iatrogenic instability<br>4. Facet joint injury<br>5. Acquired spondylolysis | 1. Decompensation<br>2. Junctional kyphosis<br>3. Pseudarthrosis | Infection |
| Progression of degenerative process | 1. Recurrent stenosis<br>2. Adjacent level disk degeneration<br>a. Disk herniation<br>b. Stenosis<br>3. Stenosis above or below a fusion | Degenerative instability in adjacent level | Degenerative arthritis in adjacent level | Disk disruption |

and balance are the chief complaints, the causes are more obvious.

The physical examinations are as vague and are often less productive than the history and the presenting symptoms.[8] Neurologic deficits found in these patients may be a residual from the primary operation or de novo from the operative procedures. Considering the difficulty of distinction, it is extremely important to gather all available information concerning the preoperative status of the particular patient.

Imaging studies are important means to clarify the causes of failure. But it must be kept in mind that its role should be confirming, rather than seeking a probable diagnosis. Plain radiographs should include the standing anteroposterior (AP) and lateral projections to check the coronal and sagittal balances, and motion studies comprising flexion and extension studies to determine the presence of instability. Cone-down views and tomography may be helpful for determination of pseudarthrosis. Multiplanar computed tomography (CT) scans are the most helpful means for the diagnosis of bony pathology, and may be combined with myelography for the detection of pathology affecting the spinal canal. However, in the presence of metallic devices used for internal fixation, it may be less helpful. Magnetic resonance imaging (MRI), enabling a distinction between recurrent pathology and scarring, is also a very helpful diagnostic tool.[24,29] Being noninvasive and effective, it is currently the most favored screening test. However, MRI may be less helpful in the presence of nontitanium metallic internal fixation devices and is less effective than CT when the pathology predominantly involves the cortical bone.[36] Other diagnostic imaging techniques include technetium bone scans and diskography. The advantages and pitfalls of each diagnostic study are detailed elsewhere in the textbook.

## TREATMENT

Before finally deciding to perform a revision surgery, the surgeon has to be aware of the following:[6,34] First, the result of revision surgery is almost always less satisfactory than a primary surgery on the virgin back. Second, the results of surgery will be increasingly less satisfactory with each subsequent revision surgery. Third, revision surgery is more fraught with complications than the primary surgery. Finally, the age and medical condition of the patient may make a lengthy and extensive procedure intolerable. It is therefore advisable that the revision surgery be reserved for spine surgeons with adequate training and extensive experience with revisions. It is by no means a job for surgeons who only do occasional spine surgeries.

For these reasons, revision surgery should be avoided except when absolutely necessary, and the surgeon is absolutely confident that the procedure will solve the patient's problem(s). Therefore, the prerequisite for revision surgery is an identification of surgically amenable cause or causes of failure clearly documented by diagnostic studies. In the absence of a definite target for surgical treatment, the revision is doomed to fail, producing a more disabled patient. For the patients with uncertain causes of failure, or with causes that are not likely to be improved by surgery, a well-programmed conservative management plan will offer the best benefits. Because the patients with failures of primary surgery are often affected by multiple problems, which might be the cause of the presenting complaints, the treatment must be designed and directed specifically to fit the individual patient.

The general principles of surgical treatment are decompression of the neural elements in neurologic compromise, stabilization with arthrodesis in instability, and correction and maintenance of correction in deformities.

Decompression in revision is much more difficult and fraught with complications than in primary surgery. Although a complete decompression at a revision surgery is more difficult than in the primary surgery, it should be adequately done because additional, or redo-revision, decompression would be more difficult. A complete decompression with wide excision of the facets and total unroofing of the neural foramen is mandatory to prevent perineural fibrosis constricting the root in a foramen.

Stabilization by a spinal arthrodesis is greatly enhanced by the use of rigid internal fixation devices.[7] As most of the primary surgery for degenerative spine disease include posterior decompression as an inherent part, the patients often present with defects of the posterior elements. In these situations, if posterior surgery is being contemplated, pedicle screws offer the best fixation.[31] They also offer the greatest holding power in osteoporotic spines, often found in these patients due to their age and prolonged protection and immobilization. Considering the postoperative evaluation, we recommend the use of titanium implants so that MRI imaging will be possible whenever needed. Sometimes, the condition of the fusion bed in the posterior column calls for an anterior fusion. Anterior fusion, in the absence of posterior rigid fixation, is best achieved by adding rigid anterior internal fixation.

Correction and maintenance of spinal deformity in revision surgery are possible only with a rigid internal fixation device and solid arthrodesis. We recommend the use of segmental pedicle screws for this purpose. The advantages are rigidity of the fixation, enhanced segmental control, enhanced restoration of the sagittal profile, and versatility that allows a long-level instrumentation from thoracic vertebrae to the sacrum. The fusion should include, in addition to the entire index deformity, all the levels with signs of instability and symptomatic degenerated disks detected on diskogram to prevent later complications.

## SURGICAL INDICATIONS

The indications for revision surgery are closely related to the etiologies of the unsatisfactory results. In general, the failures due to a wrong or misdirected operation to a surgical pathology calls for a revision. The surgical complications warrant a more deliberate approach. When the causes are mechanical, such as neural impingement by the graft, cement or fixation devices, or pseudarthrosis, revision is considered. However, it must be kept in mind that not all mechanical complications are associated with severe disability and the benefits of the surgery must be weighed carefully against the risks of revision. The causes involving the neural structures are usually not reparable by surgical treatment and should not be operated on. Complaints caused by an ongoing degenerative process should rather be considered a new disease rather than a complication, and their surgical indications are the same as for a virgin surgery. They should be managed conservatively unless they cause moderate to severe disability that is unresponsive to prolonged conservative measures.

## WRONG OR MISDIRECTED OPERATIONS

### WITH NEUROLOGIC COMPROMISE

***Wrong Preoperative Diagnosis.***

TUMOR. Considering the age of the patients with degenerative spine disease, the misdiagnosed tumor is more often a malignancy. The most likely location of a missed tumor is the sacrum, which, owing to its anatomy deep in the pelvis, is often not well-visualized on plain films and usually escapes the routine lumbar axial CT scans (Fig. 29-1). Tumors at this location and in this age group are frequently metastasis and chordoma. When a tumor is suspected, a CT-guided aspiration biopsy is helpful in establishing a diagnosis. Once a diagnosis is established, subsequent treatment for the neoplasm is instituted with consultation of relevant specialists.

METABOLIC DISEASES. Metabolic diseases causing peripheral neuropathy may be misdiagnosed as degenerative spine disorders with neurological symptoms because both commonly affect the elderly population. The most common etiology causing this failure is diabetes mellitus. Because this is not a surgical indication in the first place, it is best to avoid such a situation by careful history taking, physical examination, and relevant diagnostic studies.

***Delayed Decompression.*** If the patient had a long preoperative history of compressive neuropathy such as a chronic cauda equina syndrome or radiculopathy with single leg-raising limitation lasting for more than 6 months, there may be considerable root scarring, and the patient's neurologic recovery may be short of the expectations following the primary surgery.[25] This situation is diagnosed on the basis of detailed clinical history. As stated earlier, the failure from the causes involving the neural tissue are not reparable by surgery and, as repeat decompression in this situation is usually futile, conservative treatment including physical therapy and bracing, if necessary, are the mainstays of treatment.

***Technical Errors.***

MISSED LEVEL OR LEVELS. This refers to the primary operation being performed on the wrong level or levels. Besides human error on the surgeon's part, a missed level may occur when the patient's obesity or large size hinders the adequacy of the intraoperative radiographic evaluation, or when there are segmentation abnormalities causing discord (errors in evaluation of the levels of neurologic involvement and their respective motion segments) in levels of neurologic involvement and motion segments. When this mishap is the cause of failure, reoperation on the appropriate level is indicated.

FAILURE TO PERFORM AN ADEQUATE DECOMPRESSION. This is by far the most common technical cause of failures in primary surgery for degenerative lumbar spine.[17,33] It is most commonly caused by inadequacy of foraminal decompression, which is often difficult to accomplish when the facet joints are preserved to maintain posterior stability (Fig. 29-2, *A-D*). Inadequate decompression is also commonly found in patients with multilevel stenosis. The determination of the extent of decompression in these patients may pose difficulty, but in addition to preoperative evaluation, intraoperative confirmation of restoration of dural pulsation may reduce this complication. Inadequate decompression may also occur in short-level decompression for degenerative spondylolisthesis, isthmic spondylolisthesis, and degenerative scoliosis. In degenerative spondylolisthesis, the roots proximal to the level of the slip are compressed in the narrowed lateral recess and are often missed. In the isthmic listhesis, the roots proximal to the level of the slip are invariably compressed by the fibrocartilaginous mass at the site of the isthmic defect, and it is necessary to keep in mind that four roots, proximal and distal to the level of the slip, are to be checked. In degenerative scoliosis, the roots in the concavity of the curve are often compressed in the narrowed foramen. Though correction of the curvature may relieve the compression to a degree, the roots need to be checked for adequacy of decompression after the correction of the curvature.

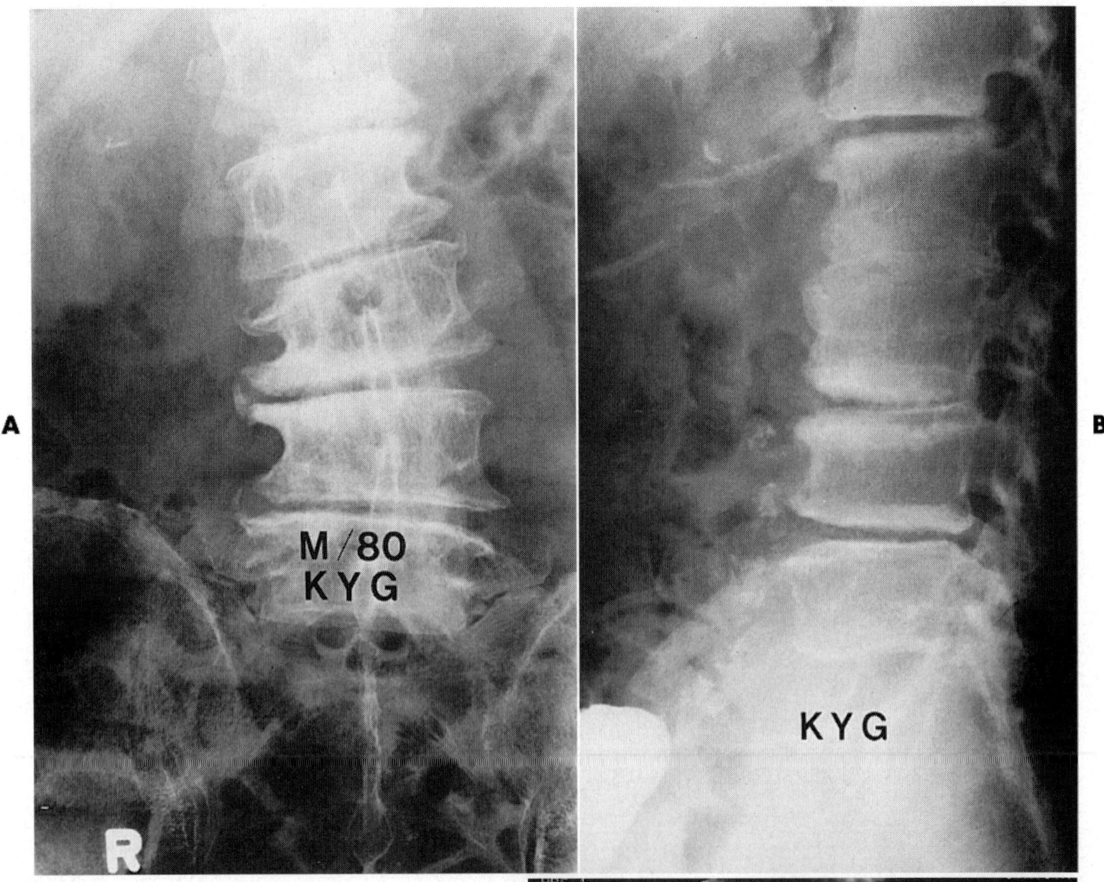


A B

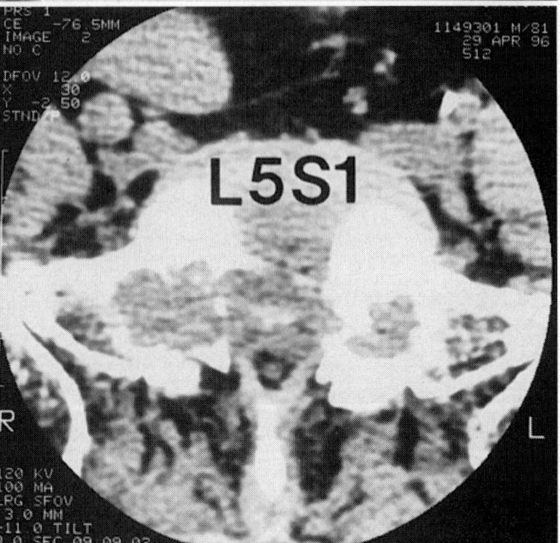


C

**FIGURE 29-1**

An 80-year-old man with typical neurogenic claudication of a long duration. **A, B,** Plain radiographs demonstrate severe degenerative change with degenerative scoliosis and subfacetal narrowing. Sacrum is not well visualized, obscured by abdominal gases and the iliac crest. **C,** Bony destruction of sacrum was incidentally discovered on routine preoperative CT.

*Continued*

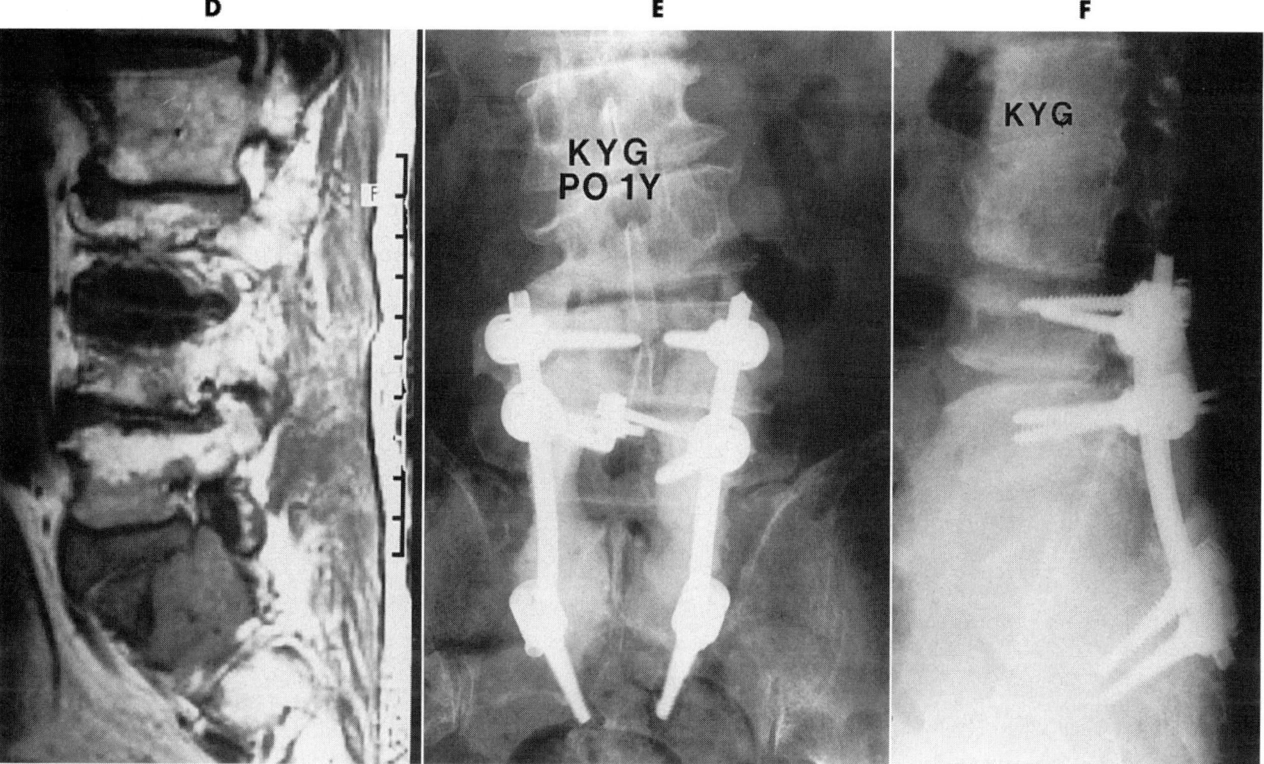


FIGURE 29-1, CONT'D

**D,** The lesion viewed on sagittal MRI. Needle aspiration biopsy revealed a sacral chordoma. **E, F,** Because of the age of the patient, the tumor was treated by sacral laminectomy, curettage, and cementation followed by a stabilization procedure with pedicle screw instrumentation to promote early ambulation.

The diagnosis of inadequate decompression is made on the basis of clinical failure in improvement of the patient's neurologic symptoms and demonstration of residual neural compression on imaging studies. Though CT and MRI are handy and helpful diagnostic tools to accomplish this, they tend to be less accurate in the presence of metallic internal fixation devices. Because myelography is less affected by the presence of internal fixation devices and allows imaging from several different views, it may offer greater help in determining the sites of residual compression. As inadequate decompression results in partial relief of the symptoms, reoperation is indicated only when the severity of the patient's residual neurologic symptoms warrants a surgical treatment. The residual compressive lesions identified on imaging studies have to be removed. Because this calls for a wider decompression, fusion is recommended (Fig. 29-2, *E* and *F*).

## WITH INSTABILITY

### *Technical Errors.*

MISSED INSTABILITY. Instability neglected during the primary operation may cause back pain during the subacute period when the patient begins ambulation. Though the main symptom is back pain, the patient may sometimes complain of radiating pain, vague in nature, to the buttocks and posterior upper thigh. The diagnosis is made on flexion and extension radiographs. It may be difficult to distinguish missed instability from iatrogenic instability or early adjacent disk degeneration. However, the presence of spondylolysis or listhesis, retrospondylolisthesis, rotary subluxation of the facets in preoperative radiographs, and the discord of the unstable segment with the segments operated on favors the diagnosis of missed instability.[30] When the back pain is severe and fails to respond to aggressive conservative therapy, fusion is indicated. Fusion should include all levels that demonstrate signs of instability.

INSUFFICIENT FUSION LEVELS. Insufficient fusion levels may result in spinal decompensation, progression of the deformity, and aggravation of the disease in segments adjacent to the fusion. As it is very difficult to diagnose, except in obvious cases with preoperative degenerative deformities, the best way to prevent it is by proper determination of fusion extent. Though difficult, it must be differentiated from pseudarthrosis to avoid unnecessary extensive procedures of pseudarthrosis repair. The diagnosis of insufficient fusion levels may be aided by diskography and facet blocks. Once the diagnosis of insufficient fusion level is made

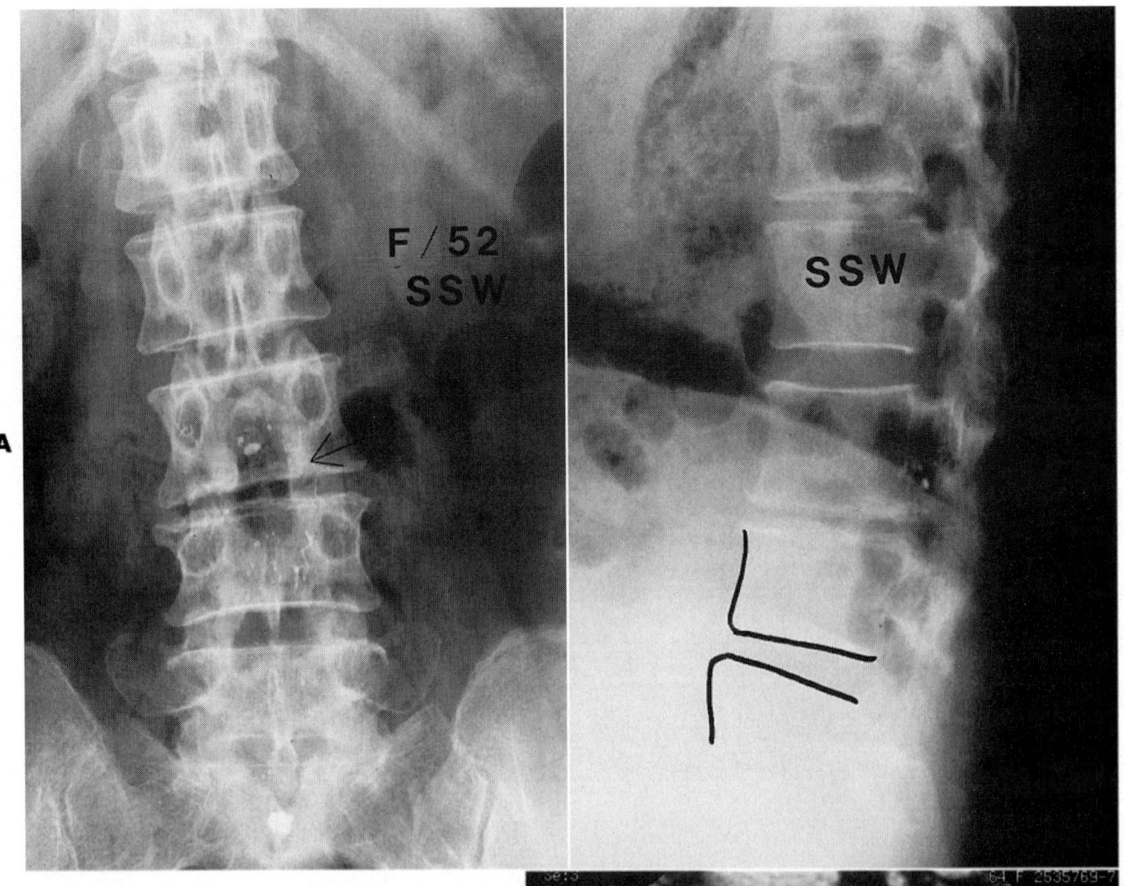


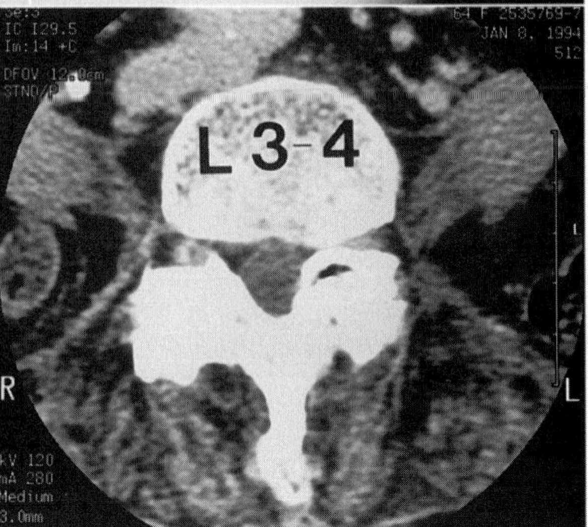


**FIGURE 29-2**

A 52-year-old woman with back pain and neurogenic claudication. She was operated on for similar symptoms 5 years prior to the visit. Following the initial surgery, her symptoms were not only unimproved, but got worse with time. **A,** Plain radiograph showing partial laminectomy of L3 and L4 and laminotomy of L5, implying a decompressive surgery done at L3-L4 and diskectomy of L4-L5. **B,** L3-L4 space narrowing and L4-L5 instability are shown on flexion lateral radiograph. **C,** CT scans of L3-L4 and L4-L5 demonstrated inadequate foraminal decompression in L3-L4 and severe lateral recess stenosis by hypertrophy of the facet joints in L4-L5. *Continued*

and surgical treatment is decided, fusion is extended to include all the pathologic levels identified.

### WITH DEFORMITY

Technical errors resulting in residual instability may cause progressive deformity if the instability is increased with time. Insufficient fusion levels in degenerative deformity may result in adding on phenomenon with extension of the deformity into adjacent segments.

### OTHERS

***Wrong Preoperative Diagnosis.***

INFECTION. The infection most commonly misdiagnosed as degenerative spine disease is early infection without significant bony destruction.[26] It may be mistaken for severe degenerative arthritis with instability, which may demonstrate a narrow disk space and zones of low signal adjacent to the disk space on MRI. Infection is diagnosed on the basis of elevated erythrocyte sedimentation rates and acute phase reac-

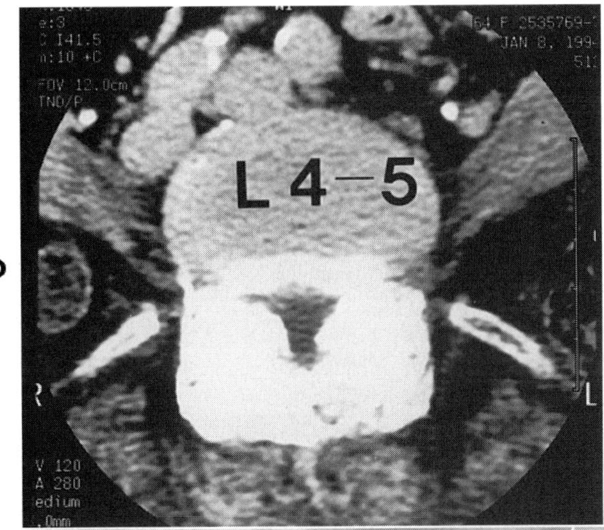


FIGURE 29-2, CONT'D

D, CT scans of L3-L4 and L4-L5 demonstrated inadequate foraminal decompression in L3-L4 and severe lateral recess stenosis by hypertrophy of the facet joints in L4-L5. **E, F,** One year after the revision, she is free of back pain and claudication.

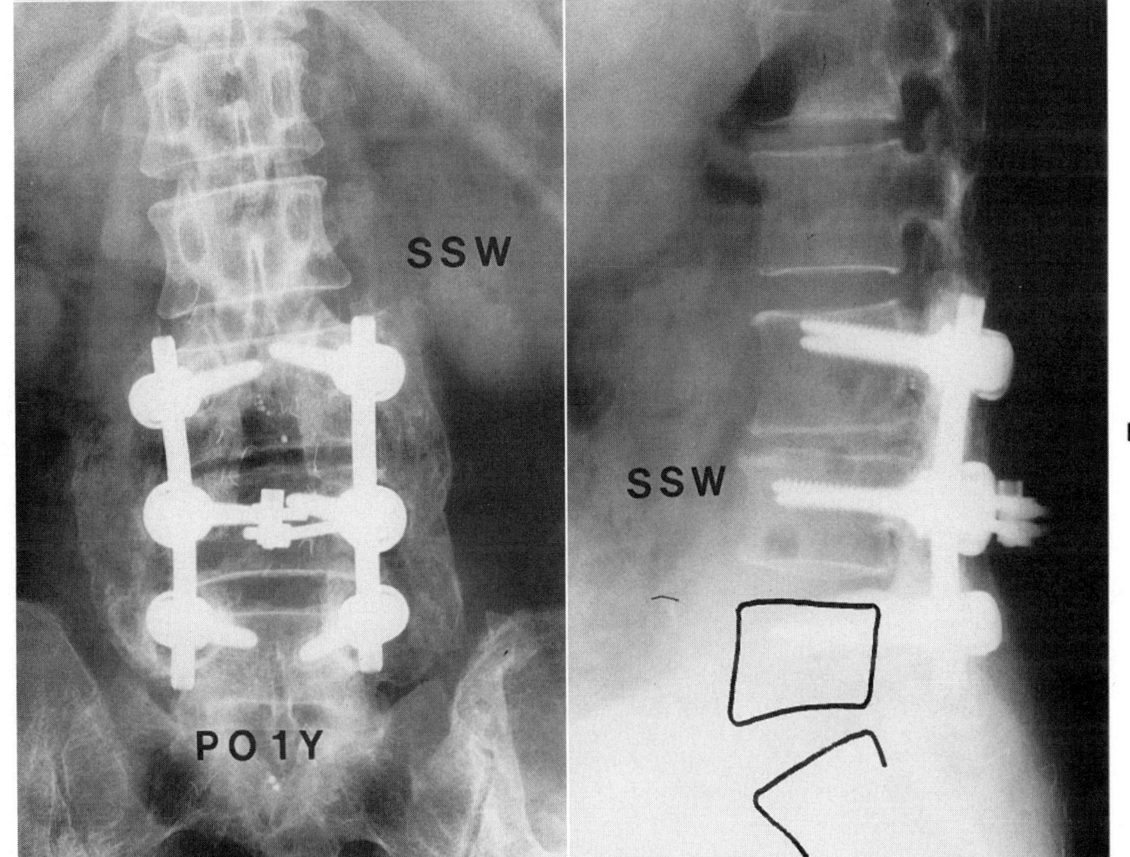


tants. When the anterior column is involved, a bone scan may be of some help. In some situations, it may be difficult to discern whether the infection was a missed diagnosis or a surgical complication. However, infection involving the disk space in a patient not subjected to diskectomy of that particular level should raise a suspicion of misdiagnosis. The treatment is based on the causative organism identified by blood culture or culture material obtained by CT-guided aspiration. Though a pyogenic infection may be managed conservatively with antibiotics and cast immobilization, it is usually better to perform an anterior debridement and fusion to reduce undue complications of neurologic deterioration and late spine deformity from destruction of the vertebral bodies and to shorten the healing period. If posterior instrumentation is used in the primary operation, it is left in place, and anterior debridement and fusion is performed through an anterior approach. A tuberculous infection is treated by anterior debridement/fusion and antituberculosis medications.

DISCOGENIC PAIN. The discogenic pain syndrome

caused by internal disruption of the disk is a rare cause of acute failure, occurring in decompressive operations without fusion.[9] However, as the pain is thought to arise from increased pressure on the disk, causing movement of catabolites via the vertebral vascular system, it is unlikely to be a cause of continuing back pain in the patient in whom rigid internal fixation was carried out. The diagnosis of discogenic pain as the cause of continued back pain after primary operation may be very difficult, especially when disk excision has been performed, as the disk is disrupted by the operation. Though the demonstration of chronic endplate changes on sagittal MRI may be suggestive, the diagnosis should be one of exclusion. If the diagnosis of disk disruption is made and surgical intervention seems appropriate, fusion with rigid internal fixation has to be carried out.[5,20]

***Psychosocial Distress.*** The importance of psychosocial determinants on the outcome of decompressive surgery has been emphasized by many authors and is indeed considered a dominant cause of failure for low back surgeries.[4,6,19,27] In patients with failed surgery, the psychosocial factors should be carefully evaluated through a detailed multidisciplinary approach. Revision in these patients is usually both unsatisfactory and inappropriate, unless a clearly demonstrable anatomic causation is present. They are to be managed conservatively with progressive exercise programs, aggressive rehabilitation, and pain clinics.[18]

## SURGICAL COMPLICATIONS

### WITH NEUROLOGIC COMPROMISE

***Root Injury.*** Roots injured during surgery may or may not cause symptoms. Symptoms of root injury range from paresthesia to motor deficit causing significant disability. Symptoms attributable to root injuries identified during surgery are accepted and are not candidates for reoperation. However, symptoms of root injury without an identified incidence warrant closer scrutiny for the cause. The unidentified causes of root injuries are traction, pressure, or thermal injuries. Traction injuries may occur in the process of retracting the roots during a disk excision or posterior lumbar interbody fusion procedure. They rarely occur during reduction of severe-degree spondylolisthesis by stretching of the nerve roots. In retraction radiculopathy, root recovery is normal and patient observation is the best choice. When stretching of the nerve roots from lengthening of the spinal column is suspected, and symptoms comprise major motor deficit, relief of the tension by shortening of the vertebral column and adequate decompression of the nerve roots is recommended.

***Neural Impingement.*** Postoperative neurologic symptoms in patients subjected to instrumentation fusion procedures may be caused by foreign materials impinging on the neural tissues. Though all misplaced instruments may impinge on neural tissue, the most common cause is a malpositioned pedicle screw. The screws, when confined within the pedicles, are separated from the neural tissue by the cortical wall of the pedicles, and are safe. However, when the screw perforates the pedicle, they are in the close vicinity of the neural tissues. Lateral and superior perforations are relatively benign and rarely cause symptoms. Medial perforations may injure the dura and the contents, whereas inferior perforation may affect the emerging nerve roots underneath the pedicle. The diagnosis of neural impingement by a pedicle screw is suspected by a malpositioned screw medial or inferior to the pedicle seen on plain radiograph; it is confirmed by axial CT scans with myelography. A combination of removal of the misplaced screw and reinstrumentation usually solves the problem (Fig. 29-3). Neural impingement may also occur by the posterior displacement of the implants placed in the disk space. Threaded fusion cages and carbon cages designed for lumbar interbody fusion, when not placed properly anterior to the axis of rotation, may be retropulsed, causing neurologic compromise. This situation is suspected when the posterior margin of the implant rests posterior to the lines joining the posterior margin of the vertebrae above and below the implant. As it is sometimes very difficult to remove the implants from a posterior approach, an anterior approach is used, and anterior fusion is performed. When spinal stability is in question, the addition of anterior instrumentation is preferable.

Neural impingement by bone cement is a complication related to the use of pedicle screws. It occurs when bone cement used for pedicle screw fixation in an osteoporotic spine leaks out through the perforations in the pedicles produced during the hole preparation. This complication is preventable by not using the bone cement in the holes in which perforation is suspected, by not inserting the cement when it is too watery, and by checking the canal and the foramen immediately after the screw insertion. It is diagnosed by axial CT with myelography. Treatment comprises removal of the cement causing neural compression. For decompression of roots in the neural foramen, wide exposure by inferior and superior facetectomy and use of a diamond burr is recommended.

Bone grafts impinging on the neural tissue may be caused by retropulsion of the bone blocks placed in the disk space for posterior lumbar interbody fusion. They may also be caused by the inadvertent slipping of bone chips used for posterolateral fusion into an inadequately decompressed spinal canal or neural foramen. They are diagnosed by axial CT with myelogra-

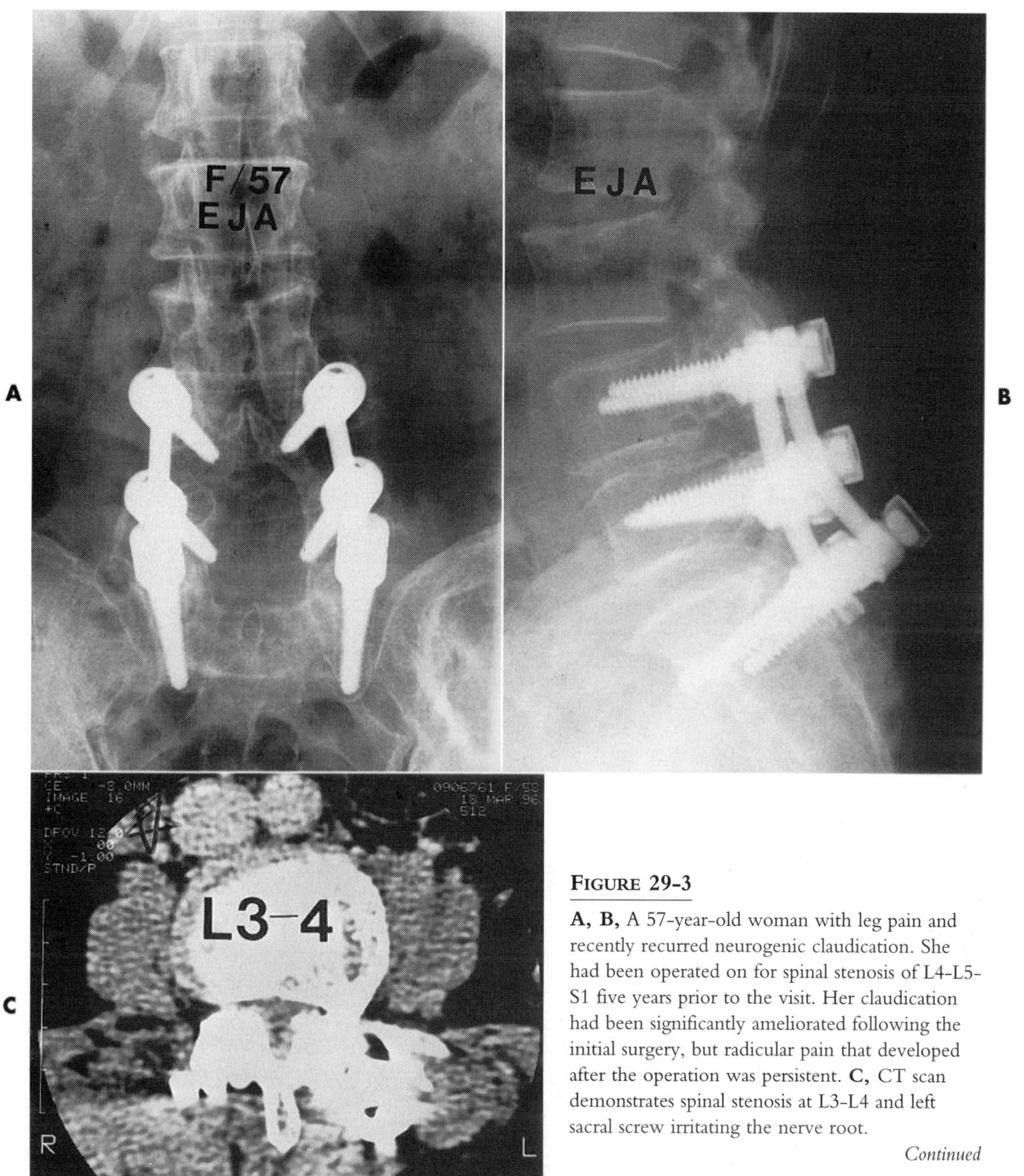


FIGURE 29-3

**A, B,** A 57-year-old woman with leg pain and recently recurred neurogenic claudication. She had been operated on for spinal stenosis of L4-L5-S1 five years prior to the visit. Her claudication had been significantly ameliorated following the initial surgery, but radicular pain that developed after the operation was persistent. **C,** CT scan demonstrates spinal stenosis at L3-L4 and left sacral screw irritating the nerve root.

*Continued*

phy. When neurologic symptoms are severe and warrant treatment, removal of the offending bone graft is performed. Unlike the implants, the retropulsed bone block may be removed piecemeal from the posterior.

***Meningeal Cyst.*** Meningeal cysts are a rare cause of acute failure resulting from a unrecognized or inadequately repaired durotomy. They are usually asymptomatic, but cause radicular symptoms when the roots are herniated into the sac and buttonholed by the opening. MRI and myelography are useful diagnostic tools. They are treated by removal and dural repair. Care should be taken not to injure the roots, which may be incorporated in the cyst.

***Perineural Scarring.*** Perineural scarring is an inevitable complication of spinal decompressive surgery and is related to the magnitude of the decompression; however, the incidence of perineural adhesion being the cause of failure for the primary operation is relatively low. When scarring is diffuse, the patient's stenotic symptoms may recur. The classic clinical pic-

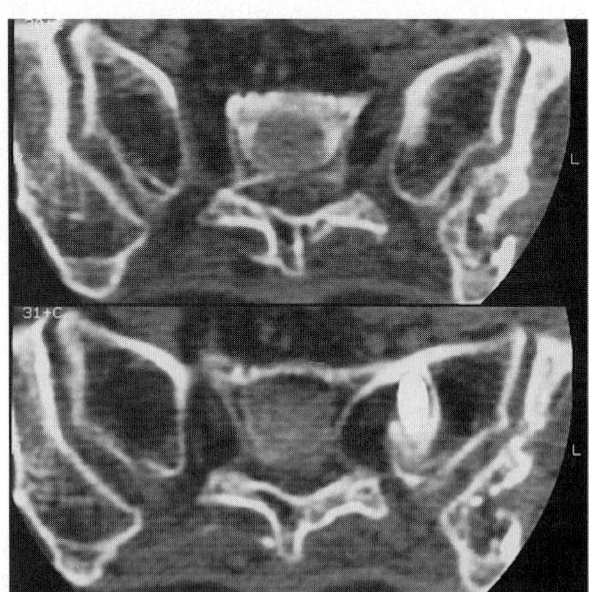

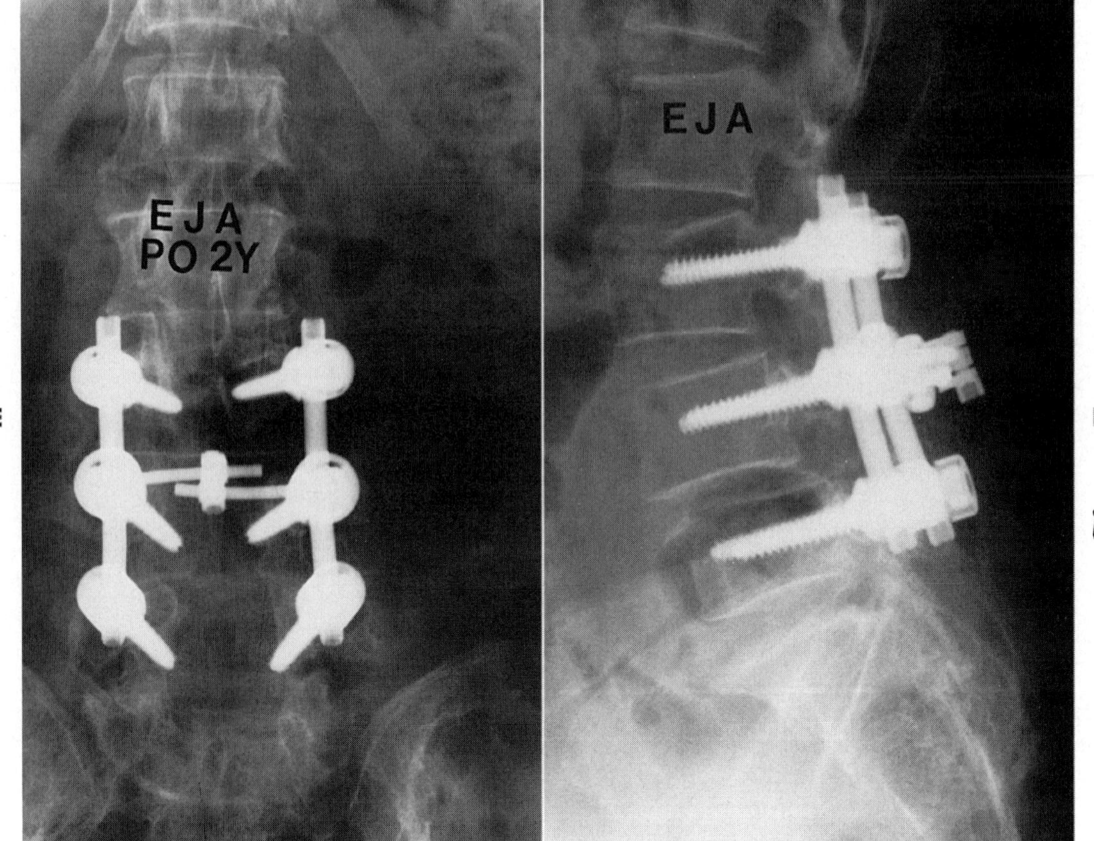


**Figure 29-3, cont'd**

**D,** CT scan demonstrates spinal stenosis at L3-L4 and left sacral screw irritating the nerve root. **E, F,** She was treated by decompression of L3-L4 and removal of the sacral screws. Fusion was extended to include L3-L4.

ture is immediate postoperative symptomatic relief followed by slowly increasing neurologic symptoms in the next 3 to 6 months. Imaging studies demonstrate a large dorsal mass of epidural scar. MRI with gadolinium enhancement is a helpful diagnostic aid in this situation, enabling differentiation between a recurrent disk and a scar. Because violating a scar results in additional scarring and most of the patients achieve adequate functional recovery with conservative therapy, surgical treatment is considered only when bony tissue entrapment of the scar-bound neural tissues is demonstrated in imaging studies. Surgery consists of decompression of the neural tissue by removal of the bony entrapment and adequate stabilization.

***Arachnoiditis.*** The most common cause of postoperative arachnoiditis complicating a modern spine surgery is surgical trauma.[21] Arachnoiditis probably becomes symptomatic by mechanical constriction of the nerve roots and by interfering with the nutrition of the nerve roots derived from the spinal fluid. The usual course of the condition is development and progression 6 to 18 months following the initial insult. The diagnosis is made on clinical manifestations of slowly aggravating neurologic symptoms and confirmed by myelography and/or MRI. The condition is managed conservatively. In some select cases, microsurgical lysis may be helpful.

### With Instability

***Pseudarthrosis.*** The mechanism of pain from pseudarthrosis is not fully understood, but it may be due in part to the persistent abnormal motion that called for fusion in the first place.[8] Pseudarthrosis following a spinal fusion has been reduced remarkably with the use of modern rigid internal fixation devices, from 40% without internal fixation to approximately 5% with pedicle screws.[16] Nevertheless, it continues to be the most common cause of failure of surgeries involving a fusion procedure. However, establishing a pseudarthrosis as a cause of failure is not an easy decision, because many patients with radiographically obvious nonunions do well without significant symptoms.[8] Because the pseudarthrosis repair, in and of itself, is a formidable procedure, has successful refusion rates much lower than that of primary fusion and even less success rates in achieving a satisfactory result, one must be absolutely sure that the failure is caused by the pseudarthrosis.[14] Trial of local anesthetic infiltration and external immobilization with cast are useful diagnostic tools for this purpose.

When one is sure that the pseudarthrosis is the cause of failure, repair should be attempted. As repeat posterior fusion for posterior fusion failure is more often futile, anterior fusion is recommended (Fig. 29-4). Addition of rigid anterior instrumentation enhances fusion and is worth trying if posterior reoperation is not considered. If there is a reason for posterior reoperation, for example an implant failure or a disk prolapse, circumferential fusion with posterior reinstrumentation (preferably with segmental pedicle screw fixation) is recommended.[32] The interbody part of the fusion may be done by posterior lumbar interbody fusion (PLIF) or anterior lumbar interbody fusion (ALIF); however, with dense scarring and adhesions, it is usually safer to perform ALIF. When the posterior instrumentation is rigid, anterior instrumentation may be omitted.

***Implant Failures.*** Implant failures usually occur within 6 months of the fusion procedure before the grafts are fully matured. They are commonly associated with pseudarthrosis, but may occur with a solid union because posterolateral fusion allows some movement in the anterior column. It is difficult to determine the role of the failed implant in the causation of failure of the primary operations because many patients with failed implants do well without symptoms. There has been speculation that metallic debris from failed implants may elicit a cytokine mediated inflammatory response and cause pain.

When instability suggestive of pseudarthrosis is demonstrated, the failed implant is removed and repeat fusion for pseudarthrosis is attempted with circumferential fusion. When the failed implant is a device using pedicle screws, previous screw holes in the pedicle may be reused, employing a screw with a larger diameter. When rigid posterior fixation with pedicle screws is feasible, repeat posterior instrumentation is performed with the addition of interbody fusion by PLIF or ALIF. If posterior internal fixation is precluded by failed implants, circumferential fusion with rigid anterior instrumentation is recommended.

***Iatrogenic Instability.*** Iatrogenic instability is caused by extensive removal of the posterior hook mechanism and disk excision.[13] It is diagnosed by flexion and extension radiographs; however, to confirm it as a specific cause of failure, external immobilization may be tried. It is treated by fusion preferably with pedicle screw fixation (Fig. 29-5).

***Facet Joint Injury.*** Proximal facet joint injuries may occur during decortication of the lateral aspect of the facet joints and pedicle screw instrumentation procedure by the screw heads and the rods inserted too close to the facets. Injured facets cause pain through instability and irritation of the pain nerve endings distributed at the capsule. The pain and tenderness is usually circumscribed and ameliorated by local anesthetic infiltration of the affected facets. When pain is severe and unresponsive to conservative measures, fusion is extended to include the affected level.

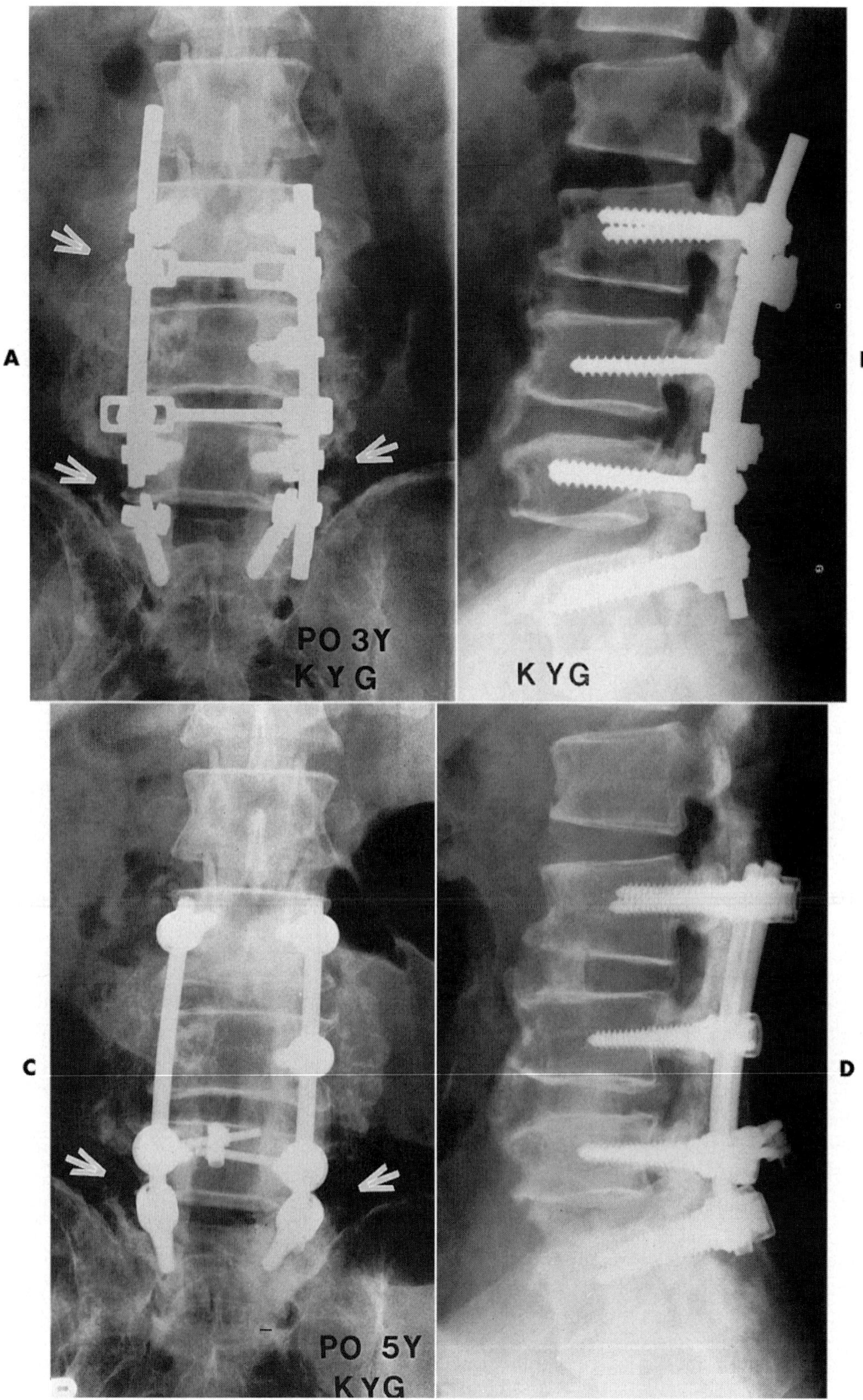


**FIGURE 29-4**

**A, B,** A 52-year-old man presenting with severe mechanical back pain 3 years after the initial operation for spinal stenosis of L3-L4-L5-S1. Rod migration and bilateral nonunion of posterolateral graft at L5-S1 is observed. On exploration, all segments subjected to previous fusion demonstrated micromotion. The implant was changed, placing larger bore screws in the holes created from the previous operation. Following repeat posterior fusion procedure with profuse amount of autogenous iliac bone graft, the patient was flipped over and anterior fusion was performed for each segment. **C,** Two years after the revision, despite the posterior repeat fusion attempt, L5-S1 is still unfused posteriorly. **D,** The solid anterior fusion, however, maintained spinal stability; the patient is back pain-free.

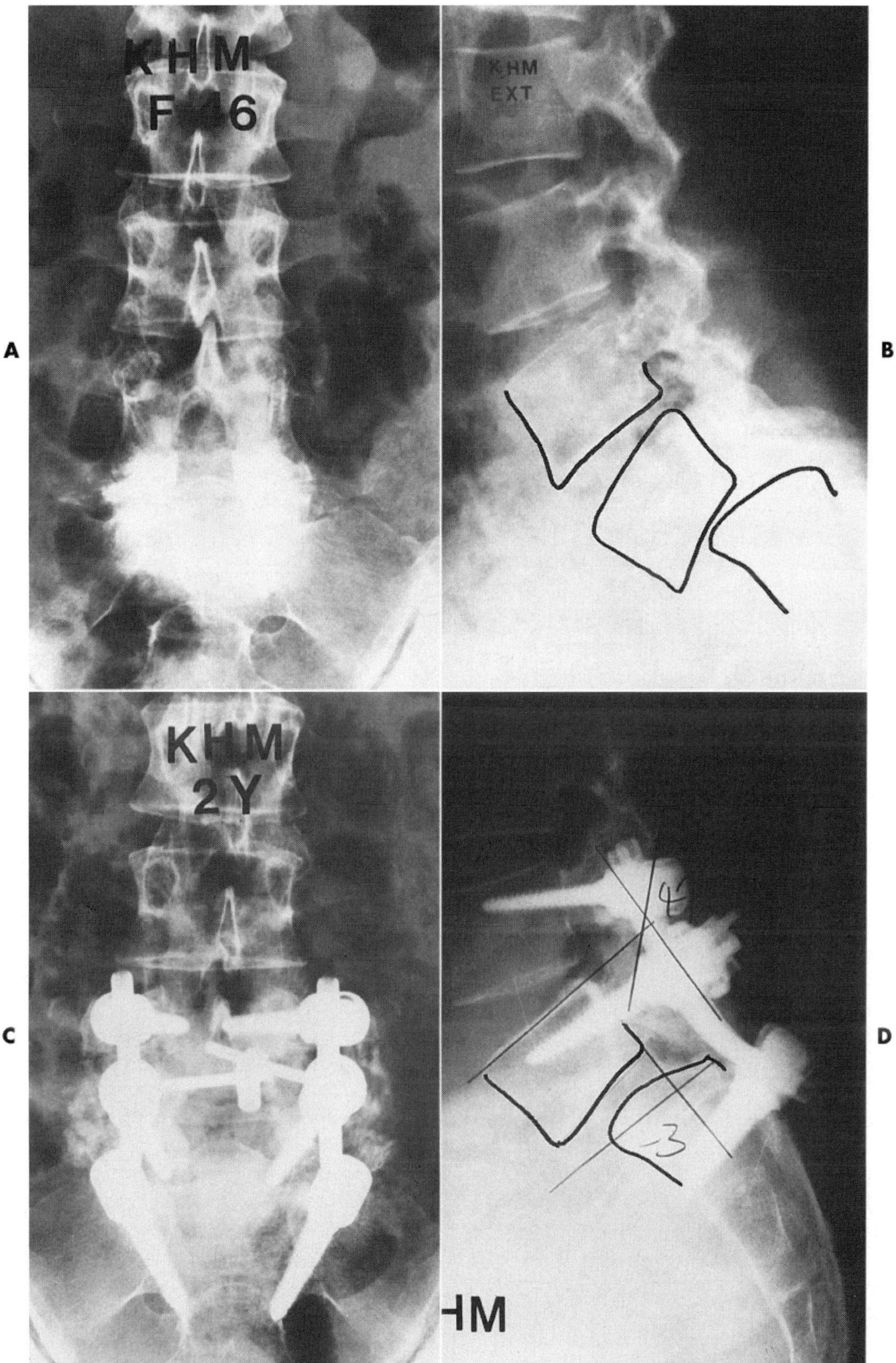


FIGURE 29-5

A 46-year-old woman with severe mechanical back pain. She had been operated on for L5-S1 disk herniation 16 years prior to the visit. **A, B,** Radiographs reveal severe degenerative change of the L5-S1 facets and anterior displacement of L5 on S1. **C, D,** She was treated by circumferential fusion with posterior segmental pedicle screw instrumentation. At 2 years, the union is solid, and the reduction gained in the revision surgery is well-maintained.

***Acquired Spondylolysis.*** This is a rare complication occurring almost exclusively following posterior midline fusion. It is caused by weakening of the neural arch and possibly by interference with the blood supply by excessive decortication.[3,8,10,22] It is treated by posterolateral or anterior fusion, preferably with instrumentation.[23]

### WITH DEFORMITY

***Decompensation.*** Decompensation from derangement of spinal balance may be a cause of unsatisfactory result in patients with degenerative spine deformities. They are usually caused by overcorrection of the instrumented segment in the presence of an uncorrected rigid curve of significant magnitude. To avoid this complication, all patients with degenerative scoliosis and kyphosis should be evaluated by preoperative standing-and-bending radiographs as in idiopathic scoliosis, and the index curve should be included in the fusion.[2] Decompensation is diagnosed clinically by head balance over the sacrum and trunk tilt, both in the coronal and the sagittal plane. When there is a significant enough trunk tilt so as to cause a discomfort when assuming a comfortable posture in standing and walking, revision is indicated (Fig. 29-6). Coronal plane decompensation with normal sagittal profile is treated by extending the fusion to include the entire length of the curve. When the sagittal profile is deranged, the sagittal curve is restored by extending the posterior instrumentation to include the entire length of the sagittal deformity with the rod contoured into a normal sagittal curve. When the sagittal deformity is rigid or severe enough as to produce a significant change in the disk spaces, osteotomy or anterior release and chip bone graft fusion of the anterior column is performed to enhance correction and prevent instrument failures.[11]

***Junctional Kyphosis.*** Reconstruction of the lumbar sagittal profile during internal fixation by a rod contoured to normal lordosis may result in junctional kyphosis when the vertebral segments proximal to the instrumented segments fail to conform to the restored lordosis.[2] This often happens in patients with decreased lordosis. The junctional kyphosis is usually asymptomatic but, when severe, may cause sagittal decompensation and back pain localized over the apex of the kyphosis. Because most of the patients do well with aggressive conservative therapy, surgical treatment is considered only in those with severe disability unresponsive to a prolonged period of nonoperative treatment. Surgical treatment consists of extending the fusion with instrumentation to at least two levels proximal to the kyphotic apex, at the same time contouring the rod into less lordosis, conforming to the patient's preoperative sagittal profile.

***Pseudarthrosis.*** Pseudarthrosis in long fusions may be the cause of recurrent deformity in primary fusions done for degenerative deformities. Pseudarthrosis is not an uncommon finding in recurrent deformity of degenerative spondylolisthesis, in which disk excision was performed during the primary operation.

### OTHERS

***Postoperative Infection.*** Postoperative infections comprise superficial and deep wound infections, discitis, osteomyelitis (involving the anterior, middle, or posterior compartment), and epidural abscess. Superficial wound infections are usually managed with intravenous antibiotics and rarely require surgical treatment. Deep posterior infections are treated by wound drainage. Two available options are closing the wound over a suction drainage for continuous irrigation and leaving the wound open for secondary closure. We prefer the latter, because the former often has problems with tube obstruction caused by clogging with necrotic debris. Deep infection in the presence of metallic internal fixation devices is treated similarly by wound drainage without removal of the instrument. The wound is closed when the discharge is scanty and granulation tissue fills the wound.

Discitis is characterized by intense back pain, presenting usually 2 weeks to 3 months after the primary operation. The diagnosis is made on the basis of aspiration of the disk space (which is more often sterile), bone scan, and MRI. If the primary operation did not include a fusion, the patient is immobilized in a plaster cast with intravenous antibiotics for 4 to 6 weeks. If fusion with internal fixation devices has been included in the primary procedure, the fixation devices are left in situ and antibiotics are administered for 4 to 6 weeks.

Postoperative osteomyelitis is characterized by systemic signs of infection and increased sedimentation rate with leukocytosis.[1] In osteomyelitis involving the anterior and the middle column, early MRI demonstrates the involvement of the vertebral bodies. The radiographic changes of vertebral destruction and collapse ensues later in the process. Although there are advocates of conservative treatment with antibiotics coverage and external immobilization, anterior debridement and fusion yield the best result. Posterior osteomyelitis is a rare complication occurring in long-standing posterior wound infection. It should be suspected when the posterior infected wound healing is delayed beyond the usual course. Aggressive debridement, 4 to 6 weeks of antibiotics, and external cast immobilization yields satisfactory results in most of the cases. If posterior instrumentation has been used in the primary operation, it is left undisturbed. It should be kept until a solid fusion is achieved (Fig. 29-7).

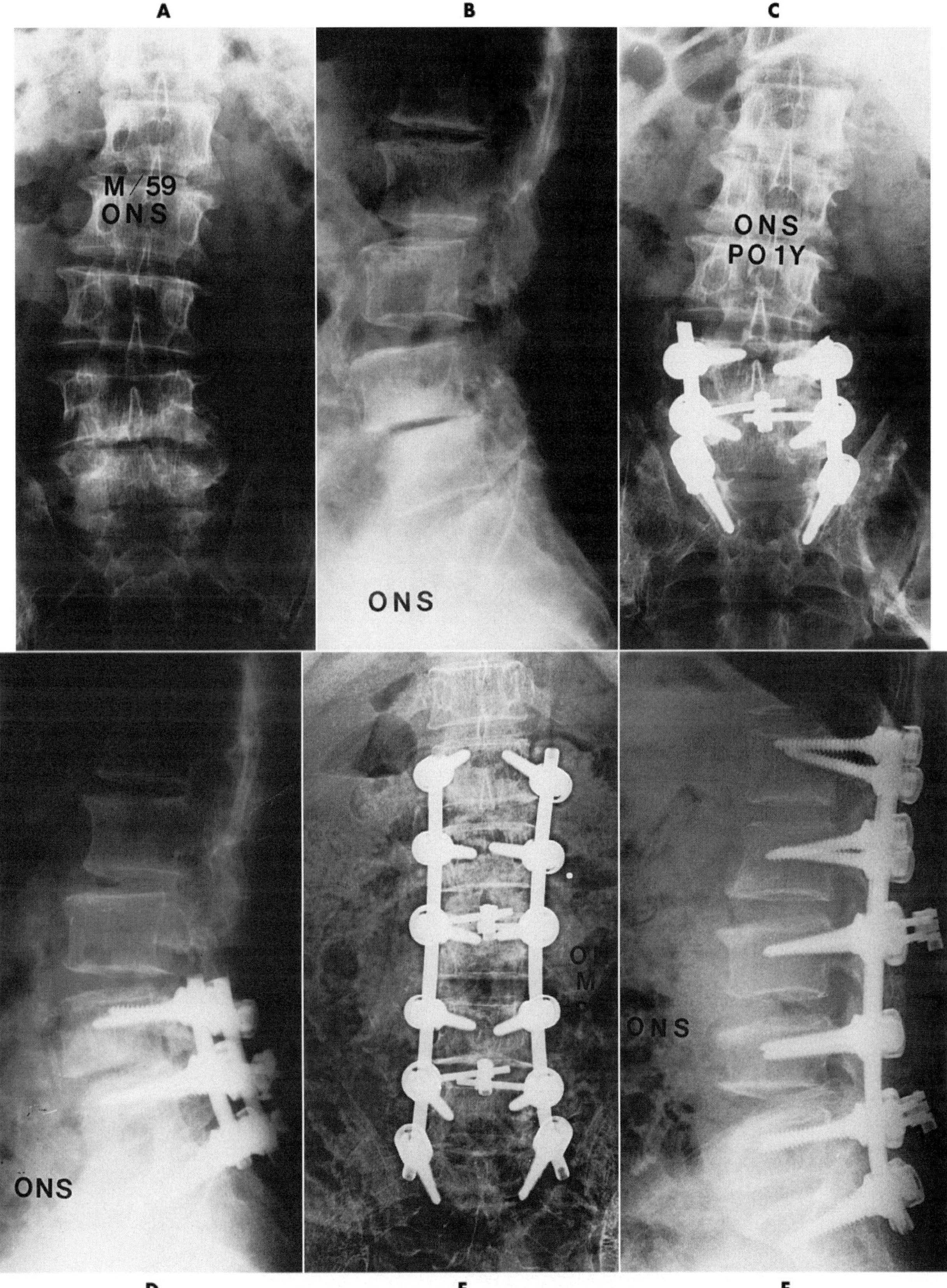


**FIGURE 29-6**

**A-D,** A 59-year-old man with degenerative scoliosis and spinal stenosis. Although the main lesion was L4-L5-S1, degenerative changes are seen at L2-L3 and L3-L4. **E** and **F,** One year after decompression and fusion of L4-L5-S1, the patient is decompensated with a trunk tilt. Radiographs demonstrate the progression of the curve with aggravation of degenerative change in the upper segments.

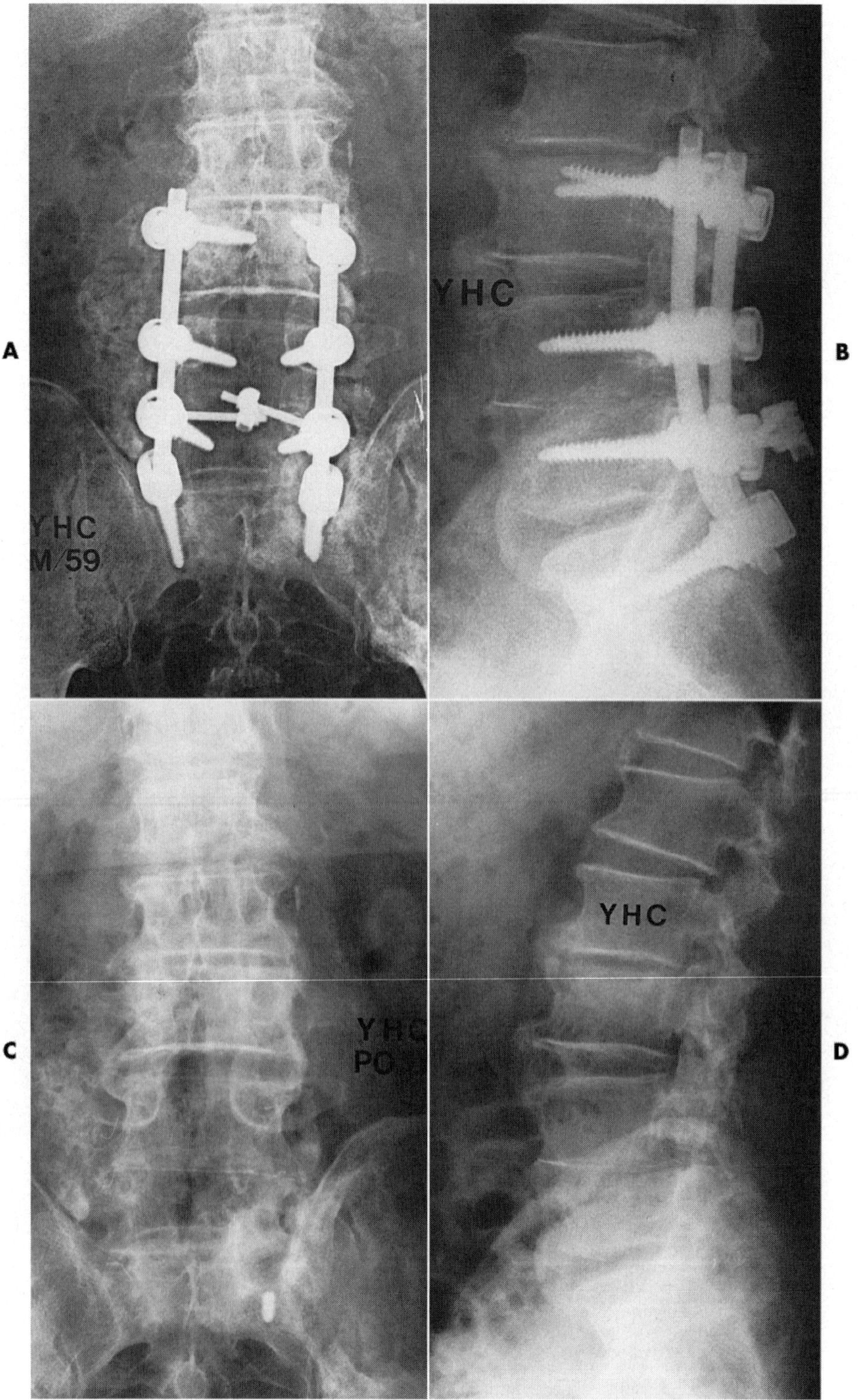


FIGURE 29-7

**A, B,** A 60-year-old man with deep posterior infection following an operation for spinal stenosis. He was managed by wound debridement and prolonged open dressing. **C, D,** At 1 year after the operation, the instrument was removed after confirming solid fusion.

Epidural abscess is a rare complication, usually occurring in association with vertebral osteomyelitis. It is suspected when the patient with suspected osteomyelitis has increasing neurologic symptoms and signs. MRI is the diagnostic method of choice, and early decompression is mandatory. Isolated epidural abscess occurring in the acute postoperative period may be difficult to distinguish from hematoma collection, and its possibility should always be kept in mind.

## PROGRESSION OF THE DEGENERATIVE PROCESS

### WITH NEUROLOGIC COMPROMISE

***Recurrent Stenosis.*** Recurrence of spinal stenosis in a level previously treated for stenosis is attributable to inadequate removal of bony components in the primary operation, resulting in regrowth of the bony components compressing the neural elements.[8,9] The clinical manifestations and radiologic findings are similar to ordinary spinal stenosis. The treatment consists of complete decompression by wide facetectomy, unroofing of the neural foramen, and fusion with rigid internal fixation.

***Adjacent Disk Degeneration.*** Degeneration of a previously normal disk adjacent to a fusion is thought to be the result of a concentration of excessive stress in a mobile segment next to a fused segment that absorbs little motion.[15,28] Although they occur late, sometimes years after the primary operation, early degeneration within months has been reported following a circumferential fusion. The degeneration may be in the form of disk herniation or collapse, with loss of disk height, narrowing of the neural foramen, and lateral recess, eventually causing spinal stenosis.[15] Surgical treatment is indicated when back and leg pain is not adequately controlled by conservative treatment. Symptomatic disk herniation and spinal stenosis are treated by wide posterior decompression and extension of the previous fusion to include the decompressed segment (Fig. 29-8). When the disk is not ruptured, simple disk excision is contraindicated, because it may cause later disk space collapse and degenerative symptoms.

***Stenosis Above or Below a Fusion.*** Stenosis above or below a fusion is usually due to progression of the degenerative process in the levels in which degenerative changes were mild, as to escape decompression at the time of the primary operation.[8] This is considered a new disease and treated as primary surgery (Fig. 29-9).

### WITH INSTABILITY

***Degenerative Instability in Adjacent Level.*** Adjacent-level instability is usually caused by disk degeneration with loss of height. It is diagnosed on motion radiographs. When symptoms are severe and fail to respond to conservative therapy, extension of the fusion to include the unstable segment is indicated.

### WITH DEFORMITY

***Degenerative Arthritis in Adjacent Levels.*** Deformity may be caused by segmental instability from disk degeneration in the levels in the vicinity of the fusion, when simultaneous facet degeneration results in failures of posterior locking mechanism. It usually takes a form of rotary subluxation of facets. When deformity is severe enough to cause mechanical back pain or trunk imbalance, extension of fusion with rigid internal fixation is recommended.

### OTHERS

***Disk Disruption.*** Disk disruption may be a cause of continuous symptoms in a patient with a solid arthrodesis, especially when the primary procedure has been a posterior uninstrumented fusion, as it allows a significant amount of anterior motion even when fully consolidated.[8,9,15] Diagnosis is made by diskography and demonstration of endplate changes on MRI. When posterior fusion is solid, the treatment is a simple anterior fusion. When there is a posterior pseudarthrosis, pseudarthrosis repair by circumferential fusion, preferably with instrumentation, is recommended.

## CONCLUSIONS

Prevention is always the best treatment. The same applies to the spine surgery. As we have reviewed, a significant portion of the causes of revision are from the errors of the surgeon performing the primary surgery and are more or less preventable by a careful preoperative evaluation and sound surgical technique.

The most common causes of failure requiring revision are incomplete decompression of bony elements and fusion failures. To reduce failures from the former cause, a complete decompression of the bony elements and total unroofing of the foramen are mandatory even for the primary operations. Of course, such a wide decompression mandates a fusion, but doing an aggressive decompression during the primary surgery is much easier than performing a repeat decompression. Spine stabilization is greatly enhanced by modern rigid internal fixation devices. However, it must always be kept in mind that the ultimate goal for an instrumentation is a solid bony union. Without an adequate environment for bony union, however hard and rigid the internal fixation devices, they are destined to fail. It needs an adequate area of well-prepared fusion bed and a large amount of graft bone, preferably autogenous can-

*Text continued on p. 413*

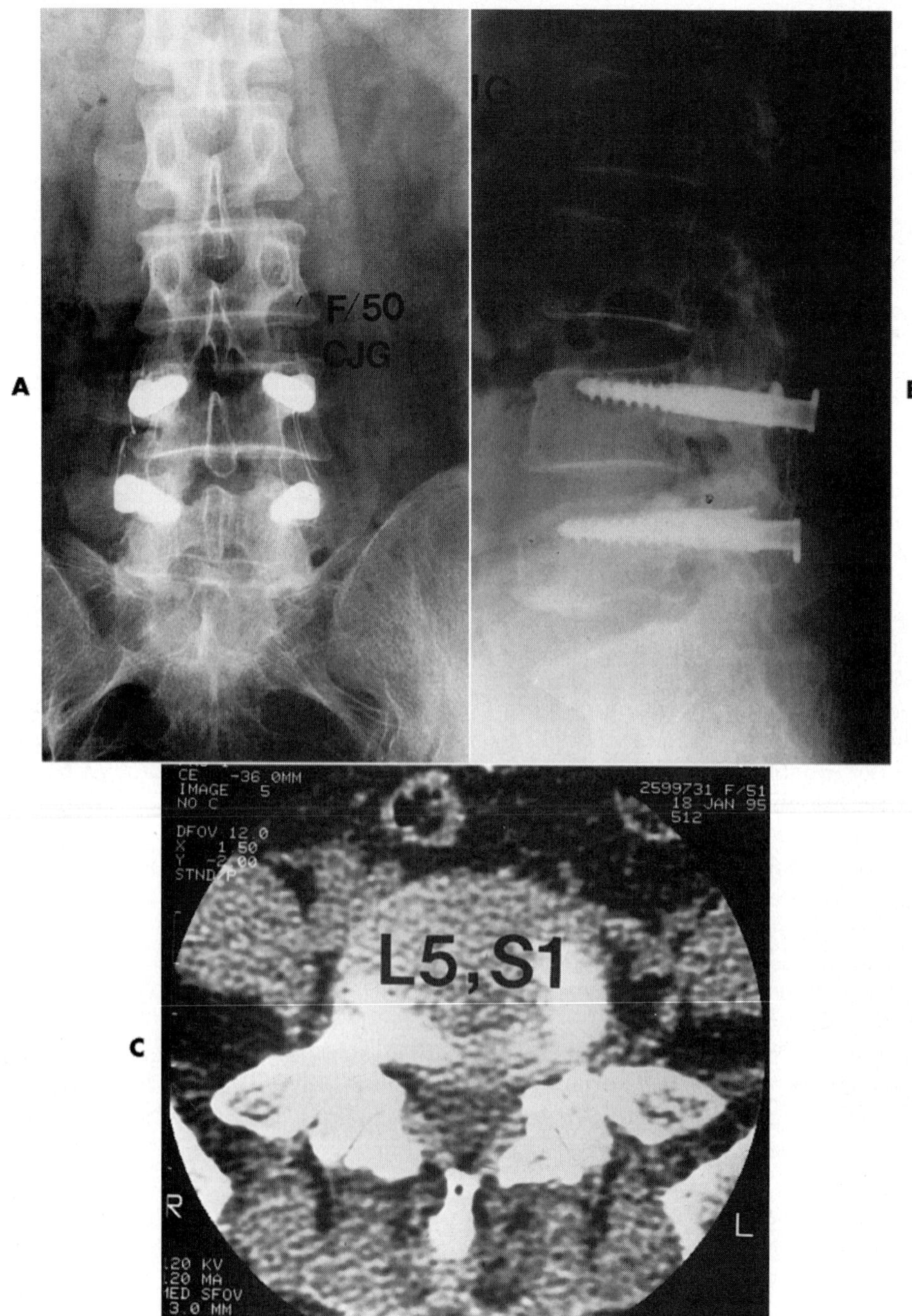


**FIGURE 29-8**

**A, B,** A 50-year-old man with recently developed radiating pain of both lower extremities. He had diskectomy and soft stabilization procedure with artificial ligaments 3 years prior to the visit. **C,** CT scan revealed herniation of L4-L5 and L5-S1 disks.

*Continued*

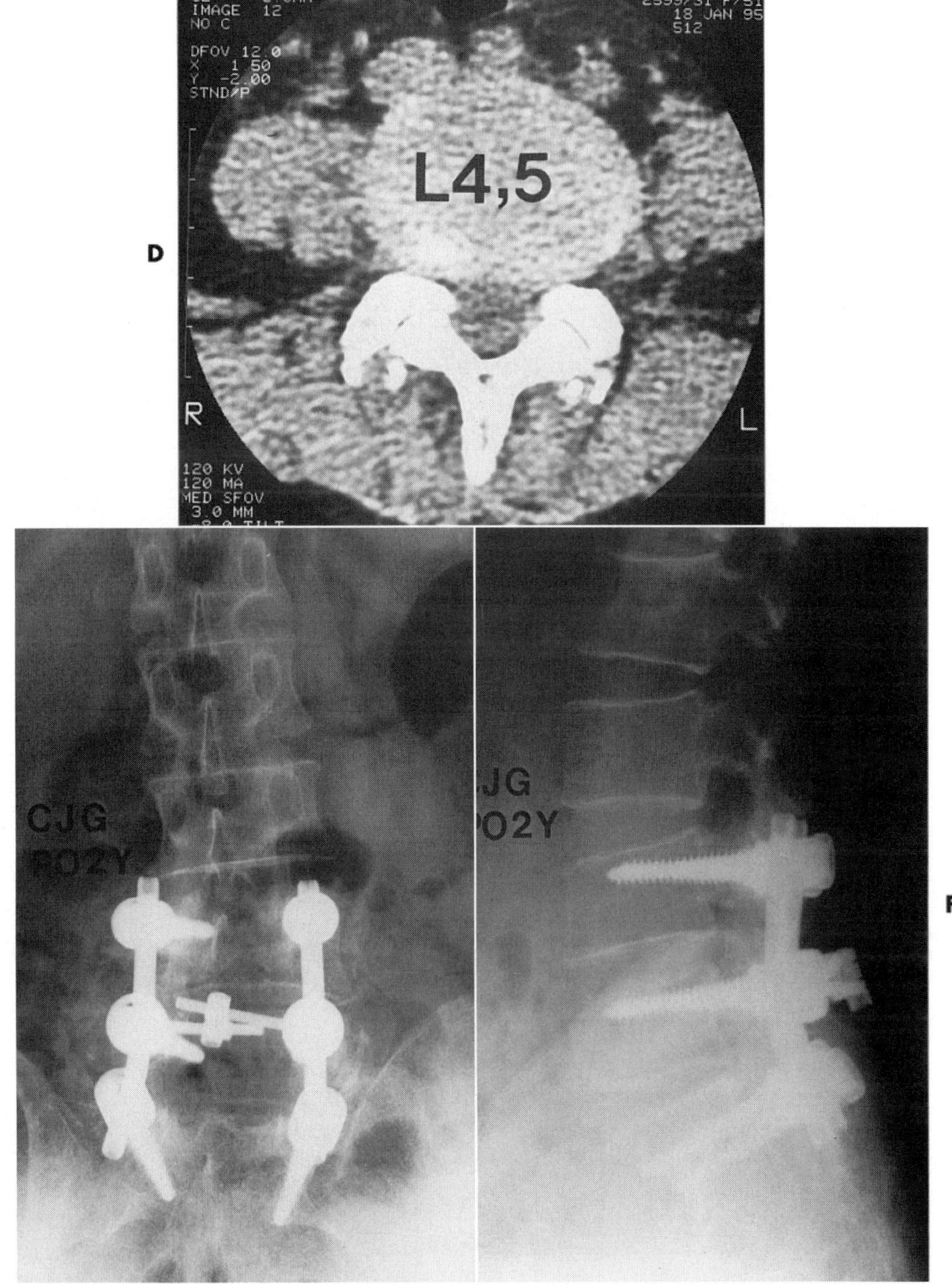


FIGURE 29-8, CONT'D

**D,** CT scan revealed herniation of L4-L5 and L5-S1 disks. **E, F,** The patient was treated by removal of the prior implant, bilevel disk excision and fusion with a pedicle screw instrument.

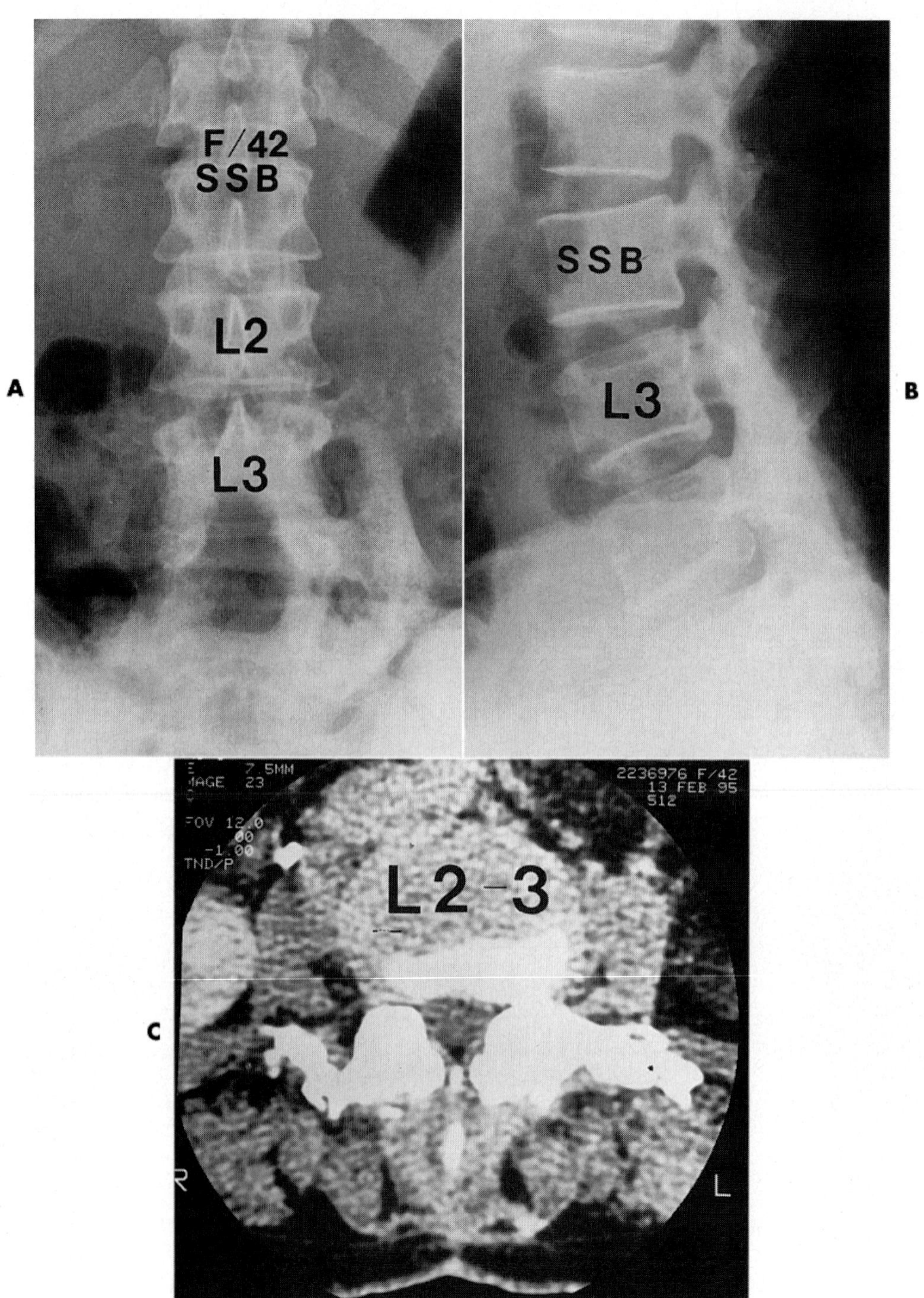


**Figure 29-9**

**A, B,** A 42-year-old woman with recent onset of neurogenic claudication. She had been operated on for stenosis of L3-L4-L5-S1 4 years prior to the visit. The posterolateral fusion was solid. **C,** CT scan revealed stenosis of L2-L3. Previously operated levels were doing well.

*Continued*

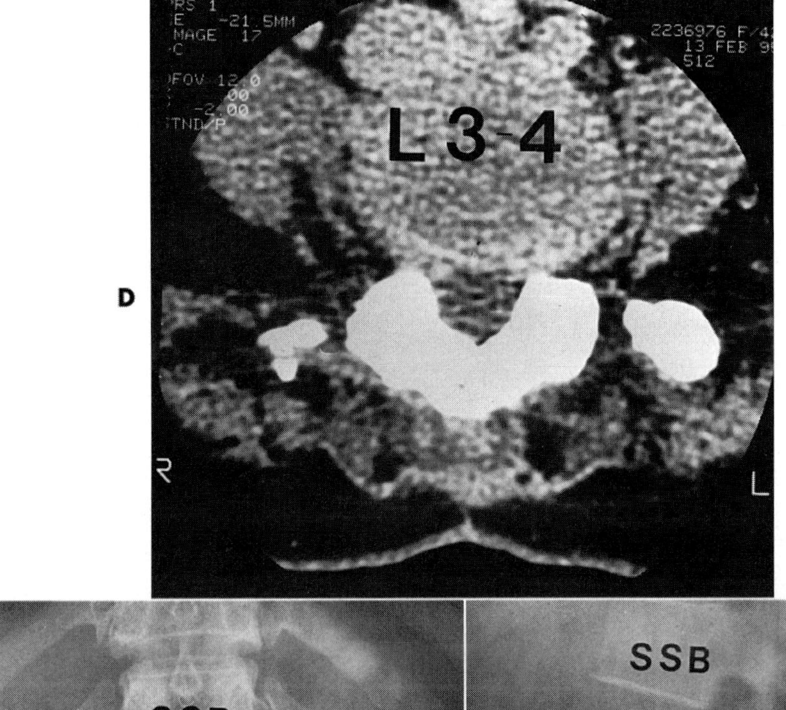


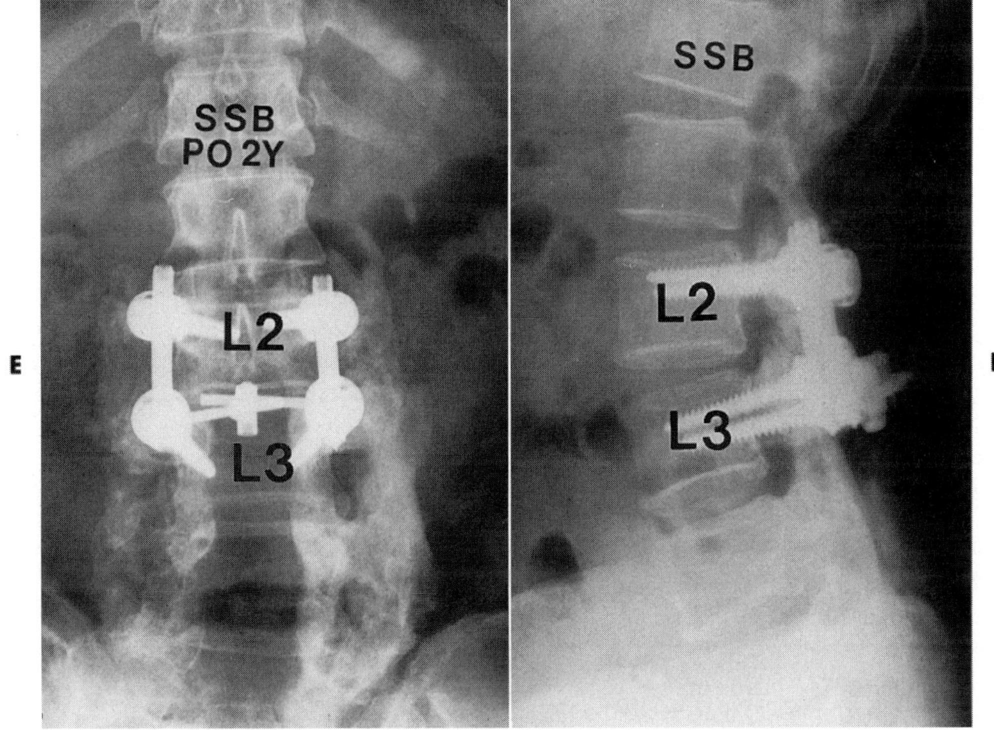


**FIGURE 29-9, CONT'D**

**D,** CT scan revealed stenosis of L2-L3. Previously operated levels were doing well. **E** and **F,** Decompression of L2-L3 followed by pedicle screw fixation. Fusion is solid after 2 years.

cellous from the iliac crests. If the posterior compartment is unable to provide such a bed, interbody fusion must be attempted. The same applies to a revision surgery to prevent another revision.

## REFERENCES

1. Arend SM, Steenmeyer AV, Mosmans PC, Bijlmer HA, van't Wout JW: Postoperative cauda syndrome caused by *Staphylococcus aureus, Infection* 21(4):248-250, 1993.
2. Bradford DS, Ahmed KB, Moe JH et al: The surgical management of patients with Scheuermann's disease, *J Bone Joint Surg* 62A:705-712, 1980.
3. Brunet JA, Wiley JJ: Acquired spondylolysis after spinal fusion, *J Bone Joint Surg* 66B:720-724, 1984.

4. Carroll S, Wiesel S: Neurologic complications and lumbar laminectomy. A standardized approach to the multiply operative lumbar spine, *Clin Orthop* 284:14-23, 1992.
5. Crock HV: Internal disc disruption: a challenge to disc prolapse fifty years on, *Spine* 11:650-653, 1986.
6. Finnegan WJ, Fenlin JM, Marvel JP, Nardini RJ, Rothman RH: Results of surgical intervention in the symptomatic multi-operated back patient. Analysis of 67 cases followed for three to seven years, *J Bone Joint Surg* 61A:1077-1082, 1979.
7. Frank JS, David GN, Faiq M, Christoper BM: Effects of spinal instrumentation on fusion of the lumbosacral spine, *Spine* 20(18):2023-2028, 1995.
8. Frymoyer JW, Hanley EN Jr, Howe J, Kuhlmann D, Matteri RE: A comparison of radiographic findings in fusion and nonfusion patients, ten or more years following lumbar disc surgery, *Spine* 4(5):435-440, 1979.
9. Hanley EN Jr, Shapiro DE: The development of low-back pain after excision of a lumbar disc, *J Bone Joint Surg* 71A:719-721, 1989.
10. Harris RI, Wiley JJ: Acquired spondylolysis as a sequel to spine fusion, *J Bone Joint Surg* 45A:1159-1170, 1963.
11. Jeffrey D, Boachie-Adjei O, Wilson M: One stage versus two stage anterior and posterior spinal reconstruction in adults: comparison of outcomes including nutritional status, complication rates, hospital costs and other factors, *Spine* 17:S310-S316, 1992.
12. Jeffery NK, Stephen JL, Sharon AL, Anne HF, Matthew HL: Seven to ten-year outcome of decompressive surgery for degenerative lumbar spinal stenosis, *Spine* 21(1):92-98, 1996.
13. Johnsson KE, Redlund-Johnell I, Uden A, Willner S: Preoperative and postoperative instability in lumbar spinal stenosis, *Spine* 14:591-593, 1989.
14. Kim S, Michelsen C: Revision surgery for failed back surgery syndrome, *Spine* 17(8):957-960, 1992.
15. Nagata H, Schendel MJ, Transfeldt E, Lewis JL: The effects of immobilization of long segments of the spine on the adjacent and distal facet force and lumbosacral motion, *Spine* 18(16):2471-2479, 1993.
16. Zdeblick TA: A prospective, randomized study of lumbar fusion: Preliminary results, *Spine* 18(8):983-991, 1993 [see comments, *Spine* 19(1):109, 1994].
17. Macnab I: Negative disc exploration: an analysis of the causes of nerve-root involvement in 68 patients, *J Bone Joint Surg* 53A:891-903, 1971.
18. Mayer TG, Gatchel RJ, Kishino N, Keeley J, Capra P, Mayer H, Barnett J, Mooney V: Objective assessment of spine function following industrial injury: a prospective study with comparison group and one-year follow-up, *Spine* 10:482-493, 1985.
19. North R, Campbell J, James C, et al: Failed back surgery syndrome: 5-year follow-up in 102 patients undergoing repeated operation, *Neurosurgery* 28:685-690, 1991.
20. O'Brien JP, Dawson MH, Heard CW, et al: Simultaneous combined anterior and posterior fusion: a surgical solution for failed spinal surgery with a brief review of the first 150 patients, *Clin Orthop* 203:191-195, 1986.
21. Quiles M, Marchisello PS, Tsairis P: Lumbar adhesive arachnoiditis. Etiology and pathologic aspects, *Spine* 3:45-50, 1978.
22. Quinnell RC, Stockdale HR: Some experimental observations on the influence of a single lumbar floating fusion on the remaining lumbar spine, *Spine* 6:263-267, 1981.
23. Raugstad TS, Harbo K, Hogberg A, Skeie S: Anterior interbody fusion of the lumbar spine, *Acta Orthop Scand* 53:561-565, 1982.
24. Ross J, Masaryk T, Schrader M, et al: MR imaging of the postoperative lumbar spine: assessment with gadopentetate dimeglumine, *Am J Neuroradiol* 11(4):771-776, 1990.
25. Rydevik B, Brown MD, Lundborg G: The pathoanatomy and pathophysiology of nerve root compression, *Spine* 9:7-15, 1984.
26. Schofferman L, Schofferman J, Zucherman J, Gunthorpe H, Hsu K, Picetti G, Goldthwaite N, White A: Occult infections causing persistent low-back pain, *Spine* 14:417-419, 1989.
27. Spengler DM, Freeman C, Westbrook R, Miller JW: Low-back pain following multiple lumbar spine procedures. Failure of initial selection, *Spine* 5:356-360, 1980.
28. Stokes IAF, Wilder DG, Frymoyer JW, et al: Assessment of patients with low back pain by biplanar radiographic measurement of intervertebral motion, *Spine* 6:223-239, 1981.
29. Suk SI, Lee CK, Kim KT, Kim WJ, Ha CW: A comparison of computerized tomography (CT), myelo-enhanced computerized tomography (MECT) and magnetic resonance imaging (MRI) in diagnosis of spinal stenosis, *J Korean Orthop Assoc* 26(1):6-11, 1991.
30. Suk SI, Lee CK, Kim KT, Kim WJ, Kim HS: The surgical treatment of spondylolisthesis, *J Korean Orthop Assoc* 26(1):334-343, 1991.
31. Suk SI, Lee CK, Lee CS, Kim EH, Huh MG: Cotrel-Dubousset pedicle screw fixation after posterior decompression of lumbar spinal stenosis, *J Korean Orthop Assoc* 25(1):161-168, 1990.
32. Suk SI, Lee CK, Lee JH, Kim WJ, Cho KI, Kim HK: Adding posterior lumbar interbody fusion to pedicle screw fixation and posterolateral fusion after decompression, *Spine* 22:210-220, 1997.
33. Suk SI, Lee JH, Min HJ, Kim HS, Ha CW, Park SE: Salvage procedure in failed low back surgery, *J Korean Orthop Assoc* 26(3):1009-1016, 1993.
34. Waddell G, Kummel EG, Lotto WN et al: Failed lumbar disc surgery and repeat surgery following industrial injuries, *J Bone Joint Surg* 61A:201-207, 1979.
35. Wiesel SW: The multiply operated lumbar spine. *Instr Course Lect* XXXIV:68-77, 1985.
36. Zinreich SJ, Long DM, Davis R, Quinn CB, McAfee PC, Wang H: Three-dimensional CT imaging in postsurgical "failed back" syndrome, *J Comput Assist Tomogr* 14(4):574-580, 1990.

# 30

# REVISION SPINAL STENOSIS

**Fabien D. Bitan, M.D.**
**Russell T. Nevins, M.D.**
**Aron D. Rovner, M.D.**
**Joseph Y. Margulies, M.D., Ph.D.**



"Congenital stricture of the vertebral canal"[44] was the first publication that clinically identified spinal stenosis as a distinct clinical entity. Sarpyener wrote the article in 1945. The literature shows that surgical treatment for stenosis had been performed for more than 140 years prior to this article. During the nineteenth century, Sachs and Frankel operated on lumboradicular pain and bent gait. Intraoperatively they found no tumor or abscess and only a thickened lamina.[42] Today this type of lamina is described as a shingled lamina. Surprisingly, a percentage of these patients had relief from the procedure. Portal in 1803 determined that thecal sac compression was correlated to spinal stenosis. Lane in 1893 performed the first decompression for cauda equina syndrome. In 1911, Russell Hibbs of New York performed the first fusion, although done for patients with scoliosis and spinal tuberculosis.[30] In the same year the "slipped" disk was recognized as a cause of low back pain and sciatica. Thirty-seven years later, Van Gelderen identified one cause of neurogenic claudication as hypertrophy of the ligamentum flavum. Verbiest, in 1954, went one step further by associating neurogenic claudication with a complete block on myelogram.[49] In 1978, Kikaldy-Willis described the three joint complex theory to explain the pathology.

Over the past twenty years an explosion of new understanding and treatment of spinal stenosis has emerged. However, even with the use of computed tomography (CT) scans, magnetic resonance imaging (MRI), hardware, and fusions, Postacchini estimated that 10% of patients who undergo initial spinal surgery for stenosis eventually need further surgery for the same condition.[37] This chapter discusses spinal stenosis with a focus on the causes of, imaging techniques for, and treatment of a patient with a poor primary surgical outcome.

## ANATOMY

The posterior column is the zone most commonly involved in lumbar stenosis. The posterior ligamentous complex consists of the supra- and infraspinous ligaments as well as the ligamentum flavum and the facet joint capsules. Each corresponding vertebral bony arch is separated superiorly and inferiorly by the foramen that gives way to the nerve roots. The superior portion of the foramen contains the nerve root of the superior level, as well as the vessels and nerves supplying the spinal canal itself.

Understanding the embryological growth of the spinal cord is vital to comprehending how the pathway that nerve roots take from the cord to the periphery plays a role in the physiopathology of lumbar stenosis. Moore explains that the cord is the entire length of the vertebral canal in the embryo.[32] However, the vertebral column and dura mater grow more rapidly than the spinal cord does, so this relationship does not persist. In fact, by adulthood the most caudal tip of the spinal cord may be found anywhere from the twelfth thoracic to the third lumbar vertebrae. The dural sac extends the entire length of the vertebral column and contains the cauda equina. The cauda equina ends at approximately the level of S1-S2.[32] Because in the adult the cord is shorter than the column the nerve roots emerge from the thecal sac above their corresponding foramen. An easy way to remember the levels, as suggested by Louis,[29] of emergence is:

-L1 root at the middle of the L1 body
-L2 root at the upper $\frac{1}{2}$ of L2 body
-L3 root at the upper $\frac{1}{3}$ of L3 body
-L4 root at the upper $\frac{1}{4}$ of L4 body
-L5 root at the upper $\frac{1}{5}$ of L5 body
-S1 root just above the L5-S1 disk

Because the nerve roots emerge cephalad in comparison to where they exit the foramina, they travel in the canal in an oblique direction. The lateral recess is a vertical canal opened medially, and it contains the level's nerve root until it exits the canal through the foramen.[28] The most cephalad roots travel in an almost horizontal direction, whereas the lower roots travel almost entirely vertically.

## LUMBAR STENOSIS: A PHYSIOPATHOLOGIC UNDERSTANDING

Spinal stenosis can be broken down into two major types: congenital and acquired. The congenital form of stenosis may be idiopathic or may be found as part of a syndrome, such as achondroplasia. In this chapter, we will focus on the more common acquired variety. There are six types of acquired stenosis: degenerative, degenerative combined with congenital, spondylolytic, iatrogenic, posttraumatic, and metabolic.

The typical patient with degenerative lumbar stenosis is the middle-aged or older person. The major cause is chronic degeneration of a disk. One concept to explain how a degenerative disk begins a cascade effect that is responsible for lumbar stenosis was described by Kirkaldy-Willis. The theory begins with degeneration of a disk. This degeneration results in decreasing disk height and possible posterior bulging of the disk. Decreasing the disk height leads to an increasing force transmitted to the facets. Because Wolff's law states "Every change in the function of a bone is followed by certain definite changes in internal and external conformation in accordance with mathematical laws,"[6] the increased force across the facets leads to the compensatory development of osteophytes. Hence, it is the increasing bone formation and its corresponding narrowing of the canal that is the cause of the stenosis.

Another important factor in the etiology of stenosis is the understanding that the osteoligamentous spine and the neural elements inside have a dynamic relationship. In flexion the nerve roots are stretched and thinned concurrently. The roots may be stretched up to 10 mm. The upper roots slide downward, the lower roots slide upward, the converging point being around L4.[29] In extension, the roots bulge. This bulging during extension may explain, at least in part, why some patients have a "bent gait."

## MAJOR TYPES OF DEGENERATIVE LUMBAR STENOSIS

### CENTRAL STENOSIS

This multilevel stable form of stenosis is directly related to the lamina compressing the thecal sac. The laminae are oblique in the sagittal plane, with the upper border slanted toward the canal, making this border of the lamina most frequently involved in compressing the neural elements. If the anteroposterior (AP) diameter of the dural sac is less than 10 mm, stenotic symptoms are likely. If this diameter is 10 to 13 mm it is considered relative stenosis.[48] Other causes for the compression of the cord include posterior vertebral body osteophytes, hypertrophic articular facets that grow in a transverse plane toward the canal (usually the superior facet of the lower vertebra), a thickened ligamentum flavum that dynamically compresses the canal with extension, and even a hypertrophic articular capsule. Epstein found that the mean diameter measured at the level of the superior border of the pedicle is from 5 to 7 mm with slight variations according to the level.

The goal of primary surgery in central stenosis is to release the dural sac. The major risks for a failed procedure and the need for revision surgery can be categorized into operative/perioperative and long-term causes.

Operative/perioperative causes for failure include: (1) inadequate central decompression of the identified pathology, (2) inadequate lateral exploration and release, thereby missing a latent asymptomatic lateral stenosis that can become symptomatic postoperatively, and (3) not identifying instability, thereby failing to use instrumentation when necessary

Long-term causes of failure include: (1) newly formed stenosis at, above, or below the level of surgery, (2) various local degenerative phenomena, and (3) pseudarthrosis after spinal fusion.

### Lateral Recess Stenosis, Foraminal Stenosis, and Extraforaminal Stenosis

These forms of unilateral and stable stenosis do not occur to the central cord but to the nerve roots, the ganglions, or the spinal nerves. Lateral recess stenosis is when compression of the nerve root occurs anywhere in the vertical canal prior to its exit through the foramen. Nerve compression occurring within the foramen or beyond the foramen is known as foraminal stenosis or extraforaminal stenosis, respectively. For a better understanding of the topographical causes of stenosis, Lee subdivides this region. His most medial zone (or entrance zone) is where the nerve root exits the canal, beneath the facet joint. Osteophytes or posterolateral disk bulging both increase the risk of compression at this site. The mid-zone is located beneath the pars and pedicle. The third zone or exit zone consists of the intervertebral foramen proper. Under normal circumstances, the intervertebral foramen is approximately 20 to 23 mm high and 8 to 10 mm wide. Osteophytes, lateral disk protrusion, and facet joint subluxation all can cause stenosis in this zone. The final region that Lee described was the extraforaminal zone. An osseous ridge along the endplates and compression by a transverse process are such causes of stenosis in this zone. Compression at this site is called *far-out syndrome of Wiltse.*[53] The L4-L5 level and therefore the L4 nerve root is the most commonly affected site of lateral recess stenosis.

Failure of primary surgery of a lateral recess stenosis can occur because: (1) the surgeon did not take into account that the nerve root compression occurred at more than one level and total decompression was not performed, (2) a foraminotomy was not complete in decompressing the hypertrophied articular process and capsule, (3) fusion was not performed with an unstable spine, and (4) late-onset pain was due to a new level of stenosis (degenerative disease) secondary to the new fusion increasing stress at the ends of the mass fusion.

## CLINICAL MANIFESTATIONS OF SPINAL STENOSIS

The classic patient with lumbar spinal stenosis is the middle-aged person. Regardless if a patient presents with a primary case of spinal stenosis or presents with a failed back syndrome, the clinical manifestations include the same spectrum of symptoms from mild low back pain to severely profound neurologic abnormalities. The three classic symptoms of spinal stenosis are intermittent neurogenic claudication, radicular pain, and lumbar pain.

In Johnsson's 1992 study, 75% of his subjects had claudication,[24] making claudication the most common complaint associated with lumbar stenosis. Symptoms may involve one or more nerve roots causing such complaints as unilateral or bilateral weakness, pain, or radicular tingling especially with ambulation. The cause of the claudication is frequently due to a central compression of the sac. Symptoms tend to decrease or resolve with sitting or bending forward. These maneuvers help because flexion opens the foramen, minimizes the bulging of the ligamentum flavum and the articular capsules, and stretches and thins the spinal canal.

Although these patients experience claudication, presentation is usually different from the vascular type. Although both types present with exercise-induced pain, numbness, and tingling, intermittent neurogenic claudication has a centrifugal pattern. A centrifugal pattern means that the patient will complain of symptoms beginning in the buttocks and proximal thigh and radiating to the distal thigh. With vascular claudication, the symptomatology begins in the distal to proximal calf. In addition, neurogenic claudication symptoms are usually less "painful" and more "bothersome," whereas a vascular claudication typically is painful. To further distinguish the two types, lying flat will relieve the vascular type but may actually worsen the stenotic type by closing the foramen and allowing the cord to bulge.

Nontraumatic radicular pain is also a common complaint in the patient with spinal stenosis. Of Johnsson's subjects, 12.5% complained of radicular pain. This pain is different from the classic radicular (sciatic) pain seen with a herniated nucleus pulposus. This radicular pain tends to be vague in its distribution, and of multilevel topography. The patient tends to report a changed location of symptoms from visit to visit. These patients complain of either radicular pain at rest, which worsens at night, or exercise radiculopathy, which is more common but less specific to spinal stenosis.

Lumbar pain is a frequent complaint from the patient with stenosis. Its spectrum ranges from annoying but nonincapacitating to severe. Because the vast majority of these patients are elderly and have multiple-system problems one can not assume all lumbar pain is stenosis, even in a postsurgical patient. The differential diagnosis includes herniated nucleus pulposus (HNP), degenerative spondylolisthesis, degenerative scoliosis, disk-related low back pain, and even an occult neoplasm. To rule out nonmusculoskeletal causes of pain, the surgeon must consider an abdominal exam to exclude such causes as an abdominal aorta and other internal causes.

Intervertebral instability also causes low back pain in the patient with lumbar stenosis. Intervertebral instability must be distinguished from degenerative back pain. Clinically pain that occurs with the same recurrent motion but is absent when at rest is a sign of instability. An example of this is when a patient has pain every time he attempts to flex forward to pick up his keys off the floor. Intervertebral instability is a major sequel of decompression, especially when bilateral foraminotomies are performed.

Distinguishing between degenerative lower back pain and intervertebral instability is important when deciding on surgical treatment, even with revision surgery. The surgeon must recall that failed back syndrome can be due to both iatrogenic instability as well as newly formed degenerative changes secondary to the stress distribution caused by a mass fusion. When lumbar stenosis is manifested by degenerative pain decompression of the nerve roots and cauda equina may be beneficial. Caputy showed that the incidence of spondylolisthesis at 5 years was higher in the surgical failures than in the surgical successes. He suggests that, because spondylolisthetic stenosis tended to recur within a few years following decompression, stabilization should be carried out at the time of decompression in patients with instability.[8]

## DIAGNOSTIC STUDIES

### PLAIN FILMS

Plain films are extremely nonspecific for lumbar stenosis. Anteroposterior and lateral films will help rule out anatomic bony changes such tumor, metabolic disease, and infections. Postsurgery plain films may show gross bony fusion, iatrogenic spondylolisthesis, hardware placement, and late degenerative changes above and below the fusion as a result of the fusion mass. These changes may include a disk that is "too high" with a widened anterior aspect on the lateral view and traction spurs may suggest instability, and conversely a narrowed disk implies stability[34] although this collapse may be the cause of a new nerve impingement.

Flexion-extension films may also be beneficial, especially when evaluating "dynamic" stenosis.

### LUMBAR MYELOGRAPHY

Over the years, myelography has become the gold standard for diagnosing and localizing the site of compression on the cord. By injecting dye into the subarachnoid space a single view will visualize the path of the radicular (dural) sleeves from the emergence through the central canal and the lateral recess down to the entrance or midpoint of the foramen, where these thecal sleeves end. Each dural sleeve contains two nerve roots, which merge in the foramen just distal to the neural ganglion (forming the vertebral nerve). All neural elements prior to exiting the foramen, from the conus medullaris to the sacrum, can be visualized. Evaluation of dynamic compression is another advantage to this procedure. By injecting the dye and taking flexion and extension views one may see subtle or unsuspected compression or instability.

Myelography is invasive. Although water-soluble contrasts are the most commonly used dyes, complications do occur. Complications include headache, pain, nausea, vomiting, meningitis, and infection. Although rare, potentially fatal seizures have been reported as well.[40]

### ENHANCED COMPUTED TOMOGRAPHY

CT has the advantage of being noninvasive. In addition, lateral lesions such as foraminal stenosis and lateral disk herniations are better visualized. CT differentiates structures according to their densities. Therefore, CT is more sensitive to identify soft tissue lesions over myelography. CT is also a very important radiographic tool for preoperative planning of revision surgery. CT with intravenous contrast differentiates vascularized bodies, such as fibrosis, from the disk. CT with intravenous contrast has an accuracy of 67% to 100% in distinguishing scar from disk. The difficulty in using CT with a patient with a failed back syndrome is the need for large contrast loads and single-plane imaging.[41] The disadvantages to CT include that asymptomatic compression at a different level may be missed. However, CT gives information caudal to the compression site, whereas myelogram does not.

Because both have advantages and disadvantages the gold standard today has become the CT myelogram.

### MAGNETIC RESONANCE IMAGING

The exact role of MRI in diagnosing and treating spinal stenosis in a patient who has been previously operated on is still evolving. MRI has the advantages of visualization of the foramen when myelogram can not, and is at least as equivalent to CT in distinguishing scar from disk[41] but without the need of contrast. Scar shows a higher signal on a T2-weighted image than disk. Ross showed that recent experience with pre-contrast and post-contrast MRI imaging in the postoperative lumbar spine indicated that it was 96% accurate in differentiating scar from disk in 44 patients at 50 reoperated levels.[41]

Disadvantages of MRI at the present time include the fact that no dynamic studies can be obtained, and sagittal cuts give only partial and fragmented views of nerve roots. This fragmentation is due to the oblique pathway that the nerve roots travel en route to the foramen. Most importantly, MRI can not be used for patients with instrumentation, including titanium, thereby excluding a large percentage of failed surgical patients.

## TREATMENT OF A PATIENT WITH FAILED BACK SYNDROME

As with any patient with primary stenosis, a patient with clinical symptomatology should always first receive a trial of conservative medical management. This includes weight control, exercise, and nonsteroidal anti-inflammatory drugs (NSAIDs). A part-time brace may also be of benefit. If these modalities fail, the surgeon must make sure a true failed back syndrome exists and secondary gain is not a factor. The surgeon must also understand why the primary surgery has failed.

The three general philosophies of primary lumbar stenotic surgery are (1) undermine the facets, thereby decompressing the nerve roots and keeping the stability of the spine intact; (2) excise the facet and risk having an unstable spine but better decompression; and (3) excise the facet(s) and add posterolateral fusion (with or without instrumentation), as a form of stabilization, compensating for the loss of the facet function.

Today, the dictum leans toward primary spinal stabilization when concomitant preoperative instability is documented or if the main elements of stability have been disrupted by the bone release. The disk and the posterolateral columns are the major stabilizing elements of the spine. When two of these elements are injured, such as a facetectomy or pars interarticularis fracture and an associated intervertebral disk excision, or facet injury to both sides, instrumentation should be performed. The need for instrumentation when only one element is disrupted is still controversial. White and Wiltse noted subluxation after decompression in 66% of patients with degenerative spondylolisthesis. They suggested that a fusion be performed in conjunction with decompression in patients younger than 60 years old with instability caused by the loss of an articular process on one side, patients younger than 55 years of age with a midline decompression for degenerative spondylolisthesis that preserve the facets, and patients younger than 50 years of age with isthmic spondylolisthesis.[47]

## REVISION SURGERY: CONSIDERATION AND PLANNING

Appropriate patient selection for decompression surgery of spinal stenosis results in good to excellent outcomes.[1,14,16,25,33] However, a percentage of patients continue to have symptoms postoperatively. This may be due to poor patient selection, treatment, or a technical error on the surgeon's part. For example, Caputy showed that spondylolisthetic stenosis tends to recur following decompression alone and stabilization should be performed at the time of decompression.[8]

Revision surgery is not ideal. Guigui et al found that in 36 patients who underwent revision, the results were mediocre at best.[17] Factors that positively affect revision surgery include: a longer asymptomatic time interval between the primary and revision surgery, a newly diagnosed herniation at a new level, and/or a separate identifiable and correctable pathologic cause.[18]

## REVISION SURGERY: OPERATIVE TECHNIQUE

The revision surgeon must have an appreciation for the previously operated spine. The posterior elements, or what were the posterior elements, may now be covered and/or replaced with scar, bony fusion, and implants. Prior to entering the operating room the surgeon must determine if the spine is stable. If the spine is unstable will a posterior approach or an anterior approach be more effective? Both techniques have advantages and disadvantages. The four main surgical procedures for revision surgery are: (1) decompression through posterior approach only, with or without fusion and with or without instrumentation, (2) a 360-degree fusion through a posterior approach using posterior lumbar interbody fusion (PLIF), (3) posterior decompression and anterior approach using anterior lumbar interbody fusion (ALIF), and (4) the option that is becoming more and more popular, reconstructing the disk height and fusion through anterior approach using ALIF. This approach is particularly beneficial in patients with pseudarthrosis.

## POSTERIOR APPROACH ONLY, WITH OR WITHOUT FUSION AND WITH OR WITHOUT STABILIZATION

The initial approach is similar to the approach used for the virgin spine. Scar will inevitably hide the normal anatomy. As one approaches the cord, caution must be taken to avoid dural tears. Dissecting from normal tissue toward the abnormal minimizes the risk of a dural tear. There is debate whether or not to remove any scar that is fixed to the dura. Steffee makes an attempt to gently remove any scar creating the "Christmas tree exposure." He also believes that solid fusion protects from scar formation. Many researchers, however, believe that scar actually makes a protective barrier and there is no reason to dissect it away. If the decompression needs to be expanded laterally this can be done by freeing the inferior edge of the laterally undissected bone from the underlying soft tissues. Once freed, successively larger Kerrison rongeurs can be used to excise this lateral bone. Upon completion of the laminectomy, and when the dural sac is decompressed, the surgeon should confirm that the lateral exposure and release is satisfactory. At this stage the stability should be reconfirmed, and if the decompression destabilized the spine, instrumentation should be employed (Fig. 30-1). One must remember that the objective of surgery is decompression, and the goal should not be compromised by stability considerations. Postoperatively, a latent asymptomatic lateral stenosis can become symptomatic if the lateral exposure and release is not thorough enough. Fusion using bone graft and/or instrumentation may or may not be performed. Sidhy and Herkowitz state that multiple revision patients are a difficult group to treat. Good to excellent results are rare and as such all beneficial tools available to the spine surgeon should be used, especially instrumentation.[46]

## USING A 360-DEGREE FUSION THROUGH A POSTERIOR APPROACH USING PLIF

As a salvage procedure Hutter had an 86% rating of good to excellent results. The advantages of PLIF include a single approach to 360-degree fusion with its great amount of stability, and concurrent excision of the pathologic disk. The procedure entails the same initial steps as discussed in the above section. Here, however, once the nerve roots are identified they should be retracted toward the midline exposing the disk, which is not an innocent surgical maneuver, especially when it is extremely difficult for even the most seasoned surgeon to differentiate between scar and native tissue. The disk is then excised and bone graft replaced.

Failure of posterior lumbar interbody fusion is not uncommon. Wetzel and LaRocca reviewed 12 patients with failed PLIF. They found 11 had extensive epidural fibrosis, 9 had pseudarthrosis of a previous PLIF, and 4 had motion segment dysfunction at a nearby level. Interestingly, seven were believed to have solid fusion but the presence of a solid fusion did not correlate with pain relief.[50]

## POSTERIOR DECOMPRESSION AND ANTERIOR APPROACH USING ALIF

Many cases of failed back surgery are due to such factors as pseudarthrosis, or broken hardware. In fact, Cleveland et al found the incidence of pseudarthrosis to be 20% after spinal fusion.[9] A posterior approach permits decompression, repair of any pseudarthrosis, and removal of hardware if necessary. Adding an anterior arthrodesis secures stability in an area that has not already proven itself insufficient, and improves stenosis in the caudal-cephalad direction.

## ANTERIOR APPROACH USING ALIF FOR THE UNSTABLE SPINE

ALIF is a viable solution for an unstable spine that has previously been operated on posteriorly. By entering anteriorly the surgeon dissects virgin tissues. Two approaches can be used for ALIF, open and laproscopic.

The more invasive open procedure begins with the surgeon using either a transabdominal approach or a retroperitoneal flank approach. After isolating the proper disk level, the surgeon incises the anterior longitudinal ligament. Creating a small flap, the disk material is then excised. Once completely removed bone graft and implants are placed.

Alternatively, a well-trained laproscopic team can enter the abdomen and proceed with the ALIF procedure in the same manner as the transabdominal or retroperitoneal procedure.

ALIF has several advantages. These include creating stability and increasing disk space height. Increasing disk space height is important because it not only corrects stenosis in the lateral directions, but it also corrects stenosis in the caudal-cephalad dimension, known as "pin-hole" stenosis. Restoring disk height is very advantageous in restoring spinal balance and lateral contour. Stewart and Sachs found five factors that statistically were associated with a successful outcome in revision surgery. These included a younger age, working outside the home, an initial period of improvement after the index operation, fewer spinal lev-

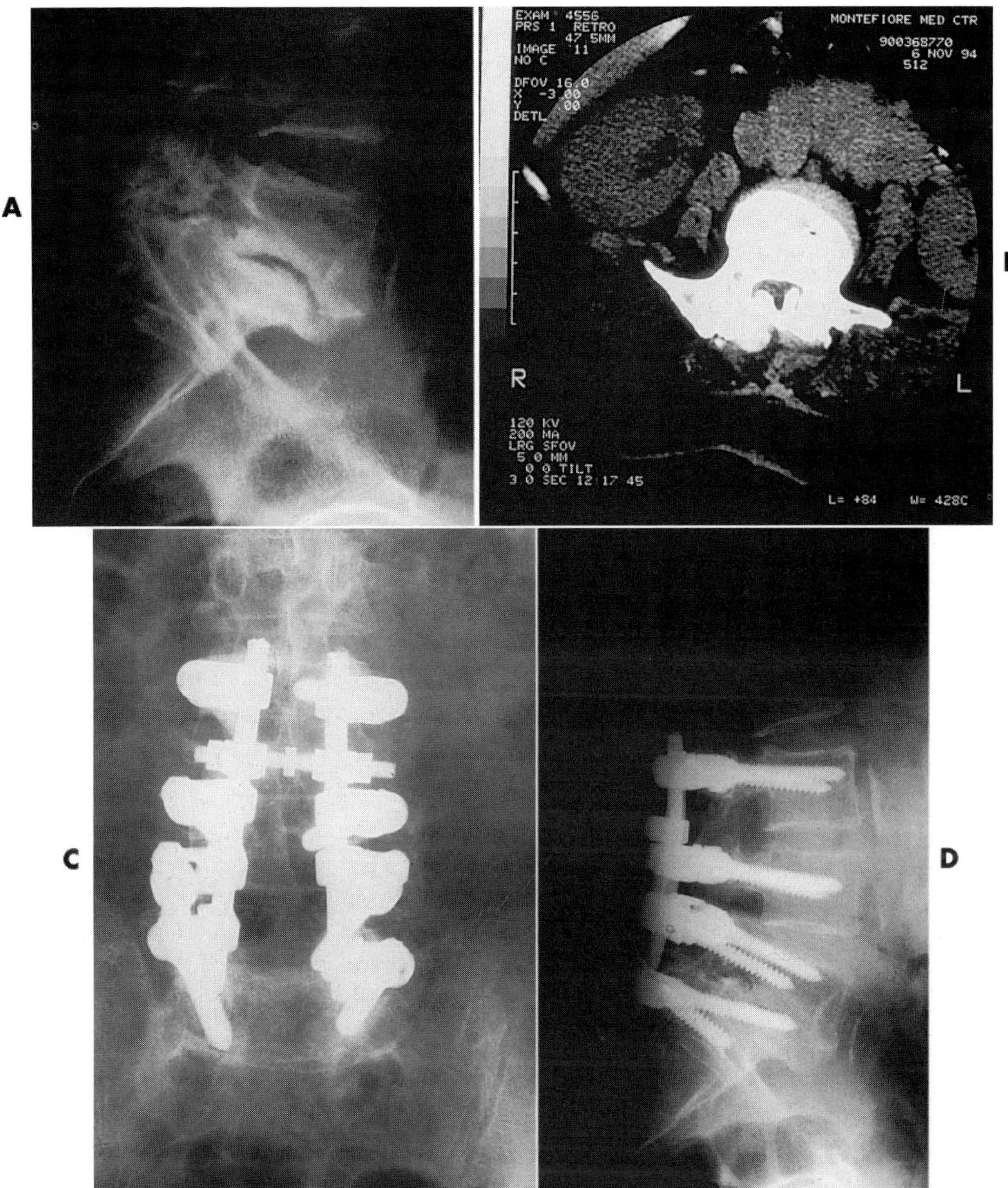


FIGURE 30-1

A lateral view x-ray film **(A)** and a CT cut **(B)** of a 63-year-old man, 7 years after laminectomy, with severe clinical spinal stenosis. Three levels are widely decompressed and fused as shown in anteroposterior **(C)** and lateral **(D)** views. A screw is placed in L5-S1 due to its degenerative appearance.

els operated on, and a revision procedure with an anterior interbody arthrodesis.[47]

## CONCLUSION

Extensive literature on the surgical treatment of patients with failed back syndrome indicates that the results are less than ideal. The most probable causes necessitating revision surgery in the short term are inappropriate patient selection, the wrong initial procedure, and intraoperative error in technique. The principal goal of surgical intervention is to relieve neural compression and assure stability. From a practical standpoint, all of the present techniques have shortcomings. Mainly, fusion and instrumentation come with the price of late-term degenerative changes, even in the ideal patient. As with the total joints of today, with anticipated longevity, the need for revision may be likely in the majority of primary surgical recipients.

The question of what salvage procedure to perform when the diagnosis of failed back syndrome is made is determined by which operation would have the greatest potential for obtaining decompression and stability. If a posterior approach is chosen the surgeon must judiciously proceed while guarding against dural tears. Dissecting from normal tissue to abnormal tissue can minimize the risk of these tears.

Currently, the consensus of spinal surgeons appears to advocate the use of the ALIF procedure as the first line of revision surgery. The ALIF procedure does have the following drawbacks: a questionable increase in the incidence of deep vein thrombosis, the risk of intraoperative visceral damage including ureteral injury,[21] and late-term degenerative changes. Despite these risks, this procedure has the benefits of operating on virgin tissue, earlier discharge and return to work secondary to being performed laproscopically,[39] and obtaining excellent stability without the increased risk of neurologic compromise that accompanies any posteriorly approached revision surgery. In the future, more research must be done to find less invasive and better means of stabilization, especially in the revision patient.

## REFERENCES


1. Altas SJ, Deyo RA, Keller RB, Chapin AM, Patrick DL, Long JM, Singer DE: The Maine lumbar spine study. Part III. 1-year outcomes of surgical and nonsurgical management of lumbar spinal stenosis, *Spine* 21:1787-1795, 1996.
2. Arct WA: Stenosis of the spinal canal after spondylodesis (iatrogenic stenosis of the spinal canal), *Arch Orthop Unfall* 83:353-364, 1975.
3. Benini A: Lumbar spinal stenosis. an overview 50 years following initial description, *Orthopade* 22:257-266, 1993.
4. Blau JN, Logue V: Intermittent claudication of the cauda equina: An unusual syndrome resulting from central protrusion of lumber intervertebral disc, *Lancet* 1:1081-1086, 1961.
5. Brodsky AE: Post-laminectomy and post-fusion stenosis of the lumbar spine, *Clin Orthop* 115:130-139, 1976.
6. Bullough P: *Atlas of orthopedic pathology,* ed 2, New York, 1992, Gower Medical.
7. Burton CV, Kirkaldy-Willis WH, Yong-Hing K, et al: Causes of failure of surgery on the lumbar spine, *Clin Orthop* 157:191-199, 1981.
8. Caputy AJ, Luessenhop AJ: Long-term evaluation of decompressive surgery for degenerative lumbar stenosis, *J Neurosurg* 77:669-676, 1992.
9. Cleveland M, Bosworth DM, Thomas FR: Pseudarthrosis in the lumbosacral spine, *J Bone Joint Surg* 30-A:302, 1948.
10. Deen HG, Zimmerman RS, Lyons MK, et al: Analysis of early failures after lumbar decompressive laminectomy for spinal stenosis, *Mayo Clin Proc* 70:33-36, 1995.
11. Einstenstein S: The trefoil configuration of the lumbar vertebral canal: a study of South African skeletal material, *J Bone Joint Surg* 62B:73-77, 1980.
12. Epstein NE, Epstein JE: *Lumbar decompression for spinal stenosis: surgical indications and techniques with and without fusion.* In Frymoyer JW, Handler NM, Kostuik JP, et al, editors: *The adult spine,* ed 2, Philadelphia, 1997, Lippincott-Raven, pp 2055-2088.
13. Epstein JA, Epstein BS, Rosenthal AD, et al: Sciatica caused by nerve root entrapment in the lateral recess, the superior fact syndrome, *J Neurosurg* 36:584-589, 1972.
14. Fast A, Robin GC, Floman Y: Surgical treatment of lumbar spinal stenosis in the elderly, *Arch Phys Rehabil* 66:149-151, 1985.
15. Finnegan WJ, Fenlin JM, Marvel JP, et al: Results of surgical intervention in the symptomatic multiply-operated back patient, *J Bone Joint Surg* 61-A:1077-1082, 1979.
16. Getty CJ: Lumbar spinal stenosis: the clinical spectrum and the results of operation, *J Bone Joint Surg* 62-B:481-485, 1980.
17. Guigui P, Ulivieri JM, Lassale B, Deburge A: Reoperation after surgical treatment of lumbar stenosis, *Rev Chir Orthop* 81:663-671, 1995.
18. Hanley EN Jr: The surgical treatment of lumbar degenerative disease. Ortho Knowledge Update: Spine. AAOS Pub, IL127-14, 1997.
19. Herno A, Airaksinen O, Saari T, Sihvonen T: Surgical results of lumbar spinal stenosis. A comparison of patients with or without previous back surgery, *Spine* 20:964-969, 1995.
20. Hutter CG: Spinal stenosis and posterior lumbar interbody fusion, *Clin Orthop* 193:103-114, 1985.
21. Isiklar ZU, Lindsey RW; Coburn M: Ureteral injury after anterior lumbar interbody fusion: a case report, *Spine* 15;21(20):2379-2382, 1996.
22. Johansen JG: Computed tomography in assessment of myelographic nerve root compression in the lateral recess, *Spine* 11:492-495, 1986.
23. Johnsson KE; Willner S, Johnsson K: Postoperative instability after decompression for lumbar spinal stenosis, *Spine* 44:107-110, 1986.
24. Johnsson KE, Rosen I, Uden A: The natural course of lumbar spinal stenosis, *Clin Orthop* 279:82-86, 1992.
25. Jonsson B, Stromquivst B: Repeat decompression of lumbar nerve roots: a prospective two year evaluation, *J Bone Joint Surg* 75B:894-897, 1993.
26. Kim SS, Michelsen CB: Revision surgery for failed back surgery syndrome, *Spine* 17:957-960, 1992.

27. Lassale B: Anatomy of the lateral recess or lumbar radicular groove, *Acta Orthop Belg* 53(2):1378-142, 1987.
28. Lassale B, Bitan F, Bex M, Deburge A: Functional results and prognostic factors in the surgical treatment of degenerative lumbar stenosis, *Rev Chir Orthop* 74(suppl):85-88, 1988.
29. Louis R: *Surgery of the spine: surgical anatomy and approaches,* Berlin, 1983, Springer Verlag.
30. Lyons A, Petrucelli R: *Medicine an illustrated history*. Japan, 1987, Abradale Press, p 599.
31. Markwalder TM: Surgical management of neurogenic claudication in 100 patients with lumbar spinal stenosis due to degenerative spondylolisthesis, *Acta Neurochir* 120:136-142, 1993.
32. Moore K: *Developing human,* ed 4, Philadelphia, 1988, WB Saunders, pp 371-373.
33. Nasca RJ: Surgical management of lumbar spinal stenosis, *Spine* 12:809-816, 1987.
34. Olsen EJ, Hanley EN Jr, Rudert MJ, Baratz ME: Vertebral column allografts for the treatment of segmental spine defects. An experimental investigation in dogs, *Spine* 16:1081-1088, 1991.
35. Pospich J, Pajonk F, Stolke D: Epidural scar formation after spinal surgery: an experimental study, *Eur Spine J* 4:213-219, 1995.
36. Postacchini F: Management of lumbar spinal stenosis, *J Bone Joint Surg* 78B:154-164, 1996.
37. Postacchini F, Cinotti G, Perugia D, Gumina S: The surgical treatment of central lumbar stenosis. Multiple laminotomy compared with total laminectomy, *J Bone Joint Surg* 75B:386-392, 1993.
38. Prager JM, Roychowdhury S, Gorey MT, et al: Spinal headache after myelograms: comparison of needle type, *AJR Am J Roentgenol* 167:1289-1292, 1996.
39. Regan JJ, Mcafee PC, Guyer RD, Aronoff RJ: Laparoscopic fusion of the lumbar spine in a multicenter series of the first 34 consecutive patients, *Surg Laparosc Endosc* 6(6):459-468, 1996.
40. Rivera E, Hardjasudarma M, Willis BK, Pippins DN: Inadvertent use of ionic contrast material in myelography: a case report and management guidelines, *J Neurosurg* 36:413-415, 1995.
41. Ross J, Modic M: Current assessment of spinal degenerative disease with magnetic resonance imaging, *Clin Orthop* 279:68-82, 1992.
42. Sachs B, Fraenkel J: Progressive ankylotic rigidity of the spine, *J Nerv Ment Dis* 27:1-15, 1900.
43. Sand T: Which factors affect reported headache incidences after lumbar myelography? A statistical analysis of publications in the literature, *Neuroradiology* 31:55-59, 1989.
44. Sarpyener MA: Congenital structure of the spinal canal, *J Bone Joint Surg* 27:70-79, 1945.
45. Schlegel JD, Smith JA, Schleusener RL: Lumbar motion segment pathology adjacent to thoracolumbar, lumbar and lumbosacral fusions, *Spine* 21:970-981, 1996.
46. Sidhu KS, Herkowitz HN: Spinal Instrumentation in the management of degenerative disorders of the lumbar spine, *Clin Orthop*. 335:39-53, 1997.
47. Stewart G, Sachs: Patient outcomes after reoperaton on the lumbar spine, *J Bone Joint Surg Am* 78(5):706-711, 1996.
48. Verbiest H: Introduction to spinal stenosis, *Spine State Art Rev* 1:361-367, 1987.
49. Verbiest H: A radicular syndrome from developmental narrowing of the lumbar vertebral canal, *J Bone Joint Surg* 36B: 230-237, 1954.
50. Wetzel FT, La Rocca H: The failed posterior lumbar interbody fusion, *Spine* 16(7):839-845, 1991.
51. White AH, Wiltse LL: *Postoperative spondylolisthesis.* In Weinstein PR, Ehni G, Wilson CB, editors: *Lumbar spondylosis: diagnosis, management, and surgical treatment,* St. Louis, 1977, Mosby.
52. Wiltse LL, Kirkaldy-Willis WH, McIvor GW: The treatment of spinal stenosis, *Clin Orthop* 115:83-91, 1976.
53. Wiltse LL, et al: Alar transverse process impingement of L5: the far out syndrome, *Spine* 9:31-41, 1984.
54. Yong-Hing K, Kirkaldy-Willis WH: The pathophysiology of degenerative disease of the lumbar spine, *Orthop Clin North Am* 14:491-504, 1983.

# 31 PEDIATRIC SPINAL DEFORMITY

**Harry L. Shufflebarger, M.D.**



The need for revision surgery connotes failure of the primary and/or subsequent procedures. On occasion, revision may be a planned event, particularly the use of subcutaneous instrumentation in the immature patient with a curve unmanageable by other methods. Revision surgery in the pediatric patient is much less frequent than in the adult population. The areas in which secondary procedures may be required are several and include pseudarthrosis, the need for implant removal (prominence, late infection, metal sensitivity), crankshaft phenomenon, imbalance, and the planned revision.

Preparation for revision surgery in the pediatric patient includes several areas. The reason for the revision should be studied by appropriate radiographic methods. An attempt to define the levels of pseudarthrosis, if present, is useful. Here, bone scan, plain tomography, and dynamic radiographs may all be of value. Adequate nutritional status for major surgery should be ensured, particularly in the neuromuscular patient. Sufficient blood, preferably autogenous, should be available. The various etiologies for which revision surgery may be necessary in the pediatric population will be considered.

## PSEUDARTHROSIS AND IMPLANT DISLODGMENT

Pseudarthrosis may occur with spinal fusion for deformity in the pediatric patient population. In idiopathic scoliosis, the incidence of pseudarthrosis with Harrington instrumentation was less than 1%.[7,9,17] With modern multiple hook/screw/rod systems, the incidence of pseudarthrosis is also less than 1%, and probably approaches zero.[23] The diagnosis may be evident with broken hardware. In the event of either persistent pain or significant loss of correction in the adolescent idiopathic patient, investigation for pseudarthrosis is indicated. This may include appropriate radiographic studies as noted earlier. Radiographic evaluation has a high incidence of false-negatives. With sufficient indications (pain or curve progression), exploration of the fusion may be necessary to determine if a pseudarthrosis is present. If it is not present, removal of the hardware may alleviate the symptoms.

If a pseudarthrosis is present, in general, it should be repaired. The repair involves removal of existing hardware if present, complete excision of the fibrous material in the area of pseudarthrosis, instrumentation in a compression direction relative to the area of pseudarthrosis,[12] and bone grafting, preferably autogenous. In the adolescent idiopathic patient with a pseudarthrosis of a previous fusion, a posterior only procedure should be sufficient. If, in the adolescent, multiple levels of pseudarthrosis are present there may be risk factors not appreciated, such as cigarette smoking. In this instance, consideration for both anterior and posterior procedures may be appropriate.

Pseudarthrosis in the pediatric patient with nonidiopathic deformity is more common. The conditions may include cerebral palsy (rare in my experience), myelodysplasia (more common), and multiple other etiologies on nonidiopathic deformity. Congenital deformity has no higher incidence of pseudarthrosis than idiopathic disease. In pseudarthrosis in the nonidiopathic group of patients, a more aggressive approach is frequently indicated and necessary to achieve union. Figure 31-1 is an example of failure of the Luque system to achieve arthrodesis in a patient with myelodysplasia. Repair was accomplished by both anterior and posterior procedures. Here, the initial procedure was posterior exploration with removal of hardware. At the same sitting, having determined the levels of failure of fusion, anterior interbody fusion of the failed levels using structural interbody grafts was done. Lastly, at the same sitting, reinstrumentation from the posterior approach was accomplished, achieving compression of both the anterior and posterior grafts.

Implant dislodgment was relatively frequent with Harrington instrumentation, due to only two levels of spinal anchorage, proximal and distal. With the advent of the multiple hook/screw/rod systems, implant dislodgment has been relatively infrequent.[24] In the adolescent patient, this has generally been the distal convex implant.[24] The implant dislodgment has usually been within the first few weeks, and replacement at the same level is usually easily accomplished. Usually, the hook dislodges from the infralaminar position, and does not fracture the lamina. In the event of lamina fracture, the hook can be replaced with a screw. If the failed implant is a screw, distal extension may be required to salvage the situation. Figure 31-2 depicts the dislodgment of the distal convex hook in an adolescent, and the replacement at the same level.

## IMPLANT REMOVAL

While implant removal is not strictly a revision procedure, it is a necessary second surgical procedure, and one that was not usually planned. The indications for implant removal may be several: prominence of the posterior device, painful back with question of pseudarthrosis, late infection of a spinal procedure with instrumentation. The first two situations are self-explanatory.

Late infection (1 to 5 years after the initial procedure) was not reported with the use of the Harrington or the Luque devices. With the advent of the multiple hook/screw/rod systems, a seemingly high incidence of this condition has been reported. This author, with Dubousset and Wenger,[6] reports an incidence of approximately 1% in pediatric patients receiving the Cotrel-Dubousset instrumentation for treatment of spinal deformity. The presentation was similar in three different hospitals (Paris, Miami, San Diego), and included spontaneous drainage, negative culture, normal laboratory examination, and lack of systemic symptoms. There was no response to antibiotic treatment, and removal of the instrumentation effected cure in every instance. The surgical findings included extensive granulomatous reaction over the entire instrumentation, with the cutaneous lesion leading to either an open body implant or the DTT. Motion was always present between components of the instrumentation. The etiology was felt to represent a reaction to metallic particles due to fretting corrosion. This theory was substantiated by finding the presence of metallic fragments on polarized light microscopy.

Richards[18] reported an incidence of late infection with the Texas Scottish Rite Hospital (TSRH) device in excess of 10%, all requiring implant removal for cure of the draining sinuses. The presentation was similar to the above Cotrel-Dubousset experience. But, Richards reported positive cultures at seven days for a variety of low virulence bacteria. He postulated that these organisms were seeded at the initial placement of the implants, and became clinically significant several years later.

Regardless of the etiology of the "late infection" syndrome with the multiple hook/screw/rod systems, it does occur. And revision surgery is required. The revision required is removal of the device with exploration of the fusion mass. An adequate exploration is frequently difficult due to the large amount of fibrous and granulomatous tissue present, and the rather large amount of bleeding produced. A pseudarthrosis may be present, but, repair of this should not be attempted in the face of the extensive granulomatous or infectious condition. After removal of the device with appropriate cultures and antibiotic treatment if indicated, the status of the spinal fusion is best determined by radiographic follow-up. If a pseudarthrosis proves to be present, appropriate revision surgery may be planned. Revision surgery with instrumentation may be safely accomplished. Consideration for the use of titanium implants should be given, even in the absence of known sensitivity to nickel or chromium.

## CRANKSHAFT PHENOMENON

The crankshaft phenomenon was first reported in the English speaking literature by Dubousset, Herring, and Shufflebarger.[5] Simply, the crankshaft is the recurrence of a scoliotic deformity with an intact posterior fusion. An instrumented (or noninstrumented) fusion is performed in an immature patient. In the presence of immaturity and a relatively large residual curve, and in particular large apical rotation, anterior growth of the spine continues. This causes increase of the deformity, particularly the torsion. While large changes in Cobb angle may not occur, large changes in apical ro-

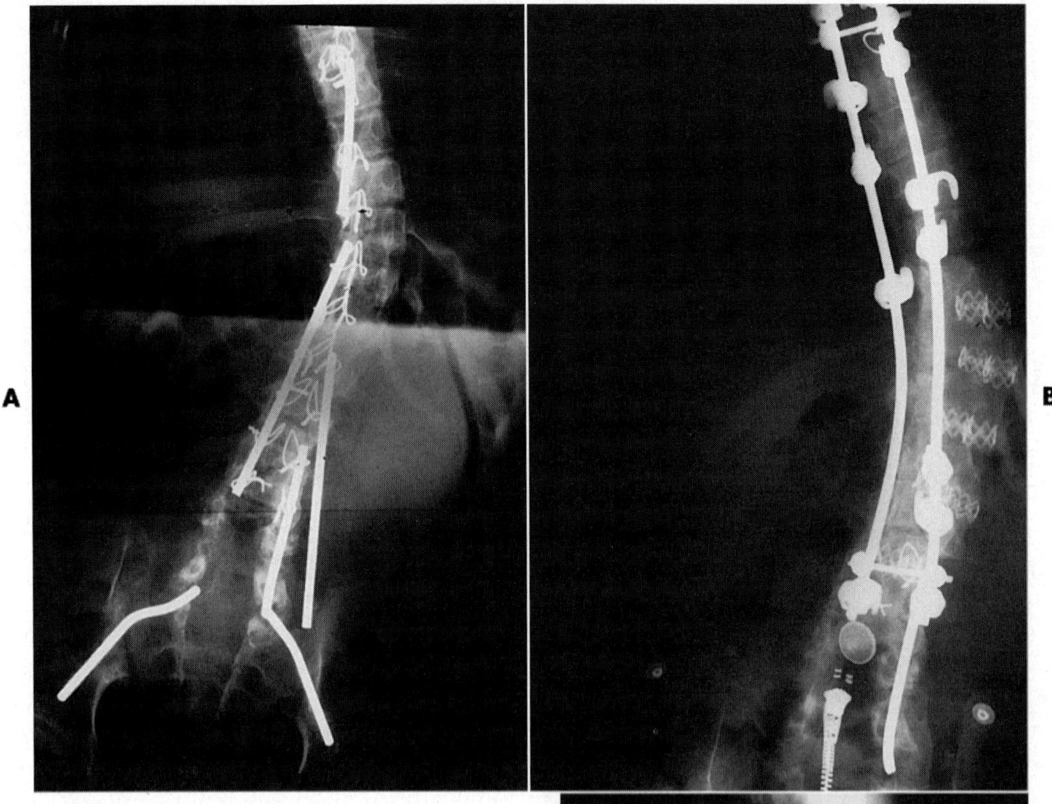


FIGURE 31-1

**A,B,C,** Failure of fusion in a patient with myelodysplasia and scoliosis is evidenced by fracture of the Luque rods in multiple places. Repair has been accomplished by a posterior/anterior/posterior sequence. This permits identification of the levels of pseudarthroses and posterior repair. Anterior structural interbody grafts supplemented with morselized autogenous bone follows. Lastly, posterior instrumentation is placed achieving stabilization and correction of the spine.

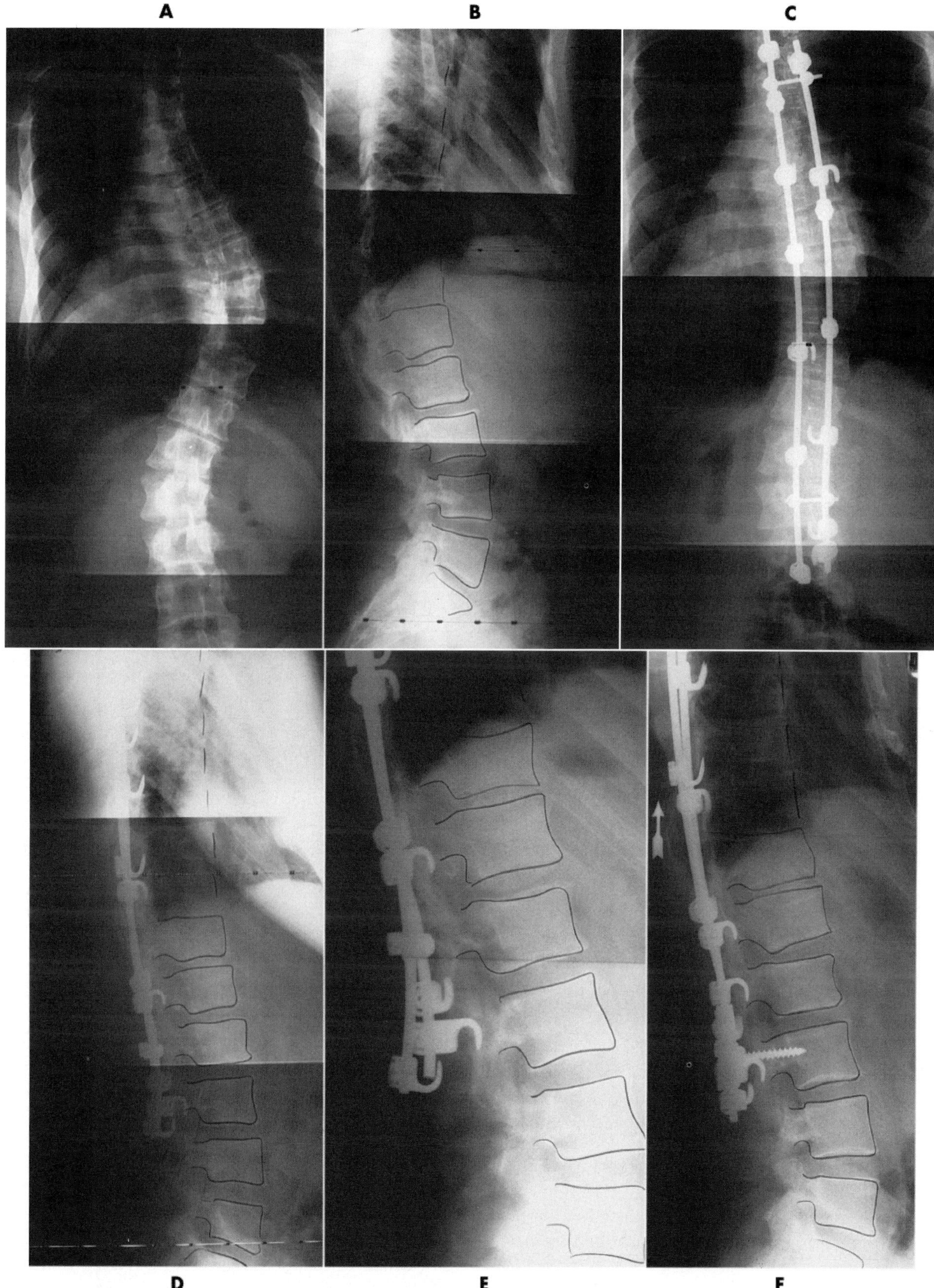


FIGURE 31-2

**A, B,** Double structural idiopathic scoliosis is present in a young adult. **C, D,** Satisfactory correction immediately after surgery. **E,** Displacement of the distal implants at six weeks after surgery. **F,** Revision at the same level using a single screw at the distal convex site and replacing the other displaced hooks. The screw is protected with an offset body hook at the same level.

tation measurements (e.g., Perdriolle torsionometer or CAT scan) frequently occur. Sanders et al[19] have defined the patient at risk to develop the phenomenon. The possibility to crankshaft relates to the timing of the spinal surgery in relationship to the peak growth velocity of the patient. Spinal fusion done prior to the peak growth velocity period has a very high risk to develop crankshaft. I have demonstrated the ability to prevent the crankshaft by joining a same day anterior growth arrest procedure to the posterior spinal instrumentation and fusion.[22]

The occurrence of the crankshaft presents the surgeon with increasing deformity and intact spinal instrumentation. The dilemma is present between the possibility of pseudarthrosis permitting the increased deformity and the crankshaft being responsible. Usually the change is not significant enough to prompt surgical intervention. Should the change in spinal alignment be significant enough to perform another spinal surgery, several options are available. If the patient is relatively mature at this point in time, exploration of the spinal fusion to ensure its integrity may be all that is required. If the cosmetic deformity is significant, thoracoplasty may improve the cosmesis sufficiently.

If the patient exhibiting crankshaft is immature, an anterior growth arrest procedure is required. In addition to diskectomy and endplate destruction, it is the opinion of the author that additional anterior procedures are required. Earlier, in-lay rib strut graft over the entire deformity was employed. With the development of anterior thoracic devices, these should be sufficient, in conjunction with anterior growth arrest and fusion, to prevent further crankshaft. Additional posterior procedures are usually required. Figure 31-3 demonstrates such a patient with crankshaft as well as adding on to the initial deformity. Here, anterior growth arrest with rib inlay graft was performed, as well as revision with distal extension of the posterior fusion. Satisfactory balance and curve stability was achieved.

## IMBALANCE

Imbalance or decompensation after spinal surgery has been recognized as a significant problem for many years in the surgical treatment of adolescent idiopathic scoliosis. Imbalance may be defined as deviation of a weightbearing axis. This has been most commonly recognized in the coronal plane. Coronal balance may be determined by the relationship of a vertical line from C7 to the center sacral line. Deviation of the C7 vertical by greater than 2 cm has been considered imbalance. Coronal imbalance may also be evident clinically. This may be indicated by inequality of the height of the shoulders or lack of symmetry of the waist. Axial plane imbalance may also occur, and is usually associated with coronal plane imbalance. This is usually seen radiographically, and is most common at the distal junctional zone (the junction of the fused and instrumented proximal spine with the unfused spine more distal). Figure 31-4 illustrates coronal and axial imbalance at the distal junctional zone.

Sagittal plane imbalance also occurs. This is determined by the relationship of a vertical line from the odontoid to the sacrum. Normally, this sagittal weightbearing axis should fall slightly anterior to the sacrum (Fig. 31-5). Posterior displacement of this axis indicates increase in lordosis. This is rarely if ever a clinical problem, as sagittal plane balance is easily accomplished by hip flexion. But, anterior displacement of the sagittal weightbearing axis is a frequent clinical problem. This connotes increase in kyphosis or loss of lordosis. The anatomic limitation of hip extension makes compensation for as anterior sagittal weightbearing axis difficult.

Coronal plane imbalance was an uncommon occurrence with Harrington instrumentation (if it ever occurred). With the advent of the multiple hook/screw/rod systems, coronal plane imbalance has been recognized as a clinical problem, and one in which revision surgery may be required. Many investigators have reported this complication,[1,8,20,25] with wide speculation of the etiology. Lonstein reported 28 cases of coronal imbalance, and polled several experts regarding their ideas regarding the etiology of the imbalance as well as their selection of fusion levels.[14] There was significant disagreement among this group. Lonstein concluded that the most common causes of imbalance were incorrect selection of fusion levels and correction of the thoracic curve to a degree greater than the lumbar curve could compensate. Dubousset reviewed the same set of problems and concluded that the causes of imbalance were several.[4] These included: improper selection of distal fusion levels, usually too short and ignoring a structural lumbar curve; improper selection of proximal fusion levels, ignoring a structural left high thoracic curve; failure to recognize a thoracolumbar sagittal plane abnormality; poor hook pattern, particularly regarding force direction in the coronal plane; no appreciation for axial plane changes on dynamic radiographs; and crankshaft phenomenon. Careful attention to the principles of selection of fusion levels as determined by static and dynamic radiographs should minimize this complication.[20,21]

Treatment of coronal plane imbalance is less of a problem than prevention. Less severe and nonprogressive instances of imbalance may be managed without additional surgery. An ocular reorientation program may be sufficient to permit compensation. The patient should spend several sessions daily (usually eight to ten 5-min sessions) observing the trunk in a mirror, and shifting appropriately to establish balance. Documen-

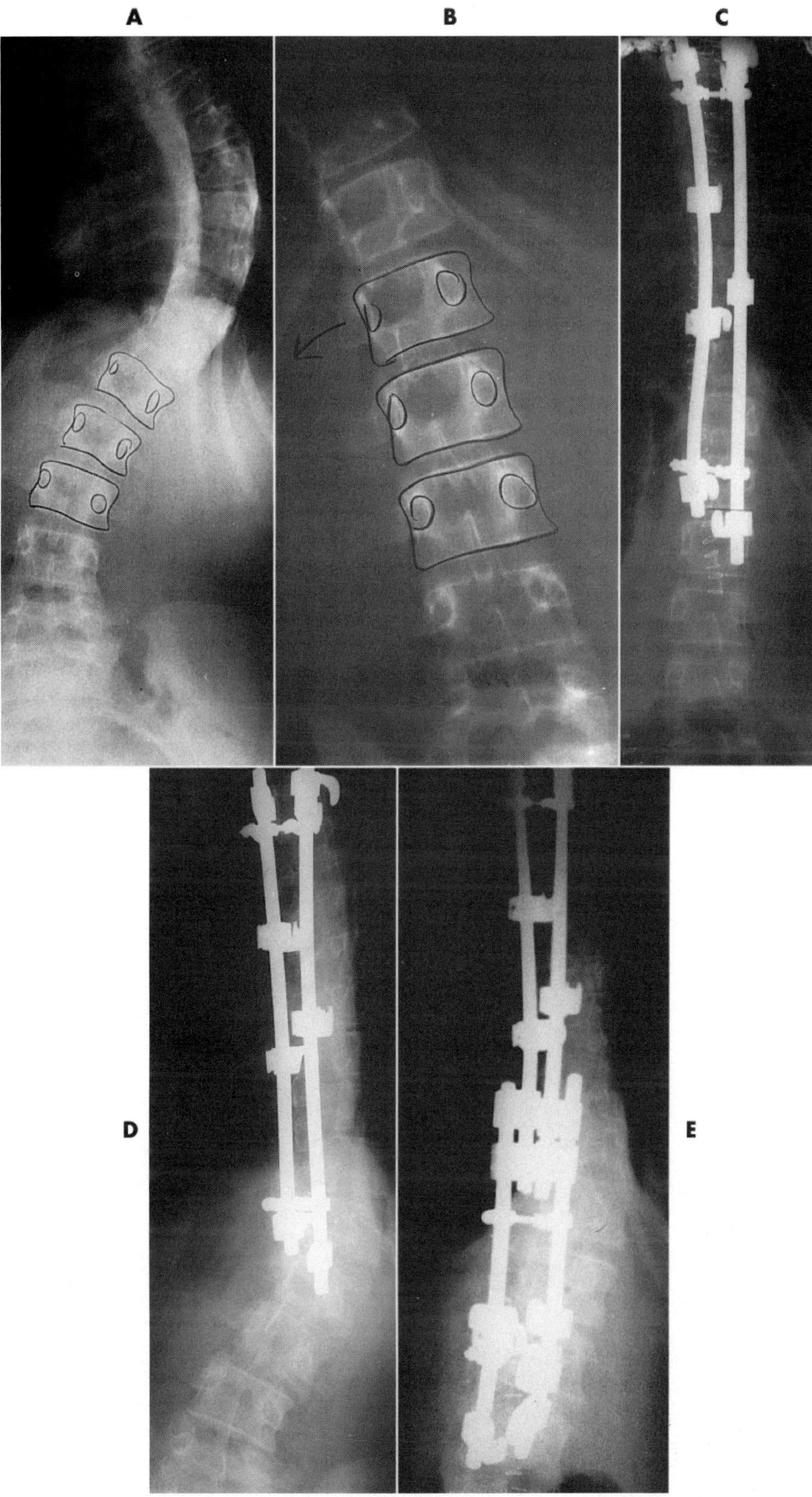


**FIGURE 31-3**

**A, B,** An adolescent idiopathic scoliosis. On the bend to the left, note that L2 and L3 join the primary thoracic curve, the Cobb measurement ending at L1. **C,** Excellent correction and balance immediately after surgery. **D,** Marked imbalance 9 months after surgery. Crankshaft phenomenon has occurred, as evidenced by the change in axial orientation of the intermediate convex hook and the diminished space between the rods. In addition, L2 and L3 have added on, as in retrospect, could have been predicted by the left bending film. **E,** The final result. Anterior growth arrest of the thoracic and lumbar curves was done, followed by posterior extension of the instrumentation. Here, the proximal instrumentation was extended with an axial extension device. Satisfactory alignment resulted.

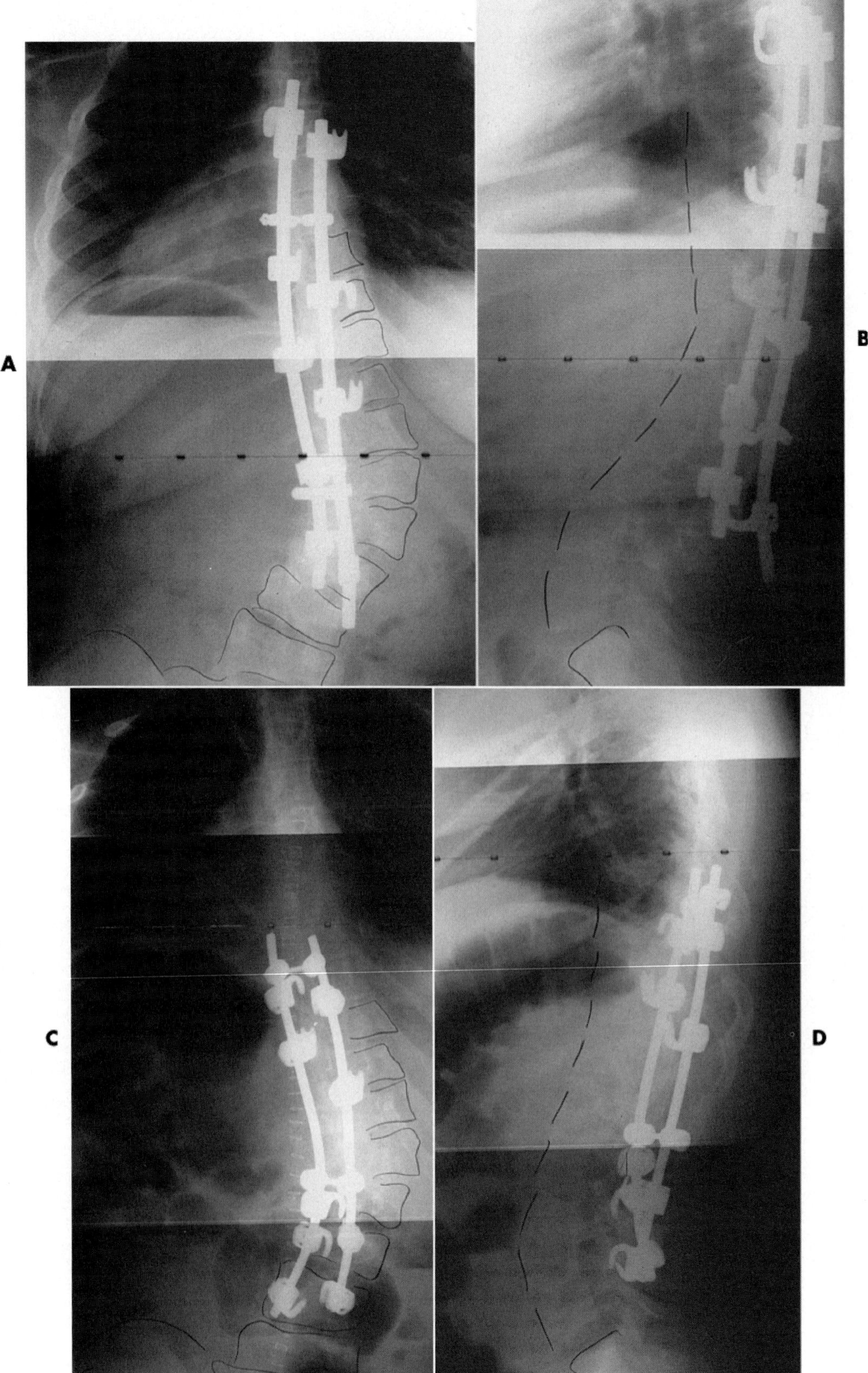


FIGURE 31-4

**A, B,** An adolescent presenting with trunk imbalance after posterior fusion. Crankshaft may have occurred. L4 was probably part of the deformity prior to surgery. On the lateral view, the distal implants appear displaced. **C, D,** The revision procedure. The existing instrumentation was removed, osteotomy of L1-L3 was done, followed by instrumentation to L4. Note the satisfactory coronal balance and improvement in the sagittal contours.

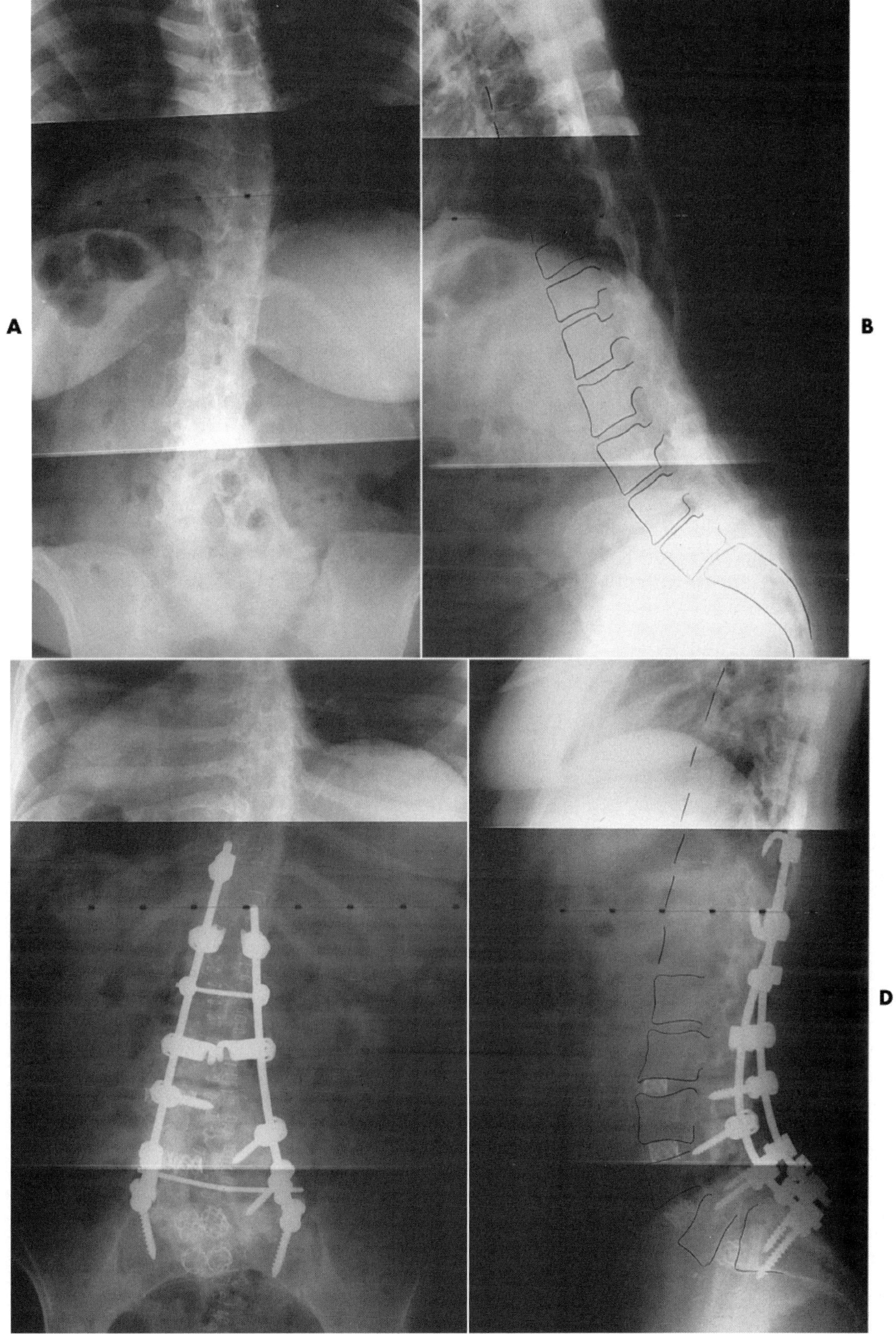


FIGURE 31-5

**A, B,** Lumbar flat back syndrome in a patient who had Harrington instrumentation to L5 20 years previously. The rods had been removed two years after surgery. Laminectomy had been done for neurogenic claudication. Note the significant forward position of the patient. **C, D,** The coronal and sagittal positions after correction. The sequence was posterior osteotomies, anterior structural interbody grafts with autogenous morselized graft, and lastly posterior instrumentation and fusion.

tation of the efficacy of this maneuver does not exist, but, it is the unsupported assumption of the author that it does aid in reestablishing balance.

In the type 2 curve of King et al, selective thoracic fusion is frequently possible.[9] The lumbar segment may not balance, remaining larger than the thoracic curve. In this situation bracing may be beneficial in reestablishing balance. Failure to include a structural left high thoracic curve may result in shoulder asymmetry, and imbalance. This may improve with time, but, if significant, may require surgical extension of the fusion.

Severe coronal plane imbalance usually requires revision surgery. Figure 31-2 demonstrates severe coronal imbalance due to both crankshaft and adding on to the initial selective thoracic fusion. Here, anterior growth arrest was done, followed by posterior extension of the fusion. The posterior procedure consisted of exploration of the fusion and removal of the distal portion of the existing instrumentation. Axial connecting implants were employed to extend the fusion distally. These axial connectors simplify extension procedures, permitting extension without removal of the entire existing instrumentation. Figure 31-3 shows another instance of coronal and axial imbalance in idiopathic deformity. Here the fusion was too short, and there was progressive deformity distal to the fusion. The treatment in this instance was osteotomy of the distal two levels of the fusion mass after implant removal and extension of the fusion one level distally. If the intended distal extension is only one or two levels, osteotomy is usually required to establish balance. Failure of the segment to balance on dynamic radiographs should indicate the need for osteotomy. In this instance, anterior release may also be considered. Again, the use of axial extension implants simplifies the revision surgery.

Sagittal plane imbalance was a frequent complication of Harrington instrumentation. This was usually not recognized until adulthood, presenting as the lumbar flat back syndrome.[2,11] This was most common in patients fused distal to L3, and resulted in distal degeneration. If symptoms warrant, the treatment is removal of Harrington instrumentation, osteotomy of the fusion mass, and usually extension to the sacrum. Anterior surgery, with structural interbody grafts of the distal lumbar spine may be employed to improve lordosis and promote union. Figure 31-5 is an example of lumbar flat back syndrome after Harrington instrumentation. Insufficient lumbar lordosis may also occur with the multiple hook/screw/rod systems. Either use of distraction direction forces in the lumbar spine or insufficient rod bend will result in insufficient lumbar lordosis, and may result in the lumbar flat back syndrome.

Sagittal plane imbalance may occur in the form of increasing lumbar lordosis in severely affected cerebral palsy patients in which fusion is limited to the thoracic spine. Figure 31-6 is an example of this situation. The initial fusion was confined to the thoracic spine in this severely affected cerebral palsy patient. After the initial procedure, the severe lumbar lordosis evolved, as well as crankshaft of the fused area. Revision was accomplished by anterior growth arrest from T5 to the sacrum, followed by extension of the instrumentation to the sacrum. In this situation, extensive posterior release (including ligamentum flavum) is required for correction of the lordosis.

Sagittal plane imbalance may also occur in the surgical treatment of Scheuermann's disease. This has been noted with Harrington and Luque instrumentation,[3] as well as with the multiple hook/screw/rod systems.[13] Distal junctional kyphosis has been the most frequent. This may result in progressive kyphosis and prominence of instrumentation. Revision may be required. Figure 31-7 is an example of distal junctional kyphosis requiring revision. Here, the axial connecting devices permit relatively easy extension of the fusion.

Proximal junction kyphosis is a less frequent complication of the surgical treatment of Scheuermann's kyphosis. Figure 31-8 is an example of this complication. Here, care was taken to preserve the interspinous ligament proximal to the proximal instrumented level. But, proximal junctional kyphosis evolved. The etiology is unclear, but may relate to the significant posterior forces with the cantilever correction of the kyphosis. An anterior procedure had not been done in this case. Here, the kyphosis is acute, and resembles a traumatic flexion-distraction injury. Revision was accomplished with the axial extension devices, extending the fusion two segments proximally.

Imbalance in the surgical treatment of pediatric deformity should be relatively infrequent with over 10-years' experience with the multiple hook/screw/rod systems. Minor imbalance usually will resolve with time or with minimal treatment. Major clinical imbalance may require revision surgery. The revision surgery consists of extension of the previous fusion, and may require osteotomy of the previous fusion and associated anterior procedures.

## PLANNED REVISION

Revision surgery may be a planned event. In the immature patient with a curve progressive despite brace and/or cast treatment, subcutaneous instrumentation without fusion may be considered. This has been most successful in the patient with idiopathic deformity, either infantile or juvenile.[10,15,16] This technique has been less successful in deformity of neuromuscular etiology. With placement of the subcutaneous instrumentation, lengthening of the construct will be required

*Text continued on p. 437*

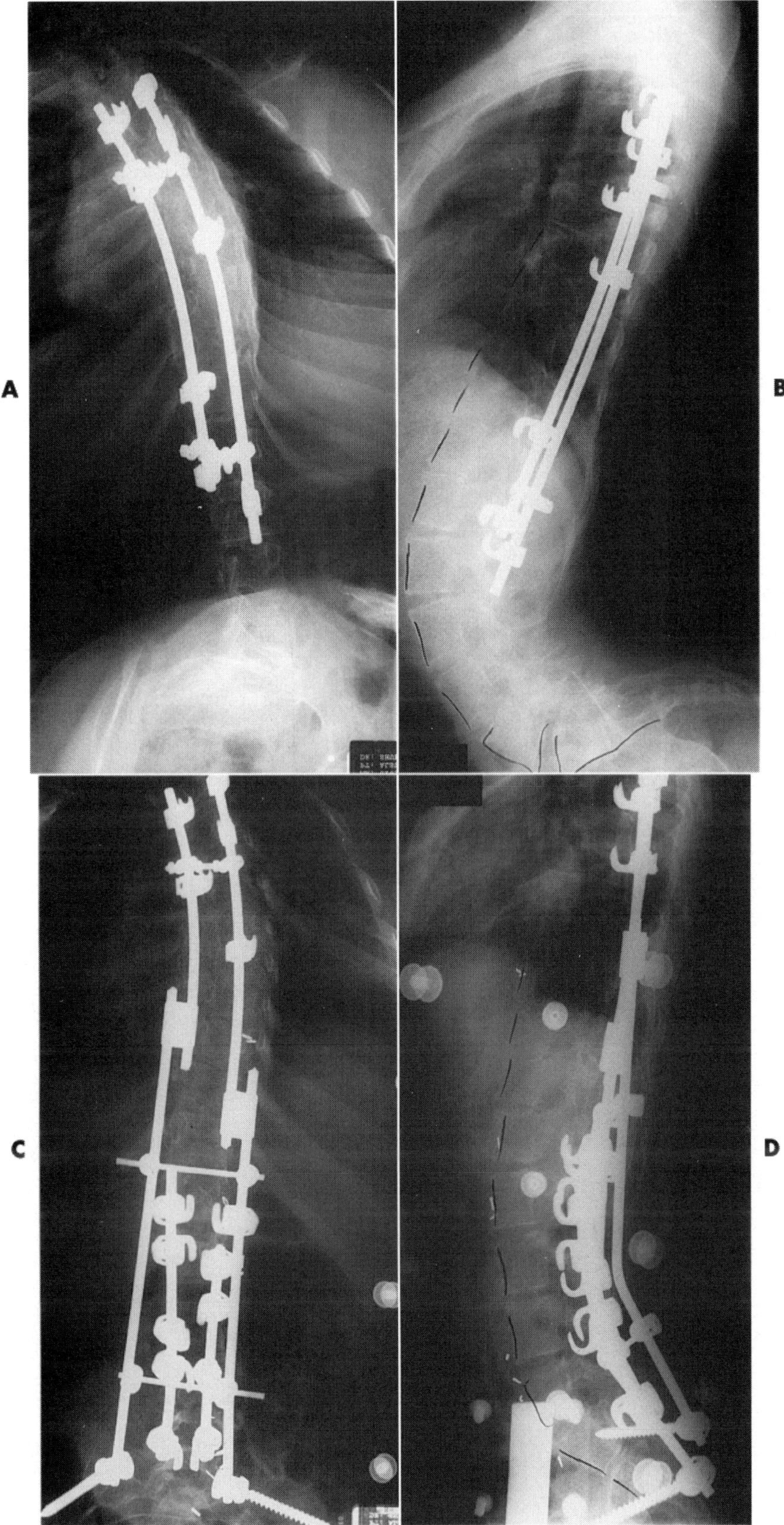


**FIGURE 31-6**

**A, B,** Quadriplegic cerebral palsy patient who had a previous thoracic fusion. The patient presented with severe lordosis distal to the instrumentation and probable crankshaft. **C, D,** The corrected position. Anterior growth arrest and fusion from T5 through the sacrum preceded the posterior extension of the instrumentation and fusion to the sacrum. Axial connectors were employed for extension. Polyaxial screws were placed in the iliac wing for distal fixation. Excellent coronal and sagittal alignment has been achieved.

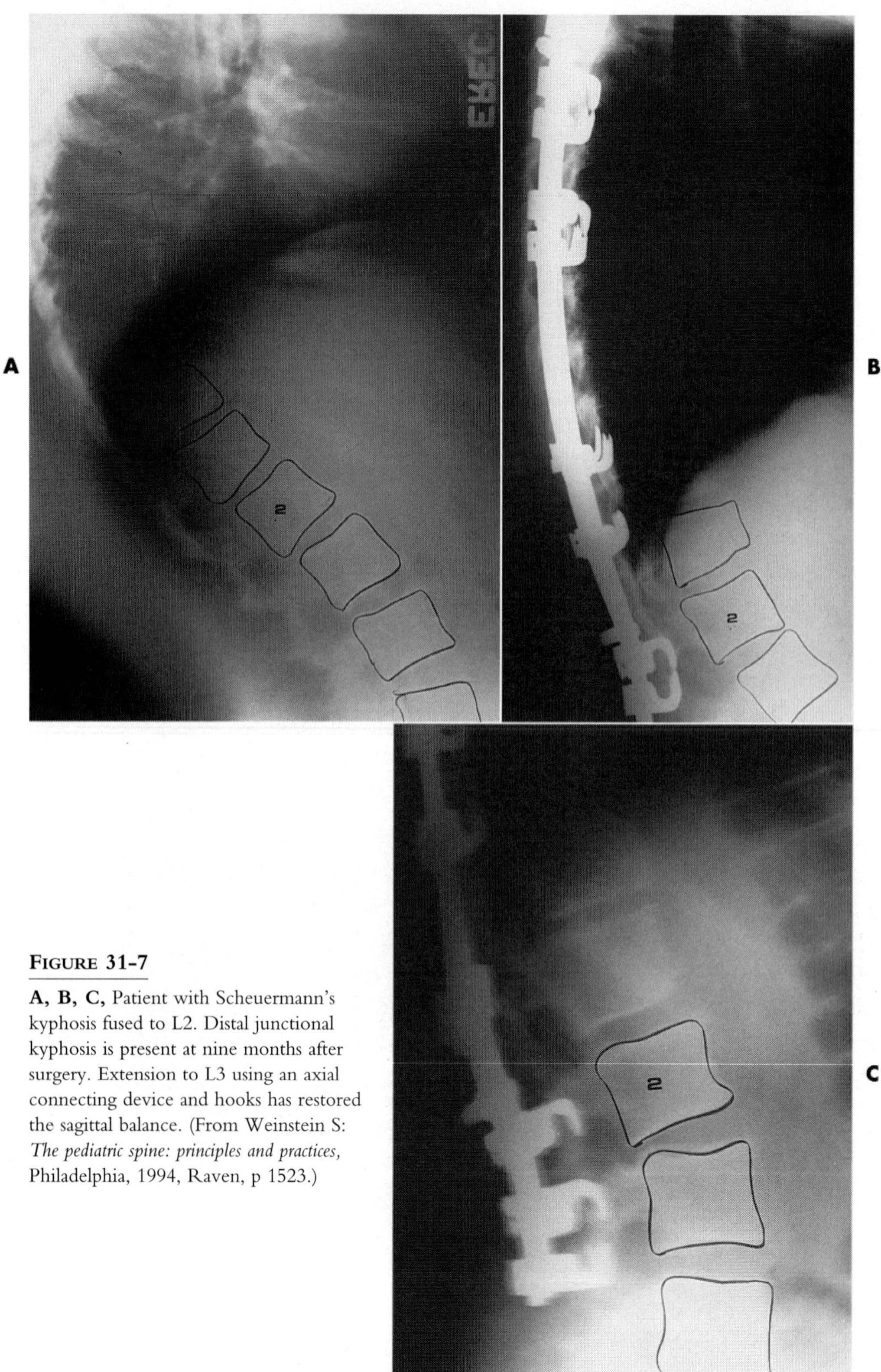


**Figure 31-7**

**A, B, C,** Patient with Scheuermann's kyphosis fused to L2. Distal junctional kyphosis is present at nine months after surgery. Extension to L3 using an axial connecting device and hooks has restored the sagittal balance. (From Weinstein S: *The pediatric spine: principles and practices,* Philadelphia, 1994, Raven, p 1523.)

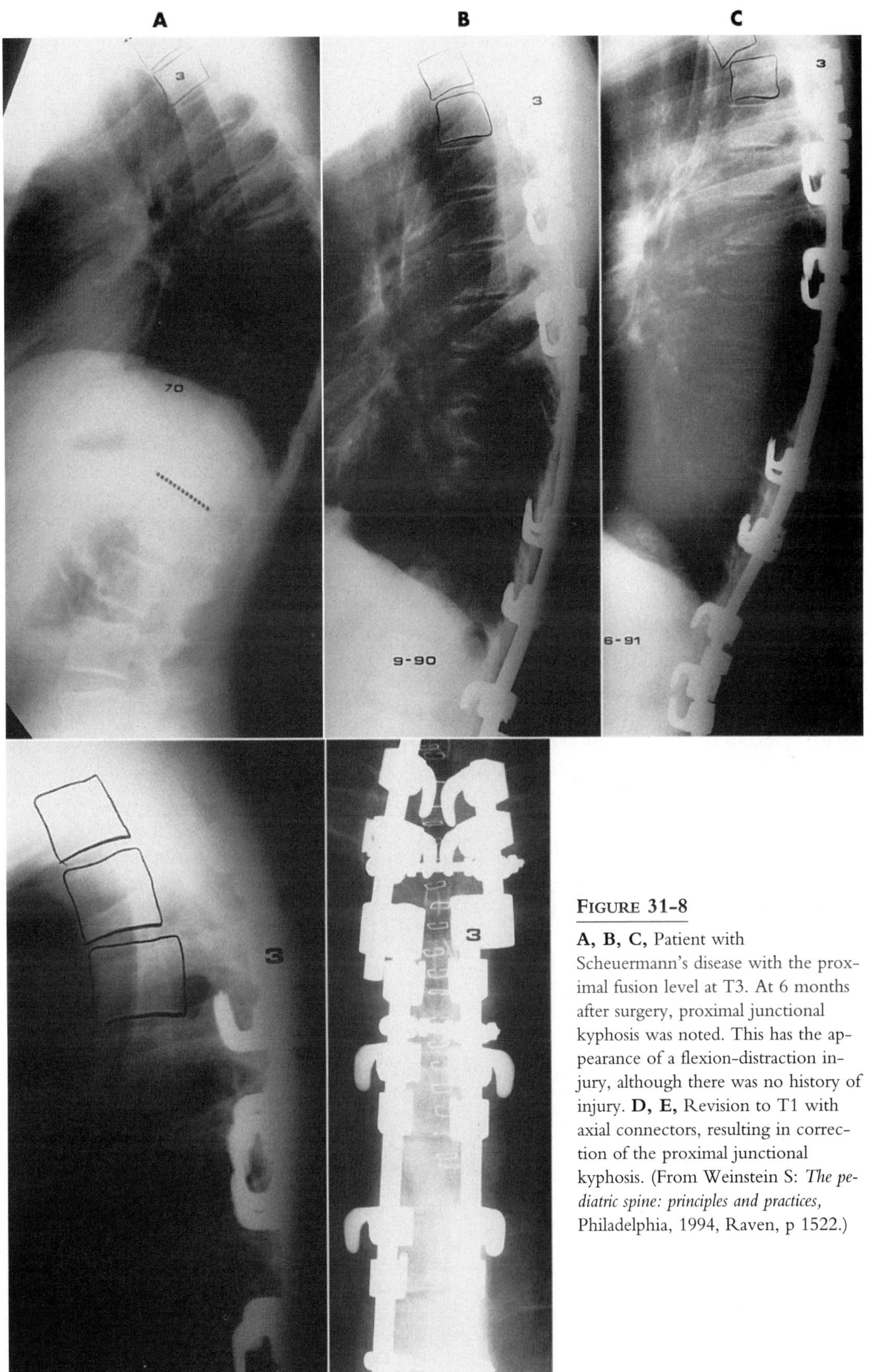


FIGURE 31-8

**A, B, C,** Patient with Scheuermann's disease with the proximal fusion level at T3. At 6 months after surgery, proximal junctional kyphosis was noted. This has the appearance of a flexion-distraction injury, although there was no history of injury. **D, E,** Revision to T1 with axial connectors, resulting in correction of the proximal junctional kyphosis. (From Weinstein S: *The pediatric spine: principles and practices,* Philadelphia, 1994, Raven, p 1522.)

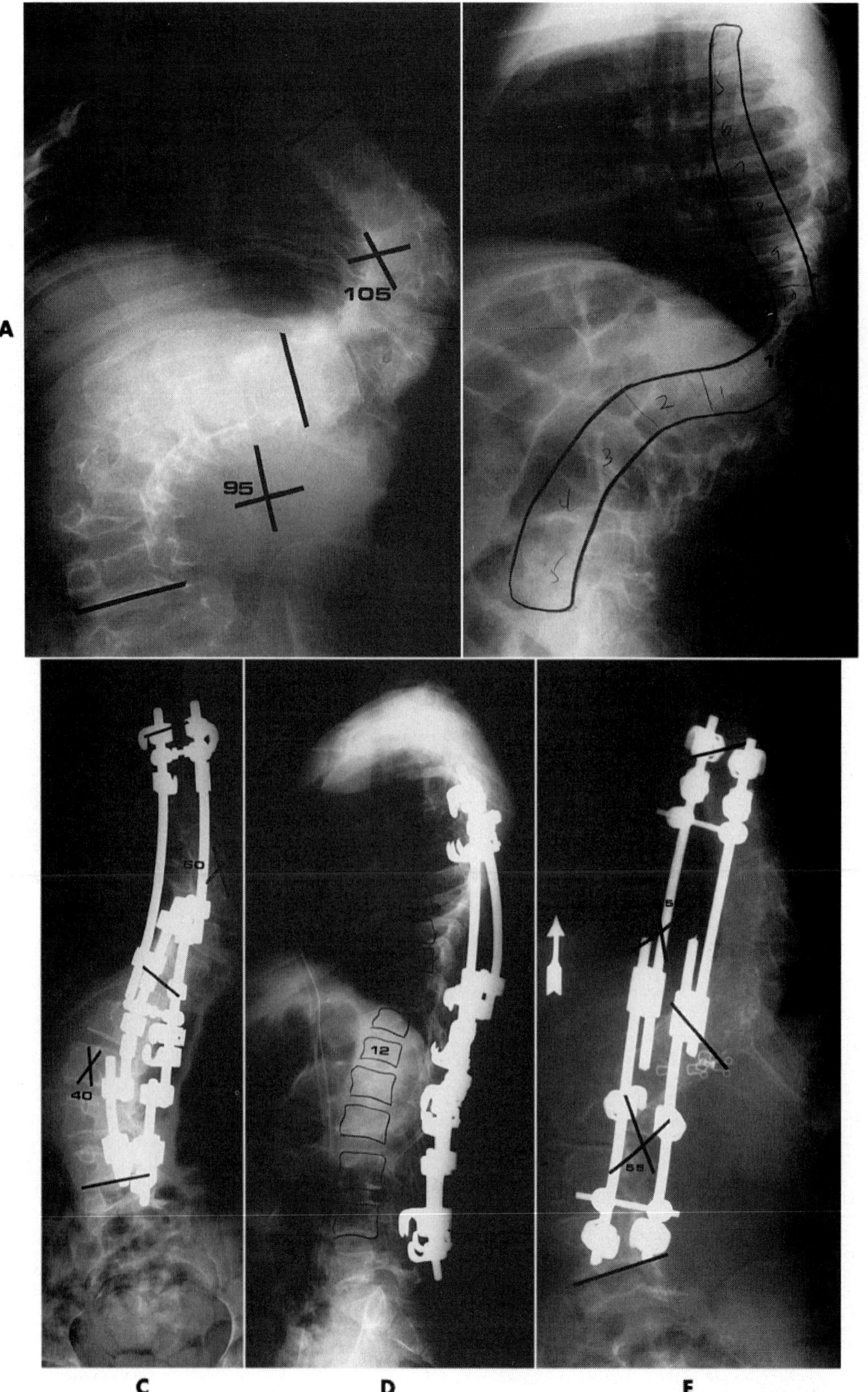


**FIGURE 31-9**

**A, B,** Patient with Ehlers-Danlos syndrome and progressive scoliosis despite brace and cast treatment. Note the kyphotic segment at the thoracolumbar junction, the junctional zone between the two curves. **C, D,** The position after the initial procedure (anterior release and fusion from T10 to L1 followed by posterior subcutaneous instrumentation). Satisfactory alignment was achieved with the Cotrel-Dubousset instrumentation. Several lengthenings were accomplished, usually by replacing the Cotrel-Dubousset device. **E,** Present condition, with Moss-Miami instrumentation and connectors that permit lengthening without removing the device. Five years have passed since the initial procedure. It is anticipated that arthrodesis will be done after puberty.

on a regular basis, usually determined by the amount of growth within a time period. Increasing deformity with intact subcutaneous instrumentation usually indicates the time for lengthening.

The final procedure, fusion, may thus be delayed until puberty, preferably after the peak growth velocity. Figure 31-9 is an example of planned revision. This patient had progressive deformity despite both cast and brace treatment. The initial procedure was anterior and posterior fusion over only the junctional zone between the two curves, this zone being quite kyphotic. Subcutaneous instrumentation was also performed. Periodic lengthening was carried out at approximately 9-month intervals. With the Cotrel-Dubousset system initially used, removal and replacement was usually required. This is due to the mechanism of attachment of implant to rod (breaking off set screw). The latter lengthening was possible without removal, accomplished via the axial connector of the Moss Miami system. This is a similar method to that advocated by Richard McCarthy with the TSRH system.[15]

The definitive fusion was accomplished at age 13, with a satisfactory final result.

## CONCLUSIONS

Revision surgery in pediatric deformity is relatively uncommon. Revision may be indicated in the following conditions: pseudarthrosis (rare); implant prominence; implant dislodgment; late infection; crankshaft phenomenon; imbalance; planned for unmanageable large deformities in young children.

Revision surgery may include several facets (depending upon the pathology): removal of existing implants, exploration of spinal fusion, extension of spinal fusion, osteotomy of spinal fusion, replacement of spinal instrumentation, lengthening of spinal instrumentation, anterior release or growth arrest and fusion.

## REFERENCES


1. Bridwell KH, McAllister JW, Betz RR, et al: Coronal decompensation produced by Cotrel-Dubousset derotation maneuver for idiopathic right thoracic scoliosis, *Spine* 16:769-778, 1991.
2. Casey MP, Asher MA, Jacobs RR, Orick JM: The effect of Harrington rod contouring on lumbar lordosis, *Spine* 12:750-754, 1987.
3. Coscia M, Bradford DS, Ogilvie J: Scheuerman's kyphosis-results in 19 cases treated by spinal arthrodesis and L-rod instrumentation, *Orthop Trans* 12:255, 1988.
4. Dubousset J: Personal communication.
5. Dubousset J, Herring A, Shufflebarger H: The crankshaft phenomenon, *J Pediat Orthop* 9:541-547, 1989.
6. Dubousset J, Shufflebarger H, Wenger D: Late "infection" with CD instrumentation, *Orthop Trans* 18:121, 1994.
7. Erwin W, Dickson J, Harrington P: The postoperative management of scoliosis patients treated with Harrington instrumentation and fusion, *J Bone Joint Surg* 58A:479-491, 1976.
8. Ibrahim K, Goldberg B: Cotrel-Dubousset instrumentation for type 2 right thoracic curves-decompensation vs compensation, *Orthop Trans* 14:780, 1990.
9. King H, Moe J, Bradford D, Winter R: The selection of fusion levels in thoracic idiopathic scoliosis, *J Bone Joint Surg* 65:1302-1313, 1983.
10. Koop SE: Infantile and juvenile idiopathic scoliosis, *Orthop Clin North Am* 19:331-338, 1988.
11. Lagrone M, Bradford D, Moe J, Lonstein J, Winter R, Ogilvie J: Loss of lumbar lordosis following surgical treatment of spinal deformities, *Orthop Trans* 11:92, 1987.
12. Lauerman WC, Bradford DS, Transfeldt EE et al: The management of pseudoarthrosis after spinal fusion for idiopathic scoliosis, *Orthop Trans* 13:116, 1989.
13. Lettice J, Ogilivie J, Transfeldt E, Cohen M: Proximal junctional kyphosis following Cotrel-Dubousett instrumentation. Presented at the annual meeting, Scoliosis Research Society, Minneapolis, 1991.
14. Lonstein J: Decompensation with Cotrel-Dubousset instrumentation- a multi-center study. Presented at the annual meeting, Scoliosis Research Society, Minneapolis, 1991.
15. McCarthy R, McCullough F: Growing instrumentation for scoliosis, *Orthop Trans* 18:126, 1994.
16. Moe J, Kharrat K, Winter R, Cummine J: Harrington instrumentation without fusion plus external orthotic support for difficult curvatures in young children, *Clin Orthop* 185:35-44, 1984.
17. Renshaw TS: The role of Harrington instrumentation and posterior spinal fusion in the management of adolescent idiopathic scoliosis, *Orthop Clin North Am* 19:257-264, 1988.
18. Richards DS: Delayed infections following posterior spinal instrumentation for the treatment of idiopathic scoliosis, *J Bone Joint Surg* 77A:524-531, 1995.
19. Sanders JO, Little DG, Richards S: Prediction of the crankshaft phenomenon by the peak growth age. Presented at the Annual Meeting, Scoliosis Research Society, Ottawa, 1996.
20. Shufflebarger HL: *Theory and mechanisms of posterior*

*derotation systems*. In Weinstein S, editor: *The pediatric spine,* New York, 1994, Raven Press, pp 1515-1543.

21. Shufflebarger HL, Clark CE: Fusion levels and hook patterns in thoracic scoliosis with Cotrel-Dubousset Instrumentation, *Spine* 15:916-921, 1990.
22. Shufflebarger HL, Clark CE: Prevention of the crankshaft phenomenon, *Spine* 16(8s):S409-S411, 1991.
23. Shufflebarger HL, Ellis R, Clark CE: Cotrel-Dubousset instrumentation in adolescent idiopathic scoliosis, *Orthop Trans* 13:79, 1989.
24. Shufflebarger HL, Thompson J, Clark CE: Complications of CD instrumentation in idiopathic scoliosis, *Orthop Trans* 16:155-156, 1992.
25. Thompson JP, Transfeldt EE, Bradford DS, Ogilivie JW, Boachie-Adjei O: Decompensation after Cotrel-Dubousset instrumentation of idiopathic scoliosis, *Spine* 15:927-932, 1990.

# 32

# REVISION PEDIATRIC SPINE SURGERY: SUCCESS AND FAILURES

**Vincent Arlet, M.D.**
**Fabien D. Bitan, M.D.**



The revision of the pediatric spine differs from the adult spine. The growth of the spine can ruin the most satisfactory initial result of spine reconstruction (Fig. 32-1). Conversely, asymmetry or lack of growth induced by a congenital abnormality or an early spine fusion can have very severe consequences on pulmonary function (Fig. 32-2), which may only be apparent later during early adulthood.[58,68] In pediatric patients, there is rarely a need for revision because of adjacent-segment degeneration. Very often the circumstances leading to revision in pediatric patients are encountered in very handicapped children with complex pediatric diseases such as congenital cardiopathy,[12] neuromuscular diseases,[3,8,14,45,47,55,57,73] or miscellaneous dysplasia.[4,10,29,36,59] The parents have to have an active part in decision making for these patients. A successful outcome of the revision will not always meet the expectations of the parents. The need for postoperative casts, extensive spine fusions, and sometimes staged procedures during the growing years needs to be explained very carefully to the parents and patients. Indications for revisions are rarely emergencies. In most cases, it is advisable to postpone the procedure until the parents understand the problems, the decisions, and the risks involved[74] because half measures are unlikely to achieve the goals of revision, which are balance and fusion. One must remember that the functional results of revisions are usually less satisfactory than primary successful procedures.

The overall rate of instrumentation failure and infections is classically low in the pediatric group but the exact rate of pseudarthrosis is still uncertain and various studies have shown ranges between 1% and 25%.[7,9,27,50,60] The advent of new sophisticated spine instrumentation in the 1980s gave the impression that any spinal deformity correction had become possible, and that a solid fusion would ensue. Old surgical textbooks insisted on decortication and fusion, whereas new manuals focus mainly on instrumentation. It appears that although modern instrumentation has dramatically improved the scope of spine surgery, it has also created several specific pathologies.[18,19,42,46,56,69,72] Similarly, new concepts of minimally invasive spine surgery, although beneficial in the immediate postoperative course, may have long-term morbidity if a meticulous arthrodesis is not carefully achieved.

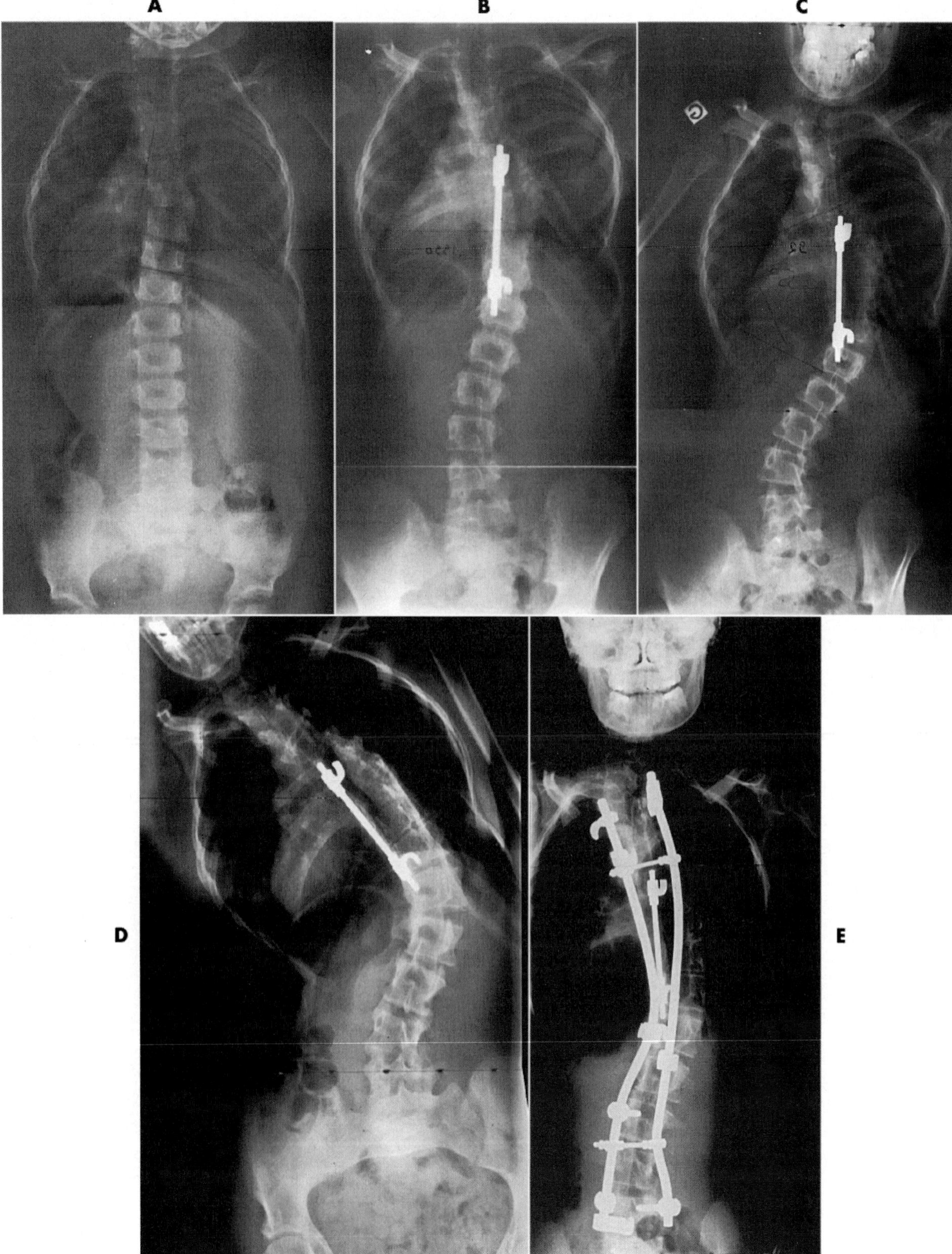


**FIGURE 32-1**

This 3-year-old patient shows a well-balanced congenital scoliosis with minimal angulation **(A).** However, at age 8, because of progression, a posterior distraction Harrington rod and a posterior fusion are carried out **(B).** At age 17, she continues to show progression of her curves **(C).** Because of the complete lack of flexibility of the lumbar curve seen on the side-bending **(D)** (one can see the transitional anomaly) fusion to L5 is decided. In order not cause an imbalance, the only correction achieved will be the one obtained after resection of the facets in the lumbar spine, the fusion is enhanced with a tibial graft **(E).** The previous Harrington rod is left in place. At two years' follow-up the patient is perfectly balanced, the fusion solid. *(Courtesy of Dr. J. P. Padovani.)*

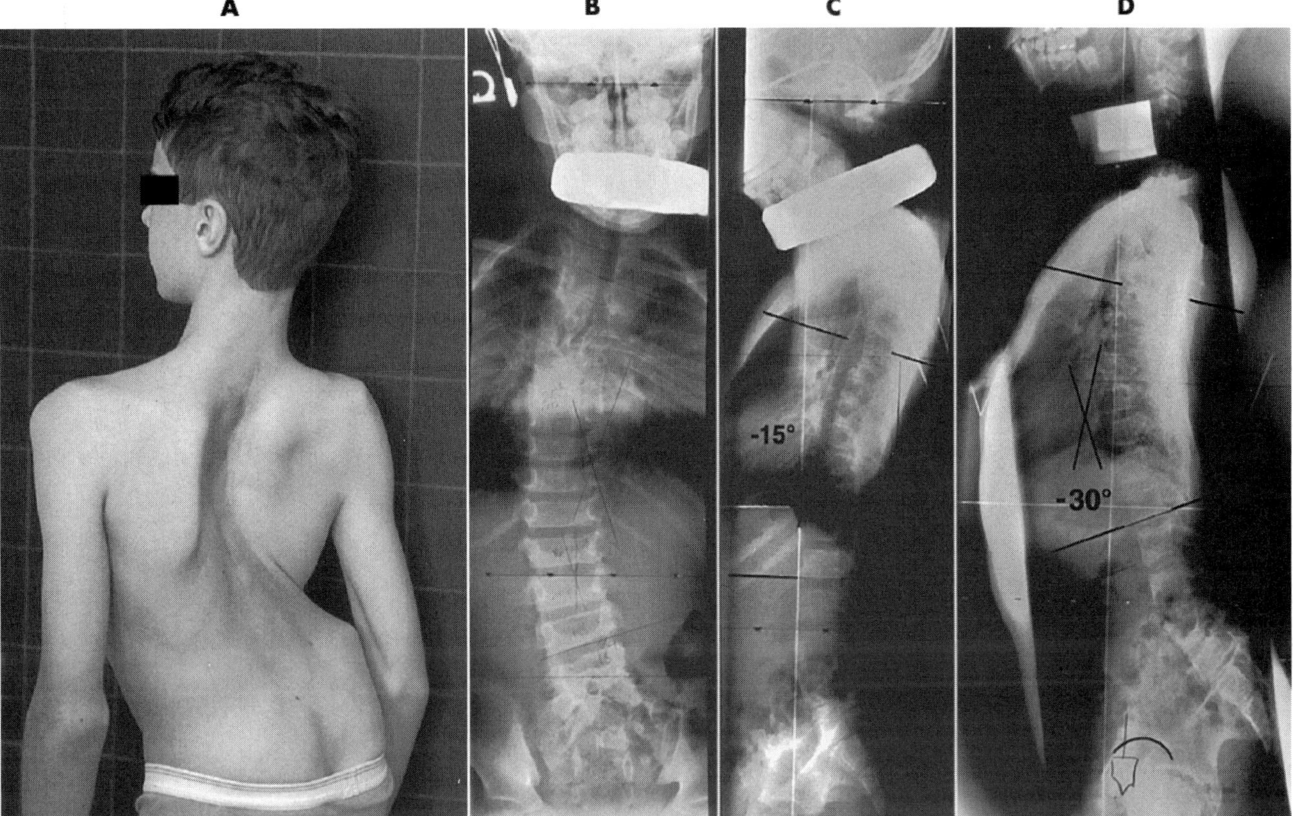


FIGURE 32-2

This 14-year-old boy is seen for a marked lordosis and shortness of breath when running **(A)**; his vital capacity is below 40%. At five years of age, he underwent division of a thoracic fibrous diastematomyelia, a posterior fusion of the thoracic spine was subsequently carried out **(B)**. The increase of his thoracic lordosis unfortunately is not recognized and the thoracic lordosis progressed from −15 to −30 degrees **(C** and **D)**. An anterior epiphysiodesis only will be carried out to prevent further worsening and deterioration; no posterior osteotomies or correction will be done because of the history of tethering with diastematomyelia. This anterior epiphysiodesis should have been done many years before to prevent crankshafting and deterioration of the lung function.

## CIRCUMSTANCES LEADING TO THE PEDIATRIC REVISIONS

We have excluded from this discussion revisions due to acute postoperative problems such as acute postsurgical infections or neurological complications. We also excluded the cases of staged procedures such as subcutaneous rod lengthening as advocated by Moe,[54] to concentrate on reconstruction or salvage pediatric spinal procedures.

Revision of a pediatric spine can be necessary to correct a functional problem. Revision can also be necessary because of a chronic infection long after a successful spine fusion by hematogenous seeding,[34] or as a late sequelae of an early postoperative infection. Functional back pain is rare in this age group and generally related to an identified mechanical problem. In other cases, the following may lead to revision: progression of the deformity, progressive restrictive lung disease, spine imbalance, instrumentation failure, late onset of neurologic signs, or a combination of the above. These conditions are often associated with one or more pseudarthroses.

## UNDERSTANDING PREVIOUS FAILURES

Understanding previous failures is, in the authors' opinion, essential for the outcome of the revision, if the mistakes of the previous procedures are not to be repeated. The etiology of the deformity is a significant factor in cases of failure.

### CONGENITAL SPINE

Progression of congenital curves is the result of an unbalanced growth of the different parts of a spine segment. Continuation of progression after surgery can be difficult sometimes to detect early by the Cobb angle method because of difficulties in picking up the appropriate levels, and also because the progression is often localized to just a few segments. Subtle clinical changes, such as progressive trunk shift, shoulder elevation, or increase of the rib hump, may alert the clinician. A retrospective and careful analysis of the history (going back to the initial x-rays as well as the postoperative ones) can help in understanding the pathological process and dictate the appropriate decision.

The progression may be explained by:

1. Progression in the fused area. The main cause observed in old cases is a posterior spinal fusion in the presence of a severe malformation (such as an hemivertebra associated with a contralateral bar). The anterior convex growth plates continue to grow leading to increasing deformity. This was coined as the crankshaft phenomenon by Dubousset.[24] The anatomy is sometimes impossible to detail when the curve has come to a severe angle. Early detection of this postoperative progression is crucial to any decision regarding performing a complementary anterior fusion (see Figs. 32-1 and 32-2).
2. Progression of associated malformations above and below, can ruin a successful initial result. This will be observed, for instance when the initial surgery that consisted in a hemivertebra resection neglected the malformed segments above. An associated malformation should never be underestimated. In some other cases, a nonsegmented bar can be missed on early films because it has not yet ossified.
3. Compensatory curves above and below the fused area can be responsible for a poor result (see Fig. 32-1). They develop early and become structural with sometimes a greater prejudice than the main curve, leading to imbalance, rib hump, or pelvic obliquity. These curves may necessitate an extension of the fusion at a later time, but it must be kept in mind that if congenital curves are nonresponsive to orthopedic treatment, it may be possible to treat them effectively with an appropriate brace.[52]

Associated neural anomalies, such as tethered cord, diastematomyelia, or syrinx, must be suspected when the deformity progresses in spite of appropriate treatments. Intraspinal investigations must be undertaken, but a previous steel instrumentation can be a major impediment to magnetic resonance imaging (MRI) investigation.

## DYSPLASTIC SPINE

The dysplastic spine can include such conditions as osteochondrodystrophia (achondroplasia, spondyloepiphyseal dysplasia, diastrophic dysplasia, mucopolysaccharidoses) with vertebral involvement, Marfan syndrome, neurofibromatosis, and associated syndromes (such as Ehlers-Danlos syndrome). Spine surgery in conditions such as these are more prone to complications than in idiopathic cases.[6,10,20,36,41,61,70] The most frequently reported reasons for these complications are frequent narrowing of the spine canal, the frequent kyphotic tendency[70] that places the posterior fusion, in the tension side of the spine, a poor biological ground to achieve a successful fusion, and defective biomechanical properties of bone that leads to poor instrumental purchase.[4,6,29,36]

The dysplastic nature of the spine may have not been obvious at the initial surgery, especially in neurofibromatosis.[20] Long after surgery fusion failure, spine collapse, and neurologic damage can be experienced (Fig. 32-3). In these cases, the revision procedure often includes an anterior fusion. This is particularly crucial if a kyphotic deformity has occurred. These cases are more prone to late neurological complications. This must lead to a specific approach in which all available approaches can be combined including cord decompression, osteotomy, and halo traction. Which combination is used is a question of experience. This surgery is marked by a high level of severe complications, and must be referred to highly trained spine surgeons.

## NEUROMUSCULAR SPINE

Neuromuscular spines have an increased incidence of pseudarthrosis.[3,8,45,50,51,54,73] This can be due to their missing posterior elements and lack of bone stock (for example, in spina bifida that consequently require anterior fusion). Neuromuscular patients regularly need long fusions, often including the lumbosacral junction. The long lever arm over a poor bone purchase is more susceptible to screw or hook pull-out. The additional stresses due to spasticity in patients with cerebral palsy are another risk factor. These patients also have the tendency to decompensate sagittally above the instrumentation, regardless of how high the fusion stopped.

Some conditions combine the problems of both categories. Down syndrome[6,23,63] or Prader-Willi syndrome,[60] for example, have a high rate of complications. These complications can include nonunions, infections, and sometimes progressive worsening despite an apparently solid fusion.

## TECHNICAL PROBLEMS

Initial surgical problems must be recognized in order to explain the failure when possible. These problems can include posterior bone graft deficiency, anterior graft deficiency, instrumentation-related complications, and other causes of failure.

***Posterior Bone Graft Deficiency.*** The promotion of new bone substitutes, though being exciting for future applications, seems to be in some cases a contributing factor to complications. It is the opinion of the authors that ceramics or bank bone grafts have a higher rate of fusion failure than autogenous bone grafts (despite some favorable reports with their use[7]). In some

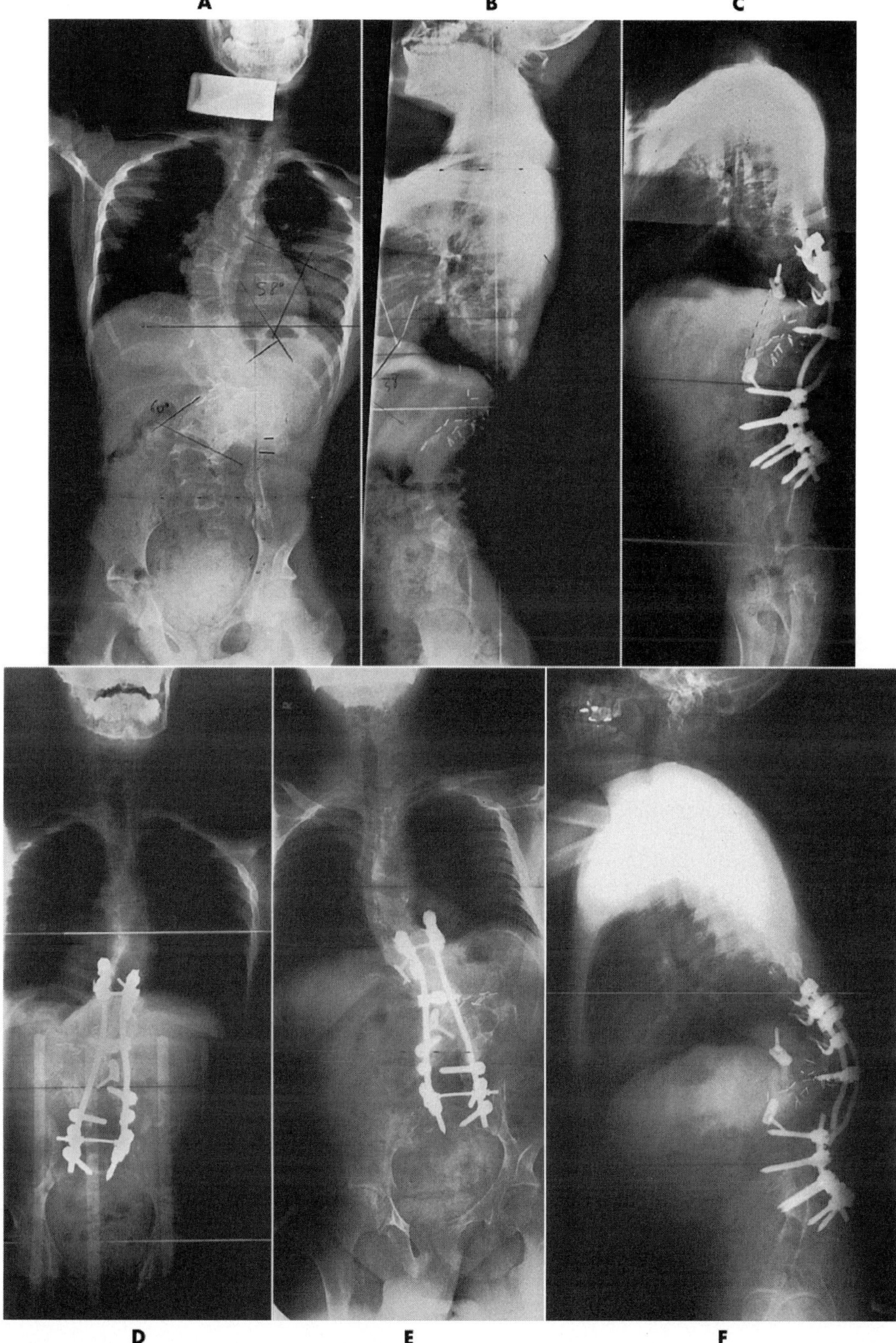


**FIGURE 32-3**

This spinal deformity **(A** and **B)** due to neurofibromatosis had already been operated 6 times including two anterior approaches to the spine. Because of progressive muscle weakness and spine instability, revision is decided. This will consist of a posterior decompression and stabilization with pedicular instrumentation once the canal had been opened with bone grafting from the two posterior iliac crests. One month later, an anterior concave approach with a fibula graft is locked in the anterior defect. During two years the balance is excellent **(C** and **D),** however, at this time the patient will experience back pain with a crack. Subsequent x-rays show the broken rods and fibula, as well as the collapse of the spine **(E** and **F).** Revision at this time is not contemplated because the patient is asymptomatic despite a loss of balance. This case illustrates that in some cases a good instrumentation with what appears to be a good biologic and mechanical fusion can fail because of the bone dysplasia.

cases, such as chondrodysplasia, neuromuscular patients, or cases of multiple revisions, the lack of adequate bone graft makes these substitutes indispensable.

Technical errors are sometime recognized, such as instrumentation without bone graft,[27] especially if the fusion extends in the lower lumbar spine.[9] Progressive failure of the graft can also occur when the graft is only disposed on the tension side of the curve (Fig. 32-4). This graft can seem initially solid but, with time, it becomes thinner and eventually breaks leading to a secondary pseudarthrosis.

The decortication technique may have been insufficient without facet excisions as seen on the oblique x-rays (facets spaces nonobliterated). The lack of decortication and bone graft under the rod or under the transverse connectors will only be observed at the time of revision. The volume of the hardware and the frequent bleeding at the end of the procedure are sometimes important factors.

***Anterior Graft Deficiency.*** Anterior intervertebral gaps after posterior correction of a flexible kyphosis, a congenital wedged vertebra, or after an anterior release, should be filled with bone graft at the time of the anterior procedure. Otherwise, an inappropriate load-sharing balance occurs, leading to posterior fixation failure. Even in immature children the expected growth from the endplates can be insufficient to prevent further collapse in kyphosis.

The quality of the anterior fusion also plays a role. When a morsellized rib or cancellous bone graft is used, the posterior instrumentation should be strong enough to support the correction during the time required for the graft to become structural. Conversely, rigid corticocancellous graft fragments, stuck in the intervertebral spaces after an anterior release, can be an impediment to efficient correction (as in correction of a lordosis).[75-77] A long anterior strut graft bridging several levels may not be sufficiently revascularized during the first months to support the correction in the absence of a posterior support.

Inappropriate placement of the anterior graft can also lead to failure. A strut graft placed too far away from the spine, or lateral from the gravity line will be more likely to break.[15] A strut graft must ideally be placed in the concavity of the tridimensional curve. This can lead to approach the spine from the concavity of the projected anteroposterior view (Figs. 32-3 and 32-4).[32,66]

***Instrumentation-Related Complications.*** It is impossible to list here all of the instrumental misuses that lead to complications. The most frequent mistakes encountered in our experience were:

1. The use of inappropriate devices, such as the small-diameter Luque rods in neuromuscular patients that led to frequent breakage, have almost disappeared now that the larger 6-mm rods are used. Sacral fixation with a single screw (not purchasing the anterosuperior cortex of S1) on each side in long lumbosacral constructs or the use of 5-mm screws at the distal end of the instrumentation (Fig. 32-5) are other examples of incorrect use of instrumentations that can lead to complications.
2. The lack of cross-links in long spinal constructs leads to torsional instability and exposes to breakage.
3. Excessive corrective maneuvers in a rigid spine without adequate anterior and/or posterior release, puts too much stress on the instrumentation and on its bony support, with a high risk of loosening.
4. An awkward accumulation of metallic devices in a particular region prevents proper decortication and grafting and fusion failure becomes more likely. This mistake should especially be avoided at the thoracolumbar junction because of the likelihood of pseudarthrosis.[48] When using multiple rod constructs, the connectors on both sides should not be located at the same level, and, if possible, not at the thoracolumbar junction (Fig. 32-5). The instrumentation of both sides of the lamina with hooks may explain the failure and must be avoided whenever possible (Fig. 32-6). When possible one of the hooks must be shifted to an adjacent level or replaced by a screw.

In other cases it will be the paucity of the instrumentation, especially if it extends in the lumbar spine that explains the failure (Fig. 32-5). Inappropriate use of instrumentation, as described by Cotrel and Dubousset,[19] can be responsible for nonoptimal fixation.

Poor purchase in osteoporotic bone should not be accepted, especially in the lumbosacral area. The Galveston technique, though often efficient,[14] can be supplemented if needed by sacral screws. In the same manner, a sacral screw can be supplemented by an iliac screw (Fig. 32-7). The Jackson technique[37] seems to be the most promising innovation. Multiple segmental instrumentation, use of pedicle screws, and supplementation with methylmethacrylate[80] are among the techniques available.

Harrington instrumentation, although a tremendous advance in spinal surgery, has produced a significant number of flat back syndromes.[1,40,42,56] Some of them that are well tolerated are simply followed until they decompensate in adulthood, while others lead to functional disabilities and have to be corrected while at a young age.[56]

In cases in which little or no instrumentation has been used, failure can be explained by the noncompliance to immobilization. Removal of a postoperative brace and early return to contact activities are frequent situations seen in the turbulent pediatric group.

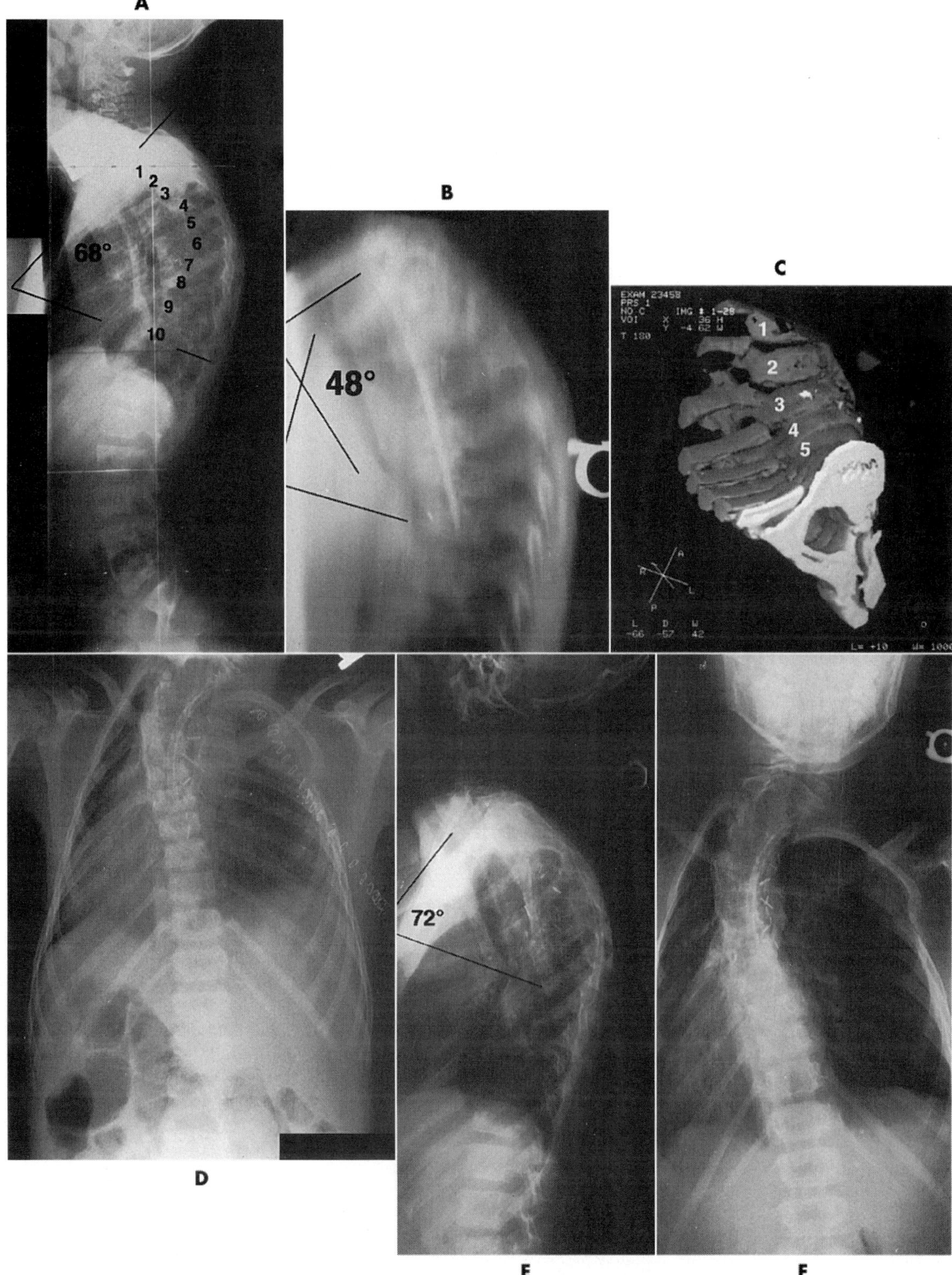


**FIGURE 32-4**

This 8-year-old patient presents with progressive kyphoscoliotic deformity **(A).** At age 2 he was operated for a neuroblastoma, and following this a total of 24 Grays was delivered to the spine. At age 5, because of a recurrence, he undergoes further neurosurgical procedure with laminectomy and arthrectomy from T3 down to T6. Postoperatively he develops a progressive deformity that is treated with an anterior convex tibial strut graft and posterior fusion **(B)** followed with halo cast application. Despite this treatment, progression of the deformity and a pseudarthrosis could be demonstrated on a 3D CT scan **(C)** 2 years later between T1-T2 and T2-T3. Revision is performed through an anterior concave approach taking the third rib **(D).** One can see two ribs between C7 and T7 used as struts. This is reinforced with a revision of the posterior fusion in which the pseudarthroses are curetted and massive iliac crest is laid. Immobilization is done with a Minerva cast for four months. At two years' follow-up **(E** and **F)** the deformity is stabilized without further progression. This case illustrates the need to put the bone graft on the concave side and along the gravity line, the necessity to bone graft these patients in an extensive fashion, and that successful revision can be achieved without instrumentation.

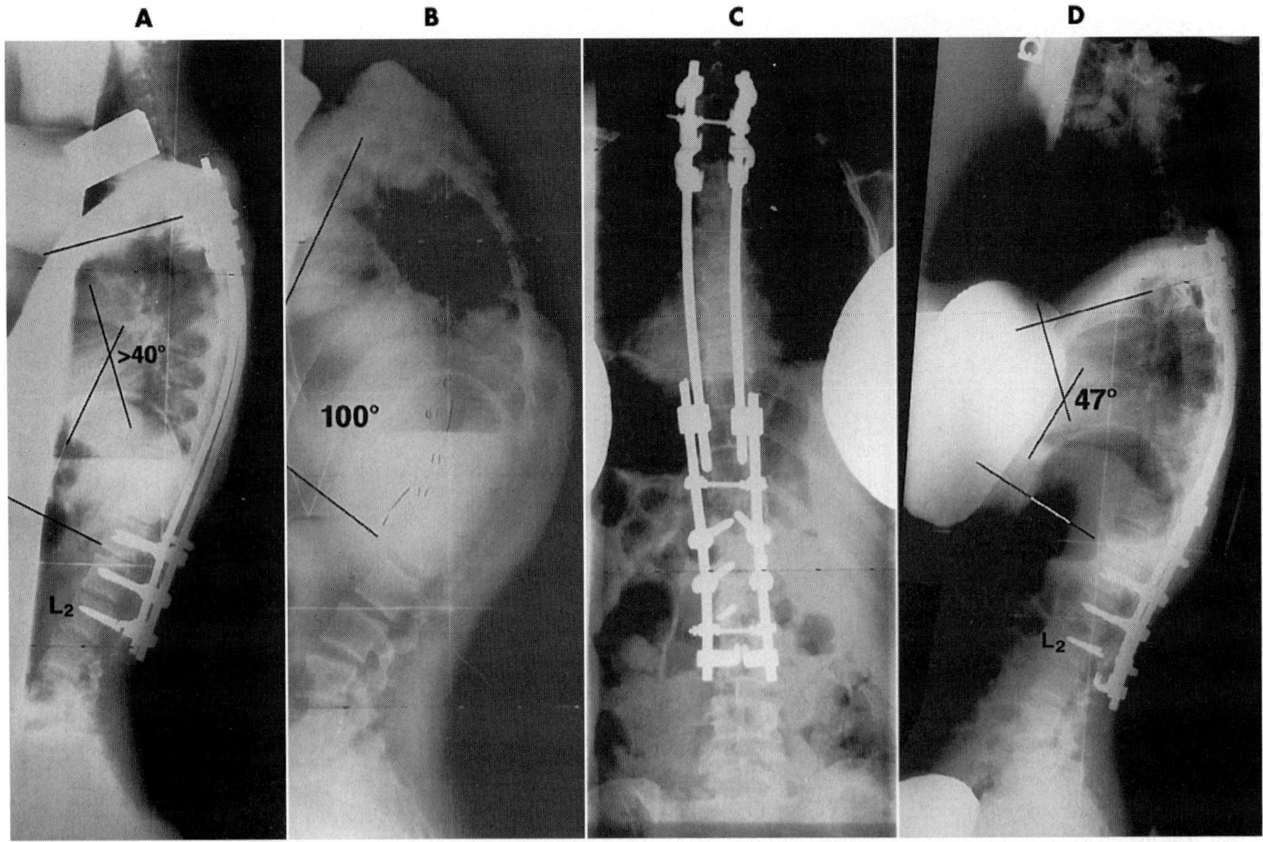


FIGURE 32-5

A 15-year-old patient presenting with sudden onset of pain in the upper lumbar spine **(A).** Her x-rays demonstrate broken 5-mm pedicle screws at the bottom of a T1-L2 posterior Cotrel-Dubousset fusion. This mildly mentally retarded patient had been treated 14 months before for a hyperkyphosis of 100 degrees **(B).** No anterior release had been done at this time. Because of the persistent pain, revision was performed. Different strategies are discussed: 1) reexploration of the fusion mass and either extension of the instrumentation to L3 or use of offset laminar screws to remain at the same level; 2) go anteriorly from T9 to L2, and carry out a diskectomy and anterior instrumentation and fusion to L2; or 3) perform a 360-degree fusion. It is decided to reexplore the posterior fusion mass first and judge if a complementary anterior fusion is necessary. Two pseudarthroses at L1-L2 and at T11-T12 are identified; the rods are cut, connected to dominos, and the instrumentation remains at L2 with the help of offset laminar hooks; a massive decortication and fresh bone graft from the opposite previously harvested iliac crest is done, no anterior fusion is done. At 4 years' follow-up the patient is asymptomatic, and there is no significant loss of correction **(C and D).** This example illustrates the possibility of remaining at the same level even when there is a failure of the most distal screws that could not be removed. However, the rods should have been cut and cross-linked at different levels, and not at the thoracolumbar junction.

## OTHER CAUSES OF FAILURES

The crankshaft phenomenon of the spine[24] around the initial posterior fusion mass is now well understood. It is now universally accepted that a posterior fusion performed in immature children warrants an anterior epiphysiodesis as well (see Fig. 32-1).[62,64] The usual indications are the timing of the surgery according to the growth spur (when a growth curve is available), the state of the triradiate cartilage, the fusion of the capitellum at the elbow, and the Risser test.[22,61] The idea of a posterior crankshafting when an isolated anterior fusion and instrumentation had been performed early can be brought forward.

Junctional imbalance can occur below or above an instrumented segment.[56] The mechanical reasons for this failure need to be analyzed because they can dictate the appropriate treatment. Multiple reasons can be found, such as an extensive exposure of the noninstrumented levels at the time of the initial surgery or too short a fusion for a kyphotic deformity. In some cases, only the etiology of the deformity will explain this junctional kyphosis (e.g., a short fusion in the thoracic spine of diastrophic dwarfism, a neuromuscular patient, or dysplastic patients will often evolve into the development of a new deformity above or below). It is well-established that in most neuromuscular scoliosis the instrumented fusion has to go up to T3 or T2.[3,14]

Another factor involved in postoperative decompensation is the status of the lower limbs, especially the hips. Performing a spine revision when the problem is actually in the hips is a certainty of failure. Mentally

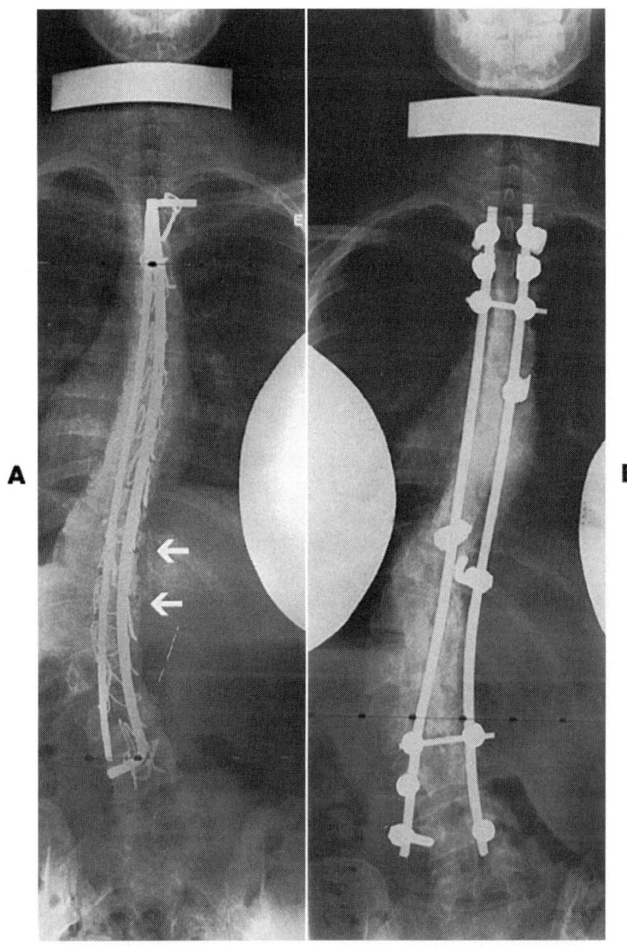


FIGURE 32-6

This 16-year-old patient had a Luque operation 2 years earlier for idiopathic scoliosis and bank bone allograft. At 2 years' follow-up, because of curve progression and pain, revision is decided in view of suspected pseudarthrosis **(A)** (*arrows*). Three pseudarthroses are identified: two at the thoracolumbar junction and one at the proximal part of the fusion. They are cleaned, decorticated, and grafted with iliac crest cancellous bone. Three years after the revision **(B)** she presents with discharge from the wound. X-rays show radiolucency along the rods. Reoperation for debridement and instrumentation removal will identify one persistent pseudarthrosis where the two laminar hooks were inserted. The failure to achieve union can be explained by a lack of compression at the pseudarthrosis level and the insertion of laminar hooks at the same lamina level, with too little room for decortication and grafting. The lack of control over the lumbar spine (not enough implant anchors) is another reason for nonunion. No instrumentation will be reinserted during this second revision; the pseudarthrosis will be simply cleaned and regrafted. One year after rod removal she complains of episodic low thoracic pain, but there is no obvious curve worsening.

retarded patients have a tendency to fall towards the sagittal decompensation, making it even worse. The complexity of a hip flexion contracture combined with a flat back syndrome can be extremely difficult to analyze especially in an ambulatory neurologically impaired patient. The questions raised are: how much is due to knee or hip flexion contracture and how much is due to sagittally decompensated fused spine?

In some cases the spine has been perfectly corrected but the patient is still not doing well. Several additional problems can complicate a nice spinal correction.

As mentioned above, persistence of a pelvic obliquity due to stiff hips can lead to a worse functional situation in a neurological patient, because a sitting position that was difficult before surgery, may become completely impossible when the spine is corrected.

The walking capabilities of some ambulatory neurologically impaired patients may deteriorate after a lumbosacral spine fusion that straightened the lumbar spine but took away the last mobile segments. The persistence of a mild sagittal imbalance may explain this deterioration, which would not have occurred if they had been perfectly balanced, or fused down to only L4 (with a persistent pelvic obliquity but a mobile lumbar spine).

A patient with a disproportionate short stature (arms shorter than trunk ) may suffer from a too beautiful correction of "providential scoliosis" (the trunk too long for arms), resulting in difficulties in hygienic care. The same consideration can be made in cases of associated congenital hypoplastic upper limbs. Missed osteoid osteoma, discovered after spinal fusion because of persistent pain, should be kept in mind.

## ASSESSMENT BEFORE REVISION

### GENERAL WORKUP

In most cases, especially neuromuscular patients due to their usual poor general condition, a general workup must be extensive enough to include nutritional status (total lymphocyte count and serum albumin).[38] A multidisciplinary approach to the workup is necessary and should involve dietitians, pulmonologists, cardiologists, and neurosurgeons. There may be an indication for a preliminary shunt revision or lengthening, feeding through a nasogastric tube or even a gastrostomy or jenunostomy to supplement nutrition, or for the surgical treatment of an unstable congenital cardiopathy.[12] The closure of a vesicostomy or enterostomy if possible may sometimes precede the spine reconstruction. This necessary workup can range from minimal in idiopathic revisions to very complex in neuromuscular patients. The results of it can even deter the surgeon or the family from the surgery and indicate the use of external means to support the trunk.

### ORTHOPEDIC WORKUP

The assessment follows the rules of all orthopedic and spine workups with specific regard to coronal and

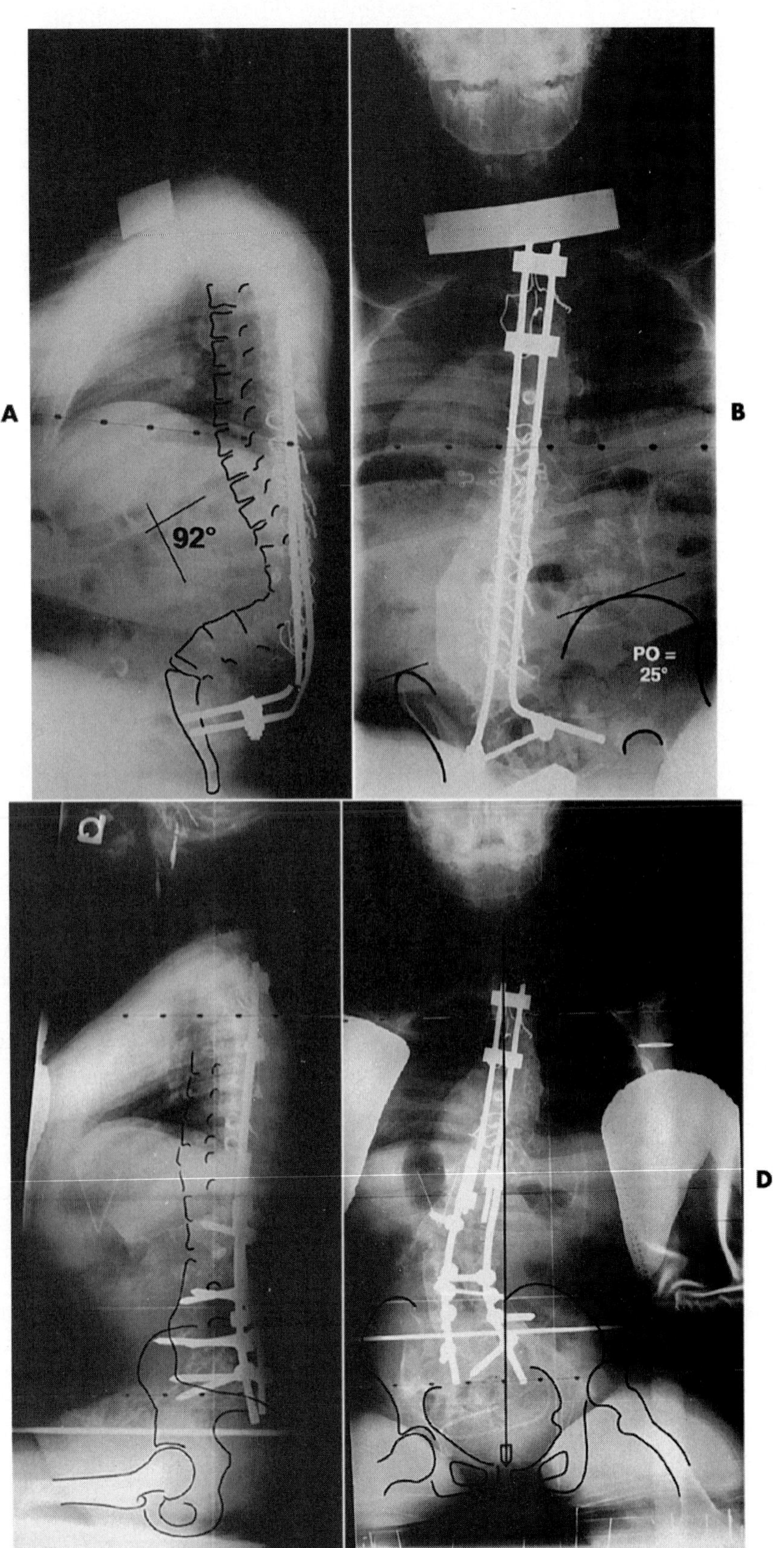


**Figure 32-7**

This 11-year-old patient has a functional T10 meningocele. She is referred for hip flexion contracture and pelvic obliquity **(A** and **B).** She underwent front and back spinal fusion with Luque-type instrumentation in the past. The revision of her spine needs to address the following problems: reduce the 90-degree kyphosis responsible for the pseudoflexion contracture of her hips, correct the sitting pelvic obliquity, and fuse the L5-S1 disk space. The deformity is considered a long bone problem. Through a posterior approach, the cauda equina is ligated at the L5-S1 disk level, the disk excised and bone grafted. A strong sacropelvic fixation is achieved with screws in S1 pedicles, and in the iliac wings, dominoes are connected to the upper part of the Luque rods and a resection osteotomy removing a wedge of 2.5 cm is done at the apex of the deformity. Correction is achieved with cantilever, compression, and distraction maneuvers. Postoperatively the patient is perfectly balanced **(C** and **D).**

sagittal imbalance and, as mentioned previously, to peripheral joints. Plain x-rays, sedimentation rate, and bending films are almost always required. Plain or oblique films or tomograms may show pseudarthrosis,[43,67] but in very severe spine deformities the pseudarthrosis will be suspected only by a thorough review of all the previous films, a 3D reconstruction computerized scanner with thin slices (see Fig. 32-4), or at surgery (in one third of the cases in Lauerman series[43]). The neural axis should be cleared before contemplating a revision. When stainless steel devices have been used, removal of the hardware must be considered first to allow for an MRI study. It is mandatory to carefully check the C-spine of all congenital and dysplastic spines (skeletal dysplasia, Marfan syndrome, neurofibromatosis) before contemplating revision of the underlying deformities.

## SURGICAL PLANNING

Assuming the decision to perform revision has been made and the patient's general health status is able to withstand it, the technical modalities require a thorough knowledge of pediatric spine surgery. Pediatric spine revision is a difficult orthopedic challenge, and the risks of complications are higher than in the initial surgery. In the surgical planning several steps must be followed.

The decision of removal of the whole hardware and new correction versus plain extension of fusion will be answered on a case-by-case basis. One must clearly define the purpose of the revision, because a plain extension of a fusion is a less dangerous procedure than performing osteotomies, especially in the thoracolumbar area. This solution is preferred when it is possible. A cosmetic problem related to a residual rib hump and without major balance problems can safely be addressed by a thoracoplasty.

Sometimes, however, vertebral osteotomies are needed because the curve needs to be recorrected. This is a demanding procedure that can be dangerous. The thicker the initial fusion and the higher the quality of the first procedure, the more difficult the osteotomy. When an initial circumferential procedure has been performed, a combined anterior and posterior osteotomy is warranted. Any simpler solution should be seriously considered before such an undertaking.

In the lumbar spine, there are wide indications for vertebral osteotomies in flat back syndromes,[1,28,40,48,78] in persistence of severe pelvic obliquity after spinal fusion in neuromuscular patients (Fig. 32-8), and in case of severe postoperative imbalance, because it is not possible to count on reequilibration in the thoracic spine.

In the thoracic spine, the indications for osteotomies are rare because of the potential for neurologic complications. Some indications exist however. This will be done for the revision of a major crankshaft or congenital scoliosis with spine imbalance when a plain anterior fusion is not sufficient, or to help maintain the trunk balance when a lumbar compensatory curve needs to be fused under a significant rigid thoracic deformity. Thoracic osteotomies to correct the thoracic curves may also be considered to save distal lumbar vertebrae if the lumbar spine is still flexible and not too structural. Somatosensory and motor evoked potential monitoring are essential during these procedures, and can be confirmed by several wake-up tests during the procedure or if any doubt subsists.

***Extension of the New Fusion.*** Extension to the sacropelvis, if sometimes inevitable (Fig. 32-9), must not be considered as a routine procedure. It implies an iatrogenic restriction to mobility of the whole trunk, and it has been shown to have the higher rate of complications. Moreover, it interferes with lower joint motion, and can deprive a neurological patient of a useful pelvic swing during ambulation. Finally, lumbopelvic fusion is challenging because no postoperative adaptation can be expected in case of residual imbalance (Fig. 32-10 and 32-11). Here again the decision is often made on a case-by-case basis. However, in some situations the decision is quite clear; extension to the sacrum is almost always required in cases of postoperative imbalance in neuromuscular patients (see Fig. 32-8).

In spondylodysplastic patients, sacral extension must never be performed because of the poor condition and limited range of motion of lower limbs, especially the hips.

In idiopathic pediatric revision patients, extension to the sacrum is rarely if ever done. Any other option must be considered because of the resulting disability and the risk of fixed imbalance that can result from this procedure, as seen in Figures 32-10 and 32-11.

Extension of the fusion in the lumbar spine is often indicated. The question therefore is where to stop the fusion. The last fused vertebrae should be neutral and transsected by the mid sacral line, provided the underneath spine is still flexible on the side-bending films, and that no specific sagittal problem dictates another procedure. This level corresponds most frequently to L3 or L4 for revision cases. If the patient experiences lumbar pain as a part of the indication of revision surgery, which is a rare situation in the pediatric age, the lower disks must be investigated by MRI or diskograms. Those different criteria can sometimes lead to the conclusion that L5 is the best level to stop the fusion (see Fig. 32-1). This decision is still a matter of controversy: should we save exposure of the lumbosacral junction and perform a further extension in adulthood, or should we fuse L5-S1 right away (see Fig. 32-11)?

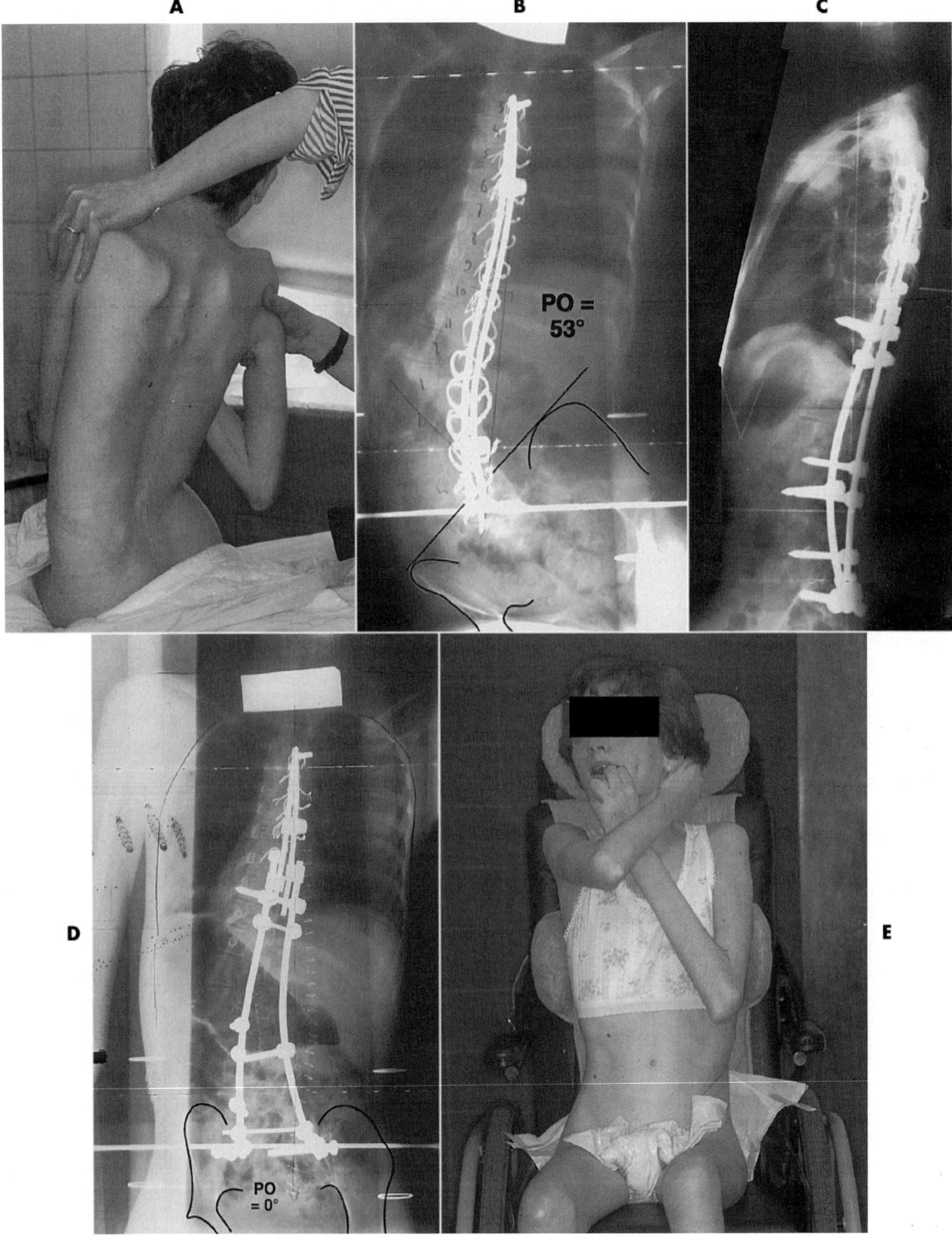


**FIGURE 32-8**

This 15-year-old patient with Rett syndrome presented to us for difficulties seating and feeding **(A).** X-rays **(B)** show a significant pelvic obliquity and what appears to be a solid fusion. Two years before she had undergone a posterior spine fusion with Luque wires and rods down to L5. Three different surgical strategies for revision were discussed: 1) posterior approach, hardware removal, multiple spine osteotomies, and reinstrumentation to the sacropelvis; 2) posterior approach, hardware removal, decancellation at the L2-L3 level removing a lateral wedge of vertebra, and reinstrumentation; and 3) anterior release, posterior approach, hardware removal, multiple spine osteotomies, and reinstrumentation to the sacropelvis. The third option is chosen. At the same time, anterior release L2 sacrum, diskectomies, and morselized bone graft, followed by posterior approach, partial rod removal, 5 spine osteotomies, reinstrumentation with iliosacral screws at the bottom and dominos at the top are performed. Postoperative course is uneventful apart from a moderate atelectasis. The sitting balance is excellent **(C and D)** and maintained at one-year follow-up **(E).**

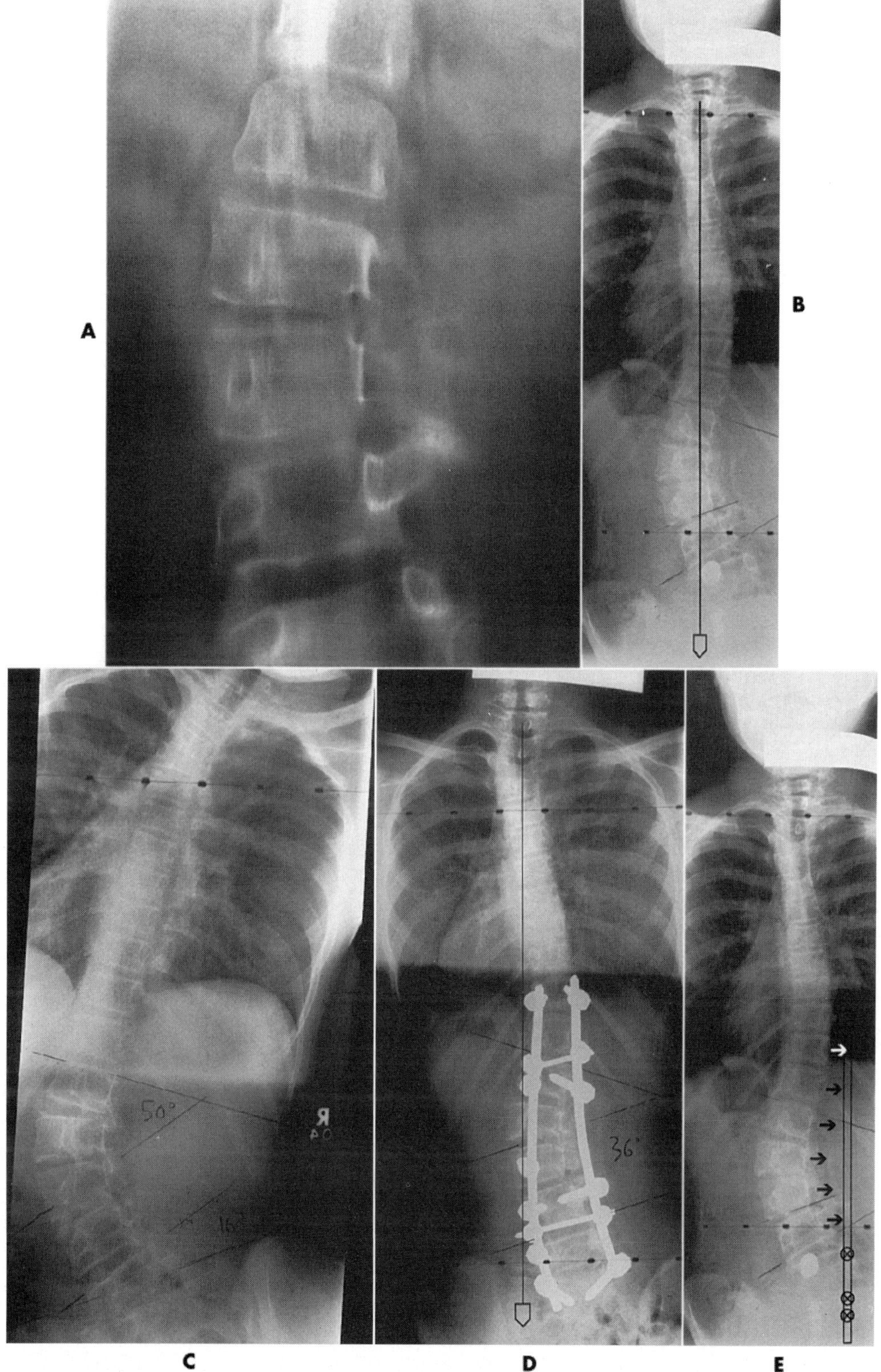

FIGURE 32-9

This 10-year-old patient has a congenital bar between the transverses processes **(A).** She first undergoes a posterior bar resection with fat interposition and brace application. Unfortunately, the scoliosis continues to progress with subsequent imbalance **(B).** Revision to the sacrum is decided because of the imbalance and the persistent and fixed obliquity of L5 on side-bending x-rays **(C).** Postoperatively, she remains unbalanced **(D)** for two reasons: proper spine x-rays could not be obtained during the surgical procedure because of the nonradiolucent scoliosis frame that was used, and a strategic mistake was made: the correction was started on the left side to preserve the lumbar lordosis, with a derotation of the rod. The concave side should have been instrumented first with S1 and in L5 pedicle screws and a sagittally fixed rod, compress between the 2 screws and then translate the spine to the right rod. Achievement of lumbar lordosis would have been done with in situ bending of the rod or symmetric compression at the end of the instrumentation **(E).**

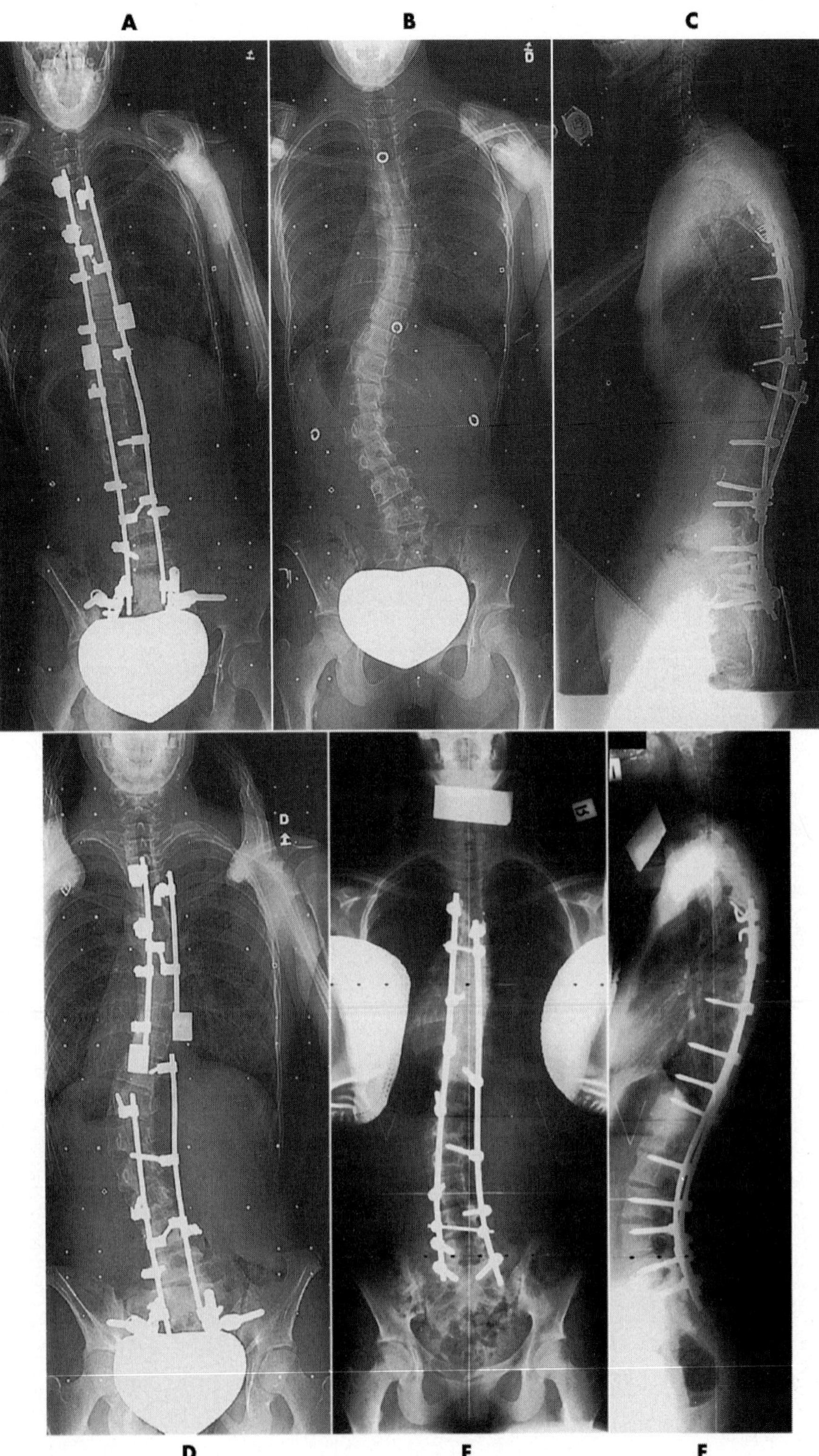


**FIGURE 32-10**

This 16-year-old patient consults for imbalance **(A)** after a posterior spine fusion with synthetic bone graft for idiopathic scoliosis that was performed six months before elsewhere **(B).** The imbalance is explained by the extension to the sacrum, and a too perfect correction of the curves (which we do not recommend). Four months later she comes back for increasing deformity, disengagement of the rods at the dominoes level, and a beginning of flat back syndrome **(C).** However, since the rods have disengaged the coronal balance is much improved **(D).** The revision is done 13 months after the initial surgery. Several pseudarthroses are identified. The instrumentation is removed; the reinstrumentation will use the same implant anchorages (with bigger screws) in the thoracic and lumbar spine but a new fixation in the sacrum without including the sacroiliac joints. The correction will be performed with the only goal to achieve both coronal and sagittal balance, neglecting completely the angular correction of the Cobb angle. No derotation at all will be used. A massive iliac bone graft will be applied after thorough decortication and facetectomies. At the last follow-up the patient is perfectly balanced **(E** and **F).**

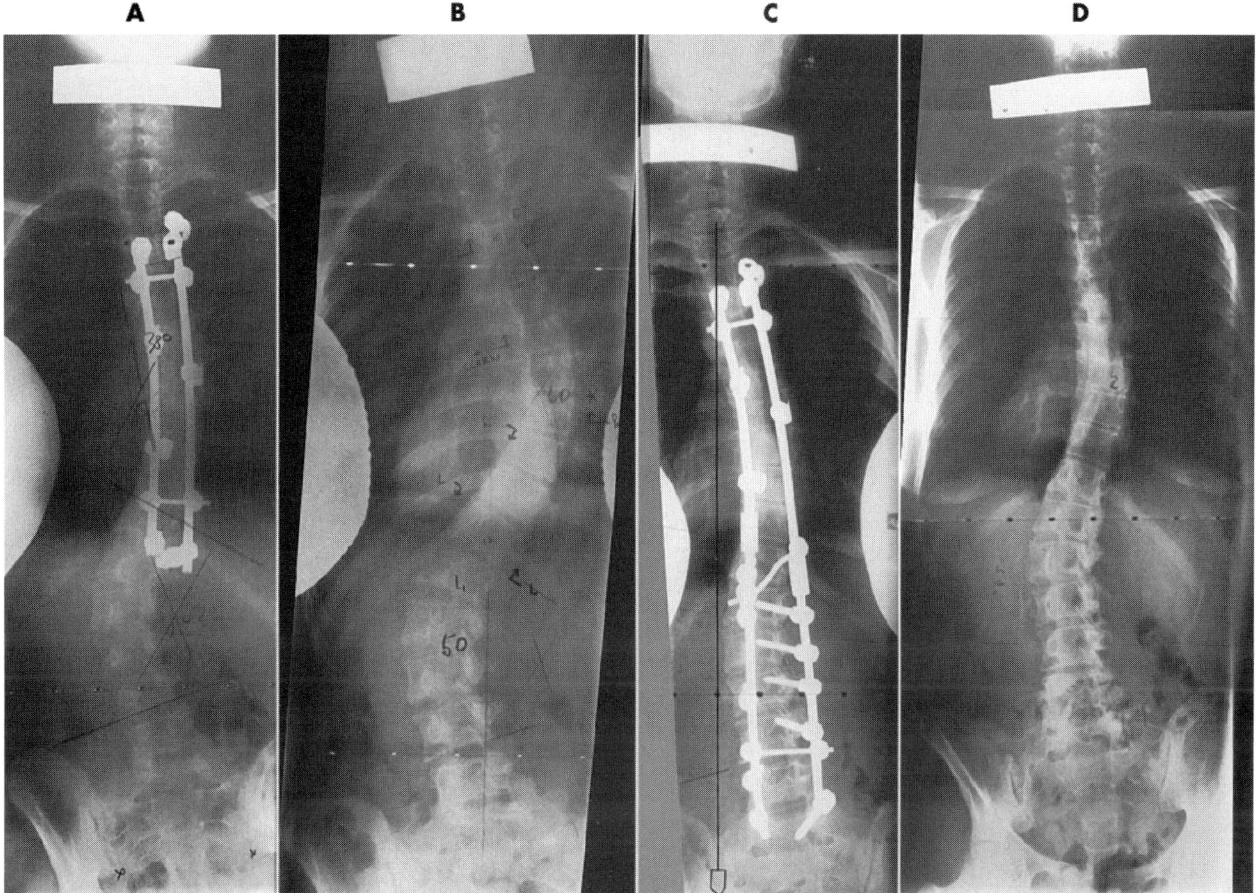


FIGURE 32-11

This 14-year-old patient had a selective right thoracic fusion **(A)** for a Kng 2 adolescent idiopathic scoliosis **(B),** unfortunately postoperatively the lumbar spine did not respond to the thoracic correction and progression of the lumbar curve as well as imbalance was observed. It was decided to extend the fusion to the sacrum. (We would have extended the fusion to L4 only.) After revision, the patient remained unbalanced **(C).** One year after her revision a draining sinus from the wound requires local debridement without hardware removal. The infection recurs within 6 weeks (*Staphylococcus aureus*) and rod removal is decided. The fusion is labeled solid at the time of the surgery. Postoperatively the infection healed uneventfully and the patient regained her coronal balance **(D)** due to the plasticity of the graft or the onset of a pseudarthrosis. This case illustrates that pseudarthroses are sometimes providential!

In revision kyphosis surgery, the most frequent situation is a junctional kyphosis under the instrumentation, which requires fusion of the whole kyphosis determined by the Cobb angle. However, the flexibility of the lower disks as mentioned previously must be taken into account and can dictate a further extension into the lumbar spine.

***Creation of a Curve to Restore Coronal Balance.*** In some very complex deformities in which spinal osteotomies are not advisable (decompensated congenital scoliosis with previous spine fusion and neural anomalies as diastematomyelia) it may be necessary to create or increase a lumbar compensatory curve to restore the balance of the patient. This can be achieved through a decancellation procedure or by conventional methods such as releases or osteotomies, or compression and distraction in the lumbar compensatory curve.

***Neural Decompression.*** A neural decompression is very rarely necessary in children. However, neural compressions are present in some rare conditions. Compression is documented by a myelogram or an MRI if the previous instrumentation is compatible. In neurofibromatosis, the compression can be due to an angular deformity (Fig. 32-3), a compressive neurofibroma, or to an incarcerated rib in the canal.[20,29,36] In achondroplasia and related syndromes, it is essentially a congenital stenosis that requires a wide decompression before reinstrumentation. An iatrogenic neural compression can be due to a hook at the lower end of the fusion or to a malpositioned screw. The decompression or the release of neural structures (in diastematomyelia or tethered cord) must be addressed by a neurosurgeon before any attempt at spinal correction is made.

***Indications for Two-Stages Surgery.*** An anterior release is indicated to correct severe sagittal deformity or to address a major balance problem either in the coronal or sagittal plane (kyphosis or lordosis). This release should always include an intracorporeal graft. This release is sometimes a plain disk excision with endplate removal, but could be a real osteotomy or in some cases an anterior wedge resection as in lordosis.

ANTERIOR FUSION. A circumferential fusion is necessary when the previous failure is due to persisting anterior gaps. This situation is encountered in Scheuermann disease or constitutional cuneiform vertebrae, as seen in congenital wedge vertebrae. Cases of missing posterior elements, such as in spina bifida, are a major indication of anterior fusion.[3,8,51,55,73] Most revisions of dysplastic spines must be stabilized by a combined fusion.

EPIPHYSIODESIS. An anterior epiphysiodesis is strongly recommended in immature patients to prevent possible crankshaft or increase of thoracic lordosis.[24,62,64] One will not regret adding an anterior fusion for a previously fused congenital scoliosis that is crankshafting rather than waiting for the time of the thoracic spine osteotomies, which are more dangerous procedures.

***Graft.*** Different sources of graft in children can be very scarce, such as in the very young patient with a skeletal dysplasia. However, in a pediatric revision case one must always try to obtain autogenous graft, because the morbidity of bone harvesting is low in this age group if correctly carried out. The two iliac crests can be used if needed; removed ribs (one or two) are positioned as struts or to fill disk spaces; a thoracoplasty provides a copious amount of autogenous bone. It can be performed by the back or by the front. A vascularized rib graft has the advantage of being incorporated faster.[17] The fibula can be taken as well in its all thickness or in its posterior half. It is the authors' preference to harvest the posterior half of the fibula via a lateral approach between the peroneus muscles and the gastrocnemius, which has the only disadvantage of leaving a long scar on the leg. The tibial crests can also be used. The main complications are tibial fracture avoided by carefully preserving the anterior and posteromedial angles and closing the periosteum meticulously. This will provide usually a strip of 10 to 20 mm wide by the necessary length. A postoperative compartment syndrome will be prevented by systematic fasciotomies of both the anterior and posterior compartments and a Hemovac in the wound. This is confirmed by the extensive experience of Zeller and coworkers with neuromuscular scoliosis.[79] We have been using this source of graft in most of our neuromuscular patients (including spina bifida patients) without significant morbidity.

When bone stock is not available on the patient, new substances must be used despite the lower fusion rate they provide. Current progress will presumably lead to new options in the future, such as bone morphogenic proteins or osteoblast cultures.

***Instrumentation.*** Most current instrumentations are available in pediatric sizes or infant sizes, and it is always possible to connect to the previous instrumentation with dominos or cross-links. In some cases custom-made cross-link dominoes need to be ordered to fit the two kinds of different rods. The use of pedicle screws is now accepted in pediatric deformities.[2,33] In revision cases, anatomic landmarks are sometime confusing and the opening of the canal with direct control of the pedicle makes their insertion safer (Fig. 32-12). The fear of crossing the neurocentral synchondrosis with a screw is legitimate in children under 5 years of age because a developmental spinal stenosis could occur. However, the growth of the spine canal has achieved 90% of its size by age 5.[22] The use of sublaminar wiring remains, in selected cases, an acceptable option except in cases of documented neurological abnormalities (such as syrinx), and in developmental spinal stenosis (as in achondroplasia). It is paradoxically safer to use pedicle screws rather than hooks in some cases of spinal stenosis.

Often, a series of details is what leads us to a choice, such as a low-profile configuration, an ergonomic shape of the instrumentation, the possibility of easy removal, the cost of the construct, and the modularity of the implants.

Titanium instrumentations have become used more frequently because several of the revision cases will require postoperative MRI.

***Immobilization.*** This is usually not desired by parents, but in a limited number of cases this may represent the best solution, especially in very young children in whom no or little instrumentation could be applied (Figs. 32-12 and 32-13). This will be achieved via recumbency, casts, orthosis, or even a halo cast.

## SURGICAL TECHNIQUES

The goal of revision procedures is to obtain a balanced spine,* a solid spine fusion, and as many mobile segments as possible above and under the fusion. According to Beaupere's new concept of the "economic spine," there is a natural tendency to maintain the body in the most economical position in terms of muscle fatigue and vertebral strain.[26] Applied to the fused spine, this means that the fusion mass has to be

*Head over the shoulders, over the trunk, over the pelvis in the coronal plane, and the gravity line dropped from the odontoid process passing between the femoral heads and S2 on a patient with the knees extended in the lateral plane.

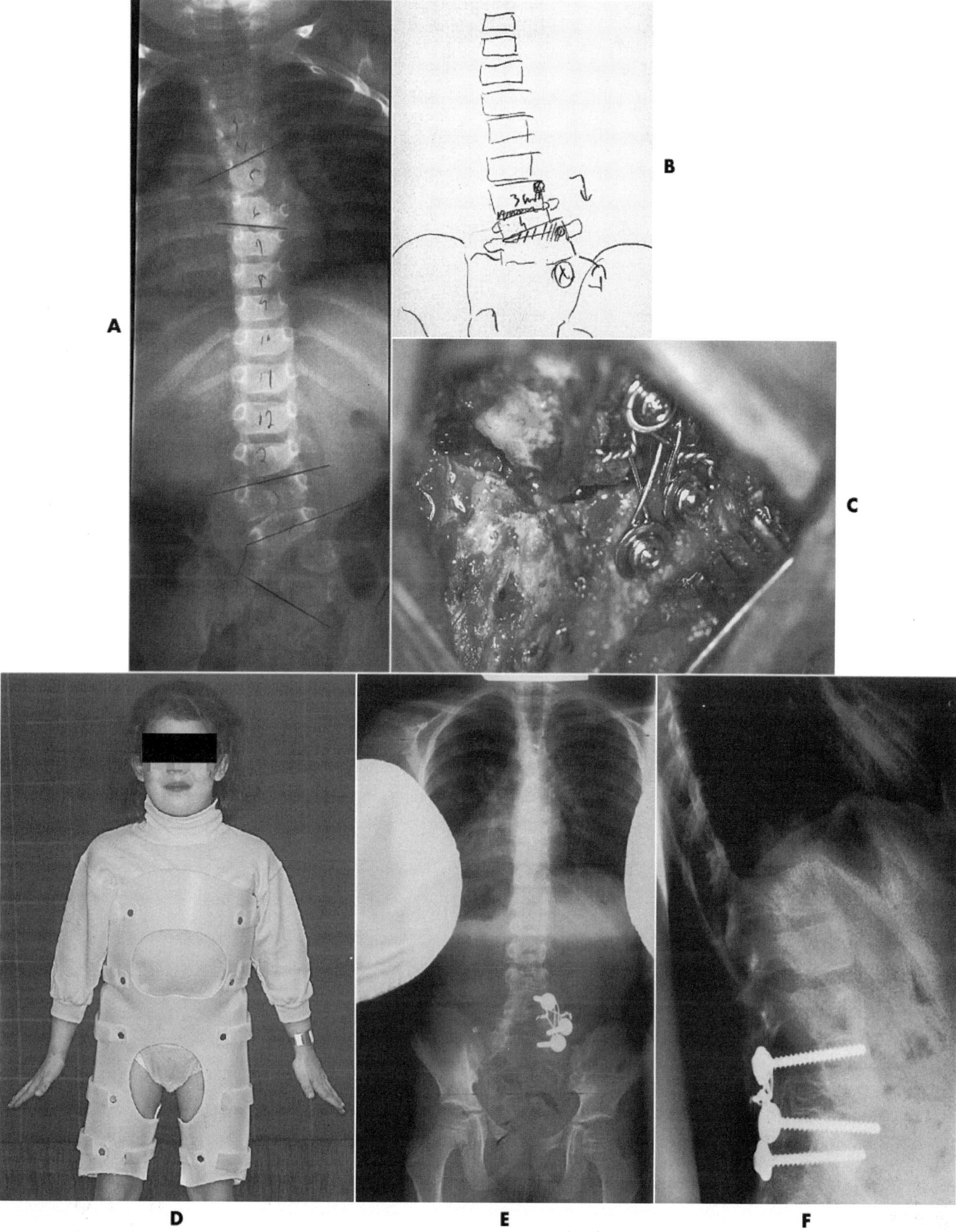


**FIGURE 32-12**

This $4\frac{1}{2}$-year-old girl presents to us with persistent imbalance after an attempted resection of an hemivertebra a year before done elsewhere **(A).** The initial surgery consisted of a vertebral excision through an anterior transperitoneal approach followed by a posterior fusion. Because of the persistent imbalance a decancellation, according to the preoperative cutout **(B)** is carried out. The intraoperative picture shows the osteotomy and the three pedicle screws with their washers and the tension band cerclage **(C)** before laying of the iliac crest bone graft. Postoperatively, a bilateral pantaloon brace is kept permanently for three months **(D).** At 1-year follow-up the balance is excellent, one can see the pedicle screws that had been put under direct control at the time of the decancellation **(E** and **F).** The hemivertebra between T5 and T6 seems to be incarcerated and nonthreatening in this case. This perfect result had four minor complications, however, all of which resolved: significant blood loss, a cerebrospinal fluid leak at the time of the surgery, a superficial infection treated with local care, and a temporary radiculopathy L5. *(Courtesy of Drs. R. B. Gledhill and M. Aebi.)*

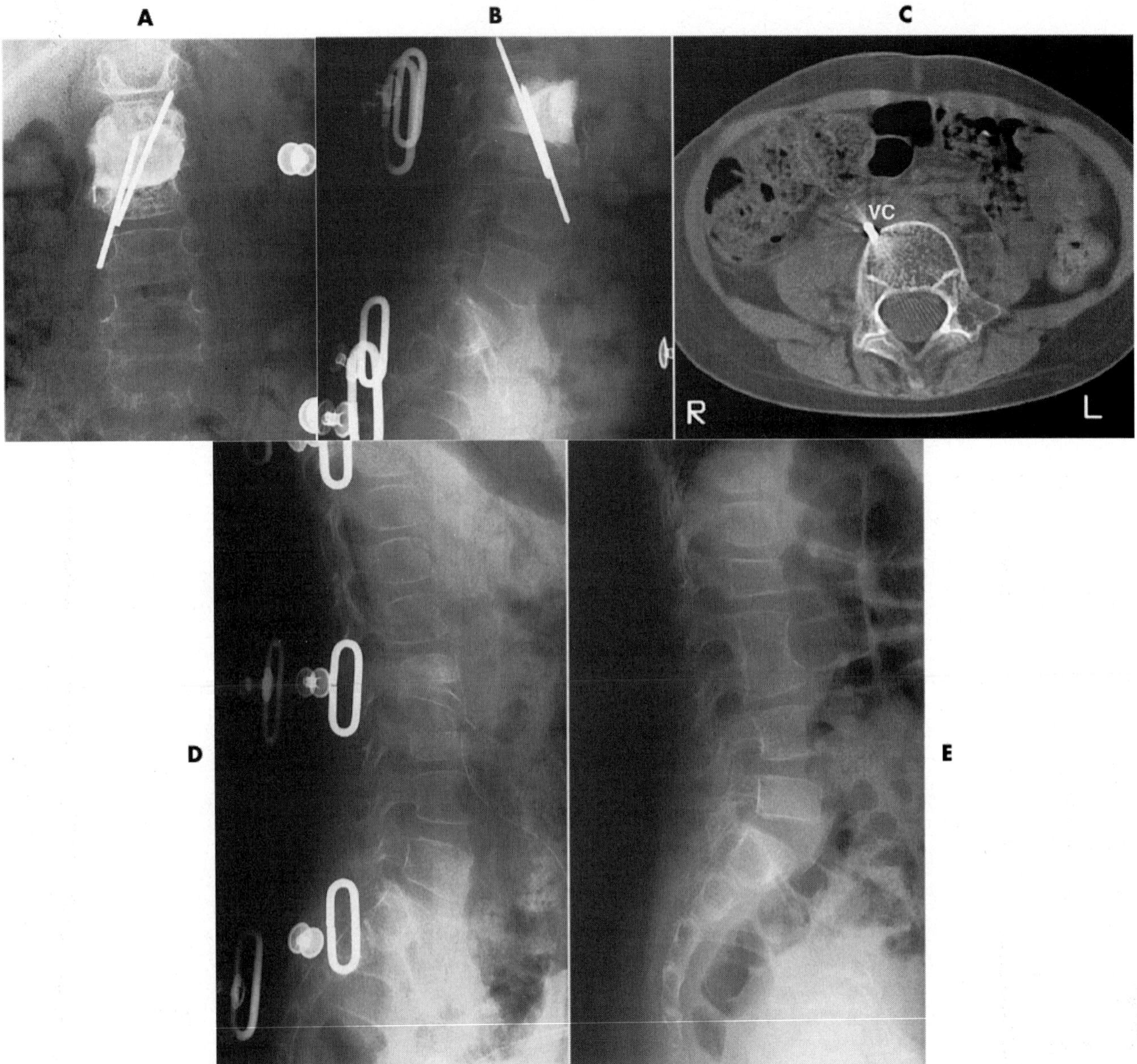


FIGURE 32-13

This 5-year-old patient who has aplastic anemia presents with a recurrent infection and migration of K-wires anteriorly **(A** and **B)**. Four months prior to this she underwent a debridement curettage of a spondylodiscitis at the L2-L3 level. Methylmethacrylate and K-wire fixation were used at the time due to the catastrophic vital prognosis (a few weeks) given at the time. Cultures grew *Candida*. Because of the recurrent infection and the risk of pin migration in the vena cava **(C)** as seen on the CT scan, revision is done. The pins and the cement are removed, the vertebrae curetted, and a massive bicortical bone graft from the iliac crest is interposed **(D)**. Brace and recumbency are followed for three months scrupulously. At two years' follow-up the patient is still alive needing only one platelet transfusion a week, and the fusion is perfectly solid **(E)**. This case demonstrates that proper bone graft with adequate immobilization can perfectly achieve the goal of successful fusion in children.

balanced and close to the gravity line. The nonfused segments must be stressed as little as possible, preventing muscle fatigue, subsequent discomfort, further imbalance, and late arthritis.

## GENERAL ASPECTS

Every strategic and technical step is challenging and needs to be meticulously prepared. The side of an anterior approach must be decided according to the previous anterior approach. Iterative vascular dissections can be dangerous, and the assistance of a general or vascular surgeon can be wise in some cases. The geometry of the deformity: although most anterior procedures require a convex approach, in some specific cases a concave approach is more logical (see Figs. 32-3 and 32-4).[32,66] Strut grafting in severe kyphoscoliosis is an example. The graft must be placed in the concavity of the tridimensional deformity. The posterior approach obviously gives less options. In spina bifida patients, skin can be a problem and requires specific plastic precautions before addressing the orthopedic problem (skin expanders for example).

Hardware removal is not always required (Fig. 32-1). A simple extension of graft can leave whole or a part of it in when it is deeply incorporated in the graft. It can even be used to anchor the new instrumentation without altering the graft (see Figs. 32-5, 32-7, 32-8, and 32-11). However, one must be cautious not to cantilever in an inappropriate direction on the former instrumentation because it could result in imbalance or worsening of the curve (Fig. 32-14). Hardware removal can be difficult especially with the early generations of segmental instrumentations such as the Luque or the first CD rods.

## PARTICULAR PROBLEMS

***Late Infections of the Spine Fusion.*** Richards[60] reported a 10% rate of late infections with modern spine instrumentation in a series of 103 adolescent patients with idiopathic scoliosis. The important steps when addressing such a problem are: assess the general status of the patient, to try to identify the germ and its sensitivity to antibiotics, and evaluate the orthopedic condition in term of balance of the trunk and quality of the graft. The procedure must be conducted under an adapted antibiotic regimen. The whole wound must be reopened and the spine entirely exposed. The hardware has to be removed no matter the difficulties (Fig. 32-11). After all infected tissues have been excised, the graft must be checked carefully. Two pitfalls are classical at this point: missing an hairline pseudarthrosis, or a very thin fusion mass that will "break" soon after the hardware has been removed. The most frequently involved germs are *Staphylococcus epidermidis,* staph coagulase negative, *Propionibacterium acnes,* and *Staphylococcus aureus.*[34,60] Maintenance of a good nutritional status, efficient and prolonged drainage, intravenous and oral antibiotics, followed by clinical radiological and biological criteria ultimately lead to healing. At this point, a residual orthopedic problem can be treated. If a pseudarthrosis had been noted, for example, an anterior fusion can be performed to avoid going back into the posterior scar, especially if the condition to treat is prone to infections as in neuromuscular deformities.

***Revision for Simple Aseptic Pseudarthrosis.*** Modern instrumentation has provided better correction of complex deformities and less postoperative constraints, but seem to expose to higher rates of fusion failures. The diagnosis is difficult and pseudarthrosis will often take several years to be identified. Pseudarthrosis must be suspected in case of a progressive loss of correction, hardware breakage, loosening, radiolucent halo around a hook or screw, or increasing back pain. Once the decision to reoperate is made (and many asymptomatic nonunions do not require revision) the whole fusion mass must be reexplored every 5 millimeters.[66] Pseudarthrosis is identified by adherence of the periosteum,[48] and micromotion at the site of the nonfusion. Different situations can basically be individualized.

There is one single pseudarthrosis, in the middle of the construct, often found in a kyphotic area. The treatment consists of decorticating of the pseudarthrosis site, bone grafting, and applying a compressive system, therefore avoiding any instrumentation at the pseudarthrosis site (as opposed to the case in which two laminar hooks are at the site of the pseudarthrosis) (see Fig. 32-6). This compressive construct can be anchored in different ways. One can dig holes in the adjacent bone graft (but the canal has to be opened for a good fixation of the hooks), insert pedicle screws (but the landmarks will be difficult to identify, unless the canal has been opened), or connect to the old instrumentation via dominoes. If the purchase is not totally satisfactory, if the area is kyphotic, or if in case of iterative attempts of fusion, a complementary anterior fusion will be done.

When the pseudarthrosis is at the distal end of the instrumentation, extension of the fusion of one level is not always warranted. If the next level is healthy and if the spine and the fusion are balanced, it is possible to remain at the same level. If the bottom vertebra has been instrumented with hooks, they will be replaced with pedicle screws (Fig. 32-14). Conversely, if the bottom vertebra has been instrumented with pedicle screws that are broken, laminar hooks, possibly offset, will allow us to remain at the same level (Fig. 32-5).

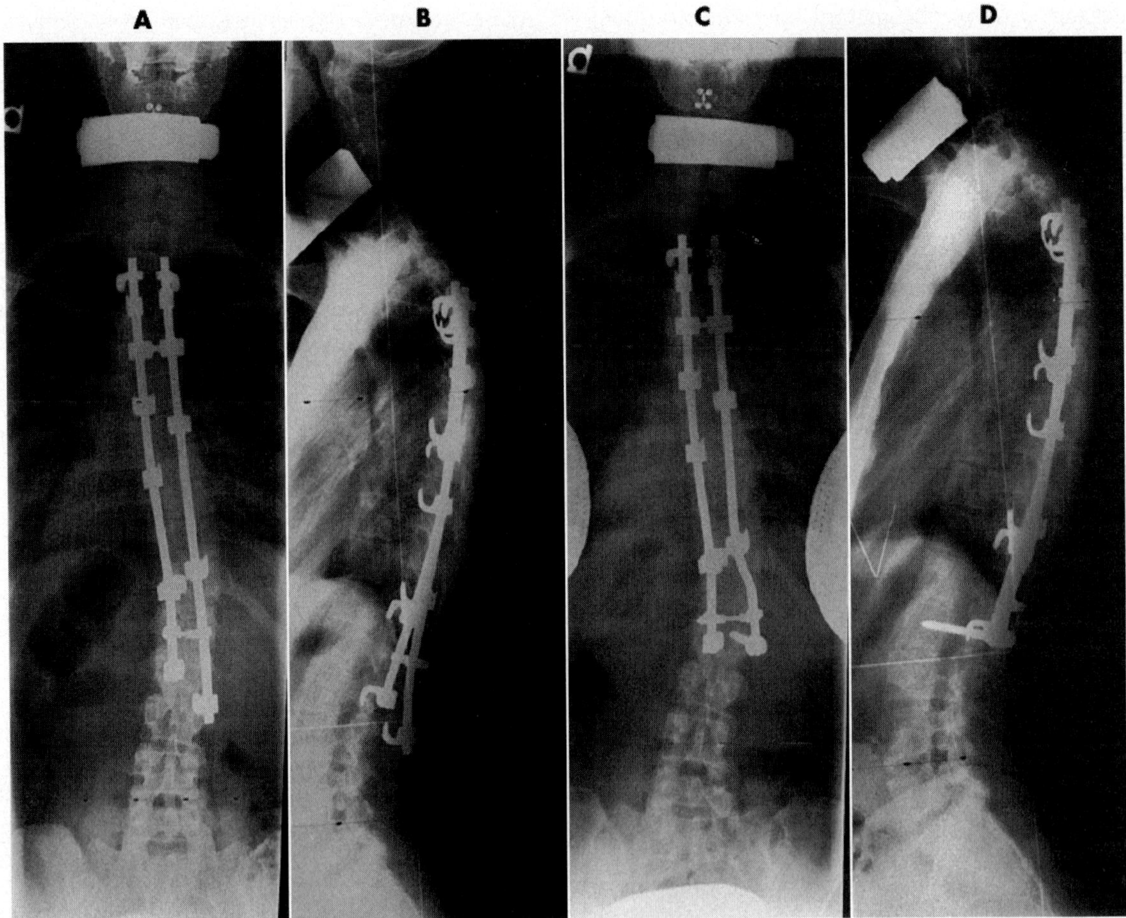


FIGURE 32-14

Because of the onset of low back pain with the sensation of a lump this 18-year-old girl comes back 13 months after her posterior Cotrel-Dubousset instrumentation for idiopathic scoliosis. X-rays clearly show that the infralaminar hook has pulled out of the lamina of L2 on the convex side **(A** and **B)**. Reexploration of the fusion mass confirms the broken hemilamina and finds an obvious pseudarthrosis at L1-L2. In order to remain at the same level a pedicular screw is used and the pseudarthrosis decorticated and grafted and compressed. However, the rod needs to be bent in a zigzag fashion to fit to the opening of the pedicle screw, translation maneuvers are even used to get the rod in the tulip screw. Postoperatively, the patient is still well-balanced but the lumbar curve had to increase to maintain the trunk equilibrium **(C** and **D)** as translation maneuvers of the rod shifted the upper spine to the left. The use of dominoes or transverse connectors and avoiding any cantilevering on the previously fused spine would probably have avoided this complication.

***Complex Pseudarthrosis.*** Complex pseudarthrosis refers to situations in which one has to deal with multiple pseudarthroses, with possible malalignment, or when the etiology is such that these cases have little chance to heal without a combined procedure. This is encountered in Charcot spine, spina bifida patients, or the dysplastic spine (neurofibromatosis), but can also happen in idiopathic cases when the first procedure has failed.

From the back, the whole protocol already described will be undertaken until the exact number of pseudarthroses, their location, and the quality of the graft in between are perfectly clarified.

Multiple pseudarthroses with a poor fusion mass, and facets still opened will require a complete reinstrumentation with the proper corrective setting of the hooks at the appropriate levels, facet excision, and massive bone graft (Fig. 32-10). In all of these cases, the spine can still end up being well balanced, with a posterior graft in a satisfactory mechanical and biologic situation to achieve fusion.

When the site of the nonunion is located in the low lumbar spine, an interbody fusion can be achieved through a posterior approach (PLIF). This technique can lead to neurological complications and has very few indications in children.

An interbody fusion through an anterior approach is indicated in cases of multiple back revisions or when the bed for the posterior graft is of poor quality. The anterior approach can be performed first, followed by posterior instrumentation and fusion, or be done as a complement. In both cases, if the anterior longitudinal ligament has been lifted as a flap, or the spine decorticated according to Stagnara, the strut can be inserted between the vertebral bodies and covered by the flap, preventing its dislodgment.[66] The anterior procedure carried out first with a good release allows a better posterior correction, but the interbody graft will not be in compression after posterior correction and is theoretically at risk for dislodgment. Therefore, if little correction is necessary, the posterior surgery done first will allow the anterior strut graft to be fit in a better mechanical condition without risk of dislodgment.

***Revision of Infected Pseudarthrosis.*** This situation is very different from an acute infection in which it has been shown that instrumentation could be left in place after thorough debridement and suction plus or minus continued irrigation.[21,30,31,33,35,49,53] Very little information is found in the literature on these very difficult cases apart from the presentation of Southern, who reported the results of primary reconstruction in a series of vertebral osteomyelitis in the adult.[65] If the principles of thorough debridement, irrigation, and drainage are well accepted, the real question is whether an immediate reinstrumentation is advisable or whether it should be postponed until an antibiotic treatment has been given for a period of time and the sedimentation rate is back to normal. This is really the issue in infected pseudarthroses as seen in idiopathic scoliosis or patients with spina bifida. In our limited experience, we chose to remove the hardware and leave the patient on intravenous antibiotics for several weeks to months. The reinstrumentation and fusion (anterior or posterior or both) were carried at a further date. This treatment, which interested two patients with spina bifida, one patient with Noonan syndrome, and one patient with idiopathic scoliosis, was successful in the four cases for both treating the infection and achieving solid fusion. However, in the pediatric spine it is sometimes possible to achieve fusion without instrumentation provided immobilization or recumbency achieve what the instrumentation would have done (Fig. 32-13). In severe soft tissue defects, muscle flap closure using either the latissimus dorsi or the trapezius could definitely be an interesting solution, as reported by Kling.[39]

***Imbalance.*** Imbalance is one of the drawbacks of pediatric spine surgery. It can be due to a wrong choice of levels, an excessive correction of a curve compared to another one (i.e., King 2 curves), or the neglect of a curve (i.e., King 5 curves).

Selective correction of the thoracic spine in King 2 curves can lead to postoperative trunk imbalance.[18,69] In such cases, after a period of observation in which the loss of equilibrium still persists, if the patient is young enough, an orthopedic treatment can be undertaken. If the patient is too old for a brace we can either wait because the situation can be stabilized in an acceptable situation, or decide to perform an extension of the fusion, usually in this context down to L4. Extension of the fusion to the sacrum is, in our opinion, not indicated in these young patients without any disk degeneration and because of the risk of persistent trunk imbalance (see Fig. 32-11).

Imbalance of the shoulders occurs when a double thoracic curve (a King 5) has not been preoperatively recognized.[44] If the imbalance is too severe and recognized postoperatively, one should revise the instrumentation, release the distraction on the concave main right thoracic curve, extend the instrumentation in the upper curve with connectors, distract the upper left curve in its concavity, and compress the convexity of this upper curve. If the imbalance of the shoulders is recognized only when the fusion is solid, extension of the instrumentation to T1 or T2 can improve the situation. Upper spinal osteotomies are in our opinion not indicated for this problem.

## SPECIFIC PROBLEMS

***Neuromuscular Scoliosis.*** In spina bifida, the cause of revision is primarily a lack of fusion or infection. The infection rate has been reported to vary between 8% and 23.6%.[8,71] The rate of union ranges between 40%[55,73] when a posterior fusion is used and 80% to 95% if a combined approach is used.[8,51] It is therefore our opinion that most revision in cases of spina bifida will require an anterior and posterior fusion. If the patient is completely paraplegic, the revision surgery can be achieved from the back only and the anterior interbody fusion will be achieved after a chordectomy or a dural sac division has been done as recommended by Lindseth for kyphectomies.[47] The whole spine can be exposed in a circumferential fashion (Fig. 32-7). However, the difficult problem will be to achieve a strong fixation in the sacropelvis. One has to be familiar with all the means of sacropelvis fixation as the classic Galveston rods may be insufficient or impossible to use if that fixation site has already been used (Fig. 32-7). One may have to use pedicle screws, Jackson sacral fixation,[37] or screws in the ilium. The graft will come from the rib or from one or both tibia if the patient is nonambulatory. If the patient is ambulatory, the procedure will be performed through an anterior approach either from the same previously operated side (if an anterior instrumentation has been inserted) or from the opposite side, which will have the advantage of an easier dissection and to put the bone graft on the concave side of the deformity. Again a tibial or fibula graft will be used. In the same setting a posterior instrumentation fusion will be carried out posteriorly. The bottom line of a successful revision in spina bifida is, more than in any other deformity, to achieve a strong fusion because a possible late infection could one day require rod removal.

In cerebral palsy patients, revision surgery is often not possible because of the poor general condition of the patient or reluctance of the parents. One may have to consider only removal of a protruding rod. If the surgery is possible (no weight loss, serum albumin above 3.5, total lymphocyte count above 1500 and no major associated conditions such as gastrointestinal reflux or uncontrolled seizures) the only goal is to balance the pelvis under the trunk to allow comfortable sitting. A combination of anterior release and spine osteotomies may be necessary to achieve the correction, or a vertebral resection[13,14] can be performed (eggshell) through the back according to the surgeon's preference. The use of iliosacral screws or a sacropelvic fixation with S1 and iliac screws, helps correction of pelvic obliquity, especially if a previous Galveston has been used. Once again, the use of tibial crest may be necessary to achieve bony fusion.

***Revision of Spondylolisthesis.*** In our experience four different situations leading to revision can be individualized: persistent or onset of sciatica after fusion of the spondylolisthesis; progression of the deformity, especially the slip angle; infection; or persistent pain with pseudarthrosis without progression. If the patient complains of neurologic symptoms (sciatica), we recommend a posterior decompression with possible sacral dome resection, neurolysis of the roots with foraminotomy, and a very thorough inspection of the fusion mass. If there is any doubt as to the solidity of the fusion, a reinforcement or complementary anterior fusion must be carried out. Our two cases of persistent sciatica did well after neurolysis and inspection reinforcement of the fusion mass, yet these two patients still had a grade 2 and a grade 4 spondylolisthesis. If there is progression of the deformity, one must consider the possibility of a pseudarthrosis or an elongation of the fusion mass. Surgical indication for revision will be based on clinical symptomatology and on progression of the slip angle rather than progression of the grade itself. Different surgical options can be performed: if one is ready to accept the deformity a repeat posterolateral fusion with massive iliac graft and careful immobilization can still give satisfactory long term results as we could observe it twice (Fig. 32-15), or an interbody L5-S1 fusion can be done through an intraperitoneal approach or through a posterior approach using the fibula after opening the sacral canal. If one wants to reduce the deformity, the use of an external fixator after spinal osteotomy will allow gradual reduction of the slip and monitoring of the neurologic function. In cases of infection if the fusion is solid, removal of hardware will solve the problem; however, if the fusion is not solid and the material exposed with skin necrosis, the following salvage solution can be performed: removal of the hardware, bilateral pantaloon cast, and anterior spinal fusion; this has been performed once with success. As to the exceptional progression of a slip under an arthrodesis for scoliosis, we strongly recommend an anterior and posterior fusion of the spondylolisthesis with reduction if possible (Fig. 32-16).[5] The technique of Padovani[5,11] is a very elegant way to achieve this goal.

***Progressive Restrictive Lung Disease.*** Progressive restrictive lung disease may be observed in patients with or without congenital scoliosis who have been fused posteriorly at a very young age, and because of continuous anterior growth, progressive lordosis will progressively lead to restrictive lung disease. This crankshaft complication must be well understood and, if observed, should be treated by anterior epiphysiodesis.[24,25,76] This simple procedure can almost be considered as an emergency so as to prevent further deterioration of the pulmonary function (see Fig. 32-2 ).[25] Other patients with previously operated complex spine deformity may have end-stage pulmonary restrictive disease. In these cases a preparation with halo and chest physiotherapy may provide a better pulmonary condition.[68] The goal of the halo is not to correct the previously fused thoracic spine but to give the patient some abdominal height to improve diaphragmatic and abdominal respiration. In some cases, one or several pseudarthroses, a few unfused disk spaces will give some additional correction during halo traction. Surgery, when possible, will ideally consist of anterior osteotomies, followed by posterior osteotomies at the same level and posterior instrumentation. However, if halo traction (prolonged until maximum correction has been achieved) gives significant improvement, a posterior fusion only can be done. The worst case scenario will be patients with a congenital or previously fused thoracic lordosis and severe lung compromise. In these patients, the treatment proposed by Winter and Bradford will consist of multiple anterior osteotomies, with convex ribs osteotomies during the anterior approach, followed by posterior osteotomies and concave rib resection during the posterior approach done in the same or different sitting.[16,75] These surgeries have a high incidence of severe complications,[76,77] but the natural history of the deformity is so severe that surgical correction may be warranted.

## CONCLUSION

For successful revision in the pediatric age group, three major goals need to be obtained concomitantly. Restore the balance of the spine by extending the fusion either proximal or distally or by doing anterior osteotomies combined with anterior releases or os-

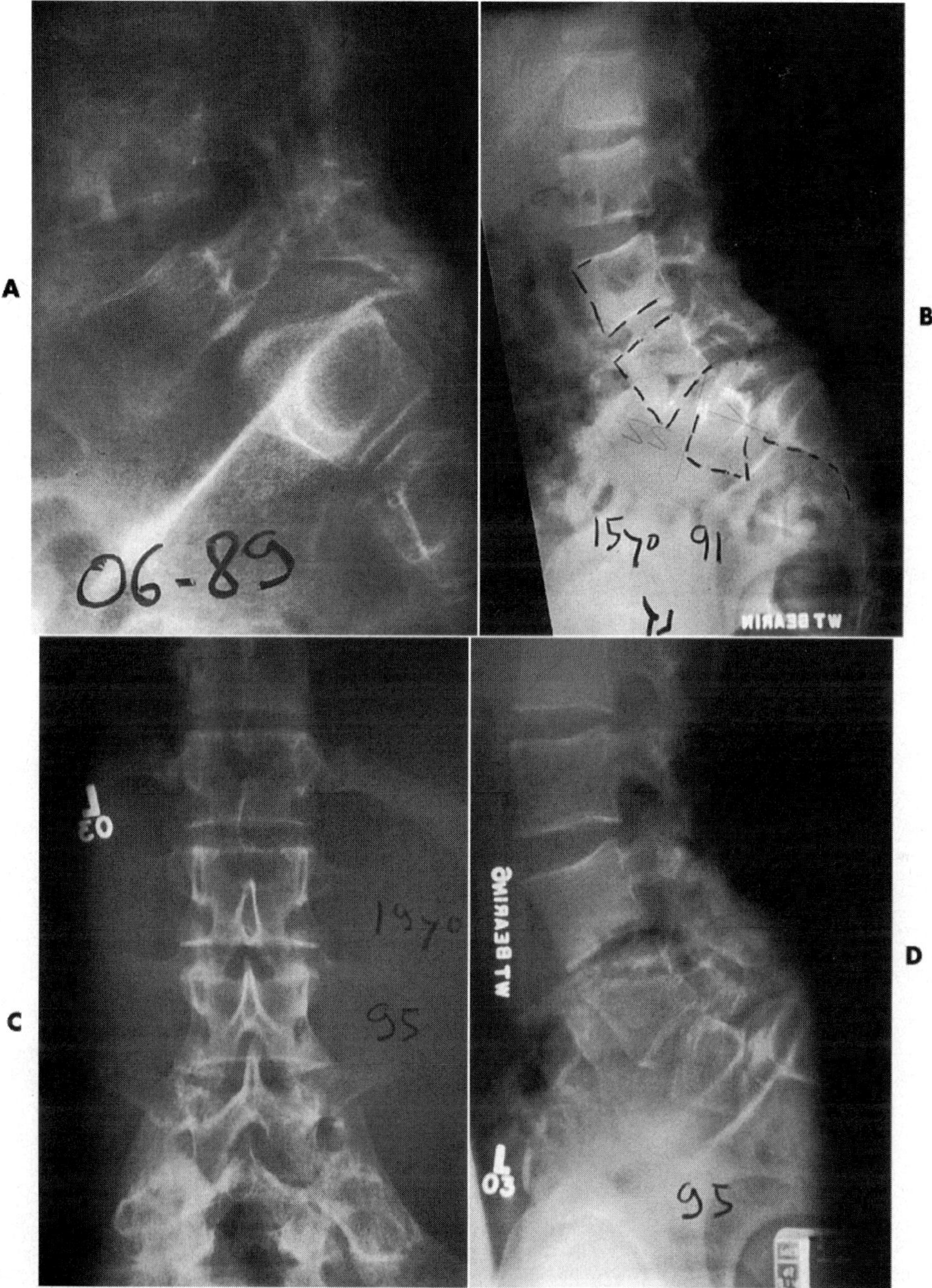


**FIGURE 32-15**

This 13-year-old patient comes two years after an in situ posterolateral fusion for spondylolisthesis **(A).** He does not complain of back pain any longer but the pain in the left leg persists. Follow-up x-rays show that the slip angle has increased remarkably **(B).** Revision is done through a repeat posterolateral fusion with iliac bone graft followed by brace immobilization; no instrumentation is inserted. Four years after the revision the patient is asymptomatic, the slip angle stable, and the fusion is solid on x-rays but extends to L3 **(C** and **D).** This case demonstrates perfectly that the most important issue in the outcome is a strong and thick fusion that will withstand the anterior shearing forces. *(Courtesy of Dr. R. B. Gledhill.)*

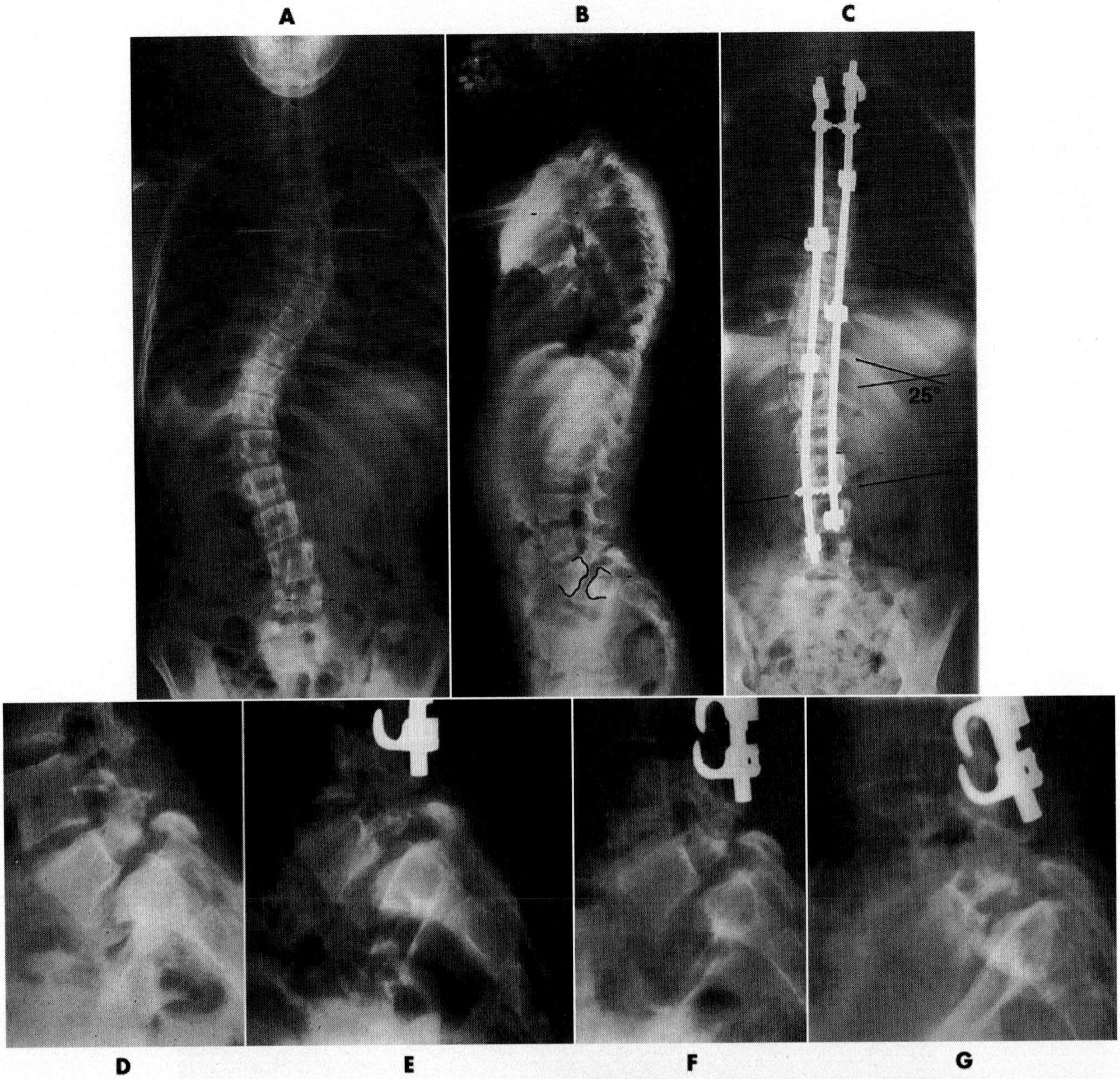

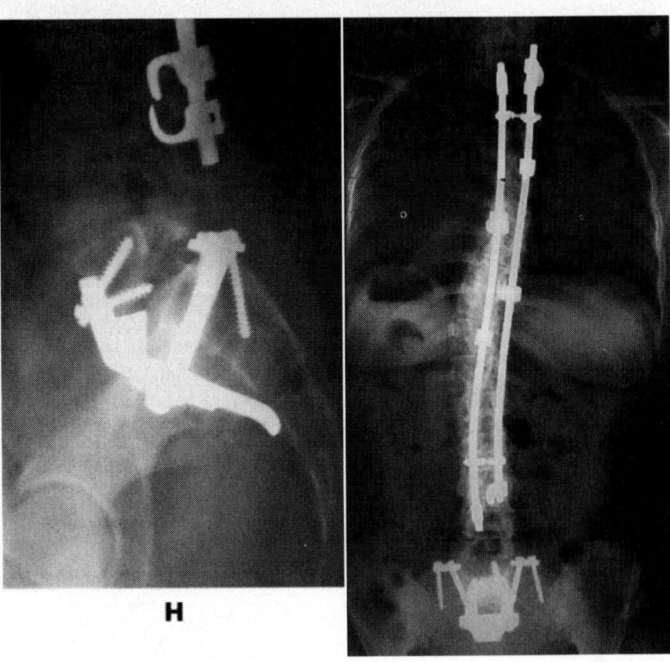

**FIGURE 32-16**

This 13-year-old girl has adolescent idiopathic scoliosis above a grade 2 spondylolisthesis **(A** and **B)**. She undergoes posterior spine fusion from T2 to L3 **(C)**. During three years no progression of her slip is observed **(D, E,** and **F)**. However, after four years she presents with acute pain and obvious progression **(G)**. She is treated with one-level anterior and posterior L5-S1 fusion using a Butress plate11 **(H)**. This leaves two mobile lumbar disks. Four years after the revision the patient is perfectly balanced **(I)** and the fusion solid. *(Courtesy of Dr. J. P. Padovani.)*

teotomies if necessary. The fusion too has to be balanced (gravity line dropped from the tragus down passing along the fusion mass and finishing in the Chopart joint of the feet). Next, achieve a solid fusion, using autogenous bone when available (one or two iliac crests, fibulae, tibial crest, one or two ribs, or decorticated pieces from the previous fusion mass). The decortication of the spine must go into the cancellous bone of the fusion mass, this is the only way to detect stratified layers of fusion that are not in continuity with the spine. The instrumentation needs to be in compression in most cases. Finally, minimize the risks of complications.

## ACKNOWLEDGMENTS

Without the help of many of my colleagues who provided us with various cases or assisted us during these revision cases this work would not have been possible. We would like to address special thanks to M. Aebi, J. P. Chaumien, R. B. Gledhill, G. Finidori, P. Janklevicz, P. Journeau, D. Marchesi, J. P. Padovani, M. Pouliquen, P. Rigault, to the audiovisual laboratory at the Shriners Hospital, Montreal Unit, and to Mark Lepik for his assistance with the illustrations.

## REFERENCES

1. Abitbol JJ, Garfin SR: *Complications associated with posterior instrumentation of the spine.* In Rothman and Simeone, editors: *The spine,* ed 3, Philadelphia, 1992, WB Saunders, pp 1846-1871.
2. Akbarnia BH, Asher Ma, Hess F, Wagner T: Safety of the pedicle screw in pediatric patients with scoliosis and kyphosis. Presented at the 31st Scoliosis Research Society Ottawa, September 1996.
3. Allen BL, Ferguson RL: The operative treatment of myelomeningocele spine deformity, *Orthop Clin North Am* 10:845-862, 1979.
4. Amis J, Herring J: Iatrogenic kyphosis: a complication of Harrington instrumentation in Marfan's syndrome, *J Bone Joint Surg* 66A:460-464, 1984.
5. Arlet V, Rigault P, Padovani JP, Touzet P, Finidori G, Guyonvarc H: Scoliose, spondylolyse et spondylolisthesis lombosacré: etude de leur association chez l'enfant et l'adolescent à propos de 82 cas, *Rev Chir Orthop* 76:118-127, 1990.
6. Arlet V, Rigault P, Padovani JP, Janklevicz P, Touzet Ph, Finidori G: Instabilité atloido-axoidienne de l'enfant trisomique 21, *Rev Chir Orthop* 78:240-247, 1992.
7. Aurori BF, Weierman RJ, Lowell HA, Nadel CI, Parsons JR: Pseudarthrosis after spinal fusion for scoliosis. A comparison of autogeneic and allogeneic bone grafts, *Clin Orthop* 199:153-158, 1985.
8. Banta JV. Combined anterior and posterior fusion for spinal deformity in myelomeningocele, *Spine* 15:946-952, 1990.
9. Bialik V, Piggott H: Pseudarthrosis following treatment of idiopathic scoliosis by Harrington instrumentation and fusion without added bone, *J Pedia Orthop* 7:152-154, 1987.
10. Birch JG, Herring JA: Spinal deformity in Marfan syndrome, *J Pediat Orthop* 7:546-552, 1987.
11. Bitan F, Padovani JP, Glorion C, Rigault P, Touzet P, Finidori G. Les spondylolisthesis a grand deplacement de l'enfant et de l'adolescent. Résultats de la reduction-arthrodèse par plaque antérieure, *Rev Chir Orthop* 76:425-436, 1990.
12. Bitan F, Rigault P, Houfani B, Sidi D, Padovani JP, Merckx J, Durand Y: Scolioses et cardiopathies congénitales chez l'enfant. A propos de 44 cas, *Rev Chir Orthop* 77(3):179-188, 1991.
13. Boachie-Adjei O, Bradford DS: Vertebral resection and arthrodesis for complex spinal deformities, *J Spine Disord* 4 (2):193-202, 1991.
14. Boachie-Adjei O, Lonstein JE, Winter RB, Koop S, Vandenbrink K, Denis F: Management of neuromuscular spinal deformities with Luque's segmental instrumentation. *J Bone Joint Surg* 71A:548-562, 1990.
15. Bradford DS, Ganjavian S, Antonious D, Winter RB, Lonstein JE, Moe JH: Anterior strut grafting for the treatment of kyphosis. Review of experience with forty-eight patients, *J Bone Joint Surg* 64A:680-690, 1982.
16. Bradford DS, Blatt JM, Rasp FL: Surgical management of severe thoracic lordosis . A new technique to restore normal kyphosis, *Spine* 8:420-428, 1983.
17. Bradford DS, Daher YH: Vascularised rib graft for stabilisation of kyphosis, *J Bone Joint Surg* 68B:357-361, 1986.
18. Bridwell KH, Mc Allister JW, Betz RR, Huss GK, Clancy M, Schoenecker PL: Coronal decompensation produced by Cotrel Dubousset "derotation maneuver" for idiopathic scoliosis. *Spine* 16:769-777, 1991.
19. Cotrel Y. Dubousset J. CD instrumentation in spine surgery. Principles, technicals, mistakes and traps. Montpellier France, 1992, Sauramps Medical, pp 133-139.
20. Crawford AH: Pitfalls of spinal deformities associated with neurofibromatosis in children, *Clin Orthop* 245:29-42, 1989.
21. DeWald RL: Revision surgery for spinal deformity. Instructionnal course lecture. 41:235-250, 1992.

22. Dimeglio A. Le rachis en croissance. Paris, 1990, Springer Verlag.
23. Doyle JS, Lauerman WC, Wood KB, Krause DR: Complications and long term outcome of upper cervical spine arthrodesis in patients with Down syndrome, *Spine* 21:1223-1231, 1996.
24. Dubousset J, Herring JA, Shufflebarger H: The crankshaft phenomenon, *J Pediat Orthop* 9:541-550,1989.
25. Dubousset J: *Congenital kyphosis and lordosis.* In Weinstein SL, editor: *The pediatric spine: principles and practice,* New York, 1994, Raven Press, pp 245-258.
26. Duval-Beaupère G, Schmidt C, Cosson P: A barycentremetric study of the sagittal shape of spine and pelvis: the conditions required for an economic standing position, *Ann Biomedical Engineering* 20 4:451-462, 1992.
27. Erwin WD, Dickson JH, Harrington P: Clinical review of patients with broken Harrington rods, *J Bone Joint Surg* 62A:1302-1307, 1980.
28. Floman Y, Norgrove P, Micheli LJ, Riseborough EJ, Hall J: Osteotomy of the fusion mass in scoliosis. *J Bone Joint Surg* 64A:307-1316, 1982.
29. Funasaki H, Winter RB, Lonstein J, Denis F: Pathophysiology of spinal deformities in neurofibromatosis, *J Bone Joint Surg* 76A:692-700, 1994.
30. Gaines DL, Moe JH, Bocklage JR: Management of wound infections following Harrington instrumentation and spine fusion, *J Bone Joint Surg* 52A:404, 1970.
31. Gepstein R, Eismont FJ: *Postoperative spine infections.* In Garfin SR, editor: *Complications of spine surgery,* Baltimore, 1989, Williams & Wilkins, pp 302-322.
32. Gonon GP, De Mauroy JC, Frankel P, Campo-Paysa A, Stagnara P: Greffes antérieures en étai dans le traitement des cyphoses et cyphoscolioses, *Rev Chir Orthop* 67:731-774, 1981.
33. Hamill CL, Lenke LG, Bridwell KH, Chapman MP, Blanke K, Baldus C: The use of pedicle screw fixation to improve correction in the lumbar spine of patients with idiopathic scoliosis. Is it warranted, *Spine* 21:1241-1249, 1996.
34. Heggeness MH, Esses SI, Errico T, Yuan HA: Late infection of spinal instrumentation by hematogenous seeding, *Spine* 18:492-496, 1993.
35. Heller JG, Whitecloud III TS, Butler JC, Abitbol JJ, Garfin SR et al: *Complications of spinal surgery. Postoperative infections of the spine.* In: Rothman and Simeone, editors: *The spine,* ed 3, Philadelphia, 1992, WB Saunders, pp 1817-1837.
36. Hsu LC, Lee PC, Leong JC, Dystrophic spinal deformities in neurofibromatosis. Treatment by anterior and posterior fusion, *J Bone Joint Surg* 66B:495-499, 1984.
37. Jackson RP, McManus AC: The iliac buttress. A computed tomographic study of sacral anatomy, *Spine* 18:1318-1328, 1993.
38. Jensen JE, Jensen TG, Smith TK: Nutrition in orthopedics surgery, *J Bone Joint Surg* 64A:1263-1272, 1982.
39. Klink BK, Thurman RT, Wittpenn GP. Lauermann WC, Cain JE: Muscle flap closure for salvage of complex back wounds, *Spine* 19(13):467-1470, 1994.
40. Kostuik JP, Maurais GR, Richardson J, Okajima Y: Combined single stage anterior and posterior osteotomy for correction of iatrogenic lumbar kyphosis, *Spine* 13:257-266, 1988.
41. Kumar SJ, Guille JT: *Marfan syndrome.* In Weinstein SL, editor: *The pediatric spine: principles and practice,* New York, 1994, Raven Press, pp 665-683.
42. Lagrone MO: Loss of lumbar lordosis. A complication of spinal fusion for scoliosis, *Orthop Clin North Am* 19:383-39, 1988.
43. Lauerman WC, Bradford DS, Ogilvie JW, Transfeldt EE: Management of pseudarthrosis after arthrodesis of the spine for idiopathic scoliosis, *J Bone Joint Surg* 73A:222-236, 1991.
44. Lenke LG, Bridwell KH, O'Brien MF, Baldus C, Blanke K: Recognition and treatment of the proximal thoracic curve in adolescent idiopathic scoliosis treated with Cotrel-Dubousset instrumentation, *Spine* 19: 1589-1597, 1994.
45. Leong JC, Wilding K, Mok CK, Ma A, Chow SP, Yau AC: Surgical treatment of scoliosis following poliomyelitis. A review of one hundred and ten cases, *J Bone Joint Surg* 63A:726-740, 1981.
46. Lettice J, Ogilvie J, Transfeldt E, Cohen M: Proximal junctional kyphosis following Cotrel Dubousset instrumentation in adult scoliosis. Presented at Scoliosis Research Society meeting Minneapolis, September 1991.
47. Lindseth RE, Stelzer L: Vertebral excision for kyphosis in children with myelomeningocele, *J Bone Joint Surg Am* 61:699-704, 1979.
48. Lonstein JE: *Salvage and reconstructive surgery.* In Bradford, Lonstein, Ogilvie, Winter, editors: *Moe's textbook of scoliosis.* Philadelphia, 1987, Saunders, pp 391-402.
49. Lonstein J, Winter RB, Moe J: Wound infection with Harrington instrumentation and spine fusion for scoliosis, *Clin Orthop* 96:222-223, 1973.
50. McMaster MJ, James JIP: Pseudarthrosis after spinal fusion for scoliosis, *J Bone Joint Surg* 58B:305-312., 1976.
51. McMaster MJ: Anterior and posterior instrumentation and fusion of thoracolumbar scoliosis due to myelomeningocele, *J Bone Joint Surg* 69B:20-22, 1987.
52. McMaster MJ: Congenital scoliosis. In Weinstein SL, editor: *The pediatric spine: principles and practice,* New York, 1994, Raven Press, pp 227-244.
53. Massie JB, Heller JG, Abitbol JJ, McPherson D, Garfin SR: Postoperative posterior spinal wound infection, *Clin Orthop* 284:99-108, 1992.
54. Moe JH, Kharrat K, Winter RB, Cummine JL: Harrington instrumentation without fusion plus external orthotic support for the treatment of difficult curvature problems in young children, *Clin Orthop* 185:35-45, 1980.
55. Osebold WR, Mayfield JK, Winter RB, Moe JH:

Surgical treatment of paralytic scoliosis associated with myelomeningocele, *J Bone Joint Surg* 64A:841-856, 1982.
56. Peterson HA: *Iatrogenic spinal deformities.* In Weinstein SL editor: *The pediatric spine: principles and practice,* New York, 19984, Raven Press, pp 651-664.
57. Ramirez N, Richards S, Warren PD, Williams GR: Complications after posterior spine fusion in Duchenne's muscular dystrophy, *J Pediat Orthop* 17:109-114, 1997.
58. Rawlins BA, Winter RB, Lonstein J, Denis F, Kubic PT, Wheeler WB, Ozolins AL: Reconstructive spine surgery in pediatric patients with major loss of vital capacity, *J Pediat Orthop* 16:284-292, 1996.
59. Rees D, Jones MW, Owen R, Dorgan JC: Scoliosis surgery in the Prader Willi syndrome, *J Bone Joint Surg* 71B:685-688, 1989.
60. Richards BS, Herring JA, Johnston CE, Birch JG, Roach JW: Treatment of adolescent idiopathic scoliosis using Texas Scottish Rite Hospital Instrumentation, *Spine* 19(14):1598-1605, 1994.
61. Robins PR, Moe JH, Winter RB: Scoliosis in Marfan syndrome. Its characteristics and results of treatment in thirty five patients, *J Bone Joint Surg* 57A:358-368, 1975.
62. Sanders JO, Herring JA, Browne RH: Posterior arthrodesis and instrumentation in the immature (Risser-Grade 0) spine in idiopathic scoliosis, *J Bone Joint Surg* 77A:39-45, 1995.
63. Segals LS, Drummond DS, Zanotti RM, Ecker ML, Mubarak SJ: Complications of posterior arthrodesis of the cervical spine in patients who have Down syndrome, *J Bone Joint Surg* 73A:1547-1554, 1991.
64. Shufflebarger HL, Clark CE: Prevention of the crankshaft phenomenon, *Spine* 16(8s):S409-S411, 1991.
65. Southern EP, Hammerberg KW, DeWald R: Complex spinal deformities in severe spinal infection. The surgical management of complex spinal deformity. GICD Ottawa Sept. 25 1996.
66. Stagnara P. Les deformations du rachis, Paris, 1985, Masson.
67. Steinmann JC, Herkowitz HN: Pseudarthrosis of the spine, *Clin Orthop* 284:80-90, 1992.
68. Swank S, Winter RB, Moe JH: Scoliosis and core pulmonale, *Spine* 7:343-354, 1982.
69. Thomson JP, Transfeldt EE, Bradford DS, Ogilvie JW, Boachie-Adjei O: Decompensation after Cotrel-Dubousset instrumentation of idiopathic scoliosis, *Spine* 15:927-931, 1990.
70. Tolo V: *Spinal deformities in skeletal dysplasia.* In Weinstein SL, editor: *The pediatric spine: principles and practice,* New York, 1994, Raven Press, pp 369-393.
71. Transfeldt E, Lonstein J, Winter R, Bradford DS, Moe J, Mayfield J: Wound infections in reconstructive spinal surgery, *Orthop Trans* 9:128-129, 1985.
72. Tredwell SJ: *Complications of spinal surgery.* In Weinstein SL, editor: *The pediatric spine: principles and practice,* New York, 1994, Raven Press, pp 1761-1784.
73. Ward WT, Wenger DR, Roach JW: Surgical correction of myelomeningocele scoliosis: a critical appraisal of various spinal instrumentation systems, *J Pediat Orthop* 9:262-268, 1989.
74. Wenger DR, Scott MD, Leach J: Managing complications of posterior spinal instrumentation and fusion, *Clin Orthop* 284:24-33, 1992.
75. Winter RB: Surgical correction of rigid thoracic lordoscoliosis, *J Spinal Disord* 5:108-111, 1992.
76. Winter RB, Leonard AS: Surgical correction of congenital thoracic lordosis, *J Pediat Orthop* 10:805-808, 1990.
77. Winter RB, Moe JH, Bradford DS: Congenital thoracic lordosis, *J Bone Joint Surg* 60A:806-810, 1978.
78. Winter RB, Denis F, Lonstein JE, Dezen E: Salvage and reconstructive surgery for spinal deformity using Cotrel Dubousset instrumentation, *Spine* 16:S412-S417, 1992.
79. Zeller RD, Ghanem I, Miladi L, Dubousset J: Posterior spinal fusion in neuromuscular scoliosis using a tibial strut graft. Results of a long-term follow-up, *Spine* 19:1628-1631, 1994.
80. Zindrick MR, Wiltse LL, Widell EH et al: A biomechanical study of intrapedicular screw fixation in the lumbosacral spine, *Clin Orthop* 203:99, 1986.

# 33

# NEUROMUSCULAR SPINAL DEFORMITY: SURGICAL TECHNIQUES AND ANALYSIS OF SURGICAL FAILURES

**Steven M. Mardjetko, M.D.**
**John P. Lubicky, M.D.**



The surgical management of neuromuscular spinal deformity is a formidable task. The surgeon is challenged by the "personality" of the deformity, characterized by long sweeping coronal plane curves that include the entire thoracic and lumbar spine. Sagittal plane deformities may vary from flexible to rigid thoracic or lumbar kyphosis, or severe thoracic and lumbar lordosis.[3,4,9,10] Complex pelvic obliquities may be related to the spinal deformity (spinopelvic pelvic obliquity), or secondary to pelvic femoral contractures, and neuromuscular hip dislocation (infrapelvic pelvic obliquity).[6,14,17,30,41] This contributes to decreased sitting tolerance due to pain associated with the spinal deformity or pressure points, and may ultimately lead to pressure ulcerations, especially in insensate children. Spinal decompensation and pelvic obliquity may also adversely affect upper extremity function when the patient must use their upper extremities for support. In its most severe form, these patients lose the ability to sit, and must remain bedridden, resulting in a host of medical and custodial problems.[3,22,33]

Typically, these children are challenged hosts, due to their numerous associated medical problems. For example, a child with cerebral palsy-related spinal deformity usually has total body involvement and presents with contractures of upper and lower extremities, muscle paralysis, spasticity, dystonia, spinal osteoporosis, seizure disorder, feeding difficulties with associated malnutrition, respiratory problems due to aspiration, gastroesophageal reflux, and decreased cognitive, perceptual, and communication skills.[24,43,46,57]

Because the underlying neurologic disorder determines the natural history of the spinal deformity, the surgeon must know the disease and understand the nature of the spinal deformity. The Scoliosis Research Society (SRS) classification of neuromuscular spinal deformity may be used to aid in decision making.[48] But, of course, each patient must be thoroughly evaluated and a rational treatment plan should be tailored to the needs of each individual. The specific etiology of a neuromuscular spinal deformity is critical to understanding the natural history and potential problems that may be encountered with surgical treatment. For example, patients with muscular dystrophy-related deformity will be at risk for cardiac arrhythmias and pulmonary-related medical complications, whereas patients with pediatric spinal cord injury-related deformity may be at risk for skin related complications, autonomic dysreflexia, and pulmonary problems depending on the neurologic level.[43,46]

The child's ambulatory status or ambulatory potential must be taken into account when determining the treatment plan. In community ambulators, the surgeon should make every effort to preserve lower lumbar levels if the deformity allows (i.e., there is no lumbosacral deformity and scoliosis-related pelvic obliquity is corrected with primary curve correction).[4,11,14,34] In addition, it is important to pay attention to the sagittal lumbopelvic alignment when deciding on where to terminate the instrumentation.

Nonambulatory patients usually require fusion to the pelvis on the basis of lumbosacral deformity or pelvic obliquity.[5,20,42] Of course, the surgeon must weigh the pros and cons of fusion to the pelvis in each patient. Cerebral palsy-related deformity usually requires fusion to the pelvis.[11,40,49,53] Some authors report good results when terminating fusion at L5 in patients with mild muscular dystrophy deformity.[9,39]

The utilization of certain techniques that work well in idiopathic scoliosis may prove to be disastrous in neuromuscular curves. For example, a surgeon may be tempted to utilize a technique such as instrumentation without fusion in a young child with neuromuscular scoliosis. Unfortunately, the results of this technique are much less predictable, and complication rates are higher based on previously published series.[16,26,35] The concept of selective thoracic fusion in the treatment of idiopathic scoliosis is well-accepted, but in neuromuscular deformity this technique has limited application.[54] It may be considered in small children in that the major curve can be stabilized and the secondary curve braced to allow further spinal growth. Ultimately, definitive revision of the deformity will likely be required.[4,12,13]

## ANALYSIS OF SURGICAL FAILURES

The goal of any surgical intervention for a neuromuscular spinal deformity should be the attainment and maintenance of a solidly fused spine with acceptable and well-balanced residual coronal plane deformity, a level pelvis, and an acceptable segmental, regional, and global sagittal balance.[8,24,34] It is always easier to attain these goals when the deformity is managed appropriately the first time around.[13] Because these children are usually followed closely for their other medical and orthopedic needs, early identification and early referral should prevent or at least minimize the need for heroic surgical interventions for ultra-severe deformity.[22,57] Each deformity has its own particular personality; it is critical to customize the surgical treatment plan based on each patient's needs.

Thorough preoperative medical evaluation by a developmental pediatrician goes a long way in decreasing medical complications associated with major spinal surgery.[19,22,25,46,57] Anesthesiologists skilled in the management of children with neuromuscular spinal disease should be sought and requested. Spinal cord monitoring is less reliable in this patient population, but nevertheless should be utilized, if available.[32]

Unfortunately, even in the best of hands problems can occur. The surgeon must be able to recognize failure and analyze the cause.[1,2,36] Surgical management involves spinal revision with the same goals in mind as the primary surgery: a solidly fused well-balanced spine, with a level pelvis.[7,8,12]

## CLASSIFICATION OF SURGICAL FAILURES

We have found it helpful to analyze problem spinal deformity cases using the following classification scheme. It is based on our clinical experience in the management of failed spinal deformity surgery. This classification is organized accordingly (Box 33-1):

(1) When failure is recognized: intraoperatively or immediately after surgery within the first 6 months (early) or after the 6-month mark (late).
(2) The location of deformity progression: within the fusion zone or outside the fusion zone.
(3) The plane or planes in which progression is noted.
(4) Residual pelvic obliquity and its clinical consequences.

### INABILITY TO ACHIEVE ACCEPTABLE CORONAL PLANE BALANCE

The ability to correct neuromuscular deformity in the coronal plane depends on curve locations, curve magnitudes, curve rigidity, and adaptive contractures of the paraspinal and truncal musculature. The surgeon needs to assess each component of the deformity to determine the relative flexibility of each curve, and the degree of fixed pelvic obliquity.[49] Forced supine bending radiographs and supine traction films provide this information.[45,55] Sitting or assisted sitting radiographs provide a reasonable estimation of the deformity when challenged by gravity. In general, coronal plane corrections of at least 10 degrees better than the bender x-rays can be reliably achieved using current techniques that combine segmental translation with wire or hook and strategically placed distraction-compression hook sequences. Residual thoracic curves of 50 degrees or less are well-tolerated. But significant residual thoracolumbar and lumbar curves of more than 40 degrees frequently contribute to pelvic obliquity and coronal plane imbalance and may represent a functionally significant residual deformity. Residual pelvic obliquities of 10 degrees or less are well-tolerated, whereas those of 30 degrees or more are poorly tolerated.

Anterior spinal releases greatly contribute to curve

### BOX 33-1. CLASSIFICATION OF SURGICAL FAILURES

**Inability to achieve acceptable deformity correction**
- (1) Coronal plane imbalance
- (2) Sagittal plane imbalance
- (3) Pelvic obliquity — mild, moderate, severe
- (4) Transverse plane displacements (residual rotatory deformity)

**Early progression of deformity within the fusion zone**
- (1) Failure of bone-implant interface
  - (a) Patient factors: osteoporosis, small vertebra, sacrum, pelvis, pelvic-femoral contractures, noncompliance
  - (b) Biomechanical factors: anterior column deficiency, posterior element deficiency, large residual deformity
- (2) Instrument failure; failure of implant, implant coupling, or rod

The plane of progression should be defined:
  - (a) Progression in the coronal plane
  - (b) Progression in the sagittal plane
  - (c) Multiplanar progression

**Late progression of deformity within the fusion zone**
- (1) Crankshaft phenomenon: growth-related apical rotatory progression
  - (a) Residual deformity acceptable
  - (b) Residual deformity unacceptable
- (2) Pseudarthrosis
  - (a) Instruments intact, acceptable residual deformity
  - (b) Instrument failure, unacceptable residual deformity

**Early progression of deformity outside the fusion zone**
- (1) Coronal plane: postoperative coronal plane decompensation of adjacent unfused curves
- (2) Sagittal plane: junctional kyphosis

**Late progression of deformity outside the fusion zone**
- (1) Coronal plane
  - (a) Independent progression of deformity in unfused regions
  - (b) "Adding on" phenomenon
- (2) Sagittal plane: degenerative kyphosis of adjacent unfused spinal segments (transition syndrome)

correction, and should be considered for all thoracic curves with benders greater than 60 degrees, and all thoracolumbar and lumbar curves with benders greater than 40 degrees.[4,49,53,56] Anterior release to the pelvis must be considered if pelvic obliquity of 25 degrees or greater is encountered on supine traction or supine bender x-rays. In our experience the most common cause for inadequate correction in the coronal plane is the failure to recognize the need for anterior release!

The utilization of halo-gravity traction has been an important adjunct in the management of severe coronal plane deformity in our practice. We have experienced substantial corrections with prolonged traction treatment utilizing up to one third of the patient's body weight. Traction treatment is frequently combined with anterior and occasionally posterior releases, which appear to enhance traction efficacy. With this technique, safe-awake correction can be achieved. Benefits include improved nursing care, and enhanced cardiopulmonary and gastrointestinal (GI) function associated with upright positioning.[49]

Pelvic obliquity may be the most important component of the coronal plane deformity to address, and the hardest to manage. Correction of the pelvic obliquity from posterior-alone surgery is usually no better than 50%, whereas the addition of anterior release increases correction to better than 80%.[23,34,41,44,52,56] Anterior release allows for improved correction of lumbar and lumbosacral curves. But other forces act on the pelvis and may affect the position of the "pelvic vertebra" in space.[14,17,37] Asymmetric contractures of the abdominal and flank musculature may impede correction of pelvic obliquity. Release of the quadratus lumborum, external obliques, and erector spinae from the iliac crest posterior to anterior on the high side may be required. Pelvic femoral contractures may also negatively affect the surgeon's ability to achieve maximal correction of pelvic obliquity.[17,30] If severe windswept and hip flexion or extension deformities are recognized it may be best to perform releases or proximal femoral osteotomies prior to or soon after spinal surgery.[6] This should allow for better correction of the pelvic obliquity and decrease the forces seen by the pelvic instruments when the patient is placed in the sitting position postoperatively.

The best way to assess the coronal plane correction of each component of the deformity is via long cassette intraoperative posteroanterior (PA) and lateral radiographs from pelvis to T1. Residual curve magnitudes, pelvic obliquity, and coronal and sagittal balance can be accurately assessed. Implant position can be checked and altered if necessary. The surgeon can leave the operating room knowing that the surgical goals have been met. All that is required are radiolucent operative frame and a long x-ray cassette holder.

### INABILITY TO ACHIEVE ACCEPTABLE SAGITTAL PLANE CORRECTION

Depending on the stiffness of the sagittal plane deformity the surgeon must decide on the best method of achieving physiologic sagittal alignment. Flexible deformity can be managed easily by appropriate rod contouring, segmental fixation with sublaminar wire translation of spine to rod, and correction utilizing hook compression-distraction sequences.[5,14,20,22,40]

Rigid sagittal plane deformity can present serious problems for the deformity surgeon. Rigid severe thoracic kyphosis requires anterior release and a posterior compression construct to achieve physiologic alignment with stable fixation. Generous facet joint excision or posterior apical osteotomies will aid in shortening the posterior column.[51] Rigid thoracic lordosis requires apical anterior release and wedge resections, followed by posterior apical translation with sublaminar wires or hooks to a physiologically contoured rod.[4,49]

Rigid lumbar kyphosis must be managed by complete anterior release and posterior column shortening via generous facet excision, or osteotomy. Opposing multihook constructs in compression mode centered at the kyphosis apex on a properly contoured rod can maintain correction of lumbar kyphosis. Alternatively, pedicle screws may be placed, and segmental compression combined with in situ rod contouring achieves sagittal plane realignment.[1,2,7,8,12,27,28]

Rod rotation maneuvers can reduce kyphoscoliosis to an acceptable sagittal position. This is best achieved through pedicle screws placed along the curve convexity. Although hooks applied in compression sequence along the convexity of a lumbar curve can produce adequate coronal and sagittal plane correction also, hooks do not control the lumbar spine well in the transverse plane because the implants are located at the axis of transverse rotation (i.e., the posterior elements). Sublaminar wiring of the lumbar curve concavity in combination with concave distraction hooks may be applied after the convex rod has been inserted. This significantly improves transverse plane stability.[14]

Although pedicle screws provide the best "fix" with regard to segmental stability and construct rigidity, they also pose significant problems. Problems with implant size, pedicle dimensions, the inherent difficulty of insertion in severely deformed spines, potential effects on spinal growth, implant-induced osteoporosis, and risk of neurovascular injury must be considered.

Lumbar hyperlordosis is quite acceptable, and even desirable, as it allows for better distribution of weight over the posterior proximal thighs. But lumbar lordosis is considered severe when the value exceeds 90 degrees and the sacrum assumes a horizontal position. These patients typically demonstrate a seal-like sitting position, may develop low lumbar pain due to facet joint syndrome, and have difficulties in sitting and seat back fitting because the trunk is displaced anterior to the pelvis. Anterior release with wedge resection, undercontouring of spinal rods, hook distraction in the concavity of the lordoscoliosis, and reduction via posterior translation with sublaminar wires have effectively allowed correction of this aspect of neuromuscular deformity in our hands.[14] The erector spinae muscles and lumbodorsal fascia may be contracted and bow strung, impeding reduction of the lumbar hyperlordosis. Transverse incision through the fascia and muscles bilaterally should be performed to aid in deformity correction.

Finally, systems that provide in situ contouring with rod benders allow the surgeon to fine-tune the sagittal plane alignment. If this technique is utilized it is best to use a system or rod type with enough ductility to avoid the need for overcontouring, which places the implant-bone interface at some risk.[14]

The inability to achieve appropriate sagittal plane alignment at the time of surgery may be due to a general lack of understanding of acceptable sagittal alignment on a segmental, regional, and global level. Currently there is a plethora of normative data to draw upon. Intraoperative radiographs are very helpful in evaluating the surgeon's success in achieving acceptable sagittal alignment.[24]

## MANAGEMENT

The best way to minimize the humbling experience of being beaten by a spinal deformity in the operating room is to remember the 6 Ps: *Proper Preoperative Planning Prevents Poor Performance (correction)!* Careful preoperative planning includes general patient assessment, deformity assessment, and construct planning. The goal is a well-balanced, stable, and fused spine in all planes. The surgeon must determine the appropriate implant size, and preoperatively draw out an instrument montage that addresses the biomechanical demands of the deformity. Detailed planning includes determining the type and location of each implant, and the appropriate application of force sequences. The need for special equipment must be anticipated and ordered. The surgeon must become familiar with these instruments prior to surgery. The operating room (OR) is no place for a "crash course" with a new instrument system. Likewise, surgeon assistants and scrub nurses should be given the opportunity to familiarize themselves with the equipment and implants.

The failure to achieve acceptable correction of a neuromuscular spinal deformity should be recognized and addressed intraoperatively. Every effort should be made to remedy the situation. Occasionally, situations arise in which implants are not available or correction cannot be achieved for any number of reasons at the time of the primary surgery. In these cases, it may be best to cut your losses and leave the operating room with the intention of returning as soon as possible to revise the deformity.

In the early postoperative period, the surgeon must evaluate the deformity correction. If there is any component of deformity correction that appears inadequate, the patient should be returned to the OR for revision as soon as it is medically safe to do so. Frequently, all that is required is a small adjustment or change in construct design. We refer to this as "fine-tuning." These adjustments are much easier now that the instrument systems currently in use have locking mechanisms that are reversible. Usually, there is a particular component of the deformity that requires revision. In our experience it is usually a residual coronal plane deformity or pelvic obliquity that is most worrisome. Small angular deviations at the foundation of a construct can result in large coronal decompensation that may affect sitting balance. Corrections can be made, and should be evaluated with intraoperative long radiographs.

## EARLY PROGRESSION OF DEFORMITY WITHIN THE FUSION ZONE

When instrument failure is identified in the early postoperative period, it is usually accompanied by progression of the spinal deformity in one or all planes. We define *early failure* as failure prior to 6 months postop because we believe that current instrument systems and technique designed for segmental fixation should, in general, be able to provide fixation to this point. Because the strength of a maturing posterior spinal fusion has been shown to improve at the 6-month mark, failures after this point in time may best be attributed to failure of the fusion (i.e., pseudarthrosis).

In general, these early failures have two main causes: failure of the bone-implant interface, or instrument-related failure. Failure of the bone-implant interface may occur due to patient factors, such as osteoporosis, associated pelvic-femoral contractures, or noncompliance. Failures may also occur due to significant biomechanical factors not addressed in the index surgery, such as large residual deformity, or significant anterior column deficiencies. Inadequate force distribution may be due to inadequate number, type, or position of implants.

Instrument-related failures may be due to implant or instrument design characteristics, or the surgeon's lack of familiarity with system nuances. Systems currently available are thoroughly tested in vitro and in vivo prior to being released for general usage. But continued reevaluation remains an important part of the process.

Early failure and progression seem to favor one plane over another. It is important to recognize the major plane of progression, search for a specific cause, and address the problem in a timely and logical fashion. A summary of these thoughts is presented in Figure 33-1.

***Inability to Maintain Acceptable Coronal Plane Correction in the Early Postoperative Period.*** The most common reason for early loss of correction is failure of the bone-implant interface. This may occur early, within the first 6 months, and should be considered a mechanical failure. Frequently the bone-implant interface fails at the deformity apex, or at the construct ends, and the deformity recurs. This failure may be due to loss of bone-hook, bone-screw, or bone-wire interface at these strategic locations. Other modes of mechanical failure include implant failure such as wire or screw breakage, failure of the implant-rod coupling, or failures of rod-rod couplers and cross connectors, and even rod failure.[1,2]

If this mode of failure is recognized, early revision should be strongly considered. Early on a consolidating fusion mass is quite plastic, and frequently correction lost can be regained without much effort.[12]

The surgeon must establish whether the construct failed due to an underestimation of the biomechanical demands that were placed on the system.[36] This may include significant unrecognized anterior column deficiencies, posterior element deficiency or failure, or large residual deformities. If this is determined to be a contributing cause of the failure, spinal destabilization and anterior column reconstruction with structural grafts and supplemental anterior instruments may be necessary. Alternatively, patient factors such as osteoporosis; small vertebral, sacral, and pelvic structures; pelvic-femoral contracture; and noncompliance may be important. Postoperative management may mandate elimination of gravity forces by application of external immobilization and enforced recumbent positioning until solid osseous healing has occurred. Usually 3 months is required.

Restoration of mechanical stability can be achieved surgically by using a number of different strategies. Removal and replacement of instrumentation requires a detailed preoperative plan based on studies that define the mode of failure. Computed tomography (CT) scans with sagittal and coronal reconstructions or conventional tomography may be invaluable in defining the mode of failure. If hook displacement without laminar failure is noted, simple replacement and augmentation with additional hook sites may be all that is required. If laminar or facet failure has occurred, either different implants (i.e., pedicle screws) must be used, or, alternatively, the construct must be extended proximally and distally to allow fixation into virgin spinal segments.[12,28]

When anatomically feasible, the addition of anterior fusion with structural grafting and anterior instrumentation provides a powerful supplement to posterior fixation. This approach is especially helpful in situations in which previous laminectomy or dysraphic states limit fixation options and provides a poor posterior fusion bed.[12,27,28]

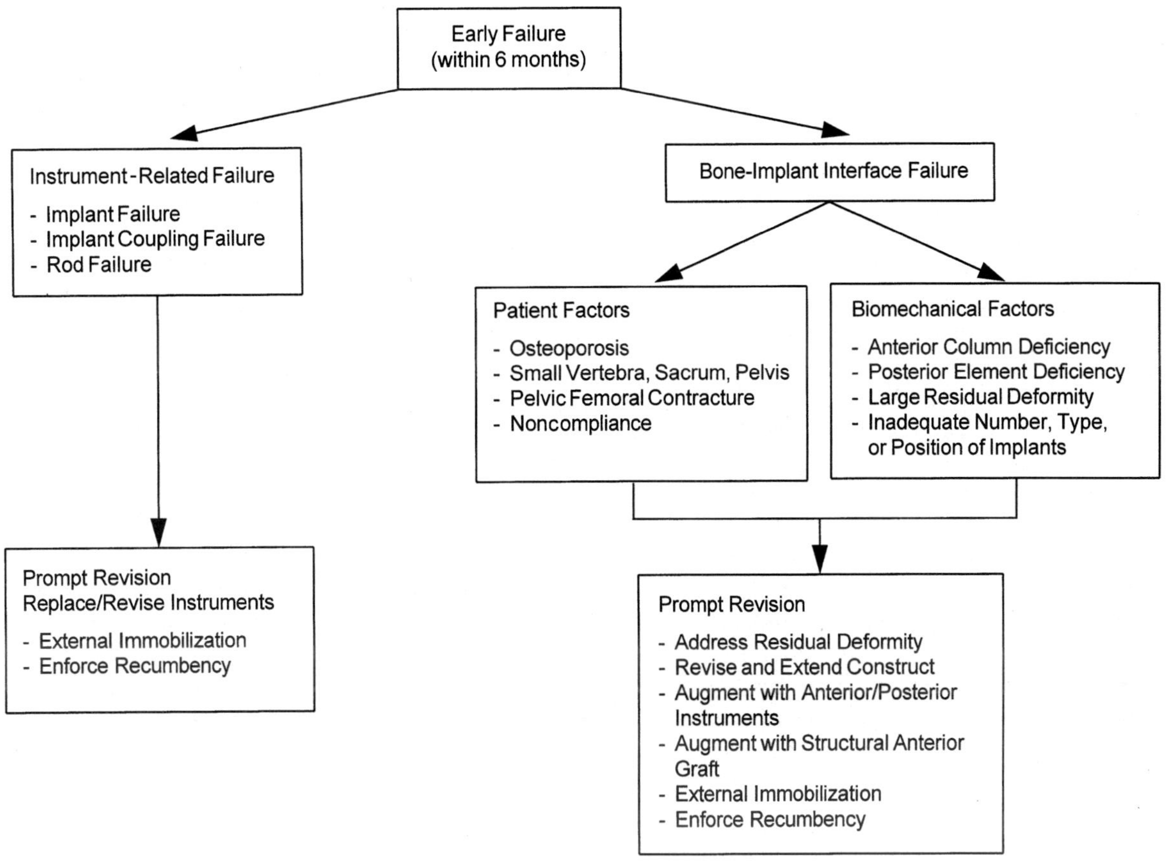


FIGURE 33-1

Early progression of deformity within fusion zone.

In neuromuscular patients fixed to the pelvis with the Galveston technique, early loss of lumbosacral sagittal alignment is rare. The intrailiac rod may rarely migrate through the medial or lateral table. The rods may displace posteriorly if the iliac wing orientation is in the sagittal plane, pathoanatomy typically seen in myelodysplasia kyphosis patients. Loss of fixation may occur when bone resorption around the iliac segment of rod becomes severe. A small halo of 1 to 2 mm is routinely seen and has no clinical consequence. But significant resorption can occur in cases of long-standing pseudarthrosis and smoldering deep infection.

Failure with other techniques of sacral fixation have been noted. The Jackson technique of sacral fixation depends on S1 pedicular fixation and intrasacral rod fixation in the sacral lateral mass region (zone III). We have encountered early failures with this technique in neuromuscular patients, probably due to sacral osteoporosis. Revision to Galveston intrailiac fixation has successfully salvaged these challenging situations.

In ambulatory neuromuscular patients fused to the lower lumbar spine, distal instrument failure will result in recurrence of the coronal plane deformity and usually a lumbar kyphosis with prominent distal hardware. This mode of failure is most frequently seen when hooks cut through or fracture the lamina. If this situation is recognized early, revision is usually quite easy. Exploration of the distal instrumented segments, removal of the lower portion of the construct, excision of fibrous tissue, and osteotomy may be necessary to regain lost correction. Revision of the instruments distal to the failure site, preferably with pedicle screws, should allow restoration of lumbar lordosis. Depending on the biomechanical demands, structural anterior grafting must be considered.

***Inability to Maintain Acceptable Sagittal Plane Alignment in the Early Postoperative Period.*** Early failure with loss of the sagittal alignment occurs when the biomechanical demands on the construct exceed the instrumentation holding power. This usually occurs at either the proximal or distal end of the instrumentation with resultant kyphosis at the construct ends extending into the unfused segments.

Proximal falloff with proximal thoracic kyphosis is very common when sublaminar wires are utilized to achieve proximal fixation. Factors thought to be important in this phenomenon include: termination of instruments in a kyphotic zone or segment (T4 or distal), removal of posterior supporting structures between the proximal fixed lamina and the adjacent segment, and proximal sublaminar wire failure.

Prevention is the best strategy! It is important to carry the instruments to a sagittally neutral segment, usually at least T2. Lamino-laminar or pedicolaminar claws provide more secure end fixation than do sublaminar wires. At least two and optimally four sets of claws should be utilized at the proximal end of the construct. The surgeon should avoid damage to the supraspinous and interspinous ligaments, and remove just enough ligamentum flavum and facet joint to insert the supralaminar hooks.

If early failure is recognized, the cause should be determined. In most cases there is a failure of the bone-implant interface. Restoration of proximal sagittal alignment by posterior-only techniques can be achieved if the failure is recognized early. In general, the proximal portion of the construct must be removed to allow a thorough cleaning of the interposed fibrous tissue that develops. Facet excision at the involved levels serves as osteotomies and aid in correction. Secure claw segmental fixation must be carried proximal to the failure site. As this is usually at the cervicothoracic junction the surgeon must have a range of implants that can be safely applied to this region. Rod connection is achieved via rod-rod connectors that allow application of compression forces across the junctional zone.

If it is determined that the proximal kyphosis is long-standing or rigid, a more aggressive strategy may be required. Posterior instrument removal with osteotomies, application of halo-gravity traction with gradual kyphosis correction, anterior release if necessary, and staged posterior reinstrumentation may be required. This dorsal-ventral-dorsal sequence is frequently necessary to achieve optimal correction for rigid revision deformity problems.[8,12,18,28] Postoperative halo cast or halo-Milwaukee bracing may be required to protect the internal fixation.

## Late Progression of Deformity Within the Fusion Zone

We have identified two main causes for progression of deformity after the 6-month postoperative period. These include the crankshaft phenomenon and pseudarthrosis. An algorithm for management has been provided in Figure 33-2.

***Pseudarthrosis.*** The loss of correction in either the coronal or sagittal plane after 6 months postop is often due to failure to achieve a solid spinal fusion.

Pseudarthrosis may occur due to arrest or failure of the biologic sequence of events that result in fusion. This may be due to lack of adequate volume and quality of autogenous bone graft or inadequate preparation of the fusion bed. Systemic causes such as malnutrition, metabolic bone disease, anti-inflammatory medications, or a local disturbance such as occult deep infection are other contributing factors. Insufficient fusion surface area may be implicated especially when dealing with posterior element deficiencies, as in

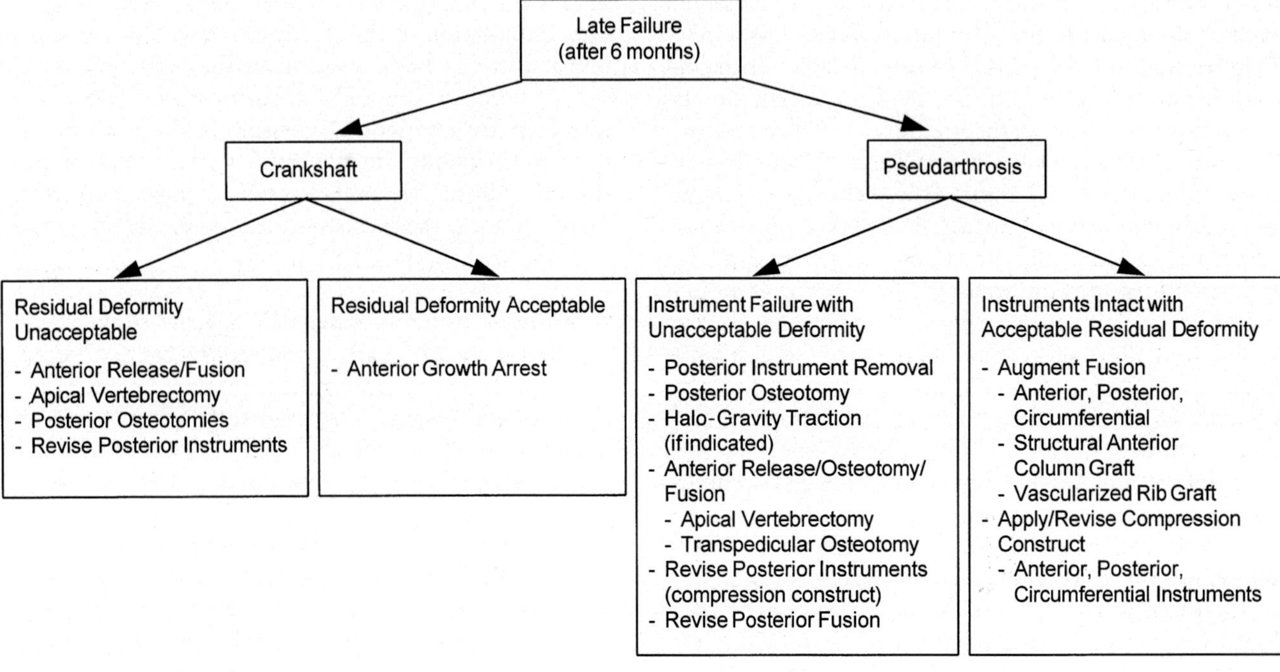


FIGURE 33-2

Late progression of deformity within fusion zone.

myelodysplasia. Residual mechanical instability that allows intersegmental strains that are greater than that tolerated by the immature fusion mass will result in pseudarthrosis. Pseudarthroses tend to occur at the apex of the deformity, and at the thoracolumbar and the lumbosacral junctions.[2,29,36]

The management of pseudarthrosis includes early recognition through routine temporal radiographic follow-up. We currently utilize the following schedule: postoperative upright anteroposterior (AP) and lateral radiographs at 4 to 7 days; 3, 6, and 12 weeks; 6, 9, 12, 18, and 24 months, 3 and 5 years; and every 5 years thereafter. Although instrument failure related to pseudarthrosis predictably occurred prior to 2 years postoperative with Harrington instrumentation, with rigid segmental fixation these failures are often delayed. In one instance instrument failure with documented pseudarthrosis presented 5 years after the index procedure. It is important to compare sequential radiograph from visit to visit to evaluate for changes in instrumentation, progression of deformity, radiographic evidence of pseudarthrosis, or changes in adjacent spinal segments. Oblique radiographs and Ferguson views may be helpful, but usually metal obscures the fusion mass, making interpretation difficult. Dynamic radio-graphs are usually not helpful if instrumentation is rigid, but motion may be evident when nonrigid instrumentation such as sublaminar wiring technique is utilized. Special studies such as AP and lateral tomograms or CT scans with sagittal reconstructions may be helpful in determining the presence of a pseudarthrosis.

Although it is estimated that up to 50% of pseudarthrosis are asymptomatic with regard to pain, the deformity surgeon must pay attention to subtle changes in spinal alignment or instrumentation position so that early revision may be performed.[47] Preemptive intervention can shorten the overall period of convalescence, and will most likely result in a better final result.

In children with neuromuscular deformity, allograft is often required due to inadequate autogenous bone sources, and in general this provides a solid fusion.[58] But if pseudarthrosis is encountered it is best to repair this with autogenous bone from ilium, rib, or tibia if necessary. The role for bone graft extenders, such as demineralized bone matrix, is not entirely clear, but appears to be working well in the children in which we've used it. In occasional cases of persistent pseudarthrosis it may be necessary to perform vascularized rib or even pedicle vascularized iliac crest grafts to enhance healing potential. Autogenous bone grafting is critical, but mechanical stability must be restored and residual deformity corrected to create an optimal environment for graft healing. The pseudarthrosis fibrous tissue should be cleaned thoroughly. This enhances healing, prevents impingement of the fibrous tissue on the neural elements, and aids in correction by mobilizing the pseudarthrosis. The defect is filled with autogenous bone graft, and compression forces applied through a compression construct. Implants should be placed as close to the pseudarthrosis as possible to prevent motion at the pseudarthrosis site. Instruments that are rigidly fixed to the spine or embedded in bone serve as great anchor points. Rods are cut with a rod cutter or high speed cutting tools. Axial connectors or dominos are applied and new implants and rods are inserted. The goal is to achieve fixation adjacent to the pseudarthrosis site and apply compression across this site. Compression is applied to the convex side a kyphoscoliotic segment first, correcting both planes simultaneously. Check radiographs in both planes should demonstrate restoration of alignment in both planes. The surgeon should check to make sure that no neural compression has occurred with the closure of the pseudarthrosis site.

In general, posterior pseudarthrosis without instrument failure or recurrence of deformity can be managed by performing exploration of posterior fusion, evaluation of spinal fixation, and revision of the posterior pseudarthrosis. This allows the surgeon to document each pseudarthrosis level. Anterior fusion with or without anterior compression instruments is performed at all pseudarthrosis levels to augment the posterior fusion. Anterior pseudarthroses are unusual, and when they occur are usually due to failure to achieve adequate mechanical stability with spinal instruments. If residual deformity is not significant, posterior stabilization and fusion should be performed. When significant anterior deficiency is not a problem, and the process is not long-standing, the stability imparted may achieve anterior column healing. But if the residual deformity is significant or is progressive then anterior and posterior revision surgery will be required. If posterior instruments have failed and there are no anterior instruments, revision should start with a posterior approach. If the anterior column prevents correction, anterior release and revision of the anterior fusion must be performed next. The surgeon may need to revisit the posterior instruments to achieve compression and optimize alignment.

Anterior revision for anterior pseudarthrosis can be a daunting task for even the most experienced deformity surgeons. It requires careful preoperative planning. In these cases it is helpful to have a general, thoracic, or vascular surgeon assist with the exposure. When broken or displaced anterior instruments are present it may be prudent to remove and revise these. This requires exposure from the same side, with a careful exploration of the instruments and pseudarthrosis site. In low lumbar and lumbosacral cases, ureteral stents may be placed preoperatively to allow easy recognition intraoperatively. In cases in which instruments do not require removal and deformity correction is not an issue, exposure from the contralateral side may also be considered.

***Crankshaft Phenomenon.*** The crankshaft phenomenon is a recently recognized cause for postoperative deterioration of an otherwise successful posterior spinal fusion.[15] It is caused by continued anterior spinal growth in situations when a solid posterior spinal fusion has been achieved. This complication has been recognized as a cause for postoperative coronal plane progression in idiopathic, congenital, and neuromuscular scoliosis.[23] The younger and more skeletally immature a child is at the time of posterior fusion, the greater the risk. Tanner one, Risser 0 children with open triradiate cartilages are at greatest risk. In general, children with idiopathic scoliosis who have these characteristics are under age eleven.[21] But in neuromuscular scoliosis the attainment of skeletal maturity is much more variable, and disease specific. Many patients with spinal deformity associated with static perinatal encephalopathy (cerebral palsy) may demonstrate significant delays in puberty. This may be due to primary abnormalities associated with pituitary function, or secondary to malnutrition. Some of these children may not reach maturity until age twenty! Conversely, children with myelodysplasia tend to undergo precocious puberty, with girls achieving menarche a full 1 to 2 years earlier than other children. The surgeon must use the physical exam and radiographic indices of maturity to estimate the skeletal age and the risk of crankshaft.

This is an insidious cause for progression within the fusion zone, and can be easily missed if serial postoperative examination is not performed, and serial postoperative radiographs are not carefully studied. On physical exam one may see gradual deterioration of coronal plane balance, worsening trunk shift, or increasing thoracic or lumbar prominences. Increasing thoracic or lumbar lordosis, although subtle, may also be appreciated. Radiographic changes occur in spite of intact spinal instrumentation and a confluent solid spinal fusion. On the AP radiograph, one may note increasing apical rotation, increasing apical deviation from the center sacral line, and a gradual migration of the curve apex toward the lateral rib borders. An increase in the Cobb angle may occur, but this is usually recognized later than the changes that are primarily related to apical rotation. On the lateral radiograph, one may find an increase in thoracic or lumbar lordosis.

If, based on the patient's skeletal immaturity and the characteristics of the deformity, the risk of crankshaft is high, then adjunctive anterior spinal growth arrest and fusion should be performed.[50] If the patient is considered to have an intermediate risk, the surgeon may choose to perform the posterior fusion and observe closely, reserving anterior growth arrest for those cases in which crankshaft is documented with careful follow-up. In low-risk patients, anterior growth arrest is not required, but of course it may be desirable to do anterior release for deformity correction.

### PROGRESSION OF DEFORMITY OUTSIDE THE FUSION ZONE

Ideal deformity correction requires spinal balance in all planes and all regions of the spine. One strives to achieve segmental, regional, and global balance for the remainder of the patient's life. The surgeon draws up a preoperative plan that determines the spinal segments to be instrumented and fused. Experience has allowed us to predict, in general, how the adjacent unfused spinal segments will respond. But unfortunately, with increasing frequency, problems adjacent to spinal fusions confront the spinal deformity surgeon. This may be characterized by progression of deformity in one or more planes, or may be related to late degenerative breakdown of adjacent spinal segments.

We have subdivided this mode of failure on the basis of the major plane of progression (sagittal or coronal), and the time to failure (before or after 6 months) (Figs. 33-3 and 33-4).

***Early Progression of Deformity.*** There are occasional neuromuscular deformities that appear more idiopathic radiographically. The surgeon may choose to treat these curves in the manner in which an idiopathic curve may be treated. As in any selective fusion technique in which the "primary curve" is addressed via instrumented correction and the "secondary curve" is allowed to respond to this correction, the ability to predict the secondary curve response is not foolproof. This is evident by the numerous reports of spinal decompensation related to selective thoracic fusion for King type II idiopathic curves. Although this decompensation was initially thought to be related to the rod rotation maneuver, the etiology is more likely related to lumbar curve characteristics and the relative correction of the thoracic curve.[54]

In general it is somewhat risky to consider this treatment course in a patient with a neuromuscular curve. We have used selective anterior instrumentation and fusion in a small number of children with neuromuscular thoracolumbar and lumbar deformity with acceptable results thus far. But the patient, family, and surgeon must realize the high potential for failure with this procedure, follow closely, and be prepared to address deterioration if encountered.

Progression of deformity in the sagittal plane outside the fusion zone usually involves the junction between the fusion zone and adjacent segments.[8] Kyphosis is the rule. There are a variety of factors that may be important. If a construct is terminated on a kyphotic segment there is a great tendency for progression of the kyphosis at the junction. Instruments

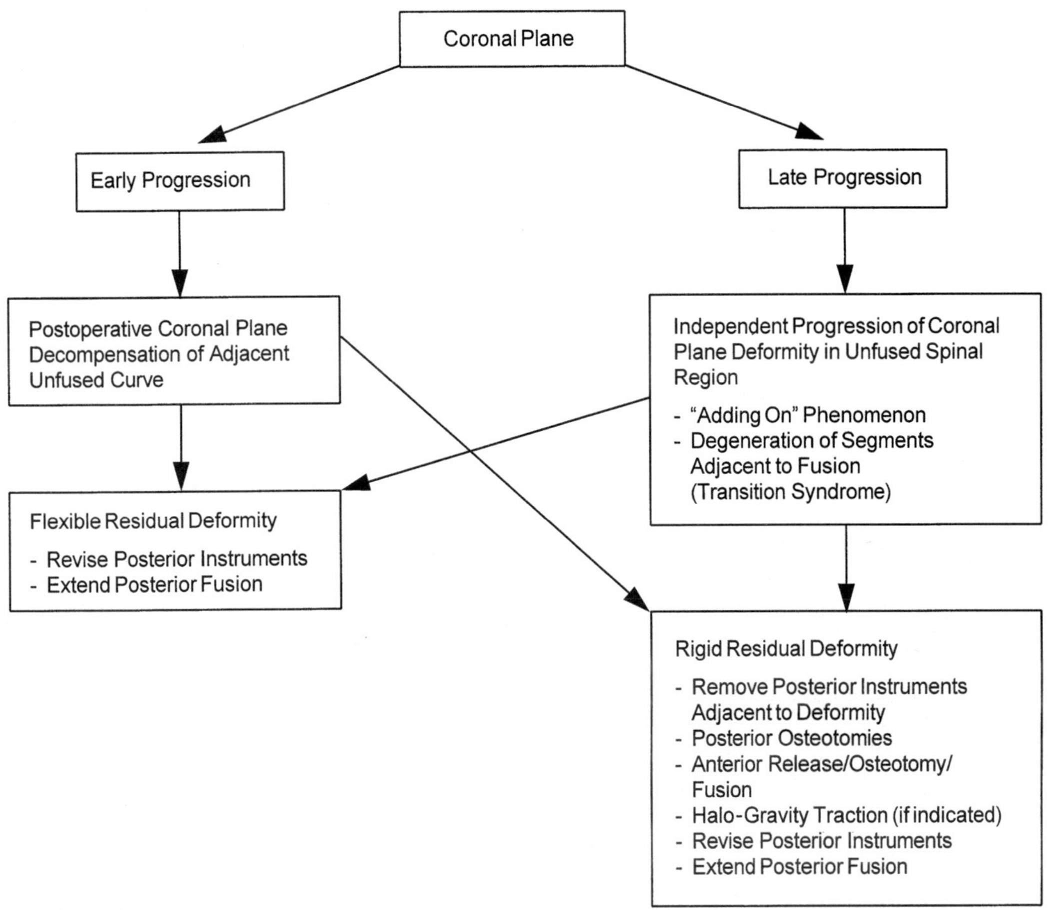


FIGURE 33-3

Sagittal plane progression of deformity outside the fusion zone.

should be carried proximal and distal to sagittally neutral or lordotic segments if at all possible. Knowledge of the normative sagittal plane data is helpful, but preoperative evaluation of the sitting or standing lateral radiograph is most important in selecting the vertebrae on which to end the construct.

If the thoracic rod is undercontoured, resulting in overstraightening of the thoracic kyphosis in the fusion zone, there is a tendency for the patient to develop junctional kyphosis in the adjacent segments. We have observed this phenomenon in both proximal and distal adjacent segments, but it appears to occur most commonly at the proximal end. Appropriate rod contouring is the key, with the goal of achieving a physiologic sagittal alignment. Intraoperative radiographs can be very helpful in this determination.

Distraction forces applied at the terminal end of a construct have also been implicated as a cause for junctional kyphosis. This creates segmental kyphosis in the last instrumented segment and appears to set up conditions for progression in adjacent segments as well.

Some patients are prone to develop proximal or distal junctional kyphosis in spite of the surgeon's best efforts. Patients with poor head control and those with connective tissue disorders such as Marfan's syndrome, Larson's syndrome, Sjögren's syndrome, or Ehlers-Danlos syndrome may be at greater risk for this complication. These patients must be observed closely for this so early intervention may be instituted.

***Late Progression of Deformity.*** Progression of deformity outside the fusion zone may occur in the coronal or sagittal plane after the 6-month mark. This progression is usually insidious and requires careful radiographic follow-up and critical comparison of radiographs from each visit.

***"Adding On."*** Definitive management of neuromuscular curves typically call for extensive fusions. But there may be cases in which fusion is terminated in the upper lumbar region. This technique presents some risk with regard to progression of the coronal plane curve with increasing tilt of the lowest instrumented vertebra and progression of the deformity distally into the uninstrumented segments. This phenomenon, known as "adding on," should be differentiated from progression by other modes such as crankshaft or

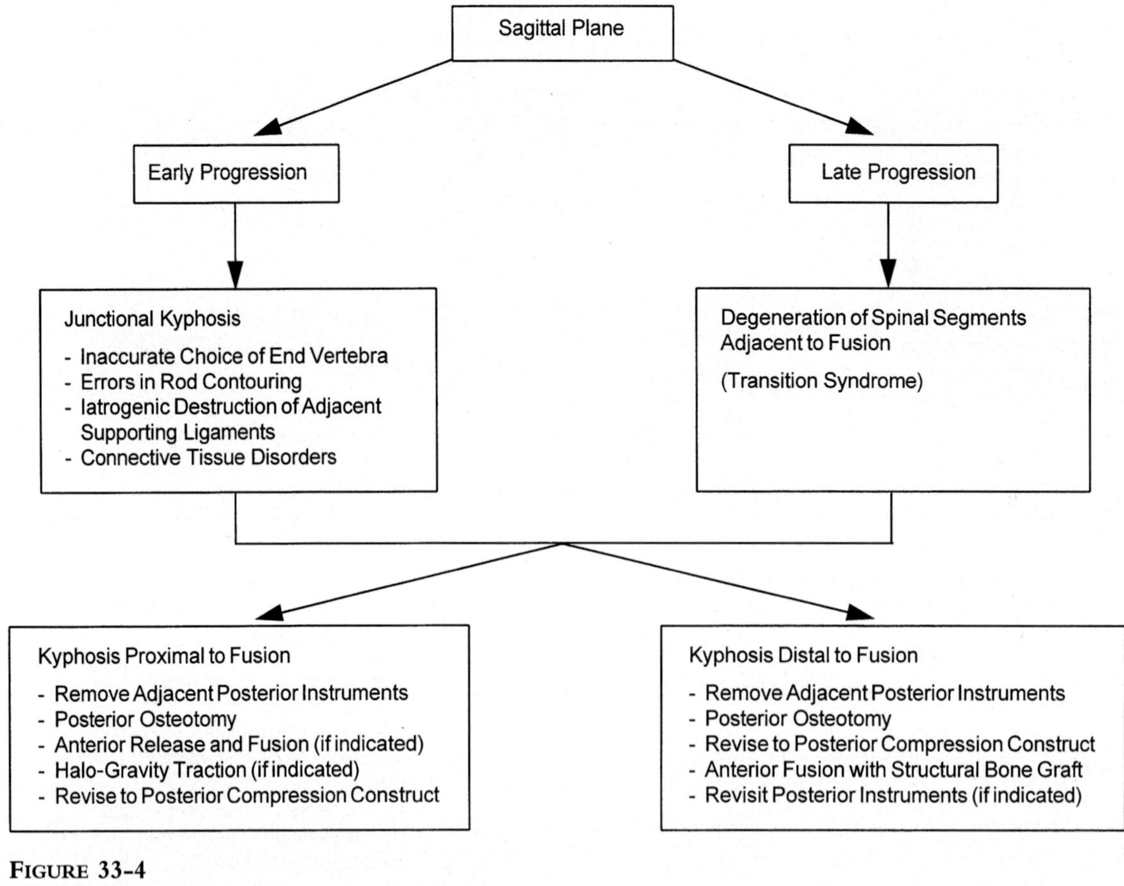


FIGURE 33-4

Coronal plane progression of deformity outside the fusion zone.

pseudarthrosis.[47,54] It is associated with loss of coronal balance, recurrence of trunk shift, and shift of the lower instrumented vertebra away from the center sacral line.[27,36] Large residual curves in which horizontalization of the lowest instrumented vertebra is not achieved are at greatest risk. Mechanical failure or degeneration of adjacent disk segments may play a role. Extension of the fusion distally is required.[2,12,27]

***Transition Syndrome.*** Degeneration of motion segments adjacent to an instrumented fusion is a major problem that usually presents many months or years after the index procedure.[8,12,27] Malalignments in the sagittal plane may hasten this degeneration, as evidenced by degeneration of lower lumbar segments distal to fusions performed with Harrington distraction instrumentation. Residual deformity in the coronal plane may also create an adverse biomechanical environment. Coronal plane tilt of the lower instrumented vertebra creates shear stresses that may result in premature demise of the adjacent motion segment. While this has not been well defined, it is known that AP tilts of greater than 10 degrees exceed the physiologic range of the lower lumbar motion segments. Residual deformity may result in degeneration of the disk with lateral listhesis.

## RESIDUAL PELVIC OBLIQUITY AFTER "SUCCESSFUL" SPINAL FUSION

Pelvic obliquity must be classified according to the etiology. Supra pelvic causes include lumbar and lumbosacral scoliosis (spino-pelvic obliquity), asymmetric contractures of truncal musculature such as the iliopsoas, or quadratus lumborum. Pelvic causes may include sacral or pelvic bony dysplasias or dissociation of the sacroiliac joints. Infra-pelvic causes include asymmetric hip contractures (windblown pelvis) in association with hip dislocations, and limb length discrepencies.

Dubousset has advanced a 3 dimensional classification that evaluates the coronal, sagittal, and transverse components of the pelvic obliquity, and provides a rationale for correction through a sequence of force applications.[14] Farcy has recently presented a somewhat simplified classification, and presents results of management with iliosacral screw fixation.[17]

The functional consequences of pelvic obliquity may be slight or severe depending on the magnitude of the deformity and patient factors. Asymmetric sitting can cause discomfort over the low ishia and buttock. Soft tissue pressures may be high enough to cause pressure ulcerations in insensate or noncommunicative patients. Pelvic flexion may occur due

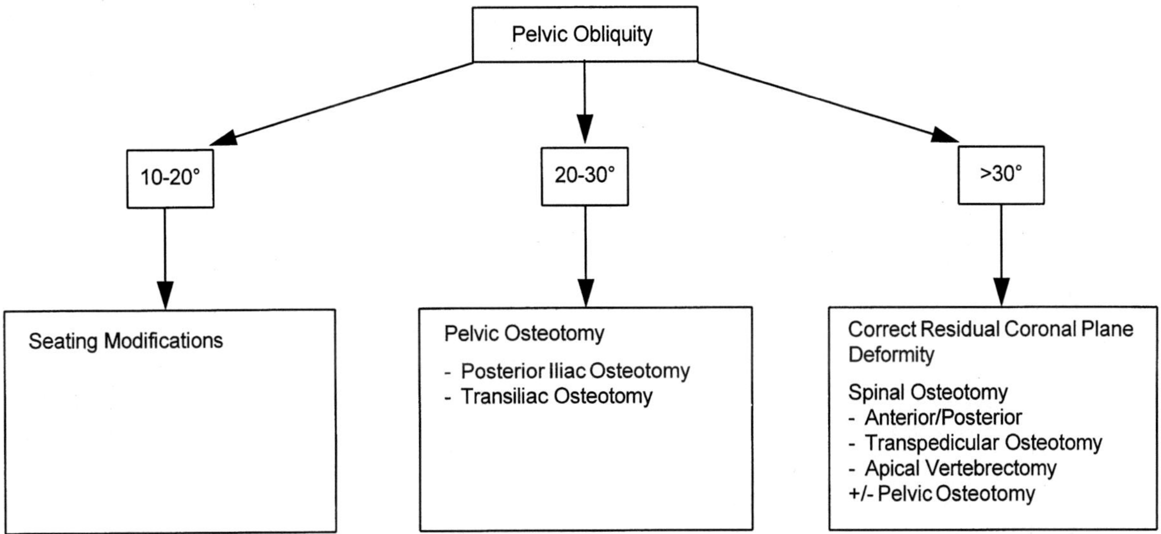


FIGURE 33-5

Management of residual spinopelvic pelvic obliquity after "successful" spinal fusion.

to lumbar or lumbosacral kyphosis or may be associated with severe hamstring contracture. This shifts the force posterior from the posterior thighs and concentrates these forces over a smaller area, including the ischiae and the sacrum, increasing the risk for pressure ulceration.

Pelvic obliquity is clearly a major problem in the unfixed spine, but significant residual pelvic obliquity after spinal fusion can be even more troublesome. The rigidity eliminates spinal compensation, and may actually increase the risk of pressure ulceration.

From a clinical perspective residual pelvic obliquities of less than 20 degrees present little clinical consequence. Seating modifications such as air or silicone seat cushions can frequently achieve reasonable distribution of weight across the ischia, buttocks, and posterior thighs. Seat wedges can be used to achieve a vertical spinal posture.

When residual pelvic obliquity exceeds 30 degrees and is causing adverse consequences, a surgical solution may be required. The surgeon must determine the most effective point of attack. If residual spinal deformity is the primary cause, and is severe, treatment will require spinal osteotomy for correction of the deformity. In a solidly fused spine this is a major undertaking.

If the residual spinal deformity is not significant, and the pelvic obliquity is less than 30 degrees, then the surgeon may have the option to correct the pelvic obliquity through a pelvic osteotomy. Lindseth described posterior iliac opening and closing wedge osteotomies for the management of residual pelvic obliquity in myelodysplasia spinal deformity.[31] Millis presents another attractive option for correction of pelvic obliquity through a transiliac lengthening osteotomy, which is basically a modification of a Salter's innominate osteotomy.[38] We have used this approach in the management of residual coronal plane pelvic obliquity, as well as residual lumbosacral kyphosis vis-à-vis anterior opening innominate osteotomies.

It is important to evaluate residual pelvic obliquity with clinical as well as radiographic criteria. Some children can tolerate relatively large residual deformity without consequence, while others may experience difficulties with a small residual deformity. We have provided an algorithm in Figure 33-5 for treatment.

## REFERENCES

1. Aebi M, Goyton M: Revision surgery of the lumbosacral spine, *Spine: State of the Art Reviews,* vol.11, no. 1, Philadelphia, January, 1997, Hanley & Belfus.
2. An H, Glover J: *Complications and revision surgery in adult spinal deformity.* In Bridwell KH, DeWald RL, editors: *The textbook of spinal surgery,* ed 2, Philadelphia, 1997, Lippincott-Raven, pp 797-820.
3. Askin G, Hallett R, Hare N, Webb J: The outcome of scoliosis surgery in severely physically handicapped child. An objective and subjective assessment. *Spine* 22:44-50, 1997.
4. Banta J: Combined anterior and posterior fusion for spinal deformity in myelodysplasia, *Spine* 15:946-952, 1990.
5. Bell D, Mosely C, Koreska J: Unit rod segmental spinal instrumenation in the management of patients with

progressive neuromuscular spinal deformity, *Spine* 14: 1301-1307, 1989.
6. Black B, Griffin P: The cerebral palsied hip, *Clin Ortho Rel Res* 338:42-51, 1997.
7. Bradford D, Tribus C; Vertebral column resection for the treatment of rigid coronal plane decompensation, *Spine* 22:1590-1599, 1997.
8. Bridwell KH: *Osteotomies for fixed deformities in the thoracic and lumbar spine.* In Bridwell KH, DeWald RL, editors: *The textbook of spinal surgery,* ed 2, Philadelphia, 1997, Lippincott-Raven, pp 821-835.
9. Brook P, Kennedy J, Stern L, Sutherland A, Foster B: Spinal fusion in Duchenne's muscular dystrophy, *J Ped Orthop* 16(3):324-331, 1996.
10. Broom M, Banta J, Renshaw T: Spine fusion augmented by Luque rod segmental instrumentation for neuromuscular scoliosis, *J Bone Joint Surg Am* 71(1):32-44, 1989.
11. Bulman W, Dormans J, Ecker M, Drummond D: Posterior spinal fusions for scoliosis with cerebral palsy: a comparison of Luque rod and unit rod instrumentation. *J Ped Orthop* 16(3):314-323, 1996.
12. DeWald RL: Revision surgery for spinal deformity, *Instructional Course Lectures,* AAOS 41:235-250, 1992.
13. Dias R, Miller F, Dabney K, Lipton G: Revision spinal surgery in children with cerebral palsy, *J Spinal Disord* 10(2):132-144, 1997.
14. Dubousset J: *Cotrel-Dubousset instrumentation for paralytic neuromuscular spinal deformities with emphasis on pelvic obliquity.* In Bridwell KH, DeWald RL, editors: *The textbook of spinal surgery,* ed 2, Philadelphia, 1997, Lippincott-Raven, pp 933-947.
15. Dubousset J, Herring J, Shufflebarger H: The crankshaft phenomenon, *J Ped Orthop* 9:541, 1989.
16. Eberle C: Failure of fixation after segmental spinal instrumentation without arthrodesis in the management of paralytic scoliosis, *J Bone Joint Surg Am* 70:696, 1988.
17. Farcy J, Weidenbaum M, Roye D: Fixed pelvic obliquity, *Spine: State of the Art Reviews,* vol 8 (3), Philadelphia, September, 1994, Hanley & Belfus.
18. Farcy J, Schwab F: Anterior posterior osteotomy with realignment, *Spine* 22(20):2452-2457, 1997.
19. Ferguson R, Hansen M, Nicholas D, Allen B: Same day vs. staged anterior-posterior spinal surgery in neuromuscular scoliosis population: evaluation of medical complications, *J Ped Orthop* 16(3):293-303, 1996.
20. Gau Y, Lonstein J, Winter R, Koop S, Denis F: Luque-Galveston procedure for correction and stabilization of neuromuscular scoliosis and pelvic obliquity: review of 68 cases, *J Spinal Disord* 4(4):399-410, 1991.
21. Hamill C, Bridwell KH, Lenke L, Chapman M, Baldus C, Blanke K: Posterior arthrodesis in the skeletally immature patient: assessing the risk for crankshaft, *Spine* 22(12):1343-1351, 1997.
22. Hsu J: The development of current approaches to the management of spinal deformity for patients with neuromuscular disease, *Semin Neurol* 15(1):24-28, 1995.
23. Jackson L, Banta J, Smith B: *Crankshaft phenomenon in neuromuscular scoliosis.* Presented at the SRS Annual Meeting, Dublin, Ireland, Sept. 18, 1993.
24. Jackson R: Spinal balance, lumbopelvic alignments around the hip axis and positioning for surgery, *Spine: State of the Art Reviews,* vol 11, no 1, Philadelphia, January, 1997, Hanley & Belfus.
25. Jaivin J, Banta J, Milanese A, Hight D, Alexander F: Perioperative jejunostomy tube feeding in reconstructive spinal surgery, *Dev Med Child Neurol* 33(3):225-231, 1991.
26. Klemme W, Denis F, Winter R, Lonstein J, Koop S: Spinal instrumentation without fusion for progressive scoliosis in young children, *J Ped Orthop* 17:734-742, 1997.
27. Kostuik J: Failures after spinal fusion, *Spine: State of the Art Reviews,* vol 11, no 3, Philadelphia, September, 1997, Hanley & Belfus.
28. Kostuik J: Spinal osteotomies in adult scoliosis surgery, *Spine: State of the Art Reviews,* vol 8, no 2, Philadelphia, May, 1994, Hanley & Belfus.
29. Laurman W, Bradford D, Transfeldt E, Ogilvie J: Management of pseudarthrosis after arthrodesis for idiopathic scoliosis, *J Bone Joint Surg Am* 73(2):222-236, 1991.
30. Lee D, Choi T, Chung C, Cho T, Lee J: Fixed pelvic obliquity after poliomyelitis: classification and management, *J Bone Joint Surg Br* 79(2):190-196, 1997.
31. Lindseth R: Spine deformity in myelomingocele, *Instr Course Lecture Series XL,* 281, AAOS, Chicago, IL, 1991.
32. Lubicky J, Spadaro J, Yuan H, Fredrickson B, Henderson N: Variability in SSEP monitoring during spinal surgery, *Spine* 14(8):790-798, 1989.
33. Majid M, Muldowny D, Holt R: Natural history of scoliosis in the institutionalized adult cerebral palsey population, *Spine* 22(13):1461-1466, 1997.
34. Maloney W, Rinsky L, Gamble J: Simultaneous correction of pelvic obliquity, frontal plane, and sagittal plane deformities in neuromuscular scoliosis using unit rod with segmental sublaminar wires, *J Ped Orthop* 10(6):742-749, 1990.
35. Mardjetko S, Hammerberg K, Lubicky J: The Luque Trolley revisited: review of 9 cases requiring revision, *Spine* 17:582, 1992.
36. Margulies JY, Bitan F, Thampi S, Deowall C: Biomechanical considerations in failed fusions, *Spine: State of the Art Reviews,* vol 11, no 3, Philadelphia, September 1997, Hanley & Belfus.
37. Miladi L, Ghanem I, Draoui M, Zeller R, Dubousset J: Iliosacral screw fixation for pelvic obliquity in neuromuscular scoliosis: long term follow-up, *Spine* 22(15):1722-1799, 1997.
38. Millis M, Ahern M, Hall J: Transiliac leg lengthening: experiences with a modified Salter osteotomy, *Othopade* 19(5):283-291, 1990.
39. Mubarak S, Morin W, Leach J; Spinal fusion in

Duchenne muscular dystrophy: fixation and fusion to the sacropelvis, *J Ped Orthop* 13(6):752-757, 1993.

40. Neustadt J, Shufflebarger H, Cammisa F: Spinal fusions to the pelvis augmented by Cotrel-Dubousset instrumentation for neuromuscular scoliosis, *J Ped Orthop* 12(4):465-469, 1992.
41. O'Brien J, Dwyer A, Hodgson A: Pelvic obliquity: Its prognosis and management and the development of a technique for full correction of the deformity, *J Bone Joint Surg Am* 57:626, 1975.
42. Ogilvie J, Transfeldt E, Wood K: *Overview of fixation to the sacrum and pelvis in spinal surgerys.* In Margulies JY, editor: *Lumbosacral and spinopelvic fixation,* Philadelphia, 1997, Lippincott-Raven, pp 191-198.
43. Padman R, McNamara R: Postoperative pulmonary complications in children with neuromuscular scoliosis who underwent spinal fusion, *Del Med J* 62(5):999-1003, 1990.
44. Perra J: Techniques of instrumentation in long fusions to the sacrum, *Orthop Clin North Am* 25(2):287-299, 1994.
45. Polly D, Sturm P: Traction versus supine side bending: which technique best determines curve flexibility? *Spine* 23(7):804-808, 1998.
46. Rochester D, Esau S: Assessment of ventilatory function in patients with neuromuscular disease, *Clin Chest Med* 15(4):751-763, 1994.
47. Sanders J, Evert M, Stanley E, Sanders A: Mechanisms of curve progression following sublaminar spinal instrumentation, *Spine* 17(7):781-789, 1992.
48. Scoliosis Research Society: *Morbidity and mortality committee report,* Rosemont, IL, 1987, AAOS.
49. Shook J, Lubicky J: *Paralytic scoliosis.* In Bridwell KH, DeWald RL, editors: *The textbook of spinal surgery,* ed 2, Philadelphia, 1997, Lippincott-Raven, pp 839-880.
50. Shufflebarger H, Clark C: Prevention of crankshaft phenomenon, *Spine* 16(suppl):409, 1991.
51. Shufflebarger H, Clark C: Effect of wide posterior release on correction in adolescent idiopathic scoliosis, *J Ped Orthop* Part B, 7:117-123.
52. Sussman M, Little D, Alley R, McCoig J: Posterior instrumentation and fusion for the treatment of neuromuscular scoliosis, *J Ped Orthop* 16(3):304-313, 1996.
53. Swank S, Cohen D, Brown J: Spine fusion in cerebral palsy with L-rod segmental spinal instrumentation. A comparison of single and two stage combined approach with Zielke instrumentation, *Spine* 14(7):750-759, 1989.
54. Thompson J, Transfeldt E, Bradford D, Ogilvie J: Decompensation after Cotrel-Dubousset instrumentation for idiopathic scoliosis, *Spine* 15(9):927-931, 1990.
55. Vaughan J, Winter R, Lonstein J: Comparison of the use of supine bending and traction radiographs in the selection of the fusion area in adolescent idiopathic scoliosis, *Spine* 21(11):2469-2473, 1996.
56. Ward W, Wenger D, Roach J: Surgical correction of myelomeningocele scoliosis: a critical appraisal of various spinal instrumentation systems, *J Ped Orthop* 9(3): 262-266, 1989.
57. Winter S: Preoperative assessment of the child with neuromuscular scoliosis, *Orthop Clin North Am,* 25(2): 239-245, 1994.
58. Yazici M, Asher M: Freeze dried allograft for posterior spinal fusion in patients with neuromuscular spinal deformity, *Spine* 22(13):1467-1471, 1997.

# 34

# REVISION SURGERY FOR KYPHOTIC DEFORMITY

**Thomas G. Lowe, M.D.**



The treatment of kyphotic deformities continues to be a challenge for the spine surgeon. Revision surgery for failed kyphosis surgery is even more problematic because of the loss of normal anatomic landmarks. This chapter will provide the reader with guidelines for normal values for sagittal curves and overall sagittal profile including balance. It also will discuss the basic biomechanical principles and instrumentation constructs necessary for restoring sagittal profile and achieving a solid arthrodesis in the surgical treatment of kyphotic deformities. One must keep in mind that no matter how good the instrumentation is, without careful preparation of the fusion bed and without the proper volume and type of bone graft material, a solid arthrodesis may not occur. For adults requiring revision surgery, autogenous bone should always be used posteriorly. For anterior revision surgery, structural allografts or cages filled with morselized allograft has been shown to work very well.[6,14] Hopefully, in the near future recombinant bone morphogenic protein (BMP) will be available and will play a major role in revision spine surgery in which prior iliac crest harvest has left very little autogenous bone available for surgery.

The surgical treatment of kyphotic deformities of the spine entails manipulation of the spine using established biomechanical principles that include: 1) lengthening of the anterior column of the spine, 2) providing for anterior column support, and 3) shortening of the posterior column (with provision for posterior stabilization).

Specific fusion levels and appropriate constructs must be carefully planned preoperatively, in order to help prevent the development of junctional deformities, sagittal imbalance, failure of fixation, and pseudarthrosis.

The surgical goals of reconstructive surgery of the spine are: 1) to provide for a stable arthrodesis with normal coronal and sagittal profile and balance and 2) to protect and/or restore neurological function.[13,17,20] As compared to the multiplanar deformity of scoliosis, the kyphotic deformity is confined to the sagittal plane. The biomechanical approach to kyphosis is thus somewhat less complicated than that of scoliosis; however, scoliosis may also be an associated deformity requiring treatment and may in itself require additional fusion levels beyond those levels dictated by the kyphotic deformity.

A prerequisite to understanding the principles of surgical correction of kyphosis includes knowledge about the normal sagittal profile of the spine. Whereas the coronal plane of the spine is normally straight, the sagittal plane normally has 3 balanced curves as shown in Figure 34-1. The cervical and lumbar cures are normally lordotic while the thoracic curve is kyphotic. The thoracic kyphosis is relatively rigid and inherently stable, largely because of the rib cage. The cervical and

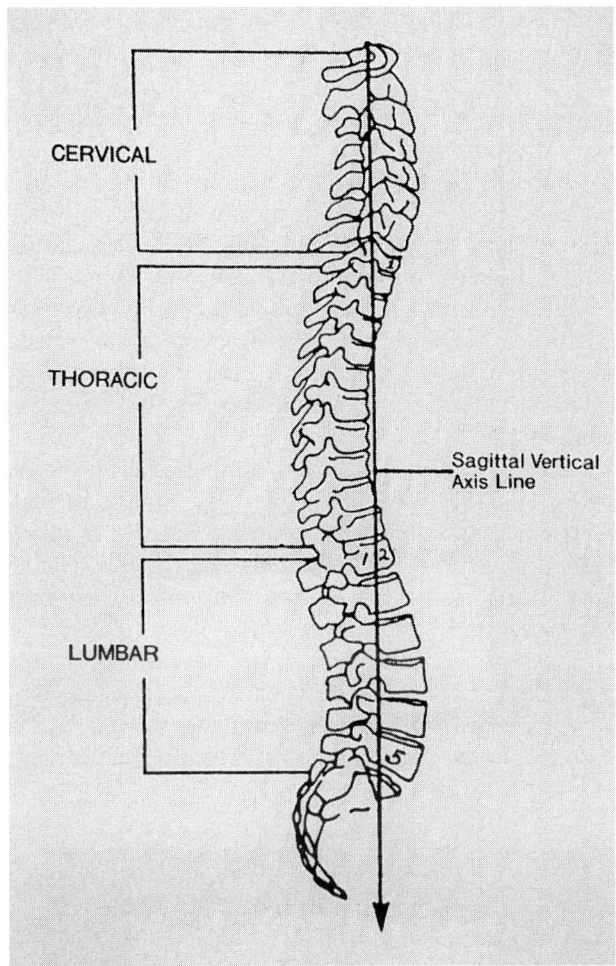


**FIGURE 34-1**

Normal sagittal profile of spine with sagittal vertical axis passing through posterior margin of body of T1 and sacral promontory.

lumbar curves are flexible, compensatory curves that are necessary to maintain balance in the upright position. Because of their flexibility, the cervical and lumbar segments are prone to instability when their structural integrity is compromised by fracture, tumor, infection, or degenerative change.

Normally, the sagittal vertical axis falls from the craniovertebral junction through the vertebral bodies of T1 and T12, and ends by passing through the sacral promontory. This axis lies anterior to the thoracic kyphosis and posterior to the lordotic curves of the cervical and lumbar spines. "Positive" balance implies that the sagittal vertical axis lies anterior to the sacral promontory. Patients with lumbar flat back syndrome are always positively balanced in the sagittal plane. We have noted that frequently patients with kyphosis secondary to Scheuermann's disease are negatively balanced.[12] It is usually best to provide for slight negative balance in revision surgery for kyphotic deformities. This usually entails providing for a lumbar lordotic curve that is approximately 15 to 20 degrees greater than the thoracic kyphosis. In patients with loss of cervical lordosis (as in patients with ankylosing spondylitis) preoperative planning must provide for additional lumbar lordosis or the patient will have difficulty with upward gaze when walking. Sagittal balance can be greatly affected by the status of the hips. It is very important to look for hip flexion contractures during the preoperative planning. When hip flexion contractures are present and not easily correctable, surgery must provide for additional lumbar lordosis at the time of surgery. If hip flexion contractures can be corrected by soft tissue release, the release should be done prior to correction of the spinal deformity.

Looking first at the sagittal curves of the spine, the normal cervical lordosis ranges between 25 and 50 degrees. The apical vertebra of the cervical spine is C4, which is horizontally oriented.[13]

The normal range of thoracic kyphosis is between 20 and 45 degrees.[7,13,19] Thoracic kyphosis is usually a few degrees greater in females.[7,13,16] It increases in both sexes with age, resulting in an upper normal level of about 60 degrees in older females. The apex of the thoracic kyphosis is T7, which is horizontally oriented. T2 is angulated 25 degrees below the horizontal and T12 is angulated 12 degrees above the horizontal. Intermediate levels having decreasing angulation as they approach T7, the apical vertebra.[1,13]

Total lumbar lordosis is normally between 40 and 70 degrees. Lordosis between L1 and L4 is usually approximately 20 degrees. Between L4 and S1 lordosis measures 45 degrees. This is roughly two thirds of the total lordosis. L3 is the apical lumbar segment and is normally angulated 5 degrees above the horizontal. The sacral promontory slope is the angle measured between the superior endplate of S1 and the horizontal. This normally ranges from 25 to 65 degrees.[10] In patients with hip flexion contractures or increased lumbar lordosis, this angulation may be greatly increased. In general, a "balanced" spine should have a lumbar lordosis that is 10 to 15 degrees greater than the thoracic kyphosis and the vertical sagittal axis should lie just posterior to the sacral promontory (measurements ± 1.0 cm are acceptable).[1,10]

The thoracolumbar junction, from T10 to L2 is a transitional zone between the thoracic and lumbar sagittal curves. This transitional area is normally from 0 to 5 degrees of lordosis. Any degree of kyphosis in this segment of the spine is abnormal and may result in sagittal malalignment.[2]

These numbers are good rules of thumb to remember when sagittal malalignment is suspected prior to surgery and when evaluating postoperative results. Mechanical loads on the spine are best tolerated when the sagittal balance and profile are relatively normal. Sagittal malalignment following surgery will result in a higher risk of pseudarthrosis and degenerative disk disease in uninstrumented segments.

In the erect position with normal sagittal balance present, the anterior column of the spine, which includes the vertebral bodies, the intervertebral disks, and the anterior and posterior longitudinal ligaments, is loaded in compression. The posterior column of the spine, which includes the facets, laminae, and associated posterior ligamentous complex, is normally under a tensile load. In the balanced spine, both columns share the load equally.[13,20]

A kyphotic deformity can develop in any area of the spine when either column of the spine is unable to fully load-share and resist either of these forces.[13,17] For example, kyphosis develops in Scheuermann's disease because of a failure of the anterior column secondary to vertebral body wedging and disk narrowing.[11] Kyphosis may also develop because of failure of the posterior column of the spine following multiple level posterior decompression for spinal stenosis.[20] The kyphotic deformity that develops following thoracolumbar burst fractures usually occurs because of a combined failure of both columns.[20]

Kyphotic deformities can be divided into two basic types (see Fig. 34-2, *A*). Type I deformities are long and uniform in shape and are generally flexible on hyperextension. These deformities generally carry very little risk of neural compromise. Examples of Type I kyphosis include postural kyphosis, neuromuscular kyphosis, metabolic kyphosis, and most forms of kyphosis associated with Scheuermann's disease. Type II kyphotic deformities are short and angular in configuration (Fig. 34-2, *B*) with the major deformity involving only five or six segments. These deformities tend to be very rigid with a much greater risk of neurological compromise related to cord compression anteriorly. Examples of this type of kyphosis are seen in neurofibromatosis, congenital spine deformity, post-traumatic kyphosis, metastatic disease, and infections of the spine.

The goals of the surgical treatment of kyphosis include 1) achieving a balanced, stable spine that protects the neural elements and 2) achieving as much "safe" correction as can be obtained for the specific type of deformity and varying medical conditions of the patient with kyphosis.

The goals of treatment in Type I deformities include both correction of the deformity as well as stabilization, whereas the goals of treatment of Type II deformities are primarily that of stabilization and achiev-

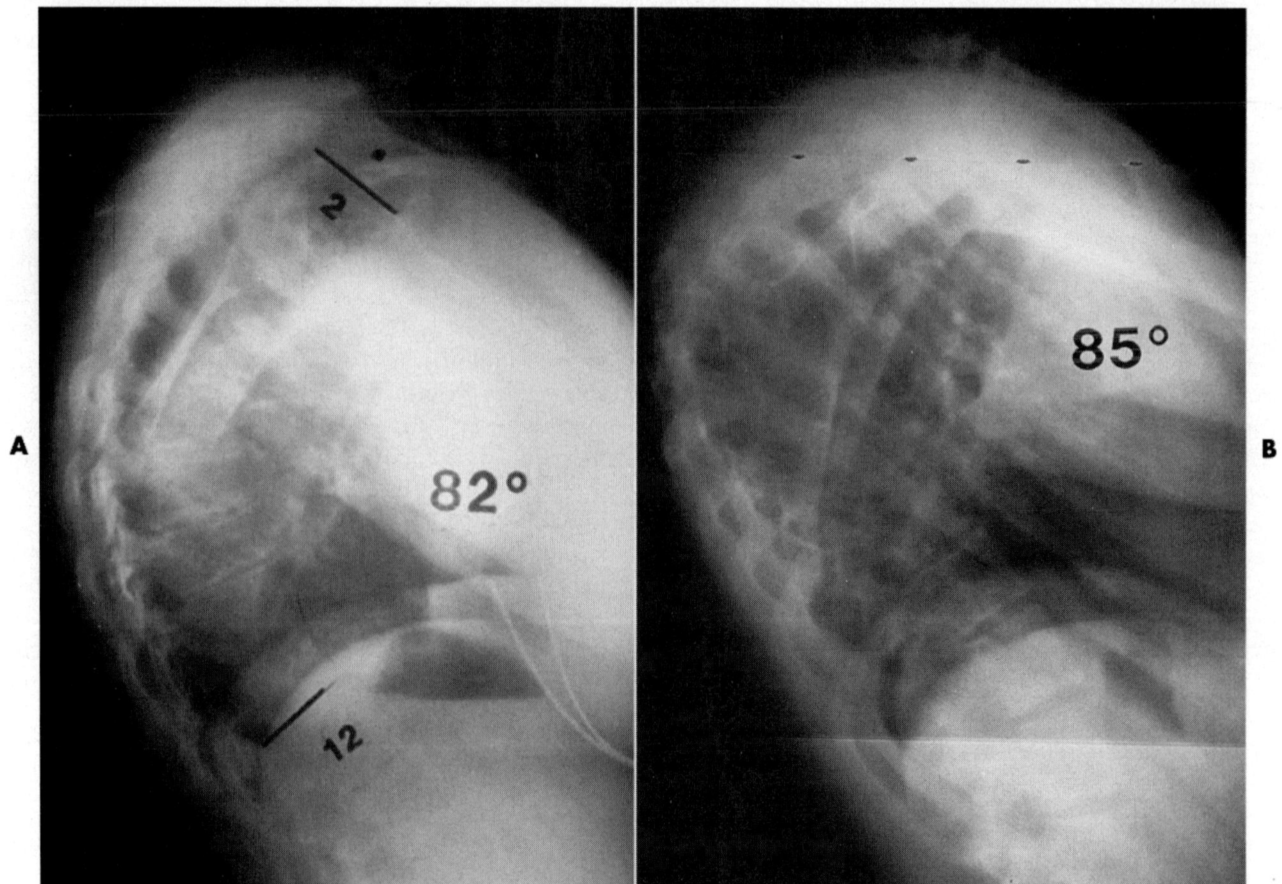


**FIGURE 34-2**

**A,** Type I kyphosis. Note uniform, large radius kyphosis. **B,** Type II kyphosis. Note sharply angular, short radius kyphosis.

ing balance with little attempt at correction because of the high risk of neurological injury unless a formal anterior decompression of the spine is done in the same setting.

The location of the kyphotic deformity is also important in decision making when surgery is being considered. (Fig. 34-3). Kyphotic deformities in the thoracic spine tend to be quite stable because of the secondary support provided by the thoracic cage. Thoracic kyphosis also tends to be less cosmetically objectionable because sagittal balance is usually maintained through increasing lordosis in the lumbar spine. Most kyphotic deformities of the thoracic spine are relatively nonproblematic until they approach 75 degrees or greater.[11, 13]

Thoracolumbar kyphosis, on the other hand, is usually of much greater concern because continuing progression of the deformity is more likely due to the lack of secondary support provided by the thoracic cage. These patients also tend to be in positive sagittal balance with associated back pain because of the inability of the lumbar spine to fully compensate for the deformity. Therefore, these patients tend to become symptomatic and require surgical intervention with less severe deformity than do those with thoracic deformities.

It is also important to remember that in the thoracic spine there is normally a kyphosis of up to 45 degrees, however at the thoracolumbar junction, any kyphosis is considered abnormal. Thus, a 40-degree increase in kyphosis of the thoracic spine would result in a thoracic kyphosis of 85 degrees, whereas a 40-degree increase in kyphosis in the thoracolumbar spine would measure only 40 degrees. It is evident that knowledge of the normal sagittal profile of the spine is extremely important when attempting to determine the significance of a specific kyphotic deformity and what treatment might be required.

## PRINCIPLES OF CORRECTION OF KYPHOTIC DEFORMITIES

As mentioned previously, the surgical goal of treatment of kyphosis is a stable, balanced spine with as much safe correction of the deformity as can be obtained.

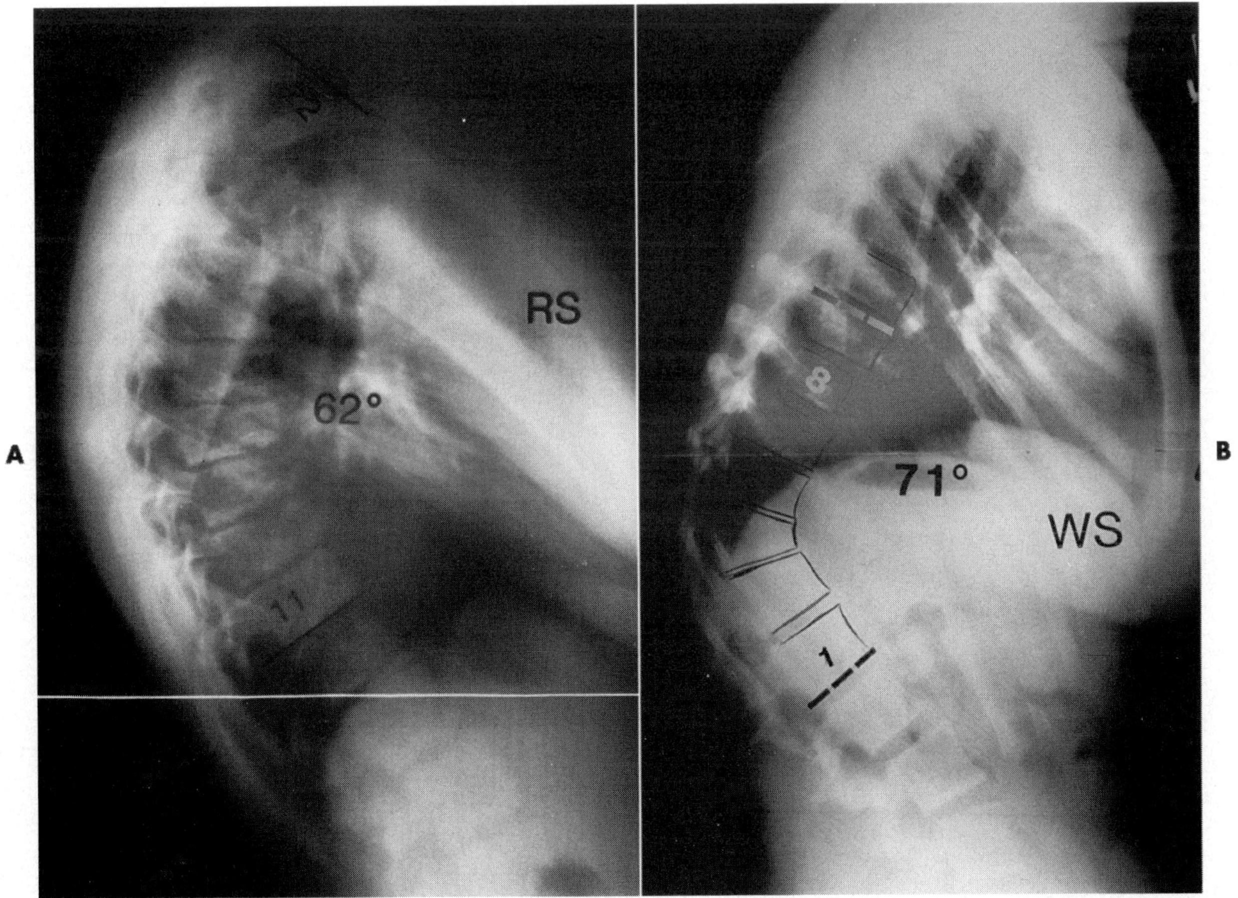


**FIGURE 34-3**

**A,** Thoracic kyphosis secondary to Scheuermann's disease. **B,** Thoracolumbar kyphosis secondary to Scheuermann's disease.

## SURGICAL CORRECTION OF TYPE I KYPHOSIS

These deformities are long and flexible with little risk of the deformity creating neural compromise. In the individual with a thoracic kyphosis greater than 75 degrees, surgery should be considered if symptoms are not manageable with nonoperative measures.[11] As mentioned previously, skeletally mature patients undergoing corrective surgery for kyphosis virtually always require a combined anterior-posterior approach in order to achieve both anterior and posterior column load sharing and a solid arthrodesis.

Surgical correction of Type I kyphosis is achieved by first lengthening the anterior column (anterior release), and providing anterior support, by either interbody fusion or anterior strut grafting. This is followed by shortening the posterior column utilizing compression instrumentation and a posterior fusion with autologous iliac bone graft. These principles are illustrated in Figure 34-4. Unless the anterior column deficiency created by correction of the kyphosis is supported with a fusion, the posterior fusion may fail because of lack of anterior load sharing. Pseudarthrosis rates of 20% to 40% have been reported in patients undergoing posterior fusion with instrumentation alone for kyphotic deformities of the spine especially if large amounts of correction are obtained in flexible curves.[3,4]

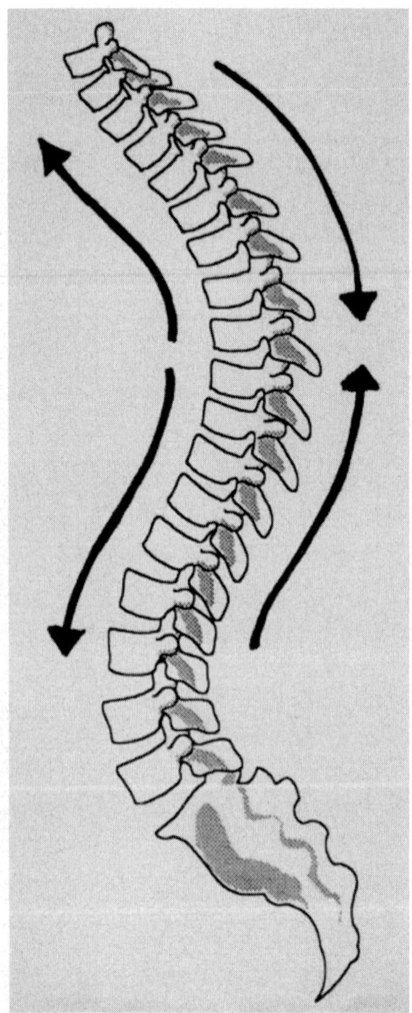

**FIGURE 34-4**

Correction of kyphosis requires lengthening of anterior column and shortening of posterior column.

On the other hand, posterior spinal fusion with instrumentation alone in skeletally immature individuals usually is effective because the anterior column deficiencies left following anterior column lengthening will usually be taken care of by the remaining anterior vertebral growth according to Wolf's law.[21] This is similar to that seen with brace treatment for Scheuermann's disease, which should successfully manage most patients with Scheuermann's disease if bracing is started when skeletally immature and there is good patient compliance. Posterior fusion alone is also utilized in older patients with hyperkyphotic deformities secondary to osteoporosis. Surgical treatment is rarely indicated in this group of patients but when severely symptomatic, a posterior instrumented in situ fusion is usually effective in controlling pain as long as spinal balance is achieved.[13]

In Type I kyphotic deformities, such as Scheuermann's disease, first an anterior release and interbody fusion are performed using tightly packed morselized rib graft. Levels of anterior fusion should include all disk levels that are not mobile on hyperextension. This usually involves the central 6 to 7 levels. When the deformity extends down to or below the thoracolumbar junction, the anterior fusion should extend distally to the level of the anticipated posterior fusion because of the increased risk of pseudarthrosis. Structural grafts or cages augmented with bone graft should be used for anterior column support where large disk spaces are present to maintain correction.[5] Usually segmental vessels in this area can be spared using vessel loops and small malleable retractors for exposure of the disk at each level.[13] Prior to diskectomy, the head of each rib should be removed to facilitate exposure of the posterior one third of the disk space. Small spreaders are available to facilitate the removal of the posterior annulus and if necessary, the posterior longitudinal ligament under direct vision.

Early results of multiple-level anterior release and fusion utilizing a video-assisted thoracoscopic approach are encouraging. It remains to be seen whether the ability to perform a thorough release and arthrodesis is possible with the development of newer thoracoscopic instrumentation.

The posterior portion of the procedure requires careful preoperative planning. In a study of patients with Scheuermann's disease,[12] it was noted that 18 of 22 patients with thoracic kyphosis greater than 75 degrees had a sagittal vertical axis that was shifted greater than 4 cm posterior to the sacral promontory (Fig.34-5).[12] This phenomenon has not been reported in patients with other types of kyphosis but probably is not limited to Scheuermann's disease. Because of the posteriorly displaced sagittal vertical axis noted in Scheuermann's kyphosis, if the kyphosis is very flexible, it is important not to attempt correction beyond 40 degrees or greater than 50% of the initial kyphosis. Attempts at greater correction will shift the sagittal balance further posteriorly, which may result in a compensatory junctional kyphosis either proximally or distally. When prebending the longitudinal rods, always leave at least a 40-degree kyphotic bend prior to insertion to avoid this complication. Figure 34-6 illustrates a proximal junctional kyphosis developing following over correction of a thoracic kyphosis.

It is also important to select the proper levels to be instrumented as shown in Figure 34-7. The upper instrumentation level should always be the upper Cobb vertebra of the measured kyphosis. In the rare situation in which the disk between the two upper vertebral levels of the kyphosis are parallel, it is preferable to instrument to the more proximal vertebra. If the instrumentation is short of the upper level of kyphosis, there is a likelihood that a proximal junctional kyphosis will develop postoperatively. The lower level of instrumentation should include the lower Cobb vertebra and the first lordotic level below it, which is usually the level below the lower Cobb level. If the first lordotic level is not included, a distal junctional kyphosis may develop postoperatively (Fig. 34-8).

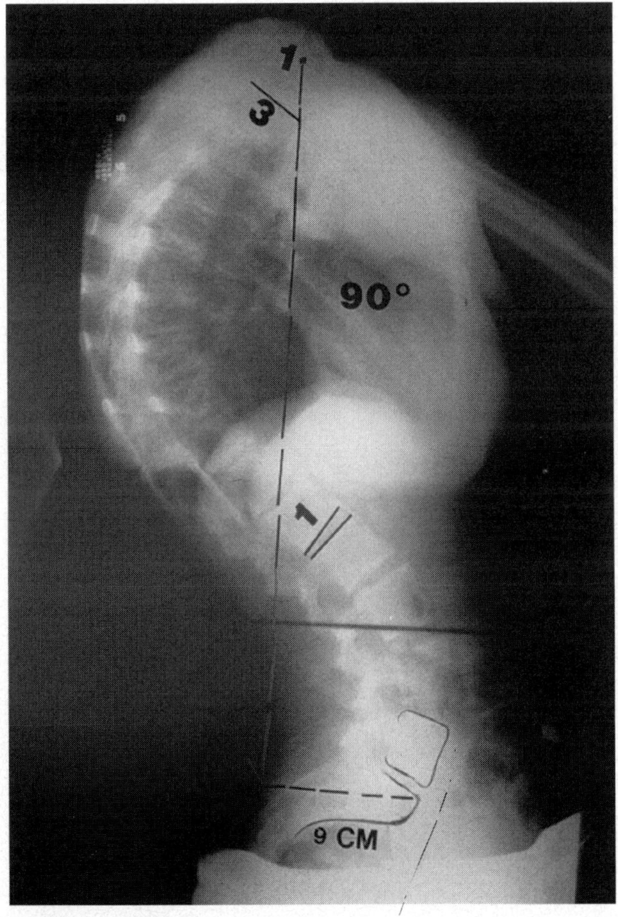


**FIGURE 34-5**

Sixteen-year-old female with kyphosis secondary to Scheuermann's disease. Note shift of vertical sagittal axis posterior to sacral promontory.

The basic posterior construct for Scheuermann's kyphosis or other Type I kyphosis should consist of a minimum of eight anchors above the apex of the deformity and six to eight anchors below as well as one longitudinal member on each side of the spine and a cross-linking device at each end of the construct. If the construct incorporates more than 12 segments, an additional cross-link should be used at the center of the construct. Above the apex, either two double-level pediculotransverse process claws (as shown in Figure 34-9, *A*) or three single-level pediculotransverse process claws (shown in Fig. 34-9, *B*) should be utilized. The former is the author's preference and is the easiest to assemble. In difficult situations with high-degree kyphosis a downgoing thoracic laminar hook under the superior lamina of the upper instrumented vertebra may be substituted for the upper transverse process hook to facilitate insertion.

Next, an upgoing pedicle or laminar hook, depending on the level, is placed one or two levels distal to the apex of the kyphosis. Pedicle hooks cannot be used below T10 because of the changing facet and pedicle anatomy at the thoracolumbar junction. Distally, either a two-level laminar claw with hooks or, alternatively and the author's preference, two pedicle screws with an infralaminar hook below on each side can be utilized as shown in Figure 34-10. Figure 34-11 illustrates the standard Scheuermann's kyphosis construct utilizing hooks only. In Figure 34-12, pedicle screws and infralaminar hooks have been substituted at the lower end of the construct, which provide the best fixation, in the author's opinion.

When there is an associated structural scoliosis present, the hook pattern is modified so that segmental distraction can be applied on the concave side of the scoliosis. In this situation, the convex rod is inserted first using the standard kyphosis hook pattern to maintain compression. Insertion of the convex rod first insures correction of the kyphosis. Insertion of the concave rod can then be used to correct any remaining segmental scoliosis without interfering with correction of the kyphosis. No more than two distraction hooks should be used (one above and one below) for correction of the scoliotic part of the deformity. Figure 34-13 illustrates the use of the modified kyphosis construct for correction of associated scoliosis.

The longitudinal rod has three specific bends as

*Text continued on page 491*

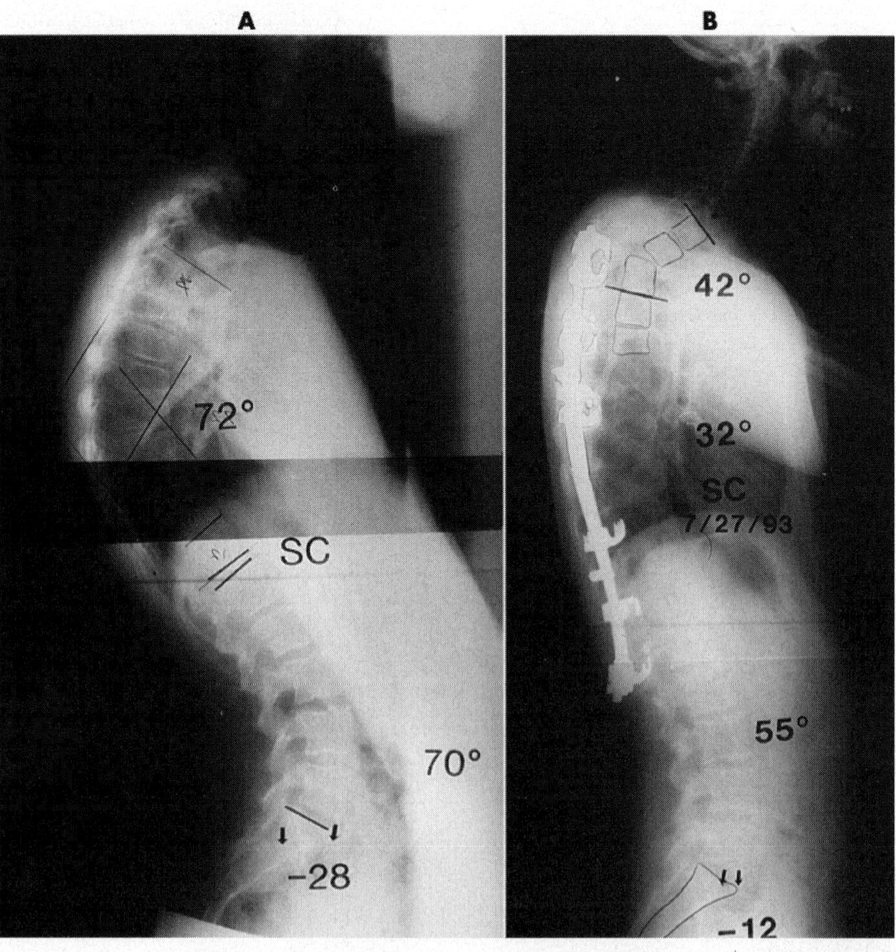


**FIGURE 34-6**

**A,** Preoperative lateral radiograph of a 17-year-old male with Scheuermann's disease.
**B,** Postoperative lateral radiograph of same patient demonstrating a proximal junctional kyphosis developing after greater than 50% correction of the deformity.

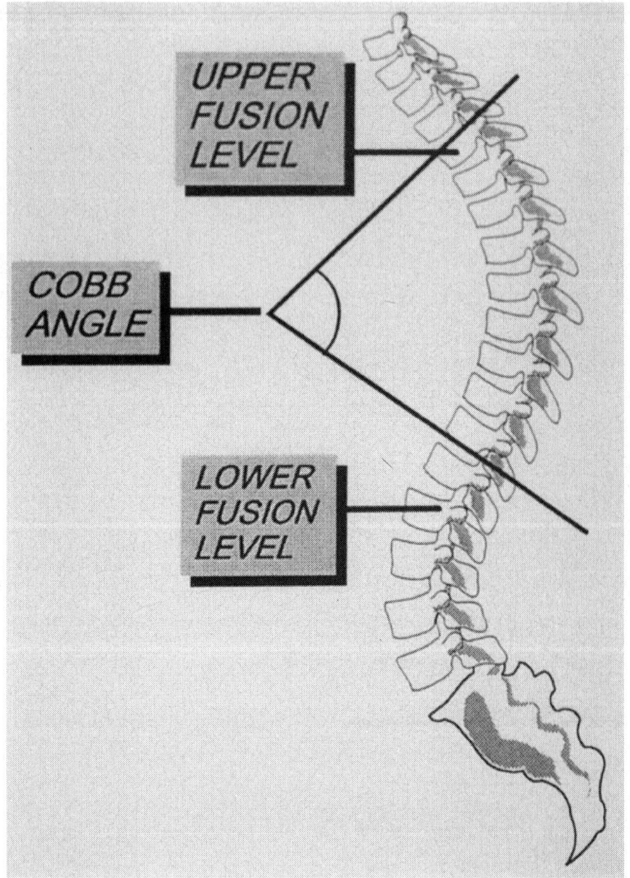


**FIGURE 34-7**

Posterior instrumentation and fusion should extend from upper Cobb level and include first lordotic level.

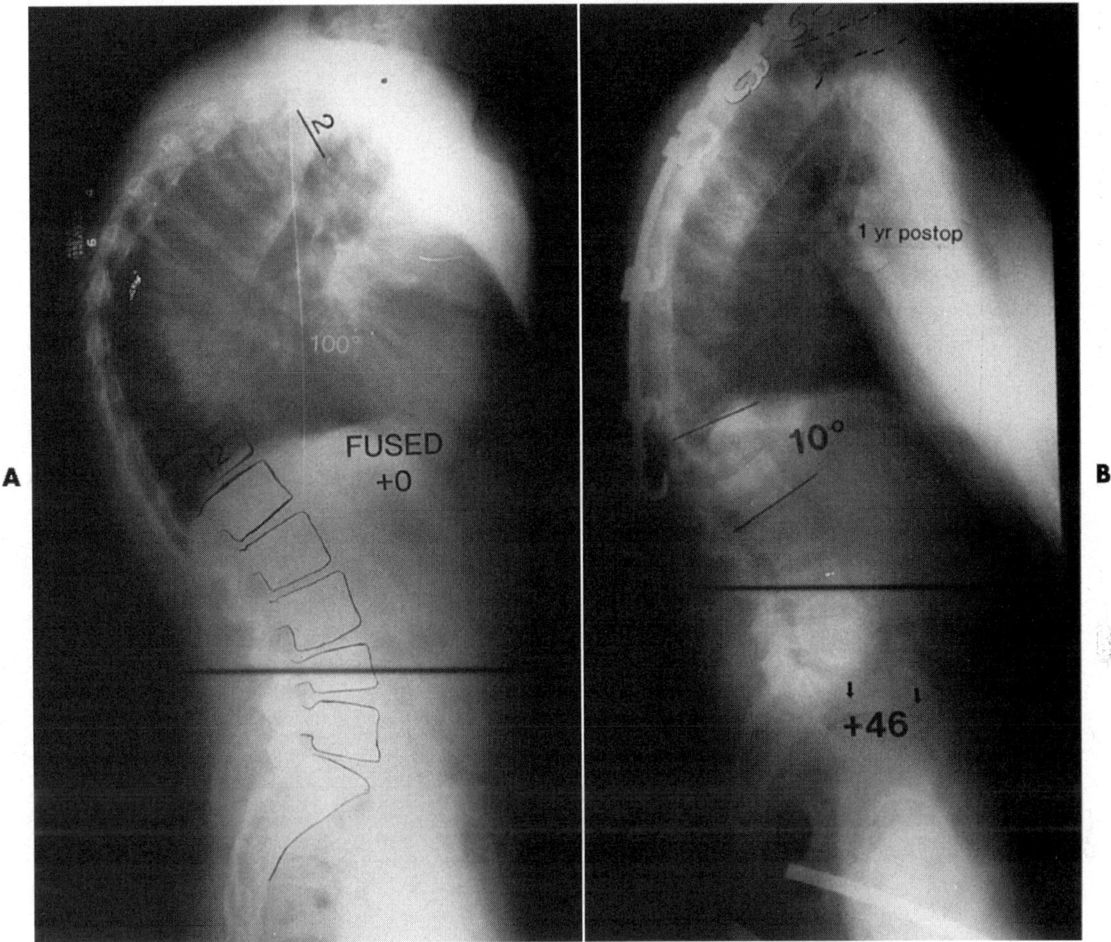


**FIGURE 34-8**

**A,** Preoperative lateral radiograph of an 18-year-old male with a 100-degree kyphosis secondary to Scheuermann's disease from T2 to T12. **B,** Postoperative lateral radiograph of the same patient following instrumentation and fusion only to T12. A junctional kyphosis developed because first lordotic level was not included.

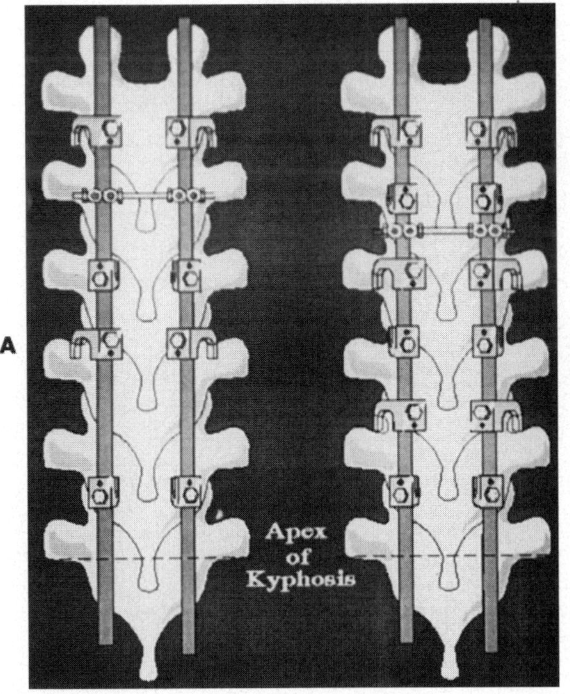


**FIGURE 34-9**

Two types of hook constructs to be used above apex of kyphosis. **A,** Double-level pedicle-transverse process claw. **B,** Single-level pedicle-transverse process claw.

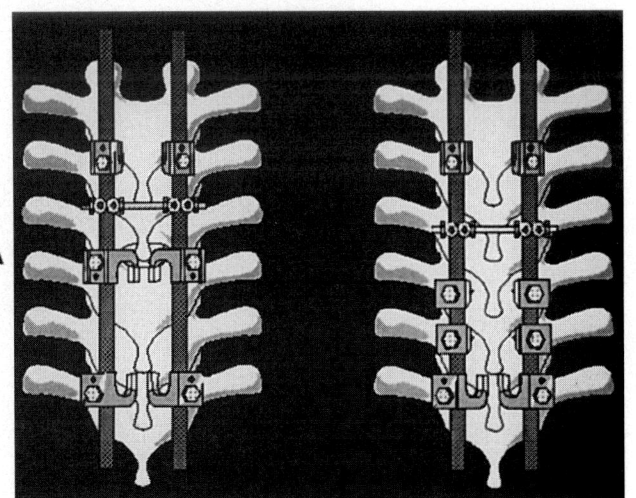


**FIGURE 34-10**

**A,** Hook construct consisting of a pedicle hook just below apex of kyphosis and a two-level laminar claw at distal end of construct. **B,** Hook-screw construct consisting of pedicle hook just below apex and or two-level pedicle screws with infralaminar hook distally.

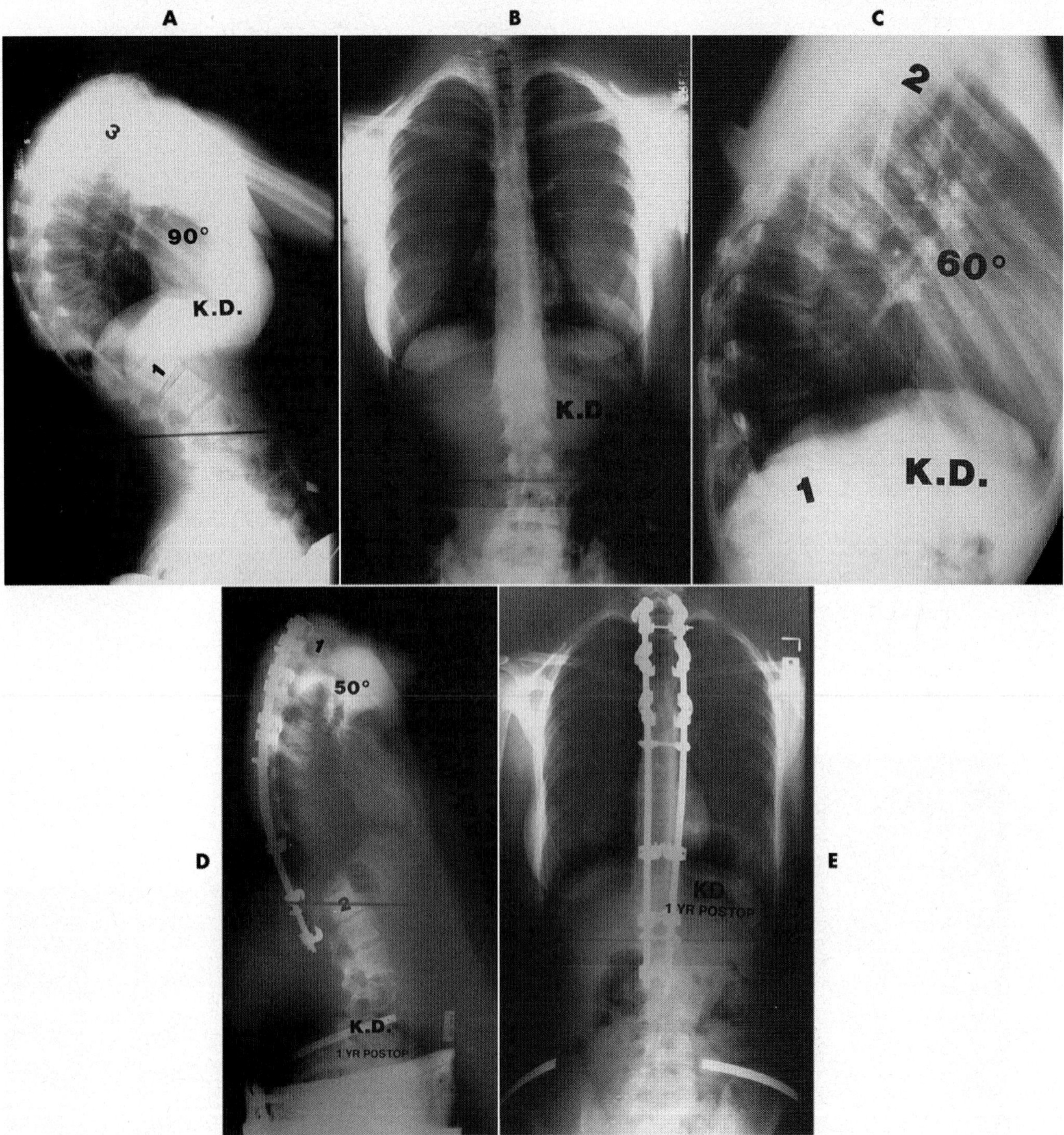


FIGURE 34-11

A 15-year-old girl with a progressive symptomatic 80-degree kyphosis secondary to Scheuermann's disease **(A-C).** Operative reatment consisted of an anterior release and interbody fusion of the wedged vertebrae and thoracolumbar junction followed by an instrumented posterior fusion T2 to L1, which includes all vertetbrae within the Cobb angle and the first lordotic level distally. **D-E,** The standard hook construct described in the text was used with restoration of normal sagittal profile.

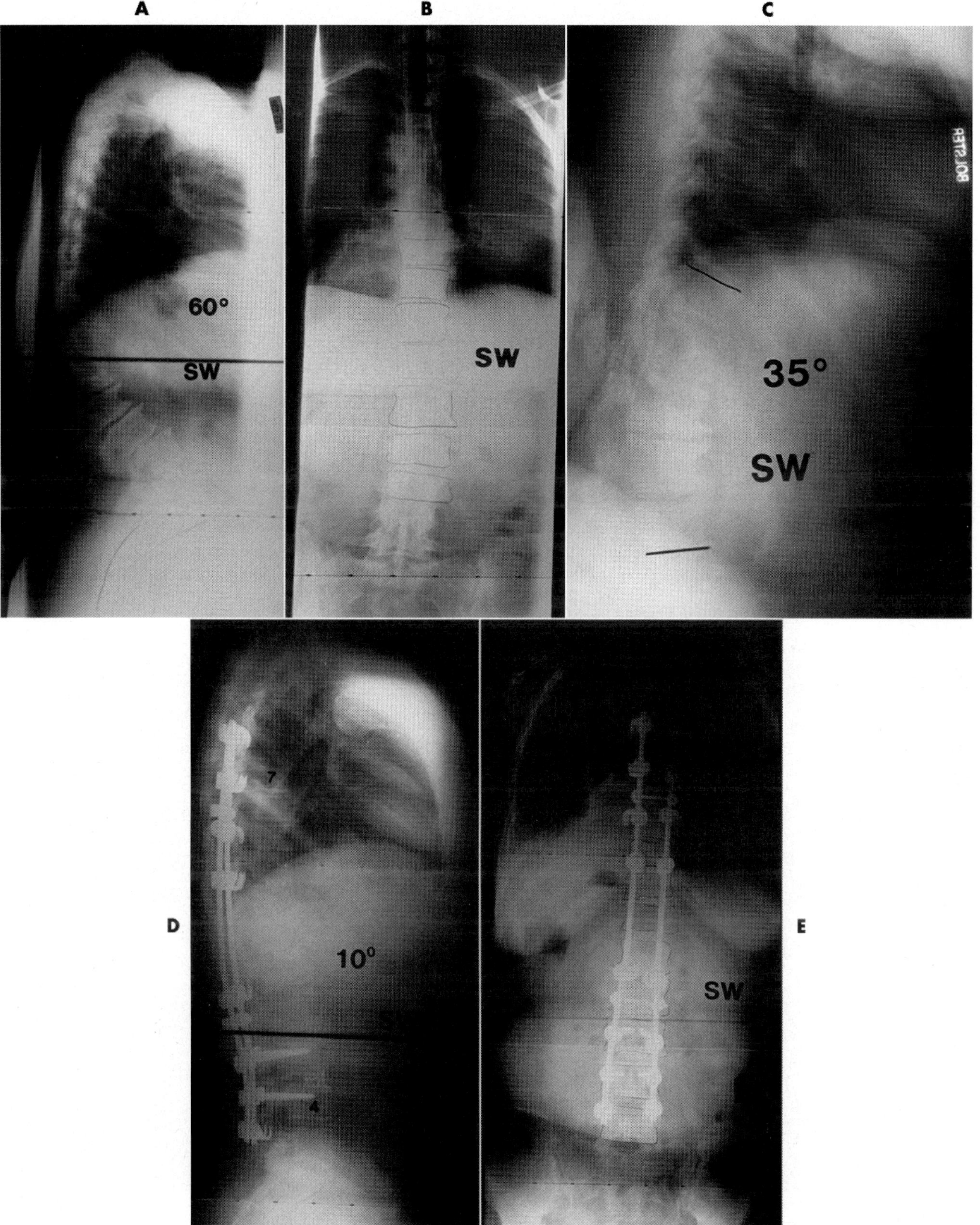


**FIGURE 34-12**

A 38-year old-woman with a progressive painful thoracolumbar kyphosis with associated degenerative disk disease. **A-C,** The patient's symptoms were not controlled with nonoperative measures. **D-E,** A combined anterior-posterior procedure was performed. An anterior release and interbody fusion were carried out from T10 to L4.

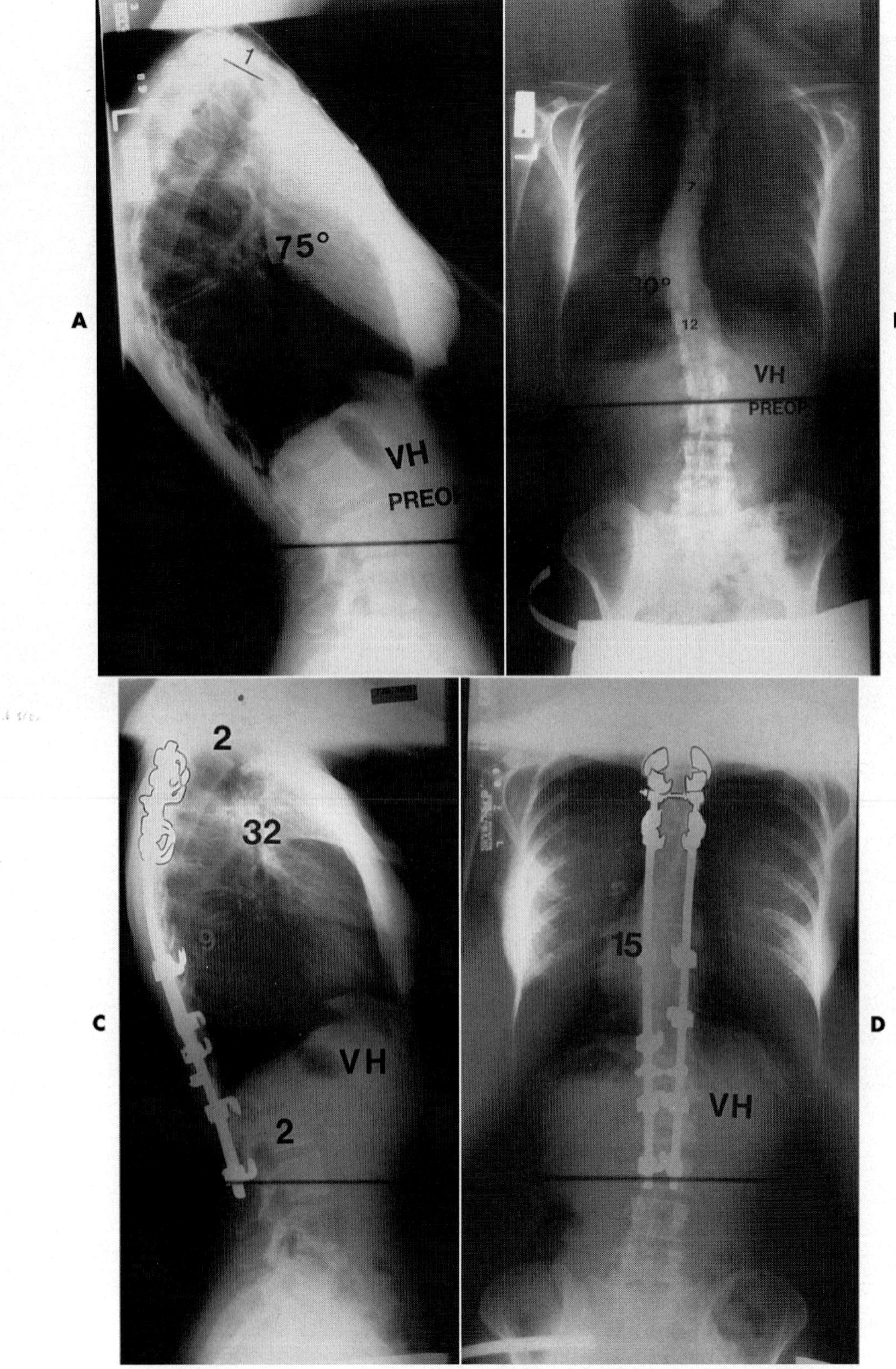


FIGURE 34-13

**A** and **B,** Preoperative radiographs of a 37-year-old woman with kyphosis and associated scoliosis secondary to Scheuermann's disease. **C** and **D,** Postoperative radiographs demonstrating distraction hooks substituted on concavity of scoliosis for additional correction of scoliosis. Note: Rod on convexity of scoliosis is inserted first for correction of kyphosis.

shown in Figure 34-14. A proximal tip bend (10 to 15 degrees) facilitates insertion into the proximal hook. A distal tip (10 to 15 degrees) lordotic bend facilitates insertion into the distal hooks or screws and the central kyphotic bend should match the hyperextension lateral radiograph. The kyphotic bend should never be less than 40 degrees to avoid junctional kyphosis. The sequence of rod insertion into the hooks and reduction of the kyphosis is very specific when systems with closed hooks are used (Fig. 34-15). The rod is first inserted into the lowest set of pediculotransverse hooks above the apex of the deformity and then advanced cephalad by rotating the rod into each hook and sequentially grasping each hook with a hook holder to facilitate rod insertion. The upper tip bend will facilitate insertion of the rod into the most proximal hook, especially if the hook is at T1. Occasionally having an unscrubbed assistant lift the shoulders is also helpful for insertion of the rod into the upper most hook if the upper part of the curve is sharply angulated. After insertion of the rod into the most proximal hook, the hook compressor is used to compress each claw to assure that each hook remains seated. Each hook set screw is then slightly tightened to provide fixation until the rest of the construct is assembled. When systems with open hooks are used, the rod is inserted in the upper hook first and then sequentially inserted into the hooks in a caudal direction toward the apex. After insertion of the hook caps, compression is applied to each claw to seat the hooks against each pedicle and transverse process. Next with the help of the spreader and rod holder, compression toward the apex of the kyphosis is applied at each level starting at the uppermost claw and continuing toward the apex of the deformity. Next, by cantilever bending of the caudal end of the rod, the rod is first delivered into the pedicle hook, which is just below the apex of the kyphosis. Compression is applied to the hook toward the apex and then by continued cantilever bending, the caudal end of the rod is delivered into the distal hooks, which are in the configuration of a two laminar claw. Again, a slight lordotic bend in the distal end of the rod facilitates hook insertion. Compression is then applied to both hooks with the hook compressor prior to final tightening. The two laminar claw helps to initiate lumbar lordosis.

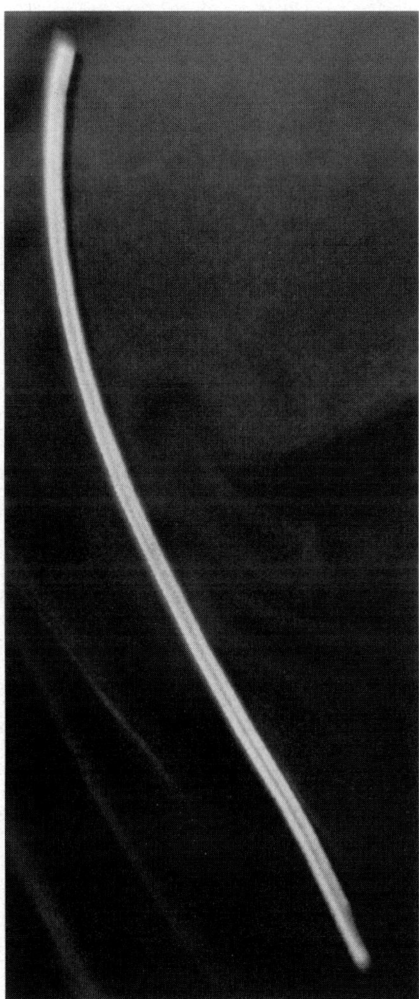

**FIGURE 34-14**

Contouring of longitudinal rod for kyphosis proximal tip bend, kyphosis bend, and lordotic bend distally.

When pedicle screws and infralaminar hooks are used distally, as demonstrated in Figure 34-10, the distal end of the rods are delivered to the spine into the two distal screws. Slight compression is applied to the screws to initiate lordosis. Once the rod has been inserted and secured to the screws, an infralaminar hook is placed on the distal end of the rod and underneath the inferior lamina of the lowest vertebra of the construct bilaterally for screw protection against pull-out. Final hook seating at each level starting at the proximal end and proceeding distally is then done sequentially with the rod holder and spreader always compressing to the apex of the kyphosis. The insertion of two or three transverse connectors completes the construct.

An alternate method for kyphosis correction involves using the same hook or hook and screw configuration but instead of using a single long rod on each side, two shorter overlapping rods are used as shown in Figure 34-16. The upper rod is contoured to the corrected upper half of the kyphotic curve and is inserted into all of the hooks above the apex of the deformity and the hook-rod plugs are inserted and tightened. The lower rod is contoured to fit the lower half of the corrected kyphosis and inserted into the hooks or hooks and screws below the apex. The overlapping ends of the rods are then brought together by cantilever bending and secured to one another with double domino-type connectors on each side. Two or three transverse connectors are applied completing the construct. The author feels that the single-rod technique results in more predictable control of sagittal

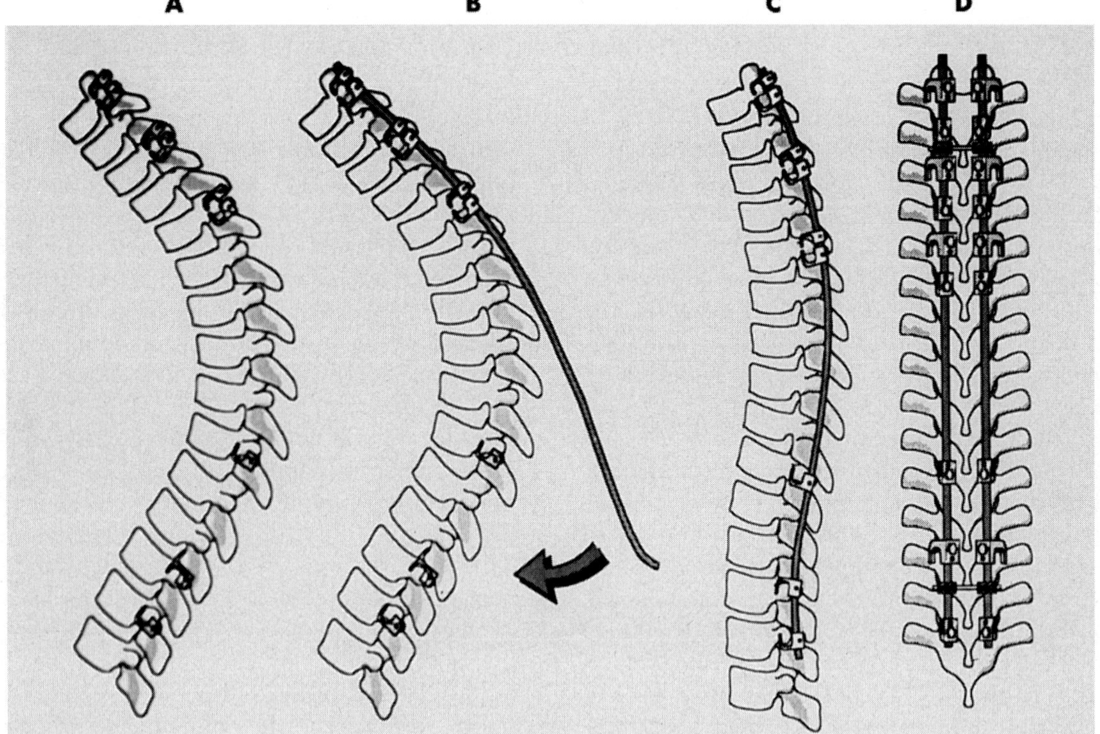


**FIGURE 34-15**

Reduction of kyphosis. **A,** Insertion of hooks or hooks-screws. **B,** Rod is contoured and inserted into hooks above the apex. **C** and **D,** By cantilever bending the rod is delivered into the lower hooks or hooks-screws. Compression is applied toward the apex of the kyphosis before final tightening. Cross-links are added proximally and distally.

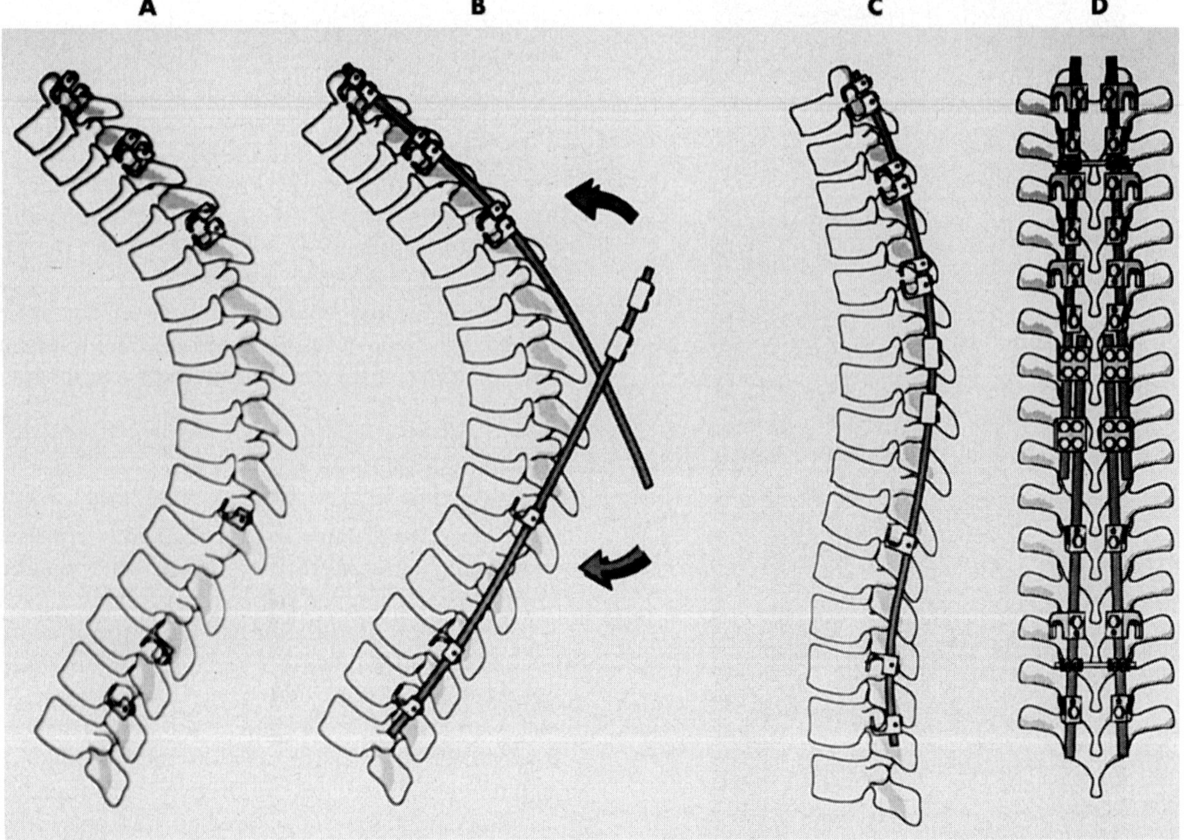


**FIGURE 34-16**

Reduction of kyphosis-alternative method. **A,** Hooks or hooks-screws are inserted in the usual fashion. **B,** Shorter overlapping contoured rods are inserted distally and proximally and are brought together. **C** and **D,** Overlapping rods are then secured to each other with domino type connectors. Transverse connectors are again used proximally and distally.

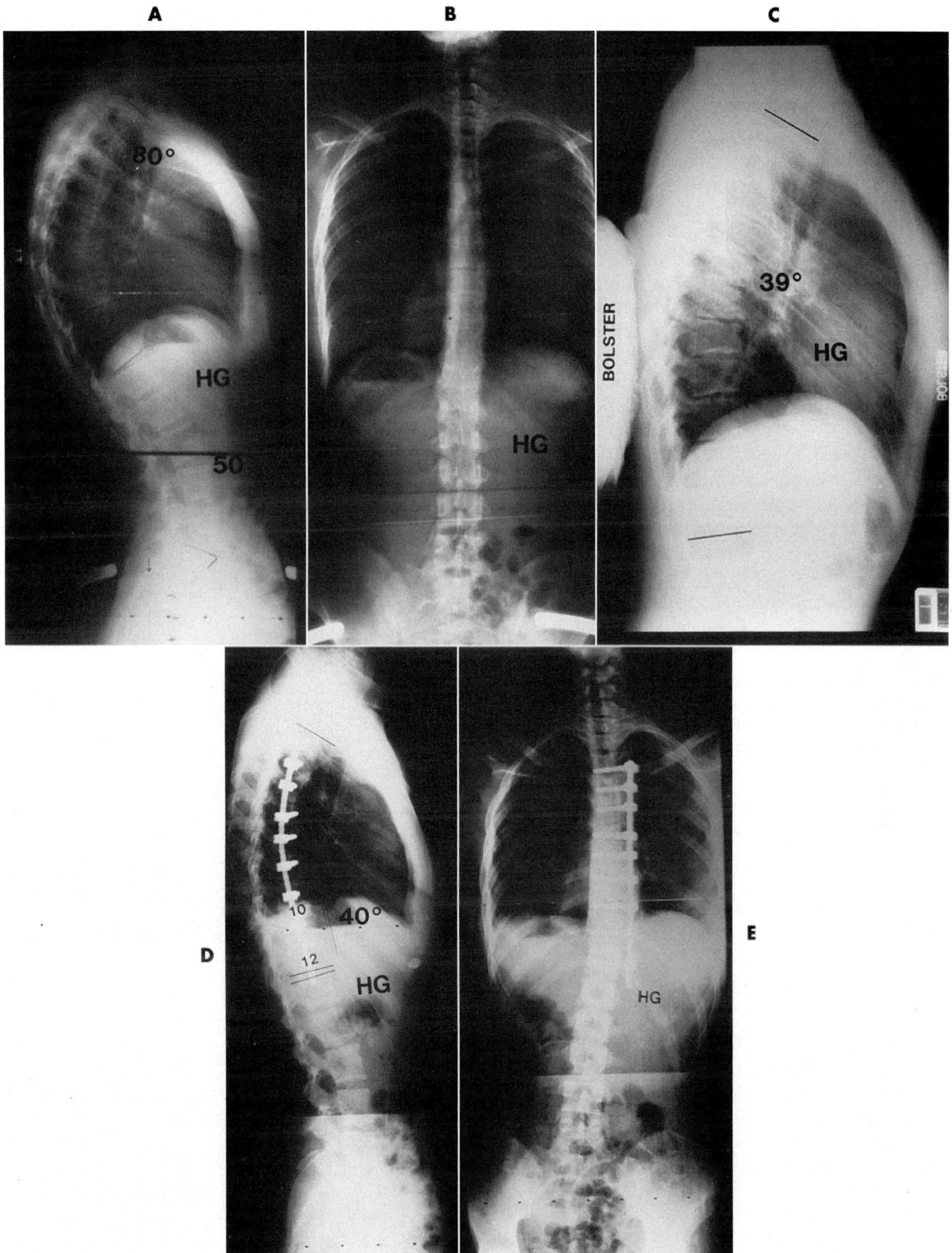


FIGURE 34-17

**A-C,** Preoperative radiographs of a 15-year-old girl with an 80-degree kyphosis secondary to Scheuermann's disease that corrects to 39 degrees on hyperextension. **D** and **E,** Postoperative radiographs demonstrating reduction of kyphosis with anterior structural grafting and single rod and screw instrumentation. Note the preoperative kyphosis extended from T1 to T12 and anterior construct extended from T4 to T12. No posterior procedure was done. Additional experience with this technique is necessary to determine whether fusion levels can be saved by this method.

curves and balance and does not use the double-rod technique. It greatly increases the amount of necessary hardware and the rod connectors, which end up near the apex of the deformity, are often prominent postoperatively. This technique is mentioned only for the sake of completeness because some spine surgeons prefer it over the standard method.

Another method of correction of the Type II deformity presently being utilized by the author involves an anterior-only method of instrumentation and fusion. Although experience with this technique is limited, it is felt that one or two levels proximally and distally can be saved with this technique and it avoids paraspinous muscle dissection. The approach is generally through a left transthoracic approach with a single incision just proximal to the apex of the kyphosis. A double thoracotomy is used with the upper just distal to the proximal level of the upper instrumented segment, and a second at about the apex of the kyphosis. This technique involves first a thorough diskectomy at all levels to be instrumented. Structural grafts or cages with autograft are placed at each level with the help of a disk space distracter. Next, bicortical screws are placed at each level adjacent to the superior endplate above the apex and adjacent to the inferior endplate below the apex. Next a 4-mm rod is contoured into the corrected kyphotic deformity and inserted into each screw and the screw plugs inserted. The structural grafts (femoral ring allografts or titanium mesh with autograft) are then impacted tightly and additional morselized rib graft is packed into each space. Final tightening of the screw plugs completes the procedure. A noninstrumented posterior fusion can be added in patients who are at increased risk for pseudarthrosis. Figure 34-17 demonstrates the use of anterior correction and stabilization of a severe kyphotic deformity of the thoracic spine secondary to Scheuermann's disease.

## TREATMENT OF KYPHOSIS IN THE ELDERLY

Treatment of kyphosis in the elderly patient poses a special problem. As previously mentioned, kyphosis increases with age, especially in females. For the most part, treatment of kyphosis in the elderly patient is nonoperative and includes nonsteroidal anti-inflammatory drugs, exercises, and orthotic management. Occasionally, elderly patients present with painful kyphosis unresponsive to nonoperative measures. When considering surgical intervention in this group of patients, one must be always cognizant of the risk-benefit ratio. These patients do not tolerate extensive surgical procedures frequently utilized for young, healthy patients. Because these patients are often medically compromised, the goals of treatment are usually limited to relief of pain, achieving spinal balance, and preservation of neurological function. Because of the increased risks associated with a thoracotomy in older patients, correction of the deformity is usually not a major priority. In this group of patients a balanced spine can be achieved by creating a posterior construct that places the sagittal vertical axis posterior to the sacral promontory. This usually entails creating additional lumbar lordosis in the construct as well as some modest correction of the thoracic kyphosis. Constructs in the older patient should include lamina-lamina two-level claws for greater strength as shown in Figure 34-18 and longer constructs with a minimum of ten anchors (hooks) above the apex of the kyphosis and eight anchors below the apex, which should include two pedicle screws and an infralaminar hook distally. It is also best to stagger the levels for hooks between the two sides to minimize the risk of laminar fractures. Postoperative bracing should also usually be considered until early bone incorporation is visible on postoperative radiographs. Figure 34-19 illustrates the longer construct used in older patients with kyphosis. When the apex of the kyphotic defor-

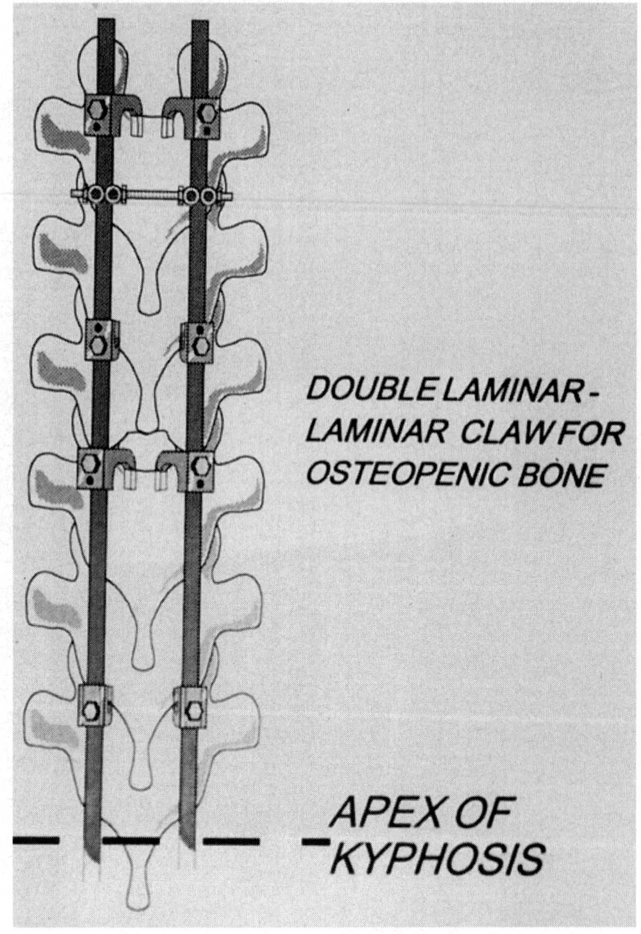


**FIGURE 34-18**

Hook construct above apex of kyphosis recommended for osteopenic bone. Hooks are placed under the lamina where the bone is of better quality. It also may be helpful to stagger levels of hook insertion.

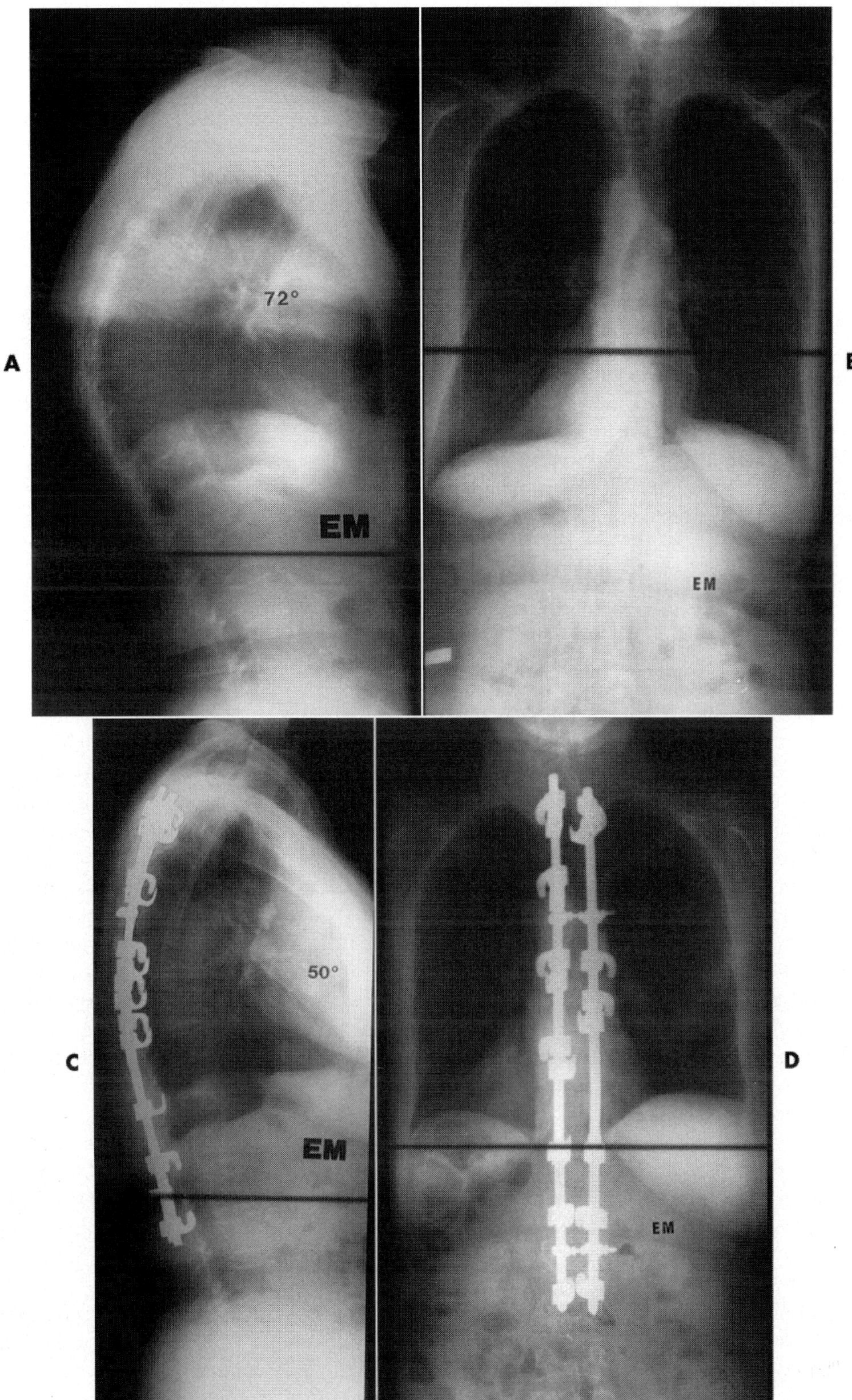


FIGURE 34-19

**A, B,** Preoperative radiographs of a 74-year-old woman with postmenopausal kyphosis. Patient is severely limited because of thoracic back pain that did not respond to nonoperative treatment. **C, D,** Postoperative radiographs following a posterior-only fusion with instrumentation. Notice the use of additional hooks in the construct and staggering hook levels to avoid laminar fractures and hook pullout. Goal of surgery is to control pain and improve sagittal profile and balance.

mity is at the thoracolumbar junction, there is a greater need for structural grafts or cages because of the large disk spaces that result in large anterior column defects with correction of the deformity. In this situation, anterior column support should be provided when the patients' medical condition is satisfactory through a retroperitoneal approach below the diaphragm.

## SURGICAL TREATMENT OF RIGID KYPHOTIC DEFORMITIES

In patients with Type II kyphoses, which are short, angular, rigid curves as seen in neurofibromatosis and congenital spine deformity, the major goals are similar to those in elderly patients, namely to 1) balance the spine, 2) provide modest "safe" correction, 3) achieve a solid arthrodesis, and 4) protect the neural elements. These patients should always have a preoperative MRI or CT myelogram to evaluate any stenotic areas in the neural canal and, if present, a formal decompression of the cord may be required at the time of treatment for the kyphosis. Surgical treatment in this group of patients is best achieved by first performing an instrumented posterior fusion utilizing one of the standard kyphosis constructs with correction. The amount of correction is dependent on the severity of the kyphosis, the correctability on the hyperextension lateral radiograph, and the status of the neural canal based on the MRI or CT myelogram. Certainly, no more correction than is obtained on the hyperextension lateral should be attempted at the time of surgery. Following posterior instrumentation and fusion, anterior stabilization is provided by a combination of anterior interbody fusion and strut grafting. Interbody fusion is performed centrally close to the apex of the deformity and strut grafting is generally utilized peripherally. When rigid posterior instrumentation is in place, a vascularized rib pedicle graft is an excellent strut that is rapidly incorporated (12 to 36 weeks) and hypertrophies with load sharing with little risk of fracture.[2,14] Nonvascularized autogenous ilium, fibula, femur, and rib can also be used for strut grafting. Allograft strut grafts never are completely incorporated and as such never remodel but large allograft struts such as femoral rings may provide significant load sharing.[5,14] It should be remembered that when there is an associated scoliosis, the anterior approach should be on the side of the concavity of the curve if a strut graft is to be used. If an anterior cord decompression is needed, the approach must be on the side of the convexity of the scoliosis in order to obtain exposure of the apical segment of the kyphosis. The patient in Figure 34-20 had a rigid, short radius kyphosis secondary to neurofibromatosis. A preoperative MRI showed a patent neural canal. A posterior fusion with instrumentation was performed first followed by a vascularized rib strut graft and interbody fusion. Partial correction of the deformity and excellent balance were achieved postoperatively and maintained at last follow up.

Another method of dealing with rigid kyphotic deformities, which carry a higher risk of neurological complications, entails shortening of the spine by transpedicular vertebrectomy or decancellation of the apical one or two vertebrae.[2,9] Once the vertebral body has been decancellated by the transpedicular route, the posterior elements of the same vertebrae are removed. Following this shortening procedure of both columns of the spine, the kyphotic deformity can be aligned and stabilized using one of the standard kyphosis constructs. This procedure has been popularized by Bradford and may be an option in selected preadolescent patients with severe kyphosis not treatable by other conventional methods.[2] This is a very technically demanding procedure and should not be attempted without appropriate training.

## REVISION SURGERY FOR HYPERKYPHOSIS

Revision reconstructive surgery for a failed kyphosis procedure is always a difficult undertaking. The basic principles and constructs for primary hyperkyphosis surgery apply to revision surgery for kyphotic deformities. Revision surgery for sagittal plane deformities is indicated because of one or more complications resulting from the initial surgical treatment. These complications include 1) pseudarthrosis, 2) a fusion that is too short, 3) loss of lumbar lordosis, 4) persistent kyphosis, and 5) disk degeneration below a previous spine fusion for kyphosis creating either back pain or spinal stenosis.

Goals of salvage reconstructive surgery following failed surgery for kyphosis include: 1) a solid fusion, 2) coronal and sagittal balance, 3) rigid internal fixation, and 4) the need for little if any external support postoperatively.

Considerations for preoperative planning should include: 1) the presence or absence of osteopenia, 2) the location of the kyphotic deformity, 3) whether there is an associated scoliosis, 4) whether the deformity is fixed or flexible, and 5) whether the deformity is balanced or unbalanced in either the coronal or sagittal planes or both.

## REVISION SURGERY FOR PSEUDARTHROSIS

Indications for reconstructive surgery following pseudarthrosis include pain unresponsive to nonoperative treatment or an increasing kyphotic deformity.

Pseudarthrosis following surgery for kyphosis has

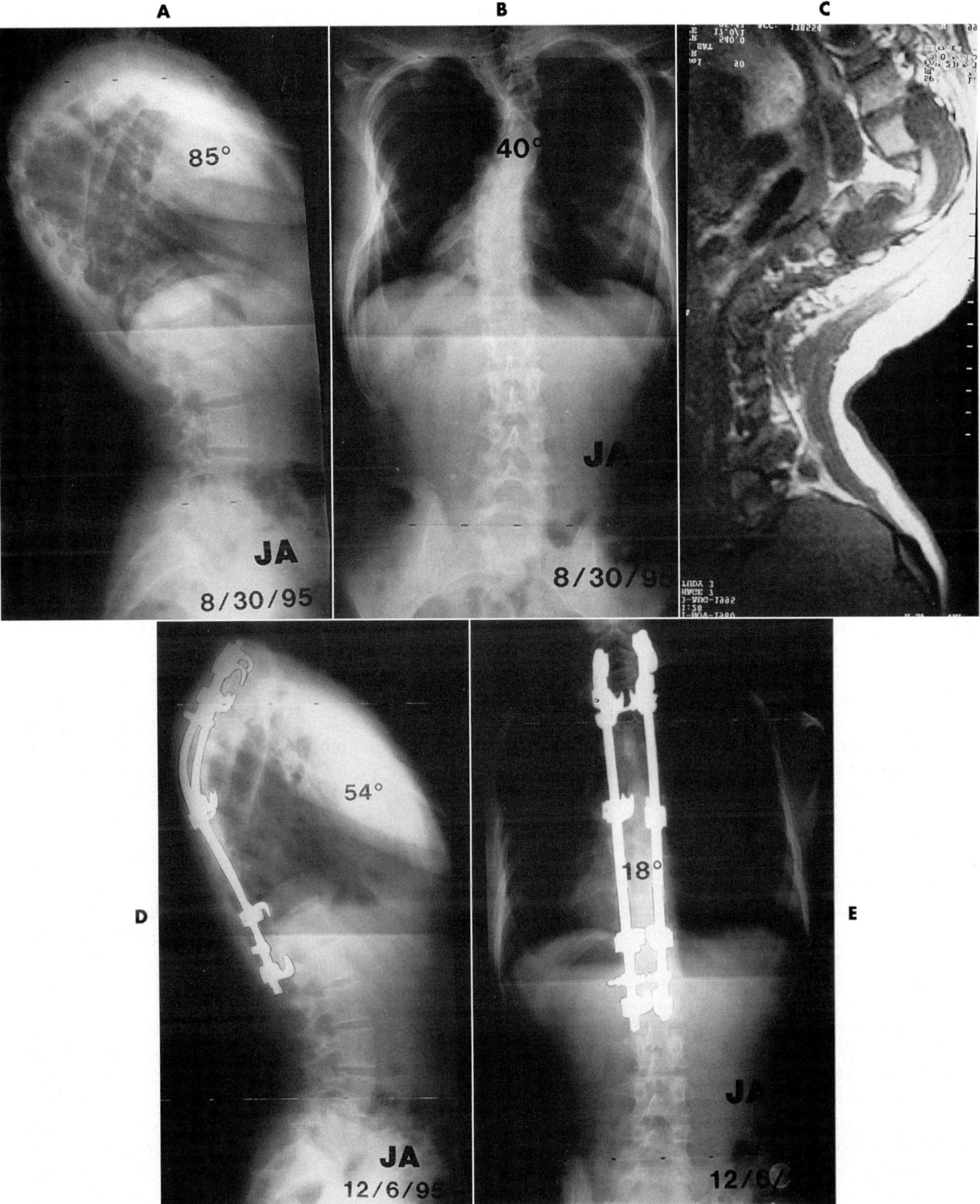


**FIGURE 34-20**

**A-C,** Preoperative radiographs and MRI of a 15-year-old girl with kyphoscoliosis secondary to neurofibromatosis. Radiographs demonstrate a rigid short radius kyphoscoliosis of the thoracic spine. The MRI shows that there are no stenotic areas in the spine. Surgical treatment consists of a posterior instrumented fusion from T1-T12 with only a modest attempt at correction of the deformity because of risk of neurological complications. This is followed by an anterior diskectomy and interbody fusion with rib graft and a vascularized rib strut graft. A solid arthrodesis occurs. **D** and **E,** Postoperative radiographs demonstrate adequate sagittal and coronal balance.

been noted to occur in 5% to 27% in several large series.[14] Pseudarthrosis following primary surgery for spinal deformity is usually associated with several common denominators. The most common cause is insufficient internal fixation. Anything less than eight anchors above and below the apex is probably inadequate fixation for most kyphotic deformities. Another cause of failure of fusion related to instrumentation is the use of distraction within the construct. Distraction creates a fusion under tension, which results in a high failure rate. Posterior constructs for kyphosis should always be in compression.

The use of allograft bone for posterior fusion is also associated with a high pseudarthrosis rate in adults.[14] Allograft appears to work well in pediatric patients, however.[6] Its use in adults should be limited to augment autogenous bone graft posteriorly or as a source of bone graft for anterior interbody fusion.

Finally, the true incidence of pseudarthrosis with an isolated posterior instrumented fusion is known to be high, except in skeletally immature patients, approaching 20% to 30% in some series.[3,14,15] The incidence of pseudarthrosis in combined anterior-posterior procedures utilizing Harrington compression instrumentation dropped to 5% in a series by Bradford et al.[4] There have been no published results with long-term follow-up utilizing the large diameter double rod-hook systems as of this writing. In a personal series of 35 patients with a 3- to 5-year follow-up, we have not had any known pseudarthroses so far using a combined anterior-posterior procedure with Cotrel-Dubousset instrumentation, although realizing that pseudarthrosis utilizing these more rigid fixation systems may not show up for 5 years or more. Stress shielding continues to be a concern for many spine surgeons with the large 7.0-mm rods; this has led to the use of 5.0- to 5.5-mm rods over the past few years.

When revision surgery is necessary because of a pseudarthrosis, it is usually because a posterior instrumented fusion alone was done primarily. Because there is no anterior column load sharing, the fusion is under tension, which results in a high failure rate. Frequently in this situation the instrumentation fails with subsequent loss of correction. These patients often will not have significant pain even though a pseudarthrosis has been present until the instrumentation fails. Another manifestation of pseudarthrosis that is more difficult to recognize is the presence of persistent pain without implant failure or loss of correction. This is often the result of a single-level pseudarthrosis that usually can not be seen on plain or flexion-extension radiographs. Occasionally, a radiolucent line or ring can be seen along a portion of the implant, which indicates motion. Diagnosis usually requires tomography, CT, or single photon emission computed tomography (SPECT).

If an asymptomatic pseudarthrosis without loss of correction is found, treatment is not usually necessary. When a single-level painful pseudarthrosis is identified in the thoracic spine without loss of correction or motion on flexion-extension radiographs, the usual treatment is merely repairing the pseudarthrosis posteriorly with fresh autologous bone graft. All fibrous and devitalized tissue (including bone) must be removed down to healthy bleeding bone prior to bone grafting. If instrumentation is present and providing stability, it can be left in place or replaced with a shorter compression construct with a minimum of six anchors above and six below the pseudarthrosis. The best anchors are usually hooks placed in the previous fusion mass. The area where the hooks are placed should not be decorticated because of the risk of weakening hook purchase sites. Anterior interbody fusion is another option if the posterior soft tissue and/or fusion bed is compromised. This should probably include a spacer such as a cage or femoral ring allograft combined with a plate or rod and screws to provide stable fixation.

When pseudarthrosis has resulted in loss of correction and implant failure, a combined anterior-posterior procedure is necessary (Fig. 34-21).[13,14,15] If the deformity corrects well on a bolster hyperextension radiograph, this author would do the posterior procedure first. The broken instrumentation is removed and the entire fusion area is explored. All pseudarthroses are curetted to bleeding bone and repaired with fresh autogenous bone. New posterior instrumentation is then inserted with eight anchors above and below the apex of the kyphosis. Hooks in the fusion mass are used unless previous pedicle screw holes can be utilized. Two claws above and below the apex on each side into the fusion mass are created and rods are inserted. Compression is then applied toward the area of pseudarthrosis. Transverse connectors are added at each end of the construct for extra fixation.

Following the posterior procedure, an anterior interbody fusion is performed at all levels of pseudarthrosis. Structural grafts (femoral allograft rings) or cages filled with morselized graft are used for anterior column support. In general, structural anterior support should be used below T9, and packed, morselized graft at T9 and above.

If the deformity is fixed on the bolster hyperextension radiograph, then the anterior procedure should be performed first to provide correctability of the deformity, otherwise, the procedure is done in an identical manner. If considerable additional correction is anticipated during the posterior procedure, then packed morselized graft should be used anteriorly rather than structural grafts which may dislodge during the posterior procedure.

## JUNCTIONAL KYPHOSIS

The major postoperative complication seen following corrective surgery for Scheuermann's disease as

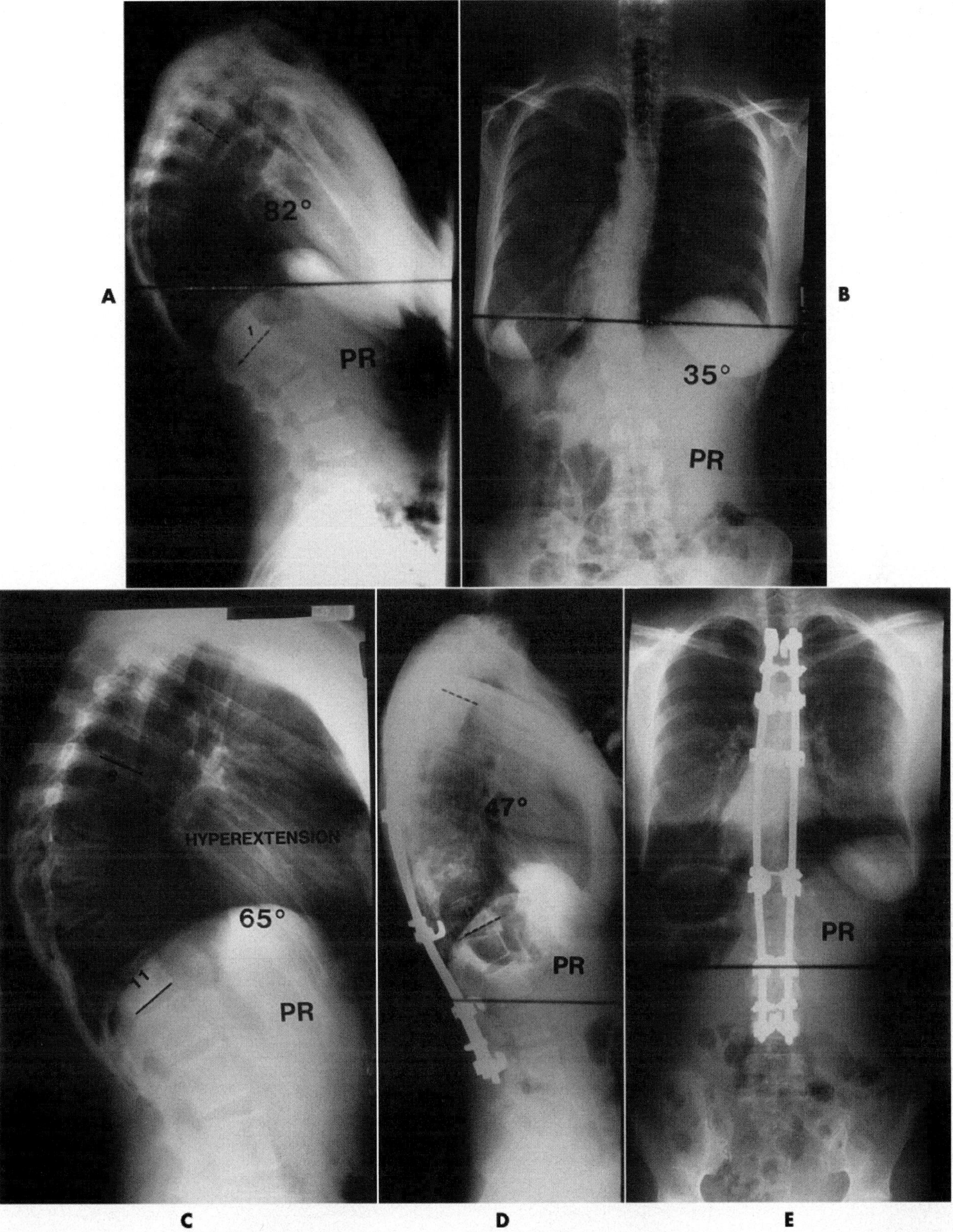


FIGURE 34-21

A 34-year-old woman who underwent a noninstrumented posterior fusion for a thoracolumbar burst fracture. She developed a painful pseudarthrosis with a progressive kyphotic deformity. **A-C,** Preoperative radiographs prior to pseudarthrosis repair. Pseudarthrosis is easily seen on the preoperative PA radiograph. Because the projected goals of treatment were to correct the deformity as well as repair the pseudarthrosis, an anterior release and interbody fusion of the apical segments were performed, first utilizing morselized rib graft followed by repair of two pseudarthroses with iliac bone graft and extension of the fusion proximally and distally the full length of the deformity utilizing a hook-screw compression construct with eight anchors above and eight anchors below the apex. Excellent correction of the deformity was achieved through the pseudarthrosis as well as relief of back pain. **D** and **E,** Postoperative radiographs of same patient following combined anterior and posterior surgery.

well as most other kyphotic disorders has been the development of junctional kyphosis.[12] Proximal junctional kyphosis, which was noted with alarming frequency following Luque instrumentation, was felt to be related to the loss of ligamentous structures proximal to the instrumentation necessary for passage of sublaminar wires. We have also recently noted proximal junctional kyphosis developing in patients with multisegmented posterior instrumentation when (1) the fusion did not include the proximal vertebra in the measured kyphosis (i.e., extending the fusion only to T3 when the measured kyphosis included T2 [see Fig. 34-6, *A* and *B*]) and (2) in patients in whom excessive correction of the kyphosis is achieved (greater than 50%) as shown in Figure 34-7. In those patients with the thoracolumbar pattern of kyphosis the upper end of the fusion should extend proximal to the end vertebra to include the first lordotic disk. If the proximal junctional kyphosis is mild, it probably will not cause any long-term difficulties. If the kyphosis above the fusion is symptomatic or cosmetically unacceptable, consideration should be given to extending the fusion proximally using axial or domino connectors because of the risk of degenerative spondylolisthesis resulting from shear forces on non horizontally oriented disks, which could result in spinal stenosis.

It is now apparent that many patients with kyphosis tend to be in negative sagittal balance, (i.e., their vertical plumb line from C7 lies more than two centimeters behind the sacral promontory). Following correction of the deformity, there is a corresponding decrease in lumbar lordosis so that sagittal balance is usually unchanged. In a few patients in whom excessive correction is obtained, a significant proximal junctional kyphosis has developed. This may represent a compensatory response to maintain sagittal balance when decreasing lumbar lordosis alone is unsuccessful. Attempts at greater than 50% correction of the deformity should be avoided to circumvent this potential problem.

Distal junctional kyphosis also has been noted when the fusion is not carried far enough distally (Fig. 34-22). The fusion must not only include all of the

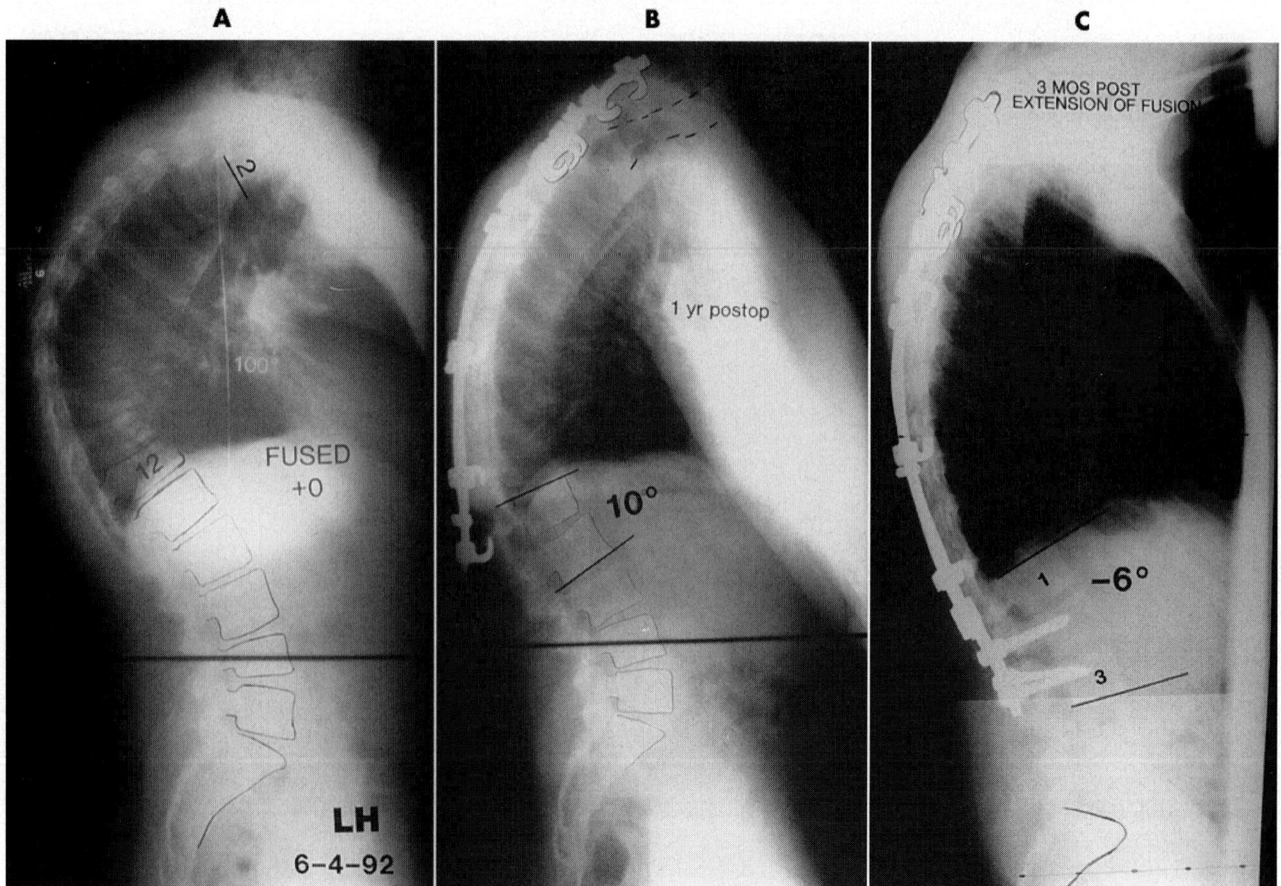


**FIGURE 34-22**

**A,** A preoperative lateral radiograph of an 18-year-old male with a kyphosis of the thoracic spine of 100 degrees secondary to Scheuermann's disease. Note Cobb vertebrae T2-T12. **B,** Postoperative lateral radiograph of same patient whose instrumentation and fusion did not include the first lordotic level, which was L2. A junctional kyphosis resulted postoperatively. **C,** Postoperative lateral radiograph of same patient following revision surgery with extension of the fusion to L3 using domino connectors and pedicle screws. Excellent restoration of sagittal balance occurred.

vertebra in the measured kyphosis but must also include the first lordotic disk distally. If these guidelines are followed distal junctional kyphosis can usually be avoided.[12] If distal junctional kyphosis develops and is mild, it probably can be left alone. If significant obliquity of the adjacent uninstrumented levels is present, which may lead to degenerative disk disease, it should be corrected by extending the fusion distally to include the first lordotic segment. In patients who have double rods this is easily done by removal of the distal hook or pedicle screw and extending the instrumentation further distally with bilateral domino or axial connectors. If large disks are present, then an anterior interbody fusion should be added using structural grafts or cages for anterior column support.

## LOSS OF LUMBAR LORDOSIS

Loss of lumbar lordosis following spine surgery for correction of kyphosis may develop from the use of distraction instrumentation into the lumbar spine or from disk degeneration from vertebral insufficiency fracture[5] in older patients below the instrumentation.

If the deformity is related to the use of distraction instrumentation (Fig. 34-23), then anterior-posterior osteotomies are necessary utilizing structural grafts or cages anteriorly and segmental compression instrumentation posteriorly.[18] A minimum of six anchors above and below the osteotomy are necessary for adequate fixation. If there is an associated rotational deformity in the lumbar spine be careful when performing a single-plane osteotomy, which may lead to coronal imbalance postoperatively. Make sure that a postoperative x-ray in the operating room is obtained prior to closure to ensure proper coronal alignment.

If the loss of lordosis is related to disk degeneration, then the fusion must be extended distally. First an anterior interbody fusion utilizing structural grafts or cages is performed to increase lordosis. Then a posterior fusion with compression segmental instrumentation contoured into lordosis is performed. Usually the instrumentation can be attached to the previous instrumentation with domino or transverse connectors.

## DISK DEGENERATION BELOW SPINAL FUSION WITHOUT DEFORMITY

When disk degeneration develops below a spinal fusion (Fig. 34-24), the patient experiences either mechanical back pain or radicular pain related to spinal stenosis or both. When mechanical back pain alone is present, diskography is often helpful in localizing the level(s). If diskography demonstrates a radial tear and there is severe worsening of the patient's chronic pain complaints, then extension of the fusion to incorporate the symptomatic level is likely to lessen the symptoms.

If the patient has radicular symptoms consistent with stenosis, a CT myelogram scan should be obtained. If stenosis is present then decompression alone should be considered as long as a wide decompression is not needed. If an extensive decompression that may lead to instability is necessary, then the fusion should be extended distally with pedicular instrumentation.

## RECORRECTION OF PERSISTENT KYPHOTIC DEFORMITY

Most of the time mild hyperkyphosis of the thoracic spine is well tolerated unless there is a painful pseudarthrosis present. The treatment of symptomatic pseudarthrosis with hyperkyphosis has previously been discussed in this chapter. When symptomatic hyperkyphosis of the thoracic spine is present following a previous fusion, revision surgery is indicated to (1) achieve proper sagittal balance or (2) correct the deformity.

Attempts at correction of previously fused kyphotic deformities is fraught with considerable risk of neurological injury.[2,9] Before undertaking such a procedure, a clear understanding of risks versus benefits must be provided to the patient. A preoperative MRI or CT myelogram should always be obtained to evaluate stenotic areas in the canal. Recorrective surgery for kyphosis always requires a combined anterior-posterior procedure. The anterior procedure is always done first. Any stenotic areas must be thoroughly decompressed by anterior vertebrectomy.

First an anterior diskectomy should be performed through a level where the posterior portion of the disk is clearly visible at a level near the apex of the kyphotic deformity. Occasionally, more than one level will be required adjacent to the apex of the deformity. If the resulting diskectomy defects are small, morselized bone is used. If the defects are large or if a partial vertebrectomy is needed, then structural grafts or cages may be required.[8]

Careful neurological monitoring including somatosensory evoked potentials, motor evoked potentials, and a wake-up test should be performed during both procedures.

The posterior procedure is performed next by first inspecting the entire fusion area. If a pseudarthrosis is found, it should be curetted to healthy bone and repaired with autogenous bone. A posterior chevron closing wedge osteotomy is then performed at the apex directly behind the anterior diskectomy or diskectomies.[18] The under surfaces of the osteotomy should be beveled so that the dura can not be compressed when the osteotomy is closed.

*Text continued on page 506*

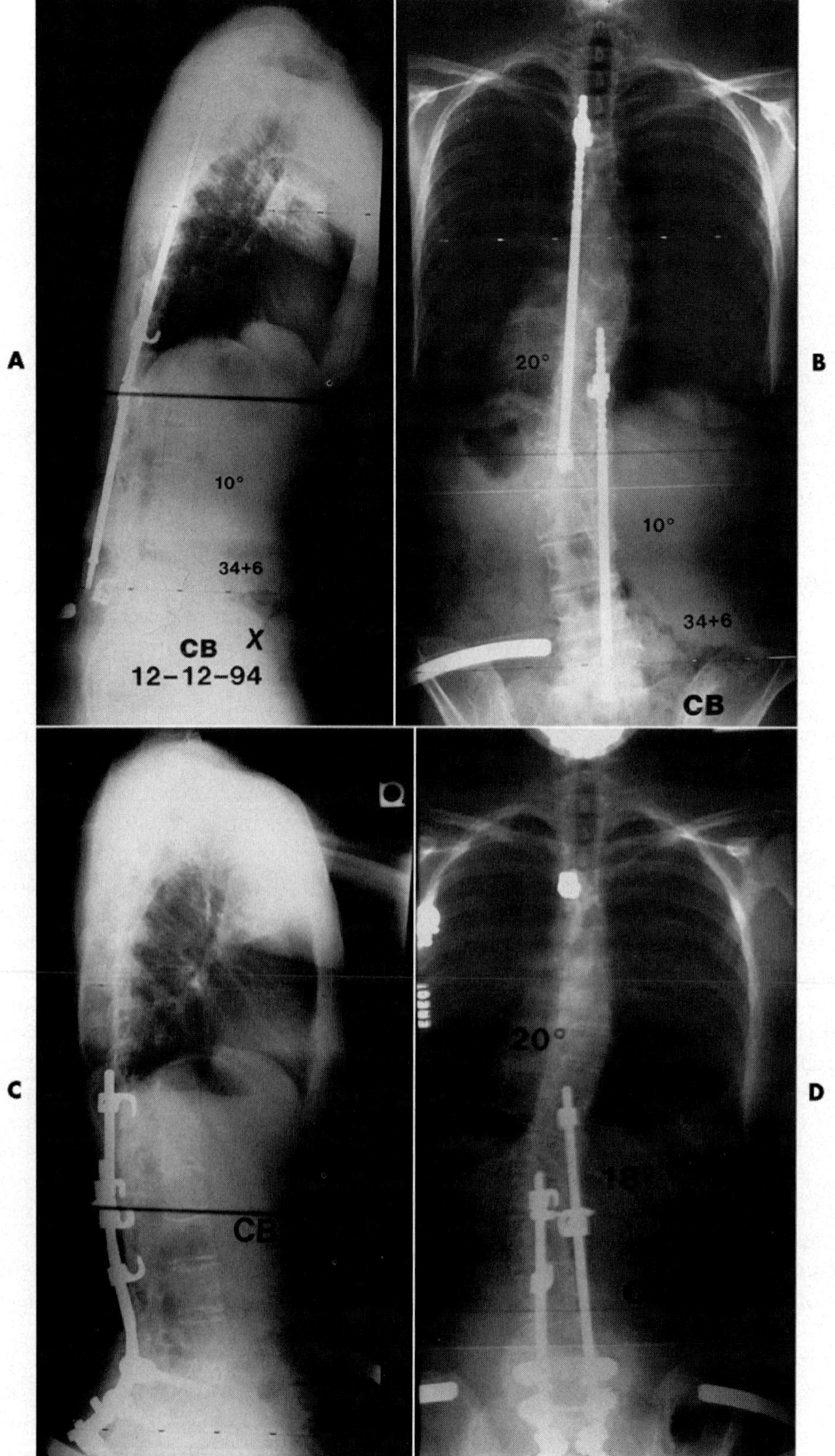


FIGURE 34-23

**A, B,** Preoperative radiographs of a 33-year-old woman who underwent a posterior fusion with double Harrington rods as a teenager for kyphoscoliosis. The use of distraction instrumentation into the lumbar spine (L5) resulted in a flat back syndrome. She also developed a painful degenerative disk at L5-S1. **C, D,** Subsequent reconstructive surgery consisted first of an anterior diskectomy and fusion with titanium mesh at L4-L5 and L5-S1 followed by removal of Harrington instrumentation, repair of pseudarthrosis L4-L5, and extension of the fusion to the sacrum using S1 and S2 pedicle screws and a compression hook and screw construct with iliac bone graft. Excellent restoration of sagittal balance and relief of back pain occurred.

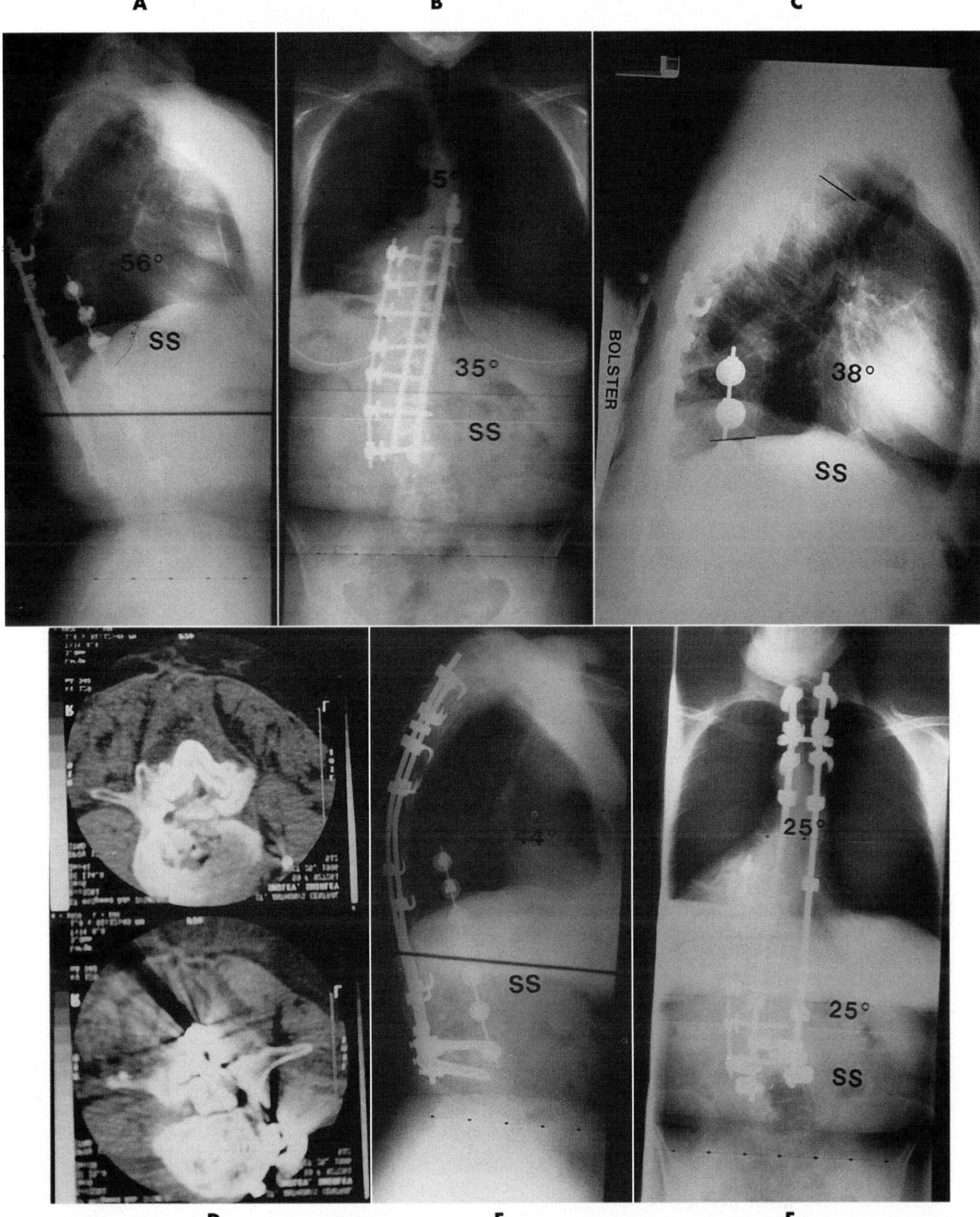


FIGURE 34-24

A 48-year-old woman who underwent an anterior-posterior instrumented fusion for scoliosis at age 40. She began developing claudicatory symptoms in both legs after 1 year and she presented a progressive kyphosis of the thoracic spine. Erect x-rays of the spine **(A-C)** reveal a hyperkyphosis of the thoracic spine of 38 degrees above a previously healed instrumented fusion from T1 to L3. A CT myelogram reveals marked spinal stenosis below the lowest fused vertebra. **D, E,** Revision surgery consisted of removal of the posterior instrumentation, a decompression of L3-L4, and insertion of new instrumentation extending from T3 to L4. **F,** Postoperative view. The kyphosis is reduced and the claudicatory symptoms disappear.

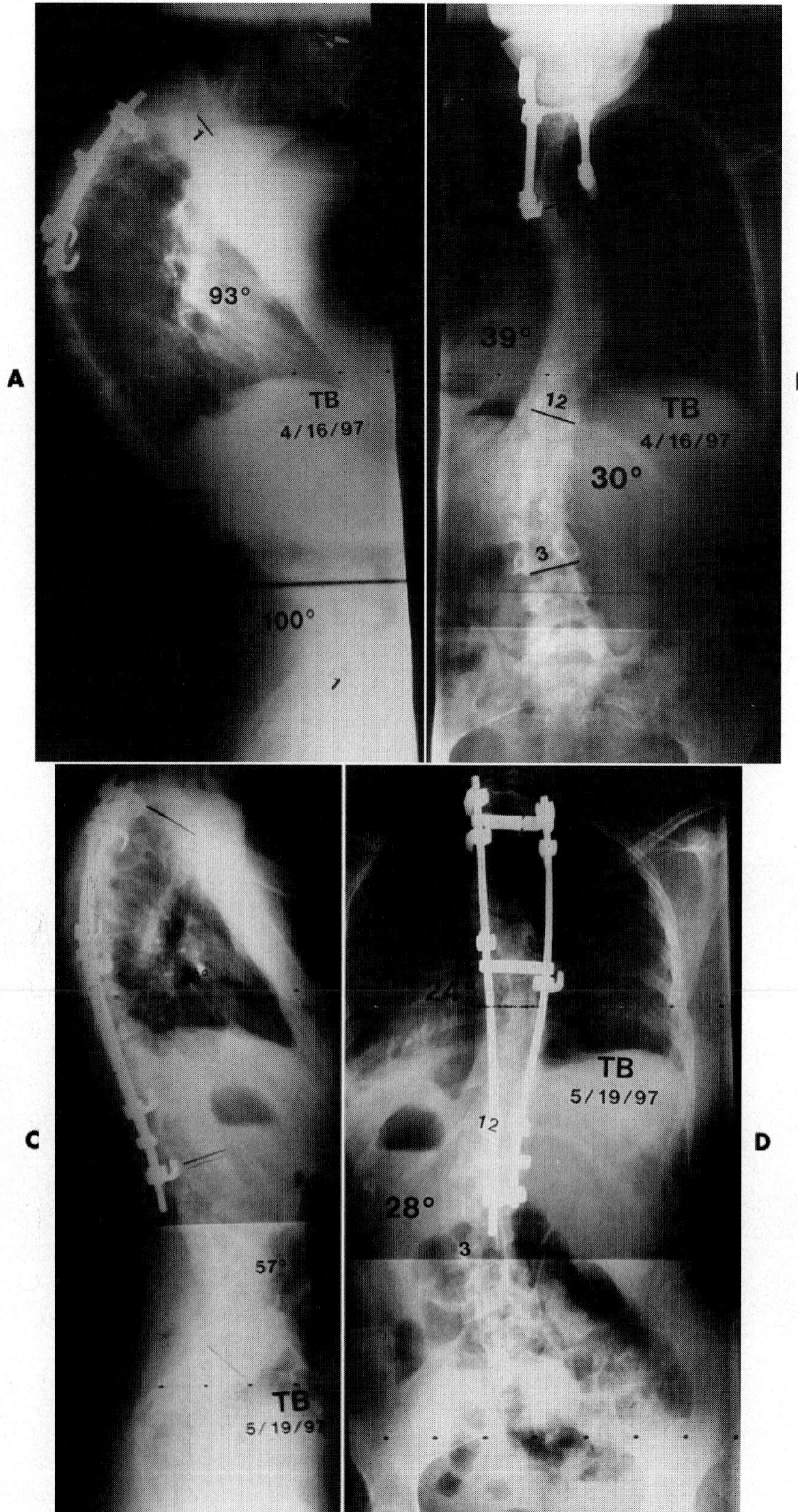


**FIGURE 34-25**

A 16-year-old girl who underwent two previous posterior spinal fusions for adolescent idiopathic scoliosis. **A, B,** Initially, an instrumented posterior spinal fusion T5-T12 was carried out and 2 years later the instrumentation was removed and the upper left thoracic curve was instrumented and fused from T1-T6. Postoperatively, she developed a progressive thoracic kyphosis that became painful and cosmetically unacceptable to the patient. Surgical revision surgery consists of an anterior diskectomy and fusion with morselized rib graft from T5-T11 followed by posterior osteotomies at T6-T7 and T9-T10 followed by posterior compression instrumentation from T1-L2 with hooks into old fusion mass. Good restoration of sagittal profile and balance is postoperatively achieved **(C, D)**.

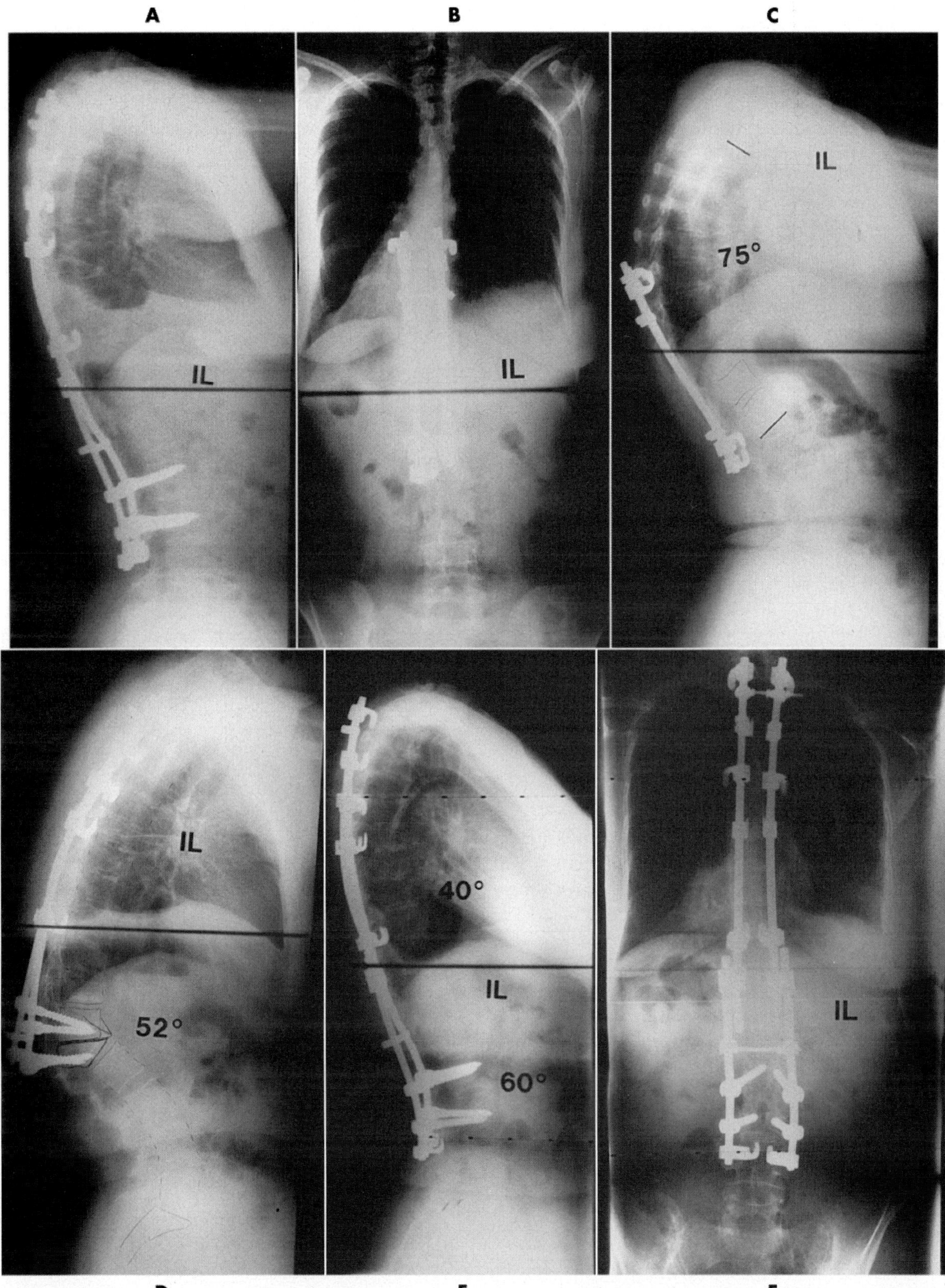


**FIGURE 34-26**

This is a 51-year-old woman who sustained a burst fracture of T11, which was treated with a posterior hook only, one-level claw construct. **A, B,** A progressive kyphotic deformity developed both within the construct as well as above the instrumented fusion. **C, D,** Because of increasing pain unresponsive to physical therapy, the patient first underwent an anterior release and interbody fusion with morselized rib graft from T5-T12 followed by removal of posterior instrumentation with repair of pseudarthrosis and extension of fusion from T3 to L1. The distal end of the instrumented fusion did not include the first lordotic disk, which shifted the sagittal plumb line anterior to the sacral promontory and because of associated osteopenia resulted in an anterior wedge fracture of the lowermost instrumented vertebra. **E, F,** This was salvaged by extending the fusion distally into the lordotic part of the lumbar spine using domino connectors. This resulted in restoration of normal sagittal balance and relief of symptoms.

A minimum of three hooks above and three hooks below the osteotomy are placed in the fusion mass on each side in a compression mode. A copious amount of autogenous graft is applied on either side of the osteotomy to insure a solid fusion. The longitudinal rods are attached to the hooks above the osteotomy with compression being applied to the apex. Then by cantilever bending, the osteotomy is closed being careful that the under surfaces do not compress the dura. The lower end of the rods are delivered into the lower hooks or screws and again compression is applied toward the apex. Transverse connecting rods are inserted above and below the osteotomy. A wake up test should always be performed at this stage of the procedure. Figure 34-25 demonstrates a two-level thoracic osteotomy performed for a persistent kyphosis following two previous posterior fusions in a 17-year-old female.

In the older patient with hyperkyphosis of the thoracic spine with loss of lumbar lordosis, extending the fusion distally into the lumbar spine to provide sagittal balance by creating increased lordosis may be all that is necessary. If large amounts of correction are necessary at individual disk levels than an anterior interbody fusion with structural grafts will be necessary also.

## VERTEBRAL "INSUFFICIENCY" FRACTURES

Occasionally in the older patient with osteopenia when a long instrumented fusion has been performed for kyphosis or scoliosis, an anterior compression fracture can develop at the distal end of the construct. This is usually the result of loss of lumbar lordosis, which leads to an anterior shift in sagittal balance and may result in an anterior wedge fracture of the distal vertebral body in the construct because of excessive load on the anterior column. This problem is well demonstrated in Figure 34-26. The solution to this problem includes extending the fusion and instrumentation distally and providing for adequate lordosis in the lumbar spine to shift the sagittal balance behind the sacral promontory. This may also require anterior interbody arthrodesis with structural graft or cage if a large anterior column defect results from increased lumbar lordosis.

## CONCLUSIONS

Revision surgery for spinal deformity continues to be a challenge for the spine surgeon. The techniques and instrumentation now available allow us to treat most of these deformities and complications resulting from previous failed surgery. This chapter has been an attempt to provide the reader with some solutions to many of the difficult problems involved with patients having kyphotic problems either de novo or as a result of previous surgical intervention for kyphosis.

Most of the revisions necessary for kyphosis are related to the fact that posterior only fusions were performed as a primary procedure with no provision for anterior column support with subsequent pseudarthrosis. Additionally, the use of distraction instrumentation and/or allograft posteriorly is fraught with a high failure rate.

The next most common reason for revision surgery is related to improper selection of fusion levels which may result in a junctional kyphosis either proximally or distally. Careful preoperative evaluation of radiographs and following principles for fusion levels out lined in this chapter will usually prevent this problem.

The development of structural grafts or spacers for anterior column reconstruction in the thoracolumbar and lumbar spines has resulted in the ability to provide for a normal sagittal profile while at the same time a high success rate of arthrodesis.

## REFERENCES


1. Bernhardt M, Bridwell K: Segmental analysis of the sagittal plane alignment of the normal thoracic and lumbar spines and thoracolumbar junction, *Spine* 14:717, 1989.
2. Boachie-Adjei O, Bradford, DS: Vertebral column resection and arthrodesis for complex spinal deformities, *J Spinal Disord* 4(2):193-202, 1991.
3. Bradford DS, Moe JH, Montalvo FJ, Winter RB: Scheuermann's kyphosis. Results of surgical treatment by posterior spine arthrodesis in twenty two patients, *J Bone Joint Surg* 57A:439, 1975.
4. Bradford DS, Ahmed KB, Moe JH, Winter RB, Lonstein, JE: The surgical management of patients with Scheuermann's disease. A review of twenty four cases managed by combined anterior and posterior spine fusion, *J Bone Joint Surg* 62:705, 1980.
5. Bridwell KH, Lenke LG, McEnerny KW: Anterior fresh frozen structural allografts in the thoracic and lumbar spine: do they work if combined with posterior fusion and instrumentation in adult patients with kyphosis or anterior column defects? *Spine* 20:1410, 1995.
6. Dodd AF, Fergusson CM, Freedman L: Allograft versus autograft bone in scoliosis surgery, *J Bone Joint Surg Br* 70:431, 1988.

7. Fon GT, Pitt MJ, Thies AC Jr: Thoracic kyphosis: range L normal subjects. *AJR Am J Roentgenol* 134:979, 1980.
8 Gurr KE, McAfee PC, Shih CM: Biomechanical analysis of anterior and posterior instrumentation system after corpectomy, *J Bone Joint Surg* 70A:1982, 1988.
9. Hodgson AR: Correction of fixed spinal curves, *J Bone Joint Surg* 47A:1221, 1965.
10. Jackson RP, McManus AC: Radiographic analysis of sagittal plane alignments and balance in standing volunteers and patients with low back pain matched for age, sex and size, *Spine* 19(14):1611, 1994.
11. Lowe TG: Current concepts review—Scheuermann's disease, *J Bone Joint Surg* 72A:940-945 1990.
12. Lowe TG, Kasten M: An analysis of sagittal balance and profile after instrumentation and fusion for kyphosis, *Spine* 19:1680-1685 , 1994.
13. Lowe TG: Biomechanical aspects of the surgical treatment of kyphotic deformities. In Haher and Merola, editors: *Spine: State of the Art Reviews,* vol 10, no 3, Sept 1996, pp 433-454, Philadelphia, Hanley & Belfus.
14. Lowe TG: *Bone grafting.* In: Margulies JY, Floman Y, Farcy JC, Neuwirth MD, editors: *Lumbosacral and Spine Pelvic Fixation.* Philadelphia, 1996, Lippincott-Raven, pp 727-744.
15. Lowe TG: *Scheuermann's disease.* In: Bridwell KH, DeWald RL, editors: *The text book of spinal surgery,* Philadelphia, 1996, Lippincott-Raven, p 1173.
16. Milne JS, Lander IJ: Age effects in kyhphosis and lordosis in adults. *Ann Hum Biol* 1:327, 1974.
17. Schultz AB, Ashton-Miller JA: *Biomechanics of the human spine.* In Mow VC, Hayes WC, editors: *Basic orthopedic biomechanics.* New York, 1991, Raven Press, p 337.
18. Thomason E: Vertebral osteotomy for correction of kyphosis in ankylosing spondylitis, *Clin Orthop* 194: 142, 1985.
19. Voutsinas SA, McEwen GD: Sagittal profiles of the spine. *Clin Orthop* 210:235, 1986.
20. White AA, Punjabi MM: *Clinical biomechanics of the spine.* Philadelphia, 1978, JB Lippincott.
21. Winter RB, Hall JE: Kyphosis in childhood and adolescence, *Spine* 3:285, 1978.

# 35

# REVISION OF PROGRESSIVE THORACIC KYPHOTIC DEFORMITIES USING A SIMULTANEOUS ANTERIOR ENDOSCOPIC AND POSTERIOR OPEN TECHNIQUE

**Isador H. Lieberman, B.Sc., M.D., F.R.C.S.(C)**
**Paul T. Salo, M.D., F.R.C.S.(C)**



The goals of primary kyphosis correction regardless of the etiology are to normalize the sagittal contours, restore a balanced spine, and prevent progression by reducing the bending moments and achieving a solid fusion. Previous studies of surgically treated kyphosis with posterior instrumentation, correction, and bone grafting reported good initial correction but also an unacceptable progressive loss of correction and hardware failure.[1,4,9,11,16] Recurrence or progression may reflect inadequate initial correction, pseudarthrosis, anterior column structural insufficiency, or the addition of levels to the underlying curve. More recent studies recommend anterior release and bone grafting followed by posterior instrumentation and bone grafting to effectively lengthen the anterior column and provide a structural buttress, while shortening the posterior column and minimizing the tension band across the posterior elements.[2,3,5,6,8,12,13,15] Despite these recommendations, patients continue to present with recurrence or progression of previously operated thoracic kyphotic deformities. To date, there are no published reports reviewing the epidemiology of progression in this group of patients.

Patients with previously operated progressive thoracic kyphotic deformities commonly report symptoms of fatigue and back pain. These may be attributable to the abnormal sagittal plane alignment and the resulting altered force distribution at the cervicothoracic, thoracolumbar, and lumbosacral junctions. Rarely, these patients may present with neurological symptoms, but they commonly express dissatisfaction with their cosmetic appearance.

The recommended surgical treatment for revision of previously operated progressive thoracic kyphotic deformities usually involves a three-stage operative correction.[7,14] The first stage involves posterior osteotomies possibly followed by traction. The second stage involves anterior osteotomies, correction, and bone grafting, followed by a third stage involving posterior instrumentation, correction, and bone grafting.

With the availability of minimally invasive endoscopic techniques the multiple operative stages may be combined in one operative session. The technique we describe below with the patient positioned prone, permits anterior endoscopic exposure, osteotomies, and reconstruction to be undertaken with simultaneous posterior exposure, instrumentation, osteotomies, and correction all in one operative session.

## TECHNIQUE

The preoperative evaluation involves a thorough clinical assessment, documentation of curve progression, as well as documentation and discussion of the patient's expectations. To determine the extent and rigidity of the thoracic hyperkyphosis, three-foot standing anteroposterior (AP) and lateral radiographs, along with lateral supine radiographs over a bolster are obtained. A computed tomography (CT) myelogram is routinely obtained to ensure that there are no occult areas of potential spinal cord compression. Keeping in mind that during the corrective maneuver the anterior column is effectively being lengthened and the posterior column effectively shortened, with the fulcrum at the posterior vertebral margins, there is minimal risk to the spinal cord because the spinal canal itself is actually being shortened. There is, however, always the risk of occult disk herniations or degenerative osteophytes that may indirectly cause canal stenosis during the correction.

The radiographs are evaluated to determine the fusion levels and the osteotomy sites. The fusion must include all levels within the curve up to and including the end vertebrae that are intersected by the central sagittal line. The osteotomy sites are planned according to the anterior levels to be released. One must remember that the interlaminar spaces lie caudal to the disk spaces and wide laminotomies and foraminotomies are necessary to avoid any nerve root or spinal cord impingement.

In patients complaining of pain above and below the thoracic hyperkyphosis, assessment of the disk and facet integrity with magnetic resonance imaging (MRI) scan, diskography, or facet blocks may be valuable in determining the extent of the fusion. If a pseudarthrosis across the previous fusion is suspected, a bone scan, and/or CT scan with sagittal reconstructions may be valuable in identifying the level.

Intraoperatively one must create wide osteotomies and laminotomies extending out to the foramina and undercut the fusion mass to ensure that there will be no encroachment on the spinal cord or neural foramina when the osteotomies are closed. The aim of the technique is to achieve a small amount of correction at multiple levels, rather than a lot of correction at a few levels.

The preferred instrumentation is segmental transpedicular at each level across the entire curve. It is important to instrument beyond the thoracolumbar junction to provide for a solid foundation, and prevent further deterioration. The pedicular screws may be protected from pull-out with laminar hooks or sublaminar wires at the proximal and distal ends of the construct.

The surgical technique involves a two-team approach (Fig. 35-1). One team performs the anterior endoscopic release and the second team exposes the spine, performs the instrumentation, and creates the posterior osteotomies.

The surgery is performed under a general anesthetic with double-lumen endotracheal intubation and with the appropriate hemodynamic and spinal cord monitoring. The patients are positioned prone on a radiolucent table (Fig. 35-1). The function of the double-lumen tube is first checked in the supine position then once again in the prone position. The back

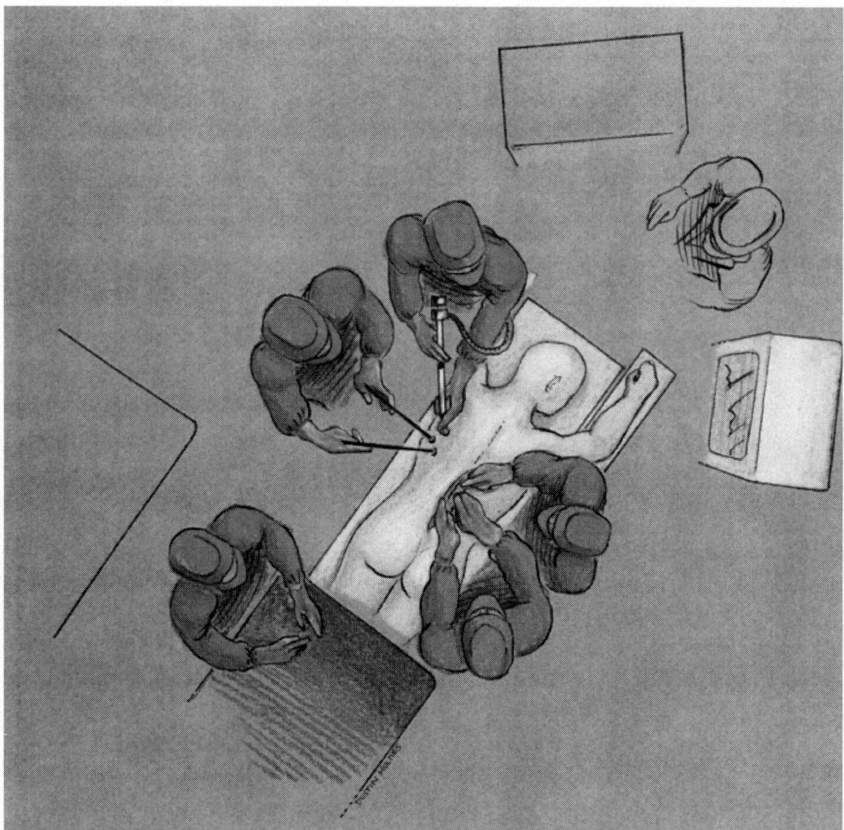

**FIGURE 35-1**

Patient position and operating room set-up.

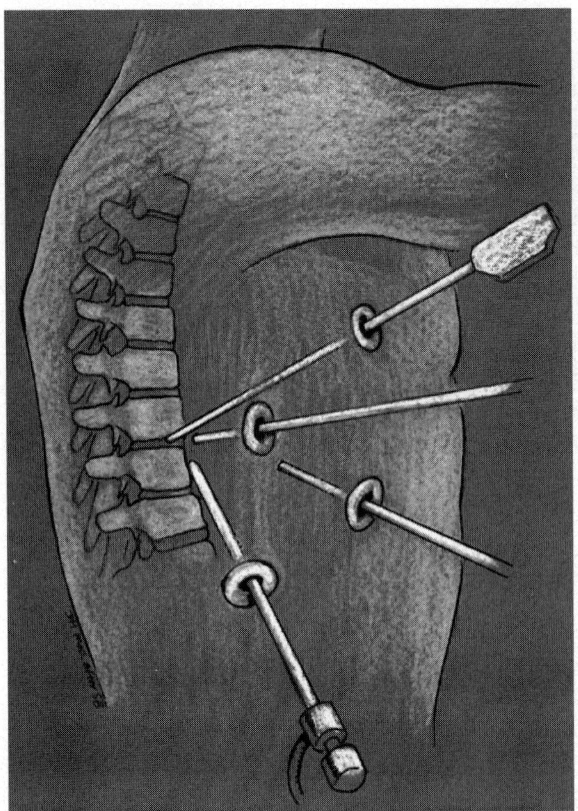

FIGURE 35-2

Portal placement.

is prepped and draped widely extending beyond the anterior axillary line on each side. The spine is first exposed through a posterior midline incision to the tips of the transverse processes over the appropriate fusion levels. Any existing hardware is removed. The posterior osteotomy sites are planned and the instrumentation is applied to the spine. Image intensifier or lateral radiographs may be used to place the implants and localize the osteotomies. The appropriate lung (right or left chest at the surgeon's discretion) is then deflated by clamping the corresponding lumen of the double-lumen tube. While waiting for the lung to deflate additional bone graft, if necessary, may be harvested from the posterior superior iliac spine through a separate incision. The first transthoracic portal is created opposite the apex of the kyphosis at the mid axillary line. A 30-degree endoscope is inserted and the chest cavity is explored. Two further working portals are created at the posterior axillary line, two interspaces cephalad and caudad to the endoscope portal (Fig. 35-2). The instruments and scope can be interchanged between the portals to facilitate work on the spine. A fourth optional portal, two interspaces cephalad at the mid axillary line can be added if necessary.

With the patient prone, the deflated lung and mediastinal structures fall out of view requiring no retraction. The spinal levels are then identified by counting ribs and confirmed with an AP radiograph. Multiple individual transverse pleural incisions are made directly over the disk spaces to be released. The segmental vessels are preserved and the sympathetic chain is bluntly dissected out of harm's way. Small gauze sponges are packed between the spine and the great vessels at each level to be released. The anterior longitudinal ligament and annulus are incised with cautery. The nucleus pulposus and cartilage endplates are evacuated with long-handled endoscopic rongeurs and curettes down to bleeding subchondral bone. The entire annulus across to the opposite side must be released to gain full mobility of the spine. If the disk space is fused it may be released with long osteotomes or high-speed power burrs. With the transpedicular instrumentation in place, the disk spaces can be levered open to expose the posterior longitudinal ligament and ensure complete evacuation of disk material (Fig. 35-3). It is important to note that the disk space is being hinged open at the posterior cortical wall (Fig. 35-4). Bone graft, either structural tricortical crest or femoral allograft ring, is inserted into the disk spaces with long bone holders and punches. The posterior instrumentation, correction, and bone grafting are then completed. The endoscope is removed from the chest and the portals closed with a subcutaneous suture and a continuous subcuticular suture. A chest tube is inserted through one portal. The posterior incisions are then closed over a subfascial drain.

## SERIES AND RESULTS

To date, four patients with previously operated progressive thoracic kyphotic deformities have undergone correction using this simultaneous endoscopic technique. The average preoperative curve measured 85 degrees. The average postoperative curve measured 56 degrees. The overall average correction was 29 degrees. All four patients had a minimum of four levels released anteriorly and osteotomized posteriorly, for an average correction of 7 degrees per level.

The total operative time varied from six to ten hours. There were no intraoperative complications as a result of the double-lumen intubation, prone positioning, or the endoscopic approach. Postoperatively, the patients were monitored in the intensive care unit (ICU) overnight. The chest tubes were removed after two days with no complications. No patient complained of symptoms consistent with a postthoracotomy syndrome, and at one-year follow-up no patient developed any problems as a result of the simultaneous anterior endoscopic and posterior open approach.

## DISCUSSION

Traditional thoracotomy requires a large incision, dissection through the shoulder girdle musculature,

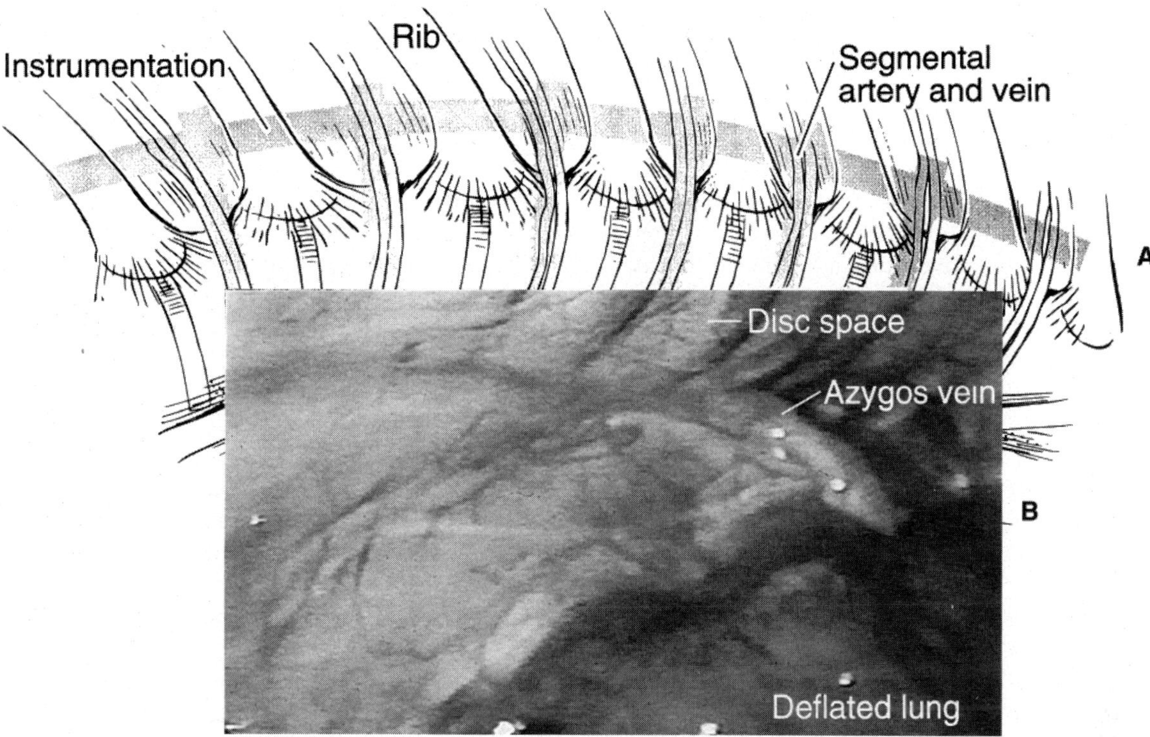


FIGURE 35-3

**A,** Endoscopic view of kyphosis. **B,** Detail of kyphosis.

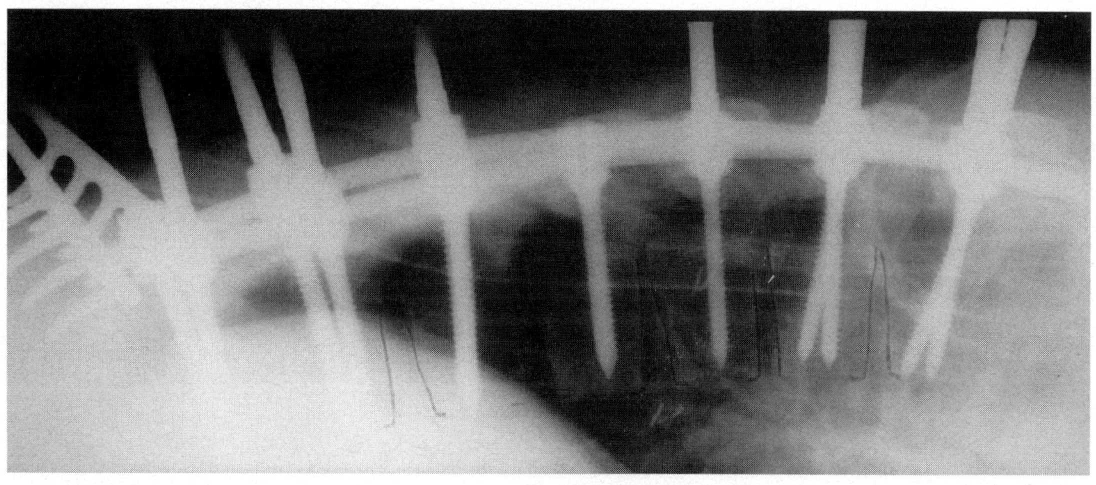

FIGURE 35-4

Intraoperative x-ray.

rib resection, and rib spreading. This can result in a compromise of pulmonary and shoulder function, significant postoperative pain, and an unsightly scar.[10] This also requires a staged procedure with either repositioning and redraping of the patient or subsequent procedures.[7,13,14]

The prone position endoscopic technique that we describe permits multiple-level anterior releases or osteotomies using only three portals, eliminating the need for a thoracotomy. By virtue of the prone positioning, this technique allows simultaneous posterior instrumentation, which provides complete control of the mobilized spine through the instrumentation system. Using endoscopic techniques, one is able to preserve the integrity of the segmental vessels, thereby maintaining blood supply to the bone, and minimizing the risk of spinal cord ischemia. Using this technique, one may apply bone graft to the anterior column, which is both biomechanically and physiologically favorable. By performing the procedures simultaneously this technique eliminates the need for a staged procedure, the added time for repositioning, and the added costs of redraping and a new operating room set-up.

The advantages of the endoscopic transthoracic techniques include a minimally invasive exposure, improved visualization of the anterior thoracic spine, the potential for reduced blood loss and a lower infection rate, and less compromise of respiratory mechanics and shoulder function. The added benefits include a reduction in postoperative pain and earlier rehabilitation, while minimizing the ICU and overall hospital stay.

The disadvantages of using endoscopic transthoracic spinal surgery techniques include a steep learning curve, a need for specialized instruments, and a unique operating room set-up. The nonendoscopic surgeon may experience initial frustration and difficulty in dealing with the diminished depth perception, and the limited tactile feedback, due to the longer instruments. The endoscopic technique may also be limited in its ability to deal with intraoperative complications (i.e., major vessel or organ injury, dural tear). The surgeon must be prepared to convert to open thoracotomy without hesitation. In the prone position this can be achieved through an extended costotransversectomy. The operating room set-up must always include easily accessible thoracotomy instruments. Experience with open anterior spinal surgery and a structured program of endoscopic technical training are essential prior to proceeding with this technique.

The single most important anesthetic concern of this technique is the double-lumen intubation with the patient positioned prone. Preoperatively, patients must be assessed to determine their suitability for single lung ventilation. Throughout the procedure the double-lumen tube must be monitored rigorously and a bronchoscope is kept in the room to allow convenient verification of tube patency and position.

The use of transthoracic endoscopic techniques in revision kyphosis surgery offers a minimally invasive alternative method of accessing anterior spinal pathology, with the benefits of excellent visualization, minimal soft tissue disruption, an improved cosmetic result, a shorter hospital stay, and subjectively reduced postoperative pain. With the simultaneous technique we describe, staged or subsequent procedures can be eliminated, and a circumferential structural release and control of the mobilized spine can be easily and safely achieved. This simultaneous technique can be extended for use in a variety of thoracic spinal pathologies, including tumour excision, trauma reconstruction, and scoliosis correction.

## CASE STUDY

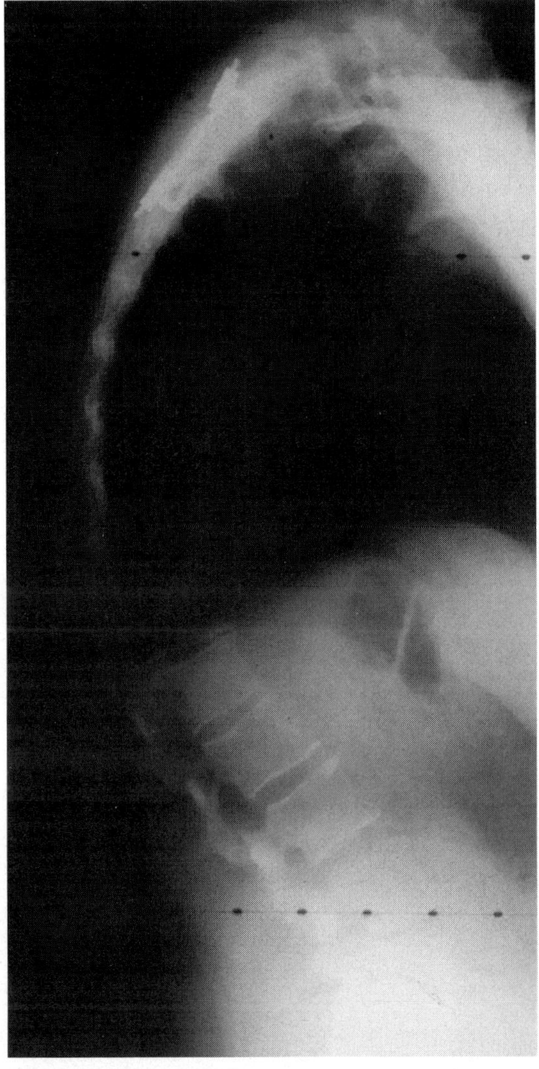

**FIGURE 35-5**

Preoperative x-ray.

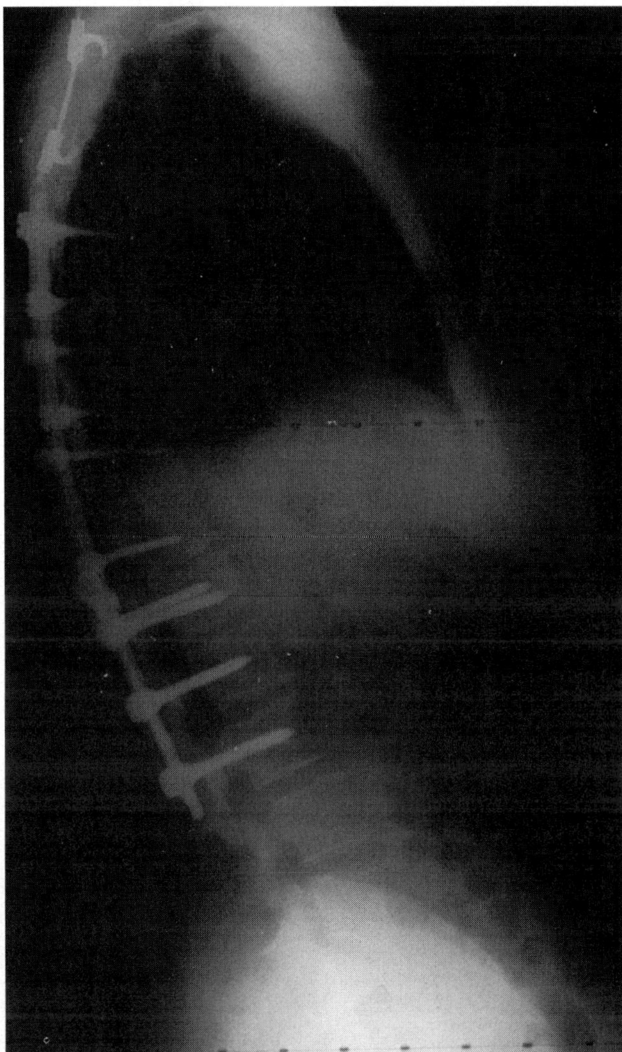

**FIGURE 35-6**

Postoperative x-ray.

This 35-year-old woman presented with cervicothoracic and thoracolumbar pain secondary to a progressive Scheuermann's thoracic hyperkyphosis. She underwent surgical correction ten years earlier, and had partial removal of the instrumentation three years later. At the time of hardware removal the fusion was assessed to be solid. Further follow-up x-rays documented that the curve progressed proximally, distally, and across the fused segments (Fig. 35-5). She was also distressed by the cosmetic appearance. Her preoperative radiographs revealed a 76-degree thoracic curve, correcting to 70 degrees on the hyperextension film. Her head was well balanced over the pelvis in the sagittal plane. The CT myelogram did not reveal any occult spinal canal encroachment. This patient underwent one-stage simultaneous anterior endoscopic releases, multiple-level structural bone grafting, posterior instrumentation, osteotomies, and posterior correction. Four levels were released anteriorly and four osteotomies were created posteriorly. Transpedicular segmental instrumentation was used at each level. The curve was corrected to 49 degrees measured at one-year follow-up (Fig. 35-6).

## REFERENCES


1. Bradford DS, Montalvo FJ, Moe JH, Winter RB: Scheuermann's kyphosis, results of surgical treatment by posterior spine arthrodesis in twenty-two patients, *J Bone Joint Surg* 57A:439, 1975.
2. Bradford DS, Ahmed KB, Moe JH, Winter RB, Lonstein JE: The surgical management of patients with Scheuermann's disease. A review of twenty-four cases managed by combined anterior and posterior spine fusion, *J Bone Joint Surg Am* 62:705-712, 1980.
3. Bridwell KH, Lenke LG, McEnery KW, Baldus C, Blanke K: Anterior fresh frozen structural allografts in the thoracic and lumbar spine, *Spine* 20(12):1410-1418, 1995.
4. Ferreira-Alves A, Resina J, Palma-Rodrigues R: Scheuermann's kyphosis, the Portuguese technique of surgical treatment, *J Bone Joint Surg Br* 77(6):943-950, 1995.
5. Hammerberg KW: *Kyphosis.* In Bridwell KH, Dewald RL, editors: *The textbook of spinal surgery,* Philadelphia, 1991, JB Lippincott, pp 501-523.
6. Herndon WA, Emans JB, Micheli LJ, Hall JF: Combined anterior and posterior fusion for Scheuermann's kyphosis, *Spine* 6:125, 1981.
7. Johnson JR, Holt RT: Combined use of anterior and posterior surgery for adult scoliosis. *Orthop Clin North Am* 19:361-370, 1988.
8. Kostuik JK: Anterior Kostuik Harrington distraction systems for the treatment of kyphotic deformities, *Iowa Ortho J* 69:77, 1988.
9. Kostuik JK: *Kyphosis surgery in the adult.* In Frymoyer et al, eds: *The adult spine,* Philadelphia, 1991, Raven Press, pp 1369-1403.
10. Mack MJ, Regan JJ, Bobechko WP, Acuff TE: Application of thoracoscopy for diseases of the spine, *Ann Thorac Surg* 56:736-738, 1993.
11. Ogilvie J, Bradford DS: Luque Instrumentation in adults with Scheuermann's kyphosis, NASS Annual Meeting, Colorado Springs, 1988.
12. Shufflebarger HL: Cotrel-Dubousset instrumentation for Scheuermann's kyphosis, *Orthop Trans* 13:90, 1989.
13. Shufflebarger HL: *Theory and mechanisms of posterior derotation spinal systems.* In Weinstein S, editor: *The pediatric spine,* New York, 1993, Raven Press, pp 1515-1543.
14. Shufflebarger HL, Grimm JO, Bui V, Thomson JD: Anterior and posterior spinal fusion: staged versus same day surgery, *Spine* 16:930-933, 1991.
15. Speck GR, Chopin DC: The surgical treatment of Scheuermann's kyphosis, *Spine* 68:189, 1986.
16. Taylor TC et al: Surgical management of thoracic kyphosis in adolescents, *J Bone Joint Surg* 61A:496-503, 1979.

# 36

# SPINE TUMOR REVISION SURGERY

**Allen L. Carl, M.D.**
**Paul Lombardi, M.D.**
**Joshua King, M.D.**



## GENERAL CONSIDERATIONS

The goal of spine tumor surgery is to maintain function and quality of life while attempting to obliterate or control disease. Revision spine tumor surgery poses even greater complexity. Treatment alternatives depend upon multiple personal factors and thus no documented algorithmic intervention directives exist. General treatment guidelines can be outlined. Making the diagnosis during the initial intervention or confirming the diagnosis during revision surgery is of significant importance. Primary spine tumors are rare and make up less than 10% of all bone tumors.[7,8] General care philosophy is to avoid contamination of surrounding normal tissue but still fully resect the lesion. On the other hand, metastatic spine tumor lesions are quite common. Forty to eighty percent of tumor patients have such involvement upon their demise. About 10% in this group require surgical stabilization for pain or neurologic dysfunction.[13] In light of limited longevity, maintenance of function is more important than complete exenteration.[19,38] The unique protective function of vertebra and its close anatomic association with spinal cord and nerve roots sometimes make it difficult for wide margin tumor resection.[5] In spite of these constraints, a multidisciplinary approach to tumors typically places these patients in the hands of well-trained spinal surgeons familiar with the most up-to-date diagnostic and treatment protocols.[2,38] The focus of care requires accurate diagnosis, staging, and prognostic assessment to tailor treatment that will allow maintenance of function and minimize morbidity and mortality. Control of pain and instability and maintenance of neurologic function are prime treatment goals. In light of the rarity of primary spine tumors and occasional tracking difficulties, little exists in the literature on revision spine tumor surgery.

Revision tumor surgery for metastatic spine disease has been described in reports focusing mainly on initial intervention and their results.[3,4,19,20,27] Reasons for spine tumor revision surgery include residual pain, instability, complications stemming from the original surgery, or neurologic dysfunction due to tumor progression.[33] Initial inaccurate diagnosis and suboptimal or inappropriate treatment may also lead to a need for revision surgery. Decompression without stabilization is known to have unsatisfactory results.[12,14,24,25] Even when a proper diagnosis is made, lesions may pose difficult treatment alternatives. On the one hand, aggressive tumor resection may result in significant morbidity and loss of function, while less aggressively treated tumors may lead to earlier recurrence and eventually greater morbidity. This treatment variability may explain the disparity in the percentage of revisions documented in the literature (Table 36-1). Individualized clinical judgment is often necessary in order to select treatment options. Age, activity level, general health, extent of disease spread, patient expectations, and neurologic function all impact outcome. These must be tailored to the patient when weighing treatment options.[13] Compromise needs to be made when complete tumor resection borders on heroics or the potential morbidity outweighs the benefits. Other reasons for revision spine tumor surgery include new or recurrent neurologic deterioration, implant failure, or new onset or recurrence of severe pain. It is often new or recurrent symptomatology or debility that

**Table 36-1. Revision Data of Primary and Metastatic Lesions***

| | Malignant Primary | Benign Primary | Metastatic | Total | Recurrence | Revision | |
|---|---|---|---|---|---|---|---|
| Turner, 1988[38] | 6 | | 35 | 41 | 16% | 1 | Primary malignant |
| Delamarter, 1990[8] | 18 | 11 | — | — | | 0 | 1 recurrence |
| Harrington, 1988[13] | | | 77 | | 8% | 3 | 5 failures only 2 w/ surgery |
| Nicholls, 1985[24] | | | 38 | — | | 0 | |
| Camins, 1978[5] | 3 | | — | | 66% | 2 | |
| Onimus, 1986[25] | | | 57 | | | 0 | |
| King, 1991[19] | | | 33 | | 27% | 9 | of 16 recurrent |
| Gennari, 1987[11] | 8 | | — | | 50% | 4 | |
| Galasko, 1991[10] | | | 55 | | 0% | 2 | none done for recurrence |
| Fagundes, 1995[9] | 204 | | — | | 31% | 63 | |
| Bridwell, 1988[4] | | | 25 | | 20% | 5 | |
| Cervoni, 1995[6] | 15 (myeloma) | | — | | 27% | 4 | |
| Bauer, 1997[3] | | | 67 | | 23% | 14 | 3 loosening-implants |
| McLain, 1991[23] | 2 | 2 | 7 | | 36% | 4 | all metastatic group |
| Rompe, 1993[27] | | | 50 | | 4% | 2 | |
| Jonsson, 1992[17] | 12 (myeloma) | | | — | 0% | | |
| Marcove, 1994[21] | 7 (sacrum) GCT | | — | | 68% | 2 | |
| Sonntag, 1992[31] | | | 6 | | 11% | | |
| Hay, 1978[15] | | ABC | — | | 13% | | |
| Kaiser, 1984[18] | | chordoma | — | | 28%–64% | | |
| Weinstein, 1987[39] | 51 | 31 | 14 | 82 | 21% | | |

*Not every recurrence led to revision. Many factors account for patient selection and revisions arise in more viable individuals. A need for more specific criteria and scoring systems in the future may be helpful.[20,36] Variability in data collection explains lack of comparable information.
GCT, giant cell tumor; ABC, aneurysmal bone cyst.

brings about the identification of lesion expansion or recurrence. Due to the rarity of primary spine tumors and the presence of multidisciplinary team involvement, revision surgery is rarely due to improper treatment. More frequently it is brought about by unforeseen circumstances arising from disease progression or the initial treatment options selected. Most cases of tumor recurrence pose problems of visualizing adequate tissue margins in order to accomplish optimal reresection. Operative summaries and studies from the original intervention, prior pathology reports, and slide evaluations are needed to provide insight into tumor histology and margins. Most frequently it is the proximity of nonresectable neurologic or vascular tissue structures that makes wide disease free margins difficult and sometimes impossible to attain.[1,5,16]

Adjuvant treatment from the initial procedure in the form of radiation, chemotherapy, and immunotherapy may cause systemic or local tissue compromise and thus increased risk during subsequent revision surgery. Scar tissue may be difficult to visually differentiate from tumor-laden tissue. Poorly vascularized scar tissue leads to a higher risk of infection. Abnormal tissue planes from prior scar formation make dissection more difficult. Plastic surgeons involved in complex soft tissue reconstruction efforts need to be included. Overall debility (altered tissues, poor nutritional status, etc.) from disease progression or prior treatment make revision surgery more taxing on the patient.[19,38] Parenteral hyperalimentation should be considered both pre- and postoperatively.

Pain can arise due to tumor recurrence, suboptimal or inadequate stabilization after the initial surgery, remodeling of bone around a nonbiologic construct, or degenerative disease due to surrounding mechanical dysfunction.[23,27]

## SURGICAL APPROACHES

Revision surgery can sometimes be performed through an anterolateral approach, which puts the surgical incision outside of the field of prior radiation.[34] This would decrease wound healing problems. Posterior midline wounds are most often in the previous radiation field and pose a greater risk to soft tissue healing.[13,35] The need for posterior or anterior surgery may occur with onset of anterior or posterior implant failure or in cases where longevity of a nonbiologic implant has been surpassed.[23] A cement construct alone led to unsatisfactory outcome.[38] Cement failure has been noted to be higher when used on the tension (posterior) side of a construct.[22] Use of cement-reinforced metallic implants anteriorly (with care taken to protect the spinal cord) has often been successful.[38]

In case of excessive neovascularity preoperative embolization prior to tumor resection should be entertained.[19]

Metastatic and benign nonaggressive spine tumors require debulking/stabilization and addressing of neurologic dysfunction or pain issues. Primary malignant and benign aggressive spine tumors pose a greater treatment dilemma. More complete resection attempts should be made to accomplish total tumor obliteration. This must be done with knowledge and recognition of morbidity potential including neurologic sequela and instability problems incurred with aggressive attempts at tumor resection.

Stabilization may be anterior, posterior, or combined. It is best to address the site of maximal involvement.[8,13,17,23,25,38] Others advocate a posterior approach regardless of site of disease involvement.[3] This may be adequate in cases that do not require anterior column support.[23] Nonbiologic implant spacers provide immediate stabilization but do not offer healing potential. In cases of increased longevity potential, biologic implants are needed. Sometimes longevity assessment is miscalculated and this sets up the need for future surgical intervention. If a biologic construct is placed and radiation is then required, healing of this graft may be curtailed leading to fibrous union or nonunion requiring later stabilization surgery.[13] On the other hand, the patient may outlive a nonbiologic implant and require surgery in the future to attain biologic healing. Either option may require a skin incision through radiated fields. Wound healing concerns and nutritional status are important when considering reoperation plans. Longevity must be taken into account when contemplating more surgery.[2] Often, patients do not survive long enough to undergo a reresection[38] or they may not have enough time to derive benefit from the procedure.[2,30] Adjuvant alternatives with further chemotherapy, immunotherapy, and radiation therapy must also be considered. Heroics in the form of complete removal of tumor must be weighed against quality of life issues. Partial tumor resection often results in earlier demise.[32] Decisions must be made regarding these complex issues. Other considerations include swiftly accomplishing mobilization, which may avoid deconditioning and associated debility. Metastatic and locally aggressive benign tumors have significant quality of life issues. Attempts at complete excision may risk neurologic function in unacceptable ways. In some cases periodic piecemeal resection may be as good as radical excision.[16] Others state that recurrence rates may be diminished by performing en bloc excisions rather than curettage and stabilization.[2,15,19,26,29,39] Tomita has introduced a saw that holds promise as a tool for en bloc vertebral resection.[37] Primary spinal chondrosarcomas have a high risk of recurrence and may benefit from this treatment.[1,5,16]

Vertebral chordomas pose a major resection problem. Their unique areas of involvement make it difficult for complete removal without significant risk of neurologic dysfunction. In the sacrum, this typically involves bowel, bladder, and sexual function. Gennari reported a 60% local recurrence.[11] When surgery is combined with proton and photon beam irradiation, a 31% failure rate has been reported.[9]

Marcove has successfully added cryosurgery to supplement marginal or intralesional resection of aggressive benign giant cell tumors.[21] This has been done to preserve lower spinal and pelvic function. Reports of lower morbidity and less resultant neurologic deficits have been reported when compared with radical sacrectomy.

As patient longevity increases with radiation, chemotherapy and immunologic manipulation revision surgery will become more commonplace (Figs. 36-1 and 36-2). Table 36-1 is a compilation of spine tumor articles that reveal a high variability of tumor recurrence dependent upon type of lesion and treatment. A far smaller subgroup of patients underwent revision surgery for recurrence or problems related to the surgical site.

## WOUND COVERAGE ALTERNATIVES

Patients who require spine surgery after planned adjuvant intervention such as failed radiation therapy pose a difficult problem for the reconstructive plastic surgeon. The relatively thin skin envelope and subcutaneous fat layer normally found overlying the spine will manifest the local subacute effects of radiation injury. These changes occur as a result of exposure to the repeated doses of radiation used in therapeutic regimens.

Initially there is skin erythema with associated edema. After several months, the skin and subcutaneous tissue become thickened and harden into a "woody induration." The skin develops a darker pigmentation. Within the radiated tissue the vessel walls become fibrotic and there is a diminution in the diffusion of nutrients, antibiotics, and humoral mediators, all essential components for wound healing. Ultimately, an obliterative endarteritis results in chronic ischemia within the irradiated tissue field.

This suboptimal state of soft tissue perfusion in irradiated tissue adversely effects the processes of wound

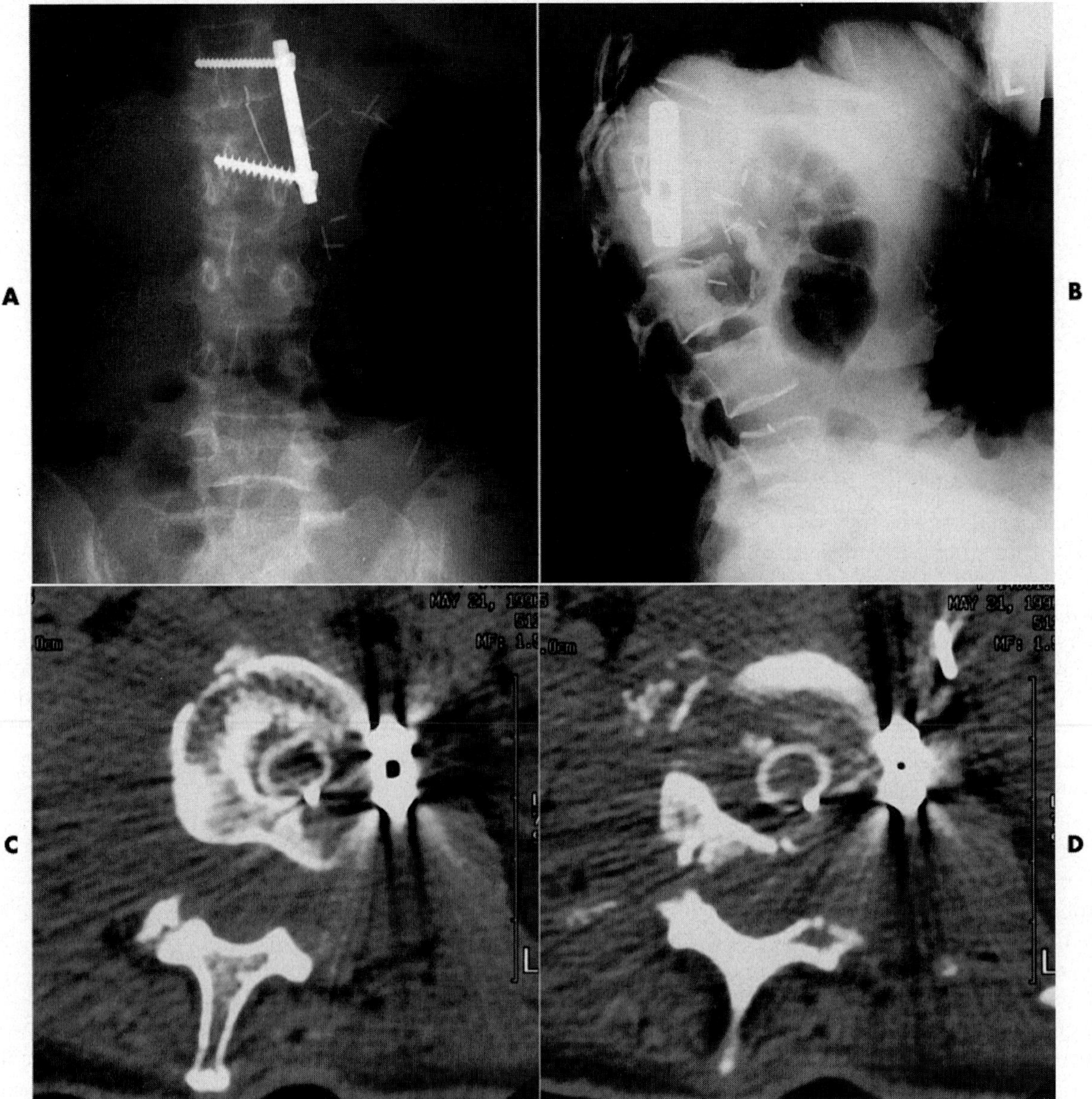

FIGURE 36-1

A 48-year-old woman, status post anterior decompression and stabilization for pathologic L1 fracture and kyphotic deformity secondary to renal cell carcinoma. Neurologic worsening and increased disease progression was noted three months after cement placement and anterior plating. **A, B,** Further disease progression and suboptimal fixation was noted. **C, D,** CT scan shows a small surface area being supported by the cement construct and a significant degree of tumor destruction.

*Continued*

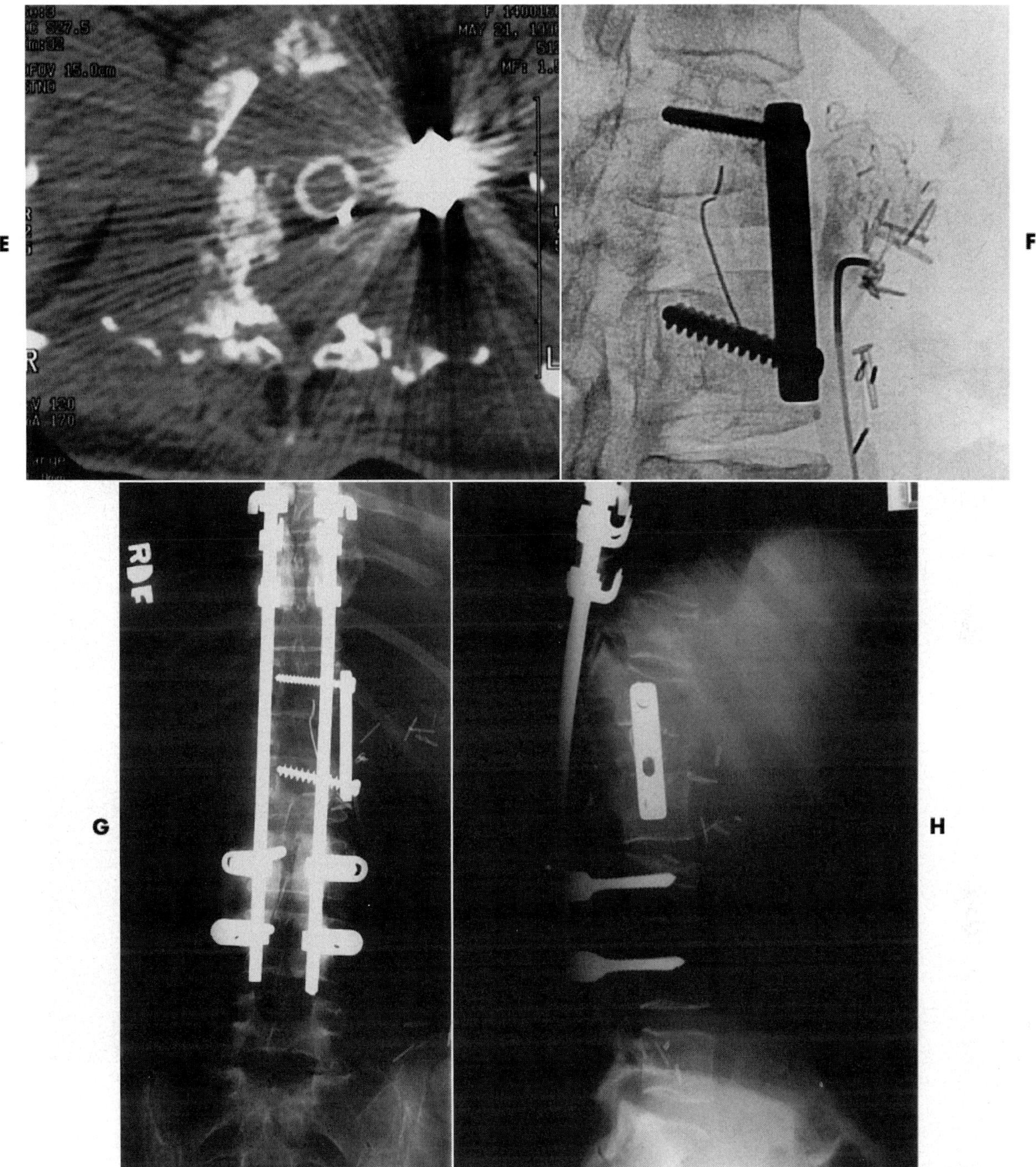

FIGURE 36-1, CONT'D

**E,** CT scan shows a small surface area being supported by the cement construct and a significant degree of tumor destruction. **F,** Angiogram and embolization were performed preoperatively. **G, H,** Posterolateral decompression and instrumentation with methacrylate fusion improved neurologic function, diminished pain, improved kyphotic deformity, and improved this patient's overall quality of life until her demise 8 months later.

healing. Clinical experience of surgery within irradiated tissue has shown a higher incidence of wound infections. Irradiated tissue cannot tolerate bacterial contamination as well as normal tissue and therefore adequate debridement of all nonviable tissue and liberal use of pulse-lavage is essential prior to closing these wounds.

In achieving wound coverage and closure following spine surgery through irradiated tissue, the reconstructive surgeon must make every effort to not further compromise the vascular status of already deficient tissue.

Several basic concepts involved in closing surgical wounds bear emphasizing in relation to irradiated tissue. Wound edges must be handled delicately to

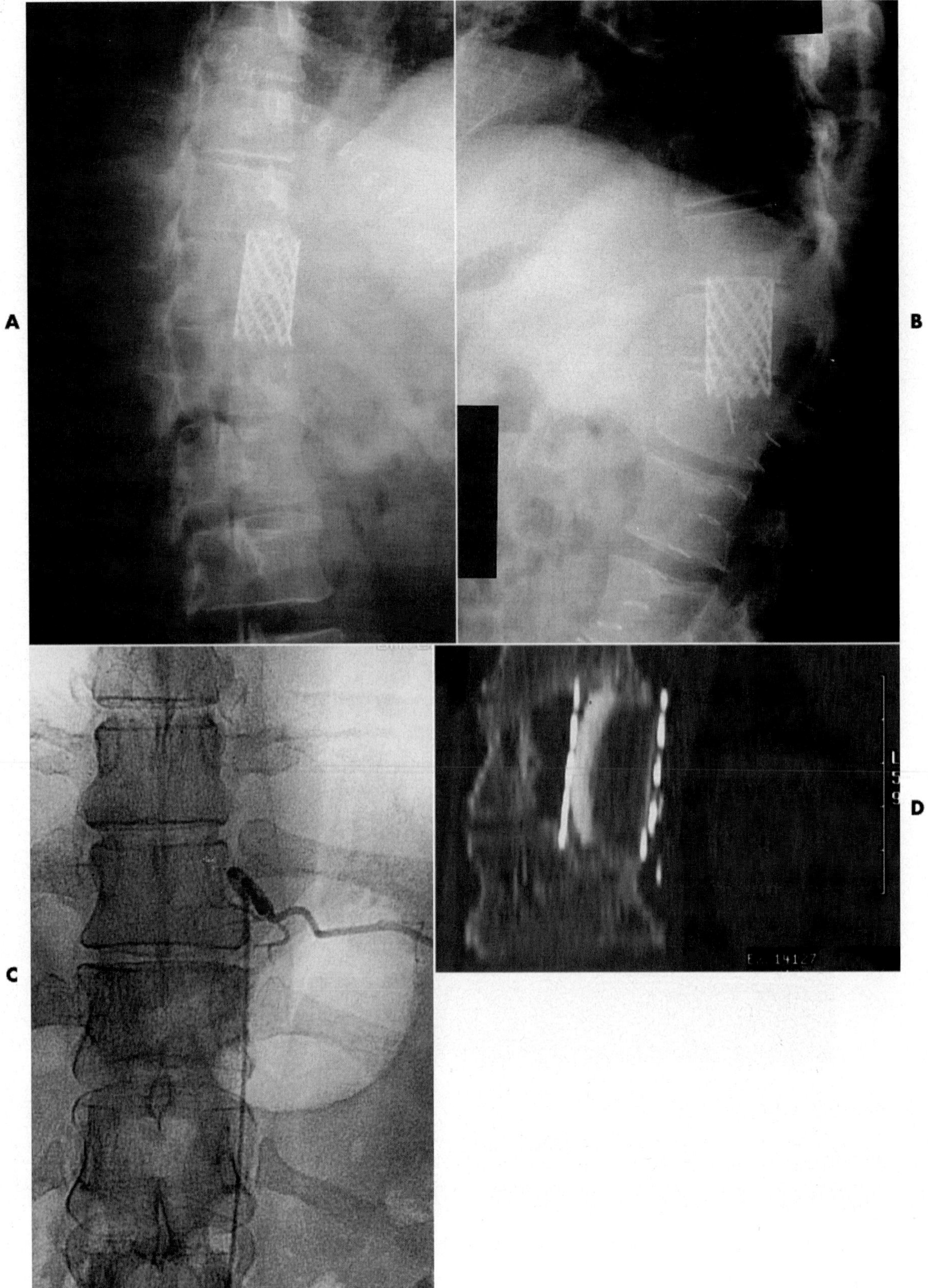

FIGURE 36-2

**A, B,** A 49-year-old man with back pain and resection of T11 chondrosarcoma, anterior tricortical autografting, and cage device support along with body casting was performed. **C,** Initial preoperative angiogram reveals artery of Adamkowitz at T10 and poses concern about the use of anterior fixation. **D,** Eight months later a 3D CT scan reveals a pseudarthrosis that is believed to be the cause of persisting pain. *Continued*

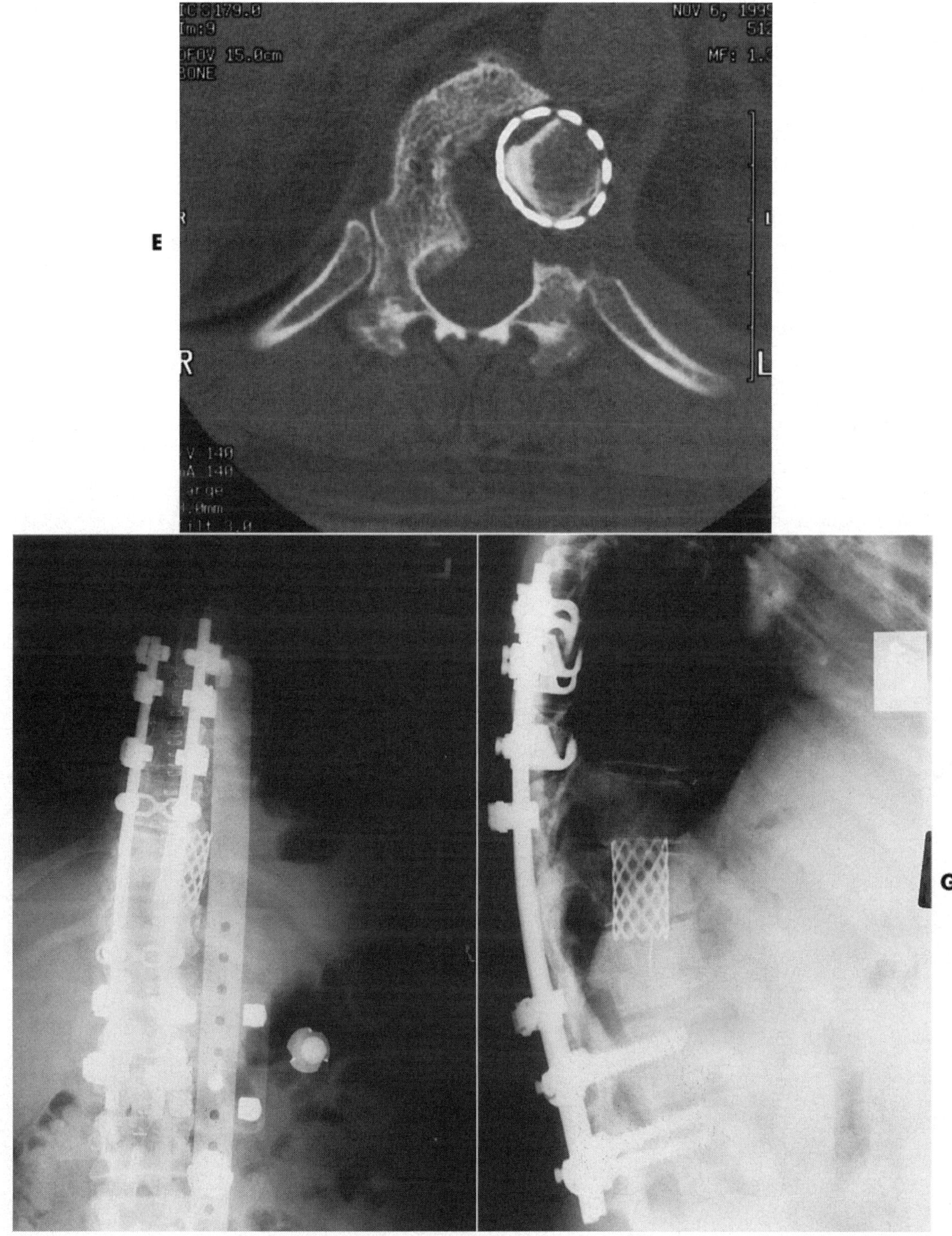


**FIGURE 36-2, CONT'D**

**E,** Eight months later a 3D CT scan reveals a pseudarthrosis that is believed to be the cause of persisting pain. **F, G,** A posterior instrumentation and autograft fusion gives stability and diminished pain. Patient remains asymptomatic at two years postoperative.

minimize local trauma, old scars should be fully excised to create relatively fresh wound edges, and as mentioned previously, thorough debridement of nonviable tissue must be performed.[28]

Wounds associated with spine surgery can frequently be closed primarily. However, radiated tissue is less tolerant to local ischemia and therefore wounds must not be closed with excessive tension across suture lines. Wide skin undermining to facilitate wound closure is unsafe and often leads to skin edge necrosis, especially if closed under tension. Longitudinally oriented relaxing incisions placed laterally on the posterior trunk can be a useful means to reduce tension in a midline back wound closure. These relaxing incisions should be carried through the fascia, essentially creating bipedicled fasciocutaneous flaps that can be advanced medially (Fig. 36-3). The resultant open wounds at the lateral sites can be covered with split thickness skin grafts.

When the deficit does not allow tension-free closure, or when there is exposed hardware and/or bone, flap tissue should be used. Flap options available for closure of the posterior midline include several reliable fasciocutaneous, muscle, and myocutaneous flaps. As is well known, even under ideal conditions, flaps can fail due to poor flap design. When designing flaps that incorporate irradiated tissue, attention to correct planning and adherence to basic principles must be applied.

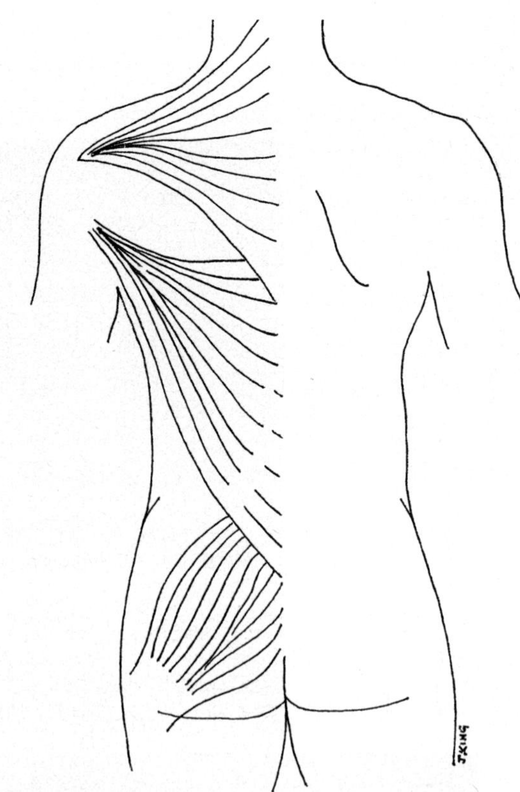

**FIGURE 36-4**

Muscles available for closure of back wounds: *Upper third,* trapezius muscle; *middle third,* latissiumus dorsi muscle; *lower third,* gluteus maximus muscle.

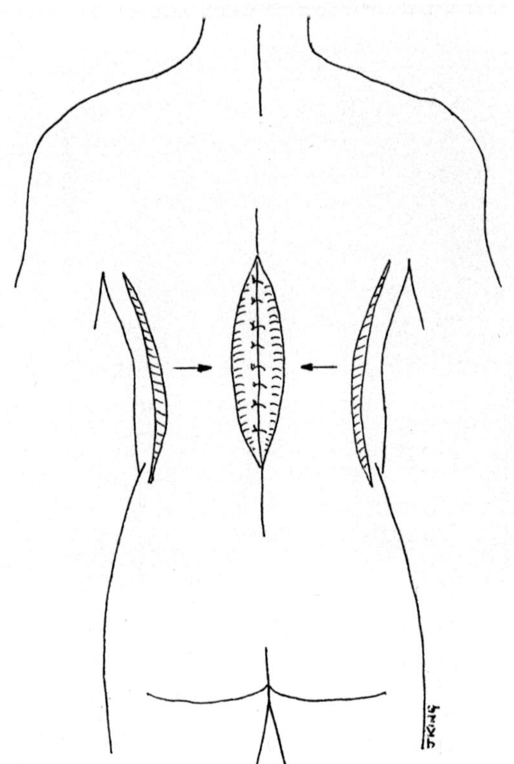

**FIGURE 36-3**

Bilateral latissimus dorsi musculocutaneous flaps with bilateral relaxing incisions to facilitate flap advancement towards midline.

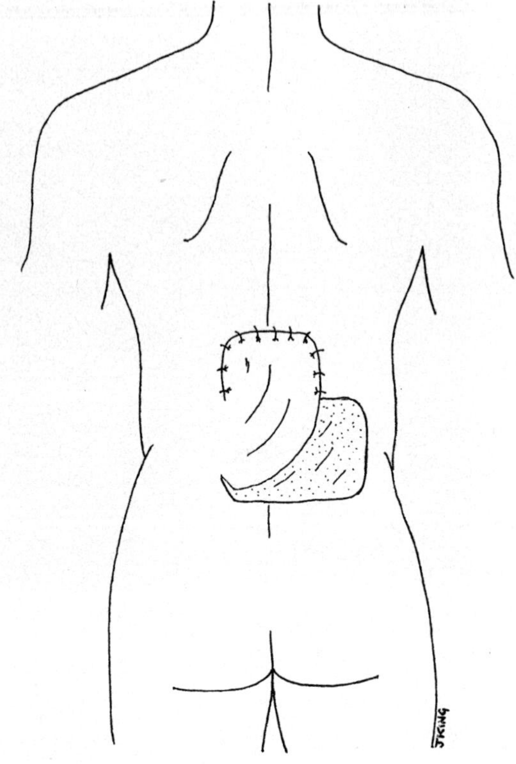

**FIGURE 36-5**

Transverse lumbosacral or transverse back flap. The flap is perfused by the contralateral lumbar and intercostal perforators. The donor site is skin grafted.

The latissimus dorsi muscle transfer is a reliable flap of adequate size and is technically straightforward to elevate. The flap may be based on either of two vascular pedicles (thoracodorsal artery or posterior perforating branches of lumbar and intercostal arteries) and can be harvested in a segmental manner for filling smaller defects. Bilateral latissimus dorsi muscle flaps can be advanced medially to fill large defects in the thoracic and lumbar regions. The latissimus dorsi flap may also be used as a myocutaneous flap. The skin paddle should be designed over the muscular portion of the latissimus dorsi to ensure its reliability. This muscle is the most versatile and useful of those available in this region.

Other useful muscle flaps include the trapezius muscle for coverage of upper one-third defects and the gluteus maximus for coverage of lower one-third defects. The paired paraspinous muscles can be raised as bipedicled muscle flaps. The arc of rotation of these muscle flaps is limited; however, they can be adequately mobilized to allow coverage of midline back defects. Frequently, movement of muscle tissue only a small distance can be invaluable in providing coverage of hardware or bone. All of these muscle flaps can be used individually or in combination with each other to suit the clinical situation (Fig. 36-4).

In regards to fasciocutaneous flaps available to cover midline back defects in irradiated wounds, the condi-

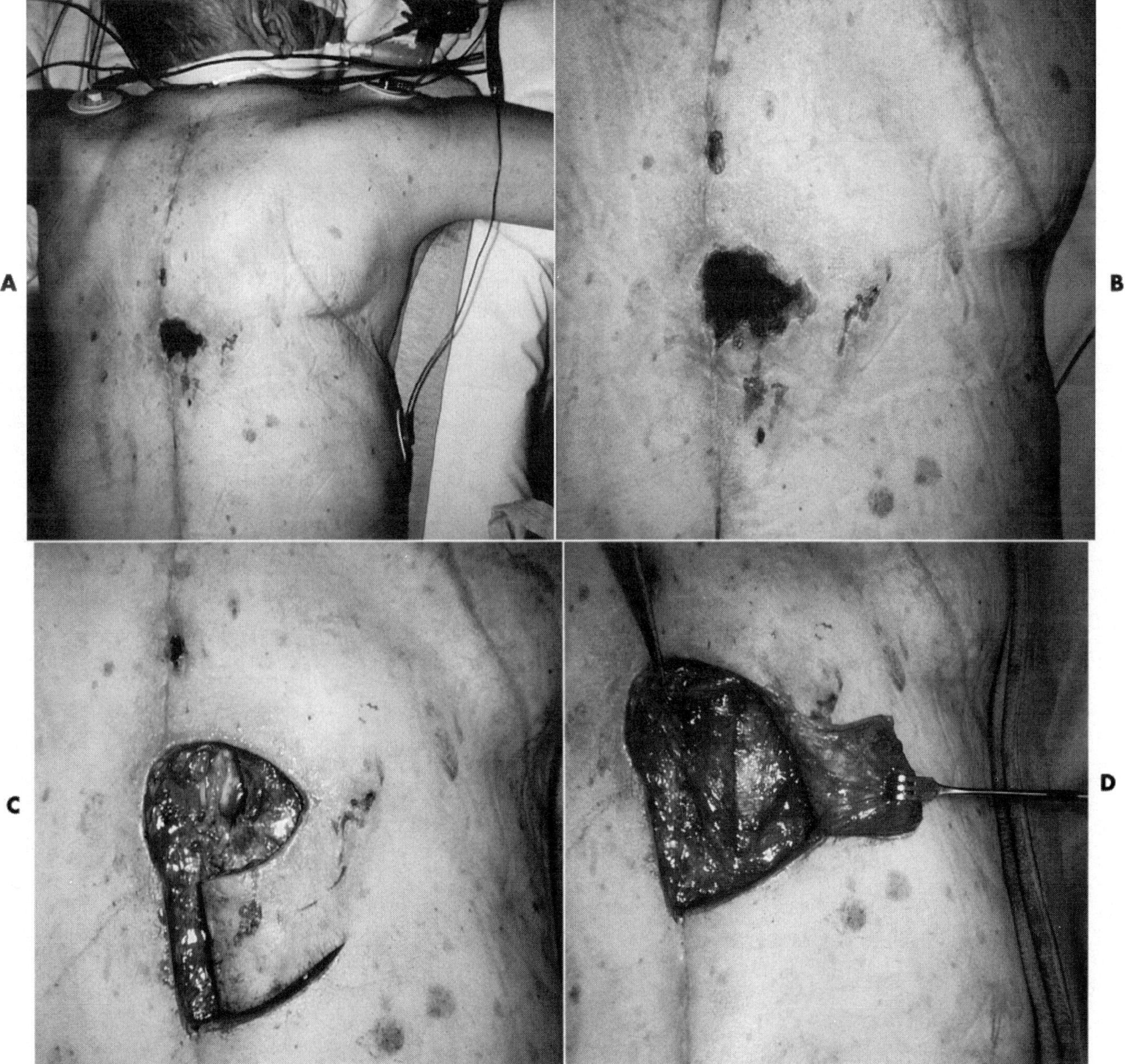


**FIGURE 36-6**

Example of a transverse back flap after full-thickness skin slough through previously irradiated tissue. **A, B,** Skin and deep tissue slough. **C,** Debrided tissue. **D,** Muscle and skin pedicle prepared. *Continued*

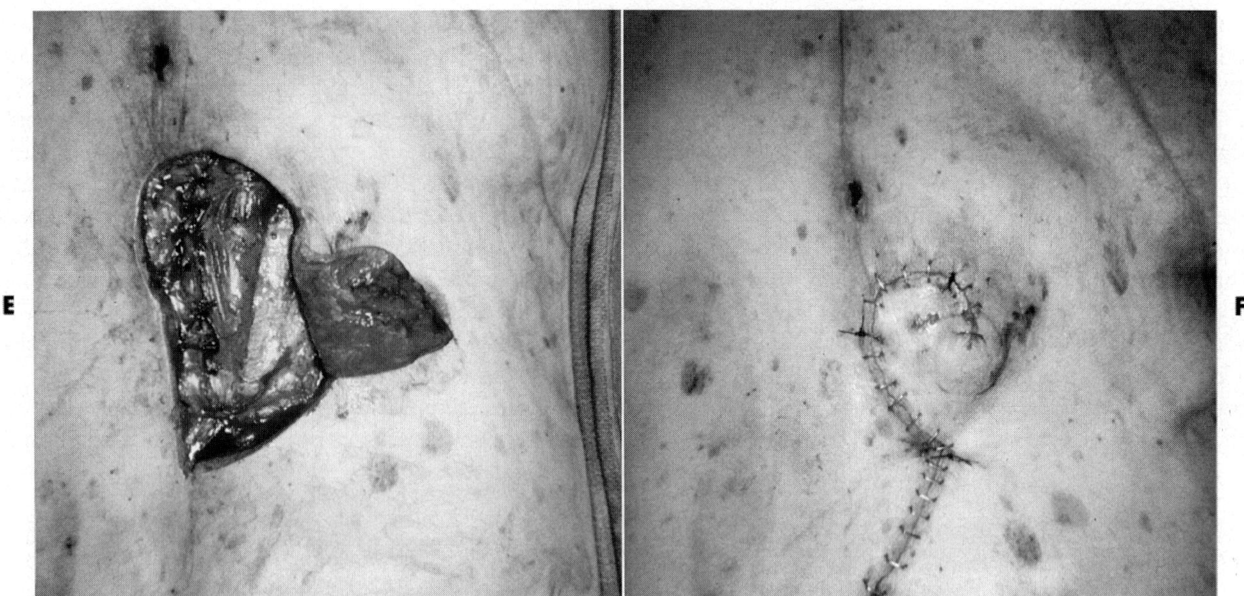


**FIGURE 36-6, CONT'D**

**E,** Muscle and skin pedicle prepared. **F,** Wound closure.

tion of the local skin and underlying fascia often preclude the design of reliable random pattern flaps. The transverse back flap is based on perforating musculocutaneous vessels through the paraspinous muscles (Figs. 36-5 and 36-6). When used in a delayed fashion, this fasciocutaneous flap can provide ample coverage in salvage situations.

Occasionally, skin closure is not possible while adequate underlying soft tissue closure has been achieved. Closing the skin under tension leads to predictable wound edge necrosis. In these situations skin grafts are useful. Split-thickness skin grafts are useful as long as the areas covered are not mobile. Bolster dressings are used to reduce shear between the graft and its bed.

Several additional technical elements must be considered when treating wounds in radiated tissue given their propensity for poor wound healing and infection. Avoid extensive undermining of flap edges to minimize disruption of the vascular anatomy of the skin. The volume of deep suture should be minimal to reduce the foreign body load. We prefer nonbraided, long-lasting absorbable sutures such as PDS for the deeper subcutaneous closure or the insetting of muscle flaps. Nonreactive suture material (monofilament or staples) is preferred for the skin closure. Skin sutures are left in place for a significantly longer period of time, often 4 to 6 weeks. Closed suction drains are placed to help avoid seromas, and antibiotics are given while the drains remain indwelling. And finally, avoidance of postoperative pressure to the repair site is accomplished using pressure relief beds and appropriate patient positioning.

## ACKNOWLEDGMENT

We thank Dr. James Hoehn for his contribution of Figures 36-1 and 36-2 and Ms. Rosemary Lombardo for her clerical assistance.

## REFERENCES

1. Alpaslan AM, Acarolgu RE, Kis M: Three stage excision of recurrent cervical chondrosarcoma, *Arch Orthop Trauma Surg* 112(5):245-246, 1993.
2. Bauer HC, Wedin R: Survival after surgery for spinal and extremity metastasis, *Acta Orthop Scand* 66(2):143-146, 1995.
3. Bauer HC: Posterior decompression and stabilization for spinal metastasis, *J Bone Joint Surg* 79A(4):514-522, 1997.
4. Bridwell KH, Jenny AB, Saul T, Rich KM, Grubb RL: Posterior segmental spinal instrumentation with posterolateral metastatic thoracic and lumbar spine disease: Limitations of the technique, *Spine* 13(12):1383-1394, 1988.

5. Camins MB, Duncan AW, Smith J, Marcove RC: Chondrosarcoma of the spine. *Spine* 3(3):202-209, 1978.
6. Cervoni L, Celli P, Salvati M, Tarantino R, Fortuna A: Solitary plasmacytoma of the spine: relationship of IGM to tumour progression and recurrence, *Acta Neurochirurgica* 135:122-125, 1995.
7. Dahlin DC: *Bone tumors: general aspects and data on 6,221 cases,* Springfield, IL, 1978, Charles C. Thomas, p 11.
8. Delamarter RB, Sachs BL, Thompson GH, Bohlman HH, Makley JT, Carter JR: Primary neoplasms of the thoracic and lumbar spine, *Clin Orthop* 256:87-100, 1990.
9. Fagundes MA, Hug EB, Liebsch NJ, Daly W, Efind J, Munzenrider JE: Radiation therapy for chordomas of the base of the skull and cervical spine patterns of failure and outcome after relapse, *Int J Rad Oncol Bio Phys* 33(3) 579-584, 1995.
10. Galasko CSB: Spinal instability secondary to metastatic cancer, *J Bone Joint Surg* 73B:104-108, 1991.
11. Gennari L, Azzarelli A, Quagliuolo V: A posterior approach for excision of sacral cordoma, *J Bone Joint Surg* 69B(4):565-568, 1987.
12. Hall AJ, Mackay NNS: The results of laminectomy for compression of the cord or cauda equina by extradural malignant tumor, *J Bone Joint Surg* 55B(3):497-505, 1973.
13. Harrington KD: The use of methylmethacrylate for vertebral body replacement and anterior stabilization of pathological fracture dislocations of the spine due to metastatic malignant disease, *J Bone Joint Surg* 63A(1): 36-46, 1981.
14. Harrington KD: Anterior decompression and stabilization of the spine as a treatment for vertebral collapse of spinal cord compression for metastatic malignancy, *Clin Orthop* 233:177-197, 1988.
15. Hay MC, Paterson D, Taylor TK: Aneurysmal bone cysts of the spine, *J Bone Joint Surg* 60B(3):406-411, 1978.
16. Hirsh LF, Thanki A, Spector HB: Primary spinal chondrosarcoma with eighteen year follow-up: case report and literature review, *Neurosurgery* 14(6):747-749, 1984.
17. Jonsson B, Sjostrom L, Jonsson H, Karlstrom G: Surgery for multiple myeloma of the spine, *Acta Orthop Scand* 63(2):192-194, 1992.
18. Kaiser TE, Pritchard DJ, Unni KK: Clinicopathologic study of sacrococcygeal chordoma, *Cancer* 54:2574-2578, 1984.
19. King GJ, Kostuik JP, McBroom RJ, Richardson W: Surgical management of metastatic renal carcinoma of the spine, *Spine* 16(3):265-271, 1991.
20. Kostuik J: The development of a preoperative scoring assessment system of metastatic spine disease diagnosing impending pathologic fracture, 32d Scoliosis Research Society Annual Meeting abstract, September, 1997.
21. Marcove RC, Sheth DS, Brein EW, Huvos AG, Healey JH: Conservative surgery for giant cell tumors of the sacrum, *Cancer* 74(4):1253-1260, 1994.
22. McAfee PC, Bohlman HH, Ducker T, Eismont FJ: Failure of stabilization of the spine with methylmethacrylate. A retrospective analysis of twenty-four cases, *J Bone Joint Surg* 68A(8):1145-1157, 1986.
23. McLain RF, Kabins M, Weinstein JN: VSP stabilization of lumbar neoplasms: technical considerations and complications, *J Spinal Disord* 4(3):359-365, 1991.
24. Nicholls PJ, Jarecky TW: The value of posterior decompression by laminectomy for malignant tumors of the spine, *Clin Orthop* 201:210-213, 1985.
25. Onimus M, Schraub S, Bertin D, Bosset JF, Guidat M. Surgical treatment of vertebral metastasis, *Spine* 11(9):883-896, 1986.
26. Reif J, Graf N: Intraspinal mesenchymal chondrosarcoma in a three-year-old boy, *Neurosurg Rev* 10(4): 311-314, 1987.
27. Rompe JD, Eysel P, Hopf C, Heine J: Decompression stabilization of the metastatic spine. *Acta Orthop Scand* 64(1):3-8, 1993.
28. Shektman A, Granick MS, Solomon MP, Black P, Nair S: Management of infected laminectomy wounds, *Neurosurgery* 35(2):307-309, 1984.
29. Shinomiya K, Furuya K, Mutoh N: Desmoplastic fibroma in the thoracic spine, *J Spinal Disord* 4(2):229-233, 1991.
30. Siegal T, Tiqua P, Siegal T: Vertebral body resection for epidural compression by malignant tumors, *J Bone Joint Surg* 67A(3):375-382, 1985.
31. Sonntag VK, Herman JM: Reoperation of the cervical spine for degenerative disease and tumor. *Clin Neurosurg* 39:244-269, 1992.
32. Steib JP, Pierchon F, Farey JP, Lang G, Christmann D, Ghassia JP: Epitheloid sarcoma of the spine, *Spine* 21(5):634-638, 1996.
33. Stener B, Johnsen DE: Complete removal of three vertebra for giant cell tumor, *J Bone Joint Surg* 53B:278-287, 1971.
34. Sundaresan N, Galicich JH, Bains MS, Martini N, Beattie EJ: Vertebral body resection in the treatment of cancer involving the spine, *Cancer* 53:1393-1396, 1984.
35. Sundaresan N, Galicich JH, Lane JM: Harrington rod stabilization for pathological fractures of the spine, *J Neurosurg* 60:282-286, 1984.
36. Tokuhashi Y, Matsuzaki H, Toriyama S, Kawano H, Ohsaka S: Scoring system for the preoperative evaluation of metastatic spine tumor prognosis, *Spine* 15(11):1110-1113, 1990.
37. Tomita K, Kawahara N, Baba H, et al: Total en bloc spondylectomy for solitary spinal metastasis, *Int Orthop* 18:291-298, 1994.
38. Turner PL, Prince HG, Webb JK, Sokal MPJW: Surgery for malignant extradural tumours of the spine, *J Bone Joint Surg* 70B(3):451-456, 1988.
39. Weinstein JN, McLain RF: Primary tumors of the spine, *Spine* 12(9):843-851, 1987.

# 37

# REVISIONS IN SPINE TUMOR SURGERY

William O. Shaffer, M.D.



Revisions of previously resected spine tumors are rarely undertaken but may be successful if proper evaluation and planning is done. This chapter defines a rational approach to such planning. The understanding of the biology of the tumor is of utmost importance. The surgeon must have a thorough understanding of the anatomy of the involved region. Whether a tumor can be resected is just one issue, one must then reconstruct the defect. This frequently requires the services of a plastic surgeon and other surgical subspecialists.

## CLASSIFICATION

Classification of primary bone tumors and neural tumors is extremely important to understanding the biological nature of the tumor. The character of the tumor must be appreciated to make a proper approach to the tumor. Dr. Fritz Schajowicz[10] helped develop the World Health Organization's classification of bone tumors to categorize lesions (Table 37-1). It has become one of the standard classifications for approaching bone tumors and should be used in the decision-making concerning surgical revision of previously resected primary spinal tumors. The following literature review will highlight the importance of tumor classification.

### BACKGROUND LITERATURE

In Weinstein and McLain's series,[12] 82 primary neoplasms of the spine covered over a 50-year period of spine tumor treatment of the University of Iowa. There were 31 benign and 51 malignant tumors. There were few revision resections. Follow-up of the benign lesions was 9.7 years and the malignant lesions was 3.8 years. The lesions were seen on the plain x-rays in 81 of the 82 cases, or 99%. Malignancies occurred at an older age. The 5-year survival rate for benign tumors was 86%. The 5-year survival rate in the malignant group correlated with the extent of the initial surgery and tumor type. Curettage in the malignant group had a 5-year survival rate of 0%. Incomplete resections had an 18.7% 5-year survival rate. A complete excision resulted in a 75% 5-year survival rate. Weinstein and McLain emphasized that radiograms were necessary for persistent and atypical back pain and neurological symptoms. They argued that surgical extirpation with aggressive removal of malignant and aggressively benign lesions should be accomplished.

Malawski[9] reported on a series of 72 primary spinal tumors. Fifty-seven malignant and 15 benign tumors were treated at the Warsaw Postgraduate Medical Education Academy between 1961 and 1987. Malawski emphasized principles of excision of the tumor, decompression of the nerve elements, and stabilization of the spine. Repeat resections of tumors were not discussed. There were no deaths in the benign group and clinical results were generally good. In the malignant group, 42 died, 17 dying within one year. Twenty-five patients survived over 1 year. 15 patients were alive with mean survival of 5 years and 3 months. Improvement in neurological disturbance

**Table 37-1. WHO Classification of Bone Tumors and Tumor-like Lesions**

**I. BONE-FORMING TUMORS**
**A. Benign**
1. Osteoma
2. Osteoid osteoma and osteoblastoma
**B. Intermediate**
1. Aggressive (malignant) osteoblastoma
**C. Malignant**
1. Osteosarcoma
 a. Central (medullary)
  1. Conventional central
  2. Telangiectatic
  3. Intraosseous well-differentitated (low-grade)
  4. Round-cell
 b. Surface (peripheral)
  1. Parosteal
  2. Periosteal
  3. High-grade surface

**II. CARTILAGE-FORMING TUMORS**
**A. Benign**
1. Chondroma
 a. Enchondroma
 b. Periosteal (juxtacortical)
2. Osteochondroma
 (Osteocartilaginous exostosis)
 a. Solitary
 b. Multiple hereditary
3. Chondroblastoma
 (Epiphyseal chondroblastoma)
4. Chondromyxoid fibroma
**B. Malignant**
1. Chondrosarcoma
2. Juxtacortical (periosteal) chondrosarcoma
3. Mesenchymal chondrosarcoma
4. Dedifferentiated chondrosarcoma
5. Clear-cell chondrosarcoma
6. Malignant chondroblastoma?

**III. GIANT-CELL TUMOR (OSTEOCLASTOMA)**

**IV. MARROW TUMORS (ROUND CELL TUMORS)**
1. Ewing sarcoma of bone
2. Neuroectodermal tumor of bone
3. Malignant lymphoma of bone
4. Myeloma

**V. VASCULAR TUMORS**
**A. Benign**
1. Hemangioma
2. Lymphangioma
3. Glomus tumor (glomangioma)
**B. Intermediate or Indeterminate**
1. Hemangioendothelioma
 (Epithelioid hemangioendothelioma, histiocytoid hemangioma)
2. Hemangiopericytoma
**C. Malignant**
1. Angiosarcoma
 (Malignant hemangioendothelioma hemangiosarcoma, hemangioendotheliosarcoma)
2. Malignant hemangiopericytoma

**VI. OTHER CONNECTIVE TISSUE TUMORS**
**A. Benign**
1. Benign fibrous histiocytoma
2. Lipoma
**B. Intermediate**
1. Desmoplastic fibroma
**C. Malignant**
1. Fibrosarcoma
2. Malignant fibrous histiocytoma
3. Liposarcoma
4. Malignant mesenchymoma
5. Leiomyosarcoma
6. Undifferentiated sarcoma

**VII. OTHER TUMORS**
1. Chordoma
2. Adamantinoma of long bones
3. Neurilemmoma
4. Neurofibroma

**VIII. UNCLASSIFIED TUMORS**

**IX. TUMOR-LIKE LESIONS**
1. Solitary bone cyst
 (Simple or unicameral bone cyst)
2. Aneurysmal bone cyst
3. Juxta-articular bone cyst
 (Intraosseous ganglion)
4. Metaphyseal fibrous defect
 (Non-ossifying fibroma)
5. Eosinophilic granuloma
 (histiocytosis X, Langerhans cell granulomatosis)
6. Fibrous dysplasia and osteofibrous dysplasia
7. Myositis ossificans
 (Heterotopic ossification)
8. "Brown tumor" of hyperparathyroidism
9. Intraosseous epidermoid cyst
10. Giant cell (reparative) granuloma

From Schajowicz F, McDonald DJ: Classification of tumors and tumor lesions of the spine, *State of the Arts Review* 10(1), 1-11, 1996.

after decompression was a predictor of good outcome of these patients.

Dreghorn et al[5] noted 55 cases of axial skeleton involvement in a tumor registry of 1,950 cases. Chordoma was found to be the most frequent tumor both in the cervical and sacral spine. Osteosarcoma ranked second. Pain was the most frequent presenting symptom with 50% of the patients presenting with a neurologic abnormality. Survival was poor with all malignant lesions. Neurologic involvement was a predictor of poor outcome. Neurologic involvement was seen in 68 patients with malignant tumors and 28% of those with benign tumors. In the cervical spine, the most common tumor was chordoma. Osteosarcoma was the second-most frequent diagnosis, with 63% of those cases arising in preexisting pagetoid bone. Of the patients with spinal cord decompression, 10 died at a mean of 2.3 years. Though multiple myeloma was previously noted as the most common primary spinal neoplasm, Dreghorn included only cases that were truly solitary plasmocytomas that had not later developed into multiple myeloma. Dreghorn noted that primary malignant spinal tumors were associated with very high mortality figures with a mean survival of only 7 months. Chordoma and plasmacytoma had mean survivals of more than 7 years. The most difficult tumors to define were the malignant round cell tumors including Ewing sarcoma, neuroblastoma, and intradural tumors.

Delamarter et al[3] looked at 29 primary osseous tumors of the spine, 8 occurring in children and 21 in adults. Back pain was present in 25 of the 29 patients with an 86% prevalence rate. Neurologic symptoms were present in 55% and all lesions were noted on the spine radiogram. There were 11 benign and 18 malignant lesions. Laminectomy alone frequently resulted in late instability and neurological deterioration. Resection and decompression combined with arthrodesis did not compromise spinal stability. Eight of the 18 patients with malignant disease died within 1 to 7 months after the diagnosis. An accurate histiologic diagnosis was imperative and was best achieved by open biopsy prior to definitive procedure. Adequate and aggressive resection of malignant lesions was required for tumor control.

Benign tumors frequently can be treated with intralesional and marginal excisions. Those tumors that are intermediate grade require a radical resection, and malignant tumors, even with wide and radical excisions, can be expected to recur.

Boriani et al[1] reviewed 366 primary spinal tumors, which he classified as "benign" and "aggressive" tumors. The benign tumors were further broken down into latent tumors that did not require treatment, and active tumors that were treated with curettage. Aggressive tumors were treated with marginal resection or curettage plus adjuvants. Malignant lesions were classified as low grade or high grade. Wide resection was attempted whenever feasible. Of the 216 surgically treated patients, 161 underwent an oncologic procedure. Intralesional margins were achieved in 154, a narrow margin in 4 and wide margin in 3. The procedures included vertebrectomy, corpectomy, posterior resection, and simple excision and capsular curettage. In this paper, interestingly, giant cell tumors were treated with either curettage or marginal resection. Marginal resections were found to give the best results. Benign lesions treated by intralesional resections showed satisfactory results. Excision of chordomas, and chondrosarcomas were always followed by recurrence. Boriani concluded that in the treatment of primary bone tumors of the spine, it was necessary to avoid partial removal of the tumor. However, an overly aggressive procedure could lead to risks and neural complications.

Celli et al[2] looked at malignant peripheral nerve sheath spinal tumors with six cases of malignant primary spinal schwannomas. Postoperative outcome was generally poor, especially in von Recklinghausen disease and local recurrence and metastases were possible even after radical surgery and radiotherapy. They discussed that over 50% of the patients with peripheral nerve tumors had von Recklinghausen disease. They emphasized that preoperative diagnosis of malignancy was difficult to obtain by imaging studies alone. The vertebral location in relationship to the dura could not be used as a predictor of the aggressiveness of the tumor. They discussed a poor prognosis from primary malignant schwannomas with local recurrences up to 71% and a 5-year survival of only 23%. They emphasized that incomplete removal of the tumor caused the worst prognosis. Postoperative radiotherapy was required even in those tumors that were felt to be fully excised.

Grubb et al[8] reviewed 36 patients with primary Ewing's sarcoma of the spine treated at the Mayo Clinic. This study looked at 37 years of experience of Ewing's sarcoma of the spine in 36 patients. Back pain was the most common presenting symptom. Neurologic symptoms and signs were noted in 58% of the patients. Forty-seven percent had open biopsy and underwent decompressive laminectomy. Three of the four thoracolumbar laminectomy patients showed progressive postoperative kyphosis. Thirty-two patients were treated by intensive chemotherapy. Nine patients were free of disease. The study showed 5-year survival rates of 33% with a mean survival rate of 2.9%. There was no obvious relationship between primary site, local recurrence, and disease-free survival. They felt that in the treatment of Ewing's sarcoma, the roll of surgery remained controversial. Anyone undergoing laminectomy for Ewing's sarcoma needs to be followed very closely for the development of kyphosis.

DiLorenzo et al[4] reviewed 38 primary tumors in

the cervical spine treated at the University of Rome. The aims of their surgical treatment plan were complete tumor removal, decompression of the spinal cord, conservation of spinal stability, and restoration of vertebral stability when destabilization procedures are required. They emphasized that in planning the correct surgical strategy, the biology of the lesion needed to be understood. The longitudinal and transverse involvement of the body needed to be appreciated by computed tomography (CT) studies. Preoperative stability and the likelihood of postoperative instability needed to be understood. Biopsy was frequently difficult to obtain without compromising resection. For this reason, they felt it was difficult to obtain oncologic or biologic information on spinal neoplasms. For benign tumors with low neoplastic potential and for malignant tumors with poor life expectancy, they recommended conservative removal. They recommended radical removal for aggressive benign tumors such as osteoblastoma and giant cell tumor and for malignant tumors with reasonably good life expectancy, such as plasmacytoma or chordoma. They recommended a fairly nonaggressive approach for all other malignant tumors of the cervical spine. Overall, the sarcomas had very poor results.

## ANATOMIC CONCERNS

The anatomic detail of the tumor is critical in deciding the resectability of a tumor. In revisions, this becomes even more important. When considering a reresection, the tissue planes, vascular structures, and neural components contaminated by the original resection must be clearly identified. For instance, a segmental vessel is easily included in a resection in which resection of a major vessel such as the iliac or femoral artery and vein require extensive vascular reconstruction to allow full resection. In a similar vein, nerve roots must be sacrificed if involved in the original resection bed of a malignant tumor. However, if the malignant tumor involves the intraspinal dura or cord curative radical resection may be impossible. It is important to also understand regional differences of a primary spinal tumor in etiologic terms and natural history. As an example, a chordoma arising in C2 and a chordoma arising in the sacrum share biologic behavior but require dramatically different approaches and skills to resect each tumor. These anatomic considerations are crucial in the appropriate surgical planning and approaching of a spinal tumor.

The presence of the tumor in the anterior versus the posterior aspect of the spine also dictates the approach and the planning for surgical resection. The location of the tumor within the vertebral body whether it be in the pedicle, the arch, or in the anterior body also dictates changes in surgical planning. Weinstein's zones (Fig. 37-1) are helpful in determining the approach and the extent of the spinal column resection, and help dictate reconstructive attempts. For example, the I B zone tumors frequently can be treated by traditional laminectomy and wide radical resection of the tumor. Tumors in zone II additionally can be resected with radical excision and wide margins but by necessity require reconstruction of the posterior stability of the spine. Those tumors in zone III A will allow wide marginal excision, though zone III B tumors become very difficult to manage with radical curative tumor resection because of the important neurovascular structures adjacent to the zone. Of course, one needs to fully search for regional and distal metastasis prior to undertaking reresection of the tumor. Due to the proximity of the spinal cord and neural elements, malignant Zone IV tumors are unresectable.

Regional issues must be taken into account. Thompson et al[11] discussed a group of 14 patients presenting with primary pelvic girdle malignancies with presentation suggestive of low-back pain and sciatica. The tumors included 6 chondrosarcomas, 5 osteosarcomas, and 4 malignant fibrous histiocytomas. Thompson emphasized that patients with sciatica and low back pain be evaluated for pelvic girdle malignancy with CT and magnetic resonance imaging

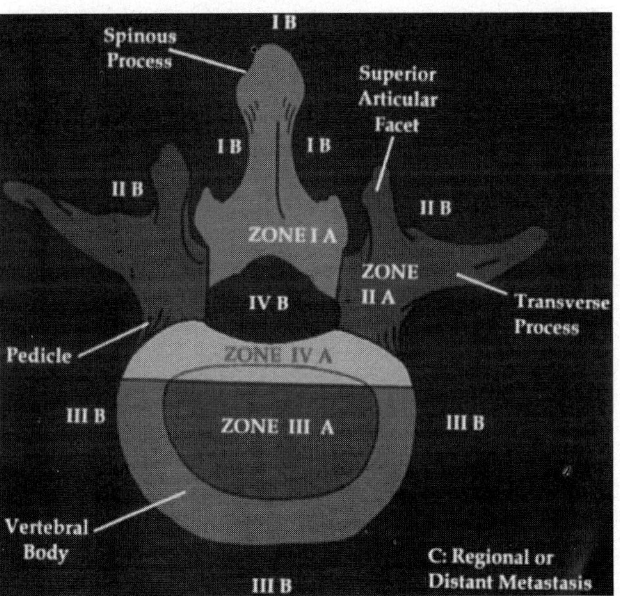


**FIGURE 37-1**

Weinstein zones. Zone I are superficial posterior elements; the lamina is zone I A, zone I B is the spinous process. Zone II are the deep posterior elements, the pedicle is zone II A and the transverse process is zone II B. Zone III B is the anterior column, the centrum of the body is zone III A, and the cortex of the body is III B. Zone IV is the middle column (IV A), the neural canal (IV B), and regional or distant metastasis (IV C). *(From Weinstein JN, McLain RF: Primary tumors of the spine,* Spine *12(a):843-851, 1987.)*

(MRI). Sacral resections require a working knowledge of the anatomy of the perineum, rectum, and sacral roots. Ebrahim et al[5] presented an anatomical study of 20 adult cadavers defining the relationship of the lumbosacral plexus to the anterior sacral spine. It is a helpful paper in sacral resections.

Grillo et al[7] discussed the problems with excising neurogenic tumors through laminectomy alone or inadvertent encounter of neurogenic dumbbell tumors in thoracic procedures. They argue that a combined thoracic and spinal surgeon approach allowed excision of both components of the tumor in a single operation through a single incision. Our center has had similar experience with neurogenic tumors. A two-surgeon approach offers better control of the tumor in this complex region.

## RISK OF BIOPSIES

In the situation of reresecting a spinal tumor, the previous surgical pathology is definitely available. It is important that all pathologic material be reviewed ahead of time for the accuracy of diagnosis and to better understand the full character of the tumor. Frequently the biopsy itself may compromise the approach to the tumor, and at this point the tumor resection becomes a revision (Fig. 37-2). When an intralesional biopsy or a needle biopsy has gone astray and has contaminated uninvolved structures, that needs to be addressed at the time of the resection. Inappropriately handled biopsy not infrequently dictates a wider resection than originally needed. Suffice it to say that all pathological material needs to be reviewed in detail in conjunction with the tumor team, the orthopaedic oncologist, the bone pathologist, and the spinal surgeon. In revision work, this team approach is essential.

## RESECTION OF TUMORS

The character of the tumor is an important consideration in understanding the ability to reresect a tumor. In Weinstein and McLain's[12] review of 82 cases of primary tumors of the spine, the presentation of the patient was identical between benign and malignant groups in terms of localized back pain and radicular pain. The presence of neurologic lesions and rapidly progressive neurologic lesions were most notable in the malignancy group. The onset of symptoms prior to presentation for the malignancy was 10.4 months and benign lesions 19.3 months. Ninety-nine percent were noted on the initial radiographs. The 5-year survival rate for benign tumors was 86%; however, 21% of the tumors recurred, and in the giant cell tumors 66% had local recurrence with adverse outcomes including a malignant transformation and death. In the malignant tumor group slow-growing, locally aggressive tumors were noted to have a greater overall survival. Solitary plasmacytoma and chondrosarcomas had the best survival rates and osteosarcoma and lymphoma showed the worst survival rates of the groups. In this paper, the survival of malignant tumors was directly related with the adequacy of the excision. There were no 5-year survivors with the curettage-only group. Compete excision of the lesion improved 5-year survival rate to 75%.

Weinstein's study documented that the character of the tumor, its aggressiveness, the resection, and the natural history of the tumor all must be taken into account prior to adequately planning the surgical

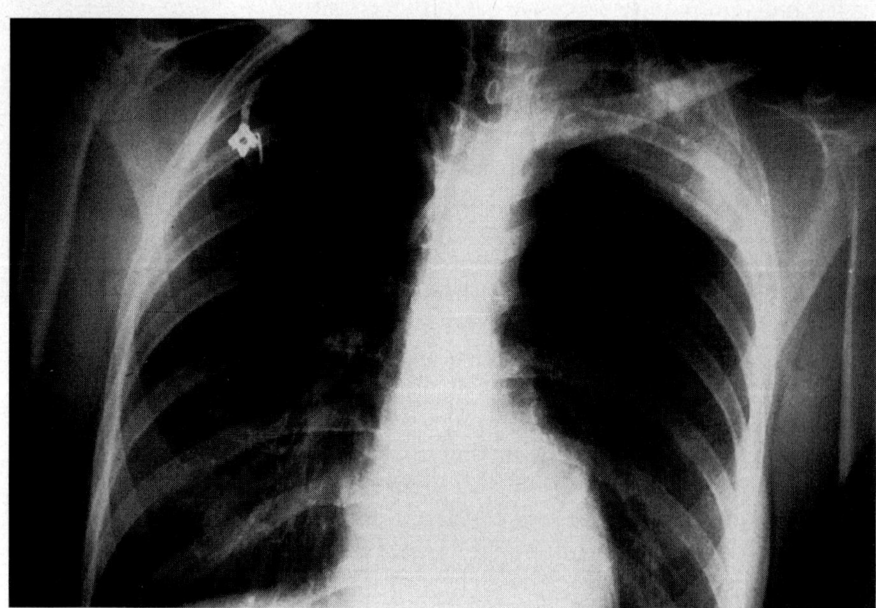

**FIGURE 37-2**

Errors in biopsy can result in a more complex resection. This case of a second-rib osteosarcoma was complicated by normal lung being noted on the biopsy slides. Note the size of the tumor involving the upper four ribs and adjacent to T1-T3. The upper lobe of the lung required resection along with the tumor mass.

approach. With this in mind, an algorithm for the approach to primary spine tumors should be used to help properly stage the tumor and to answer the question of whether or not adequate reexcision with or without adjuvant treatment will be successful (Fig. 37-3).

## NATURAL HISTORY

The natural history of the tumor is another important consideration in approaching these difficult tumors. Dreghorn, in his review of 55 cases of primary bone tumors of the axial skeleton, noted that those tumors of malignant origin, and neurologic involvement, had poor outcomes and poor survival. Their most common tumor was chordoma and the most frequent tumor in both the cervical and sacral spine and was noted to have a slow-growing character. They found that both plasmacytoma and chordoma had long-term survivals well into 7 years as opposed to other malignant tumors, which had very high mortality rates with a mean survival of osteosarcoma less than 7 months. The other important factor in this paper showed that of the 11 cases of spinal cord compres-

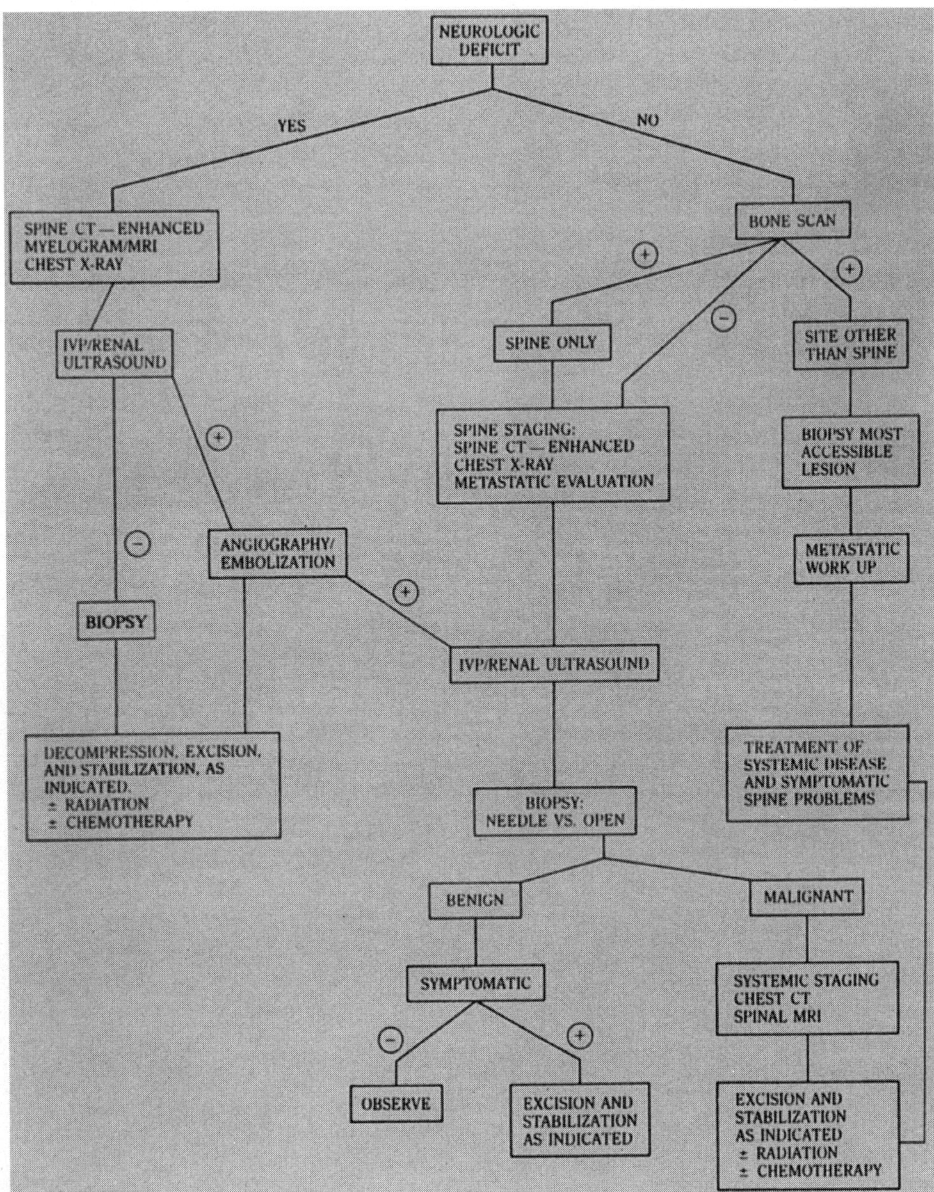


**FIGURE 37-3**

Weinstein's Algorithm. Recommended for primary spinal tumors, this algorithm is useful for revision work if one considers any tissue plans violated by the original procedure as tumor. *(From Weinstein JN: Primary and benign and malignant neoplasms. In Frymoyer, editor:* The adult spine, *1991, Philadelphia, Lippincott-Raven, pp 848-849, 851.)*

sion, 10 eventually died from their disease. The one survivor had an osteoblastoma with 7-year survival. This would seem to indicate that the location of the tumor in relationship to the neurovascular structures was also important in dictating the success or failure of adequate resection. To illustrate these concepts is a case of neurofibrosarcoma, which had been previously resected twice with local recurrence and fungating of the tumor through the excision scars. Review of the pathology showed a highly aggressive neurofibrosarcoma; however, the tumor appeared the size of a grapefruit adjacent to the spine and was limited to the erector spinae arising from neural roots. Figure 37-4 clearly shows, on MRI, the anatomic location of the tumor in relationship to the neural structures. In this case, a resection was performed by a contralateral laminectomy through an incision away from the primary tumor mass. Simultaneously, an anterior approach skirted the anterior margins of the tumor. Finally, the roots at L2, L3, and L4 were ligated and divided. An osteotomy of the L2 and L3 vertebral bodies, medial to the pedicle and the anterior lateral cortices, allowed a clear margin and block resection of the tumor. The spine was then stabilized with an anterior-posterior fusion reconstruction using allograft fibula and an anterior Kaneda device and posterior Isola rod (Fig. 37-5). The soft tissue reconstruction required surgical mesh and a latissimus dorsi flap to close the defect. The surgical margins were clear of tumor. An adequate resection of the tumor had been accomplished; however, the patient became acutely paraplegic within a month and further evaluation showed a large recurrent tumor in the midthoracic cord above the resection site. The patient subsequently succumbed to his very aggressive disease (Fig. 37-6).

## ANATOMIC RESECTION CONSIDERATIONS

One of the important decisions in resecting these tumors is whether or not neurovascular structures must be sacrificed to obtain an adequate margin. The tumor may be truly nonresectable. It is clear from Weinstein and McLain[12] and Malawski[9] that the results of surgical treatment of primary malignant spine tumors by intralesional curettage result in poor outcomes. Additionally, those patients presented with neurologic findings have poor outcomes because the tumor usually can not be resected with a wide margin; however, there are those tumors that do present in or near the spine that are amenable to aggressive surgical treatment without becoming intralesional. An example of this approach is a case of osteosarcoma of the ribs with the tumor abutting up against the zone II and lateral zone III of the upper thoracic spine (Figs. 37-2 and 37-7, *A*). This case was complicated by the biopsy that confirmed the diagnosis of osteosarcoma of the rib but normal tissue was found in the biopsy material (Fig. 37-7, *B*). In conjunction with an orthopedic oncologist, a cardiothoracic surgeon, and plastic surgeon, the spinal surgeon resected the tumor. The upper four ribs

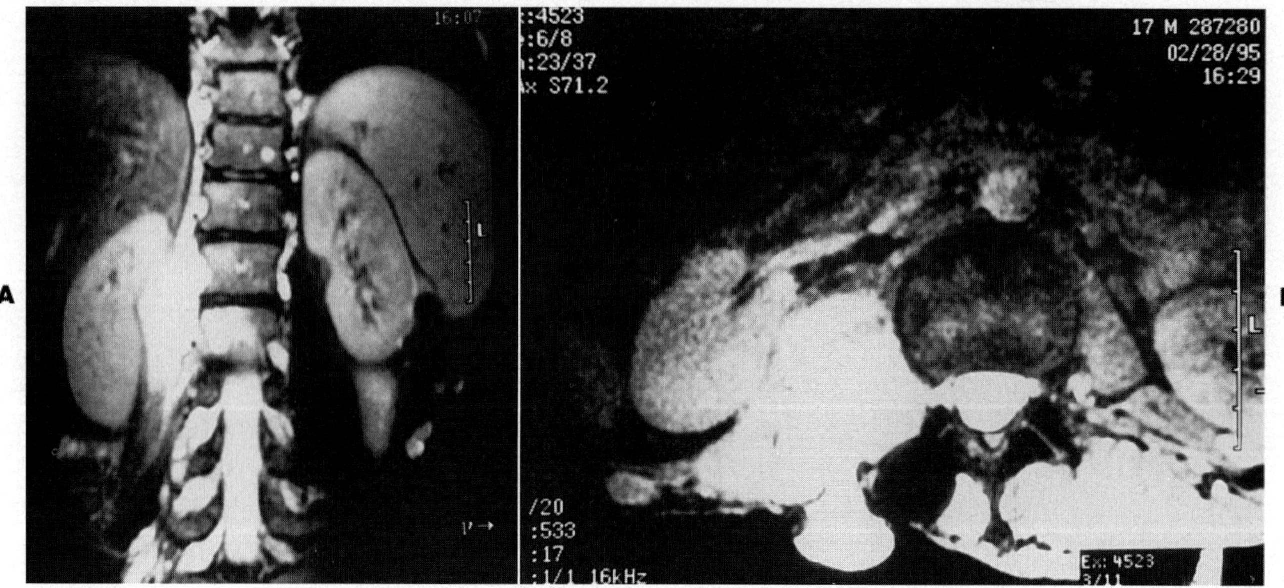


**FIGURE 37-4**

**A,** Neurofibrosarcoma, coronal view. The tumor is adjacent the spine at the level of the right kidney. **B,** Axial view: The tumor involves mostly the soft tissue adjacent to the spine though zone II B, the right transverse process, is involved. The renal capsule is not invaded. The cortex, zone III B, is intact as is zone II A. Importantly zone IV is clear of tumor. *(From Kossimic, Weinstein JN: Metastatic tumors. In Frymoyer, editor:* The adult spine, *1991, Philadelphia, Lippincott-Raven, p 864.)*

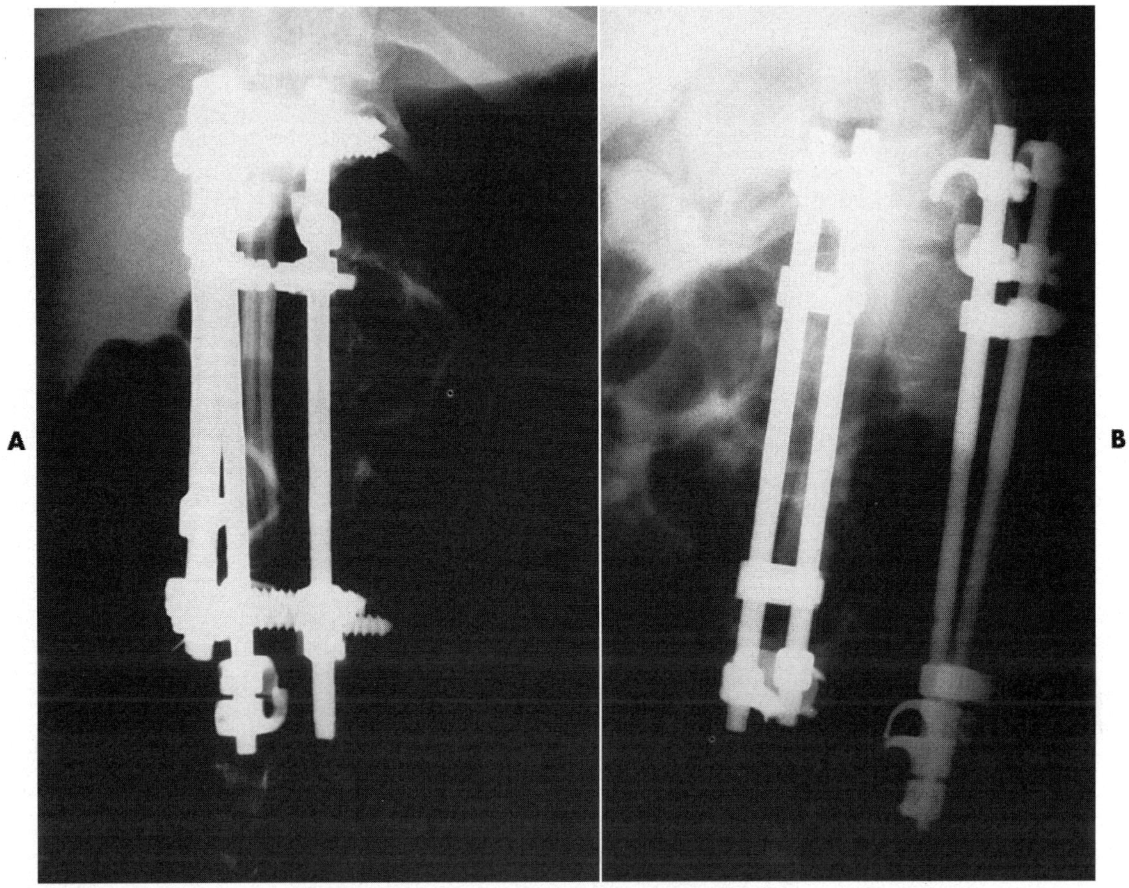

FIGURE 37-5

**A,** Reconstruction. AP view shows the fibular strut graft between L1 and L4. The graft is locked into place with an anterior Kaneda device spanning L1 to L4. **B,** Posteriorly a L1 to L5 Isola rod construct is placed by the second surgeon operating simultaneously. A posterior L1 to L5 fusion was accomplished.

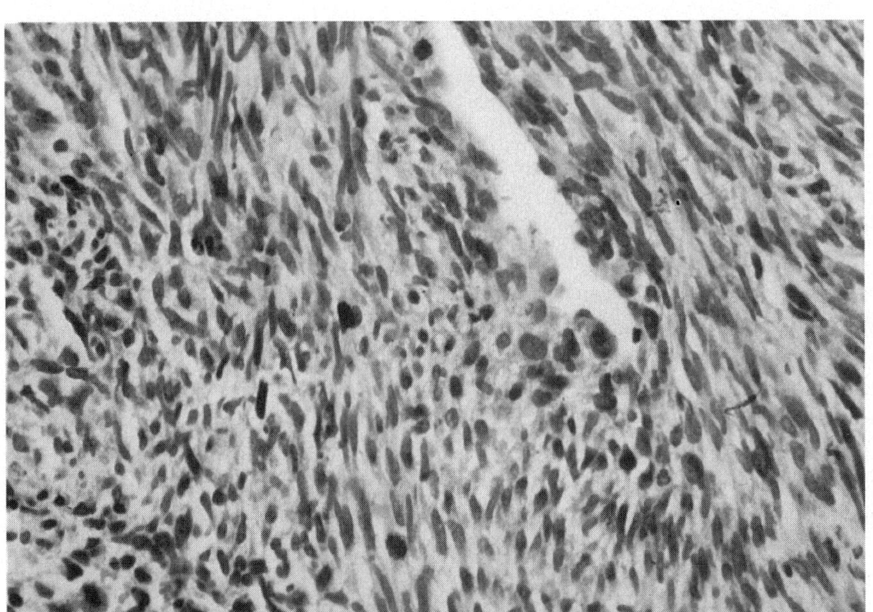

FIGURE 37-6

Photomicrograph of the resected neurofibrosarcoma. Note the aggressive appearance of the tumor with many darkly staining nuclei, mitotic figures, and pleomorphism. *(From Shaffer WO: Anterior column surgery in spinal tumors. In Devlin VJ, editor: Anterior Spinal Column Surgery,* Spine: State of the Art Reviews *12(3):611-624, 1998, Philadelphia, Hanley & Beflus, Inc.)*

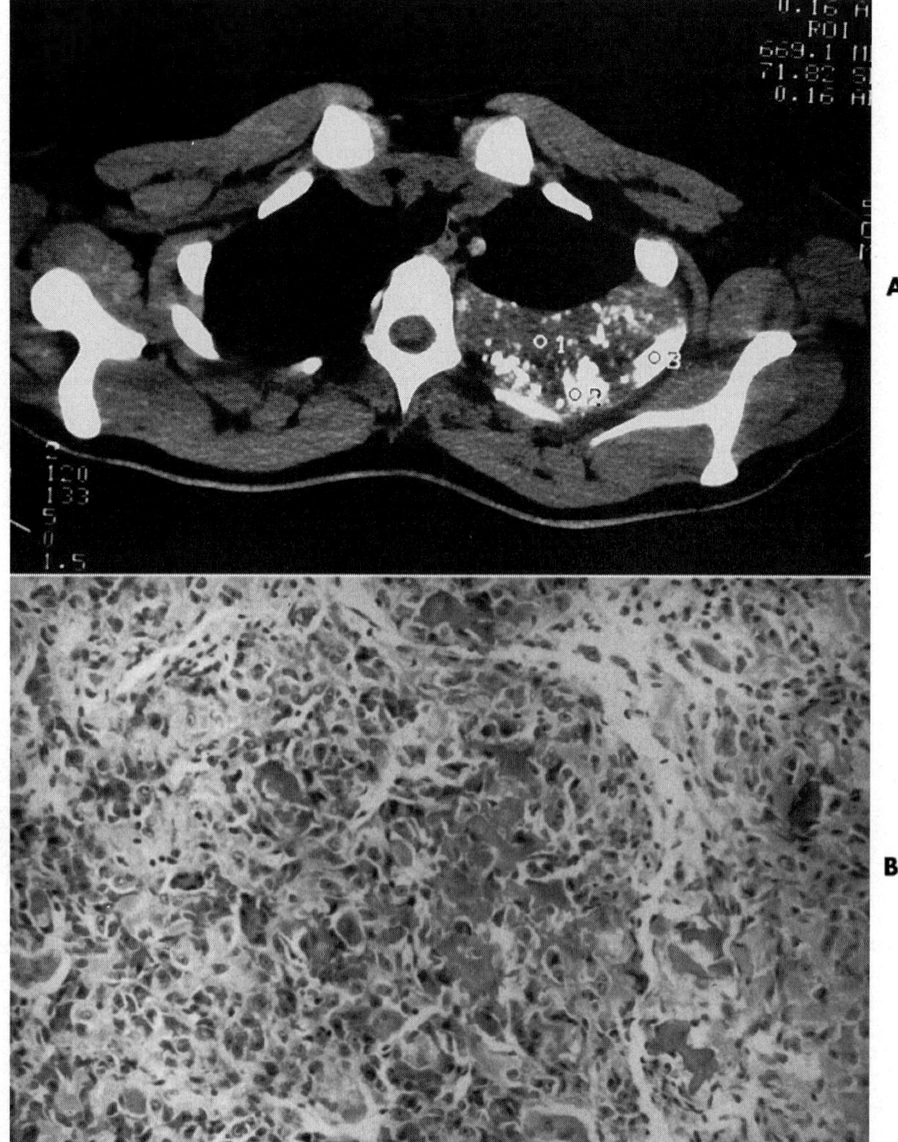

**FIGURE 37-7**

Osteosarcoma of second rib. **A,** CT scan shows the involvement of the rib and intimate association with the lung which was inadvertently biopsied by the referring institution. The tumor is adjacent to zone III B but not invading the cortex of the vertebral body. Zone II A (the Pedicle) and II B (the transverse process) are in intimate contact with the tumor. **B,** The photomicrograph of the specimen clearly shows osteoid production. *(From Shaffer WO: Anterior column surgery in spinal tumors. In Devlin VJ, editor: Anterior Spinal Column Surgery,* Spine: State of the Art Reviews *12(3):611-624, 1998, Philadelphia, Hanley & Beflus, Inc.)*

were removed attaining good anterior and lateral control of the tumor. Simultaneously, the spine surgeon performed a laminectomy of the upper thoracic spine. As the body was approached, the pedicle and lateral border of the vertebral body was used as a surgical margin. One surgeon from the front performed osteotomies of T1 through T3, another surgeon from behind ligated then divided the T1 through T3 nerve roots and osteotomized the posterior body exactly medial to the pedicle of the three bodies. The resection was then completed delivering the mass en bloc with wide margins microscopically. This case did require anterior reconstruction with a Synthes anterior cervical plate (Fig. 37-8). The chest wall was reconstructed with surgical mesh and the scapular flap was closed over the defect. The patient is now 15 months status postresection without recurrence of the tumor.

A patient with osteosarcoma of the sacrum further illustrates this concept. The patient was felt to have a low-grade osteoblastoma. He underwent an intralesional excisional biopsy (Fig. 37-9). On pathologic review, the tumor proved to be an osteosarcoma. The revised resection of the tumor required laminectomy through the posterior sacrum. An iliac osteotomy was performed. The sacral roots 2-5 on that side were sacrificed. The S1 root was saved and dissected away from the tumor mass. Osteotomy of the sacrum, such as one would do for a chordoma, was then accomplished. The roots were excised distal to the sacrum and the mass removed en bloc. This patient had been treated with adjuvant chemotherapy preoperatively and on examination of the material a full wide resection of the tumor was accomplished and no residual tumor was identified within the confines of the resection. This patient required an extensive lumbosacral iliac reconstruction and fusion of the ilium to the sacrum (Fig. 37-10). The patient is now 21 months status postresection with no evidence of recurrent tumor.

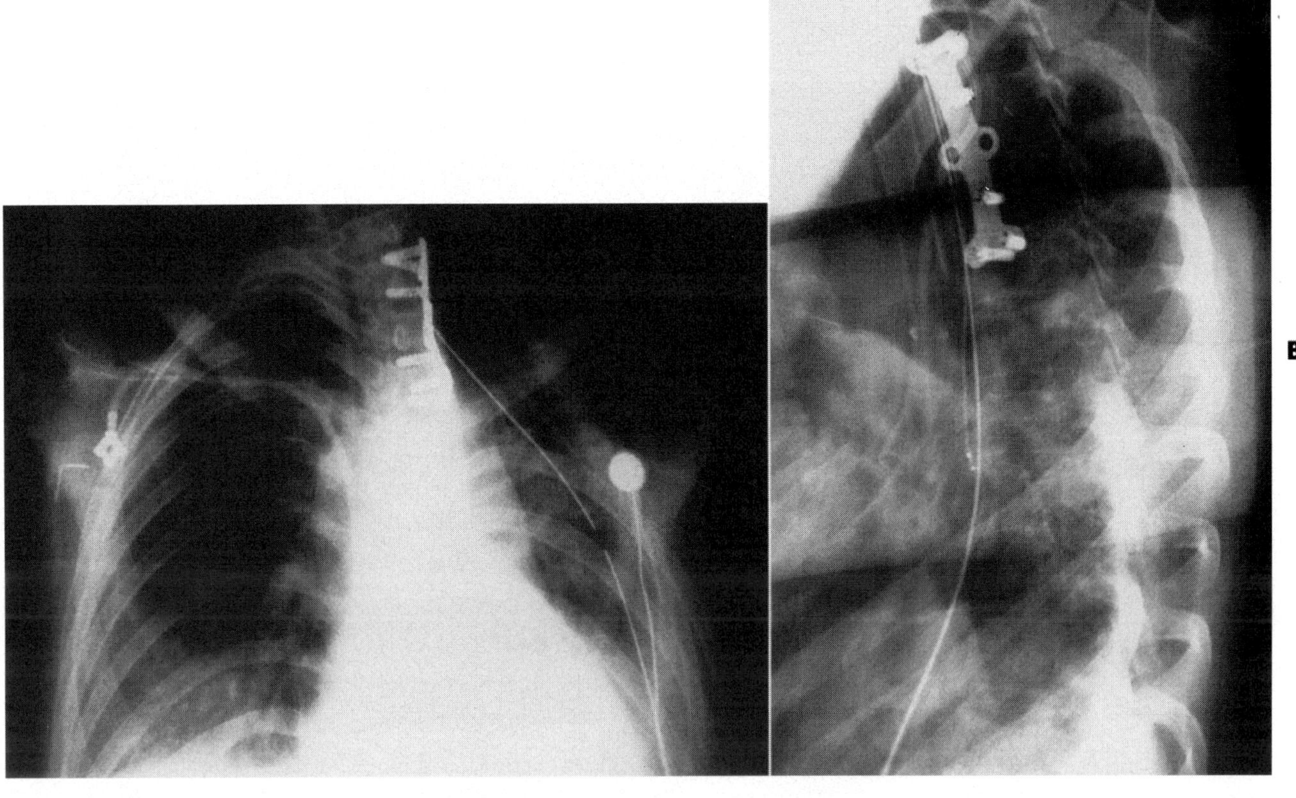


**FIGURE 37-8**

**A,** AP view of the reconstructed upper thoracic spine. **B,** Lateral view. Note the resected upper four ribs. The plate is placed laterally as one would place a Z plate or University plate from T1 to T4. One screw is placed in T2 and T3 with structural grafts in the disk space T1-T2, T2-T3, and T3-T4. The patient was nursed in a cervicothoracic Malibu brace. *(From Shaffer WO: Anterior column surgery in spinal tumors. In Devlin VJ, editor: Anterior Spinal Column Surgery,* Spine: State of the Art Reviews *12(3):611-624, 1998, Philadelphia, Hanley & Beflus, Inc.)*

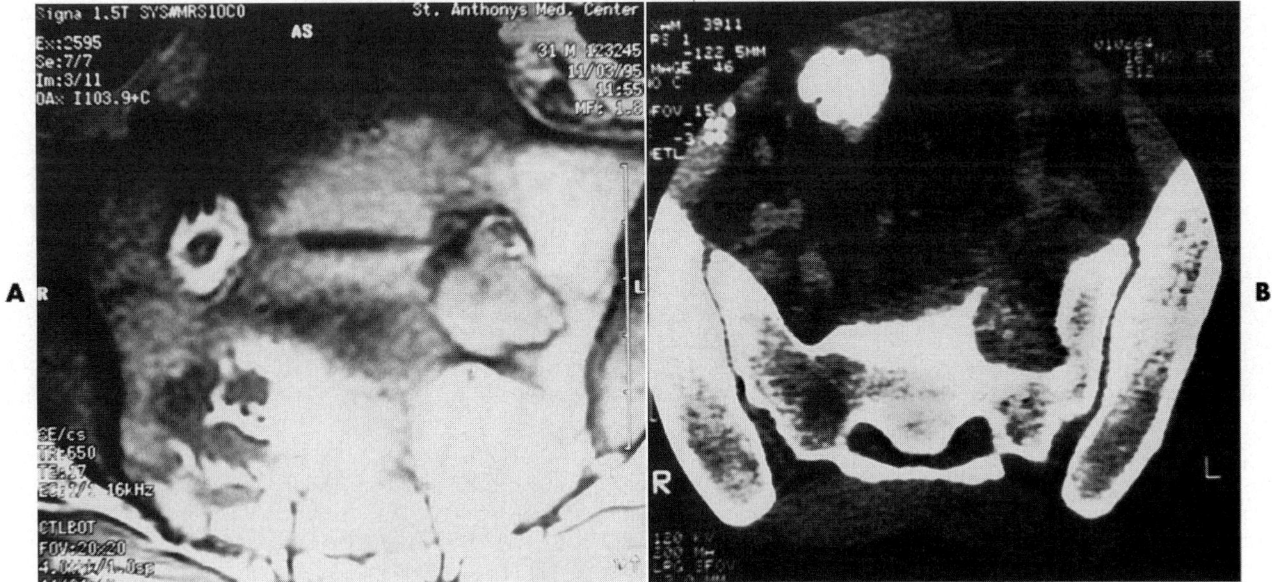


**FIGURE 37-9**

**A,** MRI view of the sacrum prior to original procedure. Mass is anterior to root canal. Involves primarily the sacral alar at S2 without involving zone 4 or the sacroiliac joint. **B,** The CT scan shows calcification in the mass. Prior to the original procedure the working diagnosis was osteoblastoma.

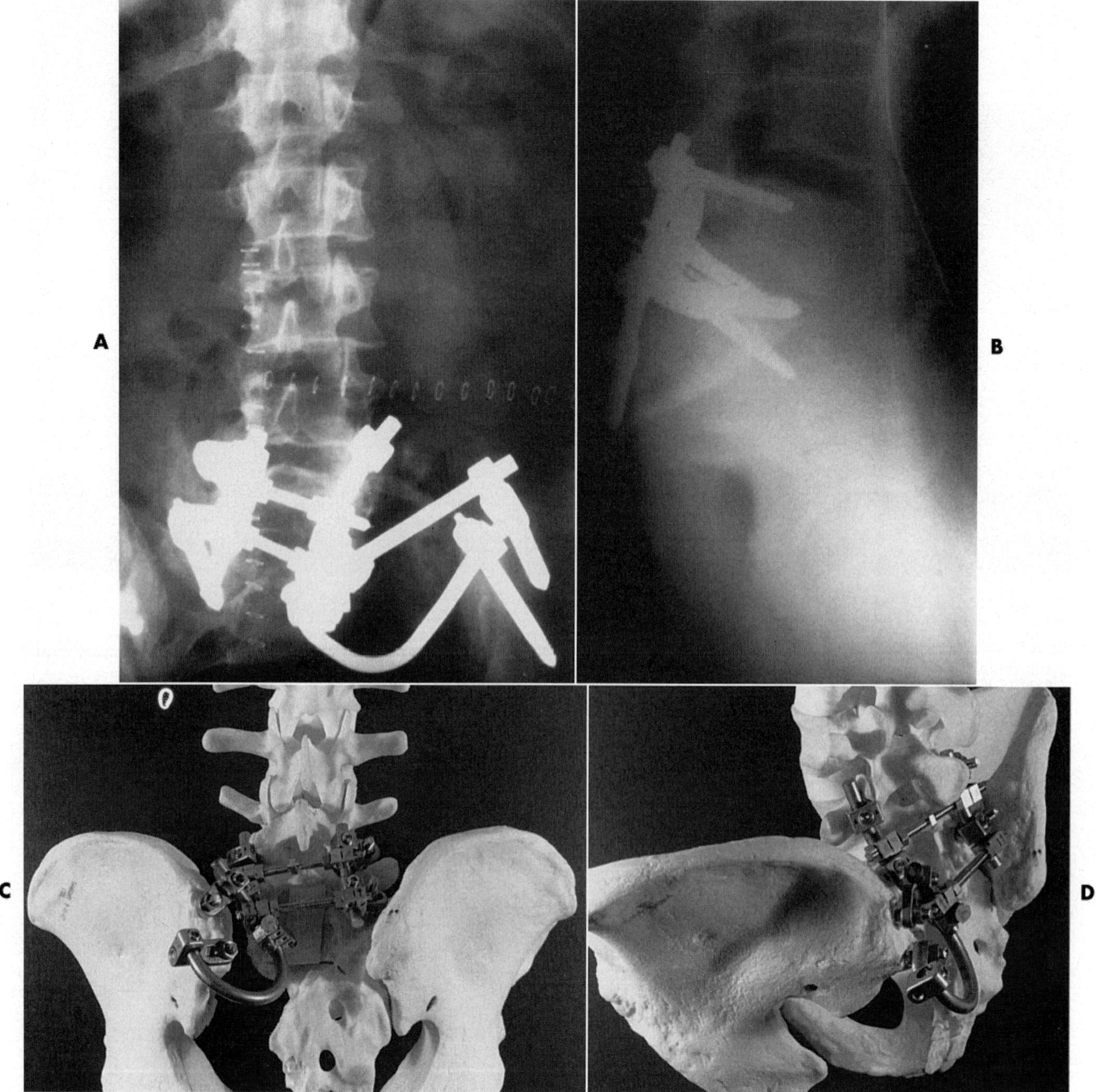


FIGURE 37-10

**A,** Reconstruction. The L5-S1 facet was taken in the resection as was the entire left sacrum. The sacroiliac joint and pedicles served as margins. The reconstruction consists of L5 and S1 Isola screws. Iliolumbar fixation is accomplished with two iliac bolts attached to a U-shaped rod between the left L5 and S1 pedicle screws and the lower iliac bolt. An L-shaped rod connects the upper iliac bolt to the U-shaped rod by a transverse connector. **B,** Lateral view. **C,** Model of construct posterior view. **D,** Model of construct lateral oblique view.

Very difficult tumors can be reresected with wide margins but a degree of aggressiveness is required. The use of normal bone as a margin frequently allows the tumor to be excised without violating the tumor capsule. Therefore, one must think of the pedicle and vertebral cortex as a potential margin. The sacroiliac joint and the ilium itself can be resected and used as a margin to obtain complete resection of the tumor. For this approach to work, resection of the roots is necessary and proper for the treatment of malignant lesions and aggressive benign lesions such as chordoma. Sacral resections usually can be accomplished by a posterior or a posterior lateral approach. Other regions of the spine almost always require a combined anterior-posterior resection to control the tumor. In our institution this requires two surgeons, one working from behind and one working from the front simultaneously to adequately direct the osteotomy paths and to assure full complete resection of these tumors.

## ADJUVANT THERAPY

Adjuvant treatment is important in controlling these tumors. Boriani et al[1] felt that angiography and embolization of highly vascular lesions was quite helpful. Aneurysmal bone cyst was treated by selective embolization and excision of all of the residual tumor. This patient had been treated for eosinophilic granuloma (Fig. 37-11, *A, B*). Six months later a very large aneurysmal bone cyst was noted arising in the anterior body of C3 with posterior extension (Fig. 37-11, *C, D*). A posterior biopsy showed a blood-filled cystic lesion and pathology confirmed an aneurysmal bone cyst (ABC). In this circumstance, to get adequate control of the tumor, a preoperative angiogram and embolization of the tumor allowed us to perform an aggressive, thorough intralesional resection of the tumor (Fig. 37-12). Skeletonizing the vertebral artery anteriorly, the spine was reconstructed with a strut graft. Then posteriorly we resected the entire lamina and lateral mass forward to the vertebral artery, stripping the vertebral artery of all tumor tissue. The neck was controlled in a halo brace and went on to solid fusion anteriorly and posteriorly with no evidence of recurrence now 15 months following resection (Fig. 37-13).

Celli et al[2] emphasized that incomplete removal of the tumor caused the worst prognosis and that postoperative radiotherapy was required even in those tumors that were felt to be fully excised. At our center we have reserved radiation therapy for intralesional resections and in tumors with known radiosensitivity such as plasmacytoma.

Patients with osteosarcoma benefit from preoperative chemotherapy. They undergo their chemotherapy between biopsy and excision as in the case discussed previously. At resection, the effectiveness of the chemotherapy then can be analyzed in terms of tumor kill and cell death (see Figs. 37-8 and 37-9).

## RECONSTRUCTIVE ISSUES

At the lumbosacral junction, excision of the sacrum and/or the L5-S1 articulation requires anchorage to the pelvis. This frequently requires innovation on the surgeon's part for obtaining adequate anchorage into the pelvis. Options include the Jackson intrasacral rod to anchor the rod securely to the sacrum with screws passed through the S1, S2, and L5 pedicles. A combination of a modified Galveston rod with an iliac anchor connected to L5 and a sacral pedicle, if one still remains, can be of help. Depending on the extent of the excision or concomitant degenerative disease, proximal fixation to L4 or L3 may be required. Figure 37-14 shows a complex iliosacral fixation in a case of a hemangiopericytoma treated previously as a L4-L5 herniated disk. The patient had a degenerative spondylolisthesis as a result of two previous disk excisions. Only later was it discovered that the cause of his radiculopathy was the tumor in the sacrum. The CT scan shows the involvement of the L5-S1 joint and the sacroiliac joint. Resection required sacrifice of the S1 root, sacroiliac joint, posterior ilium and L5-S1 articulation. Reconstruction included the L4-L5 segment to stabilize the iatrogenic L4-L5 instability.

Cervicothoracic reconstruction requires special consideration. The C7 vertebral body and posterior lateral masses are different from the upper cervical segments. The first thoracic segment is different from the lower thoracic vertebra. Its transverse process is small and obliquely oriented. We have used a special Isola rod, which is milled to drop from a $\frac{1}{4}''$ diameter rod to a $\frac{3}{16}''$ rod so that pediatric hooks can be used in the upper thoracic spine. This decreases the bulk and increases the possibility of not having to remove the hardware at a later date. Additionally, this can be combined with titanium or stainless steel cables into the cervical spinous processes to obtain intersegmental fixation of the lower cervical spine. We prefer titanium in our tumor work so that later imaging studies such as MRIs can be performed. There are hybrids available in which a rod to a lateral mass plate combination can allow anchorage into the lateral masses of the cervical spine and then fixation to the thoracic spine through a standard hook-claw construct. Danek's Horizon and Depuy's Moss Miami systems have developed such hybrids. Anteriorly, in the cervical thoracic junction, presently we don't have a particularly good fixator that addresses the needs of the area. Anterior cervical plates can be used if augmented with a posterior fixation (see Fig. 37-8).

Titanium mesh prostheses such as the Harms cage

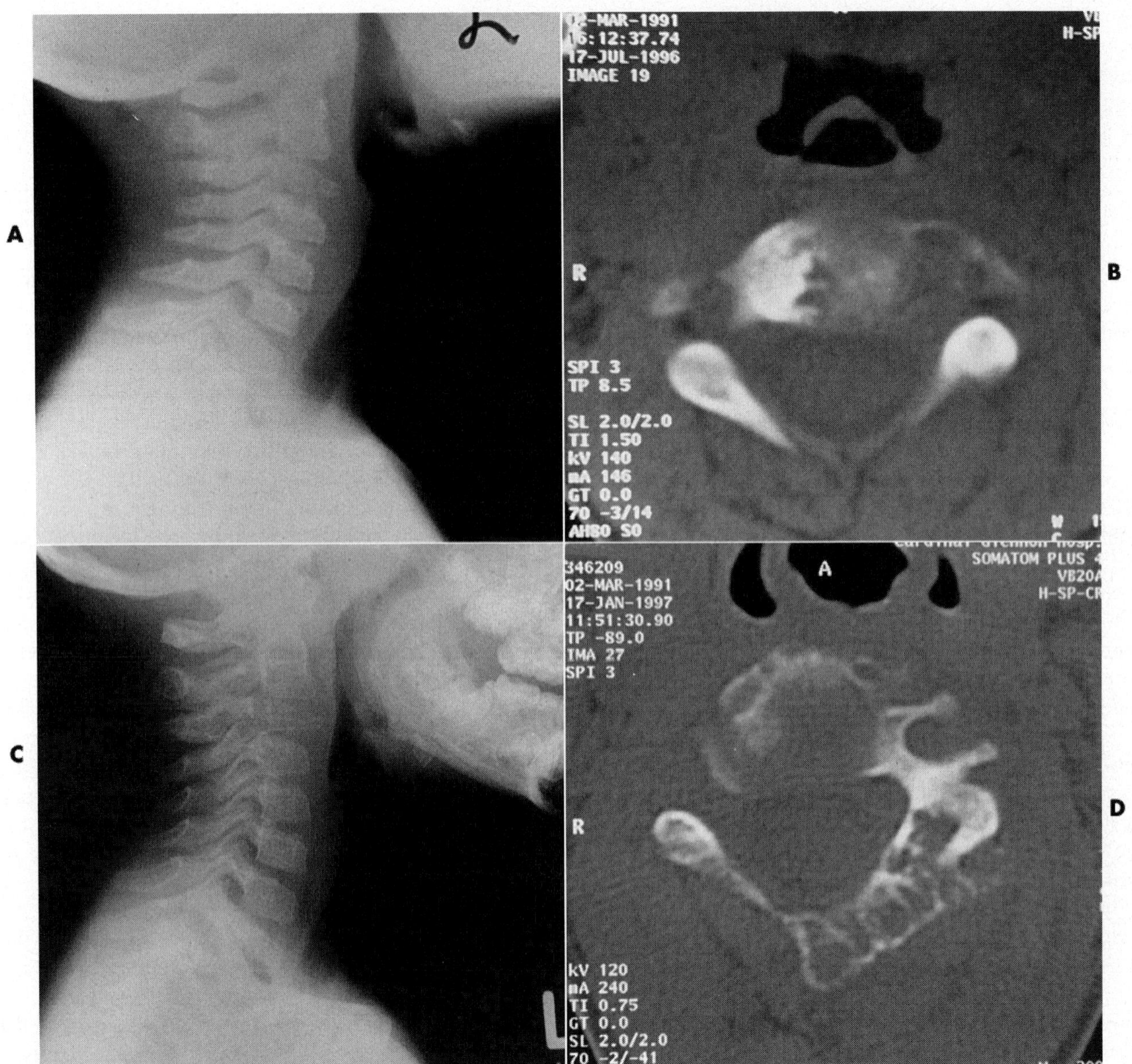


FIGURE 37-11

**A,** Vertebra plana in a child. The radiologist and pediatrician interpreted this as compatible with eosinophilic granuloma. **B,** The original CT scan showing anterior involvement and interpreted as eosinophilic granuloma. **C,** After 7 months of failure to reconstitute a repeat lateral radiogram showed an expansive lesion involving posterior elements in addition to anterior body. **D,** The CT scan now shows the expansile nature of the posteriorly developing aneurysmal bone cyst.

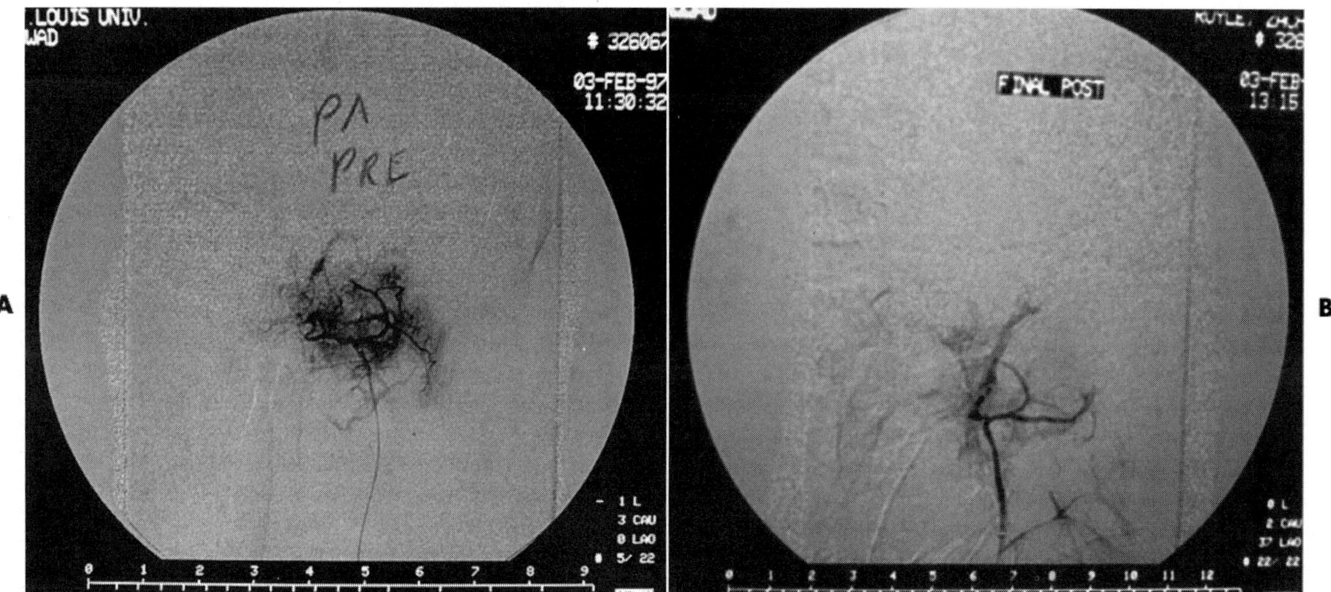


FIGURE 37-12

**A,** Angiogram shows the vascularity of the aneurysmal bone cyst. **B,** Successful embolization of the tumor blush is confirmed.

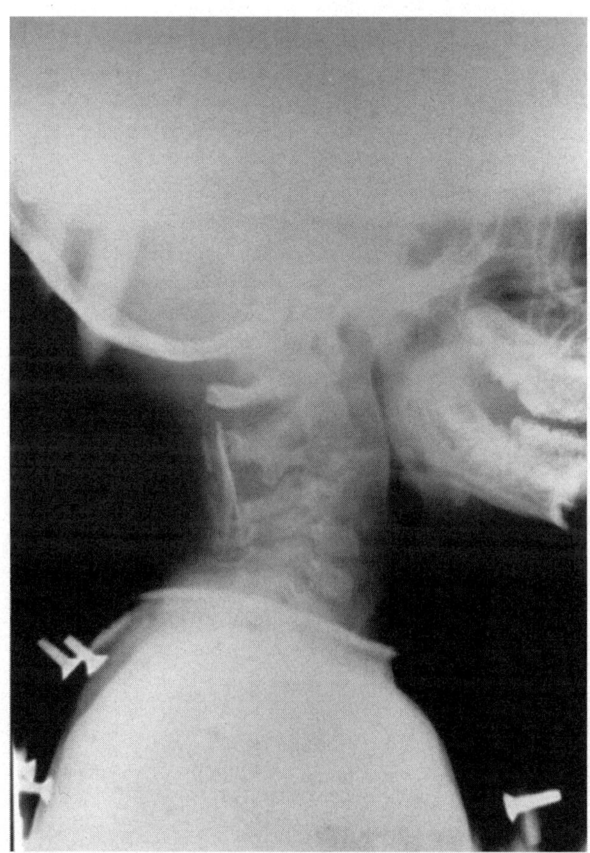

FIGURE 37-13

The reconstruction of the defect. A strut graft has been placed between C2-C4. The posterior elements are "wired" using Secure Strand (Surgical Dynamics) polyester cable and the patient was nursed in a halo vest.

have allowed a more flexible reconstructive plan. Most simultaneous anterior and posterior resections require anterior and posterior stabilization such as this schwannoma previously treated as an HNP (Fig. 37-15).

## SUMMARY

This chapter has discussed a rational approach to the reresection of spinal tumors. The tumor's biological behavior must be clearly understood. This is achieved by observing the specific patient's tumor behavior and reviewing all available pathological specimens. Imaging studies alone can not determine the behavior of a specific spinal tumor but form a frame work on which these other factors can be hung.

The anatomic involvement of the tumor and the previous resection must be carefully studied. Uninvolved normal spinal structures must be viewed as margins and nerve roots frequently must be resected to achieve a curative margin.

Reconstructive options have improved over recent years with the advent of modern spine fixation and prostheses such as the titanium mesh cage. The spine surgeon must have a thorough working knowledge of the complex fixation options. The use of a multidisciplinary team including vascular, gastrointestinal, urologic, and cardiothoracic surgeons guided by an orthopedic oncologic surgeon, radiologists, and pathologist is instrumental in the success of these reresections by the spine surgeon.

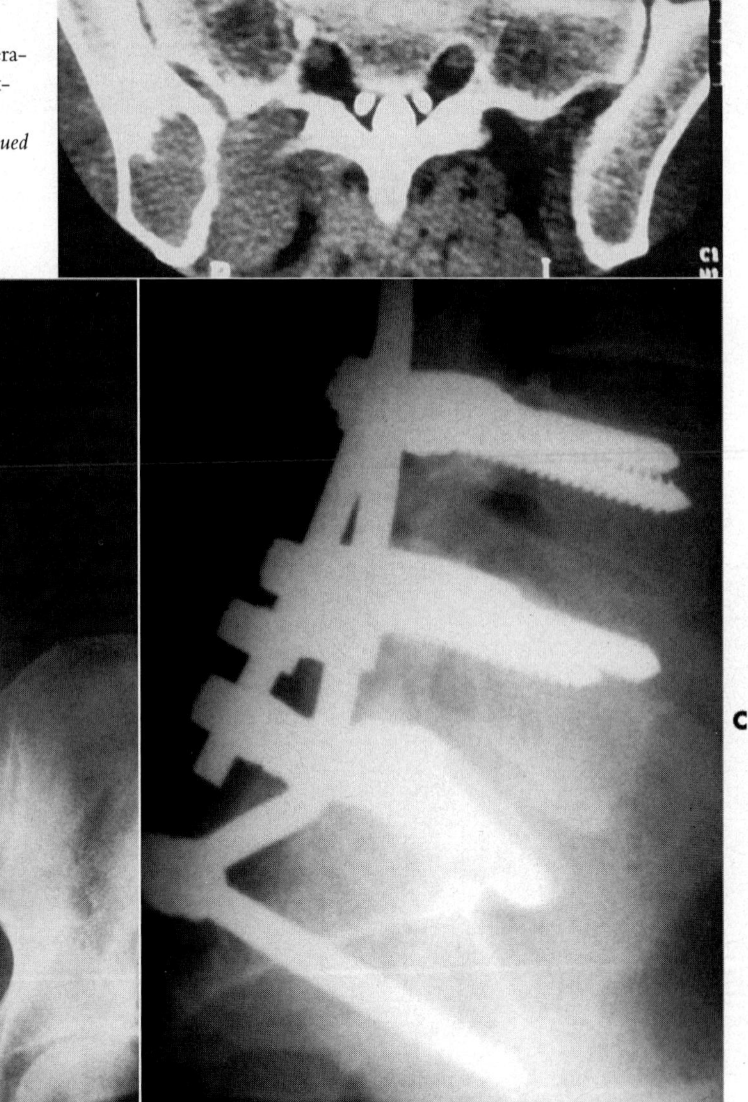

**FIGURE 37-14**

Hemangiopericytoma. **A,** CT scan shows bony involvement of the posterior superior iliac spine and soft tissue extension with involvement of zone II pedicle and facet joint at L5-S1. **B,** AP view of the reconstruction shows a iliac bolt securing the lumbar fixation to the pelvis. **C,** Lateral view showing a concomitant degenerative L4-L5 spondylolisthesis, which required extension of the fixation and fusion to L4.

*Continued*

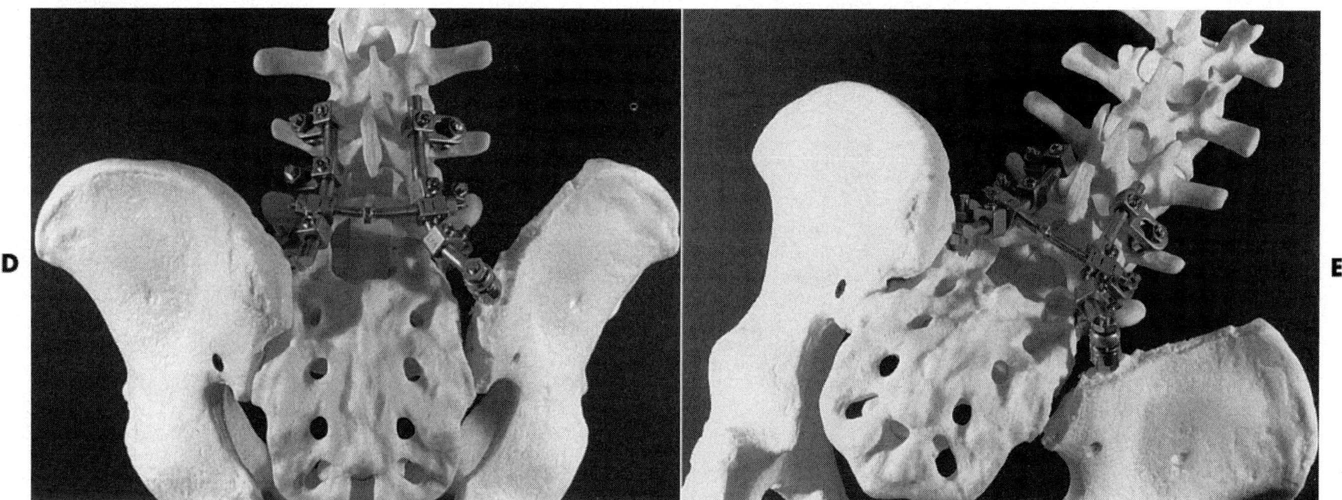


FIGURE 37-14 CONT'D

**D,** Posterior view of the modeled construct. **E,** Oblique view of the modeled construct.

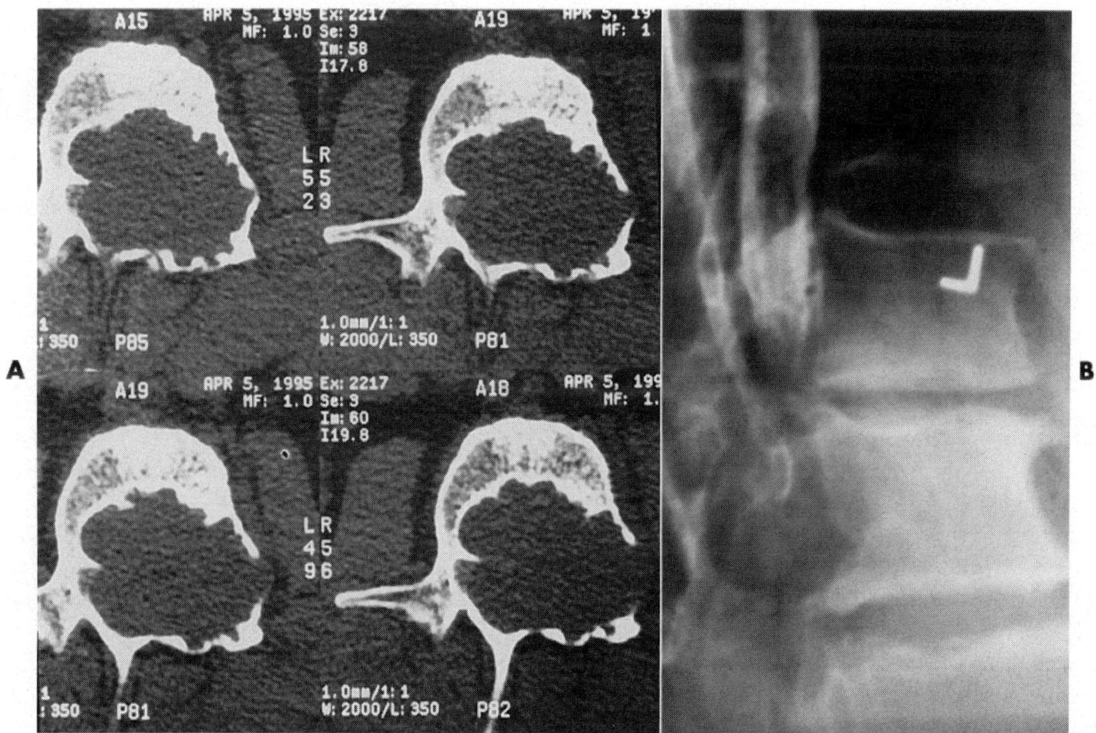


FIGURE 37-15

Schwannoma. **A,** The CT scan shows the extensive zone II and IV involvement in this benign but dangerously located tumor. **B,** Lateral view of the myelogram showing a complete myelographic block.

*Continued*

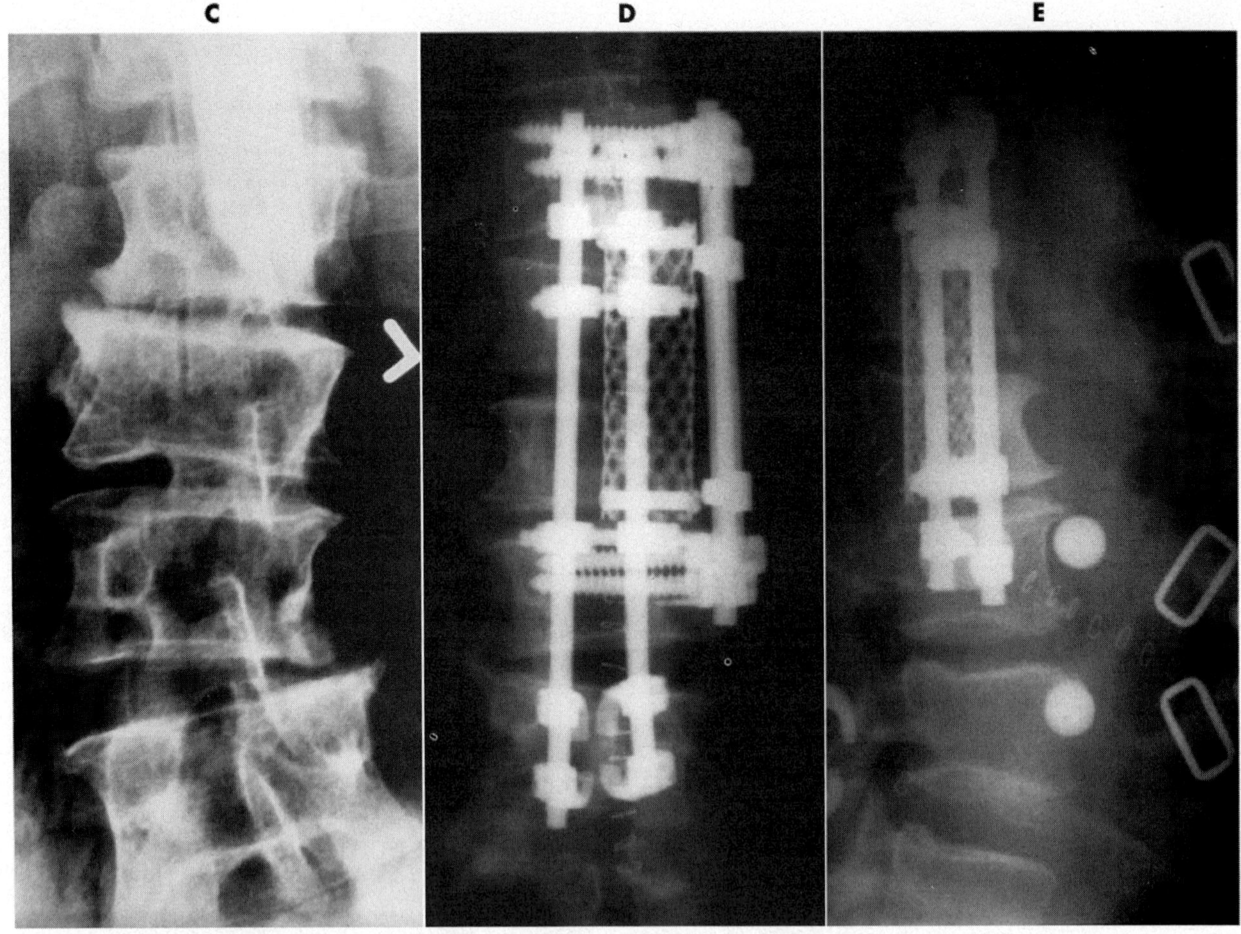


FIGURE 37-15 CONT'D

**C,** AP view of the preoperative myelogram. **D,** The Harms cage replacing L1 and L2 locked in place by an anterior Kaneda device. Posterior supplementary fixation with an Isola construct is used in multiple level corpectomies. The L3-L4 level is fixed to deal with the concomitant degenerative disease at that level. **E,** Lateral view of the construct.

## REFERENCES

1. Boriani S, Biagini R, De Iuri F et al: Primary bone tumors of the spine: a survey of the evaluation and treatment at the Istituto Orthpedico Rizzoli, *Orthopedics* 18(10):993-1000, 1995.
2. Celli P, Cervoni L, Tarrantino R, Fortuna A: Primary spinal malignant schwannomas: clinical and prognostic remarks, *Acta Neurochirurgica* 135:1-2, 52-55, 1995.
3. Delamarter RB, Sachs BL, Thompson GH et al: Primary neoplasms of the thoracic and lumbar spine: An analysis of 29 consecutive cases, *CORR* 256:88-100, 1990.
4. DiLorenzo N, Delfini R, Ciappetta P et al: Primary tumors of the cervical spine: surgical experience with 38 cases, *Surg Neurol* 38:12-18, 1992.
5. Dreghorn CR, Newman RJ, Hardy GJ, Dickson RA: Primary tumors of the axial skeleton: experience of the Leeds Regional Bone Tumor Registry, *Spine* 15(2): 137-140, 1990.
6. Ebraheim NA, Lu J, Biyani A et al: The relationship of lumbosacral plexus to the sacrum and sacroiliac joint, *Am J Orthop* Feb:105-110, 1997.
7. Grillo HC, Ojemann RG, Scannell JG, Zervas NT. Combined approach to "dumbbell" intrathoracic intraspinal neurogenic tumors, *Ann Thorac Surg* 36(4): 402-407, 1983.
8. Grubb MR, Currier DL, Pritchard DJ, Ebersold MJ: Primary Ewing's sarcoma of the spine, *Spine* 19(3):309-313, 1994.
9. Malawski SK: The results of surgical treatment of primary spinal tumors, *Clin Orthop* 272:50-57, 1991.
10. Schajowicz F, McDonald DJ: Classification of tumors and tumor lesions of the spine, *State of the Art Review* 10(1):1-11, 1996.
11. Thompson RC Jr, Berg TL: Primary bone tumors of the pelvis presenting as spinal disease, *Orthopedics* 19(12):1011-1016, 1996.
12. Weinstein JN, McLain RF: Primary tumor of the spine, *Spine* 12(9):843-851, 1987.

# VII

# SPECIFIC TECHNICAL CONSIDERATIONS IN REVISION SURGERY

# 38

# REVISION SURGERY IN THE UPPER CERVICAL SPINE

**Jürgen Nothwang, M.D.**
**Christoph Ulrich, M.D.**



## ANATOMIC AND BIOMECHANIC CONSIDERATIONS

Although the segmental construction of the cervical spine is similar to the whole spine, its function in view of its kinematic loads shows distinct differences in comparison with the thoracolumbar spine.

Under anatomical as well as kinematic aspects it makes sense to subdivide the cervical spine into three groups: the upper cervical spine with the occipitoatlantoaxial complex (C0-C1-C2), the middle cervical spine (C2-C5), and the lower cervical spine (C6-T1).[8,21,31] In the different regions we find different dominant functions. The occipitoatlantoaxial joints are the most complex joints of the total axial skeleton. While flexion and extension is the main movement in the occipitoatlantal joint, axial rotation is dominating the function of the atlantoaxial complex.

In the middle and lower cervical spine flexion, extension and lateral bending come well to the fore.[10]

Although some investigations[11,25] showed that even in the occipitoatlantal area we can perform little axial rotation (approximately 4 to 8 degrees), this movement is mainly performed of the atlantoaxial joint with an assumed instantaneous axis of rotation in the center of the axis,[32] where 60% of the total ability of rotation in the cervical spine takes place.

The operative procedure and the postoperative treatment have to take concern of those facts.

## PRIMARY MANAGEMENT OF UPPER CERVICAL SPINE LESIONS

It is well known that injuries of the occipitoatlantal joint are mostly lethal, because the displacement of the skull in relation to the atlas usually severs the medulla. To neutralize flexion and extension moments the tectorial membrane works as a stabilizer and unphysiologic rotatory forces are inhibited by the alar ligaments, which are neutralizing lateral bending forces. In cases of injury we find a ligamental lesion of those very important anatomical structures. In rare cases, the patient survived such an injury.[14,24] The instability can be verified by lateral x-ray[26] and magnetic resonance imaging (MRI). Because of this very rare entity, stabilization problems are not common.

In orthopedic patients with rheumatic disease, chronic instability may be seen.[12] In these cases, the patient has problems in balancing his head. A conservative treatment will not bring much relief for the patient considering that ligamentous lesions will heal with a loss of stability.

A craniocervical fusion after failed conservative treatment may bring an improvement in symptoms, although at quite a high price of functional loss. The fusion can be achieved by special devices or a reconstruction plate in addition to a posterior cancellous bone graft. Under biomechanical aspects, this atlantooccipital fusion is stressed by flexion and extension movements. Therefore, we recommend an additional stabilization by an external device (i.e., a stiff neck until bony fusion has taken place).

The treatment of odontoid fractures must be separated into two groups: conservatively treated patients

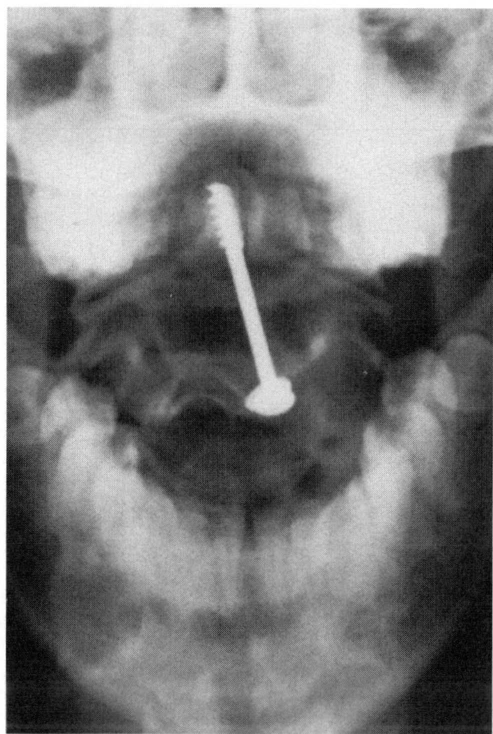

**FIGURE 38-1**

Postoperative x-ray of a 16-year-old patient with odontoid fracture type Anderson II and screw fixation (AP view).

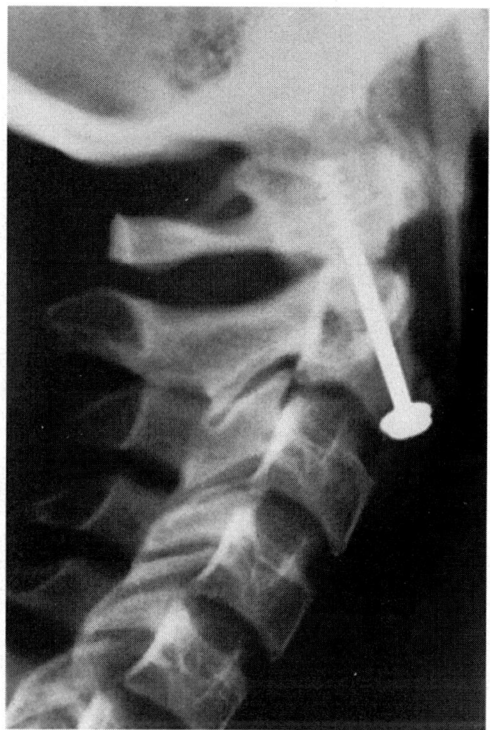

**FIGURE 38-2**

Postoperative x-ray (lateral view): an anterior gap can still be observed.

and those patients that have undergone operative stabilization. The decision for the treatment depends on the kind of fracture type according to the classification of Anderson and d'Alonzo.[3,7] The three types of this classification are important for the understanding of the clinical biomechanics of this injury. Regarding the operative treatment the Anderson II fracture type can be divided into three different subtypes respecting the direction of the fracture line.[15] Several investigations have led to the conclusion that hyperextension, hyperflexion, and horizontal shear may cause fracture types that correspond to common fracture types.[29] On the other hand type II fractures can be created either by distraction of the head tensioning the alar ligaments and the apical ligaments,[20] or by applying an experimental force vector from an anterolateral direction in a combination with horizontal shear and vertical compression.[1] The combination of rotatory and translational forces may cause a deep type III fracture through the massae laterales[20] and a combination of compression and shear force vector applied directly in the sagittal plane.[1] With some certainty our treatment should respect all these different patterns.

For conservative treatment, it is well known that the failure rate depends on the type of fracture. A comprehensive multicenter study showed a nonunion rate of 36% for type II fractures and 15% for type III fractures.[7] As in all fields of traumatology, the grade of displacement is a factor for developing pseudarthrosis.[4] Other factors are osteoporosis and angulation of the fragments.[22] Experimental investigations of Schatzker to induce pseudarthrosis demonstrated that the probability of developing pseudarthrosis depends on the fracture line in relation to the ligamenta accessoria.[30] If an osteotomy was performed below those ligaments bony healing could be seen within 12 weeks. On the other hand, the osteotomies above the ligamenta accessoria produced a pseudarthrosis in any case, although this reaction could not be founded on a deficiency of vascularization.

Böhler has previously reported that nonunions can also be caused by insufficient reduction of the fracture or a too short period of immobilization.[5] We had the same experience even after primary anatomic reduction. In one case we did not achieve a tight compression between the fragments (Fig. 38-1), but the reduction was well (Fig. 38-2). After the operation, the 16-year-old female patient received a semirigid cervical collar for about 3 weeks. This period seemed to be too short, because three months later the radiological follow-up showed a nonunion. We made functional x-rays and observed a respective motion of the dens (Fig. 38-3). The new analysis of the pretraumatic x-rays showed that this patient had suffered a compression/shear lesion. This was supported by the diagnosis of a fracture of the sixth cervical vertebrae, a flexion/compression injury previously unnoticed, which required no stabilization. The screw fixation reduced the frac-

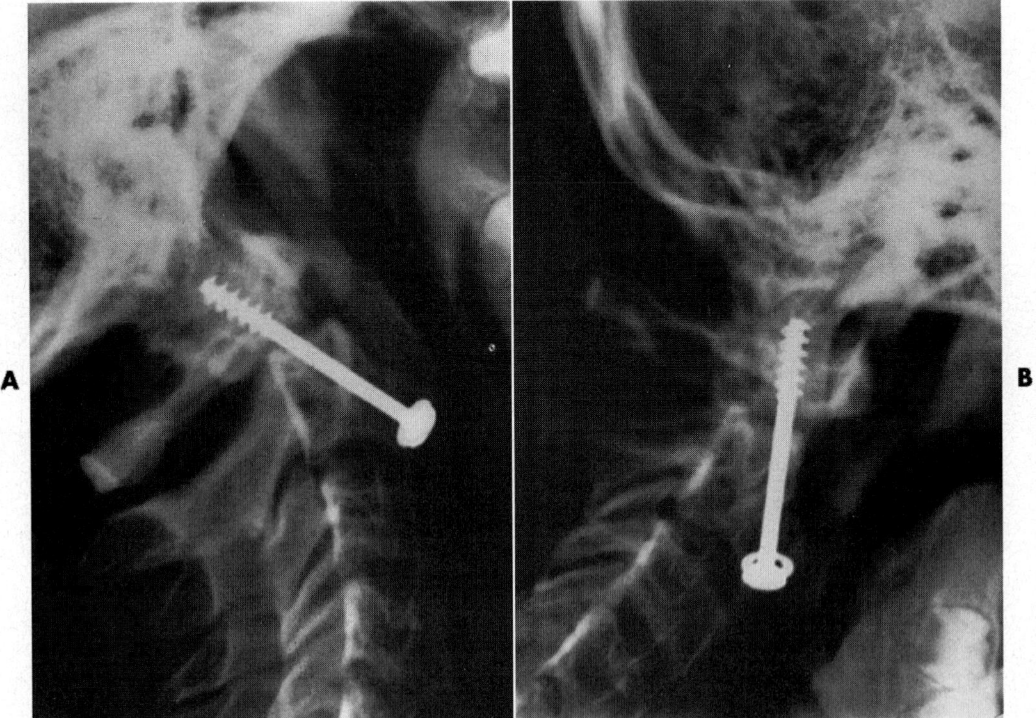


FIGURE 38-3

Follow-up three months after screw fixation; x-rays in active motion, demonstrating instability. **A,** Reclination. **B,** Inclination.

ture but we did not succeed in closing the gap between the fragments totally. The anatomical basis of this well-known problem is that the ligamenta alaria and apicis effect a cranial extension force on the odontoid.[30] This causes a distraction of the fragments and even if vascularization is well the resulting gap is too large to be bridged. This constellation occurs quite often in type II fractures. If osteosynthesis is not able to compensate, a pseudarthrosis may develop. The fibrous material that becomes part of the bony healing in this situation will prevent the consolidation. Another biomechanical aspect should be stressed regarding the biomechanical forces acting on the dens during cervical movement, and the instantaneous axis of rotation needs to be noted. For flexion and extension it is located in the region of the middle third of the dens and for axial rotation this point lies in the central portion of the axis.[16] As a result, we have to expect that Anderson type II fractures are more influenced by flexion and extension movements, whereas type III lesions can be irritated more by axial rotatory forces.

Another important prerequisite for a successful osteosynthesis is the bony contact between the fragment's presupposed normal bone quality. The presented case shows that the close contact of the odontoid fragments is mandatory for bony healing. But even in cases with a good contact between the two fragments a small necrotic area between the two fragments can be produced by interfragmentary compression of a screw. The resorption of this area during the bony healing may lead to a situation in which the dens is highly sensitive to flexion and extension momentum. Any type of external stabilization can be used to avoid those loads. Because of the quite small contact zone and the fact that the spongiotic vascularization is interrupted by the fracture and additionally irritated and perhaps damaged by the application of one or two screws, we have to expect a prolonged bony healing almost totally initiated by the periosteum. The extension of the resorption of the interfragmentary contact zone depends on the movement of this zone during the first weeks. As shown in this case a sufficient time of immobilization could be another important factor of a successful treatment. We can not expect an interfragmentary locking that may resist flexion/extension loads as well as axial rotatory force vectors. Only in cases of type III dens fractures is the spongiotic surface of the two fragments large enough for interlocking consequently. These fractures normally cause no major problems in treatment.

Nevertheless, we have to respect that the fixation of the odontoid fragments by screws, even under the condition of optimal reduction, can not create a stability that is comparable to a normal dens.[28] Under this point of view it seems to be of lower interest whether to use one or two screws. The biomechanical investigations of Sasso showed that the achievable stability of the odontoid is half of the stability of the in-

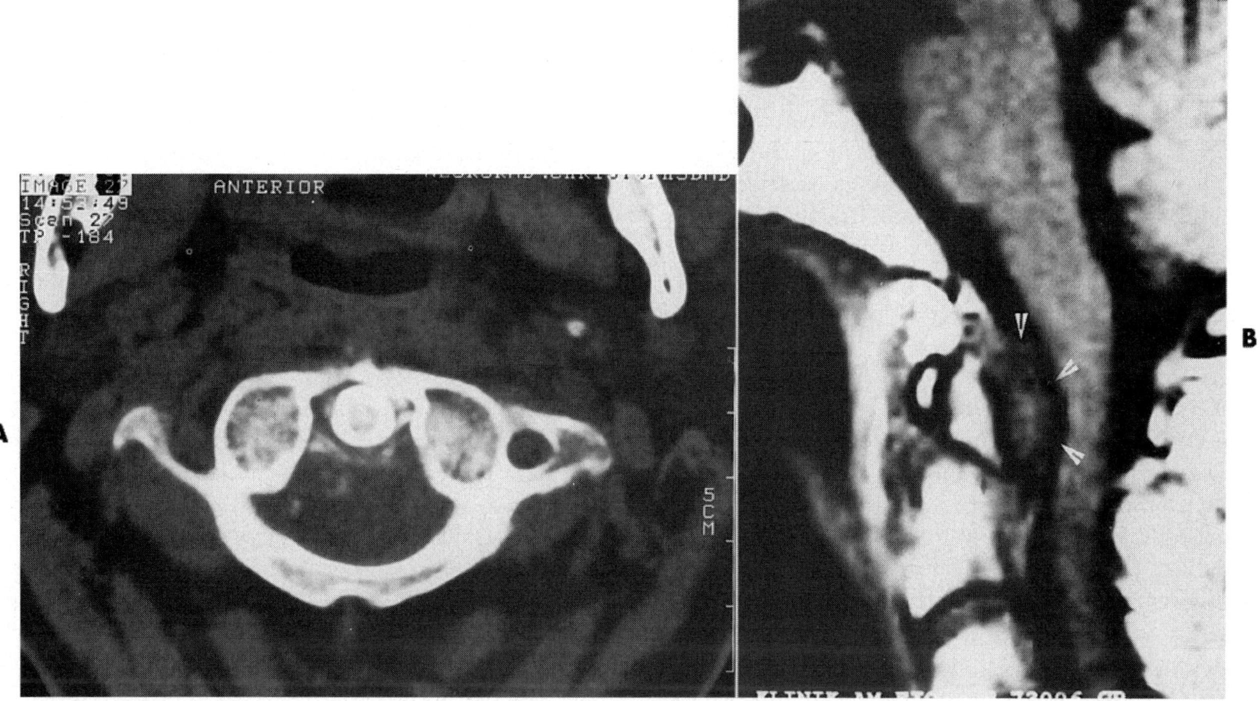


FIGURE 38-4

**A,** A 76-year-old woman with elder dens pseudarthrosis and retrodental pannus in CT. **B,** MRI shows the retrodental fibrous mass.

tact odontoid.[28] The load to failure tests showed no difference between the one- or two-screw technique. In the opinion of the authors, the motion of the upper cervical spine with its instantaneous axis of rotation is the reason for a loosening or a failure of the screw implant that can be expected in about 20% to 30% of cases after a time period of 3 months if consolidation of the fracture has not taken place before that time.

## CLINICAL PERFORMANCE OF REVISION SURGERY

Revision surgery is indicated if operative fixation or a conservative treatment after 8 to 12 months results in nonunion.

Although some authors declare that the odontoid pseudarthrosis is mandatory for operation in any case,[5,15] we believe that we first have to prove the type of instability of the dens. This can be verified by functional x-rays in reclination and inclination. If translational movement of the dens can not be observed but opening of the anterior gap is visible, a conservative attempt is justified in elderly patients with poor bone quality.[27] There is no question about the necessity of stabilization in cases of neurological deficiency and young patients. If we decide to treat the patient conservatively we have to be aware of the problem that the duration of instability may cause a fibrotic mass posterior to the odontoid (pannus), which may lead to neurological symptoms itself (Fig. 38-4). At this time, it can not be forecasted which patient will develop such a phenomenon.

If we decide in favor of operation, the quality of the bone needs to be analyzed and technical reasons in case of screw failure need to be excluded. This means in detail that the application of the anterior screws through the anterior part of the endplate is the most important presupposition for a reliable fixation[9,34] because the anterior wall of C2 is too weak to prevent cutting-out of the screws. If two screws were used for primary fixation the chances are very poor for correction because of the reduced bone material in the odontoid fragment. In Anderson Type II fractures especially, osteoporosis can be a complication. The diminution of the bony mass near the basis of the odontoid can reach 64%.[2] One cannot expect a good holding strength of the screws either for primary operation or for treatment of pseudarthrosis in those patients. For these reasons the exclusive anterior fixation by screws[13] does not seem to be sufficient in revised surgery of odontoid pseudarthrosis. Therefore, stabilization by means of posterior devices, especially in elderly people with reduced bony quality, is preferred.

Obviously there are different possibilities in reaching a posterior fusion. The principles of posterior C1-C2 fixation are the same in all of the operative procedures: segmental fixation of C1-C2 and bone transplantation until solid fusion has taken place. Gallie first described this method of C1-C2 fixation by wire in 1939 and Brooks modified this technique with a specially shaped tricortical graft.[6] Fielding presented a one-wire technique.[17] The highest grade of stiffness can experimentally be reached by a transarticular screw application in the technique of Magerl[23] in addition to a C1-C2 fixation by Fielding or Brooks.

The age of the patient must be considered when deciding on the type of treatment. In elderly patients, the transarticular fusion in the technique of Magerl may fortify the posterior fusion with a corticocancellous bone. Nevertheless, we must be aware that even a successful posterior fixation does not give the certainty for bony healing.[29] Our experiences with a single posterior fusion without transarticular screw fixation confirm this phenomenon. None of our patients reached a healing of the pseudarthrosis, although clinical symptoms of instability as evidenced by increasing neurological symptoms in retrodental fibrous tissue could not be observed. This might depend on the interfragmental gap. The smaller it is the earlier and faster a consolidation of the fracture might be achieved. All our patients showed a radiological gap of at least 2 rmm (radiol. millimeters), in the majority of the cases more than 3 to 4 rmm. But is the bony fusion of the pseudarthrosis the declared aim of our treatment? The main aspect that has to be fulfilled by the operation is elimination of the translatory displacement of the dens that threatens the patient.

The posterior fusion of C1-C2 by wires has been tested previously and the construction was not considered to be very reliable.[18] On the other hand, the specially shaped corticocancellous bone graft of Brooks and Jenkins in combination with a wire construction seems biomechanically sound[33] and has been shown to be effective with several trials.[6,19] To ensure proper separation between the posterior elements Brooks proposes a vertical diameter of the graft in place of 1 cm.[6] In contrast to the technique of Brooks, Fielding only uses one wire.[17] This reduces the operative risk of spinal cord injury. Although we are not aware of any biomechanical studies this construct might not be as stable as the double-wire technique of Brooks, and some authors do not advocate its use for rheumatoid patients and in cases with a high risk for nonunion.[33] In our experience there is a correlation between the age and the mobility of the patient. In the case of an elderly patient with pseudarthrosis of the odontoid we decided to perform an operation in the manner of Fielding. Nevertheless we disclaimed to add a transarticular screw fixation the follow-up showed a complete and biomechanically sufficient bridging between C1 and C2. Although we could observe a delayed union of posterior fusion in two cases the follow-up proved the fusion radiologically after $2\frac{1}{2}$ years (Fig. 38-5). In the previously mentioned case of the 16-year-old female, the x-rays show at least partial absorption of the bone graft with the result of a minor stability. Because of the young age of the patient we had decided not to fix transarticularly to avoid the damage of the facet joint. This young patient showed normal activity in her surrounding, not limited by the protective semirigid collar.

Clinically the patients with bony healing of their posterior fusions were free of symptoms and satisfied with the achieved stabilization, even if pseudarthrosis of the odontoid could still be verified in the x-rays. Regarding this clinical experiences we conclude that the major aim of any operative procedure should be the stabilization of the injured functional spine unit.

With a posterior approach we can relieve the patient of pain that is caused by instability, but we should not rely on a bony healing of odontoid pseudarthrosis. In consideration of the well-being of the patients, the failed bony fusion does not correspond with bad clinical results.

What we had to learn is that the activity of the patient and the circumstances of his living style may influence the follow-up of the fusion. To reach the highest certainty of stable posterior fusion it seems to be necessary to fix C1-C2 by transarticular screws.

Böhler proposes an additional anterior bone grafting.[5] In this procedure there is a risk of a secondary dislocation of the dens especially if an indirect cancellous grafting is performed. Alternatively it is possible to perform the bone grafting after an open exposure of the odontoid basis. In this case, iatrogenic trauma has to be taken into account. It may cause a diminution of the vascularization, which may lead to a failure of the cancellous bone graft. Because of the different approaches—anteriorly and posteriorly—an extension of the operation time and an increase of intraoperative blood loss must be kept in mind, a problem that becomes of importance in middle-aged and elderly patients.

## CONCLUSION

The treatment of odontoid nonunions requires good preoperative planning with clear x-rays including functional x-rays in patients without neurological deficiency. In elderly patients with high operative risks, in absence of translatory dislocation of the odontoid fragment, conservative treatment must be taken into consideration. There is no guarantee of success if the decision for operative management is made. Posterior fusion with a wedged corticocancellous bone graft in addition to a wire technique might be sufficient in most patients. Different wire techniques are described, but biomechanically the Brooks procedure might be the most stable one. Its disadvantage is the higher risk of injury to the medulla because of the two wires. The best outcome can be achieved with a transarticular screw fixation in combination with a posterior bone graft. The additional transarticular screw fixation is

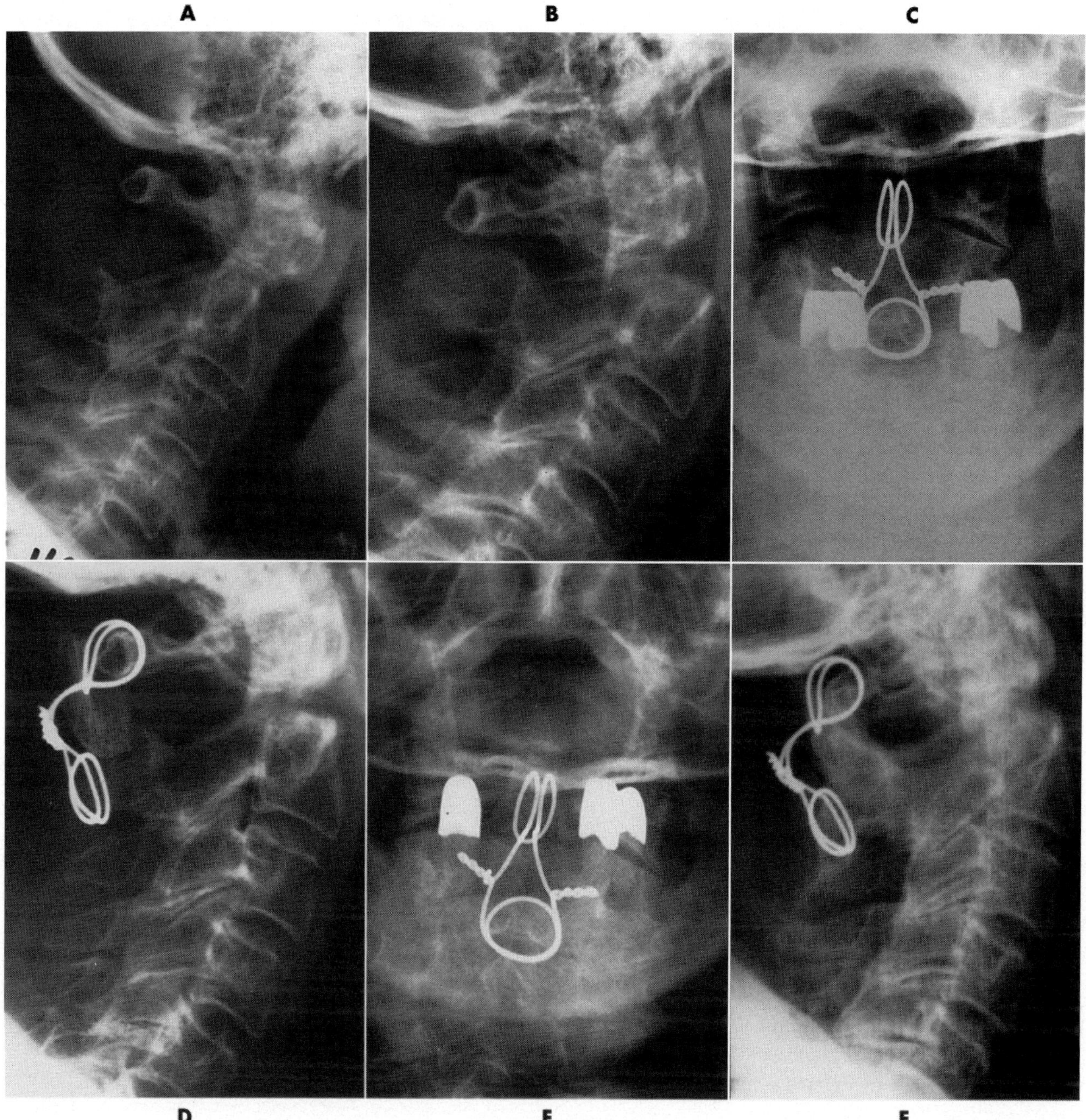


FIGURE 38-5

**A,** Lateral x-ray of Anderson II fracture treated conservatively with Minerva plaster. **B,** Secondary dislocation during plaster immobilization. **C, D,** Three-month follow-up after posterior dislocation. **E, F,** Final radiological result with sufficient posterior fusion after $2\frac{1}{2}$ years.

problematic in adolescent patients because of iatrogenic trauma of the facet joints. In young patients it might be justified to disclaim transarticular fixation. An external stabilization at least with a semirigid collar is mandatory not only in all patients.

The success of posterior fusion cannot be overrated, whether the surgeon chooses a technique of Gallie or Brooks. The bony healing of the pseudarthrosis might only be possible if the interfragmentary gap is less than 2 rmm. Because of the fibrous masses that are interpositioned in the gap between the two fragments, one can not expect to be able to reduce the dislocation totally and close this gap by a posterior procedure. On the other hand, the aim of treatment is to relieve the patient of pain. This pain depends on the instability in the functional spine unit C1-C2. After bony healing of the posterior fusion many patients report their well-being. The loss of function does not stress these patients severely.

A semirigid collar should be worn until radiological signs of osseous consolidation are observed. Whether this device supports the bony healing of the posterior fusion can only be guessed. Without doubt, it reminds the patient of his operation and might help to reduce exaggerated activity.

Contrary to the treatment of pseudarthroses in other regions of traumatology the primary aim in the treatment of odontoid pseudarthrosis is not the interlocking of the odontoid fragments, but the stabilization of the injured functional spine unit.

In patients with atlantoaxial instability by rheumatoid disease the posterior fixation in combination with a transarticular screw application should be recommended. The instability of the whole atlantoaxial complex is the main problem in these patients and is responsible for their pain. The instability involves the ligaments and the facet joints of C1-C2 because of degenerative changes. Any type of treatment has to consider these two different sources of instability.

## REFERENCES


1. Althoff B: Fracture of the odontoid process. An experimental and clinical study. *Acta Orthop Scand* 177(suppl):3-94, 1979.
2. Amling M, Wening VJ, Grote HJ, Hahn M, Delling G: Die Struktur des Axis - Schlüssel zur Ätiologie der Densfraktur, *Chirurg* 65:964-969, 1994.
3. Anderson LD, DÁlonzo RT: Fractures of the odontoid process of the axis, *J Bone Joint Surg Am* 56:1663-1674, 1974.
4. Apuzzo MLJ, Heiden JS, Weiss MH, Ackerson TT, Harvey JP, Kurze T: Acute fractures of the odontoid process.An analysis of 45 cases, *J Neurosurg* 48:85-91, 1978.
5. Böhler J: Anterior stabilization for acute fractures and non-union of the dens, *J Bone Joint Surg Am* 64:18-27, 1982.
6. Brooks AL, Jenkins EB: Atlanto-axial arthrodesis by the wedge compression method, *J Bone Joint Surg Am* 60:279-284, 1978.
7. Clarke CR, White AA: Fractures of the dens. A multicenter study, *J Bone Joint Surg Am* 67:1338-1348, 1985.
8. Coffee MS, Edwards WT, Hayes WE, White AA III: Mechanical response and strength of the human cervical spine, *Trans Cerv Spine Res Soc,* 1986.
9. Doherty BJ, Esses SI, Heggeness MH: A biomechanical study of odontoid fractures and fracture fixation, *Spine* 18(2):178-184, 1993.
10. Dvorak J, Panjabi MM: Functional anatomy of the alar ligaments, *Spine* 12:183-189, 1987.
11. Dvorak J, Panjabi MM, Gerber M: CT-functional diagnostics of the rotatory instability of the upper cervical spine; an experimental study in cadavers, *Spine* 12:197-205, 1987.
12. Dvorak J, Panjabi MM, Hayek J: Diagnostik der Hyper- und Hypomobilität der oberen Halswirbelsäule mittels funktioneller Computertomographie, *Orthopäde* 16:13-19, 1987.
13. Esses SI, Bednar DA: Screw fixation of odontoid fractures and non-unions, *Spine* 16(suppl):483-485, 1991.
14. Evarts MC: Traumatic occipito-atlantal dislocation. Report of a case with survival, *J Bone Joint Surg Am,* 52:1653-1660, 1970.
15. Eysel P, Roosen K: Ventrale und dorsale Spondylodese der Densbasisfraktur—eine neue Klassifikation zur Wahl des chirurgischen Zuganges, *Zentralbl Neurochir* 54:159-165, 1993.
16. Fick R: Handbuch der Anatomie und Mechanik der Gelenke, Jena, S Fischer Verlag 1904, 1911.
17. Fielding JW, Hawkins RJ, Ratzan SA: Spine fusion for atlanto-axial instability, *J Bone Joint Surg Am* 58:400-406, 1976.
18. Fried LC: Atlanto-axial fracture dislocations: failure of posterior C1 to C2 fusion, *J Bone Joint Surg Br* 55:490-495, 1973.
19. Griswold DM: Atlanto-axial fusion for instability, *J Bone Joint Surg Am* 60:285-292, 1978.
20. Hohmann D, Liebig K, Thull R, Haas P: Stabilität der Schraubenosteosynthese von Frakturen der Dens axis, Presented at the 11th Munich Symposium 1989, pp 10-11.
21. Jones MD: Cineradiographic studies of the cervical spine, *Calif Med* 93:S293-S296, 1960.
22. Lind B, Nordwall A, Sihlbom H: Odontoid fractures treated with Halovest, *Spine* 12:173-177, 1987.
23. Magerl F, Seemann PS: *Stable posterior fusion of the atlas and axis by transarticular screw fixation.* In Kehr P, Weidner A, editors: *Cervical spine,* vol 1, Vienna, 1985, Strasbourgh, pp 322-327.
24. Pang D, Wilberger JE: Traumatic atlanto-occipital dislocation with survival: case report and review, *Neurosurgery* 7:503-508, 1980.
25. Panjabi MM, Dvorak J, Duranceau J, Yamamoto I, Dvorak J, RauschningW, Bueff HU: Three-dimensional movements of the upper cervical spine, *Spine* 13(7):726-730, 1988.
26. Powers B, Miller MD, Kramer RS, Martinez S, Gehweiler JA: Traumatic anterior atlanto-occipital dislocation, *Neurosurgery* 4:12-17, 1979.
27. Räber D, Münch TH, Morscher E: Pseudarthrosen im Bereich der Wirbelsäule, *Orthopäde* 25:435-440, 1996.
28. Sasso R, Doherty BJ, Crawford MJ, Heggeness MH: Biomechanics of odontoid fracture fixation.

Comparision of the one-and two-screw technique, *Spine* 18:1950-1953, 1993.
29. Schatzker J, Rorabeck CH, Waddell JP: Fractures of the dens (odontoid process): an analysis of thirty-seven cases, *J Bone Joint Surg Br* 53:392-405, 1971.
30. Schatzker J, Rorabeck CH, Waddell JP: Non-union of the odontoid process. An experimental investigation, *Clin Orthop* 108:127-137, 1975.
31. Torg J, Truex R, Marshall J, Hudgson VR, Quedenfeld TC, Spealman AD: Spinal injury at the level of the third and fourth cervical vertebra from football, *J Bone Joint Surg Am* 59:1015-1018, 1977.
32. Werne S: Studies in spontaneous atlas dislocation, *Acta Orthop Scand* 23(suppl):1-84, 1957.
33. White AA, Panjabi MM: *Clinical biomechanics of the spine,* ed 2, Philadelphia, 1990, JB Lippincott.
34. Wilke H-J, Fischer K, Kugler A, Magerl F, Claes L, Wörsdörfer O: In vitro investigation of internal fixation systems of the upper cervical spine I. Stability of the direct anterior screw fixation of the odontoid, *Eur Spine J* 1:185-190, 1992.

# 39

# PSEUDARTHROSIS TREATMENT IN HIGH-GRADE SPONDYLOLISTHESIS

**Dante G. Marchesi, M.D.**
**Max Aebi, M.D.**



## HIGH-GRADE SPONDYLOLISTHESIS

The management of severe spondylolisthesis with slippage greater than 50% continues to pose a major problem for the orthopedic surgeon. In situ posterolateral fusion from the sacrum to the fourth lumbar vertebra, with or without resection of the loose posterior arch of L5, has been the accepted standard operative treatment, providing satisfactory long-term results.[12,14,17,24,25,26] The main arguments against posterior arthrodesis have been the reported high rates of nonunion ranging up to 44%, the rate of slip progression of as much as 26% despite a solid fusion, and the persistence of the cosmetic deformity.[4,12,14,15,17,20,26,27,29]

Reduction of severe spondylolisthesis improves biomechanical orientation of the lumbosacral junction and thereby facilitates arthrodesis and may prevent some of the drawbacks of in situ fusion such as high incidence of pseudarthrosis, bending, or elongation of the fusion mass and the persistent lumbosacral deformity.[4-7,12-14,17,20,21,23,26] The restoration of the sagittal alignment also allows the patient to stand fully upright with extended knees and hips and reduces the causes of back fatigue and pain.[7] Because loss of the initial correction is not uncommon after reduction,[4,5,12,28] it has been recommended to perform a combined anterior and posterior fusion.[1,6,9,22] The rational of the interbody fusion is that it provides in this critical area a mechanical load-sharing support against additional slippage and maintains any corrections that were obtained.[2,7,30]

The introduction of new pedicular instrumentations with rigid and angle stable fixation further improved the opportunity to reduce and stabilize high-grade spondylolisthesis, sometimes using a posterior approach only.[7,10,16,23,30,32] Despite these powerful spinal fixations, the difficulty to achieve solid arthrodesis in these particular conditions persists and it has demonstrated the necessity to associate the posterior instrumentation with an interbody fusion.[3]

As previously mentioned, the complications concerning spinal fusion in the management of severe spondylolisthesis persist despite the treatment used and the lumbosacral deformity tends to return to its preoperative condition. Patients with failed fusion complain about severe lower lumbar pain, most of the time radiating in one or both lower extremities as pseudoradicular pain or sometimes as true dermatomal symptoms. The classical upright position with flexed hip and knee is habitually present, sometimes associated with mild neurological deficits.

## PSEUDARTHROSIS

In a few patients there is still significant instability in the previously operated lumbosacral junction and the nonunion is easily assessed with flexion-extension lateral radiographs. For the majority of cases, the diagnosis of pseudarthrosis is not simple and it is made with the clinical symptoms, frequently associated with the recurrence of the lumbosacral deformity. Lateral x-rays in flexion-extension, computed tomography (CT) scan with reconstruction, and scintigraphic evaluation usually confirm the pseudarthrosis.

The management of this complicated situation is definitely a surgical revision. Most studies of the treatment of severe spondylolisthesis have focused on the primary treatment and very few of the studies have included patients who had secondary treatment after a failed arthrodesis.[3,5,7,10,18,19,31] The exact surgical technique used is generally not reported and data about fusion rate and complications in salvage procedures are difficult to be evidenced. Some of these authors propose a revision of the fusion mass, decortication of the pseudarthrosis, and augmentation of the posterolateral fusion. The majority tends to recommend a combined in situ interbody arthrodesis obtained with fibular graft associated with a posterolateral fusion.[3,5,7,19]

## OPERATIVE MANAGEMENT

Our preferred treatment of these patients is to manage them as if they had a primary high-grade spondylolisthesis and undergo partial reduction of the deformity with a circumferential arthrodesis. In those cases with radiological instability and partial reduction of the deformity we recommend a posterior decortication of the fusion mass, nerve root decompression, and posterior pedicular instrumentation from L4 to S1 trying to restore adequate lumbosacral lordosis. Interbody fusion from a posterolateral approach (PLIF) or from an anterior approach completes the procedure.

In patients with rigid and severe displacement, because of the high risk of neurological injuries due to the reposition maneuver and the possible scar tissue surrounding the nerve structures, we suggest a progressive reduction. This is obtained performing a first surgery in which the posterior elements of the spine are exposed from L3 to S1. Nerve decompression is carried out with careful dissection of the dural sac in respect of L5 and visualization of both L5 and S1 nerve roots laterally until their exit from the intervertebral foramen. The procedure is continued with a progressive resection of the L5-S1 disk and osteotomy of the sacral dome. The previous posterolateral fusion mass is also revised and osteotomized in order to create as much movement as in the lumbosacral junction. Schanz screws are then inserted through separate skin incisions in the L3 or L4 pedicles and in the posterior iliac wing entering from the posterior iliac spine in order to preserve the pedicle of L5 and S1 for the further definitive posterior instrumentation (Fig. 39-1).

### Reduction

After skin closure, the Schanz screw extensions are connected with the AO-external fixation frame. In the following days the device allows slow and progressive reduction of part of the deformity. This is obtained with the patient awake in order to control every possible neurological change. Daily distraction and progressive rotation of the pelvis using the screws inserted in the ilium allow the correction of the sagittal angle. During this time the patient is kept hospitalized but able to walk without external support. A special mattress with a hole in respect of the external fixator is used at rest.

### Internal Fixation

Once satisfactory partial correction is obtained, usually after 7 or 10 days of daily manipulations, the patient is brought back to surgery. In prone position, the external fixator is removed and the same posterior incision is used to expose the lumbosacral spine. AO-USS pedicular screws of appropriate dimension and length are now placed in the pedicles of L4 and S1 while Schanz screws are inserted in L5. A 6-mm hard rod is bent for an appropriate lumbosacral lordosis and then fixed to the screws. Mild distraction is applied between L4 and S1 using the distraction forceps. An appropriate reduction device specially developed for the reposition of spondylolisthesis and connected to the L5 Schanz screw allows the L5 vertebra to be pulled back almost to a full reduction of the deformity (Fig. 39-2). During this maneuver the nerve roots need to be constantly kept under visual control to avoid injury. Somatosensory evoked potential assessment is recommended during this operation time. At the end further lordosis can be obtained by compressing between the screws using the tension band concept. Autologous bone is added to the previous posterolateral intertransverse fusion after adequate decortication.

### Circumferential Fusion

Interbody fusion is mandatory in these revision surgeries in order to increase fusion chances.[3] This could be obtained with a fibula graft impacted from the sacrum into L5 or with a PLIF using autologous bone or cages during the same procedure, but we prefer combine a standard anterior approach. During the same surgery the patient is placed supine. Through a transperitoneal approach done in the suprapubic area the L5-S1 segment is identified after previous ligature of the descending sacral vessels. The anterior L5-S1 annulus and the remaining disk material are resected, the adjacent endplates are decorticated and a tricortical bone graft is introduced. Further stability can be obtained with a screw starting in the anterosuperior

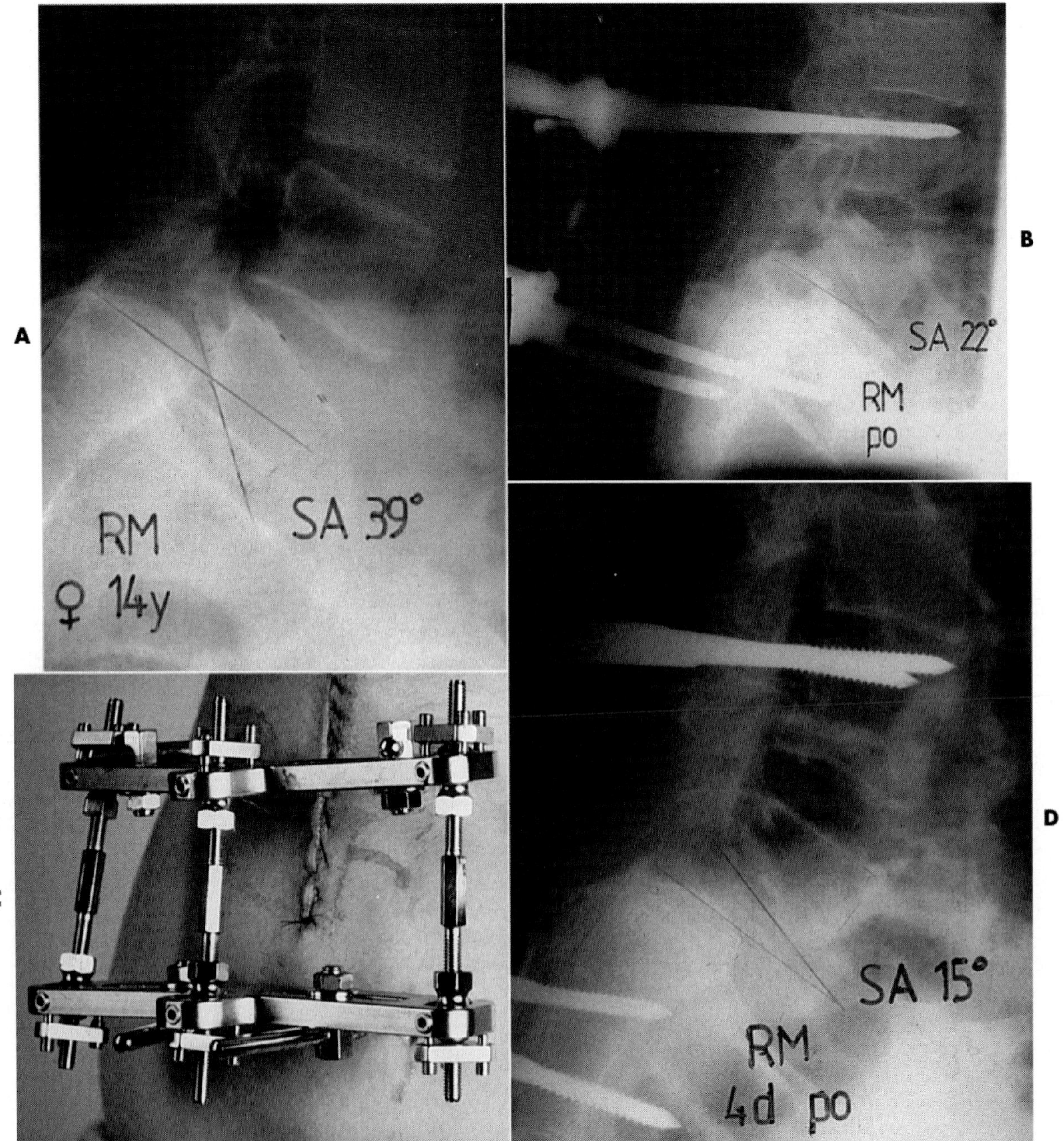


**FIGURE 39-1**

**A,** Lateral x-ray of a14-year-old female patient with grade IV spondylolisthesis and failure of previously performed L4-S1 posterior fusion. A first surgery is performed using a posterior approach, nerve decompression, L5-S1 diskectomy, resection of the sacral dome, and revision of the fusion mass. **B** and **C,** Schanz screws are placed in the pedicles of L4 and in the posterior ilium and then fixed to the external fixator frame. **D,** Daily progressive distraction and rotation of the pelvis is performed over one week. The slipping angle (SA) could be corrected from −39 to −15 degrees and the grade IV slippage to a grade II spondylolisthesis.

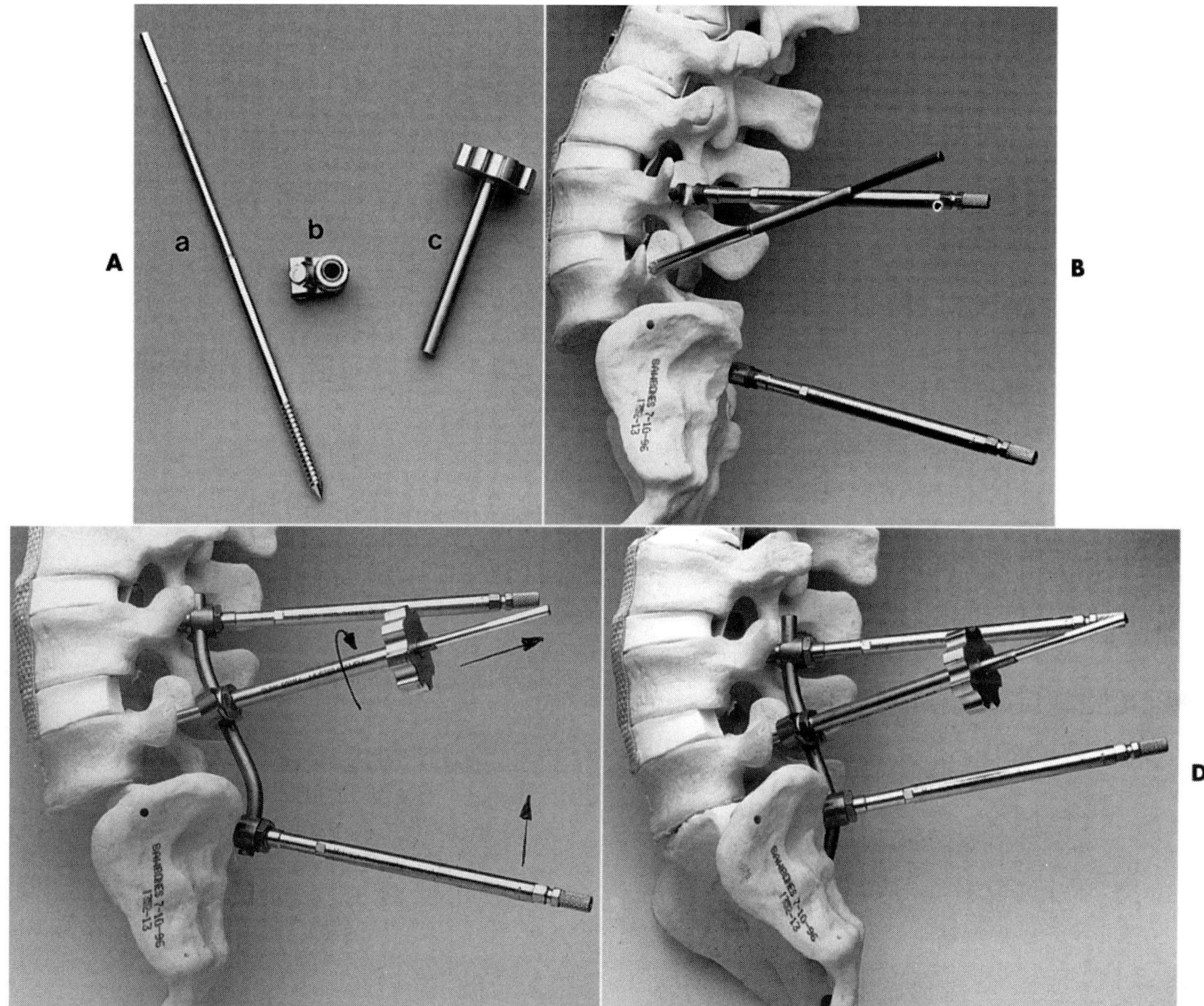


**FIGURE 39-2**

**A,** The instrumentation allowing reposition of the spondylolisthesis consists of a special Schanz screw with additional threaded zone in the mid shaft (*a*), a conventional AO-ASIF USS fractures clamp allowing multidirectional Schanz screw manipulation (*b*), and the inside threaded reduction device (*c*). **B,** As seen on this model, in a second surgery USS pedicle lateral open screws are placed in S1 and L4 while the special Schanz screws are inserted in the pedicles of L5. **C** and **D,** After connection with the rods the definitive lumbosacral manipulation is started with the help of the special reduction device allowing posterior translation of L5. Further correction of the slipping angle is obtained by manipulation of the sacrum using the lever arm of the S1 screw.

corner of L5 and running through the disk space into the body of S1 (Figs. 39-3 and 39-4). The anterior procedure may be performed using a minimally invasive spinal technique. Mobilization is started the first or second postoperative day with a lumbar orthosis at approximately 10 weeks.

Using this technique, six patients have been successfully treated. All presented with failed posterior fusion for severe spondylolisthesis. The mean age was 17 years (13 to 29 years) and 4 were females. In four cases no instrumentation had been used during the original surgery, whereas in the other two there was breakage of the S1 screws following posterior L4-S1 instrumentation and fusion. In three cases there was a grade III and in three grade IV displacement. Mean slipping angle was −26 degrees (−39 to −18 degrees).

The patients have been surgically revised as previously described and the deformity could be reduced to less than 50% spondylolisthesis. All underwent circumferential fusion, in two cases with a single posterior approach and in four cases with a combined posteroanterior surgery. One patient was found postoperatively with a foot drop complication, which progressively but only partially recovered in the following 3 months. Solid spinal fusion was obtained in all six cases without further instrumentation failure or

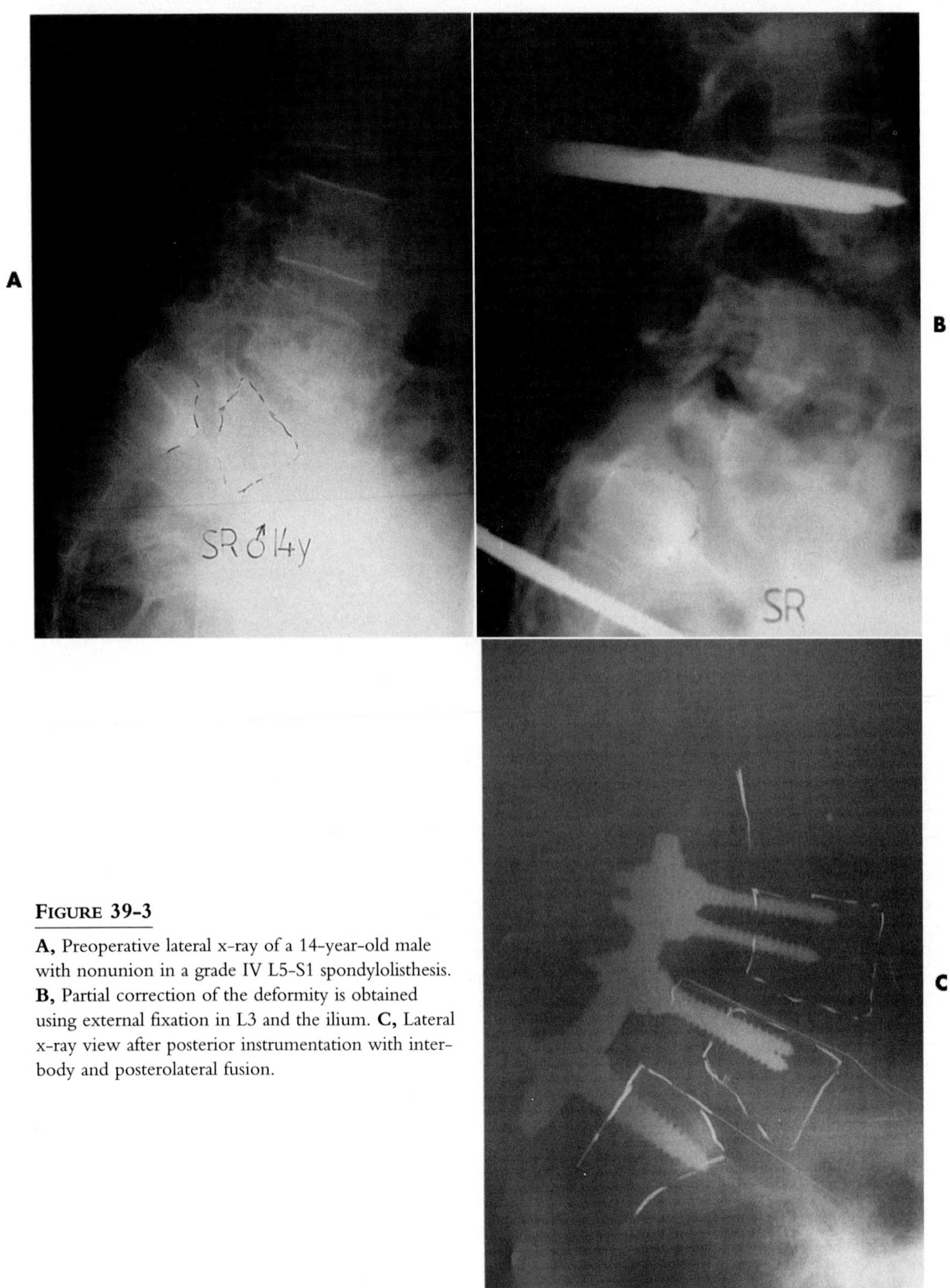


**FIGURE 39-3**

**A,** Preoperative lateral x-ray of a 14-year-old male with nonunion in a grade IV L5-S1 spondylolisthesis. **B,** Partial correction of the deformity is obtained using external fixation in L3 and the ilium. **C,** Lateral x-ray view after posterior instrumentation with interbody and posterolateral fusion.

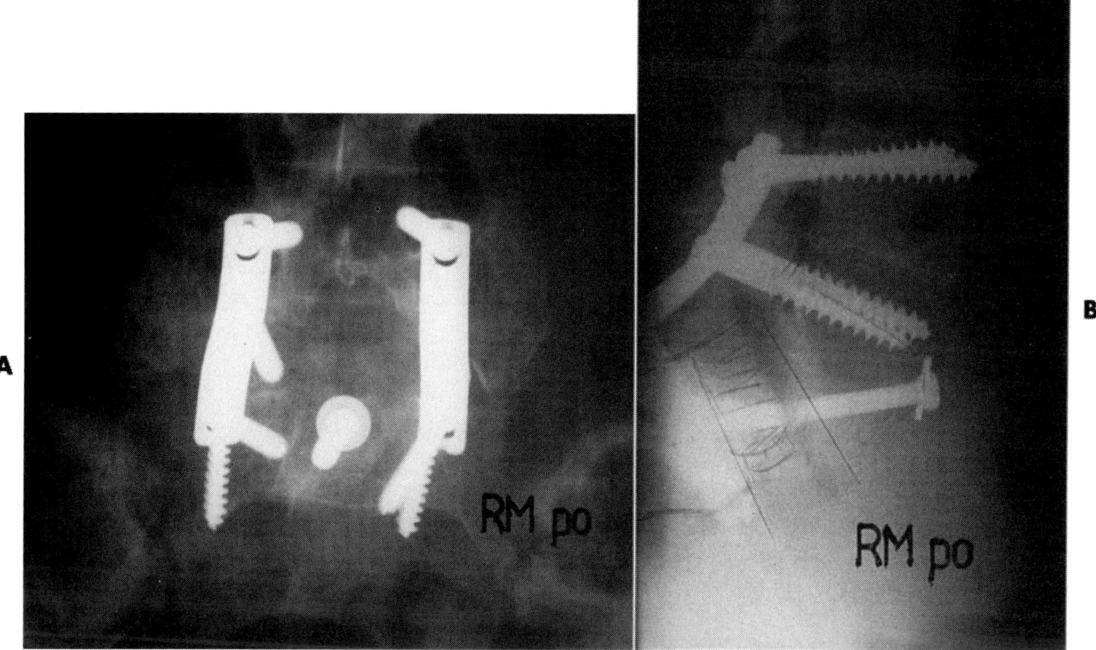


FIGURE 39-4

**A, B,** Postoperative AP and lateral x-rays of the patient presented in Figure 39-1. A posterior plate-screw fixation has been performed because the small size of the pedicles. Transperitoneal anterior interbody fusion with additional L5-S1 screw has been performed in the same operation time. The deformity has been reduced to almost an anatomical condition.

loss of correction. Pain symptoms significantly improved in five cases while remaining unchanged in one.

Based on our limited experience, failed fusion after surgical treatment for high-grade spondylolisthesis can still be managed. As it would be the original surgery, we believe these deformities need to be aggressively treated with partial correction of the lumbosacral kyphosis and of the anterior vertebral slippage. This can be performed only with accurate revision of the previous fusion mass to obtain adequate vertebral mobility. To avoid neurological complications, we recommend a progressive reduction using an external fixator. Solid arthrodesis will be obtained in a second surgery with posterior pedicular instrumentation and circumferential fusion.

## REFERENCES


1. Ani N, Keppler L, Biscup R, Steffee A: Reduction of high-grade slips (Grades III-IV) with VSP instrumentation: report of a series of 41 cases, *Spine* 16:S308-S310, 1991.
2. Bohlman H, Cook S: One-stage decompression and posterolateral and interbody fusion for lumbosacral spondyloptosis through a posterior approach, *J Bone Joint Surg* 64A:415-418, 1982.
3. Boos N, Marchesi D, Zuber K, Aebi M: Treatment of severe spondylolisthesis by reduction and pedicular fixation: a four to six year follow-up study, *Spine* 18(12): 1655-1661, 1993.
4. Boxall D, Bradford D, Moe J, Winter R: Management of severe spondylolisthesis (Grade III and Grade IV) in children and adolescents, *J Bone Joint Surg* 61A:479-495, 1979.
5. Bradford D: Treatment of severe spondylolisthesis: a combined approach for reduction and stabilization, *Spine* 4:423-429, 1979.
6. Bradford D, Gottfried Y: Staged salvage reconstruction of Grade IV and V spondylolisthesis, *J Bone Joint Surg* 69A:191-202, 1987.
7. Bradford D, Boachie-Adjej O: Treatment of severe spondylolisthesis by anterior and posterior reduction and stabilization: a long-term follow-up study, *J Bone Joint Surg* 72A:1060-1066, 1990.
8. Cheng C, Fang D, Lee P, Leong J: Anterior spinal fusion for spondylolysis and isthmic spondylolisthesis: long-term results in adults, *J Bone Joint Surg* 71B:264-267, 1989.

9. De Wald R, Fant M, Taddonio R, Neuwirth M: Severe lumbosacral spondylolisthesis in adolescents and children, *J Bone Joint Surg* 63A:619-626, 1981.
10. Dick W, Schnebel B: Severe spondylolisthesis: reduction and internal fixation, *Clin Orthop* 232:70-79, 1988.
11. Dimar J, Hoffman G: Grade IV spondylolisthesis: two-stage therapeutic approach of anterior vertebrectomy and anterior-posterior fusion, *Orthop Rev* 15:504-509, 1986.
12. Freeman B, Donati N: Spinal arthrodesis for severe spondylolisthesis in children and adolescents: a long-term follow-up study, *J Bone Joint Surg* 71A:594-598 1989.
13. Harrington P, Dickson J: Spinal instrumentation in the treatment of severe progressive spondylolisthesis, *Clin Orthop* 117:157-163, 1976.
14. Harris I, Weinstein S: Long-term follow-up of patients with Grade III and IV spondylolisthesis: treatment with and without posterior fusion, *J Bone Joint Surg* 69A:960-969, 1987.
15. Hensinger R: Spondylolysis and spondylolisthesis in children and adolescents, *J Bone Joint Surg* 71A:1098-1107, 1989.
16. Herman S, Pouliquen J: Spondylolisthesis à grand déplacement chez l'enfant et l'adolescent: résultats de 12 cas de réduction-fixation postérieure, *Rev Chir Orthop* 74:614-621, 1988.
17. Johnson J, Kirwan E: The long-term results of fusion in situ for severe spondylolisthesis, *J Bone Joint Surg* 65B:43-46, 1983.
18. Jones A, McAfee P, Robinson R, Zinreich S, Wang H: Failed arthrodesis of the spine for severe spondylolisthesis: salvage by interbody arthrodesis, *J Bone Joint Surg* 70A:25-30, 1988.
19. Kimm S, Denis F, Lonstein J, Winter R: Factors affecting fusion rate in adult spondylolisthesis, *Spine* 15:979-983, 1990.
20. Laurent L, Ôsterman K: Operative treatment of spondylolisthesis in young patients, *Clin Orthop* 117:85-91, 1976.
21. Lehner S, Steffee A, Gaines R: Treatment of L5-S1 spondyloptosis by staged L5 resection and fusion of L4 onto S1 (Gaines Procedure), *Spine* 19:1916-1925, 1994.
22. Louis R, Marescu C: Stabilisation chirurgicale avec réduction des spondylolyses et des spondylolisthésis, *Int Orthop* 1:215-225, 1977.
23. Matthiass H, Heine J: The surgical reduction of spondylolisthesis, *Clin Orthop* 203:34-44, 1986.
24. Peek R, Wiltse L, Reynolds J, Thomas J, Guyer D, Widell E: In situ arthrodesis without decompression for Grade II and IV isthmic spondylolisthesis in adults who have severe sciatica, *J Bone Joint Surg* 71A:62-68, 1989.
25. Pizzutillo P, Merenda W, MacEwen G: Posterolateral fusion for spondylolisthesis in adolescence, *J Pediat Orthop* 6:311-316, 1986.
26. Seitsalo S, Osterman K, Hyvarinen H, Schlenzka D, Poussa M: Severe spondylolisthesis in children and adolescents: a long-term review of fusion in situ, *J Bone Joint Surg* 72B:259-265, 1990.
27. Smith M, Bohlman H: Spondylolisthesis treated by a single-stage operation combining decompression with in situ posterolateral and anterior fusion, *J Bone Joint Surg,* 72A:415-421, 1990.
28. Stanton R, Mechan P, Lovell W: Surgical fusion in childhood spondylolisthesis, *J Pediat Orthop* 5:411-415, 1985.
29. Stauffer R, Coventry M: Posterolateral lumbar spine fusion. Analysis of Mayo Clinic Series, *J Bone Joint Surg* 54A:1195-1204, 1972.
30. Steffee A, Sitkowski D: Reduction and stabilization of Grade IV spondylolisthesis, *Clin Orthop* 227:82-89, 1988.
31. Transfeldt E: The cause of neurologic deficit in acute spondylolisthesis (listhetic crisis) and in reduction of grades III-IV spondylolisthesis, *J Pediat Orthop* 7:365-370, 1987.
32. Transfeldt E, Dendrinos G, Bradford D: Paresis of proximal lumbar roots after reduction of L5-S1 spondylolisthesis, *Spine* 14:884-887, 1989.

# 40

# BONE-IMPLANT FIXATION FAILURE

**Marco Brayda-Bruno, M.D.**



On many occasions we can observe loosening or dislodgement of spinal implants from their insertion sites in or on the bony structures; that means a failure of a solid bone-implant fixation, the essential factor to assure stability of the devices and to achieve fusion of the instrumented spinal segments.

Everybody agrees upon the fact that any newer modality for spinal instrumentation and fusion must compare favorably with "gold standards," and that in the last 15 years Cotrel-Dubousset instrumentation (CDI) has become the new gold standard for spinal instrumentation because of its undoubtful advantages such as multiple hook/screw placement and sagittal profile correction with minimal or no postoperative bracing.[3]

The new segmental spinal instrumentations of third generation (such as CD Horizon, Isola, Moss-Miami, Synergy, etc.) are very solid and stable, and it is possible to achieve the correction of any deformity with these powerful tools, using combined strategy of segmentary compression/distraction, translation, and/or rod rotation, achieving more correction and stability. Nevertheless, apart from the specific differences among them, there are some common features of implant assembly configuration that could cause a fixation failure: the upper thoracic claw (or foundation), the distal level of fusion and its claw, and the sacropelvic fixation.

Early series with classic CDI demonstrated a 2.5% hook dislodgement of the upper claws and 1% rate of early hook displacement and 0.5% of prominent hardware.[3,11] In the author's opinion, adult deformities and the more complex forms of scoliosis still have somewhat different risks and complication rates, and some common complications such as infection, hardware prominence, or displacement and pseudarthrosis persist also in the currently most advanced systems. This is a difficult surgery, which requires hands-on training and the ability to anticipate and treat complications, also through a revision. The spinal deformity patient who had previous surgery and who now has new or continuing problems and complaints may be a candidate for further surgical treatment. Hopefully this event should rarely occur, but some authors consider an overall reoperation rate of approximately 12% acceptable.[12] It is then a surgery to be considered and well known in any important spine center.

Before discussing "what and how to do" during revision for a bone-implant fixation failure, we should focus on the causes, diagnostic criteria, and the clinical symptoms of that unexpected event.

## ETIOLOGY

A bone-implant fixation failure could be secondary to surgical mistakes or due to specific preexisting conditions of the patient.

### SECONDARY TO SURGERY

The most common reasons for "iatrogenic" implant fixation failure are the wrong choice of fusion area or the wrong strategy in implant distribution, causing an overload of single spinal segments (Fig. 40-1).

The former cause is generally connected to a mistake in fusion level selection (the end vertebrae out of the stable zone), and to the fixation in a non-neutral level, both in sagital or coronal view (at the apex of kyphosis, at the apex of a curve, in junctional thoracolumbar levels), without preserving or restoring the sagital profile. In younger patients all these factors could be complicated by the physiological growth of the spinal column, progressing with time onto crankshaft phenomena or too short fusions.[5] In older patients, a wrong lumbar strategy (namely implants on junctional kyphosis or out of stable zone) and a wrong thoracic strategy (namely unrecognized double thoracic curve pattern or kyphosis above fusion) could produce coronal or sagital plane decompensation or both, with trunk and shoulder imbalance. At the lumbosacral level, for instance, the sacral fixation by a single screw is often connected to implant loosening and failure, pseudarthrosis, and concurrent pain. The alar screw extensions, used with some modern instrumentation, also give frequent problems at follow-up.

The use of Dubousset iliosacral screws is then preferable when a complex spine deformity requires fixation to the sacrum.[3] It is our sacral fixation of choice in sitting patients, but sometimes the long-term follow-up of ambulatory patients shows some complaint for prominent and mobilized screw, often with a solid fusion. More rarely that failure could be due to an incorrect preparation of bone site for the implant or to a wrong maneuver during implant insertion, problems not detected during surgery and that can favor an implant's early mobilization and possibly a pseudarthrosis.

### SECONDARY TO PREEXISTING CONDITIONS

Preexisting conditions that may cause bone-implant fixation failure include: an intrinsic bone weakness with reduced resistance to stress of bony structure, as we can observe related to age (in younger and older patients), sex, some systemic diseases, osteoporosis, neurofibromatosis, or postradiation bone (Fig. 40-2).[6] Under particular stress, these conditions could then cause bone breaking with implant dislodgement.

Although in the author's opinion pseudarthrosis is most often secondary to an early implant mobilization, sometimes a late implant displacement could be preceeded and caused by a pseudarthrosis due to inadequate bone grafting. In this latter event the lack of fusion brings a loss of correction with possible implant fixation failure. Generally the pseudarthrosis rate in idiopathic adolescent scoliosis should be in the 1% to 2% range when an accurate facet excision with massive bone grafting is performed and the modern devices are used.[7,10] Of course, this rate is somewhat higher in adults.[12]

Finally, this kind of failure is more likely to occur in patients with severe and stiff trunk and/or pelvic imbalance, namely adult or neurologic ones, because of the enormous stress on the device. Sometimes a too active postoperative mobilization in adults, or the iterative, sudden movements in some cerebral palsy (CP) or ataxic patient, could bring a loss of tension especially in open implants, with their consequent mobilization through micromovements and loosening of bone fixation (Fig. 40-3).

These complications, often described in neurologic patients,[9] include hook displacement inferiorly, which may occur from inadequate contouring of the rod, improper placement of the laminar or pedicle hooks, prominent device for transverse traction (DTT), or osteoporotic bone allowing multiple hook cut-outs with loss of correction.

When it occurs within the first few months postoperatively, a complete revision should always be performed.

## DIAGNOSIS

The diagnosis of a bone-implant fixation failure is generally done by clinical observation and radiographic findings.

### CLINICAL ASSESSMENT

A detailed and comprehensive history and physical examination are essential. The most common symptoms are pain or discomfort, sometimes imbalance, and eventually bursitis. Pain syndromes and patient complaints vary from a mild burning hump pain to a rather specific low back and radicular pain. Pain can be located above the fusion mass, but is most common below the fusion mass, in the lower lumbar area, and it is generally caused by degenerative disk disease, spinal stenosis, disk rupture, instability, or nerve root entrapment.

Low back pain could be also caused by a loss of coronal or sagittal balance and any attempt to alleviate pain without restoring sagittal alignment to the spine will usually fail. On occasion, a spondylolysis will develop at L5, usually secondary to a flat lumbar spine.

A careful physical examination must be performed to control patient's stance and gait for imbalance (namely hip and knee flexion, leg length discrepancy, sagittal axis, plumb line, etc.), as well as a neurological assessment to verify any radicular involvement (muscle strength, toe and heel walk, deep tendon reflexes, sphinteric control, sensitivity, etc.).

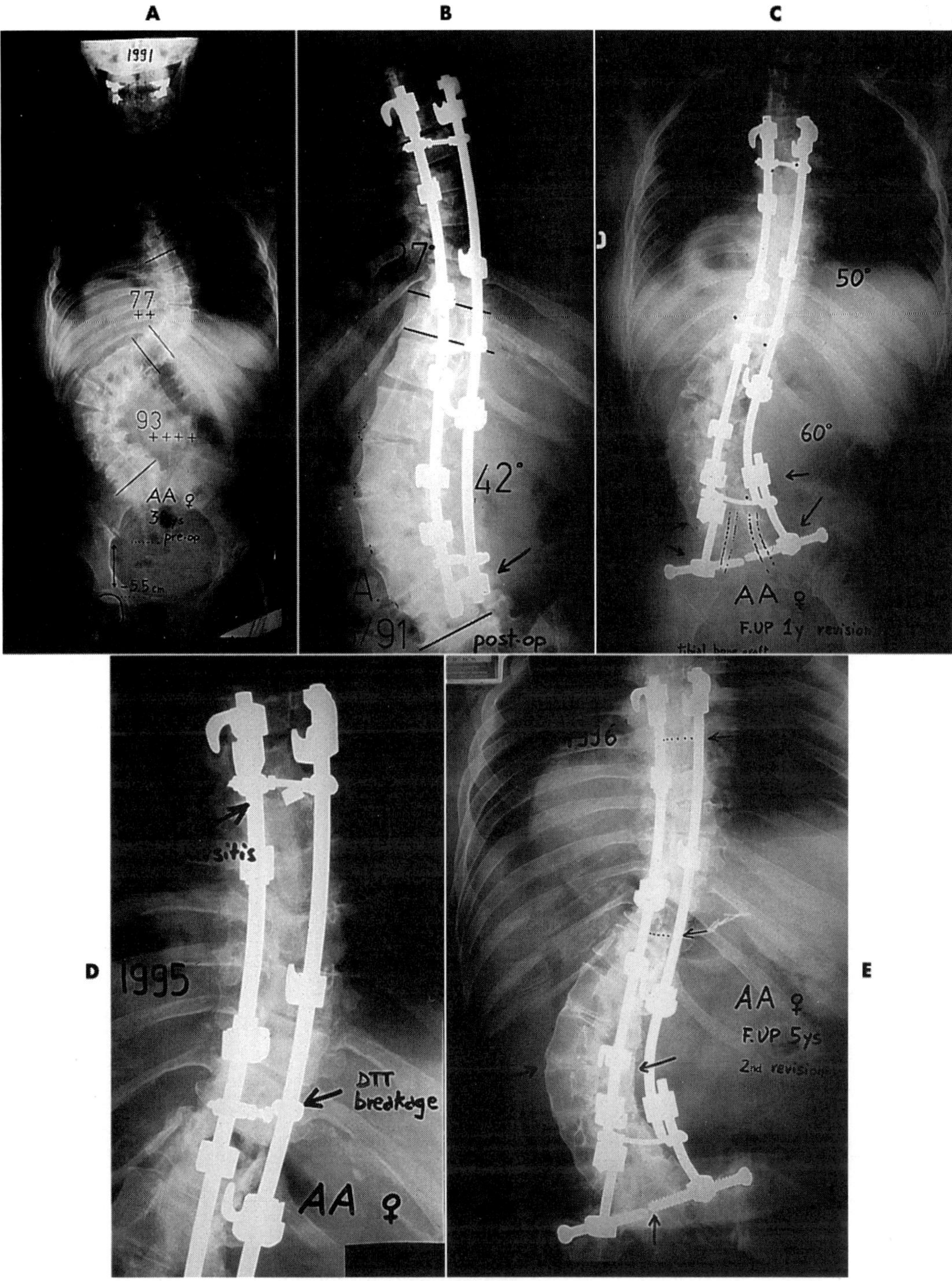


**FIGURE 40-1**

The patient is a 32-year-old woman with a progressive postpolio painful thoracolumbar scoliosis. The patient walks with spica and crutches, placing a lot of effort on her upper arms because of the severe lower limb paralysis. The first surgery was performed in May 1991, when we were not yet using pedicular screws at lumbar level. A staged anterior-posterior approach was planned, with anterior T12-L4 diskectomy and fusion and posterior T5-L5 fusion with segmentary fixation by CDI hooks. **A,** Preoperative coronal view. Note the pelvic obliquity and the leg length discrepancy. **B,** Note, in this immediate postoperative coronal view, the double laminar hook fixation on L5. There is too much stress on a single, hypoplasic posterior arch like that of L5. After 2 months it broke with bone-implant fixation failure and pain when walking. **C,** Coronal view at one-year postrevision follow-up. In July 1991, we performed a revision surgery with extension to sacrum, using the Dubousset iliosacral screws, connectors with the old frame, and tibial strut grafts to ensure a strong fusion at lumbosacral level. **D,** After 3 years, the patient was complaining of painful bursitis corresponding to the two thoracic DTTs. It was due to the important stress on the thoracic area solely using the upper arms for walking. Coronal detail of thoracic region, with a DTT breakage and bursitis. **E,** Coronal view at last follow-up after the second revision minor surgery. The two DTTs have been removed, and the thoracic fusion area has been revised without observing nonunions. Note the massive lumbar anterior and posterior fusion. Now the patient is totally pain-free.

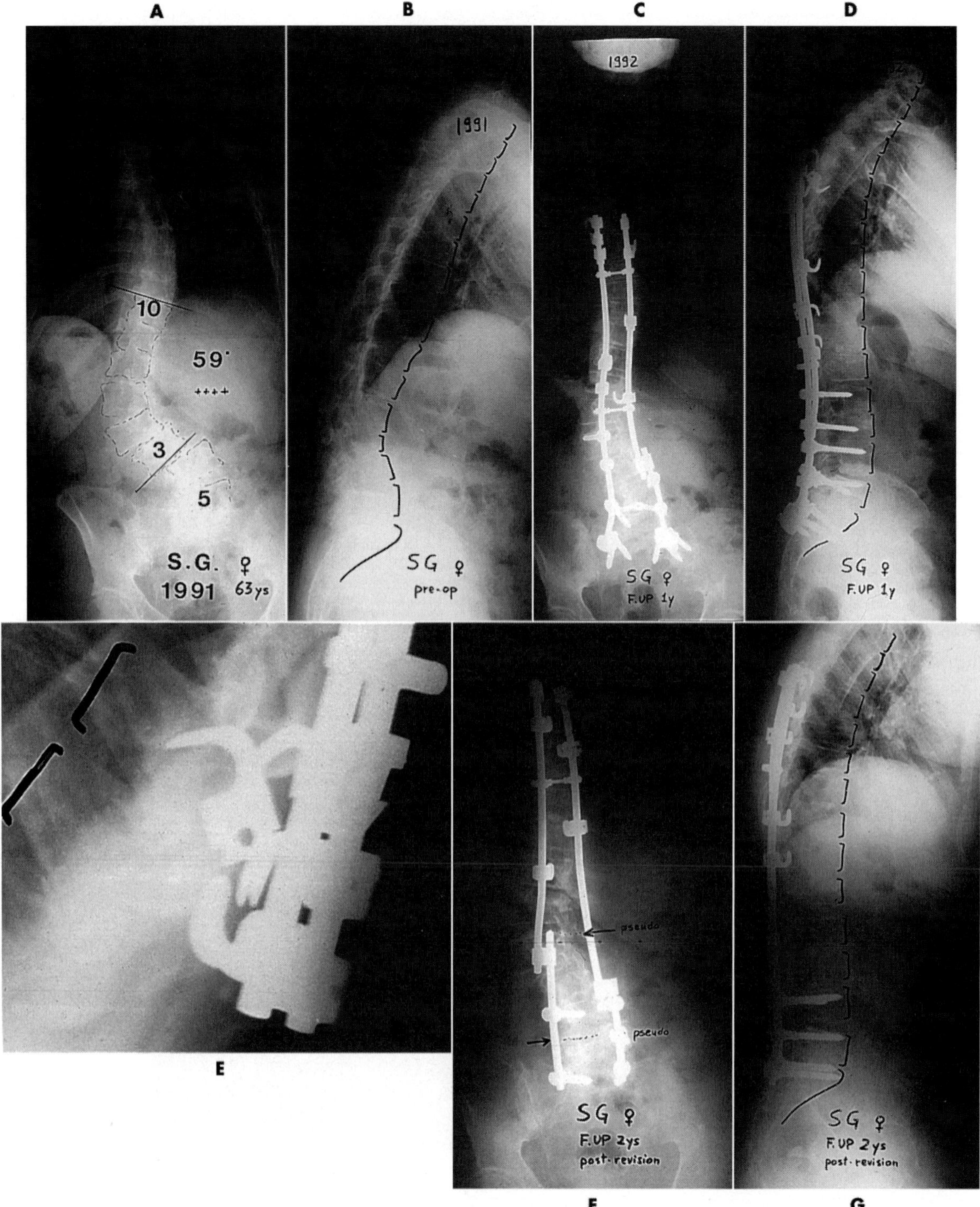


**FIGURE 40-2**

A 65-year-old woman with a severe degenerative scoliosis and a very significant forward and left trunk imbalance. The patient's complaint was severe lumbar pain when standing and recurrent leg pain. A single-stage posterior fusion T6-sacrum with CDI hooks and pedicular screws was performed in 1992. Preoperative x-ray: The coronal view **(A)** shows the imbalance to the left with rotational subluxation of L2, L3, L4; in the sagital plane **(B)**, a severe thoracolumbar kyphosis with imbalance is evident. Postoperative x-rays at 1-year follow-up: good improvement in balance both in coronal **(C)** and in sagital **(D)** views. Despite that, because of a too short proximal instrumentation of the osteoporotic bone, an implant fixation failure happened at thoracic level. **E,** Particular to bone-implant fixation failure at T6-T7 level. Another mistake was to instrument a single level with a bilateral transverse-pedicular claw. The stress was too much for an osteoporotic posterior arch. Since then, the author has begun to use thoracic bivertebral claws, which allows for a better distribution of forces. Revision surgery was performed in 1993, repairing two nonunions at thoracolumbar and lumbar level, and reimplanting the proximal part with a bivertebral T5-T6 claw. The coronal **(F)** and sagital **(G)** views at 2-year follow-up show good trunk balance without any patient discomfort. A body brace was applied postoperatively for 8 months.

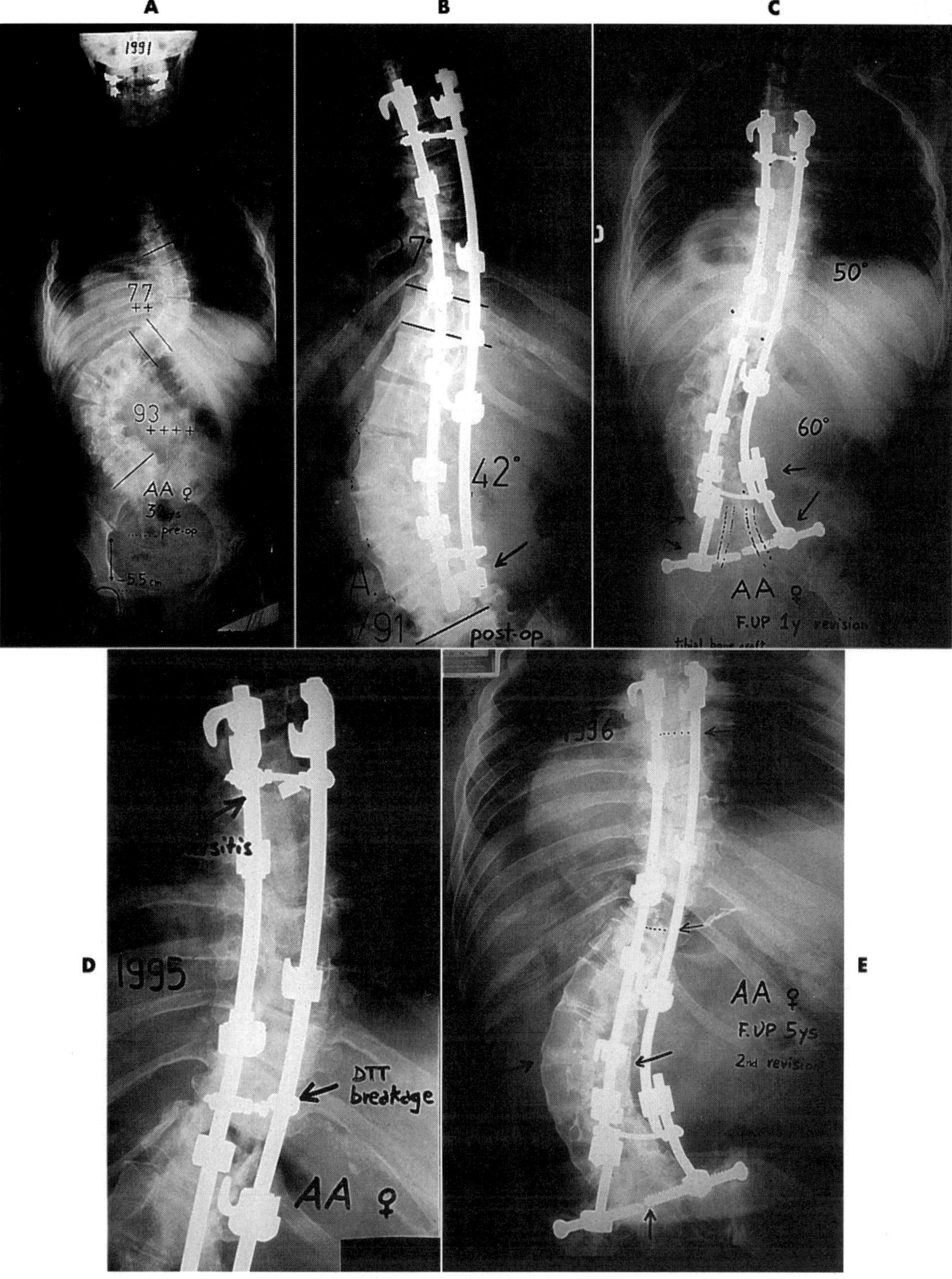


**FIGURE 40-1**

The patient is a 32-year-old woman with a progressive postpolio painful thoracolumbar scoliosis. The patient walks with spica and crutches, placing a lot of effort on her upper arms because of the severe lower limb paralysis. The first surgery was performed in May 1991, when we were not yet using pedicular screws at lumbar level. A staged anterior-posterior approach was planned, with anterior T12-L4 diskectomy and fusion and posterior T5-L5 fusion with segmentary fixation by CDI hooks. **A,** Preoperative coronal view. Note the pelvic obliquity and the leg length discrepancy. **B,** Note, in this immediate postoperative coronal view, the double laminar hook fixation on L5. There is too much stress on a single, hypoplasic posterior arch like that of L5. After 2 months it broke with bone-implant fixation failure and pain when walking. **C,** Coronal view at one-year postrevision follow-up. In July 1991, we performed a revision surgery with extension to sacrum, using the Dubousset iliosacral screws, connectors with the old frame, and tibial strut grafts to ensure a strong fusion at lumbosacral level. **D,** After 3 years, the patient was complaining of painful bursitis corresponding to the two thoracic DTTs. It was due to the important stress on the thoracic area solely using the upper arms for walking. Coronal detail of thoracic region, with a DTT breakage and bursitis. **E,** Coronal view at last follow-up after the second revision minor surgery. The two DTTs have been removed, and the thoracic fusion area has been revised without observing nonunions. Note the massive lumbar anterior and posterior fusion. Now the patient is totally pain-free.

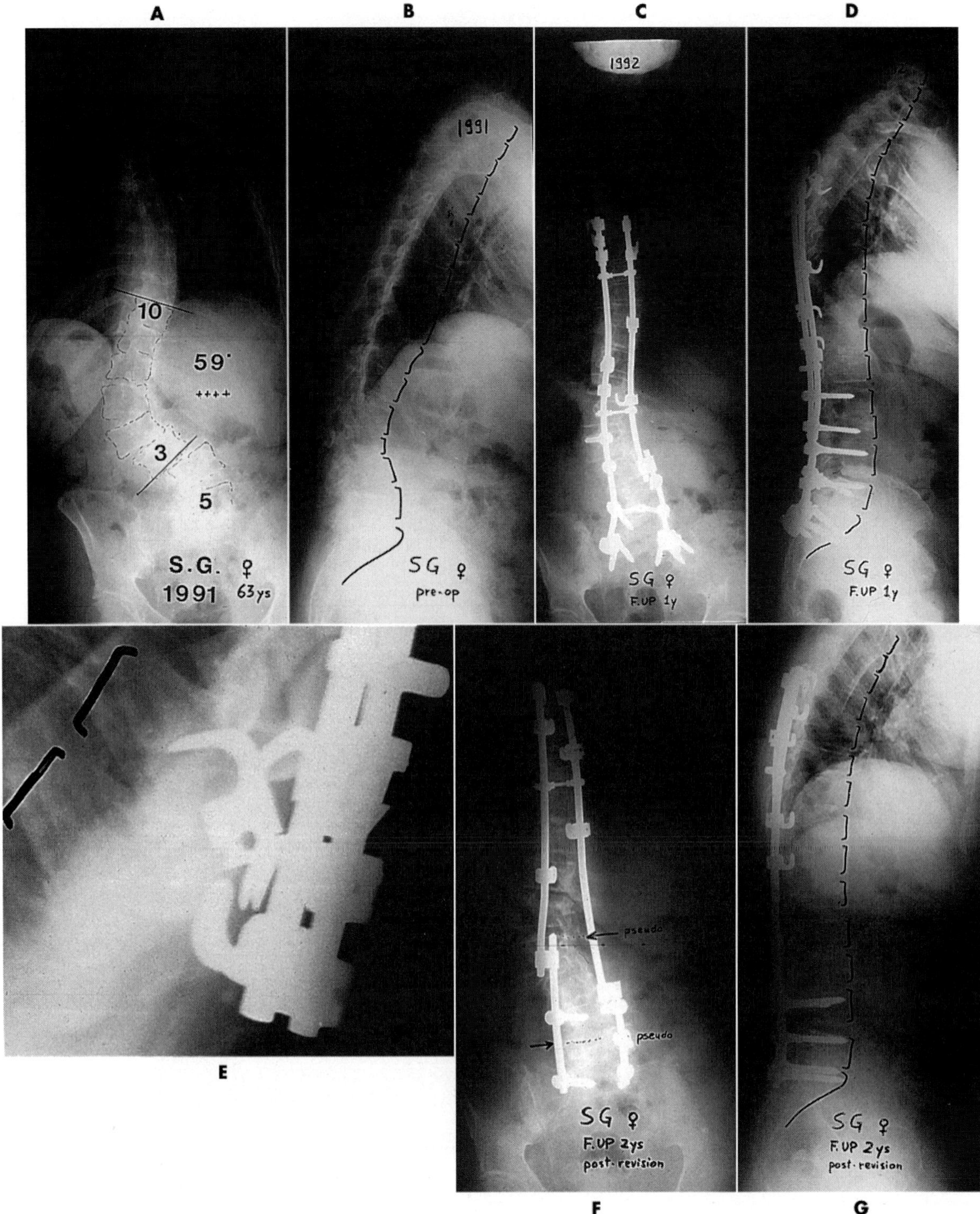


FIGURE 40-2

A 65-year-old woman with a severe degenerative scoliosis and a very significant forward and left trunk imbalance. The patient's complaint was severe lumbar pain when standing and recurrent leg pain. A single-stage posterior fusion T6-sacrum with CDI hooks and pedicular screws was performed in 1992. Preoperative x-ray: The coronal view **(A)** shows the imbalance to the left with rotational subluxation of L2, L3, L4; in the sagital plane **(B),** a severe thoracolumbar kyphosis with imbalance is evident. Postoperative x-rays at 1-year follow-up: good improvement in balance both in coronal **(C)** and in sagital **(D)** views. Despite that, because of a too short proximal instrumentation of the osteoporotic bone, an implant fixation failure happened at thoracic level. **E,** Particular to bone-implant fixation failure at T6-T7 level. Another mistake was to instrument a single level with a bilateral transverse-pedicular claw. The stress was too much for an osteoporotic posterior arch. Since then, the author has begun to use thoracic bivertebral claws, which allows for a better distribution of forces. Revision surgery was performed in 1993, repairing two nonunions at thoracolumbar and lumbar level, and reimplanting the proximal part with a bivertebral T5-T6 claw. The coronal **(F)** and sagital **(G)** views at 2-year follow-up show good trunk balance without any patient discomfort. A body brace was applied postoperatively for 8 months.

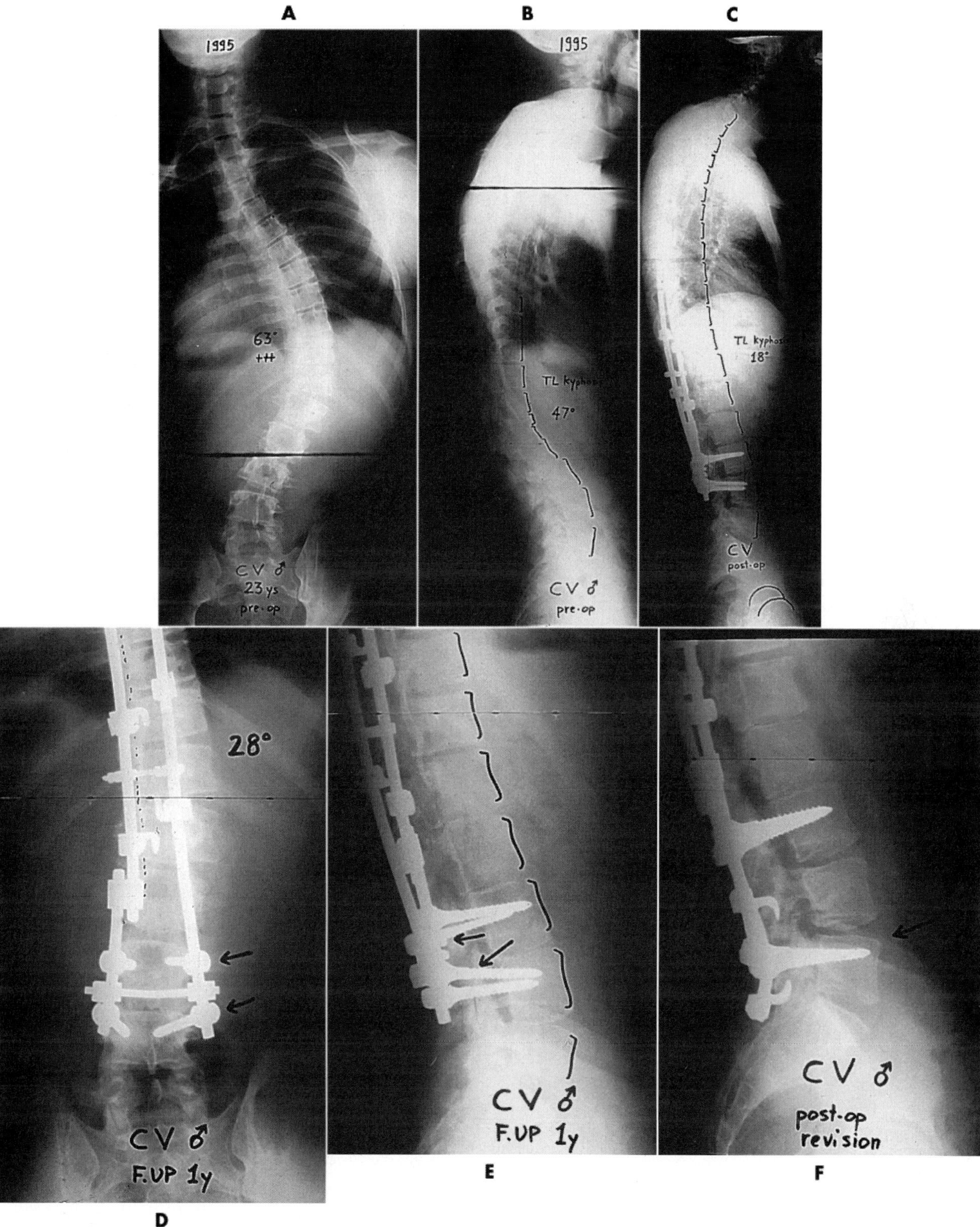


**FIGURE 40-3**

The patient is a 23-year-old man with severe thoracolumbar kyphoscoliosis due to cerebral palsy, secondary to head trauma at 6 years of age. The deformity was painful and disabling. The patient was used to walking with a crutch and with a peculiar and sudden forward tilting of the trunk. The patient underwent an operation by a single posterior approach with a T5-L4 fusion in April 1995. **A, B,** Preoperative coronal and sagital x-rays: note the thoracolumbar stiff kiphus. **C,** Immediate postoperative sagital view: note the correction of patient's profile, with a bilateral L3-L4 pedicular screw fixation in compression. At 1-year postoperative follow-up, the coronal correction is still stable **(D),** but the two pedicular screws on the right side have become loose, as seen in the sagittal view **(E),** with light pull-out movements during forward flexion and screw fixation failure. The patient complains of lumbar pain when walking and sitting. **F,** Sagital view after revision surgery. The fusion was extended to L5, after nonunion repair in L3-L4. Note the two laminar hooks put as protection of L5 screws. The patient is very well at 1-year follow-up.

Very often an early implant dislodgement can produce bursitis and painful swelling of subcutaneuos tissues due to friction of muscles and fascia on the prominent device. Bursitis could appear also without an implant dislodgement, generally at the thoracic level between the two scapulae over a DTT or over the convex implants that are more prominent on the rib hump.

### Radiographic Examination

All of the old x-rays must be examined, and compared with new standing posteroanterior and lateral radiographs. It is then possible to check the amount of fusion, disk degeneration, or the possible presence of pseudarthrosis in increasing deformity.

An eventual myelogram could be performed to show any nerve root entrapment, because the presence of metal can interfere with computed tomography (CT) scan or magnetic resonance imaging (MRI). Occasionally, a chest CT scan could be useful to control rib hump and lung situation, or a 3D CT scan reconstruction of the spine is helpful to verify the fusion mass.

Instability may be demonstrated on flexion-extension radiographs, whereas pseudarthrosis most commonly becomes evident through a curve progression or instrumentation failure rather than pain. Patients should have oblique views and cone-down views at suspected levels. A bone scan may be helpful but false-positives or false-negatives are common.

## TREATMENT

### Assessment and Selection of Patients

When a bone-implant fixation failure is diagnosed, it is necessary to verify with accuracy its real severity and its consequences on patient daily living, before any revision surgery. Furthermore it is very important to assess the ability of the patient to withstand again a heavy spinal operation. The patient's past medical history and social history, as well as psycological assessment, help also to decide if the patient could be a good candidate for this kind of surgical procedure. Be sure to always discuss with the patient all possible outcomes of the surgery to prevent a postoperative depression, very often present in those persons who are experiencing a second or third spine operation. Besides the routine preoperative tests, it is very important to perform an accurate pulmonary function test and arterial blood gas analysis before every revision surgery.

Diagnosis and prognosis are also extremely important when considering revision. Idiopathic scoliosis has usually an excellent prognosis after revision, whereas congenital scoliosis is generally rigid, difficult to correct, and has a high risk of neurological complications. Paralytic scoliosis patients (neuromuscular, CP) are also not good candidates for revision surgery.

The quality of bone also must be considered because osteoporosis is a limit for the amount of forces to be applied to correct the spine, and the use of allograft for fusion could be useful, if no autogenous bone is still available. Moreover, the surgeon should be careful also about age and health of the patient. Often it is better to rehabilitate these patients physically, mentally, and nutritionally before undertaking a spinal revision surgery.

With all these variables to consider, it is a challenge to select the patients the surgeon could really help. The best candidates for revision in bone-implant fixation failure are those patients with an associated sagittal plane deformity. They can greatly improve by creating a harmonious lumbar lordosis, sometimes connecting the revision implants to the former instrumention without replacing the whole device.

## CONSERVATIVE TREATMENT

Most patients seek help because they are feeling some pain, but occasionally only an incidental x-ray reveals that the spinal implant has failed, showing a displaced hook-screw or a broken rod, without any symptoms such as pain or loss of correction. For example, at the lumbosacral level it is some screw loosening frequently observed in a successful fusion. In these cases, there is no reason for surgery, because many authors don't consider as a bad result the simple hardware breakage in absence of a spinal pseudarthrosis.[8]

Initially for pain syndrome patients, a general conservative treatment, such as nonsteroidal anti-inflammatory agents, proper exercise, back school, and/or epidural steroid injections, may suffice. Subcutaneous bursitis can sometimes heal with anti-inflammatory drugs and rest, only occasionally requiring implant removal and revision. Of course, if the severe pain persists, further investigations, in addition to routine radiographs, may be indicated.

The roentgenographic diagnosis of pseudarthrosis does not mandate a surgical treatment too. With the Harrington system and with more modern instrumentations, not every patient with pseudarthrosis requires corrective surgery. Corrective surgery must be performed only on patients with significant progressive deformity or persistent pain. In this sense, the term pseudarthrosis is identifying almost a functional, rather than anatomic, entity.

If there is a slight imbalance without pain that is only a cosmetic concern, we must be careful, and try to avoid revision surgery, using modalities of physical therapy and posture (sometimes in growing patients, a brace could be useful) and taking care of psychological and socioenvironmental aspects. Surgery must be reserved only for painful implant fixation failure and major imbalance or trunk decompensation.

## SURGICAL TREATMENT

### MINOR REVISION SURGERY

As previously stated, some patients have a solid fusion but are suffering from localized pain that is unresponsive to conservative treatment; this often occurs at the lumbosacral level with alar screws or iliosacral screws in ambulatory patients fused to the sacrum. After localizing the trigger point by x-ray, the single prominent and mobilized screw could be removed easily and simply without a total implant revision by a short operation, sometimes with only local anesthesia. This kind of surgery in solid lumbosacral fusions achieves complete pain relief.

Minor surgery is generally enough when the problem is a prominent proximal part of the instrumentation (rod and/or hooks). If the fusion is good, a simple implant cut-off and removal could suffice. If there is an incomplete fusion, on the contrary, an extension one or two levels above with a stronger claw is needed.

In cases of early deep infections, even when they are successfully treated by open debridement and washing/drainage with local and prolonged systemic antibioticotherapy, it must be considered that there is an increased risk of bone-implant fixation failure and consequent pseudarthrosis at long-term follow-up. Occasionally an overinfection of a bursitis is observed, with late deep infection and fistulization that require a minor surgery with implant removal, washing/drainage, and check of fusion mass. Generally no loss of correction is observed if that operation is performed at 15 months or more after the first surgery.[2]

### MAJOR REVISION SURGERY

When the bone-implant fixation failure is important and symptomatic with significant patient complaint, and a conservative treatment or minor surgery was not successful, a complete and global revision surgery must be planned, and it is always a major surgical undertaking.

### GOALS AND INDICATIONS

Four principles must be applied. These are integrity of neural canal, alignment of the spine, stability, and support (especially anterior). It is important that the patient understands the goals of this surgery. These goals include the removal of failed implants, revision of fusion and repair of eventual pseudarthrosis, stronger and more stable fixation into/onto the bone, and then restoration of frontal and sagital balance, sometimes combined to an extended or a circumferential fusion. The outcomes of revision surgery must be judged in terms of pain relief, correction of deformity, and improved function.[4]

Patients with implant failure may be helped but it is necessary to identify and correct the cause of the failure. Posterior implants usually fail because there is a nonunion in the posterior fusion mass or an insufficient anterior structural support.

Indications are then fatigue fracture or dislocation of implants, pain, progressive deformity, eventual peripherial neuropathy. Generally, if the instrumentation failure is important, also with moderate or no pain and without clear evidence of pseudarthrosis, don't hesitate to reoperate.

When the pain syndrome for implant failure is well-defined, it is better to remove the implant and decompress, then to realign and reimplant. Pain associated with pseudarthrosis can also be relieved, but alignment must be achieved to obtain a good fusion after bonegrafting.

For implant and associated deformity problems, the surgeon must try always to improve the patient's balance, usually by removing implants, performing osteotomies, realigning, and reimplanting. The goal of surgery is to improve the coronal and sagittal profile of the spine and to improve neuropathy, if any. Before a revision for imbalance, we must consider how to rebalance and how difficult it is. Sagital decompensation is more noticeable than the coronal one, but the coronal plane deformities are more difficult to resolve, and usually require intercurrent traction (halo) to gain correction after osteotomies (the more osteotomies performed, the better the end result).[1,4]

Patients with instability and implant failure can be helped easily by creating a more harmonious lordosis and by including the unstable segment in the new instrumentation and fusion.

Anterior surgery is indicated when an anterior approach has been already performed, a good spine mobilization is needed, or a circumferential fusion is desired. This latter approach is necessary when there is a gross spinal instability and/or unbalanced kyphosis (as in Charcot spinal arthropathy, in which a 360-degree fusion is mandatory).[9]

## OPERATIVE TECHNIQUES

***Posterior Surgery.*** Posterior surgery is the most common approach, and a bone-implant fixation failure generally happens in posterior devices. A revision surgery for implant removal must be performed through the old scar with its excision, directly down to the spine. After the identification of the old implants that help for level identification, the spine must be stripped of fibrotic tissue, looking for any evidence of nonunion.

The failed implants are removed using the specific ancillary instruments of each different instrumentation. If wires are present, their removal requires a special technique by removing the bone around wire to make it free to slide out of canal, and by cutting it close to the lamina and pulling it. Generally this can avoid injuries of the dura, but the surgeon must be prepared to repair the dura because frequently dural tears and leaks occur.

A careful revision of the fusion area has to be performed, because pseudarthrosis is often present. The nonunion must be curetted, bone grafted, and stabilized to ensure the ultimate fusion.

In case of associated radicular pain syndromes, the surgical technique is similar but an additional decompressive surgery for entrapment syndromes could be necessary (such as a laminectomy or foraminotomy [in such cases, re-instrumentation is done by using pedicle screw fixation]).

To achieve a normal balance of the trunk, osteotomies of the spine are often required. The transverse process must be identified to perform osteotomy at the level of the disk in a chevron fashion where the facet joints were. These cuts are 6 to 7 mm wide, always looking at the underlying nerve root to prevent root impingement when osteotomy is closed. This kind of technique is desirable because it provides medial, lateral, and rotational stability. In case of preexisting laminectomy, it is imperative to identify pedicles and roots, for pedicle screw fixation.

It is very important to do as many osteostomies as possible, especially when a flat back problem exists, and sometimes to perform an intercurrent skeletal traction, when a staged surgery is planned, with a daily neurologic check.

The realignement of the spine is usually achieved through the extension of instrumentation and fusion to safe levels, from the last motion segment in the Harrington stable zone with a good disk below to the highest motion segment in the mid sacral line above the kyphus (to balance the coronal plane), whereas in the sagittal plane the thoracic kyphosis must be possibly equal to the lumbar lordosis. Reinstrumentation must be always performed with modern implants of third generation, but it is very important to avoid hybrid constructs to prevent any possible interactions between different metals or alloys.

As a final consideration in the posterior approach, the author prefers to avoid fusion to the sacrum if at all possible. When this is unavoidable or a previous failed sacral fixation is present and must be revised, the author favors the use of Dubousset iliosacral screws or the Galveston technique for nonambulatory patients, and the Jackson intrasacral fixation for walking patients.

***Anterior Surgery.*** Sometimes an anterior approach is needed to ensure ultimate fusion either through an anterior disk excision and fusion or through an anterior strut graft support when angular kyphosis persists.

The surgical procedure uses a standard thoracolumbar approach in which disks are removed, taking care to preserve the endplates, especially if an anterior graft or an intersomatic cage is necessary to realign the sagittal plane. In the case of a previous anterior surgery, through the old scar, the fused spine is reached, debrided, osteotomized, and mobilized, if a correction is to be obtained. The surgeon must be very careful during these maneuvers, which are very dangerous for the spinal cord, and in choosing the level of osteotomy.

When a combined anterior-posterior approach is needed, we perform a staged surgery if an intercurrent traction is necessary after the osteotomy. In all other cases, we prefer a same-day surgery because recovery is faster and patient's nutrition is better. On occasion a simultaneous approach could be planned, generally at lumbar level to restore lordosis when the spine is fused in kyphus.

During the immediate postoperative period, very often we use a brace for 3 to 6 months, as well as magnetic fields in case of pseudarthrosis or hyperbaric oxygen therapy on patients with high risk of infection.

### COMPLICATIONS

The possible complications of any revision surgery are related mostly to the longer time of surgery, therefore a higher risk of infection exists, and significant blood loss must be expected.[1,4] For the latter problem the usual precautions should be sufficient, such as patient's own blood predonations, the correct positioning on frame, and the use of cell saver during and immediately after surgery.

There is also danger for further neuropathy or paralysis, greater than at the original surgery. Wake-up test and spinal cord monitoring are mandatory. Moreover, after three or four procedures, a good result on pain is less likely: arachnoiditis is always a possible risk, as well as massive epidural fibrosis.

Bone grafts do not always heal easily, particularly when allograft is used because autografts are no longer available. Pseudarthrosis is then still possible and a subsequent implant failure could be observed.

## CONSIDERATION ON PREVENTION

An analysis about what to do and how to prevent a bone-implant fixation failure is outside the scope of this book, but some important things must be remembered before the first surgery.

An accurate 3D preoperative study of spinal deformity, the consequent operative planning for implants, and the choice of fusion area are fundamental. Dubousset principles and rules on 3D comprehension of a scoliotic deformity should be remembered.[3]

It is very important to choose an implant configuration that allows a good distribution of corrective forces and loading stress. This could be achieved through a real segmentary fixation, for instance avoiding bilateral claws at one level or adding more implants in between two divergent vectors or using sublaminar wires at lumbar concave side.

It must be remembered that the two most important roles of any instrumentation system are partial correction of the deformity and immobilization of the spine until an arthrodesis is achieved, because no instrumentation is stronger than the underlying fusion mass. Actually pedicle or laminar fixation should be thought of as a temporary spinal instrumentation method. McAfee, by means of a survival analysis study, has shown a 10-year predicted survival of 80% of implants with 90% solid arthrodesis, the real goal of spinal surgery.[8]

With the possibilty of stress distribution on multiple hooks, an early postoperative implant dislodgement is now rare, especially with current third-generation systems, because a better rod-implant fixation is obtained through the direct grip of plug on the rod. The other real advantage of the new instrumentation systems is that they are easily amenable to correction and revision compared with the older ones. But it is still basic to perform an accurate preparation of bone sites for implants, as well as prudent insertion maneuvers, and a re-check of the bony fixation of each implant before skin closure.

In adolescents with Risser <1, it must keep in mind the risk for subsequent further rotational anterior vertebral growth, despite a successful posterior fusion (crankshaft phenomenon), with increasing deformity.[4,5] An additional anterior approach combined to first surgery could prevent this outcome.

Finally, the chance for pseudarthrosis is often decreased by careful adherence to postoperative activity limitations, and sometimes by wearing of a brace. Furthermore, the postoperative brace, prescribed exercise, and activity restriction minimize the risk of early instrumentation failure and help to correct early postoperative trunk imbalance.[13] The remaining uncorrected compensatory or fractional curves may sometimes produce postoperative frontal trunk imbalance. This is obviously a risk-benefit ratio in achieving a more complete curve correction using modern segmentary instrumentations. Often, trunk balancing exercises or thoracolumbosacral orthosis (TLSO) bracing allows patient imbalance to improve. In the few unsuccessful cases, a reoperation with extension of the fusion is needed.

In any event, the use of 3D strategy is fundamental for distribution of the implant and for curve correction by rod rotation, translation, or rod in situ contouring. These principles must be adapted to each different instrumentation, and verified through a learning curve on less severe cases.

## CONCLUSION

Revision surgery for bone-implant fixation failure, particularly in spinal deformity patients, is demanding, difficult, dangerous, and emotionally draining for both the surgeon and the patient, requires hands-on training and the ability to anticipate and treat complications, but is often critical to the patient's future life.

## REFERENCES


1. Boachie-Adjei O, Bradford D: The Cotrel-Dubousset system—Results in spinal reconstruction, *Spine* 16:1155-1160, 1991.
2. Brayda-Bruno M, Steib JP, Tassin JL, Fabris D: Scoliosi-CD-infezioni: casistica, principi di trattamento, risultati, *Rachide* 18(suppl):191-197, 1995.
3. Cotrel Y, Dubousset J: CD *Instrumentation in spine surgery*. Montpellier, 1993, Sauramps Medical.
4. DeWald RL: Revision surgery for spinal deformity, Instruct Course Spine chapt. 26:235, 1992.
5. Dubousset J, Herring JA, Shufflebarger HL: The crankshaft phenomenon, *J Pediatr Orthop* 9:541-550, 1989.
6. Garfin SR, editor: *Complication of spine surgery*. Baltimore, 1989, William & Wilkins.
7. Lauerman WC et al: Management of pseudoarthrosis after arthrodesis of the spine for idiopathic scoliosis, *J Bone Joint Surg* 73A:222-236, 1991.
8. McAfee PC et al: Survivorship analysis of pedicle spinal instrumentation, *Spine* 16:9422-9427, 1991.
9. McBride GG, Greenberg D: Treatment of Charcot spinal arthropathy following traumatic paraplegia, *J Spinal Disord* 4:212-220, 1991.
10. Richards BS, Johnston CE: Cotrel-Dubousset instrumentation for adolescent idiopathic scoliosis, *Orthopedics* 10:649-654, 1987.
11. Shufflebarger HL, Clark CE: Complications of CD in idiopathic scoliosis. Presented at the combined meeting of the Pediatric Orthopaedic Society of North America and the European Pediatric Orthopaedic Society, Montreal, Canada, Sept.7, 1990.
12. Wenger DR, Mubarak SJ, Leach J: Managing complications of posterior spinal instrumentation and fusion, *Clin Orthop* 284:24-33, 1992.

# 41

# POSTERIOR LUMBAR DECANCELLATION OSTEOTOMY

**Oheneba Boachie-Adjei, M.D.**
**Federico P. Girardi, M.D.**
**Jerome Hall, M.D.**



## CLINICAL PERPECTIVES

The patient with a fixed, decompensated spinal deformity is easily recognized, but the treatment of this condition poses a difficult problem. Consideration of the potential risks and benefits, plus the patient's expectations, is critical before embarking on a significant surgical spine reconstruction.

For deformities that exist predominantly in the sagittal plane, a single-stage posterior decancellation, known as an "eggshell" procedure,[26] and posterior spinal fusion with segmental pedicle screw instrumentation are preferred by the authors. For deformities in the coronal plane, which also may present with sagittal malalignment, combined procedures are generally necessary to obtain a balanced correction in both planes. For severe, angular, rigid, multiplane deformities, vertebral column resection with shortening of the spine may be another surgical alternative.[4-6]

Patients with fixed sagittal deformities are often quite disabled. The patient may have a primary spine deformity such as ankylosing spondylitis or may have undergone multiple previous surgeries.* The usual cause is iatrogenic flat back secondary to failed previous spinal fusion with loss of lumbar lordosis. Distraction in-strumentation in the lower lumbar spine or malaligned lumbar fusion is the main cause in the iatrogenic group.† Other, less common causes are posttraumatic, neuromuscular, congenital, degenerative, or infections.‡

Nonspinal conditions, such as hip or knee flexion contractures and abnormalities, also can be present with sagittal malalignment and should always be ruled out. The patients are unable to stand with both hips and knees extended. In an attempt to compensate, patients usually present with a crouched knee/hip flexed position. Invariably the patient's complaints include decreased ability to ambulate,[24] severe back pain, and fatigue.[6] Pulmonary problems secondary to compression from the abdominal viscera have been reported.[12]

## HISTORICAL BACKGROUND

In 1973, Doherty first reported a postural complication observed in patients with thoracolumbar scoliosis treated by Harrington instrumentation and spine fusion with resultant loss of lumbar lordosis.[13] He reported a bilateral innominate osteotomy as a treatment to restore an upright posture.

The first report of spinal osteotomy for correction of sagittal plane deformity was by Smith-Peterson, Larson, and Aufranc in 1945.[54] Multiple posterior osteotomies

*References 7, 8, 12, 14, 17, 23, 25, 28, 30, 45, 46, 56, 59.
†References 1, 3, 10, 11, 13, 19, 22, 33-35, 37, 38, 48, 50, 51, 55.
‡References 18, 20, 21, 31, 32, 39, 49, 52.

were performed and subsequently closed, resulting in extension and opening through the disk spaces, rupture of the anterior longitudinal ligament, and elongation of the anterior spine producing lordosis.

Various authors have described modifications of the Smith-Peterson extension osteotomy.[5,7-9,25,36,41,44,45,53] The increased anterior vertebral body height obtained with these techniques may cause major complications, including paraplegia, and rupture of the abdominal aorta and mortality have been reported.[2,29,43,44,60] As described by Smith-Peterson, the original osteotomy and its modifications have several disadvantages. Significant force may be necessary to close the osteotomy, and the path of the osteotomy may be difficult to control.

Several authors describe complications related to lengthening that occurs at the anterior column.[2,29,43,60] In fact, one study demonstrated that the spine lengthened 2 cm with 40 degrees of correction at L2-L3.[60] This resulted in stretching of the anterior vascular structures and abdominal viscera, producing vascular compromise and gastrointestinal (GI) complications.[8,43,60] Some authors report mortality as high as 10% secondary to aortic rupture.[28,41,43] The osteotomy can be difficult to perform on patients with either prior anterior fusions or patients whose disk spaces are autofused from ankylosing spondylitis without first performing multiple osteotomies and releases anteriorly.

La Chapelle, in 1946, described a two-stage osteotomy with combined approaches.[36] Briggs, Keats, and Schlesinger in 1947 reported a posterior wedge osteotomy with bilateral intervertebral foraminotomy.[7] Most of these procedures achieved a correction through the disk space, which can incite intra-abdominal or retroperitoneal compromise. These problems were also reported by Adams.[2]

The transpedicular approach was initially described by Michelle and Krudger in 1949 for biopsy and drainage of a vertebral body.[47] Thomasen reported in 1985 the results of a corrective osteotomy by removal of a posterior wedge composed of the spinous process and the neural arch of the second lumbar vertebra, with removal of the bone inside the posterior part of the vertebral body of L2.[58] This allows correction of kyphosis by reestablishing lordosis with the fulcrum at the anterior aspect of the vertebral body. The overall effect is shortening of the posterior spinal column without excessive intra-abdominal distraction. Several authors have published results of Thomasen's techniques with correction averaging from 30 to 50 degrees at a single level.[30,57] These studies were done primarily on patients with ankylosing spondylitis who had not undergone previous surgeries.

Heinig popularized the term eggshell decancellation, which is currently applied in techniques to treat sagittal deformity.[26] In 1976, Moe and Denis reported satisfactory results in patients who had been treated by extension osteotomy of a previously fused spine for symptomatic loss of lumbar lordosis.[48] Lagrone et al[37,38] found, in their series of patients with symptomatic flat back, a thoracolumbar kyphosis of more than 15 degrees as a common etiology factor, especially if associated with hypokyphotic thoracic spine.[35]

## INDICATIONS

The lumbar spine osteotomy is performed to enable the patient to resume a more erect posture, thereby restoring a horizontal visual field, relieve compression of abdominal viscera, improve diaphragmatic respiration, and improve in appearance.

The eggshell procedure or transpedicular vertebrectomy may be used for a variety of indications. The transpedicular approach can be used open or percutaneously under computed tomography (CT) control for biopsies or drainage. The same approach can be used for total or partial cancellous bone removal and decompression of the anterior portion of the spinal canal in cases of tumor or fracture. A posterior vertebrectomy and/or osteotomy for correction of a fixed sagittal deformity is the most complex indication for this approach.

## OPERATIVE TECHNIQUE

The term *eggshell* describes the appearance of the vertebral body after the cancellous part of the vertebral body has been removed, leaving only a cortical shell similar to an empty eggshell. This operation consists of removal of cancellous bone of the selected vertebral body through both pedicles to weaken the vertebral body and create a posterior compression of the vertebral body with minimal force while the posterior arches of the adjacent vertebrae are approximated under direct vision by manipulating the operating table or spinal column and securing with internal fixation.

It is necessary that the spine surgeon understand the normal anatomy of the level involved and have a thorough preoperative understanding of the pathologic anatomy.

### PREOPERATIVE PLANNING

Before an eggshell procedure is performed, a thorough radiographic evaluation is mandatory. If there is neural compression, spinal canal evaluation can include magnetic resonance imaging (MRI) or myelogram with CT reconstruction of the involved spinal area. In patients with existent spinal instrumentation, the CT myelogram is the preferred study. A complete neurologic examination is required.

Finally, a complete system review and medical

clearance should be done to rule out possible contraindications for this major type of surgical procedure. The amount of correction should be estimated on standing lateral x-rays of the full spine. The osteotomy level is best placed at the mid-lumbar spine L2 or L3 to allow adequate proximal and distal fixation points. For salvage reconstruction pelvic fixation should be considered to provide strong distal foundation.

## ANESTHESIA

Anesthetic considerations must be based on the patient's overall condition. In severe cases of ankylosing spondylitis, preoperative fiberoptic intubation is mandatory. An elective tracheostomy should be considered in severe cases. Preoperatively, four to six units of autologous blood is donated by most patients. Hypotensive anesthesia and hemodilution techniques (70 to 80 mm Hg) help to control bleeding.

## POSITIONING

The patient is positioned prone with the operating table flexed in accordance with the deformity. The patient is placed on an independent four-posterior frame with the osteotomy site over the break in the table. Care is taken to avoid excessive pressure on the abdomen. An operating table that permits intraoperative biplanar radiographs is also necessary.

The surgical approach is posterior, and the magnitude of the exposure is dictated by the overall surgical goal. After the subperiosteal midline exposure, pedicle instrumentation is carried out first. We prefer three levels of rigid transpedicular fixation below the level of the osteotomy and three above. For an L3 osteotomy, removal of the entire neural arch of L3 and resection of any overhanging lamina from L2 or L4 is performed (Fig. 41-1). The dura and nerve roots are then completely mobilized. The transverse processes and pedicles are excised to free up the L2 and L3 nerve roots bilaterally, as well as the central dura. Copious bleeding may occur as the resection continues laterally down the pedicles, but hemostasis can be obtained with bipolar electrocautery and the application of Gelfoam and thrombin. The posterior wedge decancellation procedure is then carried out by careful elevation of the dura off the posterior wall of the vertebral body. The decancellation is extended to the anterior mid-portion of the vertebral body, with a graduated removal of cancellous bone in a wedge-shaped pattern toward the posterior portion of the vertebral body. In most cases, the entire posterior wall is removed. With angled curettes, the posterior vertebral wall is imploded with the reverse curettes and tamps. Angled feeders are used to check that complete posterior wall removal is accomplished, and the wedge is confirmed to make it extend to the anterior cortex, the fulcrum.

The level of the eggshell procedure and the amount of bone that needs to be resected should be predetermined on the basis of preoperative radiographs and the magnitude of correction that needs to be obtained. For larger corrections, the proximal level disk and a portion of the lower half of the proximal vertebra can be removed.

In some instances, a posterior lumbar interbody diskectomy and grafting[15] are recommended at the

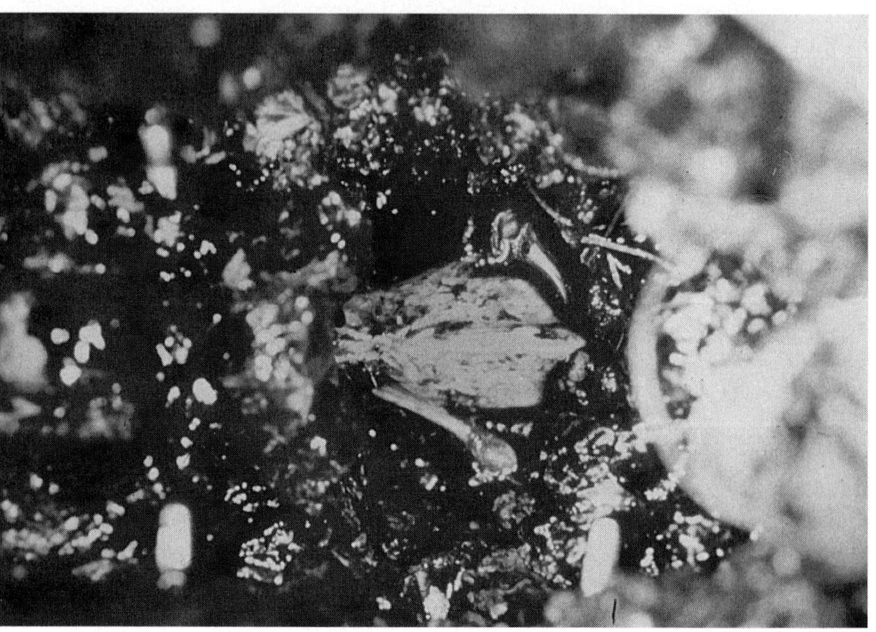

FIGURE 41-1

Wide laminectomy and facetectomy are performed in order to achieve a safe reduction of the osteotomy site.

lower level of the decancellation by extending the laminectomy inferiorly. If there is no sufficient bony apposition posteriorly, a posterior lumbar interbody graft should be added to the procedure to promote bone healing at the site of the osteotomy. A temporary fixation helps prevent premature closure of the osteotomy.

Correction is achieved by gradual extension of the operating table, closing the osteotomy site to allow the remaining superior and inferior posterior arches to have contact. Sometimes a crack is felt, and immediate post-reduction lateral and anteroposterior (AP) radio-graphs are mandatory to evaluate the reduction and alignment. The anterior part of the decancellized vertebra act as a pivot point for closure of the posterior osteotomized gap. The neurologic elements are directly visualized during closure of the osteoclasis. This maneuver is possible without causing damage to the nerves because the respective pedicles have been removed. By posterior compression, there is no stretching of the cauda equina and less stretching of the intraabdominal vessels and the aorta, compared with the osteotomy with opening the disks in front.

Bone grafting is then performed using the resected bone and supplemented with autograft from the iliac crest, if necessary. Pedicle screws are secured and attachment to a predetermined sagittally contoured rod is then carried out.

The ability to monitor the descending motor pathways of the spinal cord during surgery is a method for prevention of postoperative neurologic deficits. This is carried out using both somatosensory evoked potentials (SEPs) and motor evoked potentials (MEPs). The reliability of these two complimentary modalities has been reported.[16] However, a wake-up test to assess neurologic function in essential during this procedure.

### POSTOPERATIVE MANAGEMENT

Postoperatively, the patient is mobilized as tolerated and fitted with a thoracolumbosacral orthosis (TLSO). A leg extension may be required in some patients with weak bone. Depending on the stability achieved with instrumentation, external immobilization may not be needed and the patient can be mobilized during 1 postoperative week.

## COMPLICATIONS

In 1959, Law reported more than 100 lumbar osteotomies and eight fatal cases.[40] Intraoperative or postoperative vertebral dislocation with pressure on the nerves has been reported.[58]

Many authors have described recurrences of the deformity with the initial types of osteotomy.[17,27,28] They did not use rigid internal instrumentation, and the failures were caused by insufficient healing of the osteotomy site.

Thomasen reported no fatal complications.[58] One patient who underwent surgery had a horizontal fracture of L2 and dislocation of the upper part of the vertebra with pressure on the cauda equina. He had paresis of both legs and was operated on within 6 hours. Reposition of the upper dislocated level was achieved. Fixation with metal plates was used at this time. The patient had complete neurologic recovery.

Thiramont and Netrawichien reported no death or major complication in their series.[57] They described one dural tear that occurred during the operation, due to adhesion of the dural membrane with the ossified ligamentum flavum, while a sublaminar wire was passed.

Van Royen and Slot reported no fatal complications.[59] Instrumentation failure and nerve root compression were noticed. Lehmer et al reported 19.5% of patients had new neurologic deficits postoperatively,[42] 12.2% were minor and 7.3% were major including paraplegia.

To date, we have presented and reported on 14 consecutive patients who underwent posterior lumbar decancellation osteotomy with more than 2 years' follow-up. Preoperative diagnoses included ankylosing spondylitis (three patients), flat back syndrome (eight patients), posttraumatic kyphoses (two patients), and multiple failed surgeries with severe sagittal plane decompensation (one patient). The sagittal plane decompensation averaged 12 cm preoperatively (range 2 cm to 35 cm) and was corrected to an average of 2 cm postoperatively (range 0 to 12 cm). Preoperative lumbar lordosis averaged 6 degrees of kyphosis (range +40 degrees to −24 degrees). Postoperative lumbar lordosis averaged 59 degrees (range −30 degrees to −85 degrees). The average correction obtained was 65 degrees (range 45 to 70 degrees). The average blood loss was 3227 cc (range 1200 cc to 4600 cc; Figs. 41-2, 41-3, and 41-4).

At latest follow-up, 12 of 14 patients were satisfied. Two patients had undergone revision surgery. Three patients sustained dural tears during decompression. In all cases the dura was sutured primarily with no sequela. Three patients required revision due to broken hardware, and loss of correction.

Several authors have published results of Thomasen's techniques with correction averaging from 30 to 50 degrees at a single level.[6,14] These studies were done primarily on patients with ankylosing spondylitis who had not undergone previous surgeries.

The decancellation osteotomy has several distinct advantages. The spinal column is shortened, eliminating

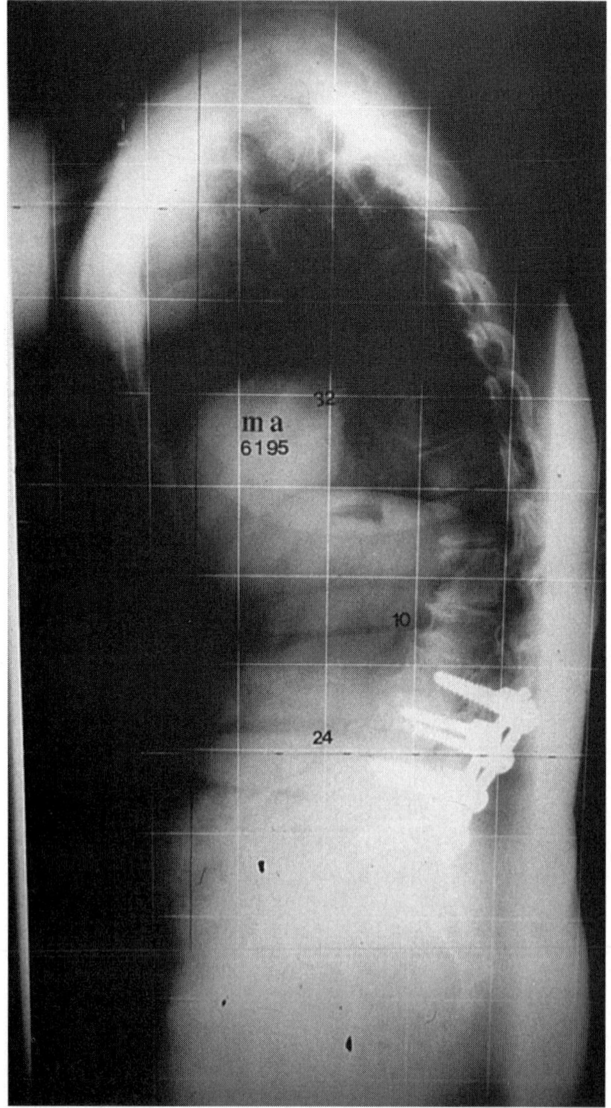


**FIGURE 41-2**

A 64-year-old woman who had previous lumbar laminectomies and developed thoracolumbar kyphosis above a well-healed fusion mass.

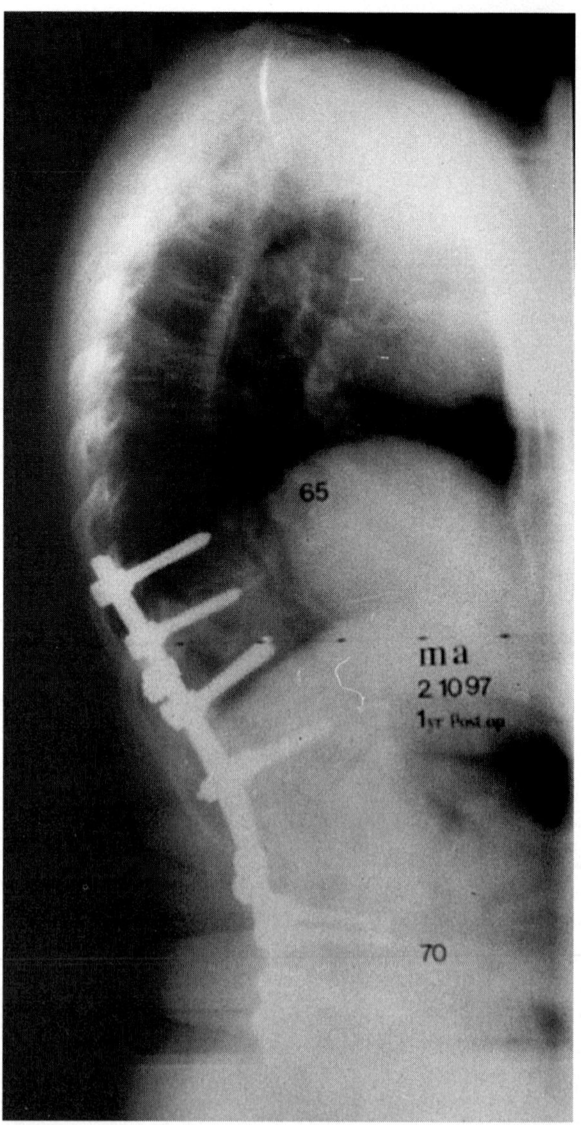


**FIGURE 41-3**

L3 decancellation osteotomy with T10-S1 PSF was performed. Restoration of normal sagittal alignment and balance was achieved.

the possibility for catastrophic vascular compromise due to lengthening of the anterior spine. The osteotomy is predictable and controlled, and compressed interdigitating cancellous bone also promotes rapid fusion. The osteotomy can be performed on previously fused patients, obviating the need for anterior release at the osteotomy site. By excising the L3 pedicle, a large foramen is created to allow the L2 and L3 nerve roots to pass freely and the neural elements and dura are completely visualized throughout the entire procedure.

Several key technical points need to be considered. Blood loss can be rapid and difficult to control once the vertebral body is decancellated. Therefore, all pedicle screws should be placed, bone graft harvested, and wide posterior decompression finished before removal of cancellous bone begins. Although excision of the pedicles creates one large foramen for the L2 and L3 nerve roots, great care needs to be taken to completely mobilize the dura and the nerve roots prior to closing the osteotomy.

This is a technically demanding, high-risk procedure and needs to be performed only by experienced surgeons. The decancellation osteotomy is a powerful procedure in the treatment of complex sagittal plane deformity. The procedure provides a mechanically stable and effective correction in selected patients with a high subjective patient satisfaction.

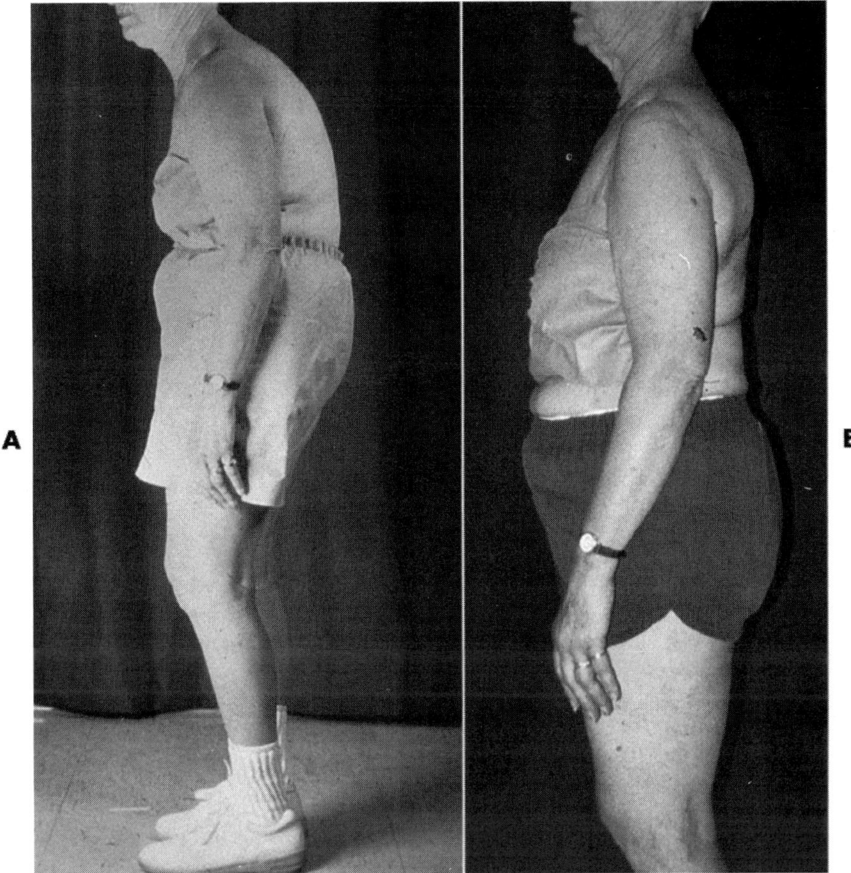


FIGURE 41-4

**A, B,** Preoperative and postoperative lateral standing clinical pictures of the patient.

## REFERENCES

1. Aaro S, Ohlen G: The effect of Harrington instrumentation on the sagittal configuration and mobility of the spine in scoliosis, *Spine* 8:570-575, 1993.
2. Adams JC: Technique, dangers, and safeguards in osteotomy, *J Bone Joint Surg* 34B:226-230, 1952.
3. Balderston RA, Winter RB, Moe JH, Bradford DS, Lonstein JE: Fusion to the sacrum for nonparalytic scoliosis in the adult, *Spine* 11:824-829, 1986.
4. Boachie-Adjei O, Bradford DS: Vertebral column resection and arthrodesis for complex spinal deformities, *J Spinal Disord* 4:193-196, 1991.
5. Bradford DS, Schumacher WL, Lonstein JE, Winter RB: Ankylosing spondylitis: experience in surgical management of 21 patients, *Spine* 12:238-243, 1987. Erratum: *Spine* 12:590-592, 1987.
6. Bradford DS, Tribus CB: Current concepts and management of patients with fixed decompensated spinal deformity, *Clin Orthop* 306:64-72, 1994.
7. Briggs H, Keats S, Schlesinger PT: Wedge osteotomy of spine with bilateral, intervertebral foraminotomy: correction of flexion deformity in five cases of ankylosing arthritis of spine, *J Bone Joint Surg* 29:1075-1082, 1947.
8. Camargo FP, Cordeiro EN, Napoli MM: Corrective osteotomy of spine in ankylosing spondylitis: experience with 66 cases, *Clin Orthop* 208:157-167, 1986.
9. Cloward RB: Posterior lumbar interbody fusion updated, *Clin Orthop* 193:16-19, 1985.
10. Cochran T, Irstam L, Nachemson A: Long-term anatomic and functional changes in patients with adolescent idiopathic scoliosis treated by Harrington rod fusion, *Spine* 8:576-584, 1983.
11. Cummine JL, Lonstein JE, Moe JH, Winter RB, Bradford DS: Reconstructive surgery in the adult for failed scoliosis fusion, *J Bone Joint Surg Am* 61:1151-1161, 1979.
12. Dawson CW: Posterior osteotomy for ankylosis arthritis of the spine, *J Bone Joint Surg* 38-A:1393-1396, 1956.

13. Doherty JH: Complications of fusion in lumbar scoliosis. In: Proceedings of the Scoliosis Research Society, *J Bone Joint Surg* 55-A:438, 1973.
14. Gerscovich EO, Greenspan A, Montesano PX: Treatment of kyphotic deformity in ankylosing spondylitis, *Orthopedics* 17:335-342, 1994.
15. Gertzbein SD, Harris MB: Wedge osteotomy for the correction of post-traumatic kyphosis. A new technique and a report of three cases, *Spine* 17:374-379, 1992.
16. Glassman SD, Johnson JR, Shields CB, Backman MH, Paloheimo MP, Edmonds HL Jr, Linden RD: Correlation of motor-evoked potentials, somatosensory-evoked potentials, and the wake-up test in a case of kyphoscoliosis, *J Spinal Disord* 6:194-198, 1993.
17. Goel MK: Vertebral osteotomy for correction of fixed flexion deformity of the spine, *J Bone Joint Surg* 50-A: 287-292, 1968.
18. Graziano GP, Hensinger RN: Treatment of congenital lumbar lordosis in adults with a one-stage single-level anterior closing-wedge osteotomy. A report of two cases, *J Bone Joint Surg Am* 77:1095-1099, 1995.
19. Grobler LJ, Moe JH, Winter RB, Bradford DS, Lonstein JE: Loss of lumbar lordosis following correction of thoracolumbar deformities, *Orthop Trans* 2:239, 1978.
20. Grubb SA, Lipscomb HJ, Coonrad RW: Degenerative adult onset scoliosis, *Spine* 13:241-245, 1988.
21. Grubb SA, Lipscomb HJ: Diagnostic findings in painful adult scoliosis, *Spine* 17:518-527, 1992.
22. Guanciale AF, Dinsay JM, Watkins RG: Lumbar lordosis in spinal fusion: a comparison of intraoperative results of patient positioning on two different operative table frame types, *Spine* 21:964-969, 1996.
23. Halm H, Metz-Stavenhagen P, Zielke K: Results of surgical correction of kyphotic deformities of the spine in ankylosing spondylitis on the basis of the modified arthritis impact measurement scales, *Spine* 20:1612-1619, 1995.
24. Hasday CA, Passoff TL, Perry J: Gait abnormalities arising from iatrogenic loss of lumbar lordosis secondary to Harrington instrumentation in lumbar fractures, *Spine* 8:501-511, 1983.
25. Hehne HG, Zielke K, Bohm H: Polysegmental lumbar osteotomies and transpedicular fixation for correction of long-curved kyphotic deformities in ankylosing spondylitis: report on 177 cases, *Clin Orthop* 258:49-55, 1990.
26. Heinig CF, Chewning SJ Jr: Eggshell procedure. In Bradford DS, ed: *The spine,* Philadelphia, 1997, Lippincott-Raven, pp 199-208.
27. Herbert JJ. Vertebral osteotomy, technique, indications and results, *J Bone Joint Surg* 31A:680-689, 1948
28. Herbert JJ: Vertebral osteotomy for kyphosis, especially in Marie-Strumpell arthritis, *J Bone Joint Surg* 41A:291-302, 1959.
29. Horton RE. Arterial injuries complicating orthopaedic surgery, *J Bone Joint Surg Br* 54:323-327, 1972.
30. Jaffray D. Becker V. Eisenstein S: Closing wedge osteotomy with transpedicular fixation in ankylosing spondylitis, *Clin Orthop* 279:122-126, 1992.
31. Kahanovitz N, Brown JC, Bonnett CA: The operative treatment of congenital scoliosis. A report of 23 patients, *Clin Orthop* 143:174-182, 1979.
32. Kao-Wha Chang: Oligosegmental correction of post-traumatic thoracolumbar angular kyphosis, *Spine* 18: 1909-1915, 1993.
33. Kohler R, Galland O, Mechin F, Michel CR, Onimus M: The Dwyer procedure in the treatment of idiopathic scoliosis, *Spine* 15:75-80, 1990.
34. Kostuik JP: Treatment of scoliosis in the adult thoracolumbar spine with special reference to fusion to the sacrum, *Orthop Clin North Am* 19:371-381, 1988.
35. Kostuik JP, Maurais GR, Richardson WJ, Okajima Y: Combined single stage anterior and posterior osteotomy for correction of iatrogenic lumbar kyphosis, *Spine* 13:257-266, 1988.
36. La Chapelle EH: Osteotomy of the lumbar spine for correction of kyphosis in a cast of ankylosing spondylarthritis, *J Bone Joint Surg* 28:851-858, 1945.
37. Lagrone MO, Bradford DS, Moe JH, Lonstein JE, Winter RB, Ogilvie JW: Treatment of symptomatic flatback after spinal fusion, *J Bone Joint Surg Am* 70A: 569-580, 1988.
38. Lagrone MO: Loss of lumbar lordosis. A complication of spinal fusion for scoliosis, *Orthop Clin North Am* 19:383-393, 1988.
39. Laroche M, Delisle MB, Aziza R, Lagarrigue J, Mazieres B: Is Camptocormia a primary muscular disease? *Spine* 20: 1011-1016, 1995.
40. Law WA: Lumbar spinal osteotomy, *J Bone Joint Surg* 41B:270, 1959.
41. Law WA: Osteotomy of the spine, *Clin Orthop* 66:70-76, 1969.
42. Lehmer SM, Keppler L, Biscup RS, Enker P, Miller SD, Steffee AD: Posterior transvertebral osteotomy for adult thoracolumbar kyphosis, *Spine* 19:2060-2067, 1994.
43. Lichtblau PO, Wilson PD: Possible mechanism of aortic rupture in orthopaedic correction of rheumatoid spondylitis, *J Bone Joint Surg Am* 38A:123-127, 1956.
44. MacEwen GD, Bunnell WP, Sriram K: Acute neurological complications in the treatment of scoliosis. A report of the Scoliosis Research Society, *J Bone Joint Surg Am* 57:404-408, 1975.
45. McMaster MJ, Coventry MB: Spinal osteotomy in ankylosing spondylitis. Technique, complications, and long term results, *Mayo Clin Proc* 48:476, 1973.
46. McMaster MJ: A technique for lumbar spinal osteotomy in ankylosing spondylitis, *J Bone Joint Surg Br* 67:204-210, 1985.
47. Michelle A, Krudger FJ: A surgical approach to the vertebral body, *J Bone Joint Surg* 31A:873-878, 1949.
48. Moe JH, Denis F: The iatrogenic loss of lumbar lordosis, *Orthop Trans,* 1:131, 1977.

49. Otain K, Satomi K, Fujimura Y, Manzoku S, Shibasaki K: Spinal osteotomy to correct kyphosis in spinal tuberculosis, *Int Orthop* 3: 229-235, 1979.
50. Peterson MD, Nelson LM, McManus AC, Jackson RP: The effect of operative position on lumbar lordosis: A radiographic study of patients under anesthesia in the prone and 90-90 positions, *Spine* 20:1419-1424, 1995.
51. Ponder RC, Dickson JH, Harrington PR, Erwin WD: Results of Harrington instrumentation and fusion in the adult idiopathic scoliosis patient, *J Bone Joint Surg* 57A:797-801, 1975.
52. Pritchett JW, Bortel DT: Degenerative symptomatic lumbar scoliosis, *Spine* 18:100-103, 1993.
53. Simmons EH: Kyphotic deformity of the spine in ankylosing spondylitis, *Clin Orthop* 128:65-77, 1977.
54. Smith-Peterson MN, Larson CB, Aufranc OE: Osteotomy of the spine for correction of flexion deformity in rheumatoid arthritis, *J Bone Joint Surg* 27:1-11, 1945.
55. Styblo K, Bossers GT, Slot GH: Osteotomy for kyphosis in ankylosing spondylitis, *Acta Orthop Scand* 56:294-297, 1985.
56. Swank S, Lonstein JE, Moe JH, Winter RB, Bradford DS: Surgical treatment of adult scoliosis. A review of two hundred and twenty-two cases, *J Bone Joint Surg Am* 63:268-287, 1987.
57. Thiranont N, Netrawichien P: Transpedicular decancellation closed wedge vertebral osteotomy for treatment of fixed flexion deformity of spine in ankylosing spondylitis, *Spine* 18:2517-2522, 1993.
58. Thomasen E: Vertebral osteotomy for correction of kyphosis in ankylosing spondylitis, *Clin Orthop* 194: 142-152, 1995.
59. VanRoyen BJ, Slot GH: Closing-wedge posterior osteotomy for ankylosing spondylitis. Partial corpectomy and transpedicular fixation in 22 cases, *J Bone Joint Surg Br* 77:117-121, 1995.
60. Weatherly C, Jaffray D, Terry A: Vascular complications associated with osteotomy in ankylosing spondylitis: report of two cases, *Spine* 12:43-46, 1988.

# 42

# PEDICLE SUBTRACTION AND LUMBAR EXTENSION OSTEOTOMY FOR IATROGENIC FLAT BACK

**Gary L. Lowery, M.D., Ph.D.**
**Atul L. Bhat, M.D.**
**A. Eugene Pennisi, M.A.**



At birth, the human spine has a kyphotic curvature that encompasses the entire spine. With progressive ambulation and eventual upright posture, the spinal column develops compensatory sagittal lordotic curves in the cervical and lumbar regions. In the upright position, however, these kyphotic and lordotic curves tend to balance out in order to position the head directly over the pelvis. There is considerable variation in the normal range of values for these curves, and the distribution of these values over the general population forms a typical bell-shaped curve.[4] From a clinical standpoint, consideration of the overall sagittal balance is beneficial.[14] A *neutral* sagittal balance is said to exist when a plumb line dropped from the body of C7 intersects the posterosuperior corner of the S1 vertebral body.[4] "Flat back" syndrome, as the name implies, constitutes a syndrome complex characterized by the loss of normal lumbar lordosis and flattening of the lumbar spine. This loss of lumbar lordosis usually leads to a well defined clinical situation comprising (1) forward inclination of the trunk, (2) inability to stand erect with the knees fully extended, and (3) pain in the low back or in the upper thoracic or cervical area. In such a situation the plumb line falls anterior to the posterosuperior border of S1 (i.e., C7 lies anterior to the sacrum).

Iatrogenic flat back syndrome is usually seen after long-segment thoracolumbar instrumentation and fusion, especially when distractive instrumentation extends to the lumbosacral junction.[11,12,14] With long-term follow-up of patients having received fusion and instrumentation for idiopathic adolescent scoliosis, flat back syndrome is now often recognized. The other causative factor of iatrogenic flat back is thoracolumbar pseudarthrosis with loss of sagittal plane correction following initial spinal fusion.[14] Hyperextension of the hips and/or the thoracic spine and flexion of the knees are two of the compensatory mechanisms by which the body tries to adjust to this loss of lordosis, with hyperextension of the hips being the most favored.[10,14]

The principal indication for surgery is a patient with symptomatic flat back presenting with continued fatigue in the thoracic or thoracolumbar area not responsive to conservative treatment. With the lumbar spine not in an anatomical lordotic position the posterior musculature is at a biomechanical disadvantage, typically leading to fatigue as the day progresses. The patient may also present with knee pain or anterior thigh pain resulting from a constant flexed position of the knee in order to facilitate forward gaze.

A standing full-length lateral view with the knees fully extended is the single most important radiograph taken preoperatively. The plumb line is established through the body of C7 and its deviation from normal is determined.

The goal of the extension osteotomy is to restore the sagittal balance such that the plumb line intersects the posterosuperior corner of the S1 vertebra. With the osteotomy stabilized using posterior pedicular instrumentation solid fusion is achieved rapidly at the osteotomy site.

## SURGICAL TECHNIQUE

The patient is placed prone on an Andrews table or a laminectomy pad with the hips fully extended. Sufficient padding is used to support the chest and pelvis, allowing the abdomen to be free in order to reduce intraoperative bleeding. Preoperative antibiotics are administered, and the lumbar area is prepped and draped in the usual sterile fashion.

Somatosensory evoked potentials are used to monitor the spinal cord function during surgery. The surgery is optimally performed at the L3-L4 level but the presence of an existing fusion at adjacent levels may affect final selection of operative level. Using a standard midline posterior incision, at least one vertebral level above and below L3-L4 junction is exposed (Fig. 42-1). The soft tissue is dissected free subperiosteally. Care is taken to preserve the facet capsules that are not to be included in the fusion site. A complete laminectomy is then performed at the L4 vertebral level. The bone is removed through the facet joint, taking out the pars interarticularis as well as the superior facet of L4 and inferior facet of L3. The dura and the nerve roots are fully exposed to permit complete visual inspection. Transpedicular screw fixation at one level above and below the osteotomy site is then performed, which is the minimal fixation required to stabilize the osteotomy. With the dura or the cauda retracted to one side the pedicle of the L4 vertebra is identified and excised completely so that it is flush with the posterior aspect of the vertebral body (Fig. 42-2). An osteotomy is extended laterally through any previous fusion mass (or incorporating any existing pseudarthrosis). It is extremely important to undercut the lamina and bone at the foramina of the vertebra above to avoid dural or nerve impingement when extending the spine during closure of the osteotomy site. A total diskectomy is then performed at the desired level, with care taken not to penetrate the anterior anulus. Strict attention should be given to removing the disk material from the inferior endplate of the superior vertebra. The vertebral endplate is abraded with a burr until punctate bleeding occurs. An osteotome is placed in the horizontal plane on the posterior surface of the vertebral body lateral to the neural elements. An angled osteotomy is then performed toward the anterosuperior corner of L4 vertebral body. This is confirmed by means of an intraoperative radiograph. A second osteotomy is performed in the sagittal plane along the edge of the dura extending from the posterior aspect of the vertebral body to the anterior vertebral border. The resultant triangular bony wedge is then carefully removed, avoiding any neural trauma (Fig. 42-3). The entire process is then repeated on the other side (Fig. 42-4). Brisk bleeding is encountered at this stage from the exposed cancellous bone, and hypotensive anesthesia is usually desirable.

The neural elements (dura, nerve roots, or cauda

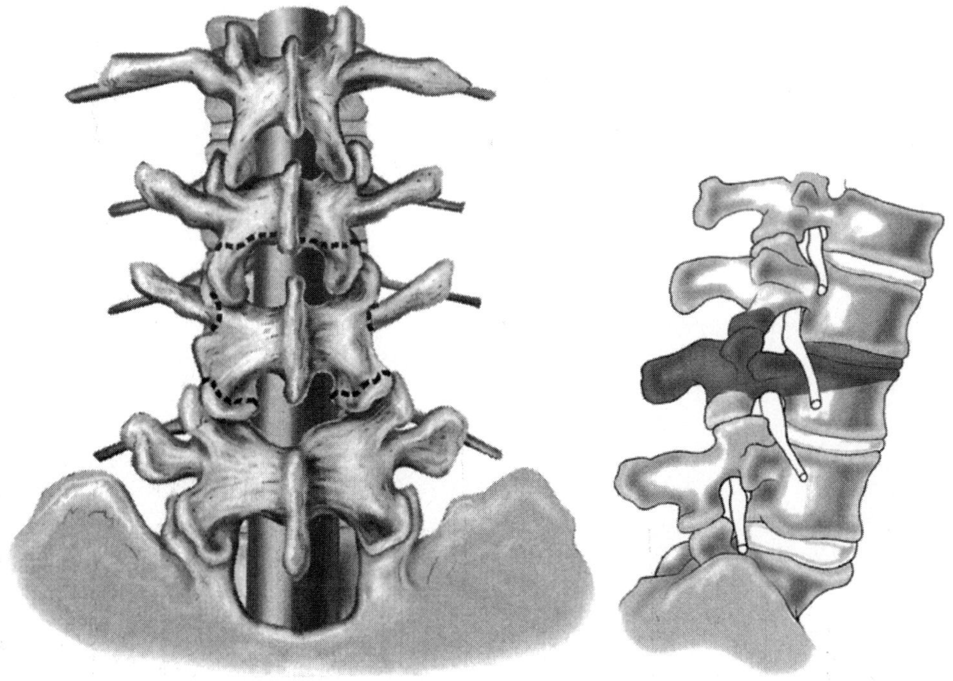

**FIGURE 42-1**

Vertebrae are exposed at appropriate levels to allow osteotomy as indicated by dotted lines and shaded portion (*inset*). Note preservation of facet joints. © Neill BioMedical Art Co.

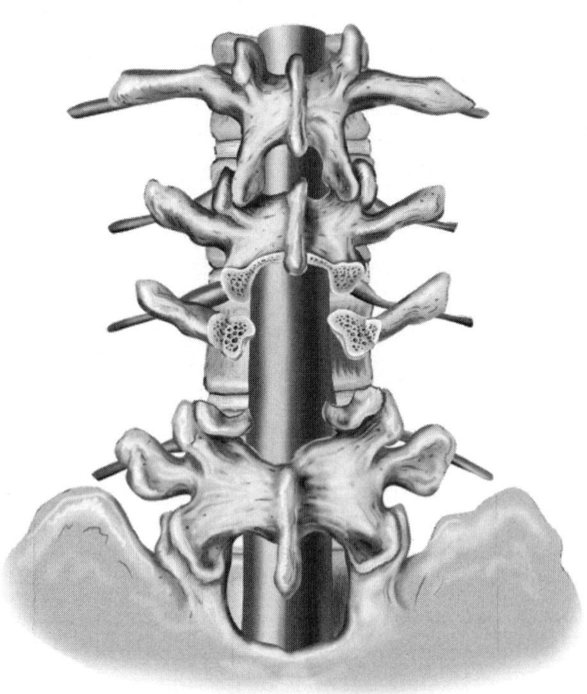

**FIGURE 42-2**

Complete laminectomy and pedicle subtraction are performed at L4. © Neill BioMedical Art Co.

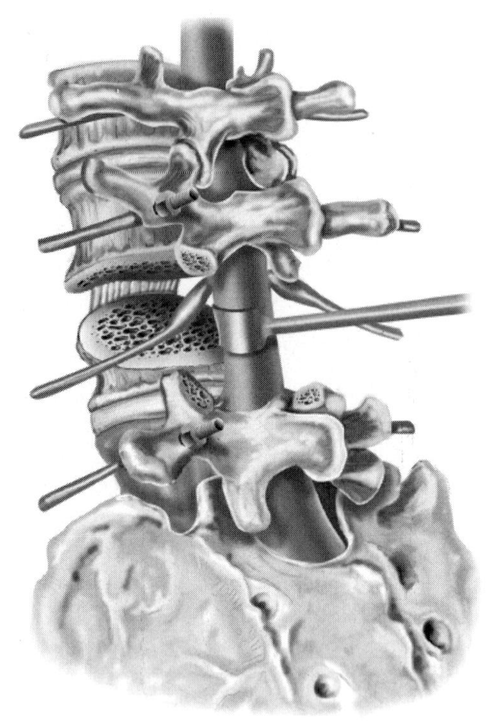

**FIGURE 42-4**

Wedge osteotomy of the entire L4 vertebral body is completed. © Neill BioMedical Art Co.

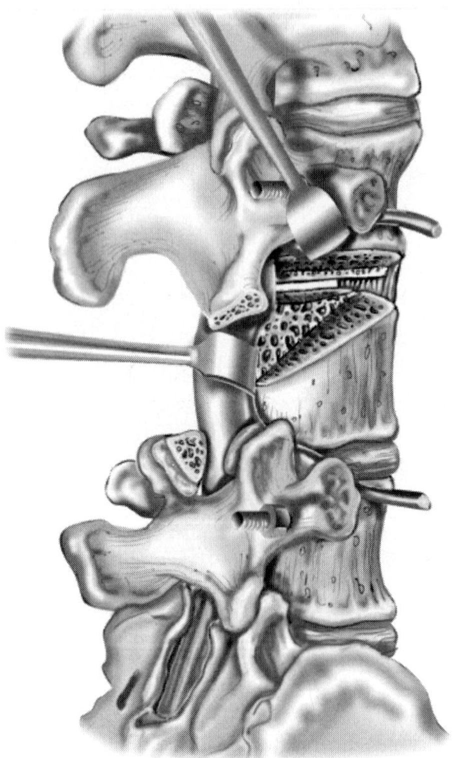

**FIGURE 42-3**

Wedge removal from right side L4 vertebral body. Note that anterior longitudinal ligament is left intact. © Neill BioMedical Art Co.

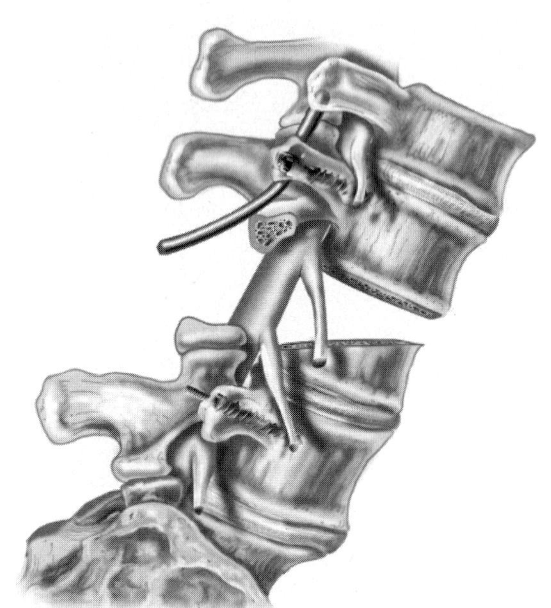

**FIGURE 42-5**

Precontoured posterior instrumentation is applied. © Neill BioMedical Art Co.

equina) are inspected for any impingement prior to closure and stabilization of the osteotomy site. The posterior rods or plates are contoured to 30 to 60 degrees depending on the amount of correction desired at the osteotomy site (Fig. 42-5). The osteotomy is then closed and the posterior compression instrumentation system is tightened (Fig. 42-6). The posterior elements of vertebrae above and below the osteotomy site are decorticated with a high-speed burr. Local laminar bone or the bone from the osteotomy site is used for bilateral intertransverse fusion. Additional autologous iliac crest bone graft is harvested and added to the fusion mass (Fig. 42-7).

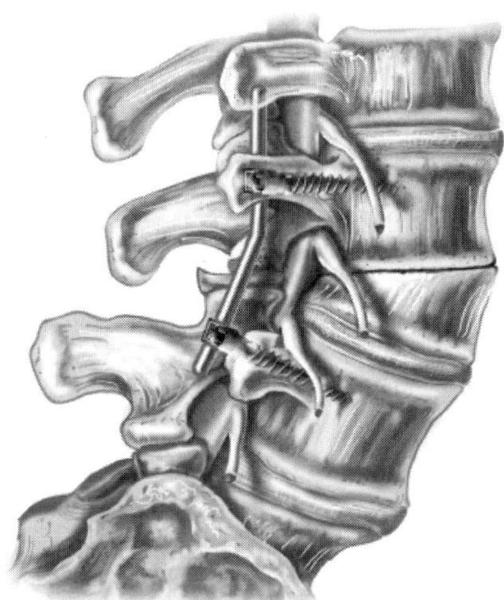

**FIGURE 42-6**

Compression of the osteotomy. © Neill BioMedical Art Co.

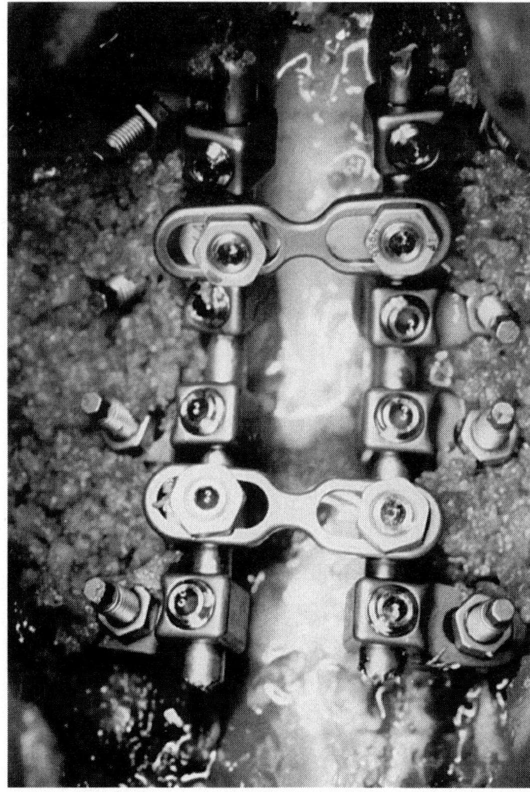

**FIGURE 42-7**

Instrumentation in place and copious posterolateral bone graft added to the area.

The lumbar wound is closed over drains, which are usually removed two to three days postoperatively. Routine intravenous antibiotics are administered 72 hours postoperatively. Patient is mobilized in a thoracolumbosacral orthosis (TSLO) on the second or third postoperative day. Postoperative radiographs are obtained in the immediate postoperative period and at 2 and 6 weeks, 3-, 6-, and 12-month intervals, and yearly thereafter. The TSLO is worn until a solid anterior fusion is apparent by x-ray examination (routinely at 3 months).

## DISCUSSION

Doherty,[7] in 1972, first reported on the loss of lumbar lordosis as a complication of spinal fusion for lumbar scoliosis. Since then there have been many reports in the literature on iatrogenic flat back.[9,11,12,14,21]

Various osteotomies, both in the anterior and the posterior spine, have been described for correction of sagittal plane deformity.[3,5,6,8,12,13,15,16,18-20,22-28,30] Early osteotomies were described principally for deformity correction after ankylosing spondylitis.[3,5,6,13,15,18-20,23-28] Smith-Petersen[25] first described a posterior osteotomy for the correction of the fixed sagittal deformity. La Chapplle[13] described a modification of this technique with an additional release of anterior structures. Osteotomy of the posterior elements of the spine followed by closure of the wedge and resultant hyperextension of the spine leads to an elongation of the anterior vertebral column or spinal lengthening. There is a theoretical chance of injury to the anterior vascular structures and the neural elements. The osteotomy of posterior elements has certain drawbacks and the surgical treatment is not without complications. Mortality rate as high as 10% has been reported, and neurological complications including paraplegia have been reported in up to 30% of patients.[15,20,24] Forceful hyperextension of the spine may result in vascular complications such as rupture of the aorta or the inferior vena cava, which are often calcified due to an extensive degenerative vascular affection especially in patients with ankylosing spondylitis.[29] With hyperextension of the spine, stretching of the superior mesenteric artery over the third part of the duodenum can lead to acute dilatation of the stomach and paralytic ileus in the early postoperative period.[19,23] Another complication of a posterior osteotomy is pseudarthrosis, especially when the osteotomy is performed without reconstruction of the anterior column. It has been suggested that addition of an anterior fusion procedure to the posterior osteotomy helps reduce the pseudarthrosis rate, and that an anterior spinal ligament release, diskectomy, and fusion should be performed one to two weeks before the posterior procedure.[14] But this entails the use of two-staged procedures or two surgeries at the same sitting. To overcome these drawbacks of osteotomies of the posterior elements, posterior transvertebral extension osteotomy has been advocated.[8,16]

Pedicle subtraction and extension osteotomy is a technically demanding procedure. Intraoperative complications can be avoided by careful preoperative planning and strict adherence to meticulous surgical technique. The L3-L4 disk space is the physiological apex of lumbar lordosis and the osteotomy can be safely performed at this level.[2] Bifurcation of the vascular structures is below this level so there is a minimal chance of vascular injury. The dura is often adherent to the surrounding soft tissues (i.e., posterior longitudinal ligament or ligamentum flavum) and careful dissection is required to avoid a dural tear. Every attempt should be made to repair a dural tear, or the defect should be covered with a fat graft. The deep muscular layer and the fascia should then be closed tightly in layers. As mentioned previously, the lamina and the bone at the foramina of the vertebra above should be adequately undercut to prevent any neural impingement after closure of the osteotomy. These neural structures should be constantly visualized for any impingement during the osteotomy closure. Somatosensory evoked potentials serve as additional monitoring for early recognition of neural injury. The osteotomy itself exposes cancellous bone and leads to a continuous bleed from the exposed surfaces. The bleeding may be potentiated by the fact that most of the region has undergone a previous surgical insult. The current surgery then disrupts the scarred soft tissues and the prior fusion area that may or may not be solid. Intraoperative bleeding is minimized by maintaining hypotensive anesthesia during the entire surgical procedure and using bipolar cautery. It is important to perform the osteotomy rapidly and also close the osteotomy site rapidly with caution. Once the two bony surfaces are closed onto each other, this helps minimize bleeding from the cancellous surfaces. This extension osteotomy shortens the posterior column without elongating the anterior column, thereby avoiding stretching of the cauda or anterior vascular structures. A single-level osteotomy extending from the base of the excised pedicle to the anterosuperior corner of the vertebral body results an approximately 30 degrees of correction.

Pedicular stabilization at least one level above and one level below the osteotomy site is the minimal stabilization necessary to maintain the osteotomy in place and promote bony fusion. The patient is also made to stand upright and ambulate early, thereby avoiding the complications of prolonged recumbency.

## CONCLUSION

Pedicle subtraction and lumbar extension osteotomy for the correction of iatrogenic flat back is a technically demanding procedure. In the erect posture, 80% to 90% of the axial compressive forces pass through the anterior lumbar column and only 10% to 20% of these forces pass through the posterior column.[1,17] This anterior osteotomy is a biomechanically superior construct as compared to a posterior osteotomy, with the fulcrum of the osteotomy now being in the anterior column. Pedicle subtraction and lumbar extension osteotomy involves the vertebral body itself, thereby creating a highly vascularized "living bone graft" in the anterior spinal column. With posterior compressive pedicular instrumentation, bone-on-bone contact is established facilitating early fusion at the osteotomy site.

The following four case examples illustrate the principles involved in the management of iatrogenic kyphotic deformity with posterior extension osteotomy.

## CASE STUDIES

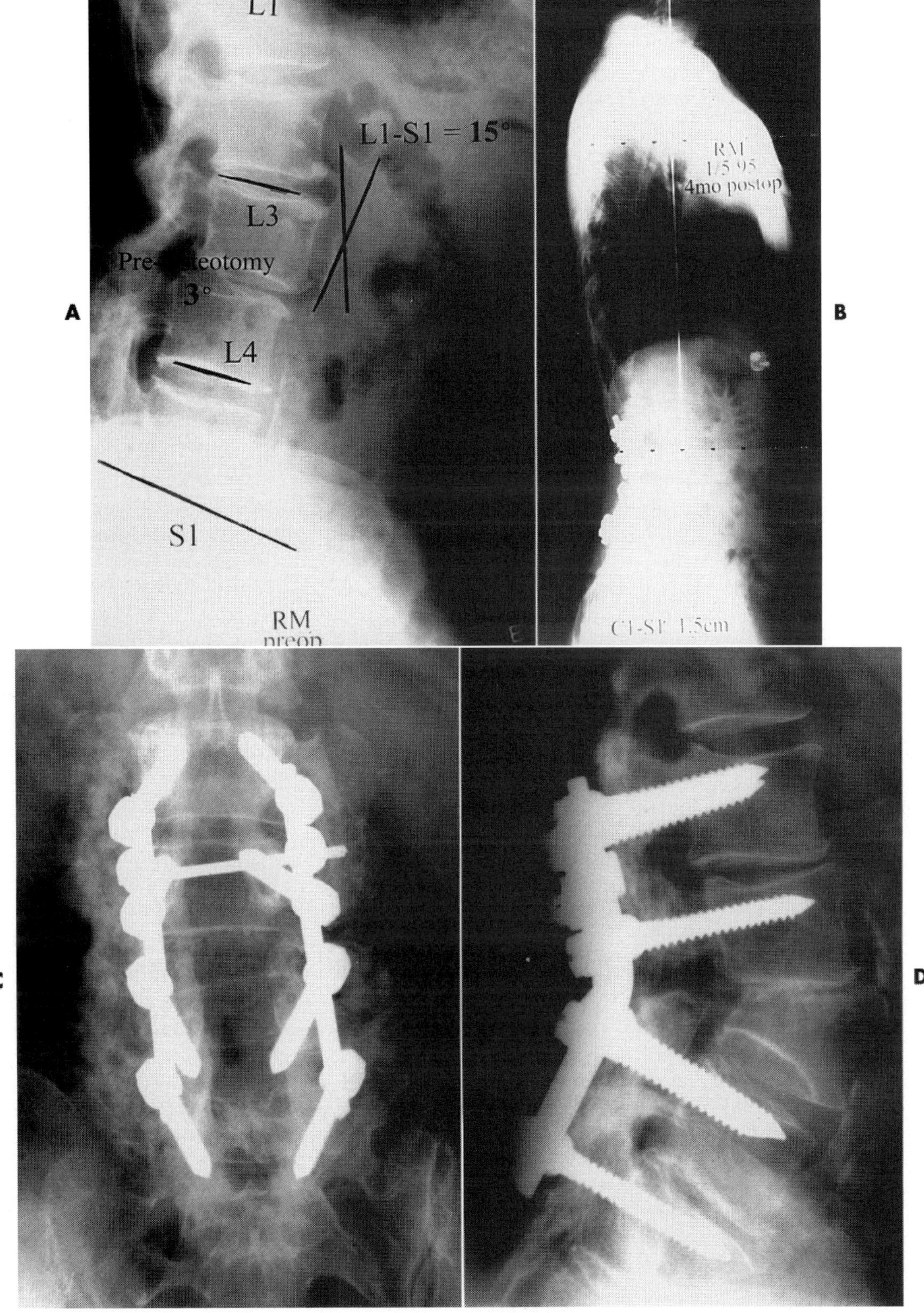


FIGURE 42-8

**A, B, C, D,** Case 1 radiographs. Intraoperative fluoroscopy images in the next five figures.

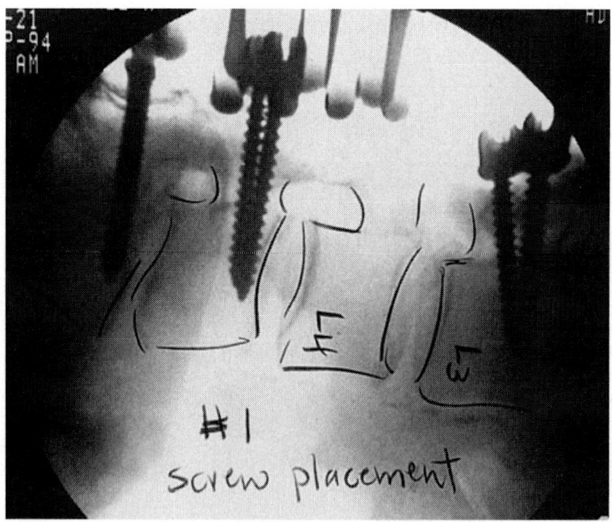


**FIGURE 42-9**

Pedicle screw placement in adjacent vertebral levels.

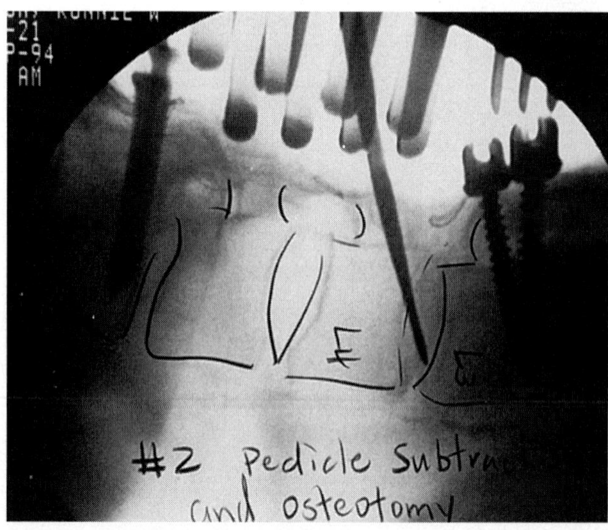


**FIGURE 42-10**

Pedicle subtraction and osteotomy at L4.

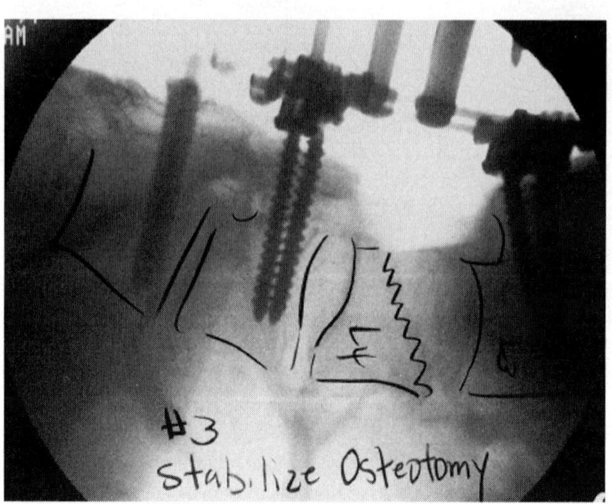


**FIGURE 42-11**

Temporary stabilization of the osteotomy with a short flexible rod.

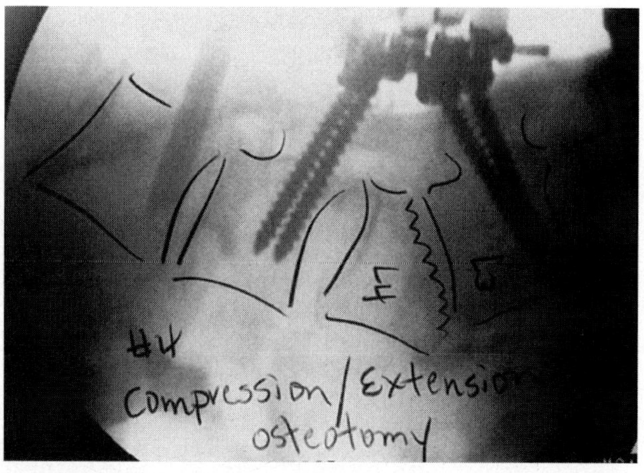


**FIGURE 42-12**

Compression of the osteotomy and extension of the spine.

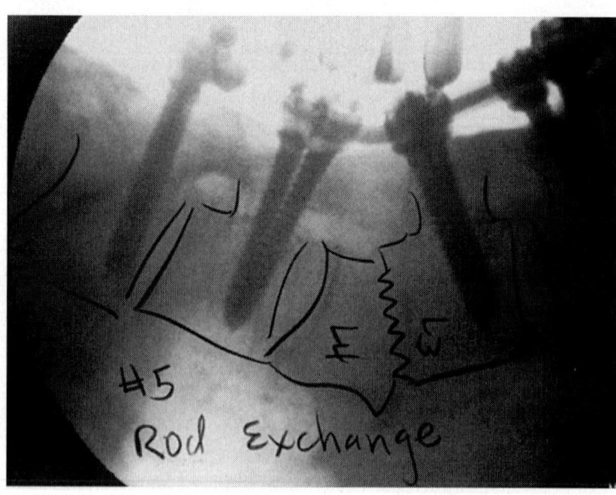


**FIGURE 42-13**

Precontoured rod is exchanged for the previous short-segment rod.

## CASE 1

This is a 51-year-old man with iatrogenic flat back from a two-level in situ posterior lumbar fusion. He presented with forward flexed posture and a 15-cm sagittal imbalance. His lumbar lordosis L1-S1 measured 15 degrees (Fig. 42-8, *A*). After extension osteotomy, C1-S1 measured 1.5 cm (Fig. 42-8, *B*). Now at 30 months postoperatively, his osteotomy is healed and his lumbar lordosis is maintained (Fig. 42-8, *C* and *D*). Figures 42-9 through 42-13 are the intraoperative fluoroscopy images of the technique in this case.

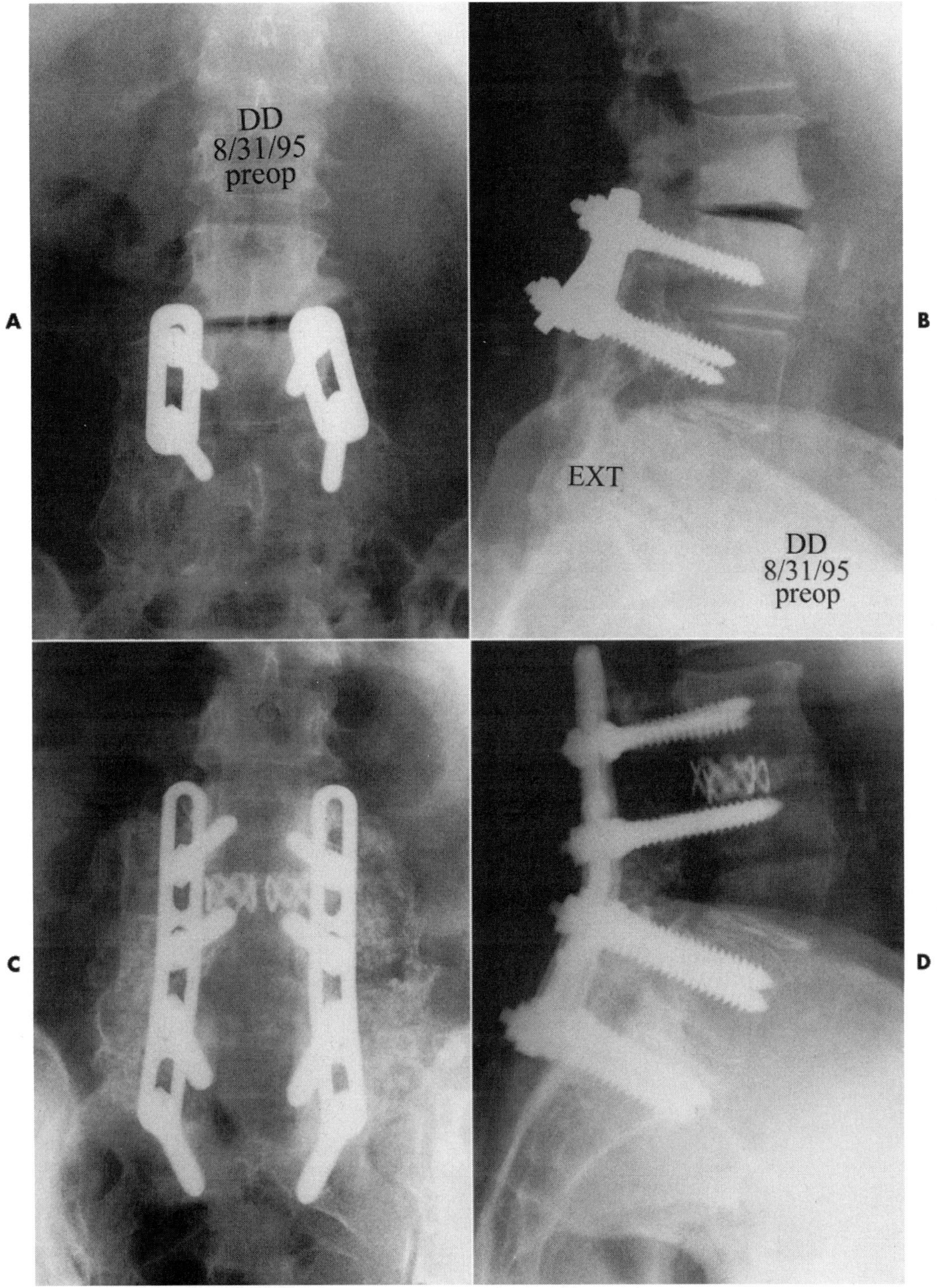


**FIGURE 42-14**

**A, B, C, D,** Case 2 radiographs. Intraoperative photographs of the technique in the next five figures.

## CASE 2

This 41-year-old woman experienced radiculopathy and sagittal imbalance of 14 cm following failed lumbar fusion. Preoperatively she had discal vacuum phenomena and degeneration at the level above her previous surgery (Fig. 42-14, *A* and *B*). She underwent extension osteotomy at L3-L4 and stabilization using Variable Screw Placement (VSP, Acromed) plating. At 18 months postoperatively, she has a solid anterior-posterior fusion and her osteotomy has healed (Fig. 42-14, *C* and *D*). She now stands in near-normal sagittal balance. The intraoperative photographs, Figures 42-15 through 42-19, demonstrate this technique.

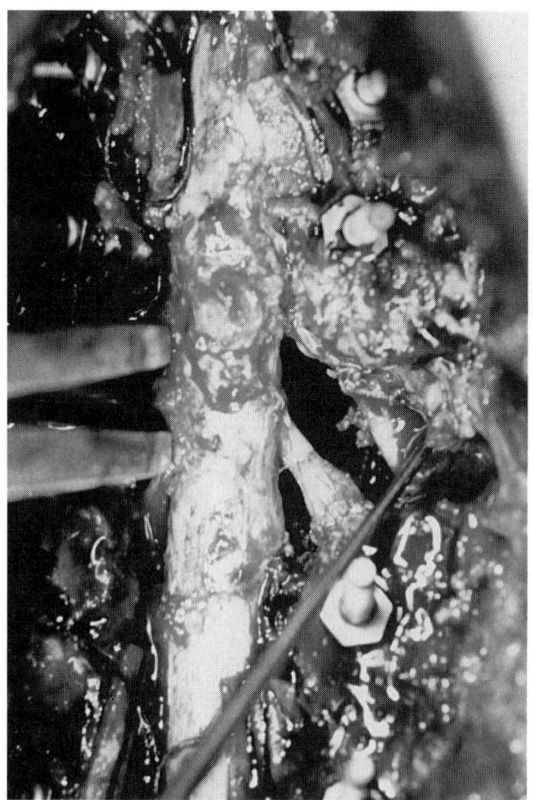

**FIGURE 42-15**

Pedicle screws in place. The distracter opening out the disk space and osteotome in place for the osteotomy.

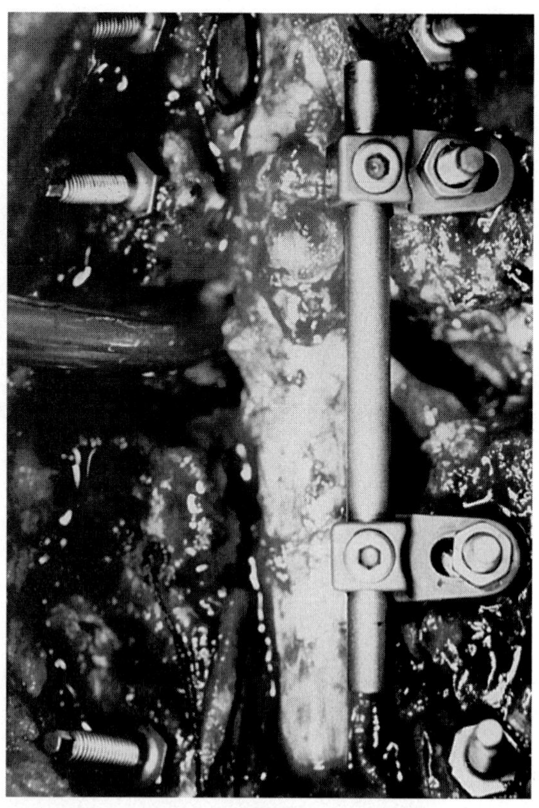

**FIGURE 42-16**

Osteotomy completed and temporarily stabilized with a short-segment rod.

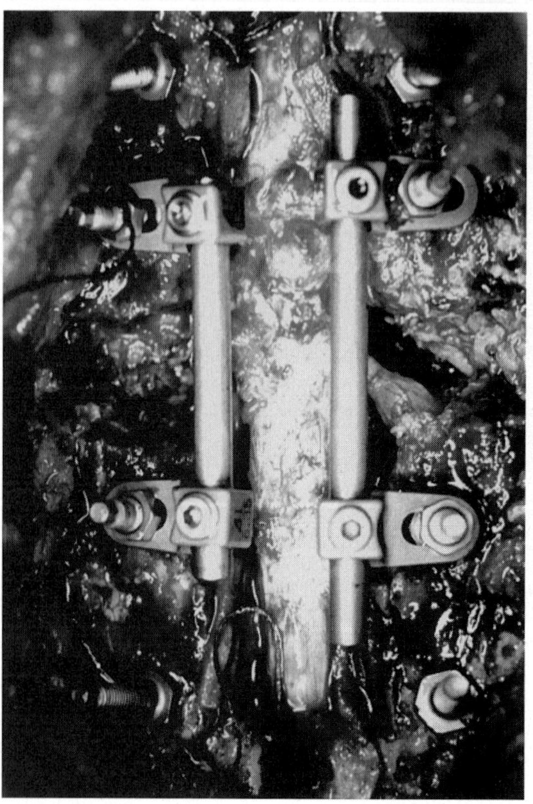

**FIGURE 42-17**

Another short-segment rod placed on opposite side.

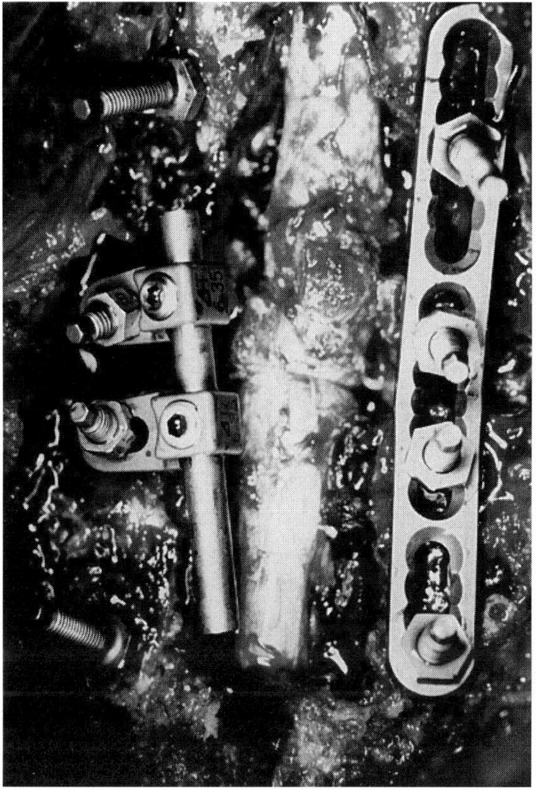

FIGURE 42-18

Osteotomy compressed and the rods are tightened to the screws. Note that the relative spacing between adjacent pedicle screws has decreased. Short-segment rod on one side is exchanged for a precontoured Variable Screw Placement (VSP) plate, which is tightened to the pedicle screws.

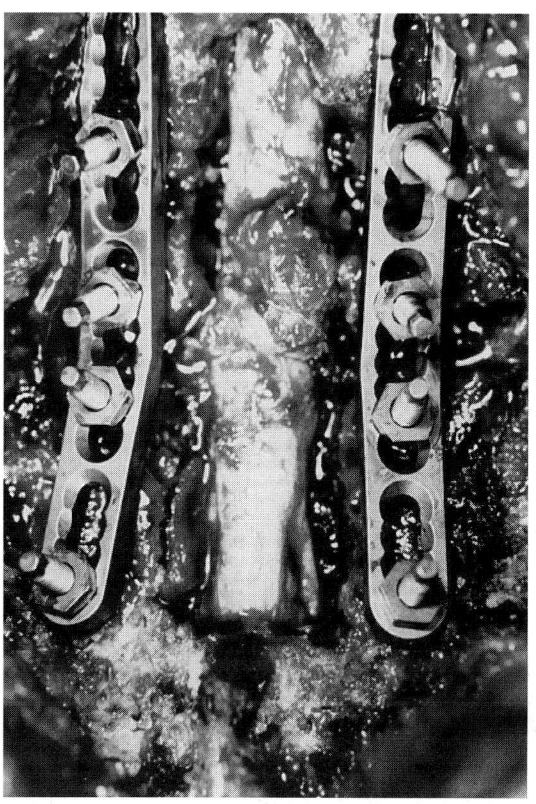

FIGURE 42-19

Another precontoured VSP plate replaces the short-segment rod on the opposite side.

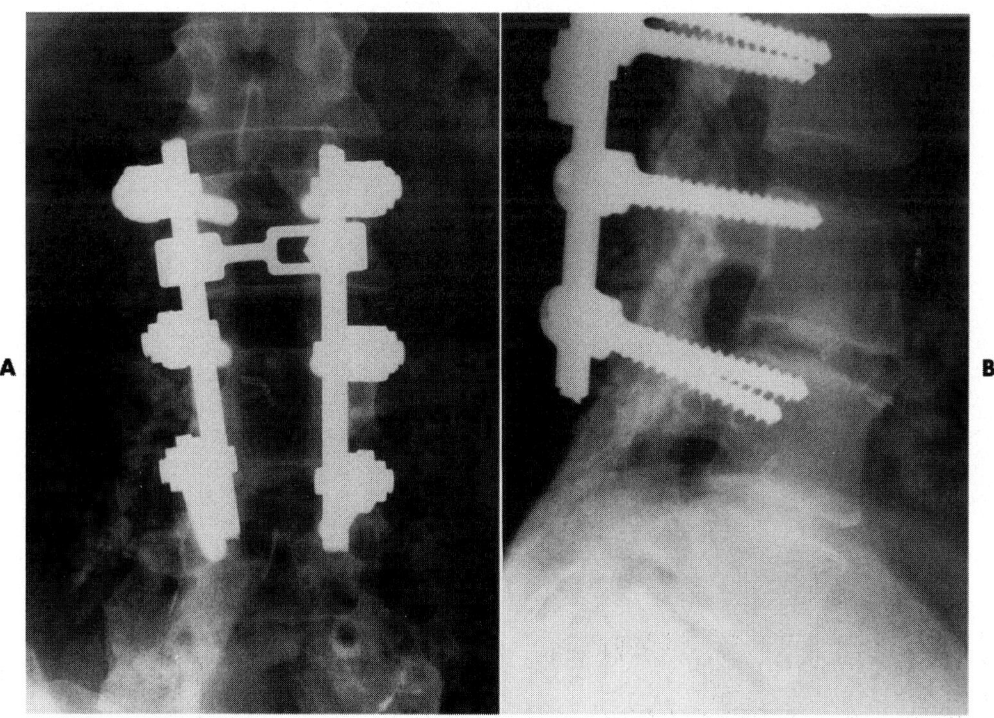


FIGURE 42-20

**A, B,** Case 3 radiographs.

*Continued*

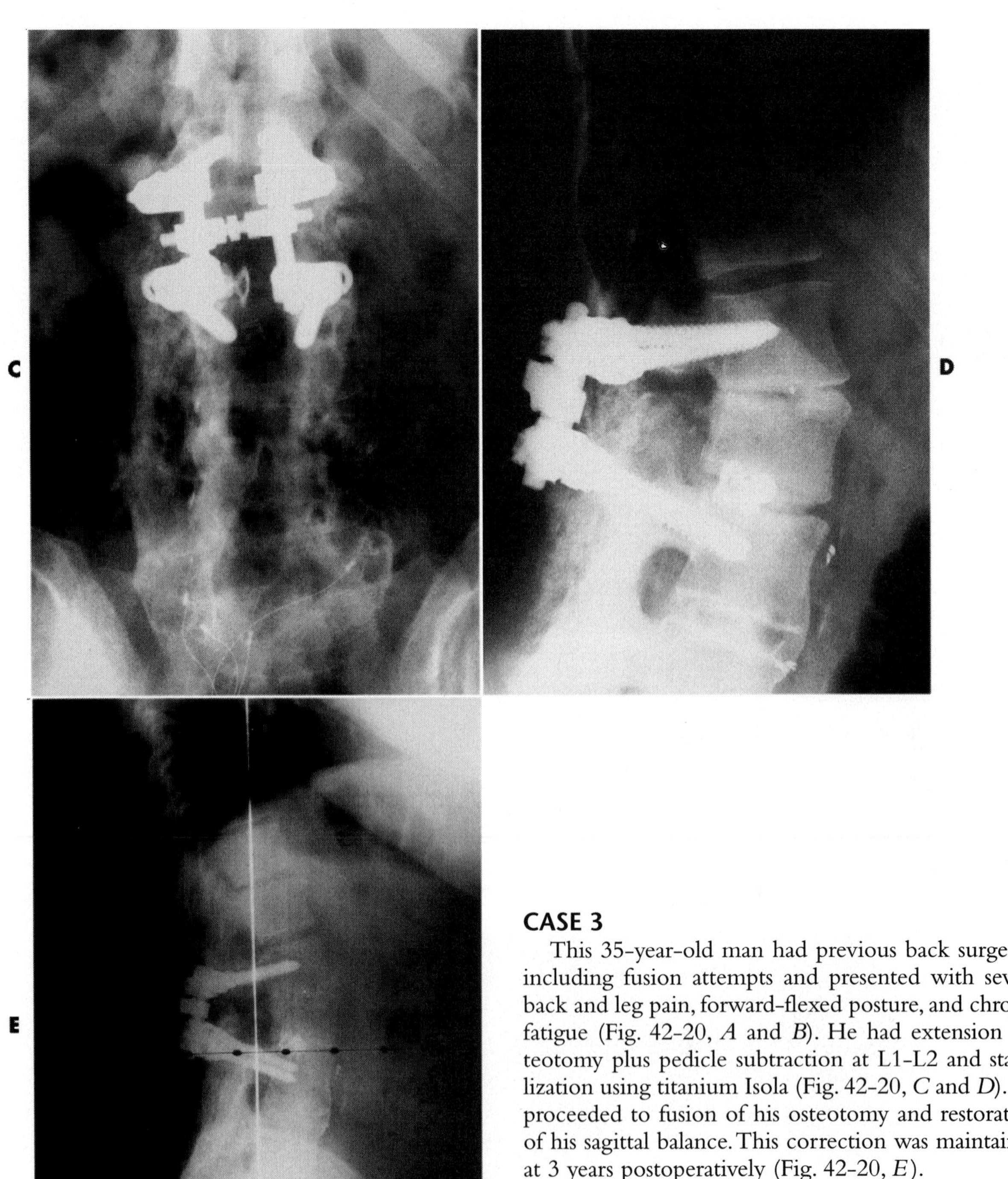


**FIGURE 42-20 CONT'D**

**C-E,** Case 3 radiographs.

## CASE 3

This 35-year-old man had previous back surgeries including fusion attempts and presented with severe back and leg pain, forward-flexed posture, and chronic fatigue (Fig. 42-20, *A* and *B*). He had extension osteotomy plus pedicle subtraction at L1-L2 and stabilization using titanium Isola (Fig. 42-20, *C* and *D*). He proceeded to fusion of his osteotomy and restoration of his sagittal balance. This correction was maintained at 3 years postoperatively (Fig. 42-20, *E*).

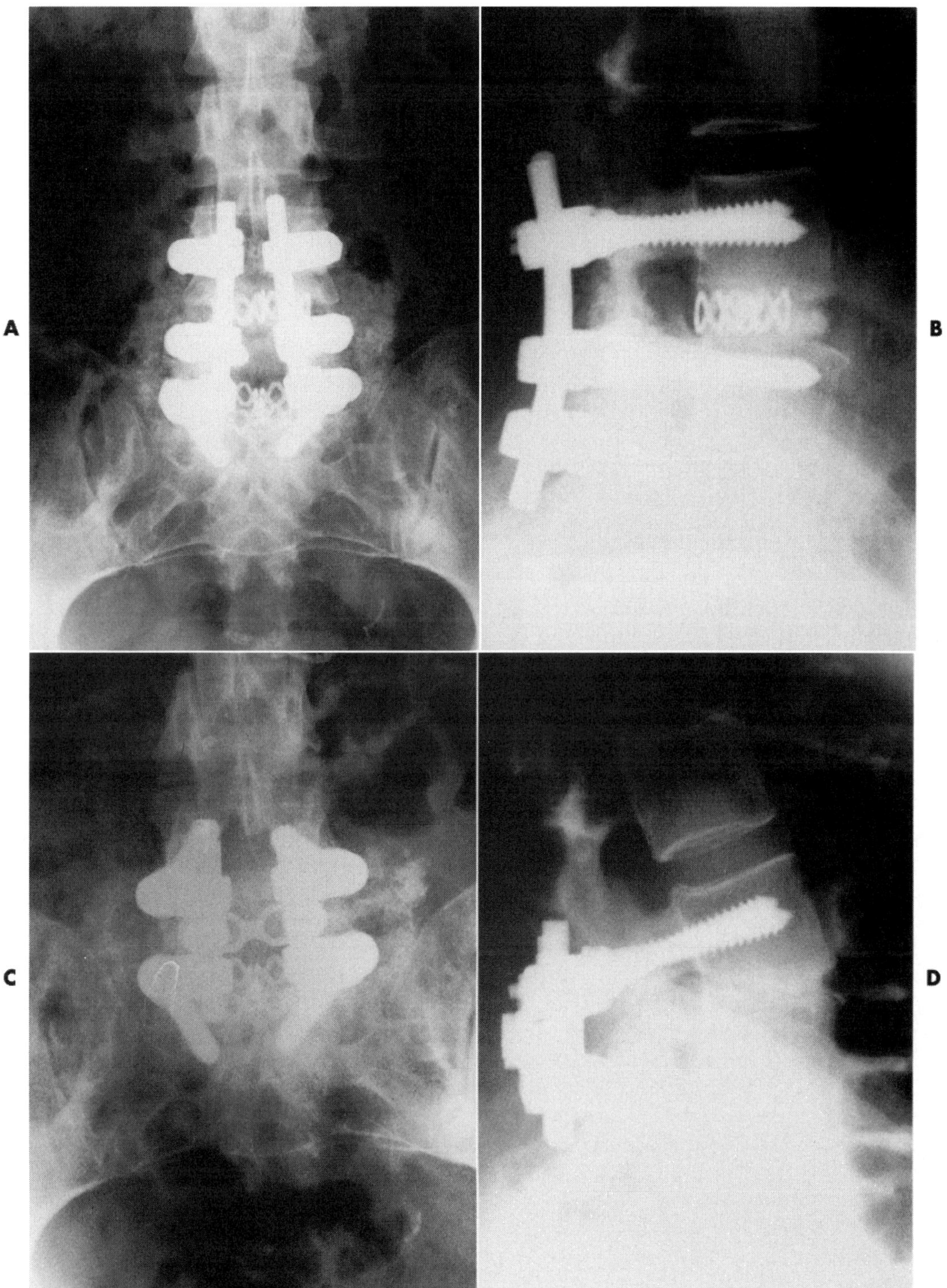


**FIGURE 42-21**

**A-D,** Case 4 radiographs.

## CASE 4

This 48-year-old woman presented with progressively increasing back pain following back surgery. Her pseudarthrosis at L4-S1 was confirmed intraoperatively (Fig. 42-21, *A*). Lateral radiographs showed flattening of the lumbar spine (Fig. 42-21, *B*). She underwent L4-L5 extension osteotomy and stabilization using titanium Isola instrumentation. She healed her osteotomy by 6 months postoperatively and is doing well at 18 months after restoration of her lordosis (Fig. 42-21, *C* and *D*).

## REFERENCES


1. Bergmark A: Stability of the lumbar spine: A study of mechanical engineering, *Acta Orthop Scand* 230(suppl): 28, 1989.
2. Bernhardt M, Bridwell KH: Segmental analysis of the sagittal plane alignment of the normal thoracic and lumbar spines and thoracolumbar junction, *Spine* 14:717-721, 1989.
3. Bradford DS, Schumacher WL, Lonstein JE, Winter RB: Ankylosing spondylitis: experience in surgical management of 21 patients, *Spine* 12:238-243, 1987.
4. Bridwell KH: Normal sagittal alignment. Presented at the Scoliosis Research Society-Sagittal Spinal Balance-Symposium No. 1, February 27, 1994.
5. Briggs H, Keats S, Schlesinger PT: Wedge osteotomy of the spine with bilateral intervertebral foraminotomy, *J Bone Joint Surg* 29:1075-1082, 1947.
6. Crawford Adams J: Techniques, dangers, and safeguards in osteotomy of the spine, *J Bone Joint Surg* 34B:226-232, 1952.
7. Doherty JH: Complications of fusion in lumbar scoliosis, *J Bone Joint Surg* 55A:438 (abstract), 1973.
8. Gertzbein SD, Harris MB: Wedge osteotomy for the correction of post-traumatic kyphosis: a new technique and a report of three cases, *Spine* 17:374-379, 1992.
9. Grobler LJ, Moe JH, Winter RB et al: Loss of lumbar lordosis following surgical correction of thoracolumbar deformities, *Orthop Trans* 2:39, 1978.
10. Hasday CA, Passoff TL, Perry J: Gait abnormalities arising from iatrogenic loss of lumbar lordosis secondary to Harrington instrumentation in lumbar fractures, *Spine* 8:501-511, 1983.
11. Kostuik JP, Hall BB: Spinal fusions to the sacrum in adults with scoliosis, *Spine* 8:489-500, 1983.
12. Kostuik JP, Maurais GR, Richardson WJ, Okajima Y: Combined single stage anterior and posterior osteotomy for correction of iatrogenic lumbar kyphosis, *Spine* 13:257-266, 1988.
13. La Chapelle EH: Osteotomy of the lumbar spine for correction of kyphosis in a case of ankylosing spondyloarthritis, *J Bone Joint Surg* 28:851-858, 1946.
14. La Grone MO: Loss of lumbar lordosis: a complication of spinal fusion for scoliosis, *Orthop Clin North Am* 19:383-393, 1988.
15. Law WA: Osteotomy of the spine, *Clin Orthop* 66:70-76, 1969.
16. Lehmer SM, Keppler L, Biscup RS, Enker P, Miller SD, Steffee AD: Posterior transvertebral osteotomy for adult thoracolumbar kyphosis, *Spine* 19:2060-2067, 1994.
17. Lowery GL, Harms J: *Principles of load sharing.* In Bridwell KH, DeWald RL, editors: *The textbook of spinal surgery,* ed 2, Philadelphia, 1997, Lippincott-Raven, pp155-166.
18. McMaster PE: Osteotomy of the spine for fixed flexion deformity, *J Bone Joint Surg* 44A:1207-1216, 1962.
19. McMaster MJ, Coventry MB: Spinal osteotomy in ankylosing spondylitis, *Mayo Clin Proc* 48:476-486, 1973.
20. McMaster MJ: A technique for lumbar spinal osteotomy in ankylosing spondylitis, *J Bone Joint Surg* 67B:204-210, 1985.
21. Moe JH, Denis F: The iatrogenic loss of lumbar lordosis, *Orthop Trans* 1:131, 1977.
22. Roberson JR, Whitesides TE Jr: Surgical reconstruction of late post-traumatic thoracolumbar kyphosis, *Spine* 10:307-312, 1985.
23. Simmons EH: Kyphotic deformity of the spine in ankylosing spondylitis, *Clin Orthop* 128:65-77, 1977.
24. Simmons EH: *Surgery of the spine in rheumatoid arthritis and ankylosing spondylitis.* In Evarts CM, editor: *Surgery of the musculoskeletal system.* New York, 1983, Churchill Livingstone.
25. Smith-Petersen MN, Larson CB, Aufranc OE: Osteotomy of the spine for correction of flexion deformity in rheumatoid arthritis, *J Bone Joint Surg* 27:1-11, 1945.
26. Thiranont N, Netrawichien P: Transpedicular decancellation closed wedge vertebral osteotomy for treatment of fixed flexion deformity of spine in ankylosing spondylitis, *Spine* 18:2517-2522, 1993.
27. Thomasen E: Vertebral osteotomy for correction of kyphosis in ankylosing spondylitis, *Clin Orthop* 194: 142-152, 1985.
28. Van Royen BJ, Slot GH: Closing-wedge posterior osteotomy for ankylosing spondylitis: partial corporectomy and transpedicular fixation in 22 cases, *J Bone Joint Surg* 77B:117-121, 1995.
29. Weatherley C, Jaffray D, Terry A: Vascular complications associated with osteotomy in ankylosing spondylitis: a report of two cases, *Spine* 13:43-46, 1988.
30. Wilson MJ, Turkell JH: Multiple spinal wedge osteotomy: its use in a case of Marie-Strumpell spondylitis, *Am J Surg* 777-782, 1949.

# 43

# ANTERIOR COLUMN SUPPORT FOR FAILED FUSION

**Parviz Kambin, M.D.**
**Mark K. Chang, M.D.**



Although at times a satisfactory clinical outcome is achieved in spite of the presence of a fibrous union, at no time should the principle of a sound surgical technique and the attempt to secure solid bony union across the unstable segments be compromised. Many factors influence the outcome of spinal arthrodesis during the preoperative stage, intraoperatively and postoperatively.

## PREOPERATIVE FACTORS

### Proper Patient Selection

Like other elective spine surgeries, proper patient selection is an important factor that affects the final outcome of spinal stabilization. A thorough medical and psychological evaluation, including work history, drug dependency, and duration of use of narcotic-based pain medications, should be taken into account prior to consideration of a second or third salvage procedure. Symptom magnification in individuals involved in medicolegal dispute is not uncommon. The subjective complaints of patients must be substantiated by objective means prior to consideration of a primary or salvage procedure. Preoperative counseling and/or a drug rehabilitation program would lessen the burden of postoperative continuous need for narcotic-based medications and failed back syndrome.

### ACCURATE DIAGNOSIS

Selection of the appropriate symptom-producing site for arthrodesis is not always easy. Although instability associated with degenerative or idiopathic spondylolisthesis may require surgical stabilization, a thorough evaluation of the adjacent intervertebral disks to make certain that they are not a pain-producing unit and a contributory factor is necessary prior to any surgical intervention. Localization of the site of arthrodesis is not difficult when disabling back pain is associated with radicular symptoms; however, extra caution must be exercised when arthrodesis is being performed merely for treatment of a stable degenerative disk disease. The selection of the symptomatic site in individuals presented with radiographic evidence of multiple disk degeneration requires prudent preoperative diagnostic workup.

Dynamic flexion and extension radiographs, selective diskography, pain provocative and analgesic testing, and, at times, temporary fixation of the spinal unit[4-12] may be helpful in localization of a symptom-producing degenerated intervertebral disk. Standing, lateral, flexion, and extension x-ray studies of the lumbar spine are a simple and inexpensive means that may be used for detection of an unstable spinal unit. The side-bending films may also provide additional information. Abnormal translation of one segment on the adjacent vertebral body of more than 3 or 4 mm is suggestive of instability of the spinal unit; however, children and adolescents may demonstrate physiologic radiographic evidence of translation of the vertebral bodies. When the patient is in severe pain, adequate analgesics must be provided prior to the dynamic studies.

In contrast, the radiographically demonstrated instability may not be the sole factor responsible for the patient's symptomatology. In the absence of associated neurological deficit, pain provocative and analgesic testing may need to be used to confirm that the patient's pain indeed is arising from the unstable segments. Diskography is commonly used to ascertain the integrity of the intervertebral disks adjacent to the unstable spinal unit and to determine whether or not it should be included in the fusion site. The role of computed tomography (CT) diskography and classification of internal disk disruption syndrome have been described.[18-21] The integrity of the posterior and posterolateral annulus, as observed in the plane lateral radiographic examination and axial CT studies following the injection of radiopaque material, provide valuable information.

The intervertebral disks (in which the integrity of the posterior and posterolateral annulus has not been disturbed, and their CT diskography demonstrates a thick and intact posterior annulus) may not require surgical stabilization. In contrast, when the posterior annulus is torn, thinned out, the injected opaque material is observed under the posterior longitudinal ligament, and the disk is pain producing, the need for inclusion of the latter into the fusion site becomes more evident.

## INTRAOPERATIVE FACTORS

### INADEQUATE SURGICAL DECOMPRESSION AT THE PRESENCE OF RADICULAR SYMPTOMS

Adequate decompression of the neural elements must precede the second attempt for surgical stabilization. Although the surgical restoration of the height of a degenerated intervertebral disk may alleviate the symptoms arising from a degenerated bulging disk, at the presence of accompanying radicular symptoms, partial facetectomy and/or annulectomy ensures the outcome of surgical stabilization of the spinal unit.

### INADEQUATE PREPARATION OF SURGICAL SITE AND BONE GRAFTING

Meticulous removal of soft tissues and ample decortication are necessary for achieving a satisfactory bony union. Although a high-speed powered drill and diamond burrs are extremely useful for removal of bone and decompression of the neural elements, they should not be used for decortication of the host bone at the fusion site. A cutting-tip burr and curette should be used to expose the bleeding cancellous bone in preparation of bone grafting.

When possible, autogenous bone graft should be used for a revision surgery. The graft should be harvested shortly prior to its transplantation. If there is a waiting period involved, the bone grafts should be kept in the patient's own blood rather than saline solution. The cortical bone should be cut in narrow strips and the corticocancellous bone grafts packed with an impactor in and around the fusion site.

## POSTOPERATIVE FACTORS

### LOSS OF REDUCTION

Postoperative recurrent translation of one lumbar segment on another may be observed. Postoperative fracture of the pedicles (Fig. 43-1), loosely seated screws (caused by repeated insertion and withdrawal during the surgery), forcefully reduced spondylolisthesis, and presence of osteoporosis are all predisposing factors responsible for postoperative loss of vertebral alignment (Fig. 43-2). It should be kept in mind that most of these patients had undergone laminotomy and decompressive procedures prior to their surgical stabilization. A satisfactory outcome in the latter group of

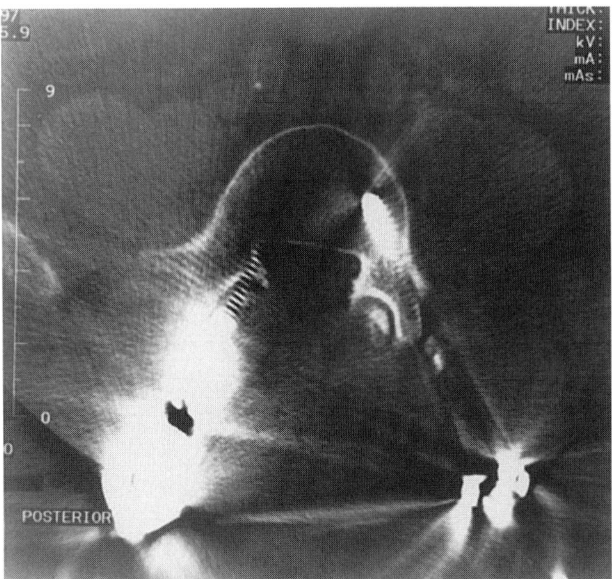


**FIGURE 43-1**

Fracture of pedicle 4 weeks following the surgery. Associated with onset of pain and weakness of the involved extremity. Required surgical extraction of the hardware with a satisfactory outcome.

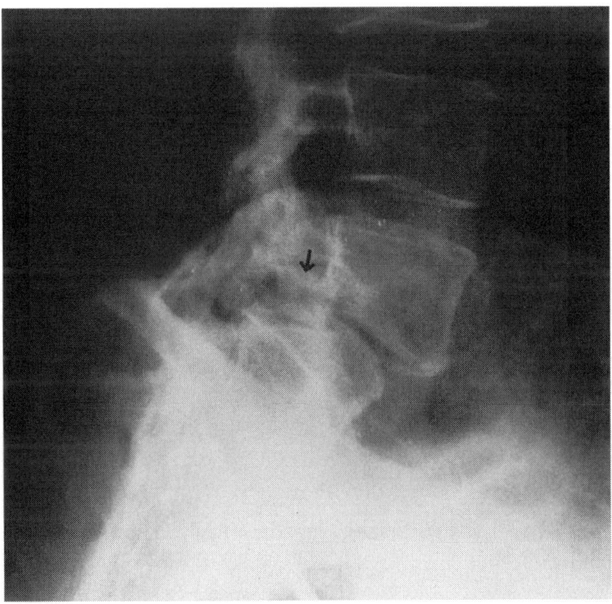

**FIGURE 43-2**

Postoperative loss of alignment of intraoperatively reduced spondylolisthesis at L5-S1. Note the posterior displacement of interbody graft.

patients may be attained when adequate in situ bony fusion is achieved without the need for additional surgery; however, if recurrence of the preoperative symptoms is proved to be caused by the traction of a specific root secondary to spondylolisthesis or retrolisthesis, then an additional surgery including anterior or posterior stabilization or both may be required. The extension of the fusion mass to include the adjacent segments and use of a long plate or rod system reduces the effect of compressive and shearing forces and may minimize the postoperative loss of reduction. The above procedure may have to be augmented with anterior retroperitoneal grafting and fixation.

## BONE GRAFT MIGRATION

The posterior migration of the interbody graft into the spinal canal (Fig. 43-2), although not common, could cause severe radicular pain and postoperative neurological symptoms.

Diagnosis is readily made by postoperative CT scan, which may need to be followed by additional surgical intervention. However, if the arthrodesis had been performed following adequate laminectomy, partial facetectomy, and decompression, the patient may remain symptom free without need for additional surgical intervention. Anterior displacement of the graft is more common when the anterior approach has been used; in contrast, posterior displacement usually occurs when the posterior interbody fusion has been performed.

The field of spine surgery has reached a sophisticated stage. The introduction of new surgical approaches and complicated devices demands better surgical training and broader exposure of surgeons to the new technologies. Although the new technological development has enhanced our rate of successful arthrodesis, it has also added a list of unwarranted complications to our previous difficulties. Casual spine surgery should be avoided. Today's spine surgeons must have a full commitment to the field in which they can expand their knowledge and skill to better serve their patients.

Because the intervertebral disks and the vertebral plates are the most common pain generators of spinal units, stabilization of the anterior column appears to be the most logical form of arthrodesis. Although posterolateral intertransverse fusion is being used most commonly for segmental stabilization, the limited available posterolateral bone surface and unavoidable interoperative insult to the paraspinal muscles and soft tissue structures make it a less desirable fusion site. In addition, the presence of radiographic evidence of posterolateral or posterior arthrodesis, a certain amount of motion that may contribute to postoperative pain, may be realized between the vertebral bodies anteriorly.

## INFECTION

An infection rate varying from 1% to 3% has been reported. In 1968, Wiley et al[21] reported the incidence of discitis to be approximately 0.6%. In contrast, Crock[2] felt that the incidence of complication was greater than previously reported. Fraser et al[7] reported the rate of infection to be 2.3% in 432 cases. Loss of height of intervertebral disks, development of lateral recess stenosis, and further displacement or loss of reduction of spondylolisthesis may be observed following wound infection. The addition of internal fixators to the armamentarium that are used during spinal fusion requires longer exposure of the wound to the external elements and a greater degree of handling of the instruments and soft tissues. This may increase incidence of surgical contamination.

Early postoperative diagnosis of infection, particularly when the patient is receiving prophylactic antibiotics, may be difficult. Although magnetic resonance imaging (MRI) is sensitive for diagnosis of postoperative discitis, it may not be helpful in early diagnosis of postoperative infection in which mechanical decortication of the vertebral plates had been performed. When the delayed closure of the surgical incision is associated with local swelling and inflammation by the sixth postoperative day, reexploration of the wound under general anesthesia, for the removal of hematoma and necrotic tissue, and vigorous lavage with antibiotic solution may prevent advancement of the infection process and its associated complications. This step then may be followed by closure of the wound and 6 weeks of intravenous antibiotic therapy pending the result of culture and sensitivity testing.

At this early postoperative stage, the internal fixators are not usually loose and may be left in place while the patient is kept under close observation. At the same operating setting, the arthroscopic visualization of the intervertebral disk for visual diagnosis,[12] extraction of necrotic tissue, debridement, and vigorous irrigation further enhance the patient's chance of rapid recovery.

### Degenerative Disk Pathology Involving the Adjacent Units

At times, a rapid progression of the degenerative process of the intervertebral disks adjacent to the previous fusion site is observed, which may or may not be symptom producing. However, in advanced stages of degenerative arthropathy, particularly when combined with abnormal translation of the vertebral bodies, pain may become a dominant factor. In contrast, the development of the degenerative process in an intact intervertebral disk adjacent to the fusion site is slow. The occurrence of degenerative changes of the adjacent segments may be more rapid when circumferential fusion or rigid fixators are used.

Deyo and coworkers[22] reported an increased incidence of failure and need for reoperation in elderly patients with advanced degenerative changes. Additionally the angle at which the vertebrae are fused may affect the biomechanics of the adjacent segments.[6] A compensatory effect and increased motion of the segment above the fusion site were observed by Frymoyer.[5] Development of segmental instability above the fusion site may complicate the long-term outcome of spine fusion.[17] Development of spinal stenosis following spine fusion may become symptom producing[1]; however, this complication is not as common following posterolateral intertransverse fusion. Acquired spondylolysis as a sequel to spine fusion, although rare, has been reported.[8] Kahanovitz and coworkers[9] reported irreversible changes in the facet cartilage of the segments adjacent to the fusion site following extraction of posterior instrumentation.

### Pseudarthrosis

The diagnosis of pseudarthrosis at times may be difficult. In addition, correlating the presenting symptoms and radiographic evidence of pseudarthrosis is not always an easy task. The diagnosis is usually established by dynamic flexion and extension lateral radiographs, presence of a defect in plane x-ray studies, and CT scan study of the fusion site, which may show the interruption of the bony trabeculae at the fusion site. The diagnosis of pseudarthrodesis may be confirmed by cessation of pain following local infiltration of the defect site by local anesthesia.

## TREATMENT

The management of a pain-producing failed fusion must be geared toward the correction of a variety of factors that are responsible for the patient's continuous symptomatology. When it is deemed that the presenting symptoms are caused by inadequate decompression of the neural elements, a combination of the extension of the laminotomy site, partial facetectomy, and impaction of posterior or posterolateral osteophytes may eliminate the patient's difficulties.

Misplaced or displaced fixators may produce pressure upon the neural elements causing pain or neurodeficit (see Fig. 43-1). The surgical extraction of the fixators may eliminate the presenting symptoms. When pseudarthrosis is deemed to be responsible for loss of reduction or stabilization of a motion segment, restabilization may be achieved via an anterior column support. Considering the broad surface of the vertebral plates, adequacy of its blood supply, and exposure of the graft to the compressive elements when the patient is ambulatory, the anterior column fusion represents an ideal site in securing bony arthrodesis.

Anterior column arthrodesis may be performed through a posterior approach following ample laminotomy, partial facetectomy, and diskectomy. Although the L4-L5 and L5-S1 intervertebral disks are readily accessible to this approach, the anatomic position of the exiting root and the content of the spinal canal preclude the use of a posterior approach for insertion of interbody grafts or cages in the mid or upper lumbar region. Open anterior retroperitoneal, transperitoneal, and laparoscopic approaches provide direct access to the vertebral bodies and the intervertebral disk at L5-S1. However the anatomic position of vascular structures limits access to the adjacent segments. A lateral open retroperitoneal approach has been used to access the mid lumbar segments.

## ARTHROSCOPIC ANTERIOR COLUMN ARTHRODESIS

Posterolateral arthroscopic access for stabilization of the anterior column was the natural progression of our earlier experience with posterolateral percutaneous arthroscopic disk surgery.[10-14] In situ and uninstrumented percutaneous interbody fusion was attempted as early as 1983 with suboptimal outcome. Failures were attributed to both the inability to reach and decorticate the concave surface of the vertebral plates and the high incidence of graft resorption. Recent technological developments,[11,13,20] namely the availability of small-caliber, high-resolution glass fiberoptics, oval cannulas, and eccentric decorticators, have added a new dimension to the field of arthroscopic posterolateral lumbar arthrodesis.

Inability to access the L5-S1 intervertebral disk via a biportal approach in individuals with elevated iliac crests is a limitation to the use of the posterolateral approach for arthroscopic arthrodesis. In addition, it may be difficult to insert an arthroscopic cannula into a severely degenerated and narrowed intervertebral disk. However, the disk height may be increased by the introduction of a blunt-end cannulated obturator into the intervertebral disk. Disk height is then maintained by insertion of an oval cannula into the disk space. Because nucleotomy and decortication of the vertebral plates are time-consuming, the arthroscopic interbody fusion can not be used when a multilevel arthrodesis is required. In addition, when a reduction and maintenance of a spondylolisthesis greater than grade I are desired, the deep positioning of the plates against the bony structures following an open procedure may be advantageous. In revision surgery, the presence of posterolateral bone grafts may preclude the proper positioning of the cannulas. The plane x-rays and CT scan study from the index level should be examined to make certain that there is no obstacle in the path of the inserted instruments.

### POSITIONING OF THE PATIENT AND C-ARM

Surgery must be performed with the patient in a prone position. A biportal approach to the intervertebral disk is necessary for ample nucleotomy, decortication of the vertebral plates, and insertion of the bone graft. Familiarity with the biportal approach for diskectomy and triangulation within the intervertebral disk is a prerequisite for the satisfactory completion of arthroscopic interbody fusion. An adjustable radiolucent frame should be used to provide adequate support under the anterosuperior iliac spine of the patient and ample space for expansion of the chest and abdomen. In contrast to the Wilson frame, the above bolsters are converged to elevate the patient's pelvis and reduce the preoperative anterior or posterior translation of the vertebral bodies.

To widen the posterior height of the intervertebral disk, the operating table may also be flexed at the onset of the procedure; however, the operating table may have to be straightened prior to insertion of the subcutaneous plates and final closure. This allows the maintenance of normal lumbar lordosis. The C-arm must be properly covered with sterile drapes and positioned for fluoroscopic visualization during the surgery. Prior to insertion of the needle, the C-arm should be maneuvered until the vertebral plates of the segments adjacent to the fusion site are seen as two parallel lines. The same principle should be exercised when the guide pins are inserted into the pedicles in preparation for insertion of the pedicular bolts. The proximal and distal boundaries of the pedicles must be seen as a single line in the lateral x-ray projection.

### INSERTION OF THE 5 × 5 CANNULAS

Steps that are taken for positioning of the cannula into the intervertebral disk at the index level are similar to those described for arthroscopic microdiskectomy.[11-14] Generally, it is advantageous to use a 5 × 5-mm internal diameter (ID) cannula on one side and a 5 × 10-mm ID oval cannula on the opposite side. The skin entry point is selected approximately 10 cm from the midline. In obese individuals with abundant subcutaneous adipose tissue, further lateralization of the skin entry site may be necessary. In contrast to arthroscopic fragmentectomy, the tip of the inserted needle may be placed lateral to the mid pedicular line as is observed in anteroposterior fluoroscopic studies (Fig. 43-3). In the lateral radiographic view, the tip of the needle is observed in alignment with the posterior boundary of the vertebrae above and below the fusion site. The stylet of the needle is then replaced with a guide wire. This step is followed by introduction of the cannulated obturator and positioning of a 5 × 5-mm ID universal access cannula into the triangular working zone.[10-14] The triangular working zone is bordered medially by the dural sac and the traversing root, anteriorly by the exiting root, inferiorly by the proximal plate of the distal segment, and posteriorly by the articular processes and facets of the adjacent

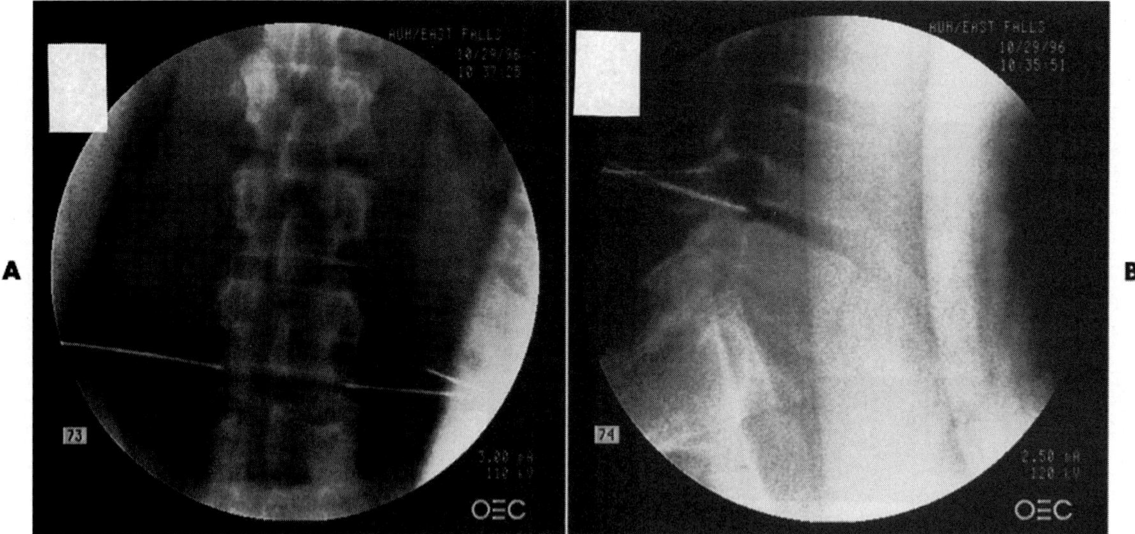

FIGURE 43-3

Intraoperative needle positioning. **A,** AP fluoroscopic view. Note that the tip of the needle is placed on the annulus at the lateral pedicular line. **B,** Lateral view fluoroscopic examination demonstrates that the tip of the needle is in alignment with the posterior border of the adjacent vertebrae.

segments. A 0-degree diskoscope or a working channel scope is used for inspection of the annulotomy site, to make certain that the contents of the spinal canal are not in the path of the instruments. It should be noted that when the cannula is properly placed on the annulus in the triangular working zone, it has already bypassed the exiting root and entrapment of this root by the inserted cannula is very unlikely. Annular fenestration is achieved either with a 5-mm trephine or with the aid of a working channel scope. While the 5-mm trephine is fully inserted into the intervertebral disk, the universal access cannula is forced into the annular fenestration for a distance of 5 to 10 mm and secured in this position by the cannula stopper on the skin surface. At this time, a manual arthroscopic diskectomy forceps, trimmer blades, and suction punch forceps are used, and the nuclear tissue is partially evacuated.

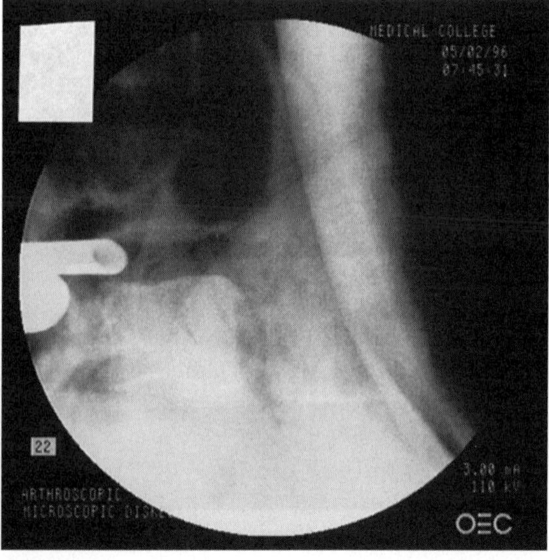

FIGURE 43-4

The position of the oval cannula is shown in lateral fluoroscopic examination.

### POSITIONING OF A 5 × 8-MM OR 5 × 10-MM INTERNAL DIAMETER OVAL CANNULA

Positioning of the oval cannula first requires arthroscopic placement of a universal 5 × 5-mm ID cannula into the intervertebral disk. This step is then followed by reinsertion of the cannulated obturator that is passed through the annular fenestration and advanced into the center of the intervertebral disk. Following the removal of the universal access cannula, a specially designed jig permits the introduction of an auxiliary obturator next to the previously positioned cannulated obturator. The distal end of the auxiliary obturator is beveled and capable of bypassing the exiting root as it enters the annular fenestration. At this time, the cannular jig is removed and the oval cannula is passed over the two cannulas and inserted into the intervertebral disk (Fig. 43-4).

### NUCLEOTOMY AND DECORTICATION OF THE VERTEBRAL PLATES

Prior to decortication of the vertebral plates, a meticulous nucleotomy is performed with the aid of a large-cup forceps, trimmer blades, and reamers.

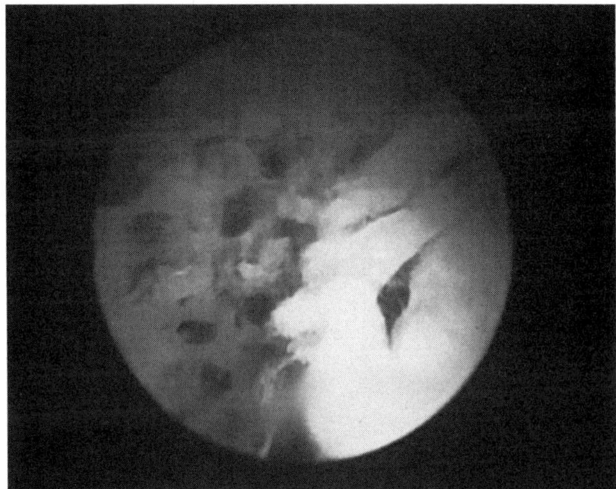

**FIGURE 43-5**

Arthroscopic view of partially decorticated vertebral plate in preparation of arthroscopic interbody fusion.

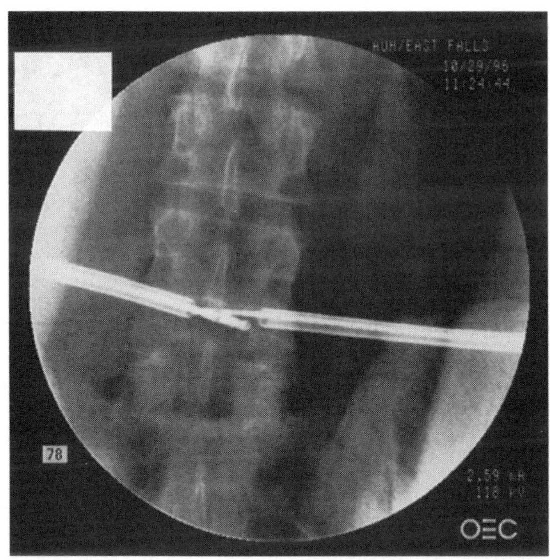


**FIGURE 43-6**

AP interoperative fluoroscopy demonstrates a biportal approach to the L4-L5 intervertebral disk for nucleotomy and decortication of the vertebral plates.

Although in the past we have used laser light for nuclear ablation under arthroscopic visualization, in recent years a radiofrequency coagulator has been employed for removal of fine nuclear tissue. The latter is more cost-effective and easier to use. The oval cannula permits the insertion of an angled-tip curette and specially designed reamers for access and decortication of the concave surface of the vertebral plate (Fig. 43-5). When the decorticators are inserted into the oval cannula and turned into a vertical position, the blades of the decorticator extend behind the boundary of the oval cannula. The nucleotomy and decortication must be performed under arthroscopic control, using a biportal approach (Fig. 43-6). Usually, the arthroscope is inserted through the 5 × 5-mm ID cannula while the decorticators are introduced through the oval cannula that has been positioned on the patient's opposite side. Bleeding from the partially decorticated plates may obscure ample arthroscopic visualization. This bleeding may be controlled by increasing the inflow pressure of the saline solution while closing the outflow valve of the saline.

## BONE GRAFTING

An ample amount of corticocancellous bone is removed from the ilium and the posterior superior iliac spine of the patient via a separate, 3-cm skin incision. The removal of autogenous bone from the external table of the ilium reduces postoperative morbidity at the donor site. Bone grafts are inserted through the cannulas and are packed between the vertebral plates of the adjacent segments. Our previous attempts to use a combination of autogenous bone and allograft for arthroscopic interbody fusion was associated with failure of arthrodesis in some cases.

## INSERTION OF THE GUIDE PINS

The proper positioning of the pedicular bolts in the pedicle is best accomplished by insertion of a guide pin in the medullary canal of the pedicle under fluoroscopic control. The "bull's-eye technique" or anteroposterior and lateral radiographs may be used.

## POSITIONING OF THE PEDICULAR CANNULAS

A longitudinal skin incision is made between the guide pins that have been inserted into the pedicles above and below the fusion site. Two small separate incisions are then made in the thoracolumbar fascia to permit the passage of 9.8-mm outside diameter (OD) cannulated obturator. The cannulated obturator is placed over the guide pins and passed through the lumbar fascia and paravertebral muscles until it reaches the articular process of the segments adjacent to the fusion site. At this time, the pedicular cannula with 10-mm ID obturator is introduced over the cannulated obturator, and the obturator is then withdrawn. It is advisable to view the position of the guide pin in the pedicle under lateral fluoroscopic examination. The undesirable cephalad or caudad position of the guide pin may be corrected at this time.

## INSERTION OF PEDICULAR BOLTS

Prior to insertion of pedicular bolts, the medullary canals of the pedicles are tapped with a cannulated bone tap that is placed over the previously inserted

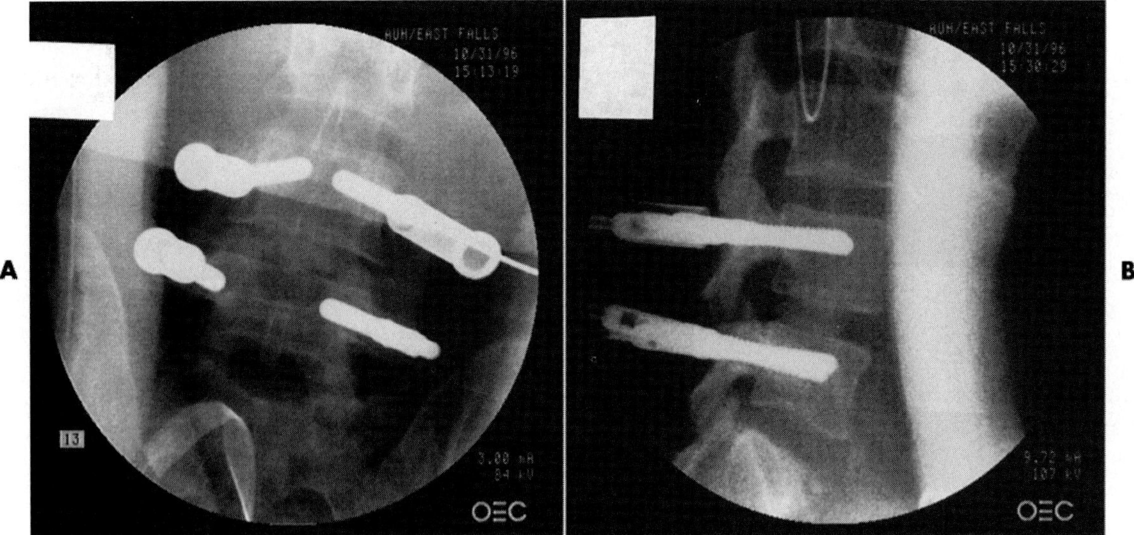

**FIGURE 43-7**

**A,** Interoperative AP fluoroscopic examination demonstrates three pedicular cannulas in place. Note properly placed pedicular bolts. **B,** Lateral view x-ray study shown in **A.**

guide pin. Withdrawal of the bone tap and guide pin permits examination of the medullary canal of the pedicle with a sonde to ensure the integrity of its cortex. At this time, a pedicular bolt appropriate in length and diameter is selected and inserted into the pedicles and vertebral bodies adjacent to the fusion site (Fig. 43-7). Most of the pedicles of the L5 and S1 segments are capable of accepting a 7-mm OD pedicular bolt. It should be noted that the pedicular bolt and the extension bars are currently under FDA feasability study and are not available for general use.

### INSERTION OF EXTENSION BARS AND SUBCUTANEOUS PLATES

Extension bars appropriate in length are selected and screwed clockwise into the proximal end of the previously inserted pedicular bolts. A specially designed wrench is used to stabilize the pedicular bolts while the extension bars are tightened. This step is then followed by positioning of the prebend plates over the thoracolumbar fascia and attachment to the extension bars via appropriate washers and nuts.

## ANTERIOR COLUMN ARTHRODESIS VIA POSTERIOR APPROACH

Most spine surgeons are familiar with this approach. Patient positioning is the same as that for a posterior fusion. Depending on the surgeon's preference, the table may need to be set to allow for interoperative fluoroscopy or portable x-ray studies. Standard midline dissection is carried down the lamina and the facets are exposed. Once the appropriate level is determined, laminectomy is performed to expose the thecal sac and nerve roots. At this time, the neural elements are decompressed, which may include partial facetectomy, foraminotomy, and diskectomy. In our experience, the use of a diamond-head burr greatly facilitates the extension of the previous laminectomy in failed fusion cases, and by carefully burring from virgin bone toward scarred tissue, we can safely delineate the margins of perineural scar tissue. The nerve root is then cautiously dissected from scar tissue and retracted medially to expose the disk space. Once satisfactory exposure is achieved, annulotomy is performed to remove disk material. Usually, an osteotome or gouge is used to cut a window in the posterior vertebral cortices. This accommodates the insertion of bone grafts or cages. The thecal sac and nerve root must be safely protected throughout the procedure.

Next the fusion site needs to be prepared. With a long-handled curette, the superior and inferior endplates are decorticated to subchondral surface. Bone graft is then fashioned to fit into the interbody space through the enlarged annulotomy. The graft should be seated at least 1 cm deep to the posterior cortices to lessen risk of extension into the spinal canal. Our practice has been to place a piece of tricortical allograft into the disk space and move it more toward the midline, so it is no longer directly in line with the annulotomy site. Further decortication of the vertebral plates and partial exposure of the host's cancellous bone in an area adjacent to the tricortical allograft are then accomplished with the aid of a high speed burr.[13] The autogenous cancellous bone graft is then placed around the allograft. Other surgeons have reported excellent results using autogenous tricortical graft and a bilateral approach toward the disk space.[16] We prefer allograft because we find it maintains disk space height while the adjacent autogenous cancellous bone is given a chance to bridge between the adjacent vertebral plates. Many investigators have reported on postoperative disk space collapse and graft subsidence with autografts[3] and allografts.[15]

Once the decision has been made to undertake revision fusion surgery, the effort should be pursued aggressively. Our experience has been to include posterolateral fusion augmented with instrumentation in addition to the interbody fusion. Although controversial, we recommend use of instrumentation because it has been shown to increase fusion rate. Wide decortication of the posterolateral structures, debridement of the facet joints, and application of abundant autogenous bone graft are steps to maximize fusion effort.

A starting hole for screw placement is made at the junction of the midlevel of transverse process and lateral facet joint. A Kirschner wire is then tapped through the pedicle and into the vertebral body. Position of the Kirschner wire must be examined in anteroposterior (AP) and lateral planes under C-arm fluoroscopy. After satisfactory placement has been achieved, the cannulated tap is used to prepare for screw fixation. The screw length can be determined from the depth of the initial Kirschner wire. The cannulated screw is then placed over the wire. Final check under fluoroscopy is performed before starting the next screw placement. After all the screws are inserted, either a plate or rod is fashioned to fit the screws and then locked into place. Before positioning the plate or rod, decortication and placement of bone graft is advised, since the hardware may partially block bony surface exposure. Again, the final construct is examined under fluoroscopy.

A last consideration in revision surgery includes the possibility of using electric stimulation, either internally or externally. Although also controversial, electric stimulation may help in the treatment of the particularly at-risk patient, such as a smoker or multiply failed patient. As a sign of current times, availability of these devices may be restricted by certain insurance and managed care policies. Two techniques are currently used to generate electric field at the fusion site. In direct current stimulation, the device is surgically implanted at the surgical site. The new bone formation occurs in negative cathode while resorption takes place in positive anode. In contrast, the pulsing electromagnetic field is used externally. However, the effect of field cell coupling in osteogenic response remains controversial.

The recent introduction of cage systems BAK (The SpineTec, Minneapolis, MN) and Ray Cage (Surgical Dynamics, Norwalk, CT) has received much enthusiasm and early results have been very promising. Most studies, however, offer at most 2-year follow-up so long-term results remain to be seen. It is not our intention to recommend specifically either bone grafting or cage systems for posterior interbody fusion because patient selection, severity of degenerative pathology, and training of the surgeon are all more important factors that affect the final outcome of anterior column stabilization; however, important distinctions are worth noting. Because cages are threaded into subchondral bone, they offer immediate stabilization postoperatively, even before fusion occurs. Moreover, in a recent animal study, cages were shown to have better capability to maintain disk space distraction over time as compared to autograft dowels.[19] Although techniques vary, interbody fusion provides support at the center of rotation in the spinal motion segment. This stabilization helps to achieve solid fusion and satisfactory outcome. Cage systems facilitate fusion bed preparation with prepackaged instruments to ream and tap the endplates for exact fit for their cages. The cages should be filled with autogenous cancellous bone graft although the sequence for filling the cages varies with each system. The SpineTec BAK system has interbody dilators that distract the disk space, and then allow the cages to be inserted with the disk space still in distraction. Because of the fixed sizes of the cages and the possible need for other instrumentation in the spinal canal, more extensive bony exposure and greater retraction of neural elements are generally required when a posterior approach is being used. This increases risk for neurologic injury and must be considered for the individual situation, particularly in cases of previous laminectomy in which adhesion may limit retraction of nerve root.

Use of cages is not, of course, without risk. Each cage system requires a prospective surgeon to attend a course and become certified before extending access to the system. Even after attending the course, the learning curve remains steep. Particularly challenging is attaining sufficient exposure to the disk space to place cannula or retractors for fusion bed preparation and insertion of cage. Failure to protect neural elements adequately may result in severe neurological injury. Moreover, because the cages come in only fixed sizes, presurgical planning is mandatory to determine whether cage application is feasible. Insertion of the correct-sized cage is critical because too small a cage may have inadequate purchase and risk of migration, and too large a cage may provide insufficient shoulder for subchondral support and lead to disk space

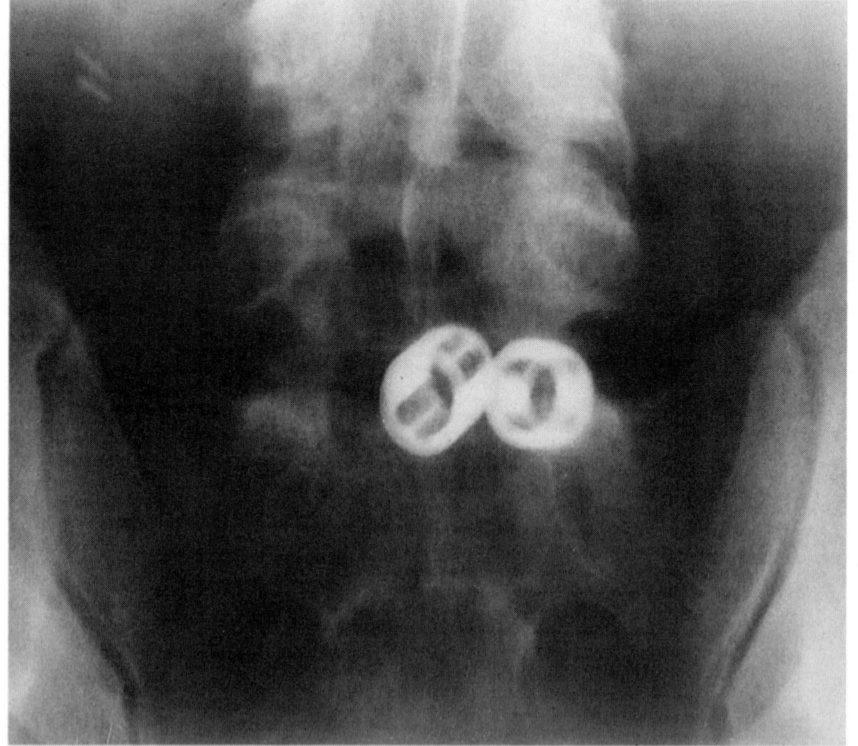


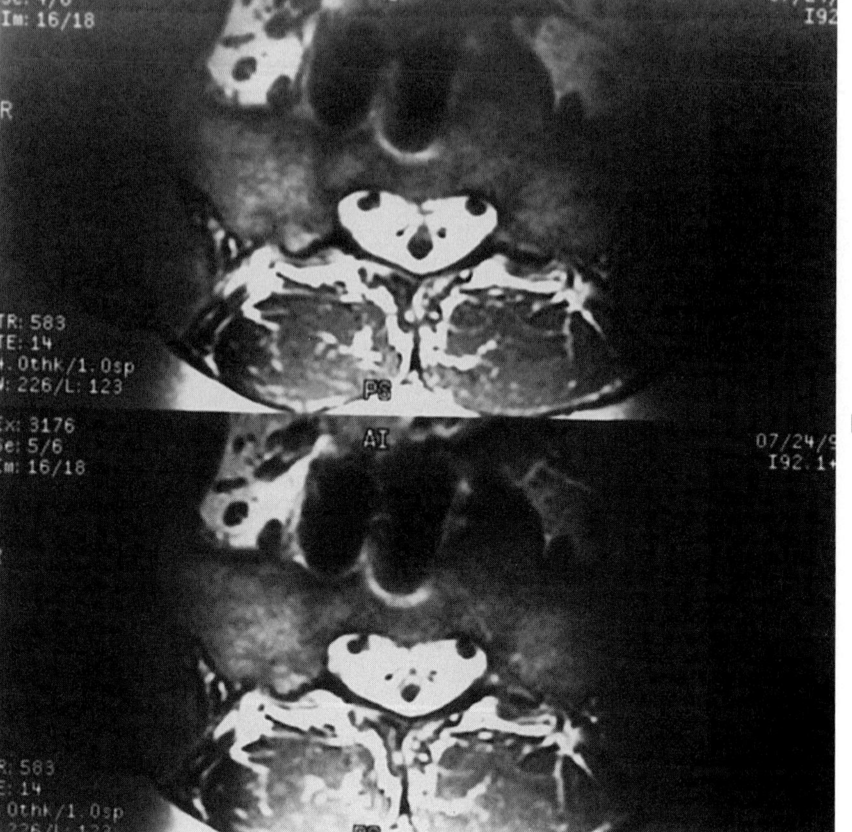


**FIGURE 43-8**

**A,** Misplaced and partially dislodged cages shown in postoperative AP radiograph. **B,** Axial view from the fusion site shown in **A.**

collapse. Since the exposure and retrieval of misplaced or displaced cages are extremely difficult, the proper positioning of the cage during the initial operative attempt is essential (Fig. 43-8).

## PARAMEDIAN ANTERIOR RETROPERITONEAL APPROACH

The key advantage of anterior approach is the avoidance of previous scar tissue and adhesion around the nerve root that may complicate revision surgery. Anterior approach to the lumbar spine has always represented a technical challenge to spine surgeons. Typically, anterolateral retroperitoneal (flank) and anterior transperitoneal approaches have been most widely used for access to this region. Each, however, has its own set of well-known limitations. In addition, new surgical techniques require greater accuracy of anatomic orientation and control of local structures than these two approaches can accommodate.

An alternative, less-known approach is the anterior paramedian retroperitoneal approach. This approach particularly facilitates surgeries for degenerative disk disease and spondylolisthesis that predominate in the lower lumbar spine, but exposure to as high as L2 can be achieved. The patient is positioned supine on the operating room table, preferably a radiolucent one to allow C-arm image both anteroposterior and lateral views. The incision starts as either oblique or longitudinal on the left paramedian abdomen. Dissection is carried down through the anterior rectus sheath. The rectus muscle is retracted medially, and an incision is made in the posterior rectus sheath through the transversalis fascia. The preperitoneal plane is developed with blunt dissection on the undersurface of transversalis fascia going down to the psoas muscle while the peritoneal contents are being retracted medially. At this point, the ureter should be identified. Additional blunt and sharp dissection medially would reveal the iliac vessels leading to the aortic bifurcation. Once a disk space has been identified, a marker can be placed for intraoperative x-ray to determine levels. From here, dissection can be carried out cephalad or caudal as needed. Mobilization of the aortic bifurcation can be achieved by ligating the iliolumbar vessels and dissecting the investing fascia. Now with full exposure of the appropriate disk space, diskectomy, and fusion can commence.

As in posterior approach, anterior interbody fusion can be achieved with bone graft or cages. Either autograft or allograft can be used, but most surgeons prefer allograft, usually fibula or femoral ring, because of the rigid structural support. For bone graft fusion, total diskectomy is required to expose as much bony surface to the graft. Cartilaginous endplates are curetted down to bleeding subchondral bone. Next, the allograft is cut to fit within the disk space. Multiple fibula sections or one femoral ring can be packed into the prepared space.

Cage systems, on the other hand, recommend subtotal diskectomy because integrity of the ligamentous and annular attachments contributes additional stability to the cages. Each system provides instruments to carry out annulotomy, fusion bed preparation, and implantation. Autogenous bone graft should be packed into the cage prior to insertion.

## REFERENCES


1. Brodsky AE: Post-laminectomy and post-fusion stenosis of the lumbar spine, *Clin Orthop* 115:130, 1976.
2. Crock H: *Practice of spinal surgery*. New York, 1983, Springer-Verlag.
3. Dennis S, Watkins R, Landaker S, et al: Comparison of disc space heights after anterior lumbar interbody fusion, *Spine* 14(8):876-8, 1989.
4. Esses SI, Botsford DJ, Kostuik JD: The role of external spine skeletal fixation in assessment of low back disorders, *Spine* 14:594-561, 1989.
5. Frymoyer JW: Failed lumbar disc surgery requiring a second operation, *Spine* 3:7-11, 1978.
6. Ha KY, Schendel MJ, Lewis JL, Ogilvie JW: Effect of immobilization and configuration on lumbar adjacent-segment biomechanics, *J Spinal Disord,* 6:99-105, 1993.
7. Fraser RD, Osti OL, Vernon-Roberts B: Discitis after discography, *J Bone Joint Surg Br* 69:26-35, 1987.
8. Harris RT, Wiley JJ: Acquired spondylolysis as a sequel to spinal fusion, *J Bone Joint Surgery Am* 45:1159-1170, 1963.
9. Kahanovitz N, Arnoczky SP, Levine DB, Otis JP: The effects of internal fixation on the articular cartilege of unfused canine facet joint cartilege, *Spine* 9:268-272, 1984.
10. Kambin P: Arthroscopic microdiscectomy, arthroscopy, *J Arthroscopic Surg* 8(3):287-295, 1992.
11. Kambin P: Arthroscopic lumbar interbody fusion. In White A, Schofferman J, editors: *Spine care,* vol two, Philadelphia, 1995, Mosby, pp 1056-1065.
12. Kambin P: *The role of minimally invasive surgery in spinal disorders.* In Stauffer RN, editor: *Advances in operative orthopaedics.* Vol 3, Philadelphia, 1995, Mosby.
13. Kambin P: *Arthroscopic lumbar intervertebral fusion.* In

Frymoyer J, Ducker T, Hadler N, Kostuik J, Weinstein J, Whitecould III T, editors: *The adult spine principles and practice,* ed 2, New York, 1996, Lippincott-Raven, pp 2037-2045.

14. Kambin P, McCullen G, Parke P, Regan JJ, Schaffer JL, Yuan H: Minimally invasive arthroscopic spinal surgery. *Instructional Course Lectures American Academy of Orthopaedic Surgeons,* 46:143-161, 1995.
15. Kumar A, Kozak JA, Doherty BJ, Dickson JH: Interspace distraction and graft subsidence after anterior lumbar fusion with femoral strut allograft. *Spine* 18(16):2393-2400, 1993.
16. Lee CK, Vessa P, Lee JK: Chronic disabling low back pain syndrome caused by internal disc derangements. The results of disc excision and posterior lumbar interbody fusion, *Spine* 20(3):356-61, 1995.
17. Lehmann TR, Spratt KF, Tozzi JE, Weinstein JN, Reinnarz SJ, Khoury GY, Colgy H: Long-term follow-up of lower lumbar fusion patients, *Spine* 12:97-104, 1987.
18. Sachs B, Vanharanta H, Spivey M, et al.: Dallas discogram description: a new classification of CT/discography in low back disorders, *Spine* 12:287-29, 1987.
19. Sandhu HSA, Turner S, Kabo JM, Kanim LE, et al: Distractive properties of a threaded interbody fusion device. An in vivo model, *Spine* 21(10):1201-1210, 1996.
20. Schaffer JL, Kambin P: *Arthroscopic fusion of the lumbosacral spine.* In Margulies JY, Floman Y, Farch JPC, Neuwirth MG, editors: *Lumbosacral and Spine Pelvic Fixation,* Hagerstown, MD, May 1996, Lippincott-Raven.
21. Wiley J, McNab I, Wortzman G: Lumbar discography and its clinical applications, *Can J Surg* 11:280-289, 1968.
22. Deyo RA, Cherkin DC, Loeser JD et al: Morbidity and mortality in association with operations on the lumbar spine: The influence of age, diagnosis, and procedure, *J Bone Joint Surg* 74A:536-543, 1992.

# 44

# RECONSTRUCTION OF THE ANTERIOR COLUMN OF THE SPINE

**Patrick J. Connolly, M.D.**
**Hansen A. Yuan, M.D.**



Although 80% of the population will have at least one significant episode of back pain during their lifetime, the vast majority never require surgical intervention. Of those patients requiring surgical treatment of the lumbar spine, the majority will be treated satisfactorily with a decompressive procedure from a posterior approach. In light of these facts, the reader should recognize that the indication for any surgical reconstruction of the anterior column of the spine is limited to a small subset of patients that require spinal surgery.

The three columns of the spine are the anterior, middle, and posterior columns.[14] Biomechanically, the anterior and posterior columns are the principal support structures with the posterior column representing the tension side and the anterior column and disk representing the compression/axial loading side. Before deciding on the specific technique of spinal surgery, the surgeon must ask and answer the following questions:

1) What is the patient's problem?
2) What is the likelihood of a successful surgical solution?
3) Does the problem require neurologic decompression alone? Structural support alone? Or a combination of both neurological decompression and structural support?
4) Are there any patient-specific requirements that need to be considered in the surgical plan (smoker, osteoporosis, elderly, morbid obesity, religious beliefs, prior surgery, history of radiation, anatomic level, etc.).

Once the physician has addressed these questions, he is able to discuss with the patient the specific goals of the surgical procedure and define in his own mind the surgical technique that will enable him to achieve these goals.

Historically, anterior column spinal reconstruction relied on bone fusion alone. Harmon[30] advocated the anterior approach to the intervertebral disk space with reconstruction, whereas Wiltberger[58] recommended a posterior interbody fusion technique. Dwyer[17] developed the first commonly accepted device for anterior fixation. This device was flexible cable and was utilized for spinal deformity only. Zielke[60] later modified the Dwyer technique to include a rod rather than a flexible cable. Humphries[36] reported on the use of an anterior plate for one- or two-level anterior spinal fusion. Werlinich[56] reported on the use of an anterior staple. Kostuik[40] is credited with developing an anterior fixation device that utilized the concept of the Harrington distraction rods and modified Dwyer screws. Although this device was successfully utilized for deformity correction, fracture stabilization, and tumor stabilization, he cautioned that the device did not provide good rotational control and therefore required supplementary external orthosis.[39,40] Harm has introduced titanium cages that are packed with bone graft and serve as a disk space or vertebral body replacement. Bagby[1] and Kuslich[61] have introduced threaded fusion cages that allow stabilization of the anterior column of the spine with subsequent fusion through bony in-growth of the cage. Lastly, investigation continues in the area of lumbar disk replacement, although these devices may represent the future of anterior column reconstruction, they remain in their preliminary stages and are beyond the scope of this chapter.

## MATERIALS AND DEVICES FOR ANTERIOR COLUMN RECONSTRUCTION

In anterior column reconstruction of the spine, the surgeon is often required to not only perform a fusion after disk excision, but often is required to perform a vertebral body replacement. The choice of materials for disk space or vertebral body replacement includes autologus or allograft bone, polymethamethacrylate (PMMA), Harm's titanium fusion cage, or carbon fiber cage packed with bone graft (Tables 44-1 and 44-2).[6,7,11,18,19,23,28,29,31,32,33,41,45–47,57]

When choosing a bone graft material for anterior column reconstruction the surgeon must take into consideration three factors, the biological requirements for fusion, the biomechanical requirements for reconstruction, and lastly bone graft donor site morbidity.[3,8,9,20,22,24,27,35,52,55,59]

**Table 44-1. Materials Available for Anterior Column Reconstruction**

| Materials | Advantages | Disadvantages |
|---|---|---|
| autograft cancellous bone | gold standard<br>osteogenic, osteoconductive, osteoinductive | limited supply<br>not as strong structural graft as cortical bone<br>donor site morbidity |
| autograft cortical bone | strong structural graft<br>osteogenic, osteoconductive, osteoinductive | limited supply<br>donor site morbidity |
| allograft bone | no donor site morbidity<br>osteoconductive, osteoinductive ?osteogenic | potential disease transmission, potential immune response<br>less osteoinductive, osteogenic than autograft |

**Table 44-2. Devices Available for Anterior Column Reconstruction**

| Devices | Advantages | Disadvantages |
|---|---|---|
| PMMA | easy and inexpensive to use as a vertebral body replacement for tumor | limited long-term stability, needs to be supplemented by additional fusion if life expectancy > one year |
| upright cage | relatively easy to use as a spacer following corpectomy or diskectomy | requires additional spinal fixation (pedicle screws, anterior plate) does not function very well as a stand-alone device; may subside or dislodge, requires autograft |
| ceramic spacer | osteoconductive; no donor site morbidity; no disease transmission; may be used with osteoinductive agent | not osteoinductive; not osteogenic, some materials have low fracture resistance; clinical efficacy has not been established |
| threaded cages | excellent fusion rate for single level; allows for restoration of normal disk height; indirect increase of neuroforamen; provides immediate stable fixation and is a stand-alone device | requires autograft designed for use in degenerated narrow disk space and is difficult to place two large-diameter cages in patients with "tall" disk space |
| vertebral body screws and single rod | allows for spinal deformity correction; provides immediate stabilization over multiple segments; relatively easy to use | does not provide the same rotational stability as vertebral body screw plate systems or double rods; screw purchase is a problem in osteoporotic bone |
| verebral body screws and anterior lateral plate | provides excellent stabilization in healthy patient<br>stand-alone device with allograft or autograft | can only stabilize short segments<br>pull-out and subsidence is a problem in osteoporotic patient |

Although autologous cancellous bone is considered the most successful bone graft material for fusion, it is not as strong as cortical bone. For this reason, cancellous bone or cortical cancellous bone (tricortical iliac crest) is not an ideal choice when bone graft alone is being utilized for anterior column reconstruction.[15,23,26,28,51,53] Although the strength advantage of cortical bone is obvious, the availability of autologous cortical bone is limited to the fibula. The routine employment of autologous fibula as a bone graft material is generally avoided because it holds a significant complication rate that is donor-site related.

Allograft bone in the way of fibula allograft or femoral ring allograft has ideal strength properties to withstand the load of anterior column reconstruction.[11,21] Femoral ring allografts eliminate the need for side by side stacking of the disk space with multiple grafts, and allow placement of autologous cancellous bone in the center of the femoral ring.[35,42,43,50] The disadvantages of allografts are that in multilevel fusions without instrumentation they have a higher pseudarthrosis rate.[41] In addition, allografts are similar to donor blood products in that they are considered unacceptable treatment materials by certain groups in American society, and they hold the potential for disease transmission and adverse immune response.[7]

Scovell[46] is credited with first suggesting the use of PMMA as a vertebral body replacement in metastatic disease. This technique is effective in the treatment of metastatic disease in the area of the cervical and thoracic spine.[29,45] This technique alone in the lumbar spine is often is inadequate because it does not provide adequate control of rotation and lateral bending.[31,32,33,47]

Both the titanium fusion cage and carbon fiber cage function initially as a vertebral body spacer, but have the potential for incorporating into a solid fusion.[6] Again, these devices alone are not ideal in the lumbar spine because of inadequate rotational control.[9,59]

The goals of any spinal implant are: (1) the device should allow correction of deformity if present and prevent further deformity during the postoperative period, (2) the fusion rate should be equal to or better than the expected fusion rate without the device in place, and (3) early mobilization of the patient should be possible with the use of less external mobilization.

Although no single implant can be utilized for every problem that requires anterior column reconstruction, there are several characteristics that each implant should have: (1) the implant should be compatible with the body, (2) the device should be at least semirigid and preferably rigid so that it can be used either with or without intact ligamentous and bony structures, (3) application of the device should allow for the ultimate goal of a solid fusion (this is not necessarily required in metastatic disease when the device can be expected to remain stable during the patient's anticipated life span), and (4) implantation of the device must be safe for the patient and user friendly for the surgeon.

Anterior spinal fixation devices are employed to: (1) help achieve initial deformity correction, (2) lock in the bone graft and/or vertebral body replacement cage, and (3) provide immediate stabilization thus allowing pain relief and early mobilization. Anterior spinal fixation devices, alone, without bone graft, are seldom utilized for anterior column reconstruction.

Anterior vertebral body screws and rods have been helpful for the correction of thoracolumbar scoliosis. They are placed on the convexity of the curve and enable the surgeon to correct spinal deformity and obtain segmental fixation over multiple spinal levels.

Anterior vertebral body screw plate fixation systems provide excellent rotational control for short-segment reconstruction.[59] They are not applicable in the treatment of most multilevel spinal deformities.

Threaded fusion cages allow distraction of degenerated disk spaces with the stabilization properties equal to segmental pedicle screw fixation.[9,12,52] They are used with autologous bone and do not require additional fixation. In patients with central disk herniations who have maintained their disk height, the requirement for a large diameter cage limits their use.

Upright cages are composed of titanium mesh or carbon fiber and, after they are packed with cancellous autograft bone, function as a disk or vertebral body replacement.[6] For the most part, they are not a stand-alone fixation device, and require either an additional anterior plate fixation or posterior pedicle fixation.

## INDICATIONS FOR ANTERIOR COLUMN RECONSTRUCTION

The following is an overview of the surgical treatment of specific problems that require anterior column reconstruction.

### DISK DEGENERATION

Patients with mechanical low back pain that has not improved with nonoperative care may benefit from surgical intervention.[28,30,38,49,53] Patients with only single-level disk degeneration that have positive results on provocative diskography are most likely to benefit from surgical intervention. Although the debate remains about the necessity of anterior diskectomy and fusion, recent reports imply that patients having anterior column fusion have the greatest tendency towards success.[50]

The surgeon has the option of performing an anterior diskectomy and fusion alone, anterior diskectomy and fusion supplemented by posterior fusion and segmental pedicle screw fixation, posterior diskectomy and subsequent posterior interbody lumbar fusion with pedicle screw fixation, and diskectomy/threaded cage anterior column reconstruction via either an anterior or posterior approach.[19,23,24,28,38]

A number of surgeons report success with the posterior lumbar interbody fusion technique. This technique holds the known complication of significant epidural bleeding and subsequent increased rate of epidural scarring.[6,19,26] The anterior approach to the lumbar spine decreases the potential for epidural scarring, however, it holds its own risks of injury to the great vessels, peritoneum, and retrograde ejaculation.[54,55] The decision to use either technique is dependent upon the experience of the surgeon. With either technique, the surgeon may be able to reconstruct the anterior column with either autograph bone, allograft bone, or threaded fusion cage.

### SPONDYLOLISTHESIS

Spondylolisthesis is the nonanatomic alignment of one vertebral body on another. Although, by definition, patients with lumbar spondylolisthesis have an abnormality of the anterior column, many patients that require surgical intervention do not require anterior column reconstruction and can be treated successfully with a posterior bilateral/lateral fusion, alone or in combination with posterior decompression and/or segmental fixation.[10,34] For patients with high-grade spondylolisthesis or those with a slip angle greater than 45 degrees, the results of bilateral/lateral fusion alone are less than optimal, and for this reason, many surgeons now recommend an additional anterior procedure to provide anterior column support.[4,48]

The specific anterior column procedure is dependent upon the requirements of the patient and the skill of the surgeon.[4,10,16,21,27] In cases of grade I and II spondylolisthesis, the positioning of the patient under general anesthesia will often provide an anatomic reduction. In these cases, utilization of femoral ring allograft packed with autologous bone anteriorly followed by posterior pedicle fixation and fusion will allow for a good result. Alternatively, the surgeon may choose to reconstruct the anterior column in a similar fashion via a posterior lumbar interbody fusion (PLIF) procedure utilizing fibular allograft or fusion cages for anterior column support followed by posterior bilateral fusion with instrumentation.[6,19]

In severe deformity or in cases of significant spondylolisthesis associated with pseudarthrosis, the surgeon is not able to obtain a reduction. The surgeon may choose not to obtain reduction of the slippage, but rather support the anterior column by placing a fibular allograft through the reamed vertebral bodies at the level of the slip.[2,21,37] Alternatively, as in the case of the spondyloptosis of L5 on S1, the surgeon may perform a total resection of the L5 vertebral body with realignment of the L4 vertebral body directly on the sacrum[25] This is followed by posterior instrumentation with pedicle fixation and fusion.

### SCOLIOSIS

Scoliosis can be defined as a spinal deformity with a Cobb angle greater then 10 degrees in the coronal plane. There are numerous classifications of scoliosis, the most common of which is idiopathic. It is a three-dimensional rotator deformity that involves the anterior column of the spine. Surgical intervention is employed in the treatment of scoliosis in order to correct the progressive deformity or to relieve pain.[5,39] The goals of the operation tend to dictate the surgery required.

In the adolescent or young adult in which correction of the thoracic curve is the goal of surgery, the anterior column is reconstructed in an indirect manner utilizing posterior segmental fixation. Patients with thoracolumbar or lumbar progressive curves in this age group may undergo a procedure with vertebral body screws and rods for a direct anterior column reconstruction and curve correction.

In the adult population,[39,43] in which pain relief is most often the significant goal of surgery, reconstructive procedures must be customized to the unique features of the patient's spinal deformity. Specifically, patients with thoracolumbar or lumbar curves and discogenic pain often require anterior release and anterior column reconstruction with a combination of structural femoral ring allograft and cancellous bone followed by posterior instrumentation and fusion. This is in contradistinction to elderly patients with de novo lumbar scoliosis and a principal complaint of pain consistent with neurogenic claudication, who may benefit from posterior decompression and posterior fusion alone.[8,39]

Therefore, in deciding the specific operation a patient requires, the surgeon must assess not only the severity and location of the curve, but also the nature of the patient's pain and the degenerative aspects of the patient's spine (disk space collapse, lateral listhesis, instability, and evidence of osteoporosis). This approach will allow the surgeon to develop a surgical plan that best addresses the specific requirements for a successful surgical outcome (Table 44-3).

## COMPLICATIONS[22,44,54,55]

The complications associated with anterior column reconstruction can be divided into four categories (Table 44-4). The first category of complications are those associated with any surgical procedure requiring general anesthesia. They are most often related to the

**Table 44-3. Indications for Anterior Column Reconstruction**

| Surgical Problem | Author's Choice |
|---|---|
| normal disk height/diskogenic pain | anterior lumbar interbody fusion (ALIF) with either multifibula allografts of femoral ring allograft packed with autogenous cancellous bone; supplemented by posterior fusion and fixation (pedicle screws or facet screws) |
| loss of disk height/discogenic pain | anterior threaded fusion cage packed with autograft |
| fracture with neurological deficit | anterior corpectomy, fibula allograft and additional autograft (rib), anterior screw plate fixation |
| fracture without neurological deficit | indirect reduction, pedicle screw fixation, autograft cancellous bone |
| removal infection | anterior corpectomy, autograft tricortical iliac crest bone graft, TLSO |
| lumbar pseudarthrosis | anterior lumbar interbody fusion (ALIF) with either multifibula allografts or femoral ring allograft packed with autogenous cancellous bone; supplemented by posterior fusion and fixation (pedicle screws or facet screws)<br>OR<br>anterior threaded fusion cage packed with autograft |
| kyphotic deformity | eggshell procedure[13] |
| adult scoliosis/discogenic pain | anterior diskectomy and fusion, autograft bone ± allograft; posterior fusion with segmental fixation |
| adult spondylolisthesis, primary surgery | posterior fusion with segmental pedicle fixation |
| adult spondylolisthesis, revision | anterior in situ stabilization with 'peg' fibula allograft,[21,48] posterior fusion with segmental pedicle fixation |

TLSO, thoracolumbosacral orthosis.

**Table 44-4. Complications**

| | |
|---|---|
| general surgical | UTI, DVT, wound infection, respiratory, cardipulmonary |
| PLIF | epidural scarring, dural tear, root/cauda equina injury |
| ALIF | iliac vein tear, iliac artery thrombosis, bowel injury, genitofemoral nerve injury, retrograde ejaculation (superior hypogastric sympathetic plexus) |
| fusion | pseudarthrosis, graft extrusion, accelerated degeneration of adjacent level, donor site morbidity |
| device-related | breakage or loosening of fixation with subsequent recurrent/progressive deformity, nerve root, spinal cord, or cauda equina injury secondary to poor placement of spinal fixation |

UTI, urinary tract infection; DVT, deep venous thrombosis; PLIF, posterior lumbar interbody fusion; ALIF, anterior lumbar interbody fusion.

age of the patient, the patient's nutritional status, duration of anesthesia, and intraoperative blood loss. Pneumonia, urinary tract infection, deep venous thrombosis, pulmonary embolism, and wound infection are examples of the first category of complications.

Complications in the second category are related to the surgical approach. These complications include epidural scarring, nerve root injury, dural tear, great vessel injury, bowel injury, and retroperitoneal injures (ureter, superior hypogastric plexus. retrograde ejaculation, and genital femoral nerve).

Complications in the third category are related to fusion, specifically pseudarthrosis, graft extrusion, accelerated degeneration of adjacent disk, and donor site morbidity. The last category of complications includes fixation device-related complications, which include breakage, subsidence, vertebral body fracture, and nerve root or spinal cord injury.

## SUMMARY

Overall, there currently exist numerous techniques the surgeon may employ for anterior column reconstruction, and the choice of techniques is ultimately dependent upon the patient's spinal problem, specific requirements of the patient, the availability of the materials and surgical devices, and the skill of the surgeon. In this chapter we have attempted to provide a rational guide for the spine surgeon in selecting one technique over another in regard to anterior column reconstruction of the lumbar spine. There is no doubt that spinal reconstruction devices and surgical techniques will continue to improve with the ultimate goal of minimal invasion and maximal predictive improvement in pain. Notwithstanding future technological advancements in spine surgery, the spine surgeon needs to remember the basic premise of successful spine surgery: choose the right operation for the right patient by the right surgeon.

## REFERENCES


1. Bagby GW: Arthrodesis by the distraction-compression method using a stainless steel implant, *Orthopaedics* 11:931-4,1988.
2. Bohlman HH, Cook S: One-stage decompression and posterolateral and interbody fusion for lumbosacral spondyloptosis through a posterior approach, *J Bone Joint Surg* 64A: 415-418, March 1982.
3. Bradford DS, Ganjavian S, Antonious D, Winter RB, Lonstein JE, Moe JH: Anterior strut-grafting for the treatment of kyphosis, *J Bone Joint Surg* 64-A: 680-690, June 1982.
4. Bradford DS, Gotfried Y: Staged salvage reconstruction of grade IV and V spondylolisthesis, *J Bone Joint Surg* 69A:191-202, 1987.
5. Bradford, DS, Boachie-Adjei, O: One-stage anterior and posterior hemivertebral resection and arthrodesis for congenital scoliosis, *J Bone Joint Surg,* 72A:536-540, 1990.
6. Brantigan JW, Steffee AD, Geiger JM: A carbon fiber implant to aid interbody lumbar fusion, *Spine* 16(S):277-282, 1991.
7. Bridwell KH, Lenke LG, McEnery KW, Baldus C, Blanke K: Anterior fresh frozen structural allografts in the thoracic and lumbar spine. Do they work if combined with posterior fusion and instrumentation in adult patients with kyphosis or anterior column defects? *Spine* 20 (12):1410-1418, 1995.
8. Bridwell KH. Load sharing principles: the role and use of anterior structural support in adult deformity. *AAOS Instructional Course Lectures* 45:109-116, 1996.
9. Brodkle DS, Dick JC, Kunz DN, McCabe R, Zdeblick TA: Posterior lumbar interbody fusion: a biomechanical comparison, including a new threaded cage, *Spine* 22:26-31, 1997.
10. Burkus JK, Lonstein JE, Winter RB, Denis F: Long-term evaluation of adolescents treated operatively for spondylolisthesis, *J Bone Joint Surg* 74A(5):693-704, 1992.
11. Buttermann GR, Glazer PA, Bradford DS: The use of bone allografts in the spine, *Clin Orthop* 324:75-85, 1996.
12. Chen D, Fay LA, Lok J, Yuan P, Edwards WT, Yuan HA: Increasing neuroforaminal volume by anterior interbody distraction in degenerative lumbar spine, *Spine* 20:74-79, 1995.
13. Chewning SJ, Heinig CF, Chapman TM: *The eggshell procedure: Segmental spinal instrumentation,* Thoroughfare, NJ, 1984, SLACK.
14. Denis F: The three column spine and its significance in the classification of acute thoracolumbar spinal injuries, *Spine* 8:817-831,1983.
15. Dennis S, Watkins R, Landaker S, Dillin W, Springer D: Comparison of disc space heights after anterior lumbar interbody fusion, *Spine* 14(8):876-878, 1989.
16. DeWald RL, Faut MM, Taddonio RF, Neuwirth MG: Severe lumbosacral spondylolisthesis in adolescents and children, *J Bone Joint Surg* 63A(4):619-626, 1981.
17. Dwyer AF, Newton NC, Sherwood AA: An anterior approach to scoliosis, *Clin Orthop* 62:192-202, 1969.
18. Emery SE, Fuller DA, Stevenson S: Ceramic anterior spinal fusion. Biologic and biomechanical comparison in a canine model, *Spine* 21:2713-2719, 1996.
19. Enker P, Steffee AD: Interbody fusion and instrumentation, *Clin Orthop* 300:90-101, 1994.
20. Esses SI, Doherty BJ, Crawford MJ, Dreyzin V: Kinematic evaluation of lumbar fusion techniques, *Spine* 21:676-684, 1996.
21. Esses SI, Natout N, Kip P: Posterior interbody arthrodesis with a fibular strut graft in spondylolisthesis, *J Bone Joint Surg* 77A(2):172-176, 1995.
22. Faciszewski T, Winter RB, Lonstein JE, Denis F, Johnson L: The surgical and medical perioperative complications of anterior spinal fusion surgery in the thoracic and lumbar spine in adults. A review of 1223 procedures, *Spine* 20:1592-1599, 1995.
23. Flynn JC, Houque MA: Anterior fusion of the lumbar spine, *J Bone Joint Surg* 61A (8):1143-1150, 1979.
24. Fraser RD: Interbody, posterior, and combined lumbar fusions, *Spine* 20:167S-177S, 1995.
25. Gaines RW: Treatment of spondyloptosis by staged resection and fusion (Gaines procedure). Presented at North American Spine Society Meeting, Boston, July 9-11, 1993.
26. Gill K, O'Brien JP: Observations of resorption of the posterior lateral bone graft in combined anterior and posterior lumbar fusion, *Spine* 18 (13):1885-1889, 1993.
27. Glazer PA, Colliou O, Klisch SM, Bradfore DS, Bueff HU, Lotz JC: Biomechanical analysis of multi-level fixation methods in the lumbar spine, *Spine* 22:171-182, 1997.

28. Greenough CG, Taylor LJ, Fraser RD: Anterior lumbar fusion: results, assessment techniques, and prognostic factors, *Eur Spine J* 3:225-230, 1994.
29. Hamilton A, Webb JK: The role of anterior surgery for vertebral fractures with and without cord compression, *Clin Orthop Internal Fixators:* 79-89, March 1994.
30. Harmon PH: Anterior excision and vertebral fusion operation for intervertebral disk syndromes of the lower lumbar spine, *Clin Orthop* 26:107-127, 1963.
31. Harrington KD: The use of methylmethacrylate for vertebral-body replacement and anterior stabilization of pathological fracture-dislocations of the spine due to metastatic malignant disease, *J Bone Joint Surg* 63A:36-46, 1981.
32. Harrington KD: Current concepts review: metastatic disease of the spine, *J Bone Joint Surg* 68A:1110-1115, 1986.
33. Harrington KD: Metastatic tumors of the spine: diagnosis and treatment, *J Am Acad Orthop Surg,* 1:02, 76-86. 1993.
34. Harris IE, Weinstein SL: Long-term follow-up of patients with grade III and IV spondylolisthesis, *J Bone Joint Surg* 69A(7):960-969, 1987.
35. Holte DC, O'Brien JP, Renton P: Anterior lumbar fusion using a hybrid interbody graft. A preliminary radiograhic report, *Eur Spine J* 3:32-38, 1994.
36. Humphries AW, Hawk WA, Berndt AL: Anterior interbody fusion of lumbar vertebrae, *Surg Clin N Am* 41:1685-1700, 1971.
37. Jones AM, McAfee PC, Robinson RA, Zinreich SJ, Wang H: Failed arthrodesis of the spine for severe spondylolisthesis, *J Bone Joint Surg* 70A(1):25-30, 1988.
38. Kim NH, Kim DJ: Anterior interbody fusion for spondylolisthesis, *Orthopedics* 14(10):1069-1076, 1991.
39. Kostuik JP: Current concepts in review: operative treatment of idiopathic scoliosis, *J Bone Joint Surg* 72A:1108-1113, 1990.
40. Kostuik JP: Anterior fixation for fractures with and without neurologic involvement, *Clin Orthop* 189:103-115, 1984.
41. Kozak JA, Heilman AE, O'Brien JP: Anterior lumbar fusion options: technique and graft materials, *Clin Orthop* 300:45-51, 1994.
42. Kozak JA, O'Brien JP: Simultaneous combined anterior and posterior fusion. An independent analysis of a treatment for the disabled low-back pain patient, *Spine* 15(4): 322-328, 1990.
43. Kumar A, Kozak JA, Doherty BJ, Dickson JH: Interspace distraction and graft subsidence after anterior lumbar fusion with femoral strut allograft, *Spine* 18(16):2393-2400, 1993.
44. Luk KD, Chow D, Evans JH, Leong J: Lumbar spinal mobility after short anterior interbody fusion, *Spine* 20 (7):813-818, 1995.
45. Malcolm BW, Bradford DS, Winter RB, Chou SN: Post-traumatic kyphosis. A review of forty-eight surgically treated patients, *J Bone Joint Surg* 63A(6):891-899, 1981.
46. Scoville WB, Palmer AH, Samara K, Chong G: The use of acrylic plastic for vertebral body replacement or fixation in metastatic disease of the spine: A technical note, *J Neurosurg* 27:274-279, 1967.
47. Siegal T, Tiqva P, Siegal T: Vertebral body resection for epidural compression by malignant tumors: results of forty-seven consecutive operative procedures, *J Bone Joint Surg* 67A:375-382, 1985.
48. Smith MD, Bohlman HH: Spondylolisthesis treated by a single-stage operation combining decompression with in situ posterolateral and anterior fusion. An analysis of eleven patients who had long-term follow-up, *J Bone Joint Surg,* 72A(3):415-420, 1990.
49. Sorenson KH: Anterior interbody lumbar spine fusion for incapacitating disc degeneration and spondylolisthesis, *Acta Orthop Scand* 49:269-277, 1978.
50. Stewart G, Sachs BL: Patient out-come after re-operation on the lumbar spine, *J Bone Joint Surg* 78A:706-711, 1996.
51. Takahashi K, Kitahara H, Yamagata M, Murakami M, Takata K, Miyamoto K, Mimura M, Akahashi Y, Moriya H: Long-term results of anterior interbody fusion from treatment of degenerative spondylolisthesis, *Spine* 15(11):1211-1215, 1990.
52. Tencer AF, Hampton D, Eddy S: Biomechanical properties of threaded inserts for lumbar interbody spinal, *Spine* 20:2408-2414, 1995.
53. Tiusanen H, Seitsalo S, Osterman K, Soini J: Anterior interbody lumbar fusion in severe low back pain, *Clin Orthop* 324:153-163, March 1996.
54. Tiusanen H, Seitsalo S, Osterman K, Soini J: Retrograde ejaculation after anterior interbody lumbar fusion, *Eur Spine J* 4:339-342, 1995.
55. Watkins R: Anterior lumbar interbody fusion surgical complications, *Clin Orthop* 284, November 1992.
56. Werlinich M: Anterior interbody fusion and stabilization with metal fixation, *Int Surg* 59:269-273, 1974.
57. Whitecloud TS, Butler JC: Anterior lumbar fusion utilizing transvertebral fibular graft, *Spine* 13(3):370-373, 1988.
58. Wiltberger BR: Intervertebral body fusion by the use of a posterior bone dowel, *J Bone Joint Surg* 39A:84, 1957.
59. Zdeblick TA, Shirado O, McAfee PC, deGroot H, Warden KE, Eng MM: Anterior spinal fixation after lumbar corpectomy, *J Bone Joint Surg* 73A(4):527-534, 1991.
60. Zielke K, Stunkat R: Derotation and fusion: anterior spinal instrumentation, *Orthop Trans* 2:270,1978.
61. Kuslich SD: Spinal instrumentation. In Regan JJ, McAfee PC, Mack MJ, editors: *Atlas of endoscopic spine surgery,* St. Louis, 1995, Quality Medical Publishing, pp 293-305.

# 45

# TREATMENT OF COMPLICATIONS OF BAK CAGES

**James F. Zucherman, M.D.**
**Stephen R. Shaw, M.D.**
**Ken Y. Hsu, M.D.**



In 1996, the BAK cage was approved by the Food and Drug Administration for general open use. Multicenter studies have shown it to be an effective fusion technique with an acceptable complication profile relative to other available fusion methods.[7] Complications do occur, however. This chapter is directed at techniques for dealing with those complications that are unique to the BAK and to some extent other interbody implants.[1,5,8]

## COMPLICATIONS OF THE POSTERIOR APPROACH

### Anterior Implant Migration and Malposition

The threaded design of the BAK implant results in a diminished chance of migration compared with the traditional types of bone graft used in posterior interbody fusions. When migration does occur, caused by reaming too far to the anterior, misplacement of the implant, improper implant sizing, or an incompetent annulus, the treatment depends on the amount of projection of the implant. Complete extrusion or large displacement (more than 60% of implant length) necessitates cage removal to prevent erosion into retroperitoneal visceral structures. Anatomically, there seem to be greater risks above the L5 level. If the implant is anterior to the posterior intervertebral space removal is more readily accomplished from an anterior approach. If the malpositioned implant is still well within the interspace it can be removed or repositioned posteriorly. This is performed by removal of the cap (if present), posterior chamber bone, and cage, using a flat-head screwdriver. The screwdriver is inserted into the BAK slot, unscrewing to the appropriate position or to removal. The reason for the cage shifting should be corrected either by replacement with a larger implant or by substitution of bone graft for the migrated cage. In our experience, reliance upon only a single central or unilateral cage for lumbar fusions has not been successful.

### Posterior Malposition

Posterior migration can be a disastrous complication if severe encroachment on the neural elements occurs. Small amounts of posterior migration are usually asymptomatic or become so with fusion consolidation. Immobilization in a rigid brace is recommended until the fusion solidifies, if symptoms are tolerable and neural element damage is definitely not ongoing. If symptoms are positional they may resolve if and when the fusion consolidates. Large and symptomatic displacements require revision surgery to remove the displaced cage or reposition it in a more anterior and thus more favorable position. A larger implant may be needed to restore stability in some cases. A general principle that must be followed for good results with all interbody implants or grafts is the attainment of maximum intervertebral distraction to minimize micromotion. As an alternative, one can consider additional posterior fixation such as wiring of the posterior elements or pedicle fixation. If the implants are properly countersunk anterior to the posterior vertebral body border by 4 mm or more, this complication is much less likely to occur.

### LATERAL MALPOSITION

In the small patient with a large disk height the width of the implants needed for good distraction may exceed the interspace width, making it difficult to fit cages side-by-side within the disk space. With the posterior approach, lateral displacement is less likely because the placement trajectory is medialized by the pedicles, but might occur due to lateral implant angulation, resulting in their exit laterally from the disk space. In most cases this is not a problem. As long as the cage is mostly within the disk space and the extraforaminal root from the level above is unimpinged there will be no symptoms, especially once the fusion has solidified.

## COMPLICATIONS OF THE ANTERIOR APPROACH

### IMPLANT MIGRATION AND ANTERIOR MALPOSITION

For various reasons, such as inadequate distraction, toggling of the reamer during reaming, cross-threading of the cage into the tapped bony pilot hole, shallow initial seating of the implant, or an unusually unstable motion segment, anterior extrusion may occur, either partially (Fig. 45-1) or totally (Fig. 45-2). If protrusion is large, erosion into the great vessels (espe-

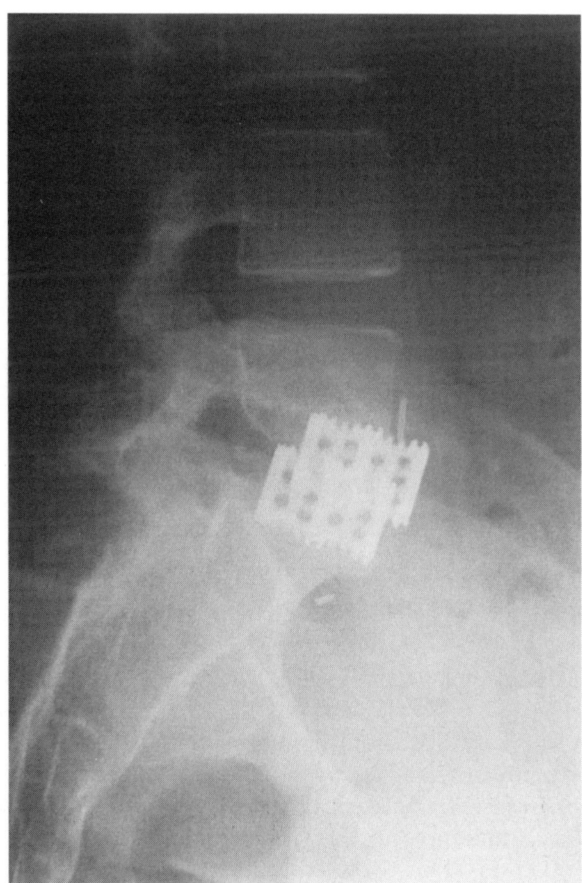

**FIGURE 45-1**

Anteriorly migrated cage in an asymptomatic patient.

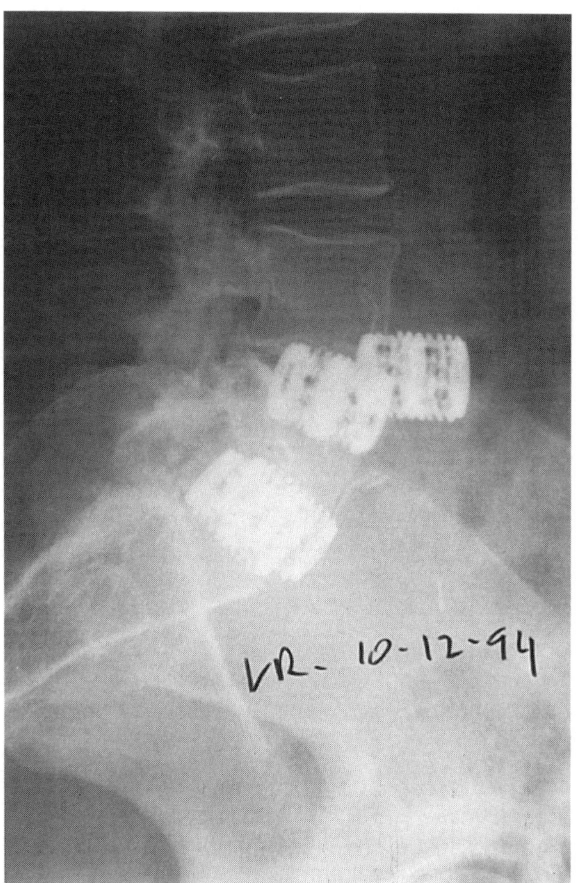


**FIGURE 45-2**

An anteriorly extruded cage prior to removal.

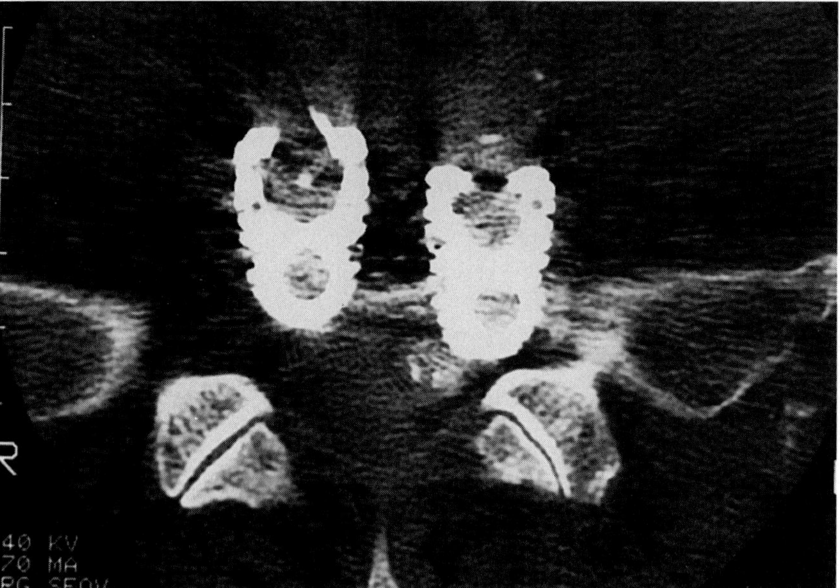


**FIGURE 45-3**

Computed tomography scan revealing posteriorly malpositioned cage and reaming debris pushed into spinal canal.

cially at the levels above L5) and ultimate pseudarthrosis from mechanical instability becomes a concern. Anterior removal and replacement should be considered in large protrusions. If the cage site is too big for the cage, a larger cage can be placed, but it should be kept in mind that if more intervertebral distraction is applied to the interspace the contralateral cage will become loose. Reseating the same cage more deeply is an option if the fit is tight, though replacement with bone graft is also satisfactory. As pointed out above, leaving only one cage on one side has usually resulted in pseudarthrosis.

### POSTERIOR MALPOSITION

Posterior displacement of implants may result in neural element entrapment not only from the implant itself but also from reaming debris that is driven ahead of the implant during insertion (Fig. 45-3). To avoid this problem, reaming and implantation should always stop several millimeters short of the posterior vertebral body border. The C-arm or x-ray must be exactly perpendicular to the patient in assessing implant depth to avoid parallax error, which may result in the actual implant depth being more posterior than is apparent from the image. If persistent neurological symptoms develop, the spinal canal will have to be decompressed. Because soft tissue, free bone, or cartilage fragments may be part of the entrapment problem, decompression is best approached from a laminotomy. The cage can also be repositioned more anteriorly from this approach by screwing it anteriorly via the transverse slot inside the cage using a flat-head screwdriver after removing the posterior chamber bone graft.

### LATERAL MALPOSITION

As with the posterior fusion this is only a problem if associated with symptoms from extraforaminal nerve irritation (Fig. 45-4). If symptoms are severe enough and persistent then implant removal is necessary from an anterior approach, as discussed above.

### POSTERIOR VERTEBRAL FRACTURE

Fracture of the posterior endplate and/or posterior vertebral body can occur from the anterior approach caused by reaming too far to the posterior, placement of the cage too far to the posterior, or undue force during reaming or cage insertion into osteoporotic bone. Treatment considerations are necessary if neurological symptoms are present and consist of posterior decompression as for posterior malposition as discussed above. If symptoms are not neurological they normally resolve when fracture healing and fusion have occurred.

## COMPLICATIONS OF THE ANTERIOR AND POSTERIOR APPROACHES

### CEPHALAD-CAUDAD MALPOSITION

The implants should engage both the upper and lower decorticated endplates. If they are too far cephalad or caudad, thus engaging only one endplate, the fusion does not solidify at the unengaged endplate (Fig. 45-5). However, even if one cage is not engaged, the other may solidify because the unengaged cage still provides a stabilizing effect. Symptomatic treat-

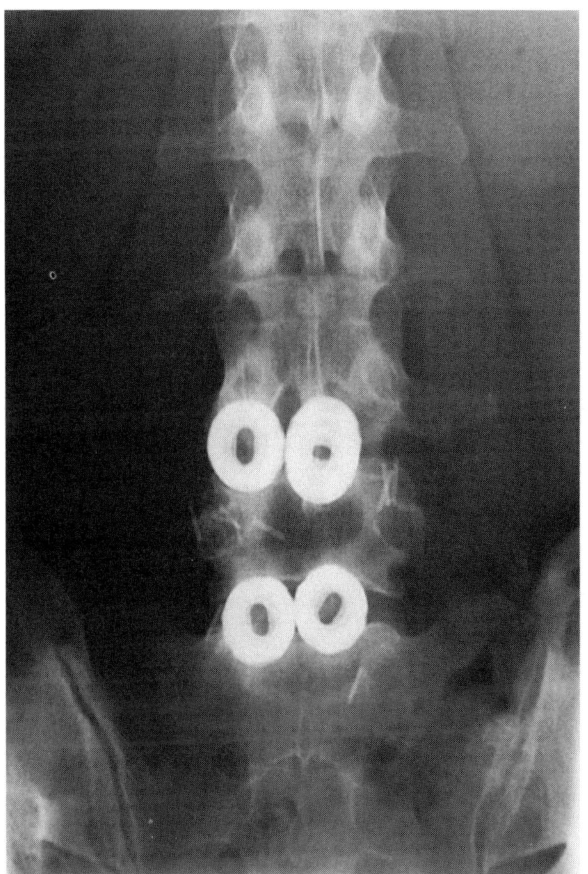

FIGURE 45-4

Malpositioned implant beyond the lateral pedicular border in an asymptomatic patient.

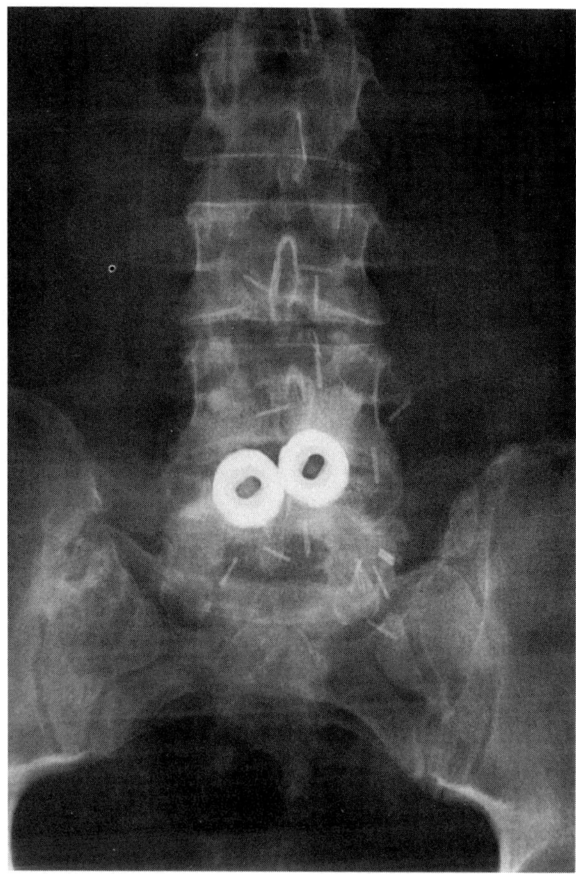

FIGURE 45-5

Cephalad-caudad malpositioning with failure of cage to fully engage superior endplate.

ment is the bottom line in these instances, since some patients are improved enough to be satisfied even in the event of nonunion. Pulsed electromagnetic field stimulators are not likely to have an effect if the endplate is unengaged by the cage. If revision of the fusion is required this can be handled as discussed in the section on pseudarthrosis.

## WOUND INFECTION

BAK implant infections are unusual.[7] Based on our experience with other spinal implants we would recommend the following: if recognized in the first postoperative week deep wound infections can often be eradicated with culture-specific antibiotics administered for 6 weeks.[2,6,9] Definitive wound cultures are most helpful for appropriate antibiotic selection. Abscess formation requires incision and drainage and probably implant removal with wound closure over tube irrigation or delayed primary closure.

Later-appearing deep infections probably can't be eradicated without removal of the implants.[6] In some cases infections can be indolent and difficult to detect. A history of chills, new-onset night sweats, general fatigue, low-grade intermittent fever, and increased back pain in the postoperative patient should be considered infectious in origin until proven otherwise.[9] Laboratory tests may be unremarkable and the wound cultures may be the only way to establish the diagnosis.

## PSEUDARTHROSIS

In our experience the most common problem with the BAK implant is failure to fuse. In patients with residual mechanical pain and static-position intolerance, fusion site motion should be ruled out. Any amount of motion may be responsible for symptoms. Flexion and extension plain x-rays will usually demonstrate motion (Fig. 45-6), but in questionable cases carefully taken lateral midline single plane sagittal tomography in side-lying flexion and extension can help delineate subtle pseudarthrosis.[4] A full year should be allowed for fusion consolidation unless patient suffering mandates earlier intervention. In those who are somewhat improved from their preoperative state indefinite observation may be appropriate, de-

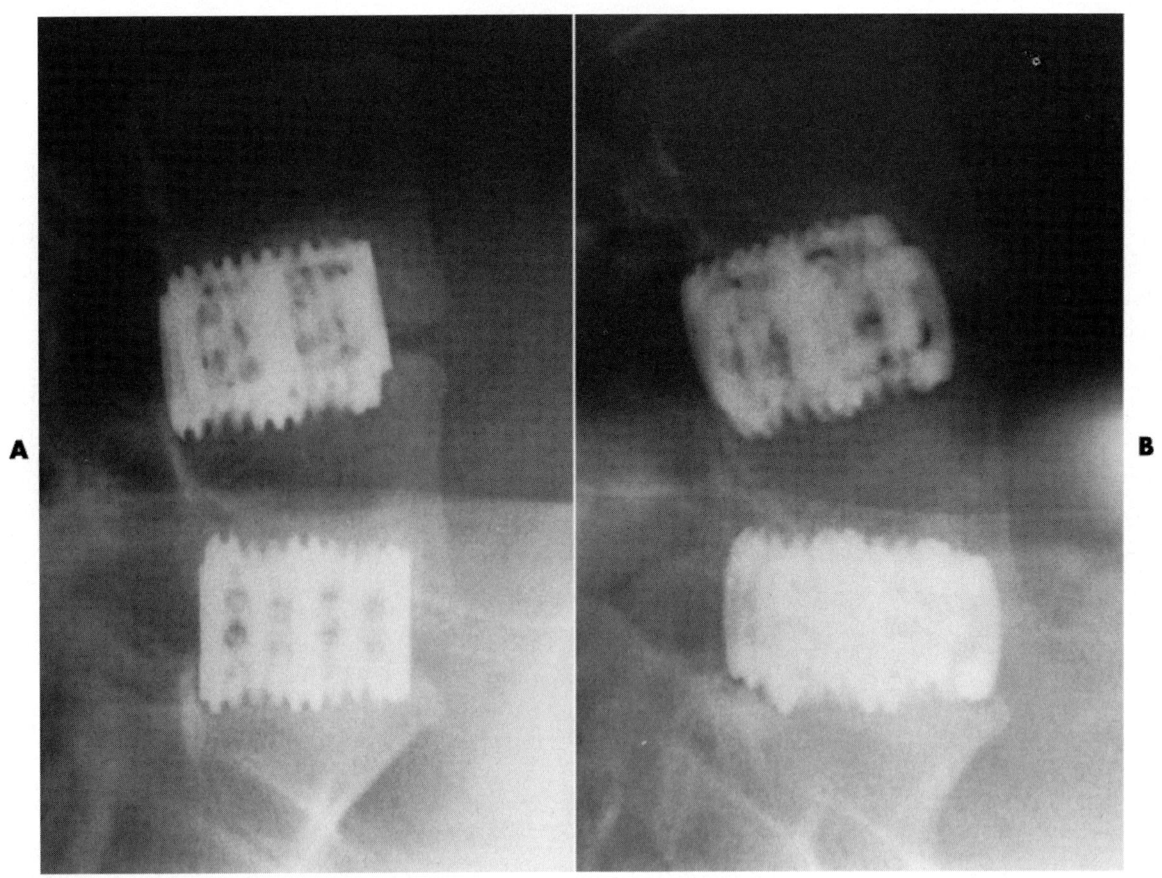


**FIGURE 45-6**

Flexion **(A)** and extension **(B)** x-rays demonstrating motion at both fusion levels.

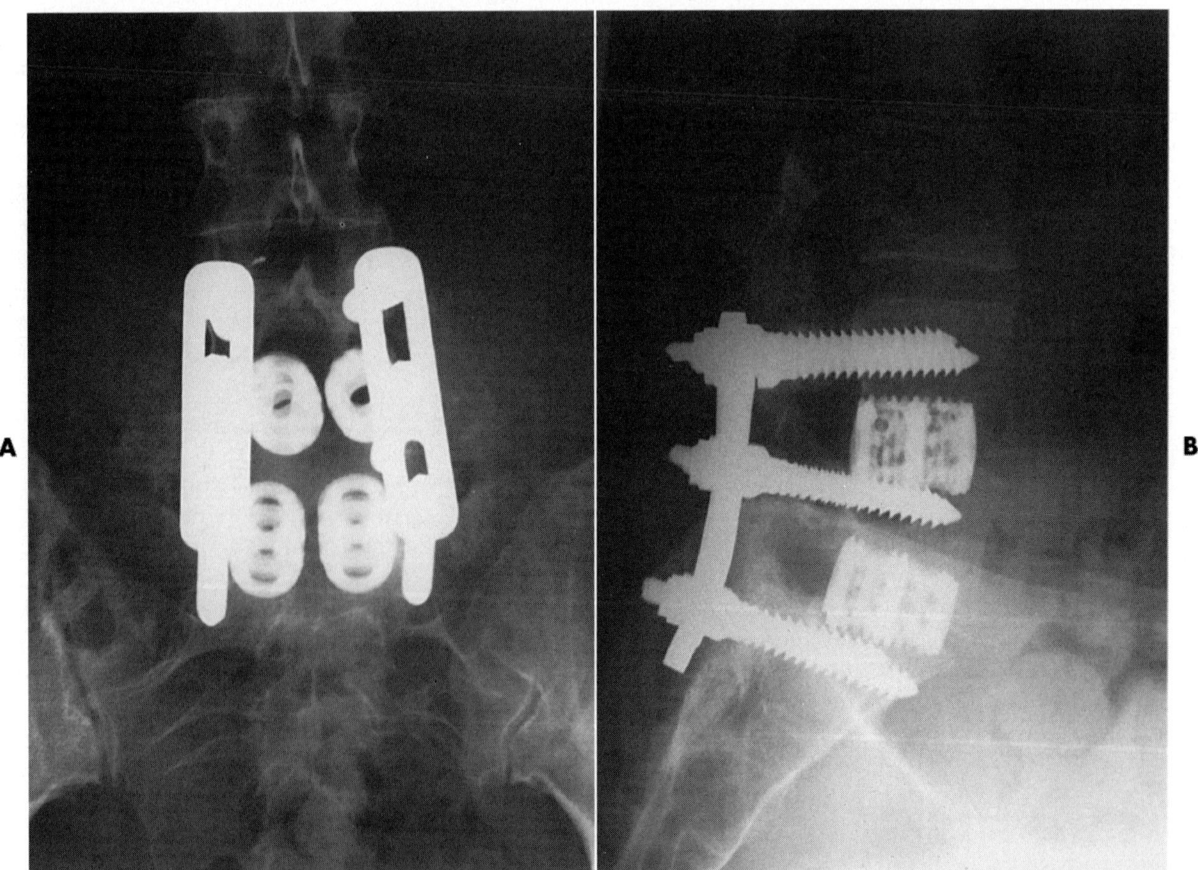


**FIGURE 45-7**

Anteroposterior **(A)** and lateral **(B)** x-rays of patients from Figure 45-6 following pedicular instrumentation.

pending on symptom severity. External electromagnetic bone stimulators may also be considered. Patients should be screened for osteoporosis and undergo a metabolic workup to determine appropriate treatment. Reversal of the metabolic bone disease state may result in fusion consolidation.

Revision options include posterolateral fusion (with or without instrumentation) and revision of the interbody fusion. The latter approach may be more difficult due to postsurgical scarring. In addition, viability of the fusion bed is compromised by the previous fusion attempt. In our own series, revision fusions without internal fixation in the same bone graft bed are successful only in 37% of patients, compared with a 66% success rate in a previously surgically unviolated fusion bed.[3] Posterolateral fusion is recommended. The fusion consolidation rate in circumferential fusions with pedicle fixation is over 95% in our experience (Fig. 45-7). One has to weigh the disadvantages of pedicle fixation, which also relates to the individual surgeon's experience and skills in choosing the revision technique.

### LAPAROSCOPIC APPROACH

Clinical trials on the laparoscopic delivery of BAK fusion cages began in September of 1993 and are still ongoing at the time of this writing.[8] The more elaborate approach entails the same possible orthopedic complications as the anterior open approach.[2,4]

## REFERENCES

1. Glassman SD, Johnson JR, Raque G et al: Management of iatrogenic spinal stenosis complicating placement of a fusion cage, *Spine* 21:2383-2386, 1996.
2. Hsu KY, Zucherman JF: Complications of pedicle screw fixation systems. In: *The adult lumbar spine.* International Society for the Study of the Lumbar Spine, Philadelphia, 1995, WB Sanders Co.
3. Hsu KY, Zucherman JF: Pseudoarthrosis of lumbar spine fusions—Origin of pain and treatment. International Society for the Study of the Lumbar Spine—Abstracts, May, 1989.
4. Kanel J, Zucherman JF, Shae B, Hsu KY: Single plane midline flexion extension lateral tomogram as a method for evaluating the integrity of lumbar spine fusion. International Society for the Study of the Lumbar Spine—Abstracts, June 1990.
5. McAfee P, Regan JR, Zdeblick T, Zucherman J et al: Incidence of complications in endoscopic anterior reconstructive surgery: A prospective multicenter study comprising the first 100 cases, *Spine* 20:1624-1632, 1995.
6. Schofferman L, Schofferman J, Zucherman JF et al: Occult infection causing persistent low back pain, *Spine* 14:417-419, 1989.
7. Yuan HA, Kuslich SD, Dowdle JA et al: Prospective multicenter clinical trial of the BAK interbody fusion system. Spinetech, Inc.
8. Zucherman J, Zdeblick T, Bailey S et al: Instrumented laparoscopic spinal fusion: preliminary results, *Spine* 20: 2029-2034, 1995.
9. Zucherman JF, Schofferman L, Gunthorpe H et al: Diptheroid and associated infections as a cause of failed lumbar instrumentation procedures. International Society for the Study of the Lumbar Spine, Abstract, April, 1988.

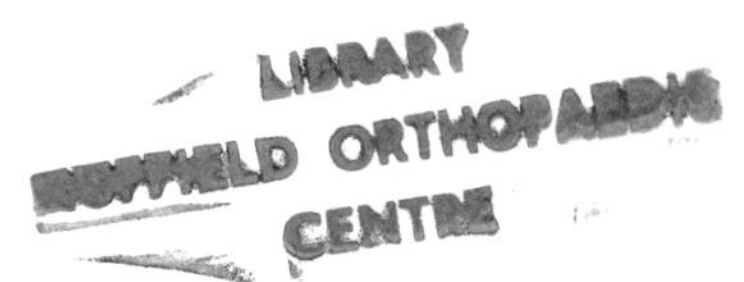

# 46

# FAILED LUMBAR AND LUMBOSACRAL SURGERY USING LAPAROSCOPICALLY INSERTED CAGES

**Robert Gunzburg, M.D., Ph.D.**
**Patrick Willocx, M.D.**
**Marek Szpalski, M.D.**



There are three main categories of spinal procedures: decompressions, fusions, and combinations of these. Surgical failure can occur after each kind of intervention. As a general rule, when failure occurs, one should avoid doing the same procedure over again. If it failed once, it will probably fail again. Indeed, failure is seldom due to bad or wrong surgical technique or instrumentation failure.

After a successful diskectomy or decompression, invalidating back pain without leg pain can occur due to progressive failure of an intervertebral disk. Conservative treatment should always be tried first: active revalidation, nonsteroidal anti-inflammatory drugs (NSAIDs), physiotherapy, and lumbar braces belong to the classic treatment scheme. However, if the pain remains invalidating, repeat surgery may be considered. It is important to perform diskography to ensure the diagnosis and to enhance the chances of success following fusion. A posterolateral fusion can be considered, but an anterior approach is a valid alternative.

After a successful spinal fusion, adjacent levels may degenerate and become painful as well. In such cases there is no need to remove or alter the instrumentation at the initial level. Surgery using a different approach often facilitates the revision operation. If a posterolateral fusion technique was used initially, an anterior approach for the second intervention presents several advantages. For the patient it is psychologically favorable to use another technique because a "failure" of the first operation was experienced. For the surgeon there is the distinct advantage not to have to work through scarred tissue.

Spinal fusion can also fail to alleviate the symptoms presented by the patient. Often fusion is acquired and no cause for failure is found. This represents a major challenge for spinal surgeons and should not lead to systematic repeat surgery. Sometimes, however, a clear nonunion of the fused vertebrae can be demonstrated. In those cases, revision surgery may be indicated, and the use of a different fusion technique advisable.

The lumbar and lumbosacral disk spaces can be approached from the back, but the anterior approach makes more sense. Indeed, a direct removal of the dysfunctional intervertebral disk with excellent graft stability is possible, with avoidance of posterior paraspinal muscle trauma and reduced blood loss.[5] It is therefore essential for surgeons dealing with the spine to be able to operate through either anterior or posterior approaches. Various devices have been proposed for these anterior interbody fusions. Autografts are usually harvested on the iliac crest. Fibular strut grafts or rib grafts have also been used. The success of the operation very much depends on the care taken to remove the cartilage and disk material, even more so when allografts or combined allo- and autografts are used. More recently, implants have been introduced. These are made of stainless steel, carbon fiber, ceramic, or titanium alloys and are generally used in pairs. The shapes of these implants vary widely, but are mostly cylindrical or rectangular. Some of the cylindrical implant devices are also threaded, which facilitates their insertion and secures a good hold. These implants are supplemented preferably with autograft, but their use allows the quantity of this autologous bone tissue to be much more limited than in implantless fusions. In this chapter, we will discuss the use of anterior fusion with cylindrical threaded cages using a laparoscopic approach in revision surgery. The implants used in the cases presented below are BAK cages, titanium threaded hollow and pierced implants, designed to promote stabilization and fusion.[1,6,11,13]

Anterior lumbar fusions with autografts have been performed since the beginning of this century. Later, allografts or combinations of auto- and allografts were utilized. Recently there has been an evolution toward the use of interbody fusion devices in combination with autografts. Modern laparoscopy started in the 1980s and by the end of that decade, laparoscopic surgery was the golden standard in general surgery. Obenchain[9] is reported to have been the first to work laparoscopically on the lumbar spine.

The laparoscopic anterior approach is usually reserved for surgery at the L5-S1 disk.[2] Higher levels can be done as well, but involves mobilization of the major vessels.

## OPERATIVE TECHNIQUE OF LAPAROSCOPIC SPINAL FUSION

The patient is placed in the supine position with a varying degree of Trendelenburg. If bone grafts are required, a separate incision has to be carried out over one of the iliac crests.

The landmarks for the incision are easily recognized. The umbilicus normally projects at the level of the L3-L4 disk space. In obese patients, however, this may vary. The pubis or symphysis can usually be recognized. Four transparent trocar sleeves are inserted. A 10-mm diameter trocar at the level of the umbilicus for the 0-degree laparoscope and two identical trocars left and right at the same level as the umbilicus and about 15 cm from the midline. In the right iliac fossa a fourth transparent trocar of 5-mm diameter is inserted. The left-sided trocar is used by the assistant who reclines the sigmoid colon with the left hand and holds the laparoscope with the right hand. The surgeon stands at the right side of the patient and uses the two trocars on his side to perform the dissection. Using a curved dissector and a unipolar cautery hook, the retroperitoneum is incised at the level of the L5-S1 disk. Careful dissection between the two common iliac veins allows exposure of the disk. The left common iliac vein crosses the spine at L4-L5 or over L5 and lies more caudal than the left common iliac artery making dissection of the left side potentially more dangerous, the vein being a more fragile structure than the artery. The medial sacral artery and vein are the only constant structures that need to be ligated either using vascular endoclips or cauterization.

Once the disk has been sufficiently exposed, a K-wire is inserted under laparoscopic and fluoroscopic vision through the abdominal wall and into the middle of the disk. Finally, an 18-mm trocar is inserted on the midline and in the prolongation with the endplates of the disk. Through this port, the instrumentation of the disk is performed: disk and endplate reaming and distraction, followed by disk fragment removal and tapping. Finally the implants containing cancellous bone graft are inserted. These are threaded, hollow, and pierced cranially and caudally, allowing bony fusion from one endplate, through the implant toward the other endplate. The rationale of the technique consists in regaining disk height by progressive perioperative distraction until the outer annulus is again placed under tension and in obtaining bony fusion between the two vertebrae.[11]

Blood loss is minimal and hospitalization shorter than with posterior or open anterior approaches. When surgery is performed carefully, there is usually no need to drain the site. If necessary, a rapid conversion to open procedure is possible and easy. Just as for any operation there is a learning curve, and, whereas operating time is initially longer than with open procedures, skilled laparoscopic hands can bring the operation time below two hours.

Recently, Faciszewski et al[3] reviewed more than 1,000 anterior fusion operations and found this procedure to be a safe one. Serious complications such as death (0.3%), paraplegia (0.2%), and deep wound infection (0.6%) were rare. The rate of complications directly attributed to the anterior spinal surgery was 11.5%. These complications include vascular laceration, neural injury, graft displacement, hardware failure, vertebral body fracture, peritoneal adhesions, urethral lesions, infection, intestinal ileus, ventral hernia, bone graft donor site complications, rectus sheath hematomata, femoral nerve palsy, and thrombotic arterial occlusions.[7,8,10]

## CONCLUSION

Anterior interbody fusion with threaded cages using a laparoscopic approach is a good alternative in revision surgery for failed posterior or posterolateral lumbar or lumbosacral fusion. It allows the surgeon to avoid having to work through scarred tissue. Hospitalization time is reduced and patients experience their surgery well. There were no major complications in this series. Finally it must be emphasized that this is a difficult procedure with a long learning curve, and that surgeons willing to use this technique should at first be familiar with open anterior techniques.

## CASE STUDIES

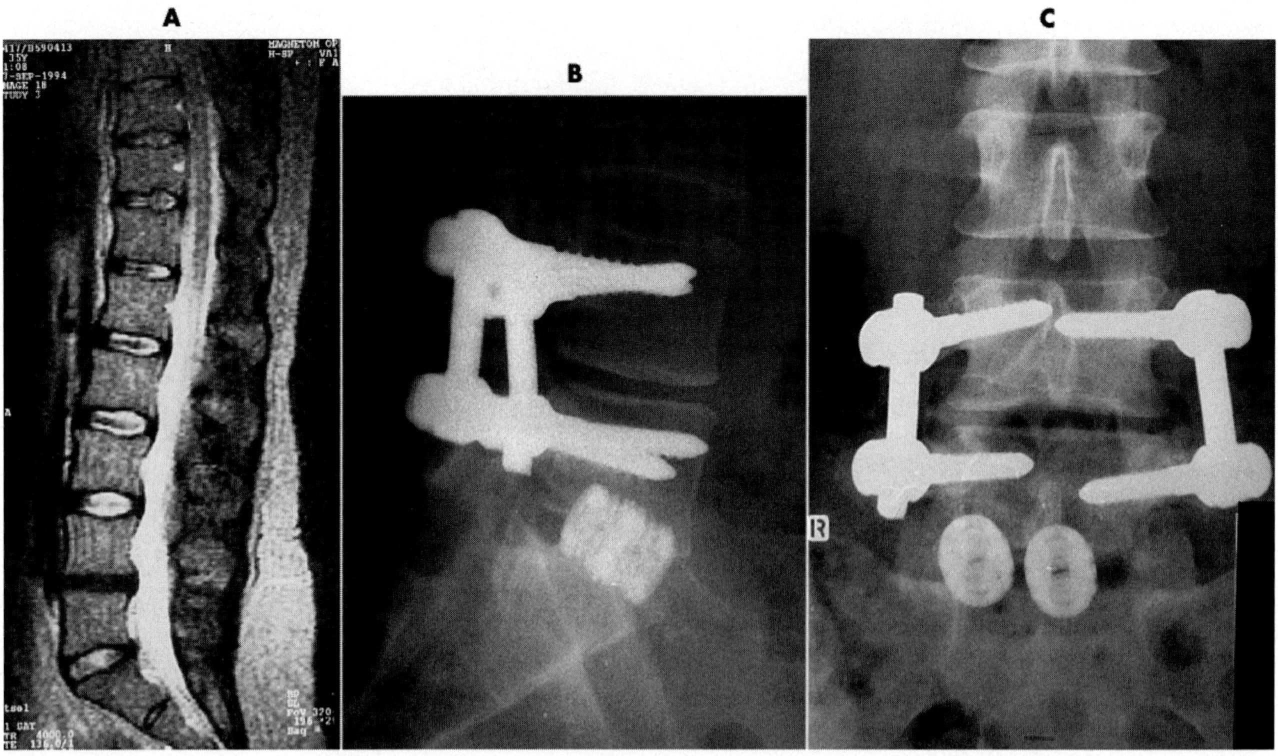


FIGURE 46-1

**A,** T2-weighted MRI showing L4-L5 disk degeneration. **B, C,** L4-L5 posterolateral fusion with Cotrel-Dubousset instrumentation and L5-S1 laparoscopically inserted BAK cages.

### CASE 1

At the age of 31, this female laborer started complaining of backache. Two years later she underwent surgery for discus hernia at the L4-L5 level. She failed to improve and surgery was repeated three weeks later. She still faired badly and was declared invalid (i.e., her earning capacity was less than 65%). Four years passed and she presented again with both back and leg pain. On the T2-weighted MRI images (Fig. 46-1, *A*), only L4-L5 showed dehydration, and diskography was positive both for pain reproduction and disk degeneration only at the L4-L5 level. At this stage, an L4-L5 laminarthrectomy with posterolateral fusion implemented with a pedicle screw/rod system (Cotrel-Dubousset) was carried out. The patient did well, solid fusion was obtained in 6 months, and a normal level of activity was regained. Because the patient had already been recognized invalid, a return to work could not be envisaged. Fifteen months after surgery, incapacitating back pain appeared again, this time without leg pain. The pain was localized at the L5-S1 level and a secondary disk failure under an existing fusion was diagnosed. Because there was no leg pain and because she had undergone failed surgery from the back three times, an anterior laparoscopic procedure was carried out (BAK cages, Fig. 46-1, *B* and *C*). A lumbar brace was worn for approximately 4 months and at 6 months the patient was pain free.

### CASE 2

L.B., a 32-year-old secretary presented with low back pain radiating toward the legs. The initial treatment was conservative and consisted of physiotherapy, NSAIDs, back school, and a lumbar support. Epidural steroids gave only partial and temporary relief. At the age of 37 she underwent an L5-S1 decompression, which cured the leg pain but not the back pain. Diskography at the L4-L5 level was normal, and one year after the decompression, an anterior spinal fusion with threaded cages (BAK) was carried out laparoscopically. Initially there was right-sided S1 nerve root pain, but this was treated conservatively and subsided after a few months. At six months she returned to her full-time secretarial occupation.

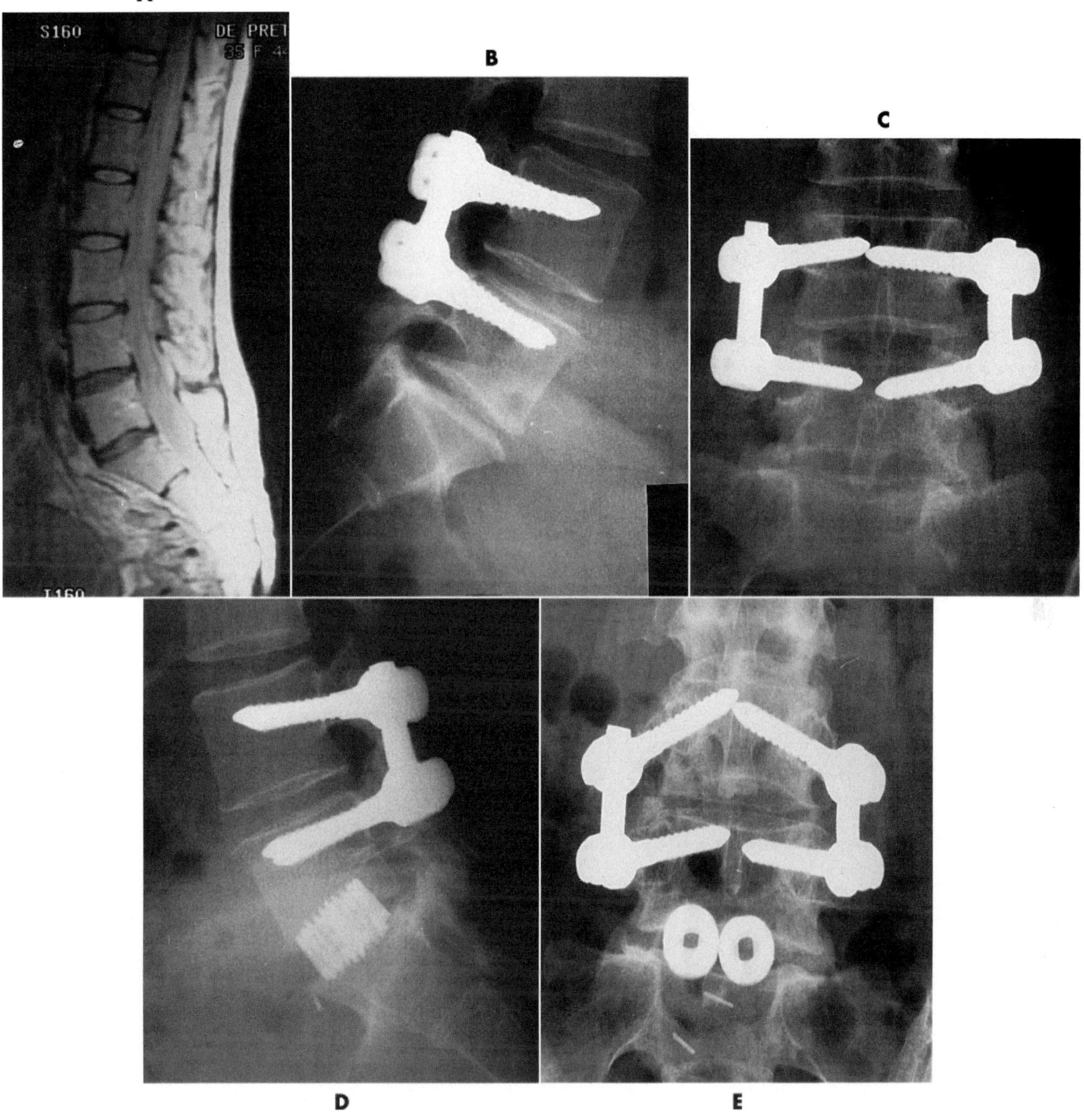


FIGURE 46-2

**A,** T2-weighted MRI showing L4-L5 and L5-S1 disk degeneration. **B, C,** L4-L5 posterolateral fusion with Cotrel-Dubousset instrumentation. **D, E,** L5-S1 laparoscopically inserted BAK cages.

## CASE 3

The patient was 35 years old when she sought orthopedic advice after having lost her job as a kitchen aid because of back pain. Standard radiography showed disk degeneration at the two lowest levels, and T2-weighted MRI (Fig. 46-2, *A*) scans indicated dehydration of the same disks with a small nonclinical protrusion at L3-L4. Diskography was carried out at the three lowest levels and only L4-L5 was positive. As a result, she was offered an L4-L5 posterolateral fusion implemented with a pedicular screw-rod system (Cotrel-Dubousset; Fig. 46-2, *B* and *C*). One year later she decompensated at the L5-S1 level. A laparoscopic anterior spinal fusion was carried out with BAK cages (Fig. 46-2, *D* and *E*). Five months after surgery she resumed work.

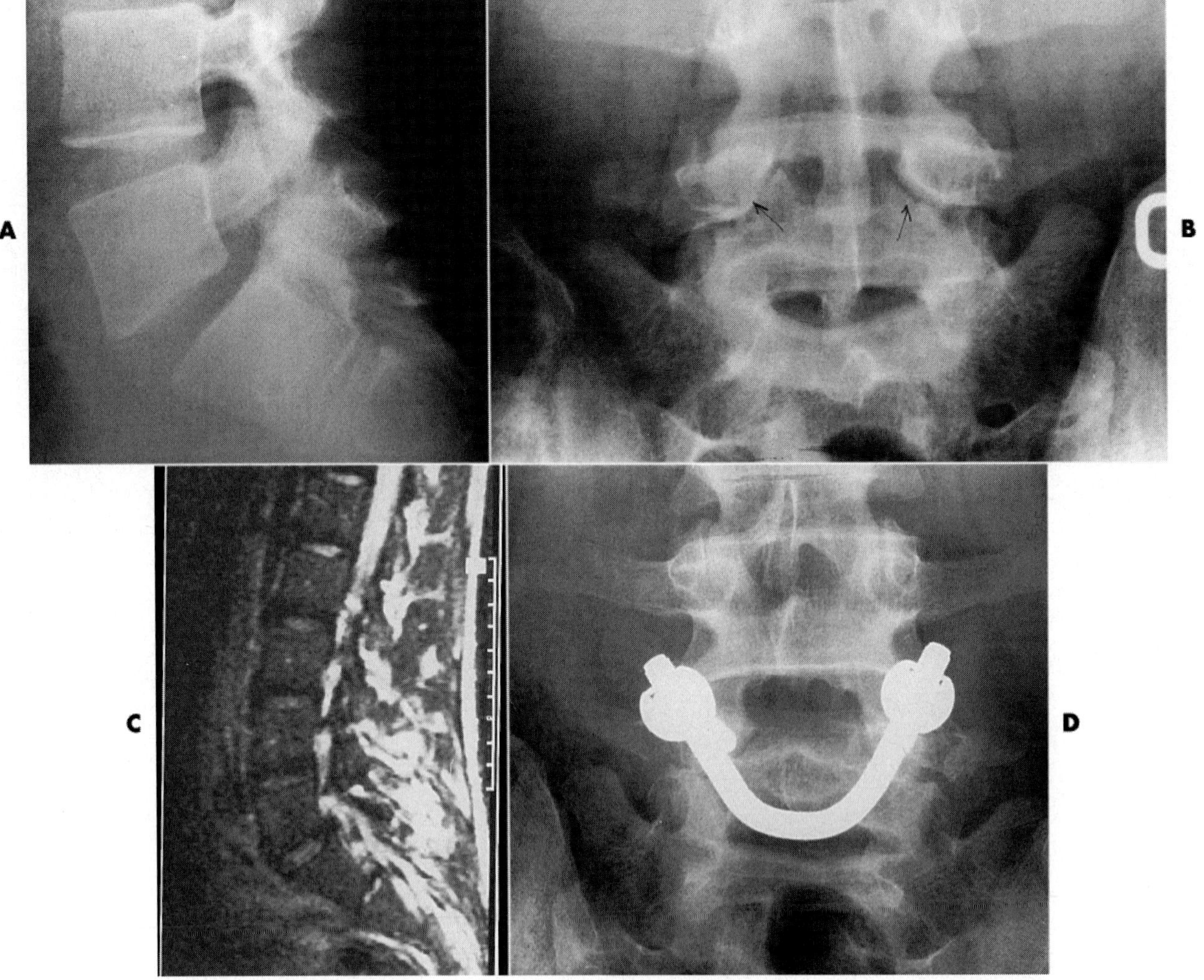


FIGURE 46-3

**A, B,** Standard radiography showing bilateral L5 pars lysis with grade 1 listhesis. **C,** T2-weighted MRI image showing L5-S1 slip and slight posterior protrusion. **D,** Lysis reconstruction and instrumentation.

*Continued*

## CASE 4

The patient is 30 years old, self-employed, and has a fish shop. He presented with progressively incapacitating low back pain, making it impossible for him to work. Standard radiography revealed an L5 spondylolysis without listhesis (Fig. 46-3, *A, B,* and *C*). After a failed conservative treatment the surgeon opted for a lysis reconstruction with instrumentation. This consisted of pedicular screws in L5 with a curved rod under the spinous process of the same vertebra to implement a bone graft at the lysis site (Fig. 46-3, *D* and *E*). The disk was left untouched and diskography was not performed in spite of a clearly degenerative disk on MRI. Postoperatively there was no improvement and the patient sought a second opinion. Diskography was carried out at the two lowest levels. L4-L5 was normal and not painful, L5-S1 reproduced the typical pain (Fig. 46-3, *F*). It was then decided to leave the posterior aspects of the spine as such and to perform an anterior approach. Threaded cages (BAK) were inserted laparoscopically (Fig. 46-3, *G* and *H*). Postoperatively the patient improved progressively and there was no sexual dysfunction. At six months the lumbar brace was discontinue and work progressively resumed.

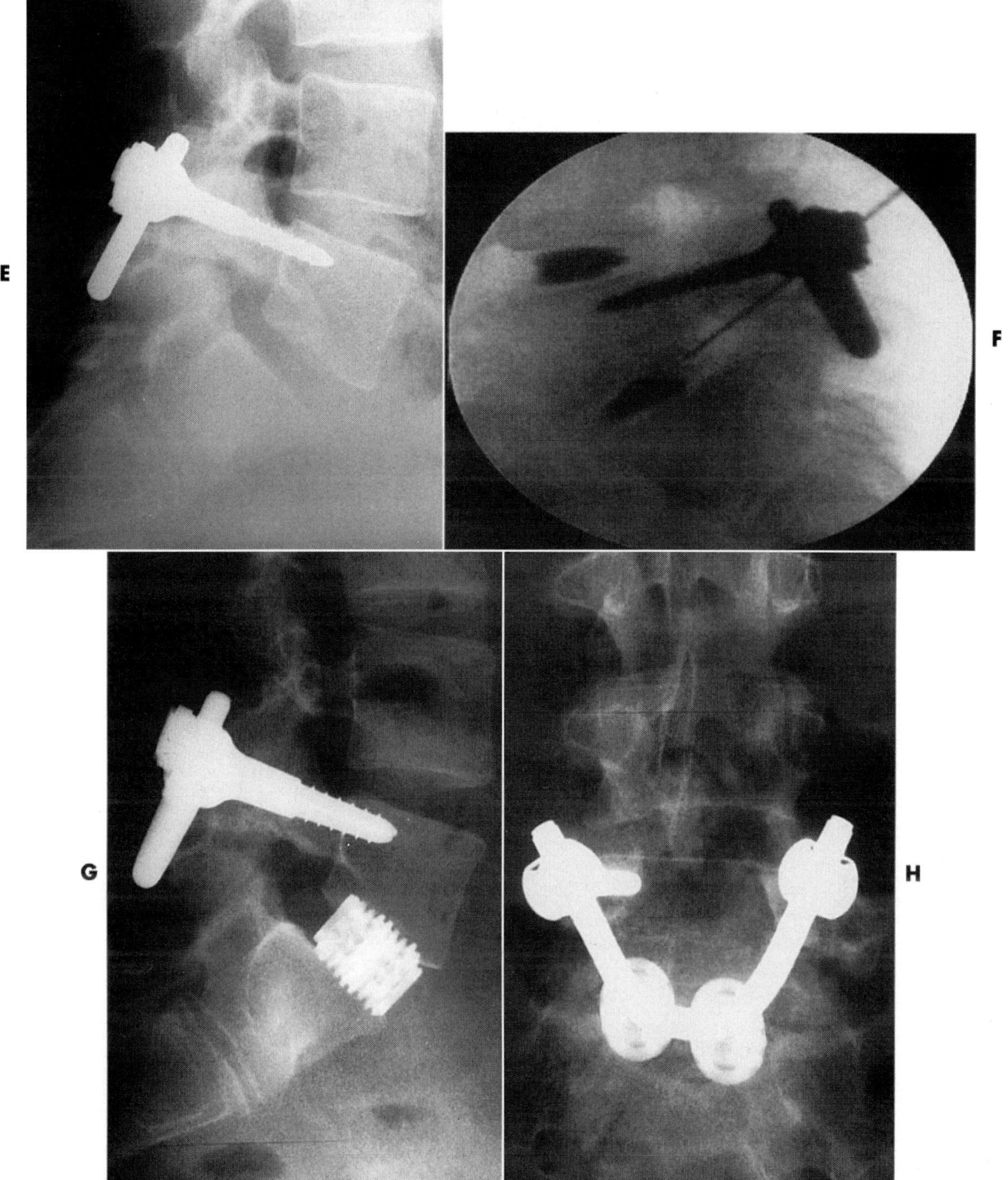


FIGURE 46-3, CONT'D

**E,** Lysis reconstruction and instrumentation. **F,** L4-L5 and L5-S1 diskography; only L5-S1 was painful. **G, H,** L5-S1 laparoscopically inserted BAK cages.

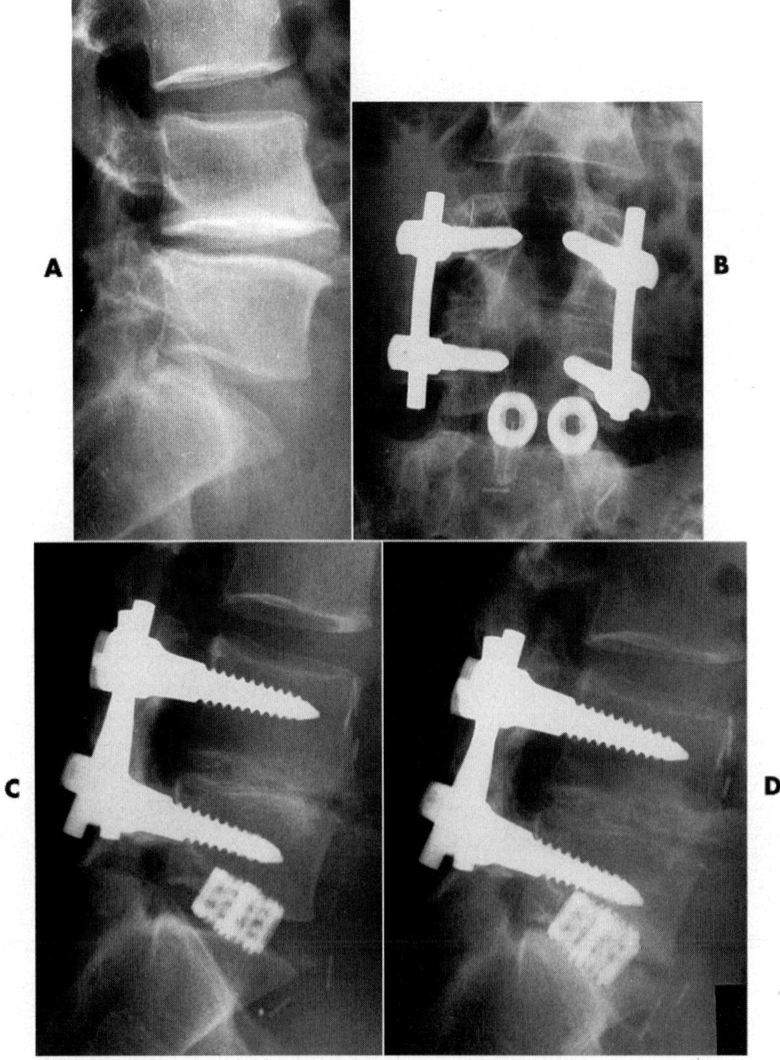


FIGURE 46-4

**A,** Standard radiography showing L4-L5 disk degeneration with narrowing and McNab spurs. **B, C,** L4-L5 posterolateral fusion with Cotrel-Dubousset instrumentation (1st operation), L5-S1 laparoscopically inserted BAK cages (2nd operation). **D,** Collapse of L5-S1 following the discitis.

## CASE 5

The patient is a factory laborer in the auto industry. He complained of progressively increasing low back pain, which failed to improve despite classic conservative management consisting of rest, physiotherapy, NSAIDs, back school, and re-education. Both standard radiography (Fig. 46-4, *A*) and magnetic resonance imaging (MRI) pointed toward the L4-L5 disk. This was confirmed both clinically and by diskography. Taking in account the anthropometric characteristics of this very tall and heavy man as well as his profession, a 360-degree fusion was performed. First, a posterolateral L4-L5 fusion (implemented with a pedicular screw-rod system [Cotrel-Dubousset]) was performed, using the Wiltse approach.[12] During the same procedure, an anterior interbody fusion was performed through a Fraser muscle-splitting retroperitoneal approach.[4] Two tricortical autologous iliac bone grafts were inserted, using Crock instrumentation. Postoperatively, the patient wore a lumbar brace for 6 months after which he resumed work in the factory. Discogenic back pain appeared again four years later, this time arising from the L5-S1 level. Diskography confirmed the origin of the pain and a laparoscopic anterior spinal fusion was carried out with BAK cages (Fig. 46-4, *B* and *C*). This operation was, unfortunately, complicated by a septic discitis. After an adequate antibiotic therapy (6 weeks intravenous and 6 weeks oral), the patient further had a normal recovery in spite of a loss of disk height (Fig. 46-4, *D*), and resumed work on a part-time basis six months after his operation.

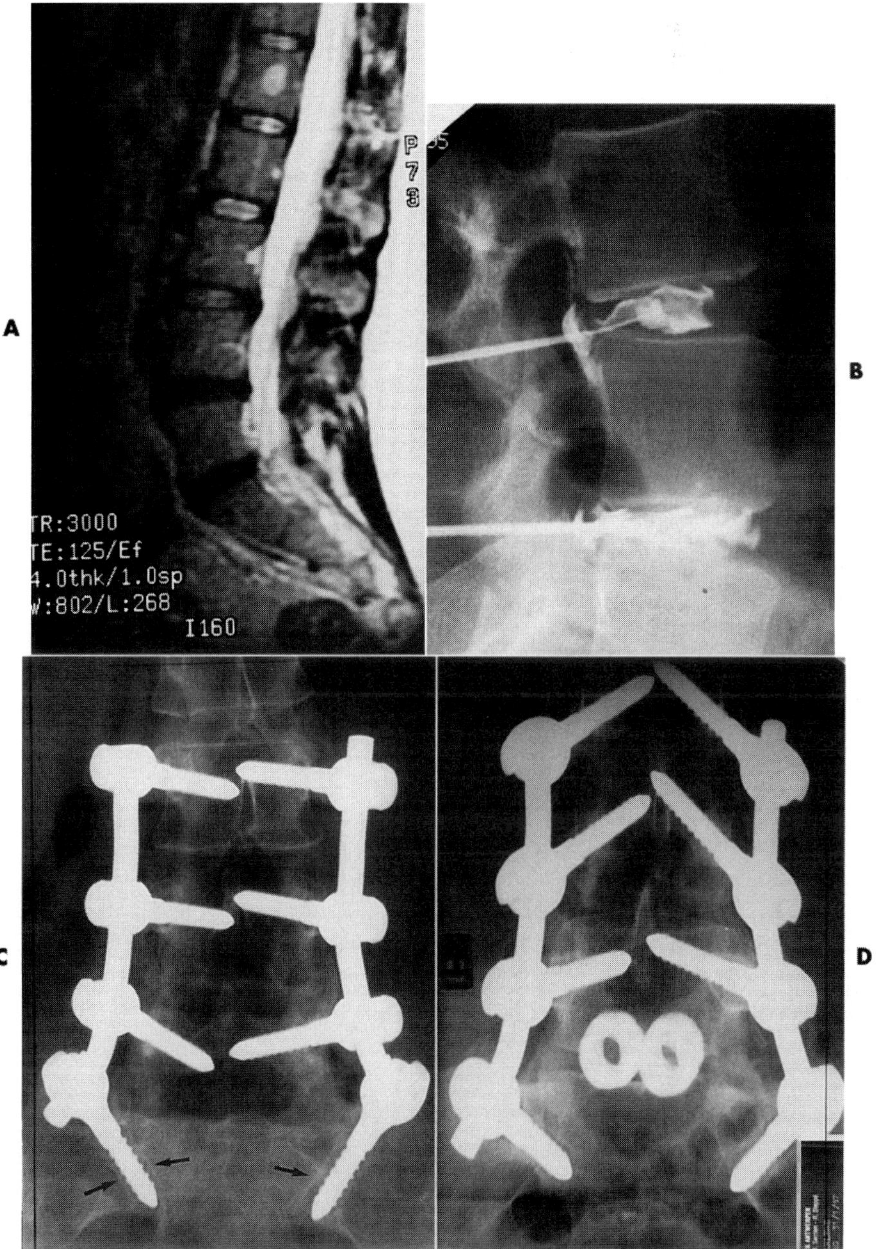


**FIGURE 46-5**

**A,** T2-weighted MRI showing dehydration at L4-L5 and L5-S1 with a slight bulge at L3-L4. **B,** Diskography showing disk degeneration at L3-L4 and L4-L5; there was a typical pain reproduction. **C,** L3-S1 posterolateral fusion with Cotrel-Dubousset instrumentation. Note the lysis around the screws in S1 and L5. **D,** L5-S1 laparoscopic fusion with BAK cages.

## CASE 6

The patient underwent an L3-S1 posterolateral fusion supplemented with Cotrel-Dubousset instrumentation. On MRI there was disk degeneration at L4-L5 and L5-S1 with a slight bulging at L3-L4 (Fig. 46-5, *A*). Diskography at these levels was positive for all levels (Fig. 46-5, *B*) and therefore L3-L4 was included in the fusion. Initially she fared well, but after about one year she began again to complain of discogenic low back pain. Dynamic lumbar radiographs showed mobility at the L5-S1 level (Fig. 46-5, *C*), and a failed fusion at that level was diagnosed. Because diskography had been positive before the first operation, this was not repeated. There was no leg pain and the pedicular screws being placed correctly, it was decided to perform an L5-S1 laparoscopic fusion using the BAK cage (Fig. 46-5, *D*). Both the procedure and the postoperative outcome were favorable, and after a period of 6 months she resumed her normal activities.

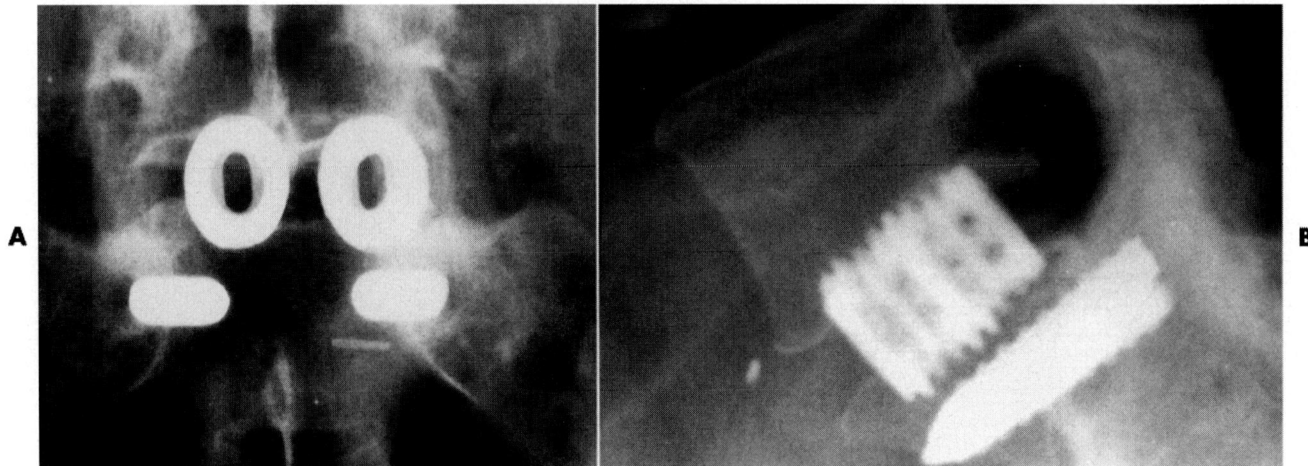


**FIGURE 46-6**

**A, B,** Laparoscopic L5-S1 fusion using BAK cages. Note the remains of fractured Cotrel-Dubousset screws in the pedicles of S1.

## CASE 7

The patient is a 38-year-old postal worker complaining of discogenic back pain. After a couple of years of conservative treatment, an L5-S1 posterolateral fusion was carried out supplemented with Cotrel-Dubousset instrumentation. Diskography at L4-L5 was normal, at L5-S1 typical pain was reproduced. After four months she returned to work and was free of symptoms for approximately one year. She then started to complain of progressively increasing back pain. Radiographs showed fatigue failure of both S1 screws. The implant was removed, but this did not make her feel any better. It was assumed that the instrumentation failure had to be the result of a nonfusion between L5 and S1. Posterior fusion having failed, a laparoscopic L5-S1 fusion was carried out using BAK implants (Fig. 46-6, *A* and *B*). She resumed work, although not as a postal worker on the street but in a post office.

## REFERENCES

1. Bagby G: Arthrodesis by distraction-compression methods using a stainless steel implant, *Orthopaedics* 11:931-934, 1988.
2. Cloyd DW, Obenchain TG, Savin M: Transperitoneal laparoscopic approach to lumbar discectomy, *Surg Laparos Endos* 5:85-89, 1995.
3. Faciszewski T, Winter R, Lonstein J, Denis F, Johnson L: The surgical and medical perioperative complications of anterior spinal fusion surgery in the thoracic and lumbar spine in adults, *Spine* 20:1592-1599, 1995.
4. Fraser R: A wide muscle-splitting approach to the lumbo-sacral spine, *J Bone Joint Surg* 64B:44-46, 1982.
5. Kozak JA, Heilman AE, O'Brien JP: Anterior lumbar fusion options: technique and graft materials, *Clin Orthop* 300:45-51, 1994.
6. Kuslish SD, Dowdle JA. Two-year follow up results of the BAK interbody fusion device. Proceedings of the 9th Annual Meeting of the North American Spine Society. October 19-22, 1994.
7. McAfee PC, Regan JR, Zdeblick T, et al: The incidence of complications in endoscopic anterior thoracolumbar spinal reconstructive surgery, *Spine* 14:1624-1632, 1995.
8. Mariscano J, Mirovsky Y, Remer S, Bloom N, Neuwirth M: Thrombotic occlusion of the left common iliac artery after an anterior retroperitoneal approach to the lumbar spine, *Spine* 19:357-359, 1994.
9. Obenchain T: Laparoscopic lumbar discectomy: a case report, *J Laparoendosc Surg* 1:145-59, 1991.
10. Papastefanou S, Stevens S, Mulholland R: Femoral nerve palsy, an unusual complication of anterior lumbar interbody fusion, *Spine* 19:2842-2844, 1994.
11. Sandhu HS, Turner S, Kabo JM, et al: Distractive properties of a threaded interbody fusion device, *Spine* 21:1201-1210, 1996.
12. Wiltse L, Bateman J, Hutchinson R, Nelson W: The paraspinal sacrospinalis-splitting approach to the lumbar spine, *J Bone Joint Surg* 50A:919, 1968.
13. Zucherman JF, Zdeblick TA, Bailey SA, et al: Instrumented laparoscopic spinal fusion. Preliminary results, *Spine* 20:2029-2035, 1995.

# 47

# REVISION OF FUSION FROM THE SPINE TO THE SACROPELVIS: CONSIDERATIONS

Joseph Y. Margulies, M.D., Ph.D.
Edouard F. Armour, M.D.
Christine Kohler-Ekstrand, M.D.
William O. Shaffer, M.D.
Samuel P. Thampi, M.D.



The pelvis consists of the ilium and sacrum. In years past, the view of the sacrum has been in isolation, without regard to the pelvic vertebra. Fusion of the spine to the sacropelvis has been a problematic issue for quite some time. The need for revision of the failed lumbosacral fusion has added still greater controversy to this issue. At least three types of problems may indicate a need for revision surgery: (1) deterioration of unfused L5-S1 distal to existing long fusion mass, (2) nonunion of previous lumbosacral fusion, and (3) clinical failure with subsequent problems in the pelvis following successful lumbosacral fusion.

The controversy stems from the lack of conclusive information on the natural history of lumbosacropelvic deterioration, and the long-term consequences of the fusion at these junctions. The Kirkaldy-Willis cascade provides the natural history of spine degeneration.[18] However, the natural history of lumbopelvic stability can not be predicted for individual patients. In lumbopelvic pathologies, such as scoliosis and spondylolisthesis, the natural history is even less well understood.

Despite numerous clinically successful lumbosacral fusions over the past two decades, these fusions have come under criticism. Long-term consequences of lumbopelvic fusions include stress fractures in the sacral ala and ilium as well as sacroiliac joint problems. These complications, though infrequent, are disastrous when they occur. The impression that fusion to the sacrum is detrimental may be statistically incorrect. Only long-term follow-up, or perhaps mete analysis can shed light on this controversy.

This chapter discusses the most recent considerations on revision fusion of the spine to the sacropelvis. This includes various indications, posterior, anterior, and mixed 360-degree fixation techniques, and a future outlook on revision surgery.

## INDICATIONS FOR REVISION SPINOPELVIC FUSIONS

### DETERIORATION OF UNFUSED L5-S1 DISTAL TO EXISTING FUSION MASS

In many cases, revision fusion of the spine to the pelvis does not pose a difficult problem to the orthopedic surgeon. The most common scenario involves a patient with a history of prior proximal lumbar spine surgery, with subsequent development of lumbosacral instability. However, other cases occur where the need for revision or fusion becomes controversial. For example, consider a patient with postlaminectomy stenosis at L3-L4 and L4-L5. The patient requires fusion to L5. However, the lumbosacral junction, while currently asymptomatic, is markedly degenerative on radiographs. Some surgeons would treat only the current symptomatology and stop the fusion at L5. Others would consider possible future deterioration and take the fusion down to the sacrum. There is no scientific evidence supporting either course. However, fusion to the sacropelvis may prevent future surgery when L5-S1 deterioration becomes symptomatic.

### FAILURE OF PREVIOUS LUMBOSACRAL FUSION

Failed fusions to the sacropelvis are a fundamentally different problem, about which little controversy exists. Reasons for failure are numerous and well-documented. The technical means to attempt repair of such pseudarthrosis requires new conceptual and technical solutions. Some of these technical solutions are discussed in this chapter.

### CLINICAL FAILURE DESPITE "SUCCESSFUL" FUSED LUMBOPELVIC FUSION

Long-term consequences of lumbosacral fusion include stress fractures in the sacropelvis, sacroiliac joint problems, and postfusion stenosis in the L5-S1 segment. Though infrequent, strategies must be developed to deal with these add-on instabilities and neural compromises despite their rarity.

## SPINOPELVIC FIXATION TECHNIQUES

There are three approaches to lumbopelvic fusion: posterior, anterior, or combined 360-degree fusions. Various techniques of spinopelvic fixation may be used with each of these three approaches. The following provides a brief overview of some of the available instrumentation for fusion of the spine to the pelvis.

### POSTERIOR CONSTRUCTS

Posterior fusion of the L5-S1 level or L4 to S1 may be performed using screws at each single level, as for example, the Bucher screw,[24] Magerl laminar screw,[17] or direct screws.[12] Some surgeons prefer the use of dowels in the same direction.[7] For single- and two-level fusions, such strategies are well-established. However, longer posterior fusions require anchors in the sacropelvis, anchors in the lumbar and/or thoracic spine, and vertical members to connect these anchors.[3] Spine anchors can consist of pedicular screws, hooks, claws, wires, and cables. As discussed, suitable sacropelvic anchors may be pedicle screws in S1 and S2 (Fig. 47-1, *A* and *B*),[11] Jackson intrasacral rods (Fig. 47-2, *A* and *B*),[15] lateral sacral alar screws (Fig. 47-1, *A* and *B*), iliosacral screws (Fig. 47-3),[9] iliac screws, Galveston intrailiac rods (Figs. 47-1 and 47-4),[1] or sacral bars (Fig. 47-5), and various sacral blocks.

As a rule, constructs that are based on single anchors are not enough to maintain the stability of spinopelvic fusion. Asher's concept of "foundation" requires solid fixation in order to manipulate the sagittal and coronal contour of the fused region in attempting to restore normal balance.

A solid foundation is built once the anchors in the spine and pelvis are in place. A good foundation consists of a combination of two rods and a cross connector hooked to the spine via solid anchors, as screws or hook-claws. This foundation allows manipulation of the spine. The foundation of the sacropelvis is created using the same concepts: rods that are connected to multiple anchors placed in the sacropelvis and cross-linked. Sacral blocks incorporate two to three screws and allow connection to a single rod.[8] The rod block interface lessens the foundation because of the single point of connection between the rod and the block. Therefore, for longer posterior fusions such as degenerative scoliosis or revision surgery, we recommend construction of a stronger foundation in the sacropelvis, a foundation in the spine, and vertical members to connect them.

### ANCHORS AND FOUNDATIONS

***Iliolumbar Fixation Techniques.***

GALVESTON FIXATION. The Galveston fixation technique involves insertion of the distal limb of the spinal rod into the posterior iliac crest intracortically at least 6 cm.[1] A number of critical aspects need to be considered: (1) avoid extending the rod into the hip joint; (2) previous iliac crest bone graft harvest decreases the availability of bone for adequate purchase and can compromise the foundation; and (3) unacceptable loosening results from the use of a roughened rod such as the standard Cotrel-Dubousset rod.

ILIAC SCREW FIXATION. The placement of 7- to 8-mm diameter threaded screws into the iliac wing provides a technically easier method of iliolumbar fixation than the Galveston technique. The screw is placed in an optimal position and then linked to the spinal rod independently. Combining the Galveston rods or iliac screws with S1 provides an excellent foundation and a solid construct around which the spine can be rotated in the sagittal and coronal planes (Fig. 47-4, left side.)

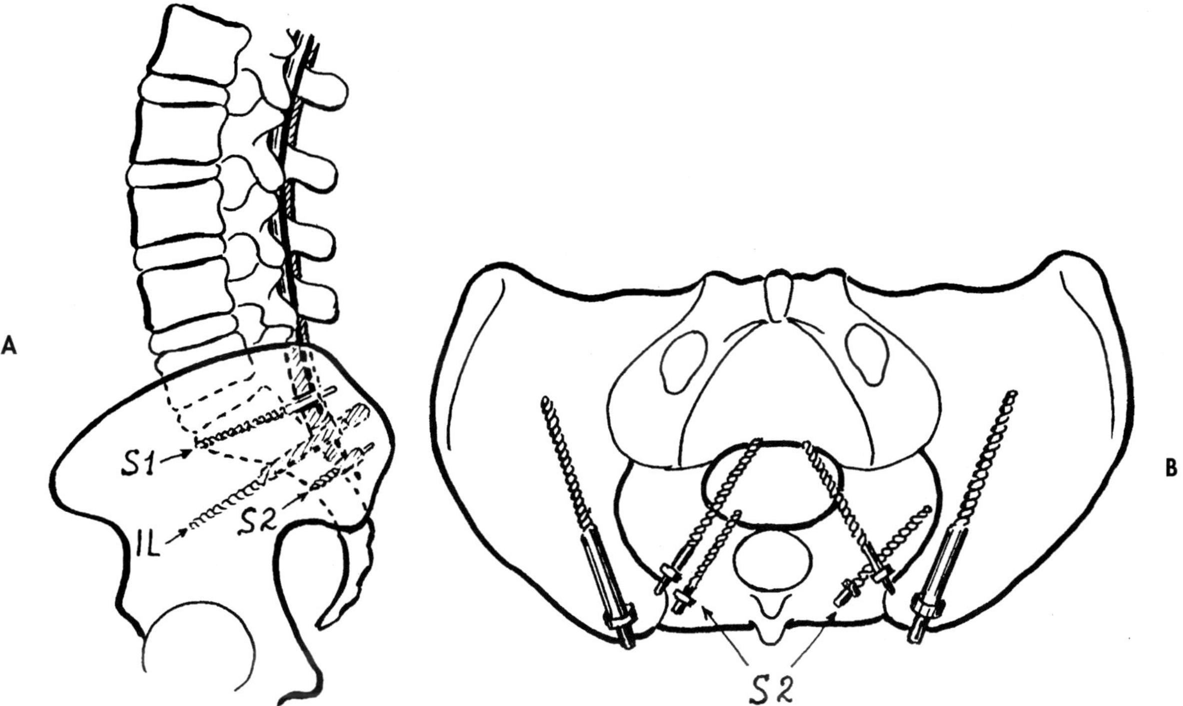


**FIGURE 47-1**

**A,** Lateral view of the lumbopelvic junction with S1 and S2 screws in the sacrum and iliac screw. **B,** Coronal top view of the pelvis with S1 screws, S2 screws in two variations, and iliac screws.

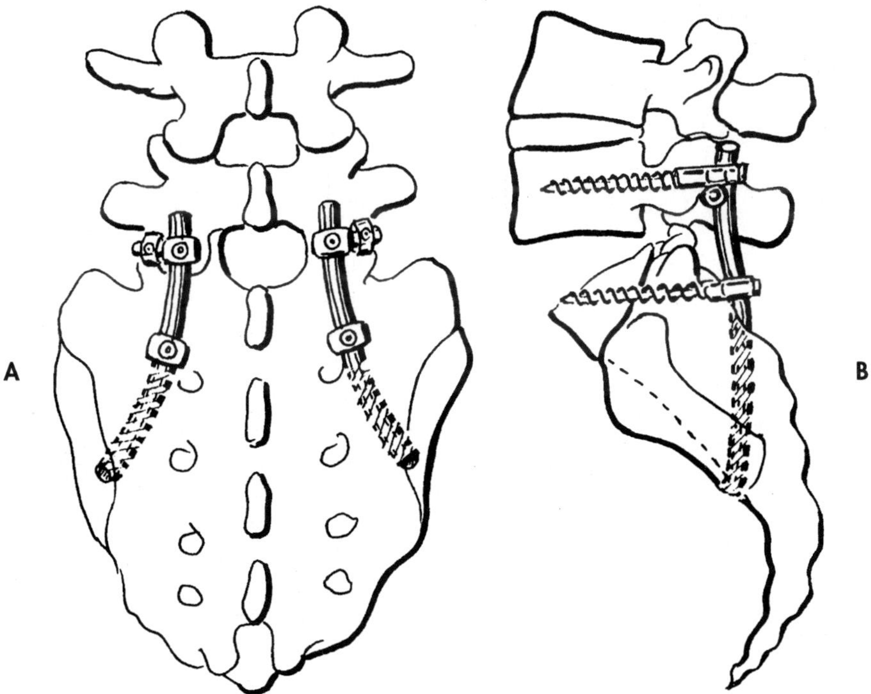


**FIGURE 47-2**

**A, B,** Anteroposterior and lateral views of the lumbosacral junction depicting the intrasacral rod placement.

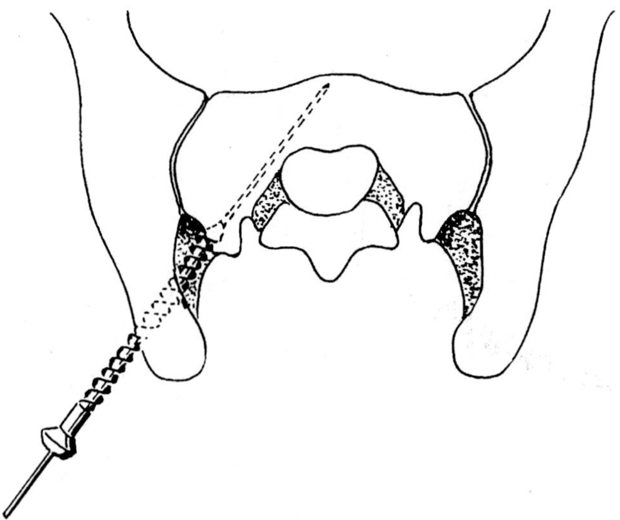

FIGURE 47-3

Coronal view of the S1 level with an iliosacral screw on its K-wire guide.

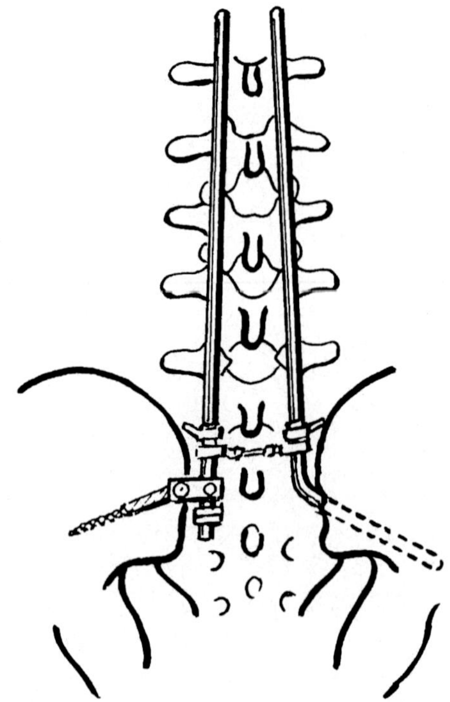

FIGURE 47-4

Posterior view of the lumbopelvic junction depicting insertion of a rod to the ilium on the right side, and a combination of iliac screw and S1 screw on the left side.

LUQUE FIXATION. Another variation, as described by Marchesi,[21] is the Luque method that involves use of a rod-sublaminar wire fixation system whereby the distal rods are driven through the pelvic wings with resulting bicortical purchase (Fig. 47-4, right side).[20] Use of this method is limited to minimally ambulatory children such as those with Duchenne's muscular dystrophy. For other uses, this fixation has proven inadequate over the long term because good axial stabilization can not be obtained. It is mentioned here because aspects of this technique could possibly be applied to revision surgery. Ideally, sublaminar wires should be considered as additional anchors between lumbar or thoracic foundation and the sacropelvic foundation to allow sagittal and coronal plane corrections.

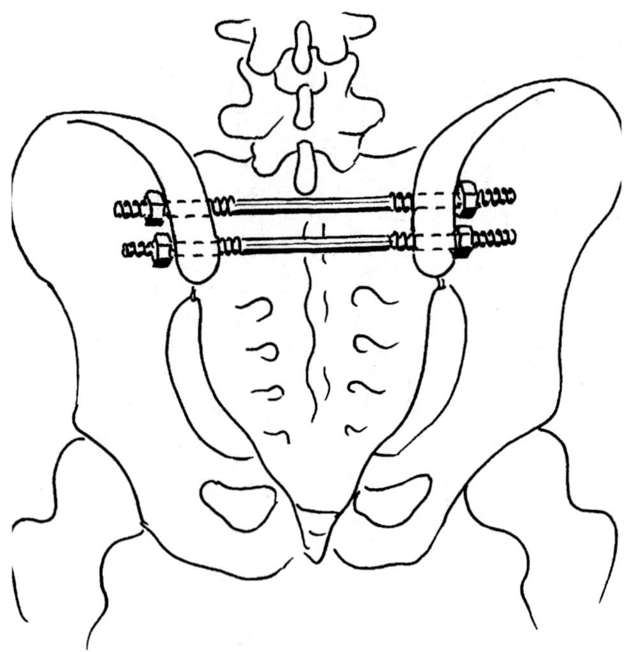

FIGURE 47-5

Sacral bars.

SACRAL SCREWS. Single pedicle screws to the sacrum can be used for instrumented short fusions such as L4-S1 and L5-S1 fusions. The large S1 pedicles can often accommodate 7- to 8-mm screws to the pelvis. If additional purchase is required, a second screw can be placed at the S2 level, directed laterally into the most lateral part of the sacral ala at an angle to the first screw. However, depending on the instrumentation system, this can result in difficulties with rod connection (Fig. 47-1).

SACRAL BLOCKS. Similar to Chopin block, sacral blocks are solid metal screw-rod connectors that accommodate two screws placed in a fixed orientation into the sacrum: one screw is directed anteriorly in the first sacral pedicle, the other screw is directed laterally in the sacral ala at 30 to 40 degrees of divergence, providing strong purchase and significant stability in its anchoring to the sacrum.[8] These devices allow easier attachment with the proximal lumbar rod. This construct results in a foundation that by itself is weaker due to its anchorage in one bone and the short distance between the points of entry. A stronger foundation should be sought for longer fusions.

INTRASACRAL RODS. This technique requires insertion of the rod intracortically within the sacrum itself, distal to the rod's connection with an S1 pedicle screw. The intraosseous extension of the rod, held by the S1 pedicle screw, provides superior fixation with excellent resistance to cantilever stresses and is buttressed by the iliac wings. This is considered one of the strongest anchors in the pelvis, and by itself placed bilaterally creates a foundation that can withstand longer constructs such as those needed for degenerative scoliosis (Fig. 47-2).

SACRAL COMPRESSION HOOKS. Sacral compression hooks are most commonly used to augment lumbosacral instrumentation in revision surgery in which there are not many options for anchors. They may be especially effective when a previous bone graft has been placed on the sacral laminae. Normal sacral laminae do not have sufficient strength to accommodate these hooks, whereas previously bone grafted laminae provide sufficient bone for adequate purchase. It should be a fall-back or secondary option to achieve a successful foundation in the sacrum.

ILIOSACRAL FIXATION TECHNIQUE. A thick cannulated "wood screw" type of screw is inserted over a K-wire guide placed from the iliac wing to the anterior aspect of the sacral promontory at the end plate of S1. The screw enters and crosses the iliac bone from posterolateral to anteromedial, inserted through a connector placed in the gap between the ilium and the sacrum, and continues into the sacrum, to the promontory anterior superior point, not crossing the midline. The connector is used as an anchor for longitudinal member going cranially to be used for fusion to the spine (Fig. 47-3).

SACRAL BARS. This type of fixation involves the use of bars spanning the sacrum from ilium to ilium. These bars have been used primarily for fixation of sacral fractures. They could also be used as alternative anchors within the pelvis and form the basis for a pelvic foundation in difficult reconstructive efforts such as severe fractures or after tumor resections of the sacrum (Fig. 47-5).

## POSTERIOR INSTRUMENTATION: BUILDING THE PELVIC FOUNDATION

The technical objective in revision spinopelvic surgery is to create two distinct foundations, one within the thoracic or lumbar spine and a second within the sacropelvis. Once the spinal and pelvic foundations are anchored, the vertical members are connected to the foundations forming a stable posterior construct. Foundations in the spine have been well-established by Asher.[3] A variation on the concept of foundation in the pelvis is presented: at least two but preferably more anchors in the pelvis should be established. These anchors are horizontally interconnected, to become a solid foundation. Vertical members are either connected or integrated into the foundation after the correction maneuver. The following

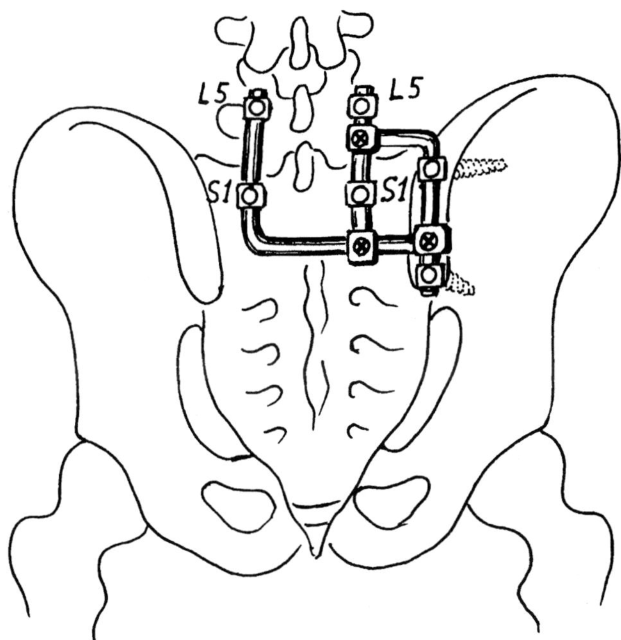


FIGURE 47-6

A foundation in the pelvis based on two L5 screws, two S1 screws and two unilateral iliac screws, all connected by rods with locking mechanism on one end.

are examples of different fixation combinations to achieve a solid foundation:

S1 and S2 screws combined with two iliac screws

L5 and S1 screws combined with two lilac screws with L5 and S1 screws on the opposite side (Fig. 47-6)

Bilateral S1 screws connected to two screws in the ilium on one side

It should be emphasized that the inclusion of the ilium in a sacropelvic foundation presupposes that a long fusion or disastrous instability of the lumbosacral articulation exists. We do not advocate the inclusion of the ilium in traditional L4-S1 fusions, because commonly accepted strategies suffice.

## ANTERIOR CONSTRUCTS

Anterior fusions of the lumbopelvic area are based on using segmental intracolumnar devices or extracolumnar constructs. Segmental implants, such as disk or vertebrectomy spacers, are placed within the confines of the vertebral column with a diameter less than the vertebral bodies. They act as load-sharing devices. The segmental devices require bone graft and/or bone substitutes for successful fusion. Polymethylmethacrylate (PMMA) or other cement can be used in cases in which the mechanical problem must be solved immediately, such as in metastatic disease. Extracolumnar longitudinal devices are very impractical due to the vital anatomy in front of the lumbosacral junction. Kostuik and others have suggested transvertebral screws. Anterior plates of various designs have been advocated but have not gained wide usage.

***Disk Space Implants.*** Implants such as the metal spacer provide structural support and undergo incorporation through porous ingrowth when placed within the disk space. In vivo however, the difference in modulus between bone and the implant becomes a problem; placed against cancellous bone, one achieves bone ingrowth at the expense of stability. Alternatively, placement against cortical bone provides stability but bony ingrowth may be sufficient. Development work continues with this and other biocompatible materials.

***Mesh Cages.*** Titanium mesh cages resist axial load and lateral displacement when placed against the vertebral endplate. When packed with cancellous bone graft, they incorporate well. These can be used in vertebrectomy as well as interbody fusions.

***Bone and Bone Substitute Struts.*** These implants provide short-term mechanical support until they are biologically incorporated into the fusion mass. They should be placed against the intact vertebral endplate in order to maintain disk height and to resist compression. If placed in contact with cancellous bone, collapse or telescoping of the implant can occur depending on the strength of the cancellous bone. Examples include autogenous, bicortical, tricortical iliac struts, and fibular and rib struts. Donor site morbidity and difficulty of harvest limit their use in longer reconstructions.

Allogenic bone grafts from the ilium, femoral shaft, fibula, tibia or calcar are an alternative to autogenous grafts. They have the advantage of no donor site morbidity, but variable biological incorporation, potential disease transmission, and brittleness raise concerns over their standard usage.

Synthetic materials of nonbiologic or nonhuman origin such as tricalcium phosphate or HA are being studied. Their short-term structural usefulness or ability for subsequent biologic incorporation and long-term support has not been proven. They are, however, readily available with minimal risk for disease transmission.

***Polymethylmethacrylate.*** PMMA is used primarily as adjunctive fixation with other instrumentation. As with disk space implants, little resistance to compressive load occurs when placed against cancellous bone. Also, as no bony ingrowth occurs, collapse is inevitable and should be confined to clinical situations that demand immediate stabilization with limited life expectancy. HA cements may offer an alternative to PMMA in the near future.

***Extracolumnar Constructs.*** In contrast to the segmental devices, extracolumnar construct fixation involves a spanning segment that lies outside the diameter of the vertebrae acting as an internal fixator. Although this method has been used as a base for distraction in the midlumbar spine and proximally, such constructs are not useful at L4-L5 and the lumbosacral junction for a variety of reasons. First, the soft bone of the sacrum offers poor fixation. Second, placement of this instrumentation at L4-L5 and L5-S1 next to the iliac vessels is both technically difficult and creates the risk of vascular erosion. Reports of rectal and ureteral injury also limit this application.

## 360-Degree Fusions

Circumferential fusions of the vertebral segment involve combining anterior and posterior instrumentation. The rationale for this treatment choice is based on the concept of Harms 20-80% rule.[14] Most of the load is transmitted through the anterior column.[13] As discussed earlier, it is known that the longer the fusion to the sacrum the higher the failure rate. Therefore, despite controversy in treatment, we suggest 360-degree instrumentation when fusion longer than L5-S1 is needed in the face of poor anterior column support, such as marked disk space collapse with gross instability of the vertebral segment, and in degenerative scoliosis.

## Anterior Versus Posterior Fusion

The question of anterior lumbar interbody fusion (ALIF) versus posterior lumbar interbody fusion (PLIF) has not been resolved.[25] PLIFs are technically demanding and carry the risk of several complications. Alternatively, ALIFs require a relatively large anterior approach with risks of compromising large vessels and other organs. Paramedian and lateral retroperitoneal approaches offer predictable exposure of the lumbosacral articulation without significant risk to the visceral structures. Video assisted techniques may further decrease the morbidity of the anterior approach to the lumbosacral junction.

Other technical aspects include variation in bone quality and bone-metal interface problems, with the obvious problem of anchoring screws in osteoporotic bone.[4]

## Balance Considerations

Adequate instrumentation of the spine requires maintenance of physiologic spinal contour and balance. Failure to maintain such alignment often results in cosmetically unattractive, painful, and functionally inadequate posture. In the sagittal plane, T1 should be centered over S1. The result of hypolordosis of the lumbar spine may be postural flat back syndrome.[19] With this altered alignment, the patient must stand with the upper body canted forward, or with hip and knee flexion if the upper body is held vertical. This often leads to development of poor posture, muscle fatigue, and axial spinal pain.

In the coronal plane, T1 must be centered over the sacrum. Deformity in this plane creates a functional limb length inequality, which is cosmetically unpleasant. The patient must align the shoulders over the pelvis.

The three-dimensional understanding of the spine and its sagittal balance is gaining momentum. Increasing numbers of surgeons are focusing on what Dubousset termed the "pelvic vertebra," that "vertebrates" between the femoral heads and the spine.[6] He discusses the balance of the spine with the pelvis while considering the pelvic balance over the lower limbs. This concept is important when positioning the patient for lumbosacropelvic fusion. Jackson illustrates that if one fuses in a limited lordotic position, one may end up with a sacrum that is more vertical with resuming hyperextended hips.[16] This certainly is not an ideal situation, especially in degenerative patients in whom hip pathology is present. Longer lumbar fusions require better control of the pelvis to prevent vertical sacrum and improved lumbar lordosis.

## FUTURE TRENDS

The role of bone morphogenic proteins (BMPs) will become more important in the near future.[23] BMP offers less extensive surgery by avoidance of the bone graft harvest. It may offer decreased reliance on solid internal constructs. In situ techniques with short-term external immobilization may result in more predictable fusion. However, the future management of lumbosacral disease may not involve fusion techniques. Strategies involving other types of mechanical solutions such as the Graf ligaments[10,11] or artificial disks are being investigated. The preliminary results await substantiation.

Unlike current spinal instrumentation, the rationale for Graf ligaments stems from the concept of restoring physiologic stability. They are designed to expedite the Kirkaldy-Willis cascade by allowing limited range of motion of the lumbar spine while restraining the unstable segment. The natural history of degenerative process in turn leads to stabilization of the motion segment.

Artificial disks are mechanical solutions that follow the path of the last two to three decades in orthopedics, namely arthroplasty instead of arthrodesis.[5] We await results of work in this area, as preliminary work is too inferential to allow analysis.

## CONCLUSION

Lumbosacral fusion, in particular revision fusion, remains a vexing problem, often with controversial indications and technically difficult fixation techniques. Coupled with issues of bone quality, bone graft technique, and creation of abnormal physiologic stresses, the problem becomes even more daunting. The use of stable foundations within the pelvis can only serve to maintain initial surgical correction to a greater degree and decrease the incidence of failed fusions over the long term. Eventually, the 360-degree fusion may assume a more important role, especially in revision salvage procedures. Ultimately, other mechanical or even nonmechanical advances may replace all fusions.

## REFERENCES


1. Allen BL, Ferguson RL: The Galveston technique for L rod instrumentation of the scoliotic spine, *Spine.* 7:276-284, 1982.
2. Argenson C: Baeses anatomique *et* experimentales de la mise en place d'une vis d'osteosynthese au nivean de la premiere vertebrae sacree, *Surg Radiol Anat* 13: 133-137. 1991.
3. Asher MA, Strippgen WE, Heinig CF, et al: Isola spinal implant system, *Semin Spine Surg* 4:175-192, 1992.
4. Coe JD, Warden KE, Herzig MA, et al: Influence of bone mineral density on the fixation of the thoracolumbar implants, *Spine* 15:902-907, 1988.
5. David T: *Lumbosacral disc prosthesies.* In Margulies JY, Floman Y, Farcy J-PC, Neuwirth MG, editors: *Lumbosacral and spinopelvic fixation.* Philadelphia, 1996, Lippincon-Raven 67:881-887.
6. Dubousset J: The pelvic vertebra—3D concept for the physiopathology classification and management of pelvic obliquities. Zielke Farewell Meeting. 1989; Bad Wildungen, Germany.
7. Esses SI, Natout N, Kip P: Posterior interbody arthrodesis with a fibular strut graft in spondylolisthesis, *J Bone Joint Surg Am* 77(2):72-76, 1995.
8. Farcy J-PC, Roye DP, Weidenbaum M: Cotrel-Doubousset instrumentation technique for revision of failed lumbosacral fusion, *Bull Hosp Joint Disord Orthop Inst* 47:112, 1987.
9. Farcy W, Rawlins BA, Glassman SD: Technique and results of fixation to the sacrum with iliosacral screws, *Spine* 17:190-195, 1992.
10. Gardner AD: *An alternative concept in the surgical manage-*

*ment of lumbar degenerative disc disease-flexible stabilization.* In Margulies JY, Floman Y, Farcy J-PC, Neuwirth MG, editors: *Lumbosacral and spinopelvic fixation.* Philadelphia, 1996, Lippincott-Raven 68:889-905.

11. Graf H: Lumbar instability surgical treatment without fusion: soft tissue stabilization, *Rachis* 4(2):123-137, 1992.
12. Grob D, Scheier HJG, Dvorak J, et al: Circumferential fusion of the lumbar and lumbosacral spine, *Arch Orthop Thauma Surg* 111:20-25, 1991.
13. Haher IR, Felmly WT, Baruch H, et al: The contribution of the three columns of the spine to rotational stability: a biomechanical model, *Spine* 14:663, 1989.
14. Harms J: Screw-threaded rod system in spinal fusion surgery, *Spine: State of the Art Reviews* 6:541, 1992.
15. Jackson R, Ebelene DK, McManus AC: The sacro iliac buttress and new methods for conection with CD pedicle instrumentation. In Proceedings of the 8th International Congress of CDI. 135-139. Montpellier, 1991, Sauramps.
16. Jackson RP: *Surgical spinal alignment and positioning of surgery.* In Margulies JY, Aebi M, Farcy J-PC, editors: *Revision spine surgery.* In press Mosby 1998, Philadelphia.
17. Jacobs RR, Montesano PX, Jackson RP: Enhancement of lumbar spine fusion by use of translaminar facet joint screws, *Spine* 14:12-15, 1989.
18. Kirkaldy-Willis WE, Farfan HF: Instability of the lumbar spine, *Clin Orthop* 165:110-123, 1982.
19. Lagrone MO, Bradford DS, Moe JL, et al: Treatment of symptomatic flat back after spinal fusion, *J Bone Joint Surg Am* 70:569, 1988.
20. Luque ER: Segmental spinal instrumentation for correction of scoliosis, *Clin Orthop* 163:192, 1982.
21. Marchesi D, Arlet V, Sticker U, Aebi M: Modification of the original Luque technique in the treatment of Duchenne's neuromuscular scoliosis, *J Pediat Orthop* 17:743-749, 1997.
22. Margulies JY, Kohler-Ekstrand C: Revision of fusion from spine to pelvis. 2nd European Consensus Conference. Cortina, Italy. Jan 1998.
23. Morone M, Boden S: Experimental posterolateral lumbar spinal fusion with a demineralized bone matrix gel, *Spine* 23(2):159-167, 1998.
24. Pennal GF, McDonald GA, Dale GG: A method of spinal fusion using internal fixation, *Clin Orthop* 35: 86-94, 1964.
25. Steffee AD, Sitkowski DJ: Posterior lumbar interbody fusion and plates, *Clin Orthop* 227:99, 1988.

# 48

# SELECTION OF SPINAL INSTRUMENTATION

Geoffrey Stewart, M.D.
Paul C. McAfee, M.D.



The breadth of spinal instrumentation has been rapidly expanding in recent years, providing the spine surgeon with increased options in the treatment of spinal instability and deformity. The first reported use of spinal instrumentation was in 1891, when Hadra reported the use of wire for stabilization of the cervical spine.[11] In 1910, Lang reported using rods wired to the posterior elements as a means of spinal stabilization.[20] The use of transpedicular spinal instrumentation was first described in the 1940s.[18,25] Development of the Harrington rod system began in 1953, as a means to provide correction and stabilization of the spine in children with neuromuscular scoliosis from polio,[12] and use of the instrumentation was reported in 1960.[13] Over the ensuing decades, experience with these techniques and refinements to these systems has led to a wide variety of instrumentation systems. The goal of spinal instrumentation remains the same: to provide for correction of spinal deformity, to enhance the stability of the spine, and to increase the rate of bony fusion.

Selection of spinal instrumentation is based on the anatomic location, surgical approach, spinal pathology, and biomechanical requirements. In revision surgery, an additional consideration is alteration of the spinal anatomy by previous surgical procedures.

## CERVICAL SPINE

### Posterior Cervical Instrumentation

Posterior cervical fusion is performed for a wide variety of cervical pathologies. The classic approach to instability has been interspinous wiring, which requires intact posterior elements. The most simple technique, a single interspinous loop as described by Rogers in 1942,[32] is still used by some surgeons in the subaxial spine. At the C1-C2 level, the sublaminar techniques of Brooks and Gallie are most commonly employed.

The triple-wire strut technique, as introduced by Bohlman, avoids the risk of sublaminar wire passage, and provides flexural and torsional stiffness superior to Roger's wiring or the use of sublaminar wires.[22] Weiland and McAfee reported fusion rates of 100% in subaxial arthrodeses, and 98% in occipitocervical or atlantoaxial arthrodeses using this technique.[37] Farey et al reported a fusion rate of 100% using this technique in nineteen patients with a symptomatic pseudarthrosis after a failed anterior cervical arthrodesis (Fig. 48-1).[8]

In recent years, braided multistrand cables have become available as a substitute for stainless steel wire. Braided cables are reportedly more flexible and stronger than monofilament wire. Weiss et al demonstrated in vitro that multistrand cables of stainless steel, titanium, and polyethylene offered superior fatigue resistance and stiffness when compared to monofilament stainless steel wire.[38] An additional benefit is that titanium and polyethylene are compatible with magnetic resonance imaging. Some surgeons remain concerned that multifilament constructs may generate

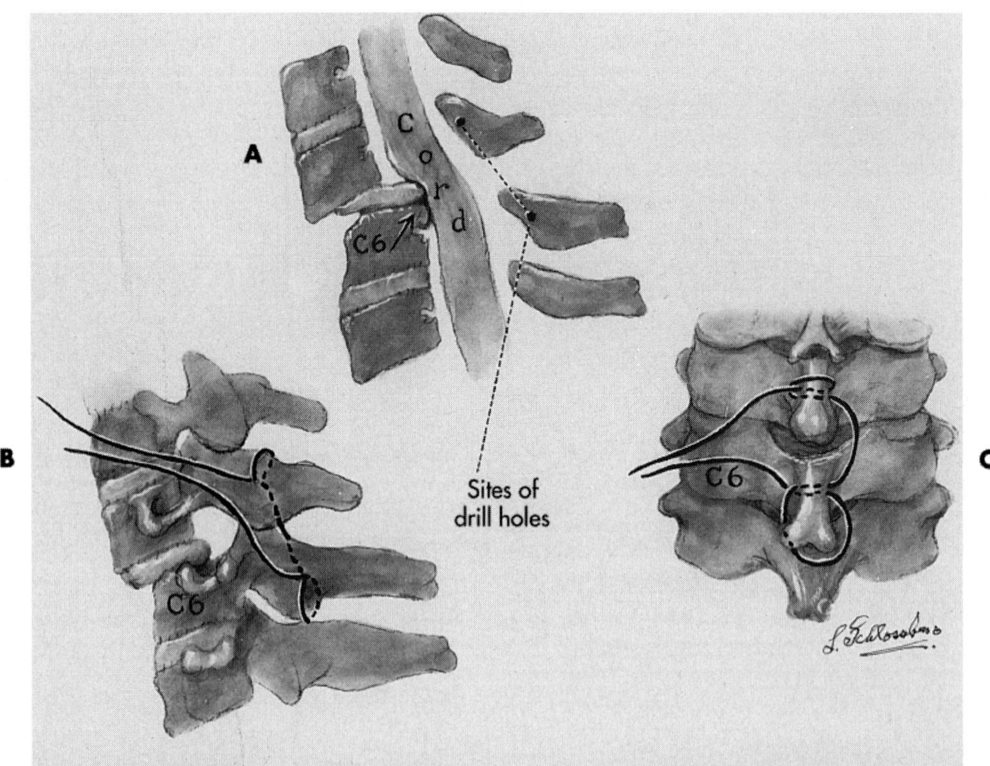


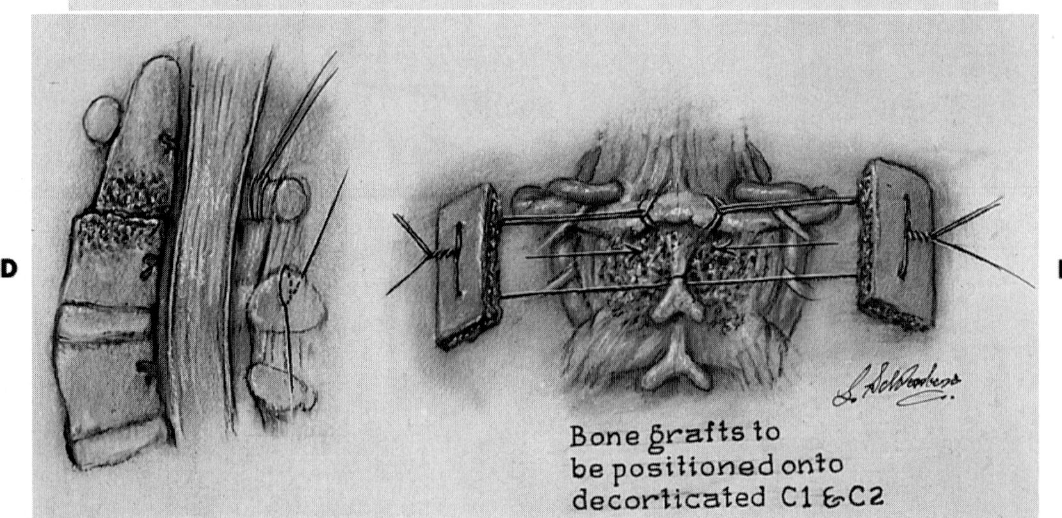


**FIGURE 48-1**

Bohlman's triple-wire method of cervical fixation. **A, B, C,** Demonstration of passage of the midline tethering wire in the case of a C5-C6 dislocation. As shown in B and C, 20-gauge wire is passed through a drill hole in the base of the spinous process, then looped over the spinous process and again passed through the hole, then into and around the next spinous process. After reduction of the dislocation and tightening of the midline wire, initial stability should be evident. Bilateral corticocancellous strut grafts are then wired to the laminae and spinous processes using 22-gauge wires passed through the same drill holes. **D, E,** Technique applied to C1-C2 fusion showing placement of corticocancellous iliac strut grafts. The addition of wired strut grafts adds to rotational stability and increases the speed of fusion due to the compressive effect of the cancellous bone against the vertebrae.

wear debris, and are more difficult to reproducibly tighten than monofilament wire.

Posterior cervical stabilization by the use of plates was reported by Roy-Camille in 1972, and the popularity of this technique has expanded rapidly in recent years, as have the number of instrumentation systems available for this purpose (e.g., Axis plates, Roy-Camille plates, AO reconstruction plates, Haid plates) (Fig. 48-2). The standard technique has been described in detail, and generally involves screw fixation into the

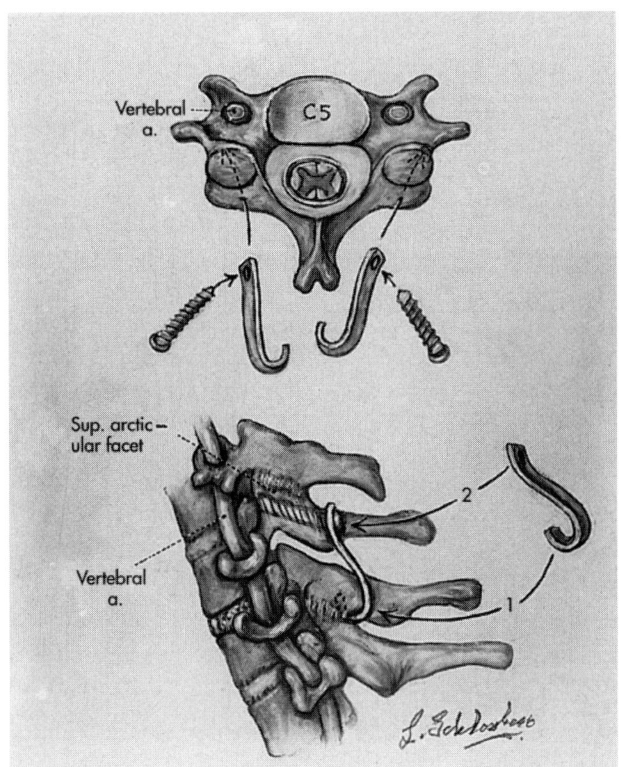


FIGURE 48-2

The Magerl hook plate technique for cervical stabilization. After reduction, the hook is secured under the lamina of the inferior vertebrae, and the upper aspect of the plate fastened by a lateral mass screw.

lateral masses of the vertebrae. The use of screw-plate systems offers a number of advantages over interspinous wiring, especially in the case of previous posterior decompression. The use of lateral mass plates does not require intact laminae or spinous processes, and thus may represent the only posterior instrumentation choice in the treatment of postlaminectomy instability or in cases of fracture of the posterior elements. Plating techniques provide greater initial stability than wiring techniques, and may eliminate or minimize the need for adjunctive postoperative immobilization. Posterior plate constructs have been shown by some to have significantly greater torsional, flexural, and extension stiffness than wire or cable constructs or anterior plates in vitro (Fig. 48-3).[36,38]

In a calf spine model of cervical instability, Kotani et al found a similar stiffness with Bohlman's triple-wire technique and posterior AO plate fixation; anterior plating methods were found to provide less stability than posterior constructs under axial, torsional, and flexural loading conditions.[19] The use of transpedicular instrumentation to achieve three-column fixation was found to offer increased stability over conventional fixation techniques.

Lowery et al reported on the use of posterior cervical articular pillar plating in the treatment of symptomatic anterior cervical pseudarthrosis.[21] A solid fusion was obtained in 16 of 17 patients treated with a posterior arthrodesis and plating, versus 9 of 20 patients treated with anterior revision and anterior plating. Hardware failure occurred in 9 of the 20 anterior revisions (45%) versus 1 of the 17 patients treated with posterior plate fixation.

The major disadvantage of posterior screw plate systems is the potential for injury of the vertebral artery, cervical nerve roots, or spinal cord during the placement of the screws. A thorough understanding of the cervical anatomy and proper screw insertion techniques is vital to avoid iatrogenic injuries. The reported incidence of complications has been lower than one might predict from anatomic considerations. Heller et al reported on 78 consecutive cases of lateral mass plating, with placement of 654 screws.[14] Complication rates per screw were nerve root injury 0.6%, facet violations 0.2%, and vertebral artery injury 0%. There was loosening or avulsion of 1.6% of screws.

A number of authors have reported a significant incidence of screw loosening. The Magerl technique of screw placement (parallel to the superior articular surface of the lateral mass in the sagittal plane) accommodates a longer screw than the Roy-Camille technique (perpendicular to the posterior cortex of the lateral mass in the sagittal plane). Lateral mass plating using the Magerl technique has been shown to result in a stronger, stiffer construct, with a higher moment to failure.[5,26,27]

## ANTERIOR CERVICAL INSTRUMENTATION

Anterior plate fixation of the cervical spine was first described by Orozco and Llovet in 1970.[30] The proposed benefits of the anterior approach are the ability to decompress the anterior spinal cord directly, the ability to apply bone graft under compression to enhance fusion, and the ability to restore and maintain spinal alignment. Most surgeons feel the anterior approach to the cervical spine is easier and less traumatic than a posterior approach, which requires stripping of the paraspinous musculature.

A number of plate systems are available for use on the anterior cervical spine. Desirable features include a low-profile construct that does not significantly disrupt the soft tissues, a means of locking the screw to the plate to prevent screw back-out, construction of titanium to allow magnetic resonance imaging, and sufficient rigidity to minimize the need for postoperative immobilization. Additionally, the system should be easy to use and versatile enough to accommodate a wide variety of applications.

Numerous biomechanical studies have examined the relative stability provided by anterior plate fixation

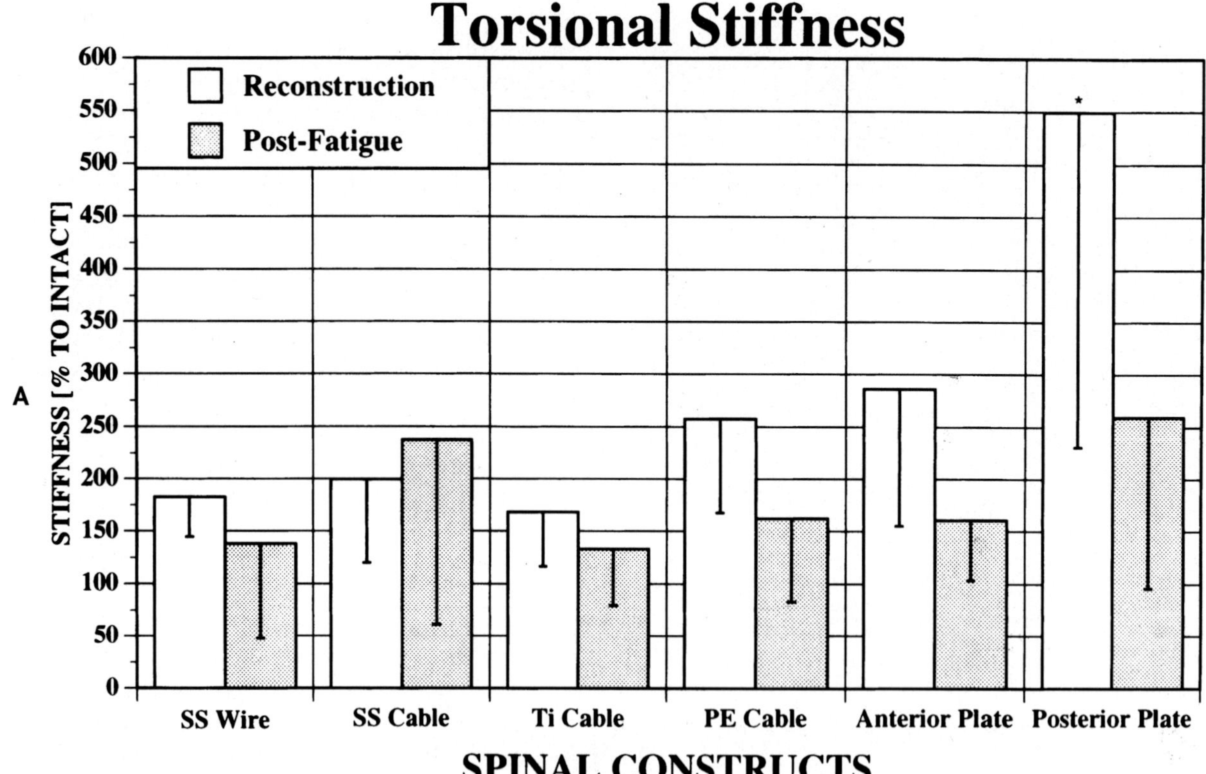


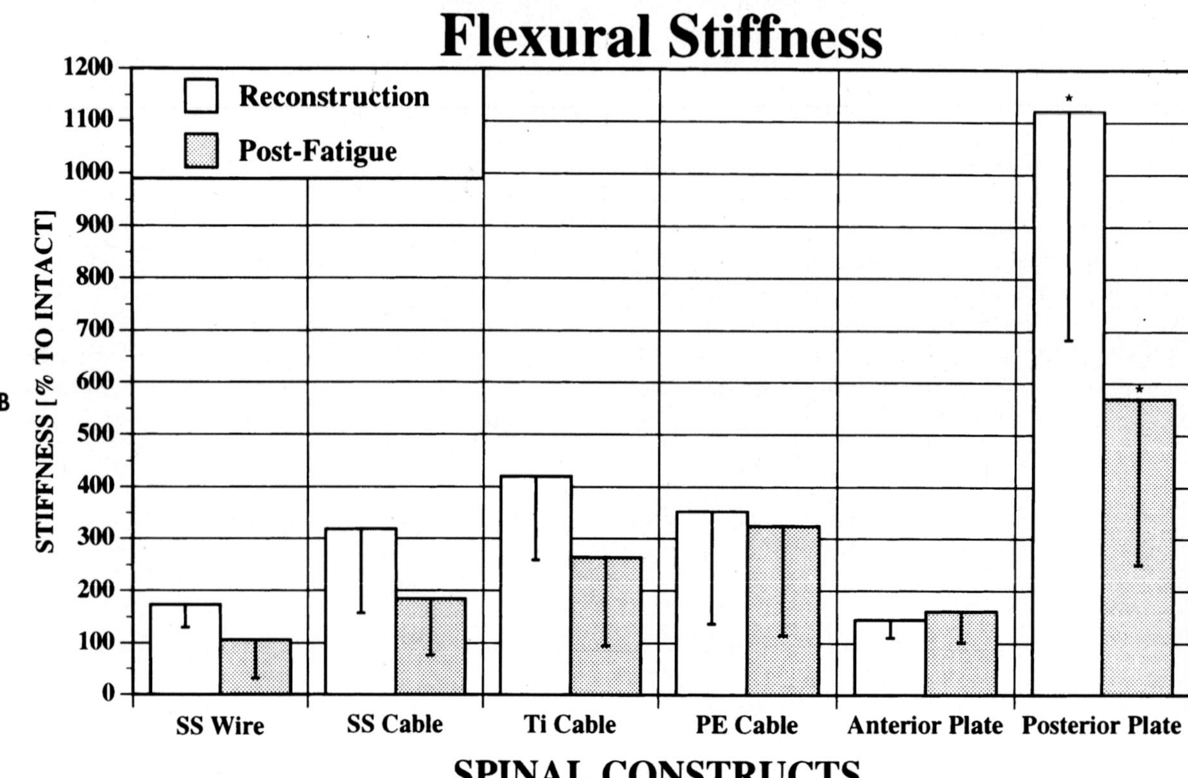


Figure 48-3

In vitro biomechanical comparison of cervical spine reconstruction techniques in an unstable calf spine model. **A, B,** Torsional and flexural stiffness of reconstruction with stainless steel wire, braided stainless cable, titanium cable, polyethylene cable, anterior plate fixation, and posterior plate fixation. Posterior plate fixation results in a significantly stiffer construct.

and posterior instrumentation techniques in models of cervical instability. In in vitro and ex vivo models of posterior ligamentous disruption or complete discoligamentous injuries, anterior plate fixation has been shown to provide suboptimal stabilization compared to standard posterior fixation techniques.[19,26,36,38] This suggests that in cases of significant posterior instability or global instability, anterior plate fixation should be supplemented by posterior fixation or rigid external immobilization (Fig. 48-4).

Aebi et al analyzed a series of 86 patients treated with anterior arthrodesis and Orozco plate fixation for cervical spine trauma.[1] Patients with three-column injuries were maintained in a Plastizote collar for six weeks postoperatively. This series included 64 patients who had predominantly posterior lesions, either discoligamentous or osteoligamentous. One patient with bilateral facet subluxation suffered a loss of reduction with loosening of the plate 10 days postoperatively; this complication was attributed to undersizing of the

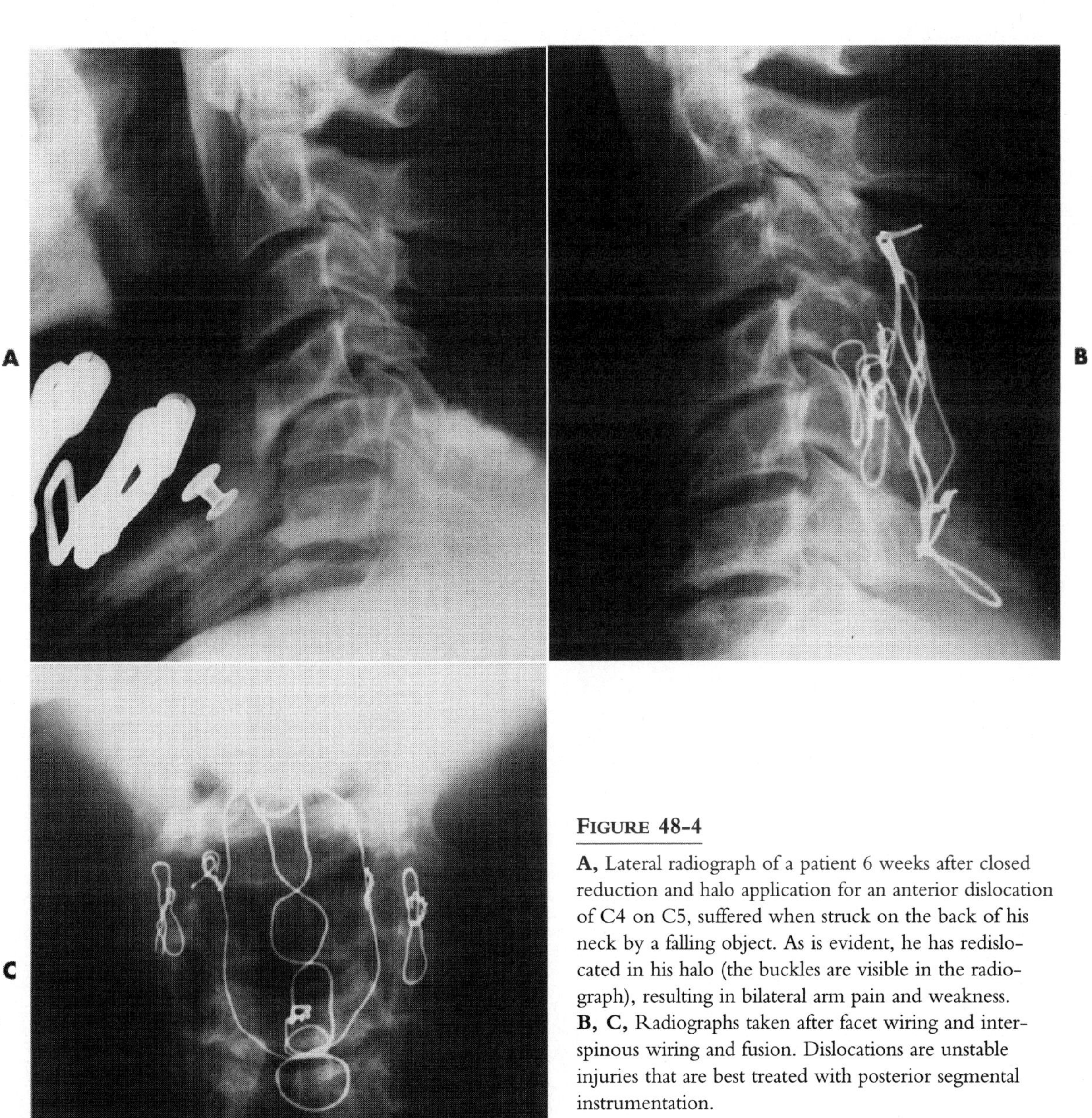


FIGURE 48-4

**A,** Lateral radiograph of a patient 6 weeks after closed reduction and halo application for an anterior dislocation of C4 on C5, suffered when struck on the back of his neck by a falling object. As is evident, he has redislocated in his halo (the buckles are visible in the radiograph), resulting in bilateral arm pain and weakness. **B, C,** Radiographs taken after facet wiring and interspinous wiring and fusion. Dislocations are unstable injuries that are best treated with posterior segmental instrumentation.

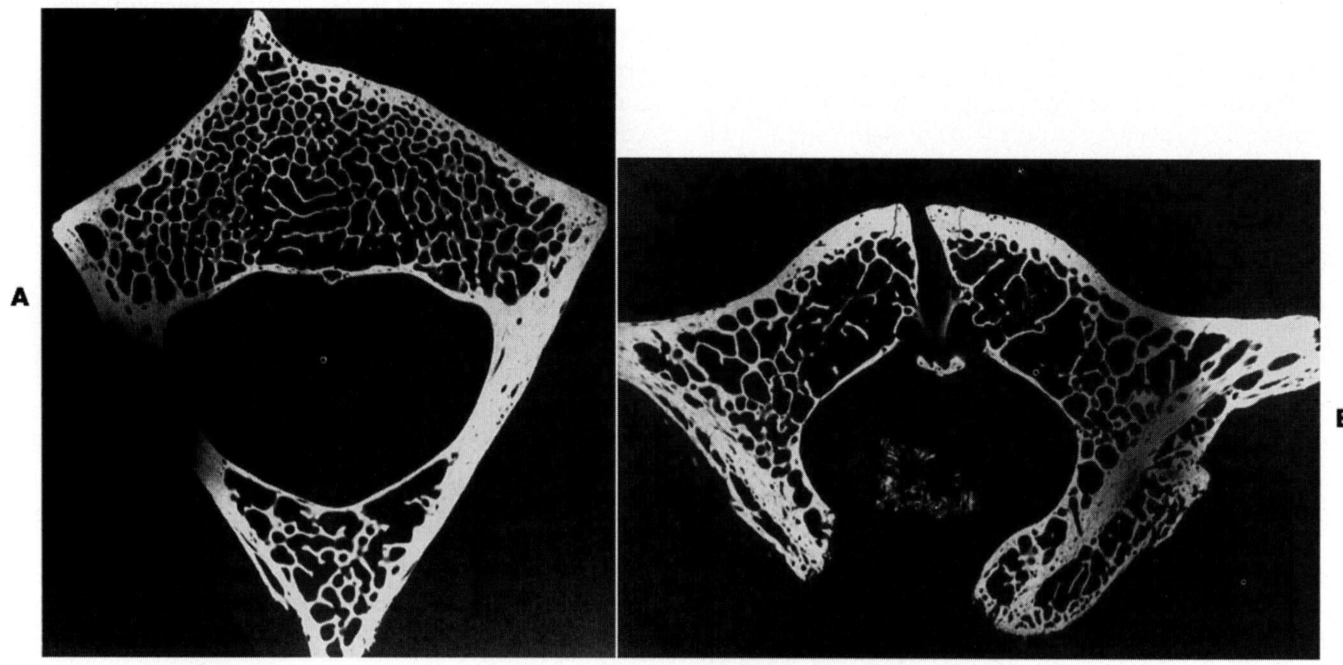


EX VIVO CANINE STUDY

FLEXURAL + AXIAL STRAIN ( % )

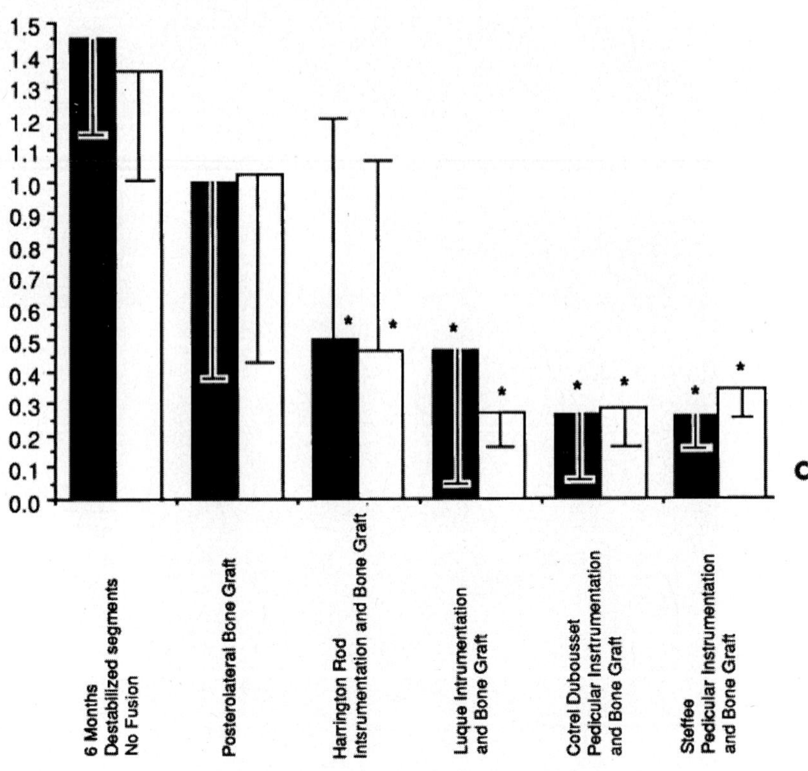


SPINAL CONSTRUCT

■ Longitudinal strain measured at L5-L6 with flexural loading

□ Longitudinal strain measured at L5-L6 with axial compressive loading

* P<.05 Significantly Different from Posterolateral Bone Graft

FIGURE 48-5

Following instrumented posterolateral fusion, canine vertebrae develop osteoporosis. **A,** The control L3 vertebra in a dog; **B,** the fused L5 level in the same dog following posterolateral fusion using Steffee pedicular instrumentation. The microradiograph shows decreased volumetric density and decreased mean trabecular diameter of the bone (localized osteoporosis). **C,** Summary of the flexural and axial strains across the fused segments in six groups of dogs. The more stable and rigid the instrumentation, the greater the device-related osteoporosis. Such osteoporosis has not been shown clinically to be deleterious; in fact, the surgeon should employ as rigid an implant as possible to maximize the likelihood of achieving a successful fusion.

bone graft. They concluded that in spite of experimental stability data, anterior plate fixation is a reliable treatment for posterior cervical lesions.

Ripa et al reviewed 92 patients treated with anterior decompression and arthrodesis with ASIF plate fixation for instability after trauma.[31] Most patients had three-column injuries. Patients were immobilized postoperatively with a SOMI orthosis for an average of three months. One patient suffered loss of spinal alignment (defined as translation <2.5 mm) postoperatively, and four patients developed screw loosening, one of which required screw removal. They report a fusion rate of 98.9%, and conclude that anterior plate stabilization of the unstable cervical spine is safe and effective.

## THORACOLUMBAR SPINE

### POSTERIOR INSTRUMENTATION

Posterior stabilization of the thoracolumbar spine is the traditional approach to spinal pathology. The use of posterior spinal instrumentation actually preceded

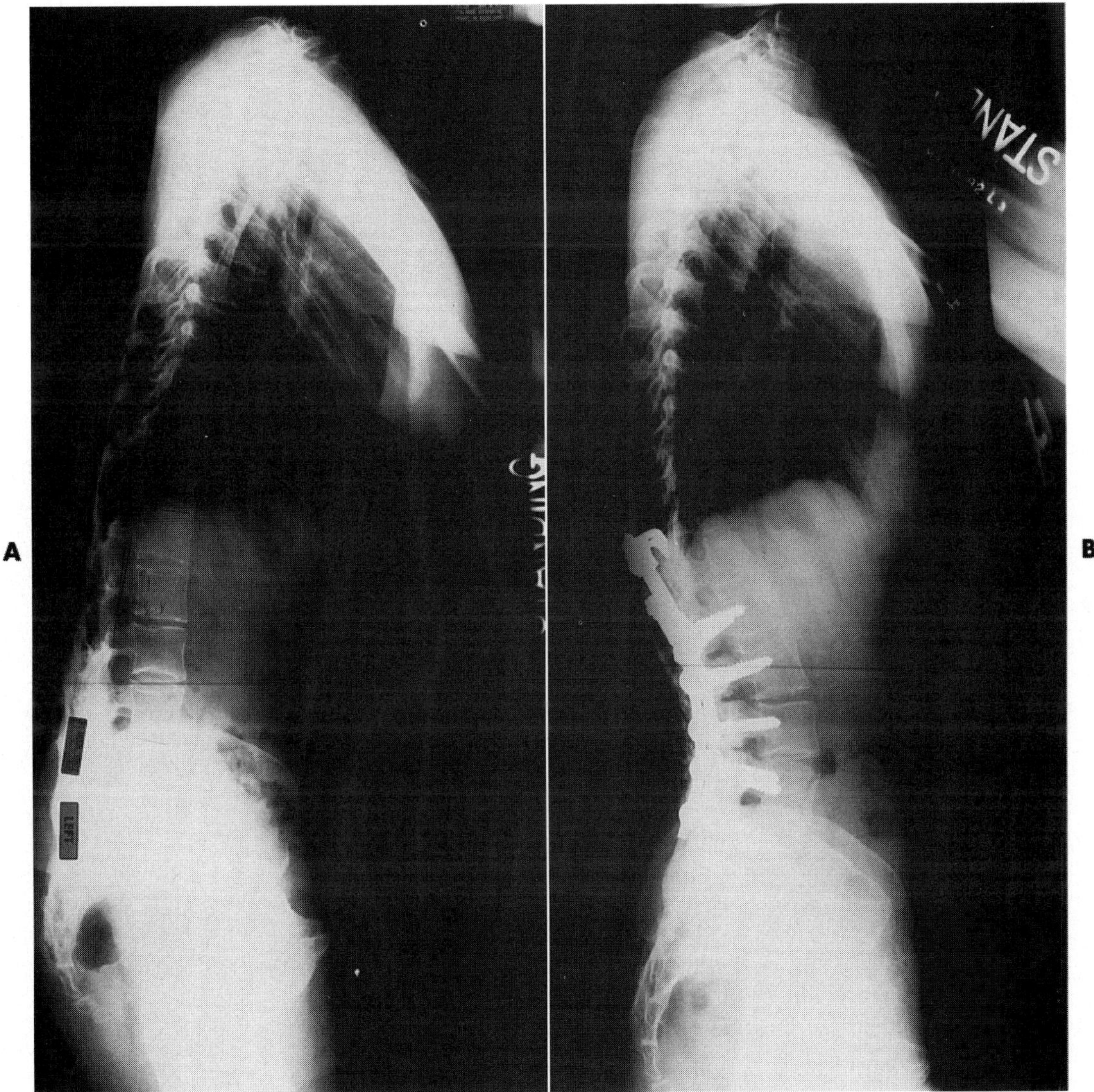


**FIGURE 48-6**

A major limitation of Harrington instrumentation is the inability to adequately control sagittal alignment. **A,** The lateral radiograph of a 42-year-old woman who had undergone posterior Harrington distraction instrumentation in the treatment of scoliosis. She had progressive back pain and the inability to stand fully erect. The radiograph demonstrates "flat back" with 4 degrees of kyphosis from L1 to L4. **B,** She underwent posterior spinal osteotomies at 3 levels, and fusion with segmental instrumentation incorporating variable angle transpedicular screws. She improved to 40 degrees of lumbar lordosis, and has had complete relief of her back pain and a marked improvement in her ability to stand erect.

spinal fusion as a means to treat instability. Today, instrumented spinal fusion is widely performed to treat deformities of the spine, degenerative conditions, postsurgical instability, and instability due to trauma.

The use of rigid spinal instrumentation has been shown by a number of authors to increase the rate of fusion in spinal arthrodesis, in both animal models and clinical studies. Additionally, rigid spinal instrumentation has been demonstrated to result in more rigid fusion mass in animal studies.[23] Device-related osteoporosis has been demonstrated in animal studies, but this has not been shown to be clinically deleterious (Fig. 48-5). Zdeblick, in a prospective, randomized study of patients undergoing lumbar or lumbosacral fusion for degenerative conditions, demonstrated a significantly higher rate of fusion and improved clinical outcome in patients treated with rigid instrumentation compared to semirigid instrumentation or noninstrumented arthrodesis.[42]

## Harrington Instrumentation

The Harrington system was the first modern spinal instrumentation system. Its first applications were for the treatment of scoliosis; however, the techniques were soon applied to the treatment of spinal trauma. Experience with the Harrington system provided the knowledge base that has served as the basis for development of the variety of instrumentation systems available today.

The Harrington instrumentation is composed of multiple hooks designed to fix to the posterior elements of the spine, and $\frac{1}{4}$-inch distraction rods. Compression rods are available in $\frac{1}{8}$ and $\frac{3}{16}$ inch. The factor that limits the force that can be applied through the system is the strength of the bone-hook interface. The system is limited by its inability to provide adequate rotational control of the instrumented spinal segments, and the inability to adequately maintain or restore sagittal alignment of the spine (Fig. 48-6). Contouring of the distraction rods facilitates maintenance of lumbar lordosis, and supplemental segmental wires added to the rods improve rotational stability and spinal stability.[24]

Harrington distraction systems tend to fail by dislodgment at the rod-hook junction, by fracture of the rod at the ratchet junction, or by failure of the lamina. The compression rods tend to fail by failure of hook attachment to bone (Fig. 48-7).

## Segmental Wiring

Luque instrumentation was introduced in the 1970s as a more rigid system for scoliosis. The instrumentation was later applied to the treatment of fractures. The system involves the use of contoured L-shaped rods (available in $\frac{1}{4}$- and $\frac{3}{16}$-inch diameters), which are attached to the spine by means of sublaminar wires (16 or 18 gauge). Segmental attachment to the vertebrae provides for increased rigidity and allows for increased control over sagittal alignment, notably maintenance of lordosis. However, the system provides little stability in the axial plane, limiting the surgeon's ability to attain or maintain distraction.[24,29]

As a means to combine the axial control of Harrington instrumentation with the rotational control and sagittal correction of sublaminar wiring, a number of surgeons began to combine the use of sublaminar wires with the Harrington rod. This provided for correction of deformity and maintenance of height through distraction, coupled with enhanced sagittal plane correction and rigidity of construct by the addition of segmental fixation.[34,35,41] This construct was shown to have superior axial load and flexion rigidity (Fig. 48-8).[24,28,29,39]

A major disadvantage of the system is the need for the

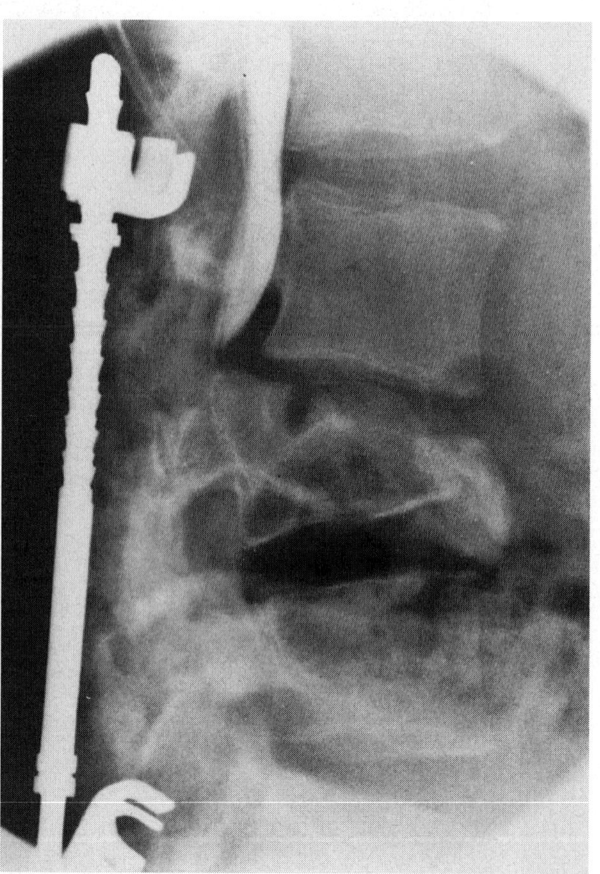

**FIGURE 48-7**

Failure of Harrington instrumentation in a fracture dislocation of L3 on L4. The construct has failed by dislodgment of the rod-hook junction, resulting in recurrence of deformity and a complete myelographic block at L3-L4. Distraction instrumentation requires intact ligaments for stability. Reliable stabilization of lumbar fracture-dislocations is best achieved with segmental transpedicular instrumentation. A patient with an incomplete neurologic deficit following stabilization may require a secondary anterior decompression to optimize neurologic recovery.

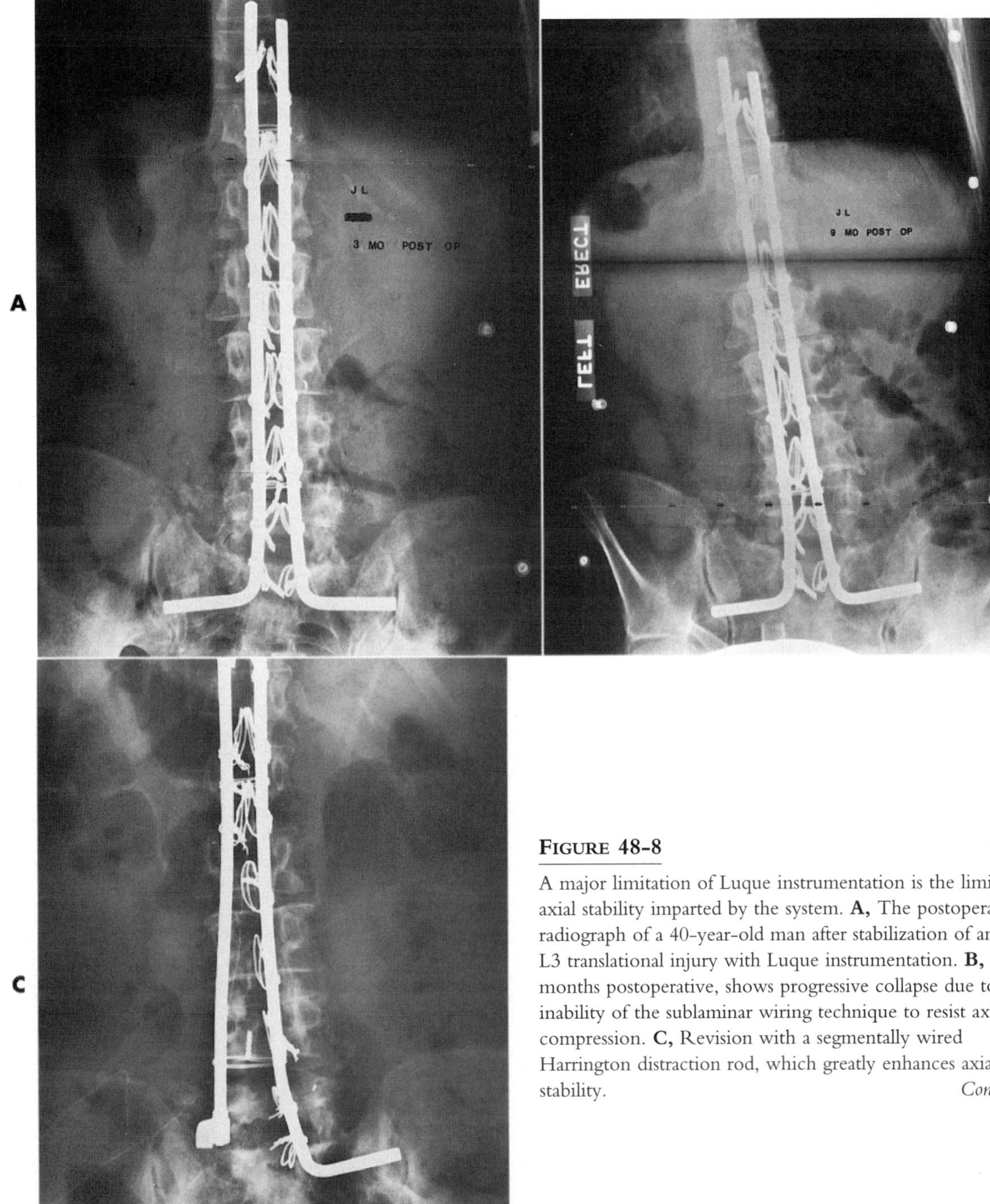


FIGURE 48-8

A major limitation of Luque instrumentation is the limited axial stability imparted by the system. **A,** The postoperative radiograph of a 40-year-old man after stabilization of an L2-L3 translational injury with Luque instrumentation. **B,** At 9 months postoperative, shows progressive collapse due to the inability of the sublaminar wiring technique to resist axial compression. **C,** Revision with a segmentally wired Harrington distraction rod, which greatly enhances axial stability. *Continued*

sublaminar passage of wires, which is associated with a high incidence of iatrogenic neurologic injuries.[15,17,40]

The Wisconsin instrumentation evolved as a means to gain segmental fixation coupled to a distraction rod, without the need for sublaminar wire passage. The instrumentation combines a contoured, square-ended distraction rod with a C-shaped Luque rod of $\frac{3}{16}$-inch diameter. The spinous processes are wired to the rod using 18-gauge wire attached through a button. The system has biomechanical properties similar to the Luque system.[3,24]

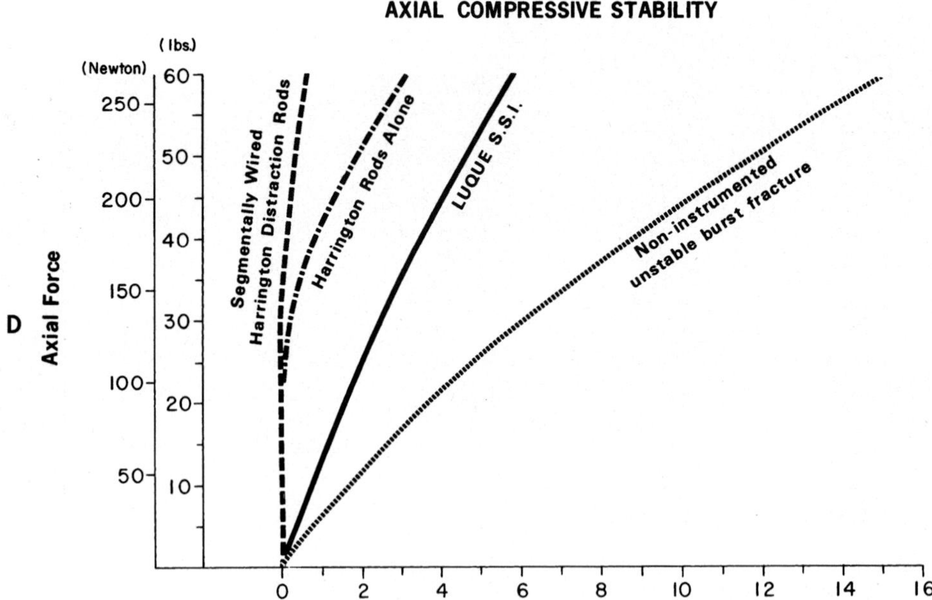


FIGURE 48-8, CONT'D

D, The relative axial stability of Harrington and Luque constructs in experimentally produced translational injuries in human cadaveric spinal segments.

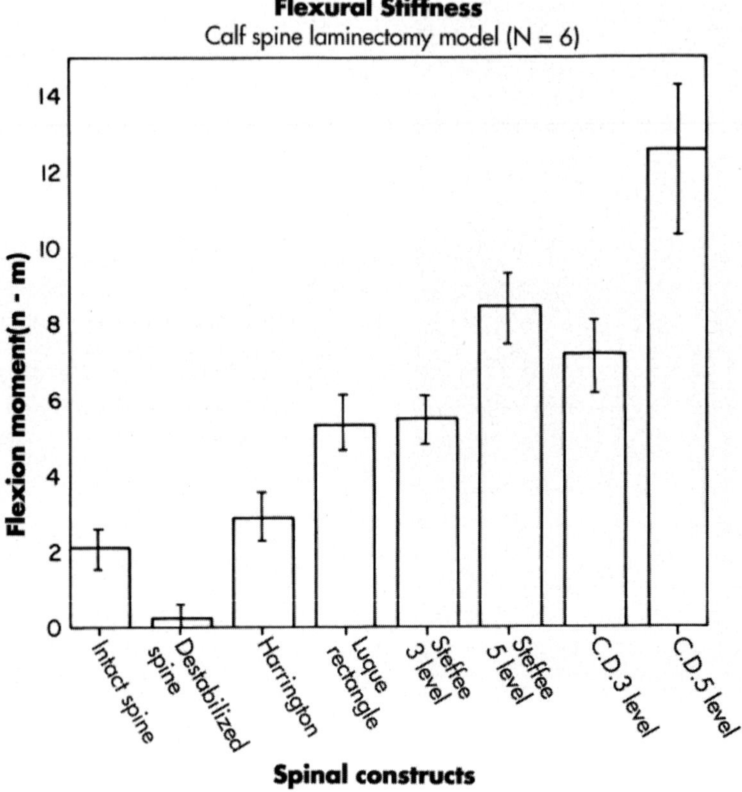


FIGURE 48-9

Flexural stiffness of instrumentation constructs in an unstable calf spine model demonstrates that CD and Steffee transpedicular systems offer a significant increase in flexural stability compared to traditional Harrington and Luque implants. Axial and torsional stability are similarly greater with segmental transpedicular instrumentation.

### RIGID SEGMENTAL INSTRUMENTATION

The Cotrel-Dubousset (CD) instrumentation system, was introduced in 1984.[6] It was one of the first rigid, multisegmental spinal fixation systems. A number of similar systems, incorporating these components and principles, have since become available. The CD system will be discussed here as an example of these rigid, segmental systems.

The goal of the instrumentation system is to provide three-dimensional correction of spinal deformity, as well as rigid immobilization, thus minimizing the need for adjunctive postoperative immobilization. CD instrumentation contains three basic elements: implants for vertebral fixation (hooks and screws), rods (available in 5 mm and 7 mm), and devices for transverse traction (DTT). The system incorporates closed and open hooks in a variety of shapes and sizes to accommodate cervical, thoracic, lumbar, and sacral placement. Pedicle screws are available in several sizes, and are usually utilized in the lumbar spine.

Correction of spinal deformity is accomplished by the selective fixation of strategic vertebrae, rotation of prebent rods, and selective compression and distraction. Rigidity of fixation is enhanced by forming a frame from parallel rods joined together by at least two transverse traction devices. DTTs are effective against torsional strains, and the system is sufficiently rigid that external immobilization is often not required.[7]

Numerous biomechanical studies have demonstrated that CD instrumentation is significantly more rigid than Harrington instrumentation or segmental wiring (Fig. 48-9).[9] A number of similar systems are now available, which incorporate rigid multisegmental fixation. Rigid spinal fixation has been shown to improve the rate of spinal fusion and the strength of fusion mass, and to result in improved clinical outcomes.[23,42]

## ANTERIOR THORACOLUMBAR INSTRUMENTATION

With advances in posterior instrumentation, particularly transpedicular constructs, the surgeon is increas-

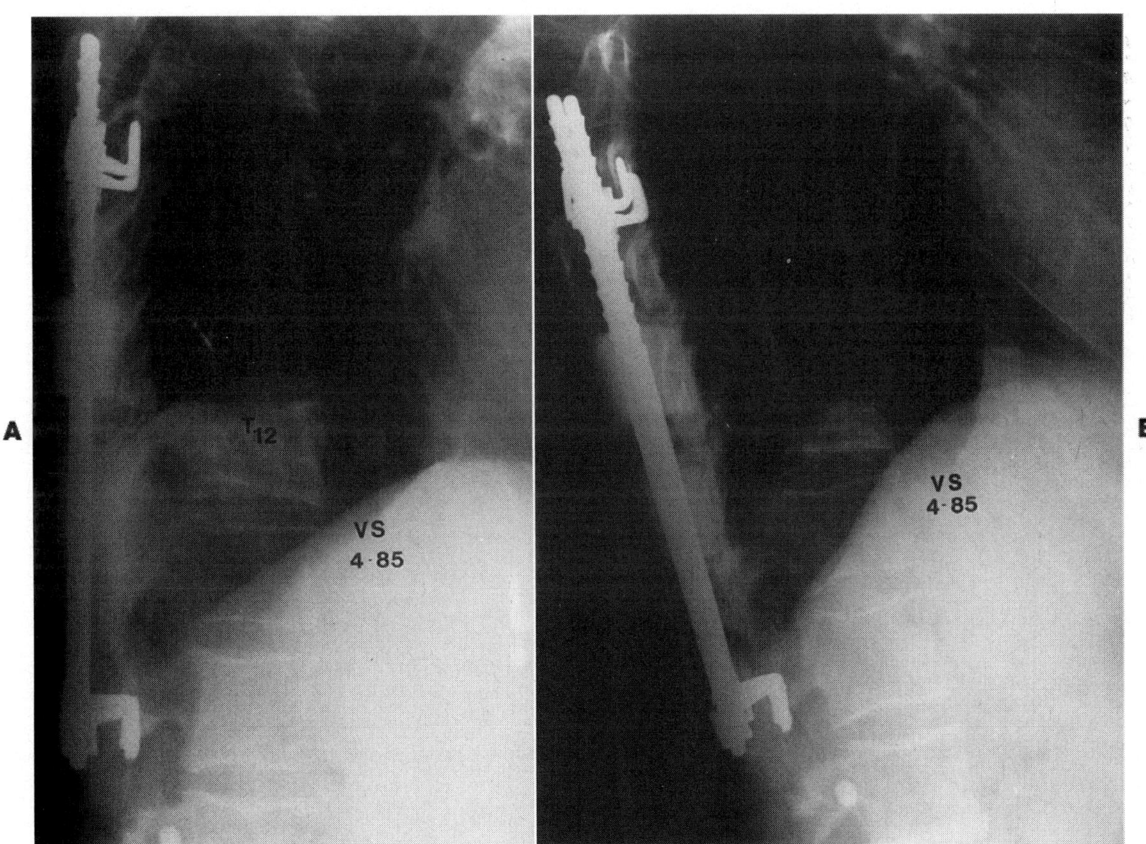


**FIGURE 48-10**

A 40-year-old man who suffered a T12 burst fracture with incomplete neurologic deficit was treated with distraction instrumentation with rod sleeves. He presented to us postoperatively with ongoing neurologic deficits. **A, B,** Excellent fixation and distraction of the fracture site have been achieved. *Continued*

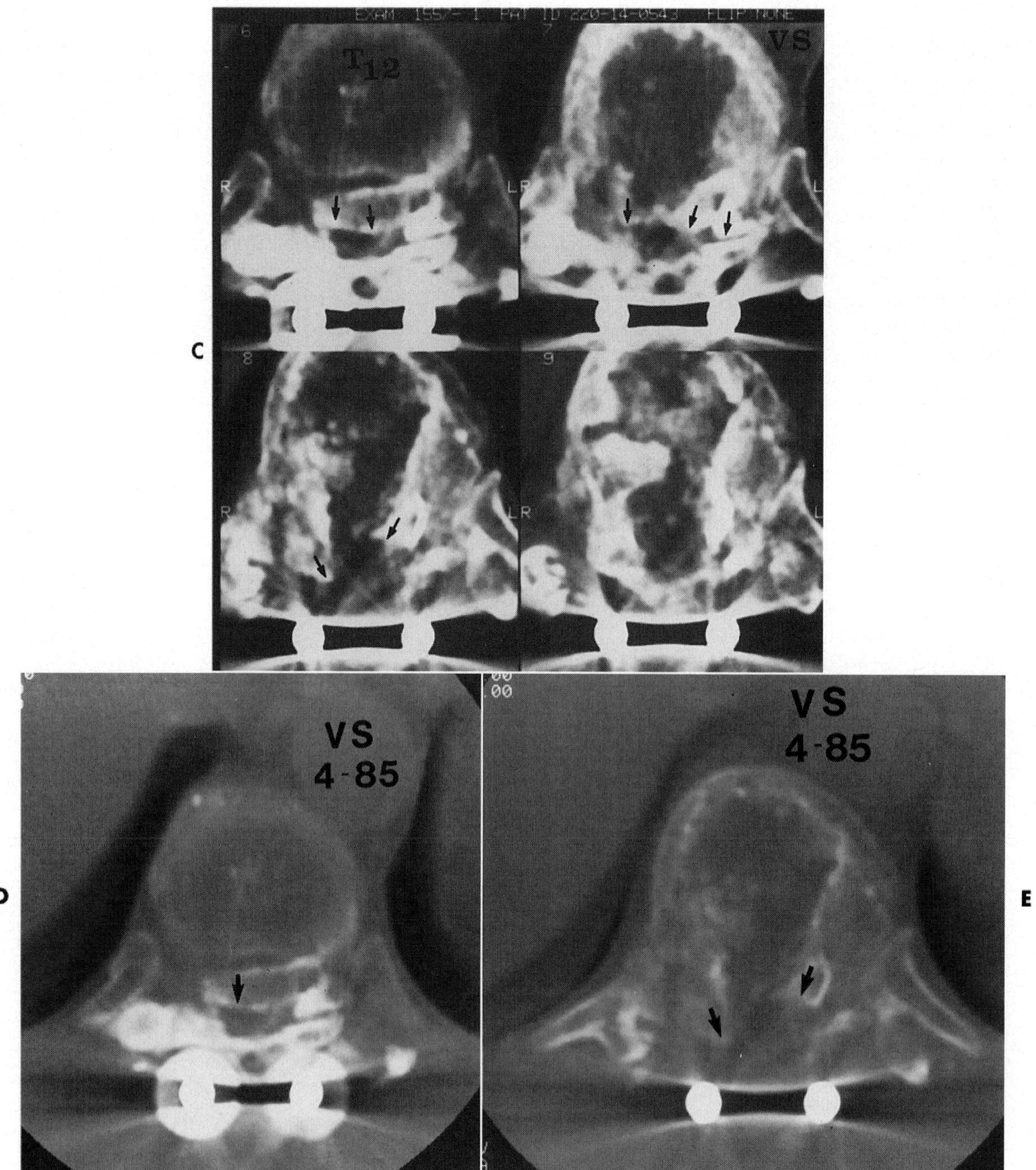


**FIGURE 48-10 CONT'D**

**C, D, E,** Significant canal compromise in spite of adequate distraction. The patient had full neurologic recovery after formal anterior T12 corpectomy. Posterior distraction instrumentation affords only an indirect reduction, and can not reliably reduce the bone fragments out of the spinal canal. In a patient with a persistent incomplete neurological deficit, postoperative CT scanning should be performed. A formal anterior corpectomy produces the most reliable neurologic recovery following burst fractures.

ingly able to achieve correction of deformity, decompression of the spinal canal, and stabilization of the thoracolumbar spine without need for concomitant anterior procedures. Anterior spinal approaches are preferred in cases of incomplete neurological deficit from anterior impingement (Fig. 48-10), for anterior release in cases of inflexible deformity, and to allow for short-segment fixation in certain cases of deformity and traumatic instability. Anterior arthrodesis allows reconstruction of the anterior and middle columns of the spine, and allows the graft to be placed under compression, which should enhance fusion rates.

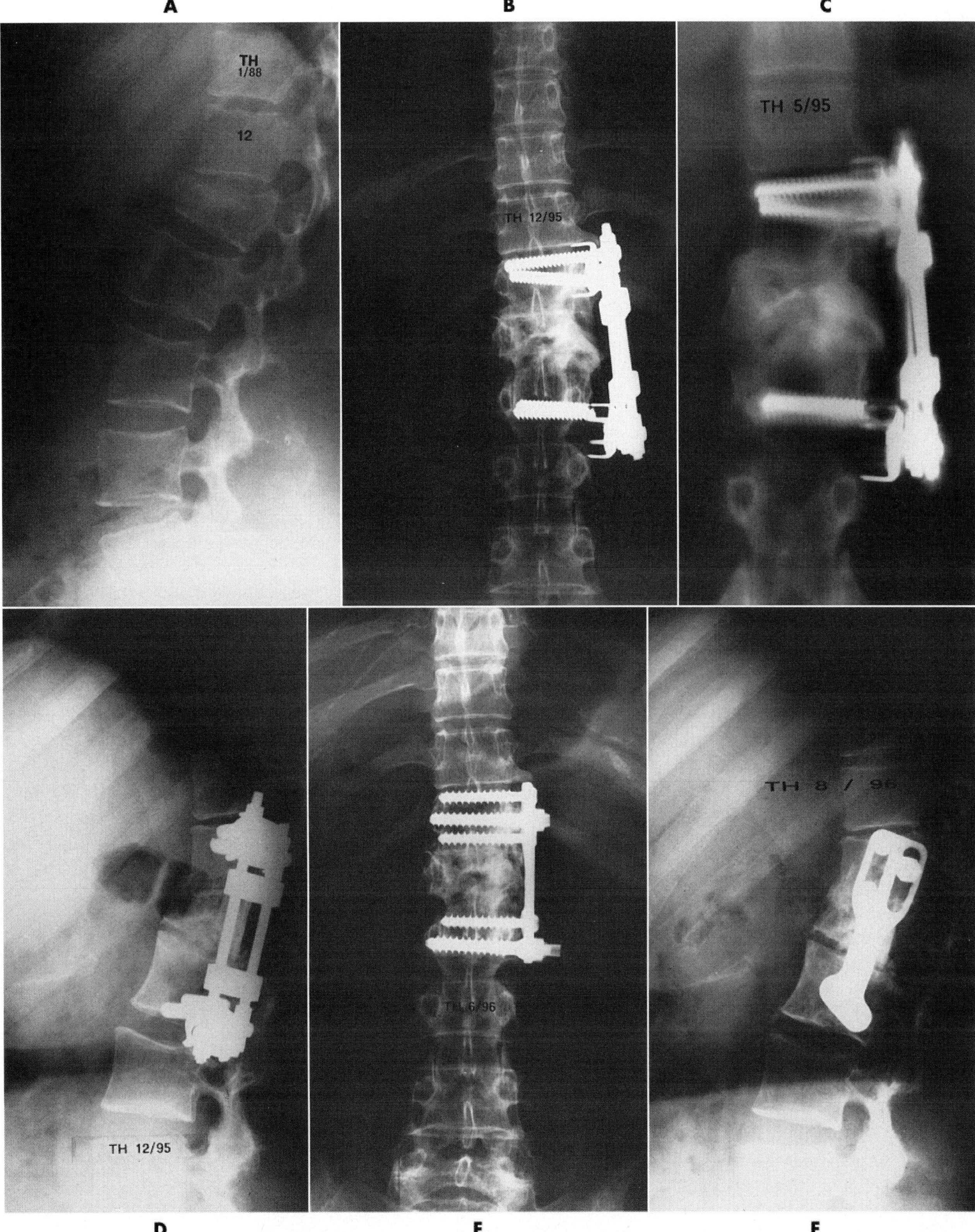


**FIGURE 48-11**

This 20-year-old woman suffered an L1 burst fracture with left leg weakness when her toboggan jumped a high mogul. **A,** Lateral radiograph of the fracture; the posterosuperior aspect of the L1 vertebrae compressed the thecal sac. She underwent anterior decompression, strut grafting, and Kaneda instrumentation. She had a full neurologic recovery; however, she presented seven years later with back pain. **B, C, D,** Anteroposterior radiograph and tomogram and lateral radiograph showing a pseudarthrosis at the lower aspect of the graft and fracture of the lower screws. **E, F,** She underwent removal of instrumentation and resection of the pseudarthrosis, and iliac crest autograft was used to graft the defect. Fixation in compression was achieved with a Z-plate. Although the Z-plate should be less susceptible to fatigue failure than the threaded rods of the Kaneda system, all anterior instrumentation devices are load sharing and rely on successful fusion for ultimate stability.

Zdeblick et al demonstrated that the use of anterior instrumentation to stabilize anterior bone grafts led to a higher rate of fusion in an animal model.[43] Instrumented spines demonstrated a significantly greater torsional stiffness than noninstrumented spines. Similarly, Shirado et al demonstrated a higher fusion rate in anterior strut grafts stabilized by the Kaneda device versus noninstrumented grafts.[33]

Anterior instrumentation is a more exacting technique than posterior spinal instrumentation. The proximity of the great vessels requires that care be taken to avoid injury during fixator implantation, and that juxtaposition of implants to the vessels be avoided to prevent late erosion of the implants into vessels. Screw purchase in the predominantly cancellous vertebral body is usually inferior to that gained with transpedicular instrumentation, and meticulous surgical technique must be maintained to ensure adequate stability. Triangulation of screws within a vertebral body will maximize resistance to pull-out. Horton et al demonstrated that screws oriented obliquely in the frontal plane have a greater resistance to loosening, because forces applied to these screws are resisted by both endplates.[16]

Anterior instrumentation devices are load-sharing implants.[4,10] Success of the technique relies on transmission of load through a graft of ample strength to provide secure fixation and long-term stability. Rod systems such as the Kaneda device and Texas Scottish Rite Hospital (TSRH) are dynamic systems that allow distraction at the operative site and compression loading of grafts prior to the final seating of instrumentation, and are thus preferable to first-generation plating systems. However, the higher profile of most rod systems increases the potential for vascular injury. Therefore, dynamic plate systems such as the Z-plate and University plate have been introduced to provide a means for compression loading of the construct while maintaining a low profile (Fig. 48-11).

An et al recently evaluated the biomechanical properties of anterior instrumentation systems, including the University plate, Z-plate, the Kaneda device, and TSRH.[2] When used with an interbody graft, all restored stability similar to the intact specimen. The Kaneda device with a transfixator was found to be superior to other systems in the restoration of torsional stability.

## REFERENCES


1. Aebi M, Zuber K, Marchesi D: Treatment of cervical spine injuries with anterior plating, *Spine* 16(suppl 3): 38-45, 1991.
2. An H et al: Biomechanical evaluation of anterior thoracolumbar spinal instrumentation, *Spine* 20:1979-1983, 1995.
3. Ashman RB, et al: Mechanical testing of spinal instrumentation, *Clin Orthop* 227:113-125, 1988.
4. Bayley JC, Yuan HA, Frederickson BE: The Syracuse I-plate, *Spine* 16(3Supp):S120-124, 1991.
5. Choueka J, Spivak JM, Kummer FJ, Steger T: Flexion failure of posterior cervical lateral mass screws, *Spine* 21(4):1996.
6. Cotrel Y, Dubousset J: New segmental posterior instrumentation of the spine, Scoliosis Research Society, Nineteenth Annual Meeting, Orlando, 1984.
7. Cotrel Y, Dubousset J, McAfee PC: Technique of CD instrumentation for spinal surgery, especially for scoliosis. In *Spine: Recent Surgical Procedures*.
8. Farey ID, McAfee PC, Davis RF, Long DM: Pseudarthrosis of the cervical spine after anterior arthrodesis, *J Bone Joint Surg* 72A(8):1171-1177, 1990.
9. Gurr KR, McAfee PC, Shih CM: Biomechanical analysis of posterior instrumentation systems after decompressive laminectomy, *J Bone Joint Surg* 70A: 680-691, 1988
10. Haas N, Blauth M, Tscherne H: Anterior plating in thoracolumbar spine injuries, *Spine* 16(3Supp):S100-111, 1991.
11. Hadra BE: Wiring of the spinous processes in Potts disease, *Trans Am Orthop Assoc* 4:206, 1891.
12. Harrington PR: The history and development of Harrington instrumentation, *Clin Orthop* 227:3, 1988.
13. Harrington PR: Surgical instrumentation for the management of scoliosis, *J Bone Joint Surg* 42A:1488, 1960.
14. Heller JG, Silcox DH, Sutterlin CE: Complications of posterior cervical plating, *Spine* 20:2442-2448, 1995.
15. Herring JA, Fitch RD, Wenger DR: Segmental spinal instrumentation: a preliminary report of 40 consecutive cases, *Spine* 7:285-298, 1982.
16. Horton WC, et al: Strength of fixation of anterior vertebral body screws, *Spine* 21:439-444 1996.
17. King AG: *Complications in segmental spinal instrumentation.* In Luque E, editor: *Segmental spinal instrumentation,* Thorofare, 1984, Slack, pp 301-330.
18. King D: Internal fixation for lumbosacral fusion, *Am J Surg* 66:357-361, 1944.
19. Kotani Y, Cunningham BW, Abumi K, McAfee PC: Biomechanical analysis of cervical stabilization systems, *Spine* 19(22):2529-2539, 1994.
20. Lang E: Support of the spondylolitic spine by means of buried steel bars attached to the vertebra, *Am J Orthop Surg* 8:344, 1910.
21. Lowery GL, Swank ML, McDonough RF: Surgical

revision for failed anterior cervical fusions: articular pillar plating or anterior revision? *Spine* 20:2436-2441, 1995.

22. McAfee PC, Bohlman HH, Wilson WL: The triple wire fixation technique for stabilization of acute fracture-dislocations: a biomechanical analysis, *J Bone Joint Surg/Orthop Transact* 9:142, 1985.
23. McAfee PC, Farey ID, Sutterlin CE, Gurr K, Warden KE, Cunningham BW: The effect of spinal implant rigidity on vertebral bone density, *Spine* 16(suppl 6): S190-197, 1991.
24. McAfee PC, Werner FW, Glisson RR: A biomechanical analysis of spinal instrumentation systems in thoracolumbar fractures, *Spine* 10:204-217, 1985.
25. Michele AA, Krueger FJ: Surgical approach to the vertebral body, *J Bone Joint Surg* 31A:873-878, 1949.
26. Montesano PX, Juach EC, Anderson PA, Benson DR, Hanson PB: Biomechanics of cervical spine internal fixation, *Spine* 16(supp):10-16, 1991.
27. Montesano PX, Juach EC, Halldor J: Anatomic and biomechanical study of posterior cervical spine plate arthrodesis: an evaluation of two different techniques of screw placement, *J Spinal Disord* 5:301-305, 1992.
28. Munson G, et al: Experimental evaluation of Harrington rod fixation supplemented with sublaminar wires in stabilizing thoracolumbar fracture-dislocations, *Clin Orthop* 189:97-102, 1984.
29. Nasca J, Hollis JM, Lemons JE, Coal TA: Cyclic axial loading of spinal implants, *Spine* 10:792-798, 1985.
30. Orozco R, Llovet J: Osteosyntesis en las fracturas del raquis cervical, *Rev Orthop Traumitol* 14: 285-88, 1970.
31. Ripa DR, Kowall MG, Meyer PR, Rusin JJ: Series of ninety-two traumatic cervical spine injuries stabilized with anterior ASIF plate fusion technique, *Spine* 16(suppl 3):S46-55, 1991.
32. Rogers WA: The treatment of fracture dislocations of the cervical spine, *J Bone Joint Surg* 24:245-250, 1942.
33. Shirado O, Zdeblick TA, McAfee PC, Cunningham BW, DeGroot H, Warden KE: Quantitative histologic study of the influence of anterior spinal instrumentation and biodegradable polymer on lumbar interbody fusion after corpectomy: a canine model, *Spine* 17: 795-803, 1992.
34. Silverman BJ, Greenbarg PE: Idiopathic scoliosis posterior spine fusion with Harrington rod and sublaminar wiring, *Orthop Clin N Am* 19:269-279, 1988.
35. Sullivan JA, Conner SB: Comparison of Harrington instrumentation and segmental instrumentation in the management of neuromuscular spinal deformity, *Spine* 7:299-304, 1982.
36. Ulrich C, Woerdoerfer O, Kalff R, Claes L, Wilke HJ: Biomechanics of fixation systems to the cervical spine, *Spine* 16(suppl 3):S4-S9, 1991.
37. Weiland DJ, McAfee PC: Posterior cervical fusion with triple-wire strut graft technique: one hundred consecutive patients, *J Spinal Disord* 4(1):15-21, 1991.
38. Weiss JC, Cunningham BW, Kanayama M, Parker L, McAfee PC: In vitro biomechanical comparison of multistrand cables with conventional cervical stabilization, *Spine* 21:2108-2114, 1996.
39. Wenger DR, et al: Laboratory testing of segmental spinal instrumentation versus traditional Harrington instrumentation for scoliosis treatment, *Spine* 7:265-269 1982.
40. Wilber SR, Thompson SH, Shaffer JW: Postoperative neurologic deficits in segmental instrumentation, *J Bone Joint Surg* 66A:1178-1187, 1984.
41. Winter RW: Thoracic lordoscoliosis in neurofibromatosis: treatment by Harrington rods with sublaminar wiring, *J Bone Joint Surg* 66A:1102-1106, 1984.
42. Zdeblick TA: A prospective randomized study of lumbar fusion, *Spine* 18:983-991, 1993.
43. Zdeblick TA, Shirado O, McAfee PC, DeGroot H, Warden KE: Anterior spinal fixation after lumbar corpectomy: a study in dogs, *J Bone Joint Surg* 73A: 527-534, 1991.

# 49

# REVISION SPINE SURGERY IN THE PRESENCE OF OSTEOPOROSIS

**Marcel F. Dvorak, M.D., F.R.C.S.C.**
**Charles G. Fisher, M.D., F.R.C.S.C.**



The prevalence of osteoporosis continues to increase as medical and scientific advances lead to major gains in life expectancy. It is known that 25% of females and 12% of males over the age of 50 are affected with osteoporosis.[20] This demographic shift brings new challenges to spine surgeons as osteoporosis is more frequently being held responsible for the failure of what would otherwise have been a successful surgical procedure. Despite their age, these patients continue to have high expectations for pain relief and functional recovery. Modern spinal surgical procedures, often including anterior and posterior instrumentation techniques, are being performed more frequently on elderly patients.

When osteoporosis is considered a contributing factor in the mechanical failure of a spinal procedure it can be manifested in several different patterns. Osteoporosis-related failure may result from intraoperative difficulties at the bone-implant interface, or the late failure of anterior or posterior instrumentation or prostheses. Furthermore, osteoporosis may lead to junctional failure, or fracture above or below a stable fused spine segment. In any of the above situations, the spine surgeon may be faced with a difficult salvage or revision situation. The surgeon must be cognizant of the various treatment alternatives, their risks and likely success rates in osteoporotic bone, and this information combined with technical expertise enables the surgeon to salvage an otherwise difficult situation.

The purpose of this chapter is to provide a detailed overview of comprehensive management strategies available to the spine surgeon when faced with a complex revision in a patient with osteoporosis of the spine.

## MEDICAL MANAGEMENT

Surgeons tend to focus intently on the technical aspects of a complex surgical problem and often fail to consider the patient as a whole. Many osteoporotic patients are elderly, functionally impaired, poorly nourished, suffer from chronic disease, and may live in a precarious environment that only serves to amplify the above problems. It is therefore essential that an interdisciplinary approach be taken in the medical management of this patient population to optimize their chances for a successful surgical result.

Osteoporosis refers to diminished density of normally mineralized bone, which leads to increasing fragility and susceptibility to fracture. The World Health Organization defines osteoporosis as a bone mineral density (BMD) measurement more than 2.5 standard deviations below peak bone mass.[11] Bone mass increases from birth until the middle of the second or third decade. The highest bone mass obtained is termed peak bone mass. It is known that the greater the peak bone mass achieved, the lower the chance of developing osteoporosis later in life.[14]

Osteoporosis is classified as either primary or secondary osteoporosis. Primary osteoporosis consists of two types: Type I (postmenopausal), characterized by rapid bone loss over an 8- to 10-year period of time; and Type II (age-associated idiopathic), affecting both males and females, due to the inevitable physiologic changes and environmental factors associated with aging.[14] It is important to remember that the prevalence of osteoporosis increases with age in both sexes. Secondary osteoporosis is the result of an identifiable agent or disease process that accounts for the change in BMD.

The diagnosis of osteoporosis is made by identifying patients at risk and then directly measuring their BMD. Patients at risk include females with early or surgical menopause; postmenopausal women not receiving ovarian hormone therapy; primary hypothyroidism; strong family history; males with hypogonadism; and exposure to numerous medications, especially oral glucocorticoids taken for more than three months.[20] Anticonvulsants, heparin, and antineoplastic drugs, smoking, alcohol, sedentary lifestyle, and low dietary calcium and vitamin D are also linked to osteoporosis.[11]

The measurement of BMD verifies the diagnosis and allows the treatment response to be monitored.[4] Numerous methods to measure BMD have been developed and tested over the years. Based on accuracy, precision error, and practicality, dual-energy x-ray absorptiometry (DXA) is currently the gold standard.[4,20] Plain x-rays have low sensitivity in detecting osteoporosis.[4] Indications for testing BMD are controversial. Currently, the indications are for diagnostic confirmation in patients with risk factors and monitoring the response to treatment. Bone mineral density does not affect fracture healing and its influence on fusion is not known.

The pathophysiology of osteoporosis is targeted at bone remodeling and the constant balance between resorption and regeneration. Cancellous bone with its large surface area is the most metabolically active region in this remodeling process. With the vertebral body being almost entirely cancellous bone it becomes quite apparent how susceptible the spine is to this disease process. It is the fundamental process of bone remodeling to which all preventative and corrective treatments are targeted.

Lifestyle modification and pharmacologic agents are fundamental to the effective management of osteoporosis. Elimination of risk factors such as smoking, excessive alcohol consumption, unnecessary medication, and sedentary lifestyle are simple concepts, often overlooked and difficult to achieve. The patient should be encouraged to participate in regular physical activity. Weightbearing aerobic exercise is effective as a preventative measure and is associated with increased BMD.[24] In terms of strengthening, resisted exercises prescribed for specific muscle groups will increase bone mineralization.[24] Immobilization should be avoided at all costs because of its profound affect on bone homeostasis. Bone mass can decrease by approximately one percent per week with bed rest.[14] Dietary supplementation, consisting of calcium (1500 mg/day) and vitamin D (400-800 IU/day), can reduce but not prevent bone loss if used in isolation.[20]

Some of the pharmacologic agents used to treat osteoporosis include hormone replacement therapy, bisphosphonates, and calcitonin. Hormone replacement therapy has been found to be effective in not only preventing BMD loss but can actually increase it.[20] The dosage, duration, and contraindications to the use of hormone replacement therapy must be carefully evaluated.

The bisphosphonates (i.e., etidronate and alendronate) inhibit bone resorption. Etidronate increases BMD 5% to 8% in the spine with the most dramatic effect occurring in the first year.[20,25] Alendronate increases BMD by 8%, appears to take effect sooner, does not inhibit mineralization, and can therefore be used daily.[15,20] Both etidronate and alendronate are ideal for the older patient, particularly if that patient is taking glucocorticoids. Alendronate appears to be the most appropriate medication for the spinal surgical patient with osteoporosis.

Finally, calcitonin can increase BMD and prevent vertebral fractures.[22] Two years of calcitonin therapy have been shown to increase BMD by 5% to 10% and the beneficial effects may be seen within 3 months.[22] Calcitonin is also an effective analgesic in osteoporotic fractures, particularly when its use is initiated early. Side effects and method of administration, however, make its use more controversial.

## SURGICAL TREATMENT

### INSTABILITY FOLLOWING DECOMPRESSION

Postlaminectomy instability is a recognized cause of late mechanical failure of the spine,[8,18] which unfortunately often occurs in patients who are elderly, have been immobile due to their back disability, and frequently suffer from osteoporosis. These patients have often had a lengthy period of inactivity following their index surgical procedure and this, combined with a wide posterior element resection leads to limited surgical options. In a review of 16 patients with iatrogenic instability, three of four patients treated with a revision posterior decompression and pedicle screw instrumented fusion failed.[30] The most common site of failure was at the screw-bone interface with screw pull-out and recurrent deformity, suggesting that osteoporosis was an etiological factor. Nine of ten patients treated with combined anterior and posterior fusion had a successful fusion.

The simple addition of a posterior instrumented fusion to a mechanically unstable spine, in which the fixation is compromised by soft bone, is likely to fail. This illustrates one of the essential principles of dealing with patients with osteoporosis and failed previous surgery. The combination of posterior scar tissue, posterior element removal, and osteoporosis leading to compromised fixation, necessitates a combined approach addressing both the anterior and posterior columns. The specific issue of how best to salvage patients with iatrogenic instability is dealt with in more detail in other chapters of this book; however, one must remember that these patients often have compromised BMD.

## LOSS OF FIXATION OF SPINAL IMPLANTS

There is a wealth of data that correlates instrumentation failure with BMD.[3,23,28] Bone mineral density is often the limiting factor in the surgeon's ability to achieve his or her surgical goal. Some surgeons view severe osteoporosis as a contraindication to surgery, specifically surgery designed to obtain a fusion involving deformity correction with instrumentation. As spine surgery becomes more frequently performed, the spine surgeon cannot avoid facing a situation in which osteoporosis has contributed to the failure of an instrumented fusion construct.

## INTRAOPERATIVE HARDWARE FAILURE

The most commonly encountered example of mechanical failure due to osteoporosis is the intraoperative recognition of poor bone-screw interface. This may become evident when the surgeon is drilling or probing the pedicle and identifies that the bone is very soft and inadequate to anchor a pedicle screw.

In the osteoporotic patient the technique used to prepare screw holes appears to have a significant effect upon screw fixation.[26] Tapping or drilling a pedicle hole appears to be inferior to using a blunt pedicle probe that compacts surrounding bone.[6] As the screw is inserted, the surgeon may appreciate the low torque required to insert the screw. Insertional torque has been correlated to both BMD and to screw pull-out and may predict early failure of pedicle screws, particularly in osteoporotic bone.[19] Insertional torque has also been proposed as a more sensitive indicator of failure through cyclical loading.[29] It is postulated that cyclical flexion and extension loading may lead to failure due to compaction of adjacent cancellous bone resulting in loosening of the screw. This better resembles the most common clinical mode of screw failure and thus insertional torque measurement may be a better predictor of poor screw fixation than merely assessing the BMD. The clinical realization that a screw may not be adequate at the time of insertion should enable the surgeon to attempt one of several salvage strategies to ensure adequate fixation at the instrumented level.

The first strategy to be considered is to improve the fixation of the suspect screw. This may be achieved by augmentation vertebroplasty, most commonly described by injecting methylmethacrylate (i.e., bone cement) into the pedicle. A two-fold increase in screw pull-out has been determined with the use of pressurized bone cement (2 to 3 ml) injected into the vertebral body through the probed or drilled pedicle.[23,31] Caution must be exercised because extrusion of cement out of the vertebral body and into the foramen, spinal canal, and even adjacent vessels is possible with this technique. Pressurized injection is contraindicated when the outer pedicle cortex has been violated. Alternative techniques to augment the cancellous bone of the vertebral body have been described. These include the insertion of matchstick cortical bone graft, a technique that is helpful in a stripped screw hole in normal density bone but is less helpful in severely osteoporotic bone.[6]

More recently, a technique of vertebral body augmentation has been described that involves vertebral augmentation by means of an injectable, biocompatible, carbonated apatite cancellous bone cement. This has been shown to increase pull-out strength and energy absorbed during cyclical loading by up to 70%.[16] This substance and other biological materials avoid the exothermic reaction of methylmethacrylate bone cement and its attendant risk to the neural elements.

Another possible salvage technique involves altering the characteristics of the screw to optimize purchase in the vertebra. Screw length may be increased, thus ensuring that the screw just engages the anterior cortex of the vertebra. Increasing the depth of insertion of the screw can significantly improve pull-out strength.[31] This is particularly important in the sacrum, where the anteroposterior diameter of the S1 vertebral body is less than most other vertebrae. Bicortical purchase in the sacrum is not fraught with the vascular risks found at other vertebral levels as long as the screw tip is directed medially. With the cancellous bone of the vertebral body more significantly affected by osteoporosis than the cortical bone, strategies that optimize purchase in the cortical bone of the pedicle may be effective at improving fixation. Increasing screw diameter to 80% of preoperative computed tomography (CT) pedicle diameter, in an attempt to optimize fit and fill of the pedicle has been shown to improve screw fixation.[1,5] The surgeon should be aware that the design characteristics of various pedicle screws do not necessarily affect their purchase in osteoporotic bone.[27] There are many variables in screw design that affect screw purchase, including screw diameter, depth, and pitch of thread,[21] however, these factors become less significant as the patient's BMD drops. Apart from varying the length and diameter of the screw there is little effect in varying screw type in an attempt to optimize screw purchase in osteoporotic bone.[10]

Nonparallel placement of pedicle screws in an upward and inward direction has been shown to better resist lateral shifting of the instrumented motion segment.[13] The addition of a laminar hook at the caudal edge of the same vertebra as the one that contains the screw may be an effective technique of reinforcing what otherwise may be a suspect screw.[2,6,7,9] The addition of a sublaminar wire or cable may also augment a suspect screw.

Pedicle screws are not necessarily the optimal bone fixation devices in severely osteoporotic vertebrae. As has been previously discussed, osteoporosis preferentially affects the cancellous bone of the vertebral body, relatively sparing the cortical posterior element bone. Laminar fixation, either hooks or sublaminar wires or cables, are potentially better choices in the face of severely compromised BMD.[3] Laminar fixation may not always be practical particularly in the lumbar spine in which a concomitant laminectomy is often required.

Finally, when fixation at a particular motion segment is no longer possible or stable, the surgeon is left with two final choices. The first is to perform an in situ fusion without instrumentation and place the patient on bedrest or in an orthosis. A further period of recumbence is best avoided because of the severe disuse osteoporosis, which may compound what is already significantly demineralized bone. The second option is to extend the instrumentation and fusion to a cephalad or caudal vertebra where adequate fixation may be achieved.

### EARLY POSTOPERATIVE HARDWARE FAILURE

Any fixation device may fail early and potentially result in sudden pain, recurrence of deformity, and subcutaneous prominence of the instrumentation. Pedicle screws may fail by means of pull-out, cut-out, or toggling, leaving a radiolucent line at the bone-screw interface, migration of the screw, or loss of reduction. Hooks and sublaminar wires may similarly cut out of bone or fracture laminae, resulting in early recurrence of deformity and postoperative instability. Occasionally, if the patient's pain and recurrent deformity are minimal, conservative treatment may be considered, thus avoiding what may be a complex surgical revision. Conservative treatment may involve placing the patient on bedrest or in an orthosis with limited activity. One must keep in mind the deleterious effects of further recumbence on patients who may already suffer from significant disuse osteoporosis.

### LATE POSTOPERATIVE HARDWARE FAILURE

When the surgeon is faced with late loss of fixation of an implant, this does not necessarily represent failure of the implant, but is more likely due to biological failure of the underlying bone to fuse. If this was to occur it would result in an underlying pseudarthrosis or delayed union. Metal fatigue with fracturing of the rod or screws is less likely to occur in the osteoporotic spine, because the weak link is almost always the bone-implant interface. When the surgeon considers revising a late failure of fixation, one must always consider why the biological fusion failed and not only why the instrumentation failed.

The contribution of the anterior column, not only to immediate stability, but also to fusion surface area, must be strongly considered. When one realizes that most late failure occurs due to the inability of the spine to withstand physiological flexion loads, then a surgical strategy that also addresses the anterior column becomes a necessary part of the revision strategy. The addition of anterior release and strut grafting to the correction of a deformity may significantly diminish the forces placed upon posterior instrumentation and thus minimize risks of further failure. The presence of anterior column support also minimizes the flexion-bending moments applied to posterior instrumentation and may minimize the risk of cyclical loading leading to windshield wiper loosening of pedicle screws.

## DEFORMITY CORRECTION

The most common indication for revision, apart from failed fixation within a fused segment, is dealing with the problem of junctional kyphosis above or below a fusion. Clinically, patients present late following an apparently successful fusion with severe pain and new deformity. It is important to keep in mind that most simple compression fractures are effectively treated with conservative and medical modalities. It is often prudent to begin with a trial of bracing, analgesics, and medical osteoporosis management prior to considering an extension of the fusion. There are several key principles involved in surgically revising these patients.

### BONE GRAFTING TECHNIQUES

The first principle relates to bone grafting to attain a solid fusion. Instrumentation alone, without appropriate bone grafting, is destined to lead to a pseudarthrosis and eventual failure. This is particularly true

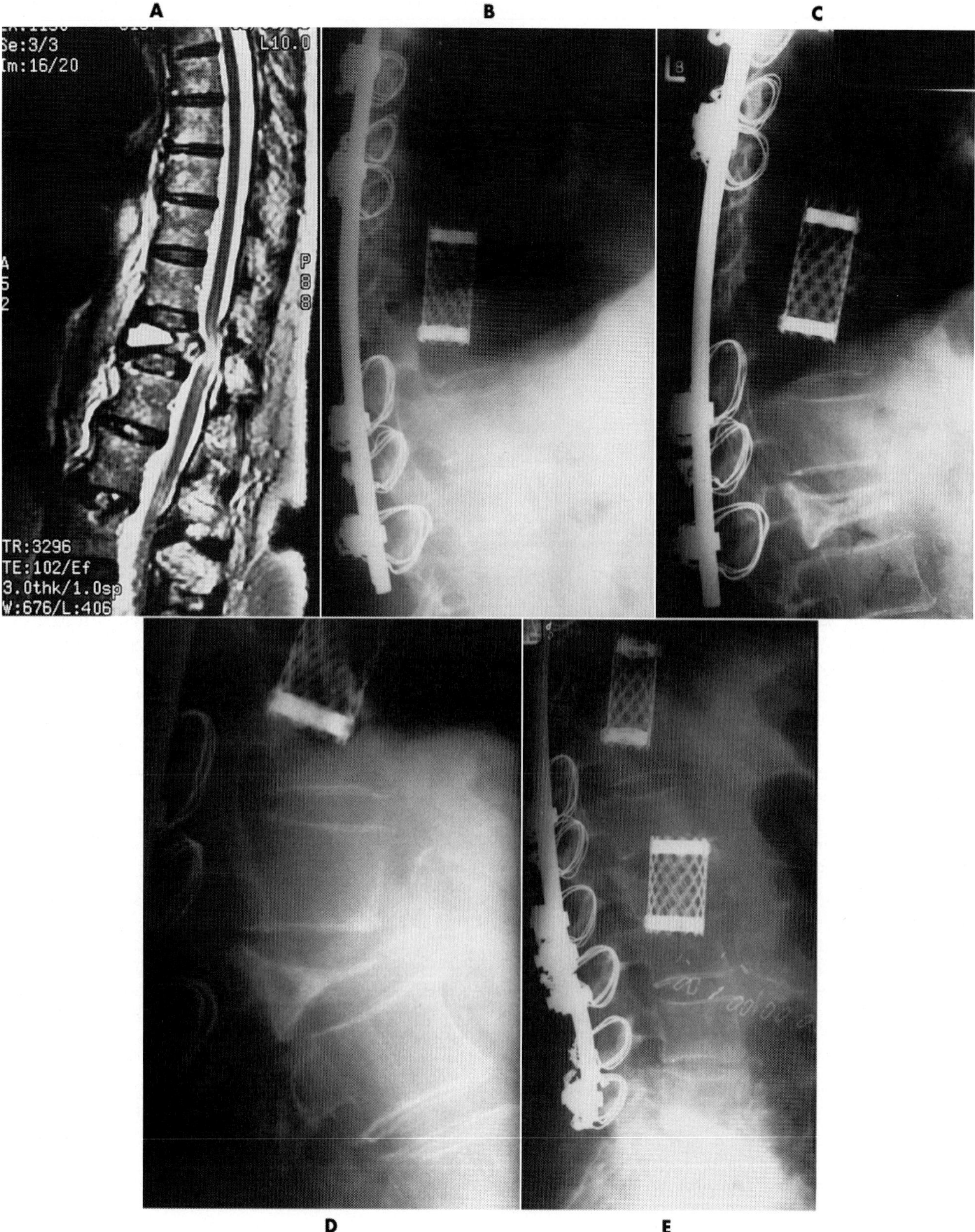


**Figure 49-1**

A 71-year-old woman with rheumatoid arthritis and a compression fracture of T12 presents with myelopathy. **A,** Sagittal T2-weighted MRI image, revealing cord compression with signal change at the site of the T12 compression fracture. **B,** Postoperative lateral x-ray following anterior vertebral body resection and cage reconstruction with posterior segmental spinal instrumentation. **C,** Six months postoperatively the patient presented with renewed back pain and deformity at the lower end of her fusion. A lateral radiograph revealed a pathologic junctional compression fracture of L3. She was initially treated conservatively with a brace. **D,** The patient's kyphotic deformity progressed and she developed neurological symptoms. **E,** Postoperative lateral radiograph following a L3 vertebral resection, cage stabilization, and extension of fusion to L5. The patient has recovered neurological function and returned to her normal level of activity.

in the osteoporotic spine where the best chance for success is at the time of the first revision. Part of the surgical planning exercise must include consideration of where the surgeon will obtain bone graft. Most patients have had at least one previous autologous bone graft harvest performed. Making note of the location of previous bone harvesting and assessing the possibility of repeat access to the same iliac crest with a preoperative CT scan is a critical component of the preoperative planning process. Mixing allograft with what autograft is available or with bone marrow aspirate may be a logical approach. Considering alternative sources of autologous bone, such as rib from a thoracotomy or thoracoplasty, or fibula, should be planned prior to surgery. The role of growth factors such as bone morphogenic protein in augmenting or obtaining spinal fusion is just starting to be explored in clinical trials. Whether they will find a substantial place in the treatment of spine patients with osteoporosis is not known.

In patients who have already undergone several posterior iliac crest harvest procedures and who have extensive fusions often to L5 or the sacrum, the presence of osteoporosis and further posterior iliac procedures may lead to insufficiency fractures through the pelvis. Most of these pelvic fractures can be treated conservatively.

## POSTERIOR REVISION PRINCIPLES

A common goal of all spine surgery should be to achieve sagittal and coronal plane balance. This becomes even more important in revision surgery in the presence of poor density bone where having achieved a balanced spine diminishes the risk of failure of the instrumentation and fusion.

General principles used in achieving successful posterior instrumentation in the presence of osteoporosis include the use of segmental fixation from one neutral vertebra to another. This necessitates performing a fusion and instrumentation over the entire kyphosis of the thoracic spine. A fusion must not end at a kyphotic segment and this often means extending the fusion up to T2, T3, or T4. Similarly, balance must be achieved in the coronal plane. If the end vertebra of a fused segment is still within the curve of a scoliosis further deformity may be expected. Often revision surgery is necessary because these basic principles have not been followed. In these cases, the revision should attempt to ensure that the end result is that of a balanced spine.

As has been mentioned above, fixation on the laminae is much better than pedicle screw fixation in the presence of severe bone mineral loss. The use of sublaminar wires is most appropriate in achieving the parallel goals of segmental and laminar fixation. Sublaminar wires allow for sequential, gradual, controlled correction of deformity, while providing the skilled surgeon with a tactile feel for the rigidity of both the deformity and the fixation. Sublaminar wiring has the disadvantage of not neutralizing compressive forces well. This shortcoming may be addressed by adding several cross-links or hooks to minimize the risk of vertical settling. When using sublaminar wiring it is common to begin and end the construct with hooks or screws. Particularly at the cephalad end of a construct, it is important not to disrupt the ligamentum flavum or the interspinous or supraspinous ligaments, because this might predispose to a kyphotic deformity developing above the last level fused. It is recommended, therefore, that the cephalad-most fixation point be a screw or transverse process hook, leaving the ligamentous attachments above intact.

## ANTERIOR COLUMN SUPPORT PRINCIPLES

One of the most common complications leading to the need for a revision in an osteoporotic spine is the failure of the weak anterior column cancellous bone to maintain normal alignment. This often results in the development of a kyphotic deformity. Whether due to osteoporotic compression fractures above a fusion or within a fused segment leading to posterior instrumentation pullout, the revision principle is the same. The surgeon must address the anterior column deficiency, achieve a balanced spine, and revise or extend the posterior instrumentation.

Correction of kyphotic deformity may be achieved in one of two ways. Either the anterior column height can be restored, or the posterior and middle columns may be shortened to obtain the same result. In the osteoporotic spine, restoration of anterior column height is fraught with complications such as graft penetration into soft vertebral bodies leading to posterior instrumentation failure and recurrence of the deformity. Potentially more successful are attempts at achieving sagittal plane balance by shortening the middle and posterior columns while providing support to what may be a shortened anterior column. Techniques used to achieve this include the eggshell osteotomy, as well as combined anterior and posterior procedures whose goal it is to attain normal sagittal plane balance by supporting a shortened vertebral body with a cage or graft while performing a posterior element closing wedge osteotomy.

There are several principles common to all procedures attempting anterior column reconstruction that become critically important in the patient with diminished bone mass. Surgical technique must be precise and gentle in an attempt to preserve what bony support is available. Because the bone is soft, anterior disk excision may lead to inadvertent violation of the bony endplates. Mechanical distraction devices and disk space spreaders may easily cut into endplates, thus damaging a vertebra that was to be counted on for mechanical support. Distraction is better achieved by an assistant pushing on the apex of the kyphosis to open the interspace.

Operating on osteoporotic bone requires techniques different from those used when operating on patients with normal BMD. In normal strength bone some authors have suggested perforating the endplates or recessing the grafts into the endplates to improve healing and fusion. In the patient with poor BMD, maintaining the integrity of endplates is critical particularly when one considers that much of the anterior graft's mechanical support may come from the endplate.[17]

Optimizing the surface area of an anterior reconstruction is critical regardless of whether the surgeon is using autograft, allograft, or a prosthetic device (e.g., cage). Allograft, such as diaphyseal tibia, provides better surface area than does smaller diameter allograft such as the fibula. Iliac crest strut grafts often provide a narrow bone surface, which tends to cut into the adjacent endplates. Some commercial prosthetic devices come with endplates that may be added to increase the surface area of the cage. Occasionally, anterior grafts or cages may sink into a vertebral body until they come to rest against an anterior screw or pedicle screw inserted from posterior but extending into the vertebral body. Allowing a graft or cage to subside until it contacts instrumentation may work as a strategy to stabilize anterior grafts and minimize the chance of further pistoning or vertical migration of the graft or cage.

In the presence of a long-standing posterior fusion, for example in revising patients with scoliosis, the effects of stress shielding and device-related osteoporosis may lead to severe vertebral body bone density loss. The majority of the bone that has maintained good structural integrity resides in the fusion mass where the majority of the weight has been transmitted, and very significant loss of bone mineral density occurs in the vertebral bodies. This may force the surgeon to consider creative reconstruction alternatives when performing osteotomies and revisions through a mature previous fusion.

Finally, the techniques of vertebral body augmentation, as discussed above, have been used to provide anterior column support in the presence of a junctional compression fracture.[12] Bone cement verteboplasty in conjunction with posterior instrumentation has recently become popular. Caution must be exercised because the long-term clinical significance of cement or biological vertebral injection is unknown at present.

## SUMMARY

Given the demographic trend toward an aging population, the expectations from patients for continued pain control and satisfactory function and the ability of modern techniques of spine surgery to achieve these expectations, it is likely that spine surgeons will be faced with the challenge of revision spine surgery in patients with osteoporosis.

The surgeon may often be the first individual to diagnose osteoporosis and suggest concomitant medical treatment. As society ages and gains in longevity continue, osteoporosis is destined to become an even more serious health care problem. Fortunately a multitude of resources are being directed towards its prevention and corrective treatment.

A comprehensive and well-planned surgical approach to revision surgery in osteoporosis should include consideration of sources of bone graft and alternative methods of fixation in the case that a bailout is needed intraoperatively. Sagittal and coronal plane balance is a critical goal in order to minimize the stress placed upon fixation and adjacent levels. The surgeon often must address the anterior column, providing mechanical support anteriorly, while establishing a tension band posteriorly. In correcting kyphotic deformity, often a posterior closing wedge osteotomy is better tolerated than an attempt to restore anterior column height back to normal. The clinical application of vertebral body augmentation techniques has yet to be proven, however, is a promising technique in dealing with some of the most complex problems in modern spine surgery.

## REFERENCES


1. Brantley AG et al: The effect of pedicle screw fit: an in vitro study, *Spine* 19(15):1752-1758, 1994.
2. Chiba M et al: Short-segment pedicle instrumentation. Biomechanical analysis of supplemental hook fixation, *Spine* 21(3):288-294, 1996.
3. Coe JD et al: Influence of bone mineral density on the fixation of thoracolumbar implants. A comparative study of transpedicular screws, laminar hooks, and spinous process wires, *Spine* 15(9):902-907, 1990.
4. Coupland DB et al: Recommendations for the measurement and quantitation of bone mineral density, *Br Col Med J* 38(5):265-268, 1996.
5. Fisher CG, Gurr K, Bailey SI: Effect of matching pedicle screw diameter on screw fixation strength: a biomechanical study, Presented at the Canadian Orthopaedic Association, Annual General Meeting, Winnipeg, MB, 1994.

6. Halvorson TL et al: Effects of bone mineral density on pedicle screw fixation, *Spine* 19(21):2415-2420, 1994.
7. Hasegawa K et al: An experimental study of a combination method using a pedicle screw and laminar hook for the osteoporotic spine, *Spine* 22(9):958-962, 1997.
8. Herkowitz HN, Kurz LT: Degenerative lumbar spondylolisthesis with spinal stenosis: a prospective study comparing decompression with decompression and intertransverse process arthrodesis, *J Bone Joint Surg Am* 73:802-808, 1991.
9. Hilibrand AS et al: The role of pediculolaminar fixation in compromised pedicle bone, *Spine* 21(4):445-451, 1996.
10. Hu S: Internal fixation in the osteoporotic spine, *Spine* 22(24S):43S-48S, 1997.
11. Kendler DL: Risk factors in osteoporosis, *Br Col Med J* 38(5):263-264, 1996.
12. Kostuik J: Personal communication. Professor, Department of Orthopaedic Surgery, John Hopkins University, Baltimore, MD, 1997.
13. Krag MH et al: Placement of transpedicular vertebral screws close to anterior vertebral cortex: description of methods, *Spine* 14(8):879-883, 1989.
14. Lane JM et al: Osteoporosis diagnosis and treatment, *J Bone Joint Surg Am* 78A(4):618-632, 1996.
15. Liberman UA et al: Effect of oral alendronate on bone mineral density and the incidence of fractures in postmenopausal osteoporosis, *N Engl J Med* 333(22):1437-1443, 1995.
16. Lotz JC et al: Carbonated apatite cement augmentation of pedicle screw fixation in the lumbar spine, *Spine* 22(23):2716-2723, 1997.
17. McBroom RJ et al: Prediction of vertebral body compressive fracture using quantitative computed tomography, *J Bone Joint Surg Am* 67(8):1206-1214, 1985.
18. Nakai O, Ookawa A, Yamaura I: Long term roentgenographic and functional changes in patients who were treated with wide fenestration for central lumbar stenosis, *J Bone Joint Surg Am* 73(8):1184-1191, 1991.
19. Okuyama K et al: Stability of transpedicle screwing for the osteoporotic spine. An in vitro study of the mechanical stability, *Spine* 18(15):2240-2245, 1993.
20. Osteoporosis Society of Canada, Scientific Advisory Board: Clinical practice guidelines for the diagnosis and management of osteoporosis, *Can Med Assoc J* 155(8):1113-1133, 1996.
21. Perren SM et al: Technical and biomechanical aspects of screws used for bone and joint surgery, *Int J Orthop Trauma* 2:31-48, 1992.
22. Siminoski K, Josse G: Calcitonin in the treatment of osteoporosis, *Can Med Assoc J* 155(7):962-966, 1996.
23. Soshi S et al: An experimental study on transpedicular screw fixation in relation to osteoporosis of the lumbar spine, *Spine* 16(11):1335-1341, 1991.
24. Swezey RL: Exercise for osteoporosis—is walking enough? A case for site specificity and resistive exercise, *Spine* 21(23):2809-2813, 1996.
25. Watts NB et al: Intermittent cyclical etidronate treatment of postmenopausal osteoporosis, *N Engl J Med* 323(2):73-79, 1990.
26. Wittenberg RH et al: Effect of screw diameter, insertion technique and bone cement augmentation of pedicular screw fixation strength, *Clin Orthop* 296:278-287, 1993.
27. Wittenberg RH et al: Importance of bone mineral density in instrumented spine fusions, *Spine* 16(6):647-652, 1991.
28. Yamagata M et al: Mechanical stability of the pedicle screw fixation systems for the lumbar spine, *Spine* 7(suppl 3):S51-S54, 1992.
29. Zdeblick TA et al: Pedicle screw pullout strength: correlation with insertional torque, *Spine* 18(12):1673-1676, 1993.
30. Zeller L, Dvorak M, Fisher C: Salvage surgery in iatrogenic instability following lumbar decompression. Presented at 12th Annual Meeting Of the North American Spine Society, New York, 1997.
31. Zindrick MR et al: A biomechanical study of intrapenduncular screw fixation in the lumbosacral spine, *Clin Orthop* 203:99-112, 1986.

# VIII

# SPECIFIC PROBLEMS IN REVISION SURGERY

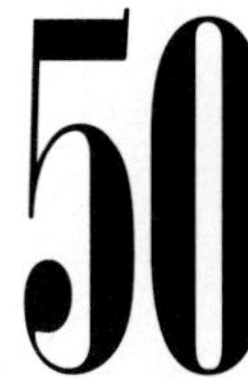

# SPECIFIC CONSIDERATIONS IN THE REVISIONS OF CERVICAL LAMINECTOMIES

**Stephen R. Freidberg, M.D.**
**Bernard A. Pfeifer, M.D.**



Since the classic report of successful cervical laminectomy for the treatment of degenerative disease by Scoville,[51] the posterior approach for decompression surgery of the cervical spine has enjoyed a long and flourishing history. It is a powerful procedure and many surgeons are comfortable performing it with good success.[16,49,52,58] However, as in any useful procedure, its success has led us to understand its limitations and it is not infrequent that some type of revision surgery must be performed for the patient who has undergone cervical laminectomy.[41,57,62] In reviewing this topic we find there are areas of little controversy and others of considerable discussion. This chapter begins with a review of our approach to the patient at the time of the index procedure. After that, the causes of early and late failure of the procedure are examined, and then a more controversial subject is discussed: the late instabilities that can result from the procedure. The chapter concludes with a discussion of our assessment of and preoperative planning for the patient who requires revision surgery and some thoughts on appropriate achievement of that surgery. The discussion centers on the subaxial spine, because the upper cervical spine is discussed elsewhere in this volume.

## CORRECT DIAGNOSIS AND APPROPRIATE PATIENT SELECTION FOR THE INDEX PROCEDURE

Operations are intended for the relief of the patient's symptoms and correction of the offending structural problem. We begin with the patient's history, the physical signs, and the review of the corroborative studies. We divide patients, if possible, into three symptom categories: those with neck and central upper back pain, those with radicular problems, and those with myelopathy.

We prefer to treat central pain nonoperatively, utilizing physical therapy and other modalities. Fusion can be considered in highly selected cases if an isolated lesion such as an arthritic facet or subluxation can be found. Laminectomy has little or no place in the care of the patient with central neck pain only.

Accurate clinical characterization of the neurologic lesion is mandatory before proceeding with any therapeutic regimen. It is critically important to rule out any overlap syndromes.[20,38,53] Unguided use of radiological studies may result in misinterpretation if one is not aware of the incidence of abnormalities in normal individuals.[6,24] Elimination of intrinsic neurologic diagnoses such as multiple scleroses or motor neuron disease is necessary but may be difficult.

It is essential in planning the surgical approach to assess the sagittal contour of the spine. Posterior decompressive surgery alone in the patient with either static or dynamic kyphosis will be ineffective in relieving myelopathy and may accelerate development or progression of the kyphos leading to progressive myelopathic symptoms. Mikawa et al[43] have reviewed the methods of measurements of cervical motion and described four types of curvatures: lordotic, straight, kyphotic, and meandering. In the Batzdorfs' review,[3] positive results of laminectomy correlated only with a lordotic spine, using a similar classification scheme. Figure 50-1 shows an example of spinal alignment that can be considered for posterior decompression alone. Figure 50-2 shows alignment in which either anterior procedure should be considered if the alignment is fixed or posterior instrumentation if mobile and posterior procedure are deemed appropriate.

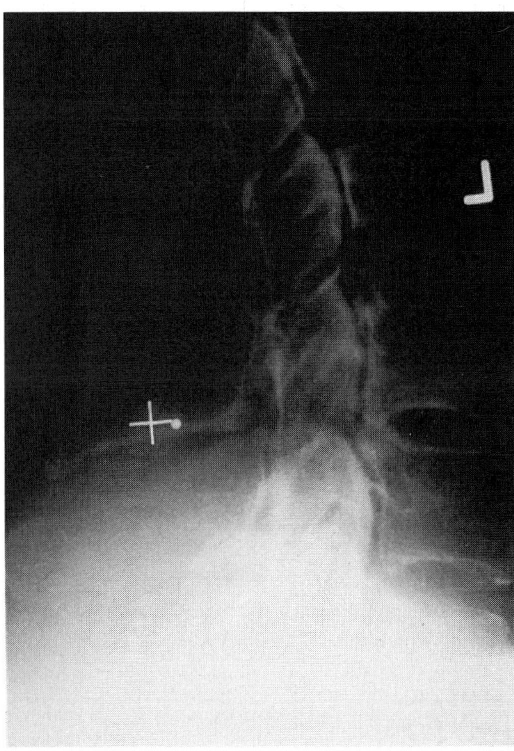

**FIGURE 50-1**

Myelograph of patient with normal lordosis in which laminectomy should be safe.

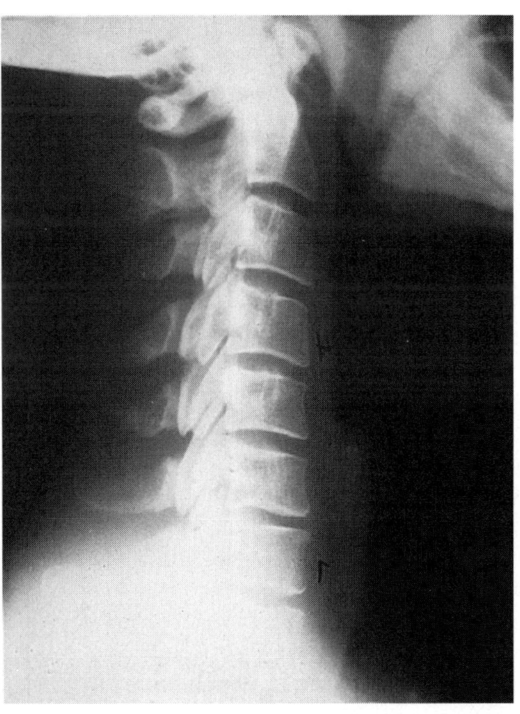

**FIGURE 50-2**

Lateral radiograph of a straight spine. Here, either an anterior procedure to recreate lordosis or posterior fusion at the time of laminectomy should be considered.

## LAMINECTOMY ALONE

With these generalizations in mind, laminectomy is indicated to correct the following specific problems.

### RADICULOPATHY WITH LATERAL DISK OR SPONDYLOSIS

We initially do posterior hemilaminectomy with facetectomy and disk removal. This provides better lateral exposure of the nerve root than can be obtained with the anterior approach. For spondylosis we curette

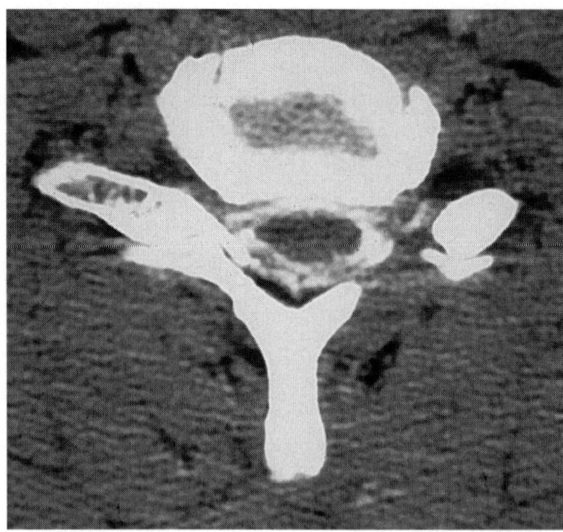

**FIGURE 50-3**

Axial CT image of a 40-year-old man who underwent laminectomy and facetectomy, without excision of the disk fragment. His symptoms persisted and an anterior diskectomy and fusion were required for relief.

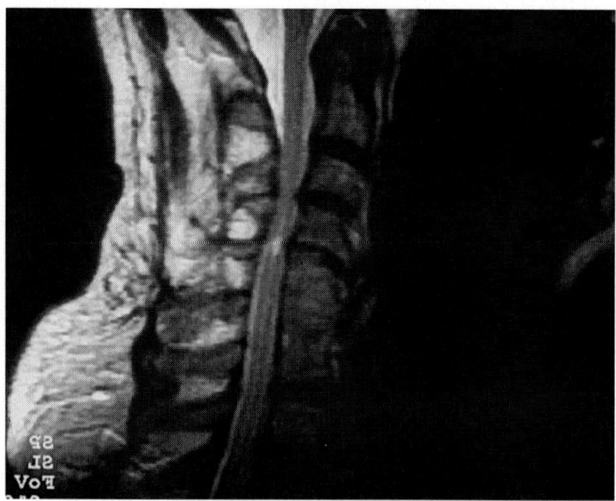

**FIGURE 50-4**

Lateral sagittal MRI of a 51-year-old man who has previously had good result with three cervical procedures. He presents with a 4-month history of root symptoms in his arm. Note the bright area in the cord.

the ventral epidural space anterior to the nerve root with small Epstein curettes. We and others[18,29,48] do not follow the suggestion of Henderson[31] that a facetectomy alone is sufficient. We also have not decompressed the nerve root using the uncovertebral approach described by Louis (Fig. 50-3).[37]

### MYELOPATHY FROM MULTILEVEL SPONDYLOSIS OR OSSIFICATION OF POSTERIOR LONGITUDINAL LIGAMENT WITH GOOD LORDOSIS

In this situation we address the narrow spinal canal.[16] If the spine is stable we will do a multilevel laminectomy, taking care not to disrupt the lateral aspect of the facets. This will allow the spinal cord to migrate posteriorly away from ventral masses.[49,50] Because there frequently is a posterior compressing component, this will be dealt with by the posterior approach. If it is felt that the patient is unstable we perform a laminectomy with a posterior plated fusion following the laminectomy. There are instances in which there is instability and an anterior resection is indicated. We will then initially do a posterior fusion and then the anterior corpectomy with plated fusion, at the same or a subsequent operation. This has been better tolerated by the patient than a prolonged period in a halo.[25,35]

## LESIONS IN WHICH LAMINECTOMY ALONE IS NOT THE PROCEDURE OF CHOICE

In treating the following conditions, either the nature or location of the pathology make laminectomy alone not the appropriate operation.

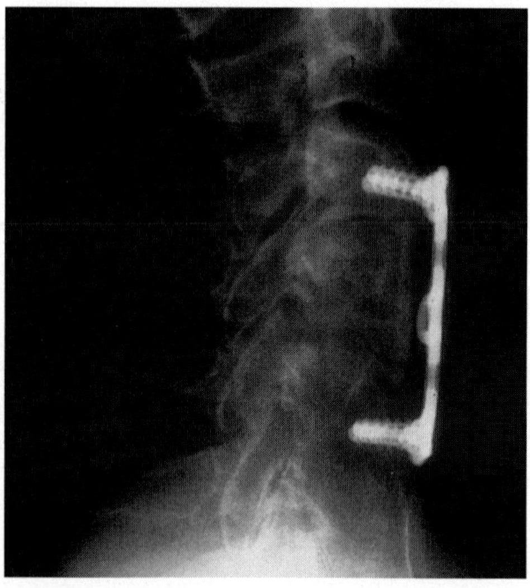

**FIGURE 50-5**

Postoperative radiograph of the same patient following anterior diskectomy and fusion with complete resolution of his numbness and pain.

### MYELOPATHY FROM ACUTE MIDLINE HERNIATED DISK

We do anterior diskectomy and fusion removing the posterior longitudinal ligament and exposing the dura. We have not performed an anterior diskectomy without fusion as supported by Dorward[40] and by Sonntag.[56] Our concern is that the relatively good short-term result will be followed by kyphotic deformity with late progressive myelopathy. Time and further study will answer this question. Figures 50-4 and 50-5 show our suggested approach for this type of lesion.

### Myelopathy with a Kyphotic Spine

In this situation, we will perform a corpectomy of the compressing levels with interbody fusion. We have not done multilevel diskectomies and interbody fusion as described by Smith and Robinson.[54] We feel this does not provide adequate decompression. We always remove the posterior longitudinal ligament and expose the dura. If there is a fusion segment that spans more than one interspace we will hold the graft in place with a plate. For long defects we consider using a microvascular transfer of a fibular graft.[3,4,21]

### Trauma

The patient with cervical trauma should not have a laminectomy alone.[10,42,44,57] In the intact cervical spine, the interaction of disk, facet joint, and capsule, and the posterior ligamentous complex limit anteroposterior translation to 2 mm at any one interspace.[60] Because virtually 90% of spinal traumas involve flexion, at least one part of this complex is usually injured. Choosing posterior approach alone for decompression will further destabilize this complex and it will not decompress neural elements draped over a kyphotic segment. Combination of fusion with laminectomy at the time of decompression can be highly useful especially in posterior lesions such as facet dislocation. Recognition of preexisting or potential instability at the time of decompression should lead one to consider fusion in any traumatic event. This discussion is expanded elsewhere in this volume.

### Metastatic Tumor

It is relatively rare for metastatic tumor to involve only the posterior elements of the spine. It is not rare for extradural metastases to circumferentially compress the neural elements. While there is some controversy, posterior decompression can be very useful for treatment especially of multilevel lesions or lesions at the cervicothoracic junction. However, given the nature of the lesion and its propensity for progression, stabilization at the time of decompression is indicated for most patients. Many patients will require anterior procedures in combination with the posterior surgery for the complete management of their lesion. Patients with incomplete paraplegia, intact sphincter control, a long duration of neurologic deficit and pain, and a gradual onset of compression will have a better prognosis than others.[45] A full discussion of this topic is beyond the scope of this chapter.

### Intradural Lesions

Intradural lesions usually require extensive exposure for adequate treatment and laminectomy is required for their management. The operating surgeon must be aware of the propensity to develop postlaminectomy kyphotic deformity in this group of patients. Patients who have not completed their growth, those with neurologic deficit, and patients who require resection of the facets for complete exposure of the lesion are especially prone to develop late deformity after this surgery. Treatment with prophylactic bracing, prophylactic fusion at the time of index procedure, and late fusion with instrumentation have been advocated to prevent this problem.

## APPROACH TO REPEAT SURGERY AFTER LAMINECTOMY

What are the indications for repeat surgery? The types of problems that require a second operation can be divided into early and late based on when the patient presents with recurrent or persistent symptoms.

### Early Repeat Surgery

***Persistent Radicular Symptoms.*** Patients whose index surgery failed to relieve their symptoms must have repeat radiological studies to determine the cause. Most commonly, magnetic resonance imaging (MRI) will suffice; occasionally a myelogram with computed tomography (CT) scan will be necessary, especially if fine bony detail is required or sagittal or three-dimensional views would be helpful. The patient may have had an incomplete resection at the correct level, operation at the wrong level, or adequate treatment of the pathology but persistent radiculopathy.

If the resection was at the correct level but the pathology was not completely addressed, repeat surgery is indicated (Figs. 50-6 and 50-7). The large patient with a short neck is especially susceptible to decompression at a level other than that intended because of difficulty in obtaining adequate intraoperative radiographs. Once the problem is recognized, repeat surgery to correct the deficiency should be carried out quickly. If the pathology was adequately addressed initially, the patient should be counseled appropriately and nonoperative modalities employed. Assuming that the initial surgical approach was appropriate, the repeat surgery should be accomplished through the same incision and tract.

***Persistent Myelopathic Symptoms.*** Patients whose myelopathic symptoms persist may have had adequate decompression and simply have myelomalacia that will not improve. Review of the synopsis provided by Epstein[13] shows that even in the best series, only 75% of patients reported improvement of symptoms. We advise our patients of this before surgery and stress the operation for prevention of progression of symptoms. Nonetheless, the patient who does not report improvement should be carefully assessed for adequacy of

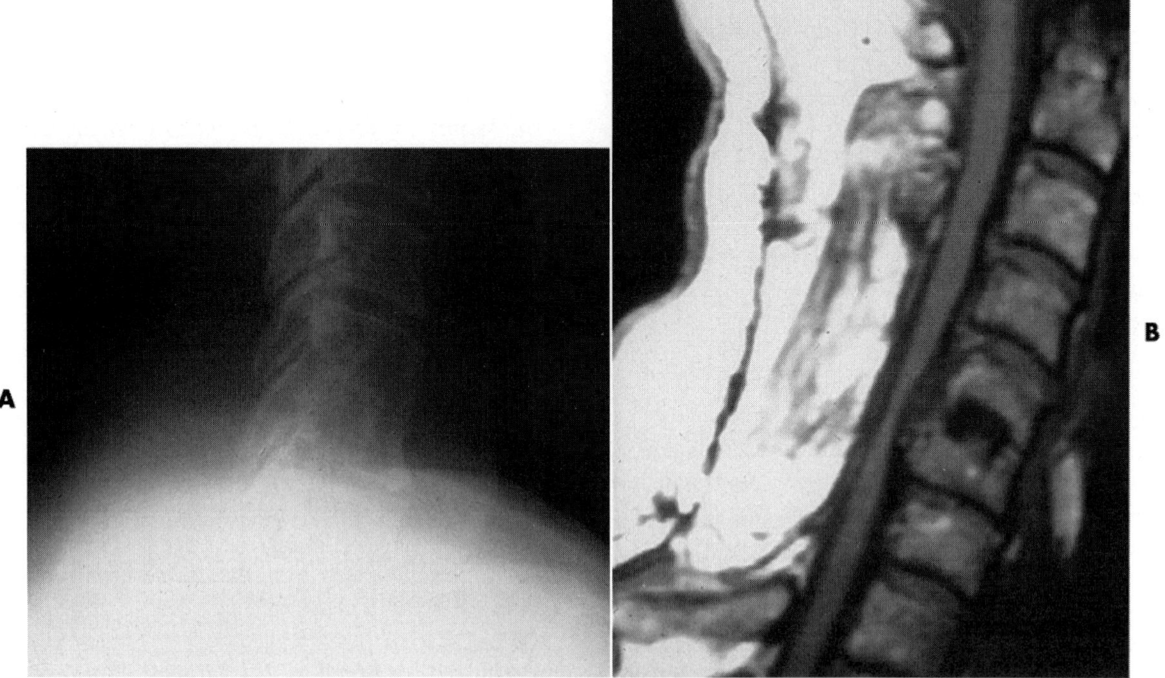


FIGURE 50-6

**A, B,** Lateral radiograph and sagittal MRI of a 58-year-old man who had undergone a laminectomy in 1983 and an anterior procedure in 1985 with persistence of symptoms in his arm. He presents with new leg symptoms and an increase in arm symptoms in 1994. Note the size of the graft used and the failure to completely resect the offending disk material.

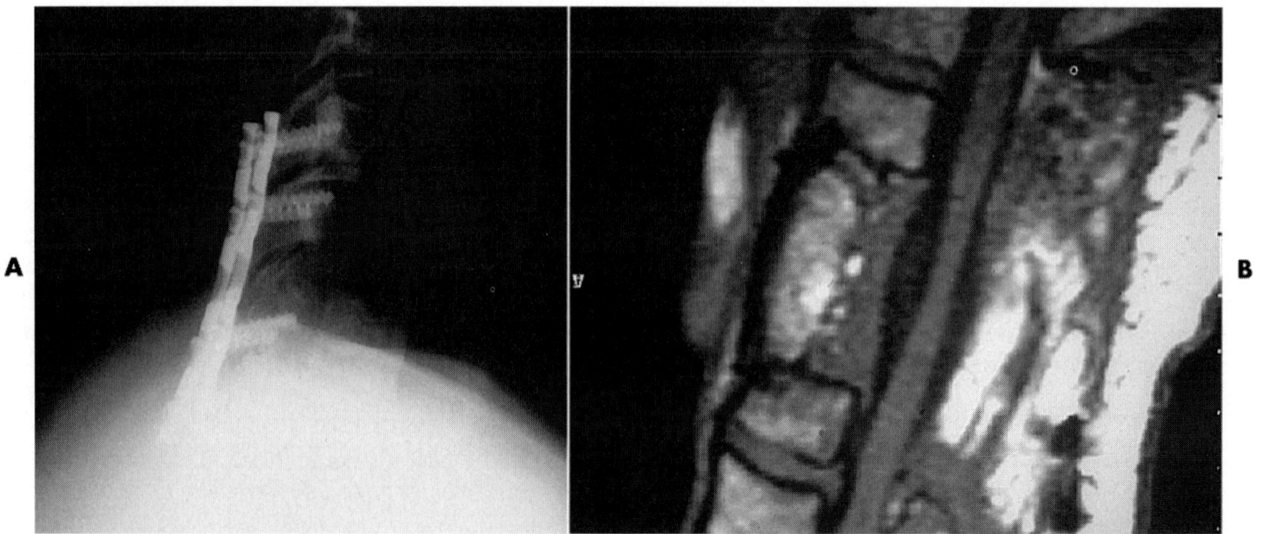


FIGURE 50-7

**A, B,** Postoperative lateral radiograph and sagittal MRI. Note that a posterior fusion and corpectomy have been carried out, and the sagittal contour has been reasonably restored. There is cord atrophy, but copious amounts of cerebrospinal fluid surrounding the spinal cord.

decompression with MRI scanning. Stability of the spine should be evaluated with controlled flexion and extension radiographs.

***Neurologic Deterioration.*** Patients should be closely followed in the immediate postoperative period. Those whose neurologic status deteriorates in the first 24 to 48 hours should have emergent study, usually by MRI, to assess the adequacy of the decompression or the presence of hematoma or other compressive element.

Early correction of the condition is mandatory through the initial approach. Hematoma evacuation should be followed by meticulous cauterization and ligation of vessels. We have seen one case in which the Gelfoam pad placed over the dura became adherent and caused further compression.

Surgery at the wrong level is possible and should be ruled out. Graft or construct dislodgment may occur with subsequent neurologic deterioration.

Infection[30] may be another source of deterioration in the early postoperative period and must be managed aggressively.[34,36] If the patient is on corticosteroids, early signs of infection may be masked. A high index of suspicion is required to appropriately diagnose and manage infection in the operated patient. Wound drainage, fever in the previously afebrile patient, and pain require investigation and may take time to present. While the white blood cell count may be normal, the erythrocyte sedimentation rate or C-reactive protein studies are usually elevated.[5,47]

Infections that occur early after surgery almost always require reoperation for drainage and debridement of necrotic and infected tissue. A high index of suspicion is required for timely diagnosis. Questionable wounds are probably best managed by early surgery. The patient should have adequate cultures before starting antibiotics. The use of oral antibiotics alone to suppress a suspicious wound is discouraged.[36]

In face of infection, the removal or exchange of hardware depends on many factors including the host defenses, the organism involved, and the length of time to treatment.

We do follow the principle of eradication of the infection followed by reconstruction, but if the graft bed is not in direct contact with purulence, we irrigate thoroughly (4 to 6 liters, pulse lavage), leave the hardware in place, close the wound over suction drainage, and if necessary, re-explore the wound in two to three days. Organism-specific intravenous antibiotics are used. Infectious disease consultation should be obtained.

## LATE RECCURRENCE OF SYMPTOMS OR NEW ONSET OF SYMPTOMS

A recurrent lateral cervical disk herniation, as opposed to lumbar disk, is exceedingly rare. If it occurs at the same level and same side, there is a possibility that the initial fragment was missed and the primary operation was inadequate. The nerve root should be re-explored in this situation. A herniation at a different level on the same or opposite side should be handled as a separate problem with a posterior hemilaminectomy and facetectomy. On the other hand, in the rare occasion in which there is extrusion of disk to the opposite side at the original level, we have performed hemilaminectomy and facetectomy but accompanied this by a posterior fusion to prevent the instability caused by bilateral facetectomy at one level.

## PROGRESSION OF MYELOPATHIC SYMPTOMS

If there is progression of myelopathic symptoms, one must be certain that the initial surgery provided adequate decompression.[14,16,27] If the initial surgery, on imaging, was inadequate, this must be corrected. On the other hand, recurrent progressive myelopathy can be related to developing kyphosis or disk herniation at adjacent levels.

## POSTLAMINECTOMY INSTABILITY

Patients who had initial resolution of their symptoms and subsequent recurrence or who present with myelopathy after prior cervical surgery need complete evaluation. Special attention to the sagittal contour of the spine is needed. This may include flexion-extension lateral radiographs and possibly cineradiography to rule out delayed onset of instability.

Preservation of sagittal contour in the cervical spine is a prime consideration for a successful result. Although the flexibility of the spinal cord is such that it can accommodate a large range of motion, a kyphotic deformity stretches the cord and additional motion, usually flexion, will compromise it. The kyphotic deformity causes anterior compression of the cord and, more importantly, compromises its blood supply. Posterior decompression alone will not change the anterior compression unless there has been concomitant resection of the anterior bone or stabilization of the sagittal contour to prevent repetitive cord trauma.

Laminectomy for degenerative conditions has been deemed safe and reported not to lead to late instability.[8,33,49,59] However, incident studies of this entity are hampered in that most of the patients are elderly and are unavailable for follow-up. In 1990, we reviewed a consecutive cohort of surgery patients for the years 1975 to 1985. Of 144 patients identified as having had greater than three-level decompressions, only 73 were available for follow-up. Of these only one case of late instability requiring surgery was noted. Thirty percent of the patients found had C2 or higher as their upper level of decompression.

Treatment of postoperative kyphosis involves decompression of the neural elements and restoration of the cervical lordosis if possible. Johnson and Southwick described fusion using individual facet wiring and fibula strut grafting.[9] A variation on this technique is described by Garfin.[23] Newer techniques using lateral mass plating have better fixation and are very effective.[2,19] If restoration of lordosis is not possible, the patient should be decompressed anteriorly and stabilized both anteriorly and posteriorly.

We recently reviewed our approach to the patient with a straight or slightly kyphotic spine at the time of index or revision surgery.[26] Thirteen patients were analyzed in which we accomplished posterior decom-

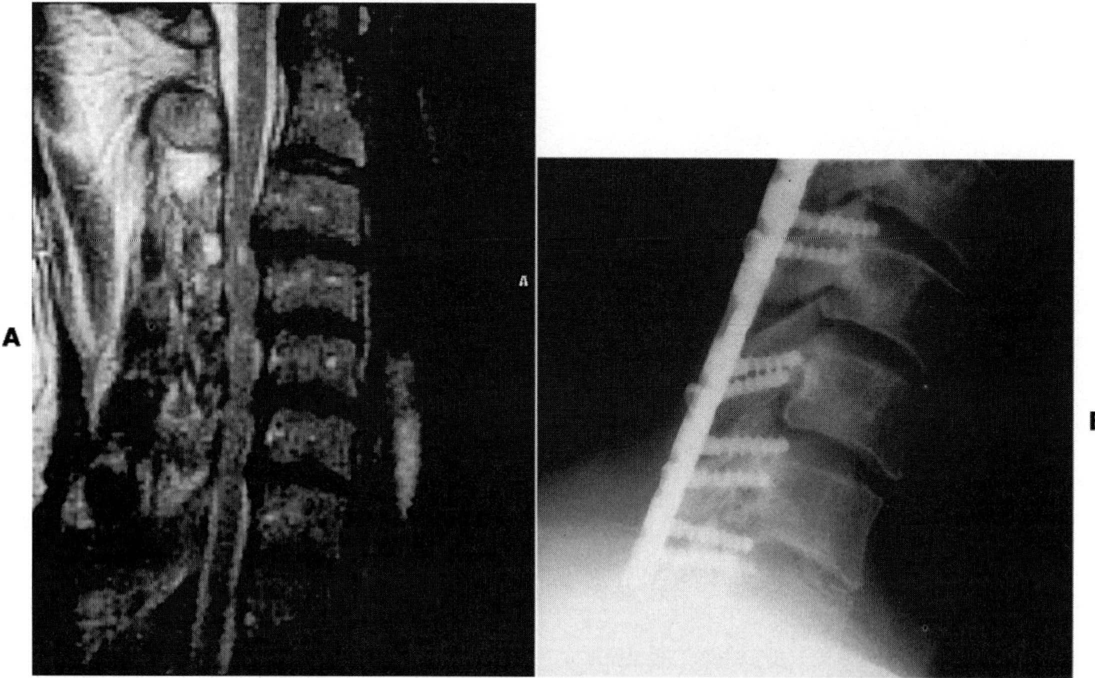

FIGURE 50-8

**A, B,** Lateral sagittal MRI of one of our early cases. A 42-year-old man with predominantly upper extremity symptoms and findings. Postoperative lateral radiograph shows maximal correction obtained. C2 screws are in the inferior portion of the pedicle verified by probing the screw hole in four quadrants at surgery. Patient returned to work at 4 months postoperative.

pression and lateral mass plate fusion as a first step to a procedure that might have included a second-stage anterior operation. We were impressed that we did not need to complete the second stage given the positive response to the first. We were not able to correct the measured lordosis, that is, we were able to correct our patients only to the preoperative maximal extension. One such case is presented in Figure 50-8. We feel that the reason for the good clinical result is that we stabilized the spine and prevented repeat minor trauma to the cord that occurred with flexion. For a fixed severe kyphosis in the face of prior laminectomy, we would do an anterior procedure to obtain extension and combine it with a posterior fixation.

## POSTERIOR RECONSTRUCTION FAILURE

Although this chapter deals with laminectomy failure, it is not uncommon to have prior fusion and/or instrumentation attempted or accomplished. Revision of that procedure may be required.

If posterior reconstruction that has failed was done with wire, reconstruction with lateral mass plates is appropriate. The residual bone stock should be adequate. If prior plating has been done and the screw hold has failed, reconstruction of the screw tract or extension to another level could be considered. We have had only two plate failures in over 50 such cases and those occurred at the end of long constructs. Each occurred late and the patients were asymptomatic so no further repair was undertaken.

Sublaminar wire failure deserves special attention. If removal of a sublaminar wire is required,[46] care must be taken to avoid injuring the dura while removing the wires that were originally placed. Drilling a trough through the lamina may be required. We have done two cases where removal of the wire was facilitated by using a heavy suture attached to the cut end of the wire, maintaining tension on the suture as the wire is removed so as to keep the wire in contact with the lamina as it is removed (Table 50-1).

## LATE POSTOPERATIVE INFECTION

In infections with a delayed insidious onset, the management depends on the setting and the same principles discussed earlier apply. Given the time since the surgery, the graft will usually be either satisfactorily incorporated or necrotic and the host bone deficient. The best option is to remove the loose graft and hardware and once eradication of the infection is accomplished, reconstruct with fresh graft and hardware.

Late hematogenous infections are rare and should be treated by thorough debridement and an assessment

**Table 50-1. Posterior Reconstruction after Failed Instrumentation**

| Failed Element | Consider for Reconstruction |
|---|---|
| Spinous process wire | Sublaminar wire, lateral mass plate |
| Sublaminar wire | Sublaminar wire, lateral mass plate |
| Facet wire | Lateral mass plate, extend level |
| Lateral mass plate | Facet wire, screw reconstruction, extend level |

of stability. If the fusion is solid, it should be left in place. Hardware can be removed if the fusion is solid. All screw holes should be curetted and cleaned of membrane and necrotic tissue. The soft tissues should be managed appropriately. If reconstruction is required, judgment similar to that for delayed onset infections should be employed.

## SURGICAL APPROACH TO REVISION SURGERY

We must be prepared to decompress the spinal elements and stabilize the cervical spine. The surgical approach must be carefully planned in advance. It is necessary to adequately decompress the neural structures whether they be spinal cord or nerve root. The stability of the cervical spine can be maintained by a halo, by anterior and/or posterior plating, or by a posterior fusion prior to a corpectomy. Cusick et al have recommended that in elderly poor-risk patients with spondylitic myelopathy, a fusion alone will provide adequate symptomatic relief.[11]

## SURGICAL TECHNIQUE

Acutely one usually goes through the initial incision, either anteriorly or posteriorly. It is almost always necessary to extend this incision longer than the initial incision. In the anterior cervical spine one may have the option of operating from the opposite side in fresh tissue. If the first surgery was remote in time, one can consider operating from posterior if the previous surgery was anterior and vice versa. This will reduce the possibility of injury to the soft tissues of the neck including the recurrent and superior laryngeal nerves, the carotid sheath, and the esophagus. However, ability to operate in fresh tissue should not be used as the sole criteria for the new approach. The approach to the cervical spine should usually be guided by firm indications.

## IMAGING FOR SURGICAL PLANNING

It has been our practice to repeat imaging in all cases of myelopathy to assess the adequacy of decompression. MRI is the imaging modality of choice to look at the cervical spinal cord. Gadolinium-enhanced MRI helps differentiate unenhanced disk fragment from enhancing scar in the postoperative spine.

For the best definition of the relationship of the spinal cord, subarachnoid space, dura, and bone in the axial view, however, we prefer myelography with postmyelogram CT. The axial images on CT scan also should be critically evaluated for bony landmarks, extent of facet resection, and location of the vertebral artery. The facets and disk spaces should be studied as well for signs of fusion whether or not there has been a previous attempt at surgical fusion.

Flexion-extension x-rays will help to determine stability as well as the maximum amount of lordosis possible. If this alignment is considered inadequate, then an anterior procedure should be entertained as a first step.

### PREOPERATIVE PREPARATION

While revision surgery has significantly more complexity than primary surgery, meticulous preparation is required for both. Special considerations for revisions include the use of spinal cord monitoring if a significant correction of deformity is being considered.[15] One may need intraoperative fluoroscopy especially if upper level fusion is being considered. We position the patient prone if there is considerable instability or a long fusion is required and use the sitting position if extensive decompression is required.[1,17,39] A surgical team should be created with head and neck specialist support for the multiply operated individual or patient in which C2 level or higher anterior procedure is needed. Similar support from the microvascular surgeon, if a vascularized graft is required for reconstruction of a three level or greater anterior corpectomy, may be appropriate. Finally a plastic surgeon may be required for appropriate management of the soft tissues, especially if a large diastasis of the paracervical muscles is present or wound closure problems are anticipated.

Prophylactic use of steroids should be considered only in the face of very severe myelopathy.[7,28,32] If infection is suspected, antibiotics should be withheld until appropriate cultures are taken.

Radiographs, scans, and other studies should be

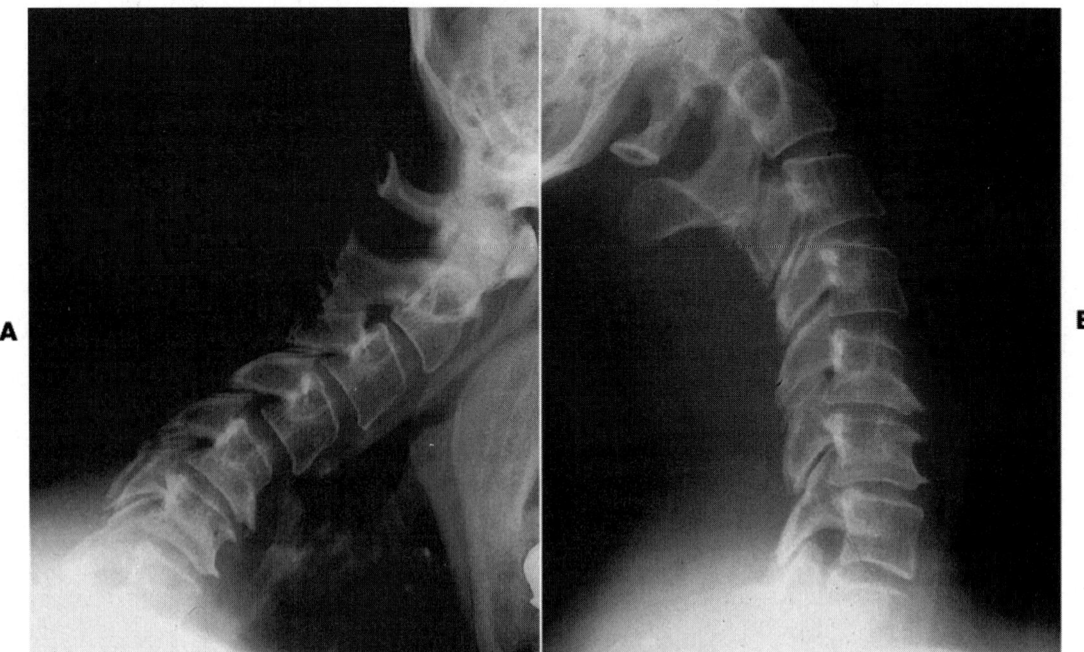


FIGURE 50-9

**A, B,** Flexion-extension lateral radiographs of a 60-year-old woman who had two laminectomies 23 years and 13 years prior to presentation. She complains of l'Hermitte phenomena, numbness, and loss of coordination.

reviewed for bony landmarks as a guide to safe approach. The axial CT images are especially important for planning the type of fixation required and any anatomical aberrations that factor in both the decompression and fusion. If secure internal fixation cannot be expected, the patient should have a halo device applied preoperatively in a manner that will not interfere either with intraoperative imaging or procedure.

Exposure follows the principles valued for all revision surgery: use of the previous incision if possible, exposure from areas of virgin anatomy to areas previously operated, use of bony landmarks for orientation, and liberal use of localizing radiographs as required for safety. We leave scar in place over areas where decompression is not required. However, if fusion is required, meticulous clearing of the scar tissue from the bony areas to be fused is done. The dura is exposed to assure that the decompression is adequate. In our institution, revision surgery is carried out as a team approach with the neurosurgeon performing the decompression he feels is adequate, and the orthopedic surgeon, performing the stabilization. We feel this approach prevents any compromise of either part of the procedure similar to that philosophy expounded by tumor surgeons.

Figures 50-9, 50-10, and 50-11 show the application of this approach to a patient with recurrent disk late after multilevel cervical laminectomy for myelopathy and a flexible neck. Figures 50-12, 50-13, and 50-14 show the approach used for a patient with recurrent myelopathy after laminectomy and a fixed kyphosis.

## COMPLICATIONS OF REVISION SURGERY

### CEREBROSPINAL FLUID LEAK

The problem of cerebrospinal fluid (CSF) leak must be dealt with. In dealing with any recurrent spinal surgery, either in cervical or lumbar area, it is necessary to first find fresh dura before proceeding to the scarred dura. This will help prevent the surgeon from suddenly finding himself in the subarachnoid space when he assumed he was epidural. Should a CSF leak develop it is necessary to expose the area adequately to repair the dura. This can be done by either direct suture, a sutured dural patch, or if necessary a dural patch with fibrin glue. Lumbar drainage for several days may be necessary to allow the repair to heal watertight.[12,22,55]

### NEUROLOGIC DETERIORATION

Neurologic complication can be expected in revision surgery as in the index surgery, though no rates comparison have been found in a literature review.

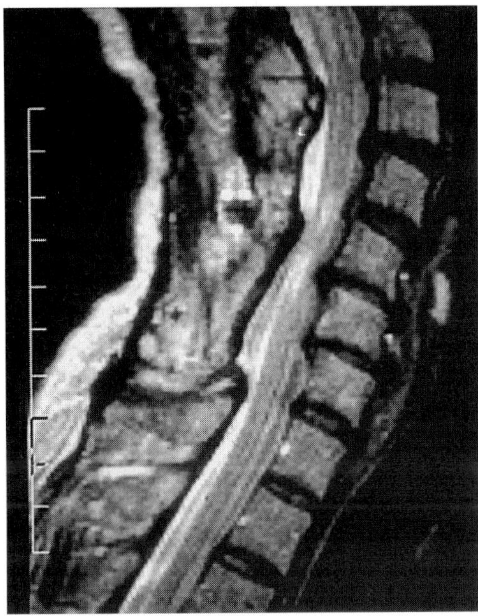

**Figure 50-10**

Lateral sagittal MRI of the same patient shown in Figure 50-9. Note the anterior impression at C5-C6 and the kyphosis at this segment.

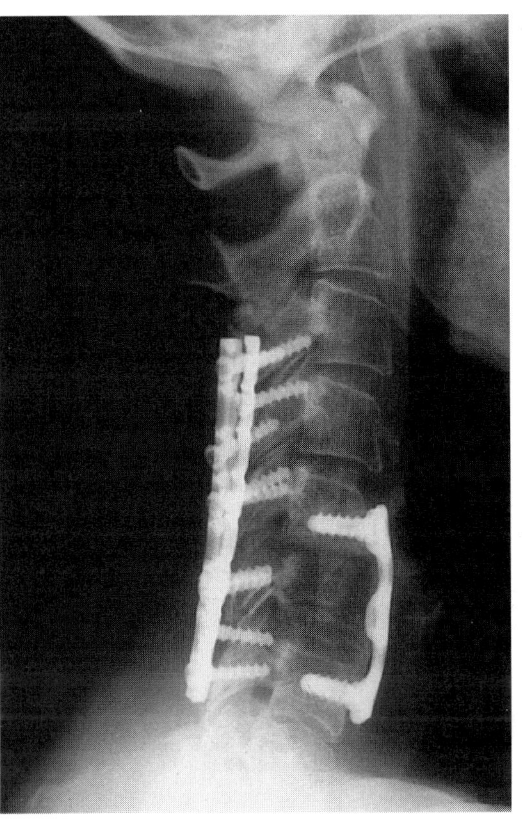

**Figure 50-11**

Postoperative lateral radiograph showing posterior stabilization and anterior corpectomy and fusion. Both are done during the same anesthesia.

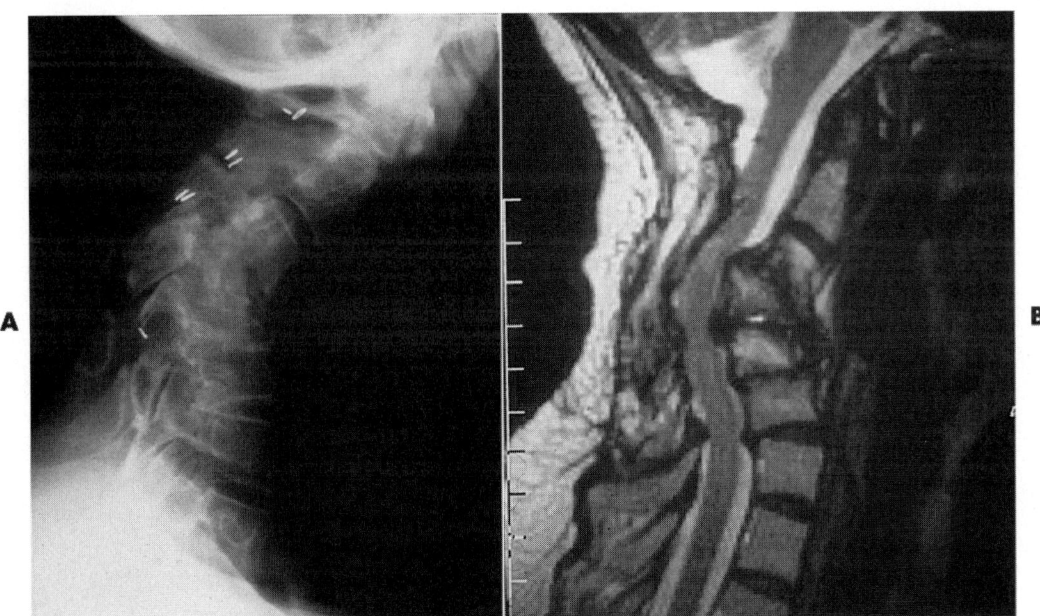


**Figure 50-12**

**A, B,** Lateral radiograph and sagittal MRI of a 59-year-old woman 10 years after laminectomy and cervical rhizotomy for pain. She has symptoms and findings in both upper and lower extremities and has urinary difficulties.

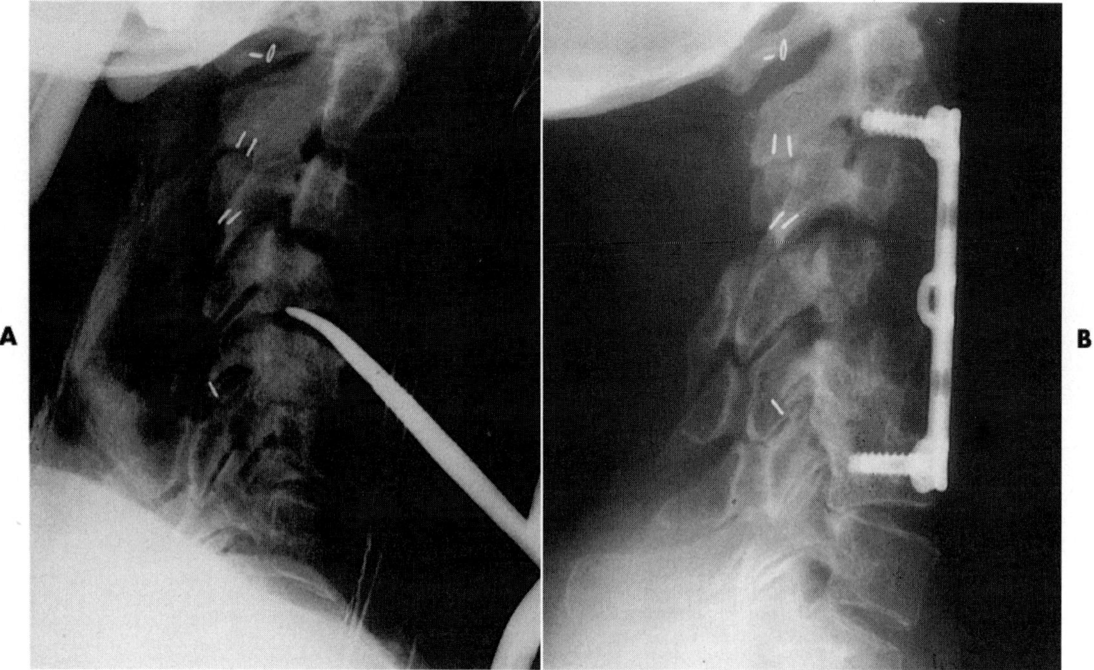

**Figure 50-13**

**A, B,** After a period of traction the patient is brought to the operating room for anterior extension osteotomy (corpectomy) and tricortical iliac crest graft and plate fixation.

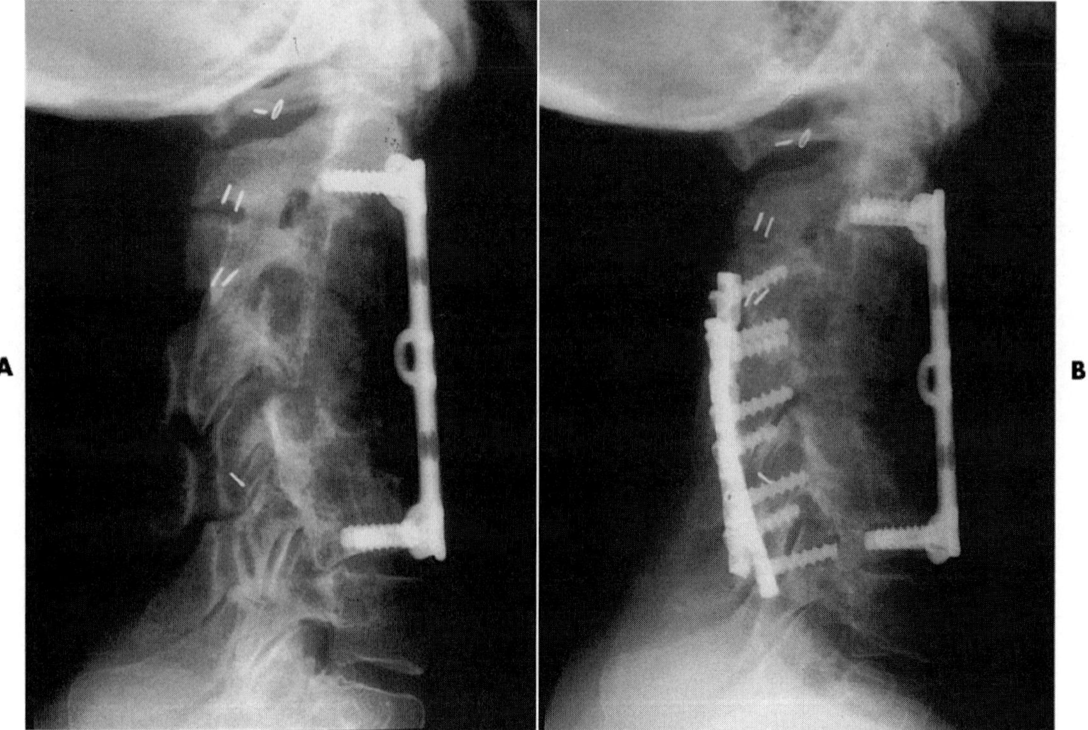

**Figure 50-14**

**A, B,** Eighteen months postoperative, after minor trauma the patient has onset of neck pain. Radiograph shows late fracture of the graft with partial reoccurrence of kyphosis. This is remedied with posterior instrumentation.

Ono et al reported that 5.5% of patients subjected to a variety of surgical approaches for treatment of compression myelopathy sustained neurologic deterioration.[61]

### HARDWARE AND GRAFT FAILURE WITH INSTABILITY

Meticulous attention to detail as outlined above should keep hardware failure to a minimum but rates of failure are not available. In a review of our series of posterior lateral mass plating for kyphosis,[26] we have had a single failure of the lower-most fused segment at 6-month follow-up of an asymptomatic individual. He has been followed now for two years and continues to be asymptomatic.

## SUMMARY

Even with the best conceived and executed primary operation on the cervical spine there will be instances in which repeat surgery is necessary. Repeat surgery usually requires very careful planning, but if done appropriately can provide a satisfactory outcome for the patient who has a failed cervical laminectomy.

## REFERENCES


1. Albin MS, Carroll RG, Maroon JC: Clinical considerations concerning detection of venous air embolism, *Neurosurg* 3:380-384, 1978.
2. An HS, Coppes MA: Posterior cervical fixation for fracture and degenerative disc disease, *Clin Orthop* 335: 101-111, 1997.
3. Batzdorf U, Batzdord A: Analysis of cervical spine curvature in patients with cervical spondylosis, *Neurosurg* 22:827-835, 1988.
4. Bell GR: The anterior approach to the cervical spine, *Neuroimaging Clinics NA* 5:465-479, 1995.
5. Bircher MD, Tasker T, Crawshaw C: Discitis following lumbar surgery, *Spine* 13:98-102, 1998.
6. Boden SD, McCowin PR, Davis DO, Dina TS, Mark AS, Weisel S: Abnormal magnetic resonance scans of the cervical spine in asymptomatic individuals, *J Bone Joint Surg Am* 72:1178-1184, 1990.
7. Braughler JM, Hall ED: Current application of "high dose" steroid therapy for CNS injury, *J Neurosurg* 62: 806-810, 1985.
8. Braun W, Lawandowski M, Handbuch D: *Neurologie* 1:1279, Julius Springer 1910.
9. Callahan RA, Johnson RM, Margolis RN, Keggi KJ, Albright JA, Southwick WO: Cervical facet fusion for control of instability following laminectomy, *J Bone Joint Surg Am* 59A:991-1002, 1977.
10. Capen D, Waters RL, Nelson R, Zeigler J, Sadlar C: Cervical decompressive laminectomy in spinal cord trauma. Instructional course lecture AAOS, 1983.
11. Cusick JF, Steiner RE, Berns T: Total stabilization of the cervical spine in patients with cervical spondylotic myelopathy, *Neurosurg* 18:491-495, 1986.
12. Eismont FJ, Wiesel SW, Rothman RH: Treatment of dural tears associated with spinal surgery, *J Bone Joint Surg Am* 63A:1132-1136, 1981.
13. Epstein JA, Janin Y: *Management of cervical spondylotic myeloradiculopathy by the posterior approach*. In Bailey RW, editor: *The cervical spine,* Philadelphia, 1983, JB Lippencott, pp 402-410.
14. Epstein N, Epstein JA, Benjamin V, Ransohoff J: Traumatic myelopathy in patients with cervical spinal stenosis without fracture or dislocation. Methods of diagnosis, management and prognosis, *Spine* 5:489-496, 1980.
15. Epstein NE, Danto J, Nardi D: Somatosensory evoked potential monitoring during 100 cervical operations, *Spine* 18:737-747, 1993.
16. Fager CA: Results of adequate posterior decompression in the relief of spondylolitic Cervical Myelopathy, *J Neurosurg* 38:684-692, 1973.
17. Fager CA: *Atlas of spinal surgery,* Philadelphia, 1986, Lea & Febiger.
18. Fager CA: Posterior surgical tactics for the neurological syndromes of cervical disc and spondylotic lesions, *Clin Neurosurg* 25:218-244, 1978.
19. Fehlings MG, Cooper PR, Errico TJ. Posterior plates in the management of cervical instability: long term results in 44 patients, *J Neurosurg* 81:341-349, 1994.
20. Feinstein B, Langton JNK, Jameson RM: Experiments of pain referred from deep somatic structures, *J Bone Joint Surg Am* 36:981-997, 1954.
21. Freidberg SR, Gumley GJ, Pfeifer BA, Hybels RL: Vascularized fibula graft to replace resected cervical vertebral bodies, *J Neurosurg* 71:283-286, 1989.
22. Freidberg SR: *Surgical management of cerebrospinal fluid leakage after spinal surgery*. In Schmidek HH, Sweet WH, editors: *Operative neurosurgical techniques,* Philadelphia, 1995, WB Saunders, pp 2049-2054.
23. Garfin SR, Moore MR, Marshall LF: A modified technique for cervical facet fusion, *Clin Orthop* 230: 149-153, 1988.
24. Gore DR, Sepic SB, Gardner GM: Roentgenographic findings of the cervical spine in asymptomatic people, *Spine* 11:521-526, 1986.
25. Goto S: Anterior surgery in four consecutive technical phases for cervical spondylotic myelopathy, *Spine* 18: 1968-1973, 1993.

26. Goulet B, Boren R, Pfeifer BA, Dempsey PD, Freidberg SR: Results of surgery to correct myelopathy secondary to kyphosis. Presented New England Neurosurgical, 1996.
27. Guidetti B, Fortuna A: Long term results of surgical treatment of myelopathy due to cervical spondylosis, *J Neurosurg* 30:714-721, 1969.
28. Hall ED, Wolf MS, Braugler JM: Effects of a single large dose of methylprednisolone sodium succinate on experimental post traumatic spinal cord eschemia, *J Neurosurg* 61:124, 1984.
29. Hardy R: The posterior surgical approach to the cervical spine, *Neuroimaging Clin NA* 5:481-490, 1995.
30. Heller JG: *Postoperative infections of the spine.* In Rothman RH, Simeone FA, editors: *The spine,* Philadelphia, 1992, WB Saunders, pp 1817-1837.
31. Henderson CM: Posterior-lateral foraminotomy as an exclusive operative technique for cervical radiculopathy: a review of 846 consecutively operated cases, *Neurosurg* 13:504-512, 1983.
32. Iizuka H, Iwasaki Y, Yamamoto T: Morphometric assessment of drug effects in experimental spinal cord injury, *J Neurosurg* 65:92-98, 1986.
33. Jenkins D: Extensive cervical laminectomy, long term results, *Br J Surg* 60:852, 1973.
34. Keller RB, Pappas AM: Infections after spinal fusion using internal fixation instrumentation, *Orthop Clin North Am* 3:99-111, 1972.
35. Law MD, Bernhardt M, White AA: Cervical spondylotic myelopathy: a review of surgical indications and decision making, *Yale J Biol Med* 66:165-177, 1993.
36. Lonstein J, Winter R, Moe J, Gaines D: Wound infection with Harrington instrumentation and spine fusion for scoliosis, *Clin Orthop* 96:222-233, 1973.
37. Louis R: *Surgery of the spine: surgical anatomy and operative approaches,* Berlin, 1983, Springer Verlag.
38. Massey EW: Coexistant carpal tunnel syndrome and cervical radiculopathy (double crush phenomenon), *South Med J* 74:957-959, 1981.
39. Matjasko J, Petrozza P, Cohen M, Steinberg P. Anesthesia and surgery in the seated position: analysis of 554 cases, *Neurosurg* 17:695-702, 1985.
40. Maurice-Williams RS, Dorward NL. Extended anterior cervical discectomy without fusion: a simple and sufficient operation for most cases of cervical degenerative disease, *Br J Neurosurg* 10:261-266, 1996.
41. Mayfield FH: Cervical spondylosis: a comparison of the anterior and posterior approaches, *Clin Neurosurg* 13: 181-188, 1965.
42. Meszaros G: Injuries to the cervical spinal cord, *Manitoba Med Rev* 46:182, 1996.
43. Mikawa Y, Shikata J, Yammamuro T: Spinal deformity and instability after multilevel cervical laminectomy, *Spine* 12:6-11, 1987.
44. Morgan TH, Wharton G, Austin G: The results of laminectomy in patients with incomplete spinal cord injuries, *J Bone Joint Surg Am* 52A:822, 1970.
45. Nather A, Kamal B: The results of decompression of the cord or cauda equina decompression from metastatic extradural tumors, *Clin Orthop* 169:103-108, 1982.
46. Nicastro JF, Hartjen CA, Traina J, Lancaster JM. Intraspinal pathways taken by sublaminar wires during removal. An experimental study, *J Bone Joint Surg Am* 68A:1206-1209, 1986.
47. Puranen J, Makela J, Lahde S: Postoperative intervertebral discitis, *Acta Orthop Scand* 55:461-465, 1984.
48. Raynor RB: Anterior or posterior approach to the cervical spine: an anatomical and radiologic evaluation and comparison, *Neurosurg* 12:7-13, 1983.
49. Rogers, L: The surgical treatment of cervical spondylotic myelopathy. Mobilization of the complete cervical cord into an enlarged canal, *J Bone Joint Surg Br* 43:3-6, 1961.
50. Rogers L: The treatment of cervical spondylitic myelopathy by mobilization of the cervical cord into an enlarged spinal canal, *J Neurosurg* 18:490-492, 1961.
51. Scoville, WR: *The surgical approach to the lateral cervical ruptured disc,* read before the Harvey Cushing Society, Boston, 1946.
52. Scoville WB: Cervical spondylosis treated by bilateral facetectomy and laminectomy, *J Neurosurg* 18:423-428, 1961.
53. Simeone FA: *Cervical disc disease with radiculopathy.* In Rothman RH, Simeone FA, editors: *The spine,* ed 3, Philadelphia, 1992, WB Saunders, pp 553-560.
54. Smith GW, Robinson RA: The treatment of certain cervical spine disorders by anterior removal of the intervertebral disc and interbody fusion, *J Bone Joint Surg Am* 40A:607, 1958.
55. Smith MD: Postoperative CSF fistula associated with erosion of the dura, *J Bone Joint Surg Am* 74A:270-277, 1992.
56. Sonntag VK, Klara P: Controversy in spine care. Is fusion necessary after anterior cervical discectomy? *Spine* 21:1111-1113, 1996.
57. Stauffer ES, Shields C: Late instability in cervical spine fractures secondary to laminectomy, *Clin Orthop* 119:144-147, 1976.
58. Stoops WL, King RB: Chronic myelopathy associated with cervical spondylosis: its response to laminectomy and foraminotomy, *JAMA* 192:281-284, 1965.
59. Teng P: Spondylosis of the cervical spine with compression of the cervical cord and nerve roots, *J Bone Joint Surg Am* 42A:392, 1960.
60. White AA, Panjabi, MM: *Clinical biomechanics of the spine.* Philadelphia, 1978, JB Lippencott Co.
61. Yonenobu K, Hosono N, Iwasaki M, Asano M, Ono K: Neurologic complications of surgery for cervical compressive myelopathy, *Spine* 16:1277-1282, 1991.
62. Yonenobu K, Okada K, Fuji T, Fujiwara K, Yamashits K, Ono K: Causes of neurologic deterioration following surgical treatment of cervical myelopathy, *Spine* 11:818-823, 1985.

# 51

# THORACOLUMBAR PSEUDARTHROSIS: GENERAL CONSIDERATIONS

**Stephen I. Esses, M.D.**
**Michael H. Heggeness, M.D., Ph.D.**
**Ramin Raiszadeh, B.S.**



Pseudarthrosis continues to be the most frequent complication of thoracolumbar spinal arthrodesis.[23] It has been considered the leading cause of failed back surgery. The number of fusion procedures carried out annually has increased dramatically. It is estimated that currently approximately 20,000 spine fusion procedures are carried out annually in North America.[8] With the increasing longevity of the population it is estimated that 4% of the population will undergo spine fusion in their lifetime.[1]

In this chapter general considerations about pseudarthroses are discussed. This includes: various modalities to identify and diagnose pseudarthroses, their histology, and a system for classifying them. It is important to have an understanding of these topics to direct intelligent management. Nonoperative and operative treatment are discussed in a later chapter.

There are a variety of indications for lumbar spine fusion. These have been well-described elsewhere. These include degenerative disk disease, deformity, trauma, and spondylolisthesis. Although the most common indication is degenerative disk disease, it is precisely this indication that has the highest clinical failure rate.[8]

The rates of reported pseudarthroses are variable and are dependent on several criteria. These include the various diagnostic criteria used to establish the presence or absence of fusion, the underlying diagnosis for the indicated fusion, patient age, the use of certain medications and tobacco, litigation and workers' compensation involvement, the number of previous spine operations, intraoperative technique, the number of levels fused, and the type of postoperative immobilization and treatment.[23]

## IDENTIFICATION

Following spine fusion, 30% to 40% of patients have persistent or recurrent pain.[20] A pseudarthrosis in the fusion mass may be the cause or a contributing factor in many of these cases. Slizofski stated that pseudarthrosis may produce persistent postoperative low back pain as was evidenced by 60% of his patients (9 out of 15 patients).[26] However, DePalma and Rothman found no significant difference between patients with pseudarthroses as compared to patients with solid fusions.[7] Similarly, Watkins et al reported that 43% of their patients with pseudarthrosis were asymptomatic.[27] Whether patients are symptomatic or asymptomatic from a pseudarthrosis, there are a variety of diagnostic techniques that can be used to identify failure of the fusion. It is generally agreed that early methods of diagnosis are able to detect pseudarthroses within 1 year of surgery. It is certainly advantageous to make an early diagnosis to prevent loss of correction, failure of instrumentation, and pain.

It may be possible to assess the state of fusion by careful attention to the postoperative history and physical findings.[21] Pain and tenderness localized over a fusion area suggest pseudarthrosis, especially when the patient is in the prone position. Localized pain may also indicate tuberculosis of the spine. However, with clinical and roentgenographic examination, in addition to blood tests, one may rule out this disease. In some cases a successful spine fusion may not result in relief of symptoms.[7] However, patients who continue to have low back pain and have a solid fusion usually do not have well-defined localization of the pain and have more diffuse tenderness.

In patients who have been fused for an infection such as tuberculosis, the patient's neurological status may give an indication to the presence of pseudarthrosis. In these instances the pseudarthrosis may allow continued activity of the underlying infective process and therefore may be associated with progressive neurologic deficits. Ralston and Thompson reported that of 21 patients who developed pseudarthrosis following fusion for tuberculosis, progression of spasticity was prominent in seven.[21]

It may be possible to detect pseudarthroses by documenting anatomical changes. Surgical fusion of the spine means that the spine is fixed by a continuous column of bone that allows no motion in any plane of the body throughout the vertebral segments involved.[21] Progression of deformity over a long period of time usually indicates failure of fusion. Furthermore, following spine fusion for scoliosis, lateral deformity indicates failure of fusion. Any increase in sagittal or frontal deformity in excess of 5 degrees should be regarded with suspicion. In addition, an increase in listhesis in the frontal or sagittal plane may be an indicator of underlying pseudarthrosis. In these instances the presence of a pseudarthrosis should be considered.

Despite the many radiographic methods used to evaluate the fusion mass, many have proven to be unreliable. Dawson and Clader reported that anteroposterior and lateral radiographs of the full spine with the patient standing were useful only in measuring spinal deformity.[6] They reported that these radiographs had a rate of correlation to the presence of pseudarthroses in only 48% of cases. They also reported that the use of oblique radiographs increased the sensitivity in identification of pseudarthrosis. They suggested an 82% correlation between abnormal oblique radiographs and the presence of pseudarthroses. Because a pseudarthrosis usually occurs through the facet joint and because these joints are best seen on the oblique views, the oblique radiographs have been recorded by many as the most reliable for visualizing the fusion mass. However, these oblique radiographs are not as reliable when used for patients with kyphosis or rotational deformity.[6]

Dynamic radiography has been used to evaluate fusions. The most popular technique is the flexion-extension lateral radiograph.[23] Because micromotion can be present without radiographic motion, one might expect a low sensitivity with this technique. Nevertheless, investigators still use flexion-extension lateral radiographs and side-bending views to help identify a pseudarthrosis. Albert et al were able to successfully diagnose 82% of pseudarthroses with posteroanterior (PA), lateral, and oblique radiographs, but only a 23% pseudarthrosis rate was found with flexion-extension films.[1] Brodsky et al, in 214 explorations in 175 patients for posterolateral fusions, also found a greater correlation with anteroposterior (AP), lateral, and oblique radiographs as compared to bending films.[2] Lauerman et al similarly did not find bending radiographs of additional assistance.[16]

Scintigraphy employing technetium is another method used to detect pseudarthroses. There is a wide variation in the reported usefulness of technetium bone scans for this purpose. Rawlings and Michelson reported that scintigraphic assessment in the diagnosis of pseudarthroses was not useful particularly in the early diagnosis where there might be some bone formation in an immature fusion.[23] The general principle of scintigraphy is that during the healing process, the increased blood supply and osteoblastic activity result in more absorption of radio nucleotide.[26] However, the bone scan should return to normal within 1 year if healing has occurred. Continued uptake presumably due to continued healing, suggests pseudarthrosis. McMaster and Merrick reported on 110 patients (6 months postoperatively) in whom routine bone scans were done to evaluate the postoperative fusion mass. They reported a 50% false-positive rate and 3% false-negative rate.[19] They added that scans performed after 1 year were more accurate than those performed at 6 months postoperatively. Hannon and Wetta reported a 82% false-negative rate.[10] Larsen found the predictive value of bone scanning was negligible.[15]

Tomograms give excellent information on the quality and location of the fusion mass. Tomography has remained extremely useful in the diagnosis of pseudarthrosis. Dawson and associates have reported that anteroposterior tomograms are the most useful radiographic test to demonstrate pseudarthrosis.[6] They reported no false-positive cases in their study and only one false-negative study in 135 patients. They reported the correlation between a known pseudarthrosis and its radiographic identification on AP tomography as 96%, as compared with 82% correlation to pseudarthrosis when AP, lateral, and oblique radiographs were used.[6] The main disadvantage of tomography is the increased amount of radiation exposure the patient receives. However, the amount of exposure is less than the amount of a series of four radiographs (AP, lateral, right, and left oblique). It is crucial when using tomography to adhere to trispiral technique, coning, diaphragms, and gonadal and thyroidal shields to minimize radiation exposure.

Lateral tomography might also be useful in analyzing

a fusion mass.[6,14] It is particularly useful in patients with primary kyphotic deformity as the fusion mass is difficult to detect in other planes. However Dawson et al reported lateral tomography is not as useful as AP tomography.[6] Computerized axial tomography (CAT) initially had limited success in identification of thoracolumbar pseudarthrosis because of its inability to reveal transverse hairline pseudarthrosis.[15] With the development of computer software that allowed reformations in the frontal, sagittal, and coronal planes, the value of CT scanning has increased. Coronal reconstructions are well suited to the evaluation of posterior, posterolateral, and interbody fusions. The usefulness and sensitivity of CT is decreased when metallic implants are near the fusion mass; this may result in artifactual blurring. Image processing techniques can be used to minimize this artifact.

In general, second-look operations have been recorded by many as the gold standard in the identification of a pseudarthrosis. The technique was first proposed by James and later championed by McMaster and Merrick.[18,19] In 1952 Cobb stated that "the only way to be absolutely accurate in a study is to explore each one, and even then one might overlook an occasional pseudarthrosis."[5] McMaster and Merrick reported that 2 of 9 patients had a pseudarthrosis that was missed at time of reexploration.[19] Subperiosteal dissection over a fusion mass at time of surgery should demonstrate smooth stripping of tissue from the bone. When this does not occur a pseudarthrosis may be present. A demonstration of motion within the fusion mass is an absolute indication that a pseudarthrosis is present. Clearly, the disadvantage of second-look surgery is the increased morbidity and mortality associated with a second procedure. At the present time a routine second operation is not indicated except in patients with paralytic scoliosis. In these cases the incidence of pseudarthroses is sufficiently high that a routine reexploration is justified.

It has been reported that instrumentation improves fusion rates. Grubb et al in 100 patients with degenerative disk disease whose spines were fused, reported 35% pseudarthrosis in patients without instrumentation compared with 6% pseudarthrosis in patients with instrumentation.[9] Similarly, Lorenz reported 58.6% pseudarthrosis in 29 patients without instrumentation compared with no pseudarthrosis in 39 patients with instrumentation.[17] Thus, failure of instrumentation may also indicate the presence of a pseudarthrosis. The classic teaching has been that a race exists between the development of a solid fusion mass and implant failure. That is, it was formerly thought that implant failure necessarily was an indication of underlying continued motion due to the presence of a pseudarthrosis. With new pedicle screw implants, however, there may be a significant mismatch between the modulus of elasticity of the implants and the fusion mass. In these cases, implant failure does not necessary indicate an underlying pseudarthrosis.

In summary, second-look surgery is the most sensitive and specific method for the detection of spinal pseudarthrosis. Of the noninvasive methods available, it would appear that AP tomography is the most reliable. The use of plain radiography, flexion-extension radiographs, CT, and bone scintigraphy for the preoperative evaluation of fusion status is neither accurate nor cost-effective.

## HISTOLOGY

We have previously published a histologic description of pseudarthroses.[12] In addition, we have presented research demonstrating nerve fibers within the fibrous matrix adjacent to thoracolumbar pseudarthroses.[13] This histologic study was undertaken based on biopsy specimens obtained at surgery from 40 consecutive patients during open pseudarthrosis repair procedures. Biopsy specimens were taken from solid areas of the fusion mass, from areas of motion, and from the lumbar facet joint remnant when identifiable (Figs. 51-1 and 51-2).

Soft tissue found between adjacent bony segments was noted to contain predominately fibrous tissue. A dense fibrous stroma was noted, often accompanied by local signs of fibrocartilaginous metaplasia within the scar tissue. Neural fibers were identified within the fibrous tissue adjacent to the pseudarthrosis, but in no instance was nerve tissue seen within the fibrous tissue located specifically between the bony surfaces. Immunohistochemical staining for the S100 protein was performed on these specimens and no positive staining for this protein (which normally stains neural tissue) was found between adjacent bony surfaces.

Small fragments of impacted nonviable bone were frequently seen embedded in the fibrous tissue between the mobile segments. These fragments of bone were sometimes noted to be undergoing active resorption and occasionally demonstrated a foreign body response. The presence of these nonviable bony fragments within the fibrous tissue matrix has not been described in long bone pseudarthrosis.[28] The histologic appearance of these areas of the specimen was strikingly similar to that of a Charcot joint. In no specimens were discrete synovial cavities seen, a feature that has been described with long bone pseudarthrosis.

The bone immediately adjacent to the fibrous areas of motion was noted to be universally sclerotic. A poorly organized mixture of woven lamellar bone was universally seen. These bony areas were noted to frequently contain enclosed islands of incompletely mineralized matrix. The endosteal bone surfaces near the areas of motion were usually covered with active

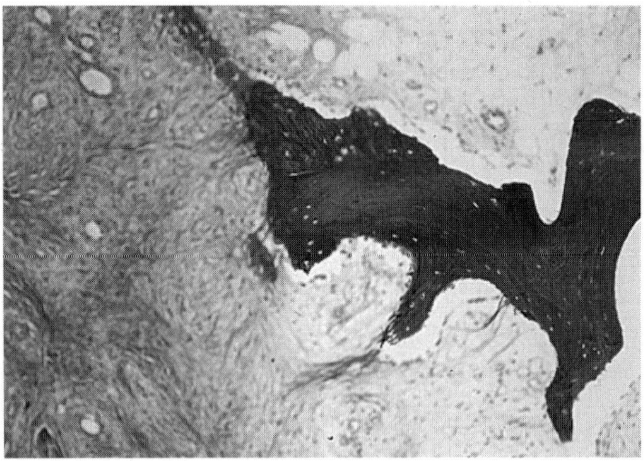

**Figure 51-1**

The histologic appearance of a typical lumbar pseudarthrosis. Fibrous tissue is present between the bone surfaces. This section demonstrates ongoing new-bone formation at the edge of the bone surface.

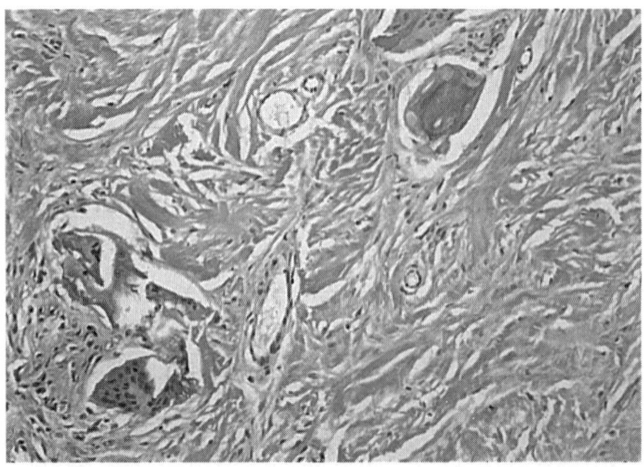

**Figure 51-2**

A typical histologic field from between the opposed bony surfaces demonstrating fragments of nonviable bone present within dense fibrous tissue.

osteoblast. Interestingly, in the cancellous bone underlying the sclerotic areas near the regions of motion, microtrabecular fractures in various stages of active healing were sometimes noted.

All of the facet joint biopsies (n = 18) were remarkable for very significant degenerative disease characterized by subchondral sclerosis, cartilage fissuring, and chondrocyte cloning.

This study demonstrated that in the majority of lumbar pseudarthroses, the primary tissue noted between the opposed bony surfaces is fibrous tissue with the frequently encountered feature of embedded fragments of nonviable bone. While it is possible the areas of this fibrous tissue may be innervated, no nerve tissue was documented in these areas in the course of this study. Nerves were frequently seen in scar tissue adjacent to these areas, a finding that may have clinical significance.

The microtrabecular fractures noted in the cancellous bone underlying the opposed bone ends suggest another possible source of pain. It might be theorized that these fractures occur as a result of incongruities in the opposed bone ends when subjected to continued motion. The presence of the severe degenerative changes in the facet joint remnants at the site of pseudarthrosis was not unexpected and indeed may also be considered a likely source of pain in some, if not many, patients.

The true clinical significance of these observations must await further work, because all of the patients in the above study had complaints of pain. No biopsy specimens were available from painless pseudarthroses. This histologic study does, however, suggest the possibility that there may be multiple possible pain sources in any given patient with a failed fusion. This may be important in the assessment and treatment of these patients.

## CLASSIFICATION

Pseudarthroses of the long bones are classified and characterized in the classic work by Weber and Ceck.[28] Their classification system, however, does not apply to spinal pseudarthroses. We have previously reviewed imaging studies and operative records on 85 surgically documented pseudarthroses.[11] We have published a classification system that is useful in understanding the reasons for graft failure. There may be significant treatment implications if the type and cause of a particular pseudarthrosis can be identified.

A spinal pseudarthrosis is defined as an absence of bridging bone between adjacent vertebrae. This may be manifest as gross atrophy and resorption of the bone graft. In these instances the failed fusions are designated as atrophic (Fig. 51-3).

In some circumstances a substantial mass of viable remodeled bone may be recognized. This bone may be continuous with the fusion mass of adjacent levels but may process a horizontal of transverse discontinuity. In those instances in which there is bone graft but there is discontinuity in the frontal plane the pseudarthrosis is classified as transverse (Fig. 51-4).

A third morphologic type of pseudarthrosis can also be classified as shingle pseudarthrosis. In this instance there is a substantial amount of fusion bone but a defect is present in the fusion mass, which passes obliquely through the sagittal plane. This type of pseudarthrosis is similar to an onion skin in which the fusion bone is solid but is not continuous with the underlying vertebral bone (Fig. 51-5).

In some instances a pseudarthrosis can not be classified as only an atrophic, transverse, or shingle type.

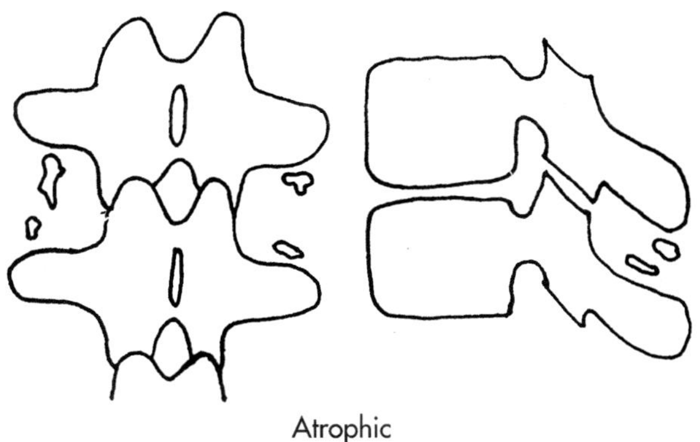


FIGURE 51-3

Schematic of atrophic pseudarthrosis.

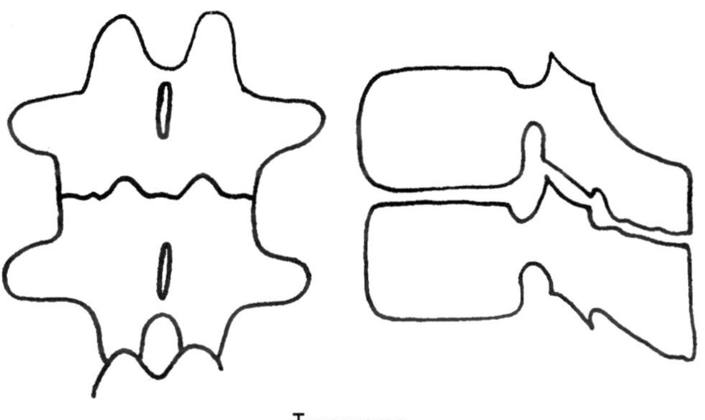


FIGURE 51-4

Schematic of transverse pseudarthrosis.

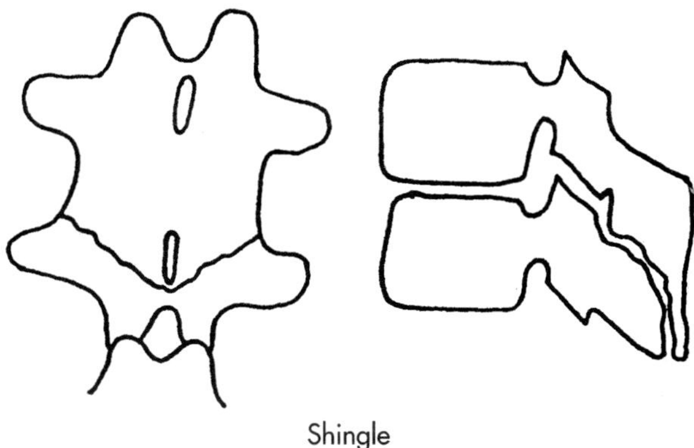


FIGURE 51-5

Schematic of shingle pseudarthrosis.

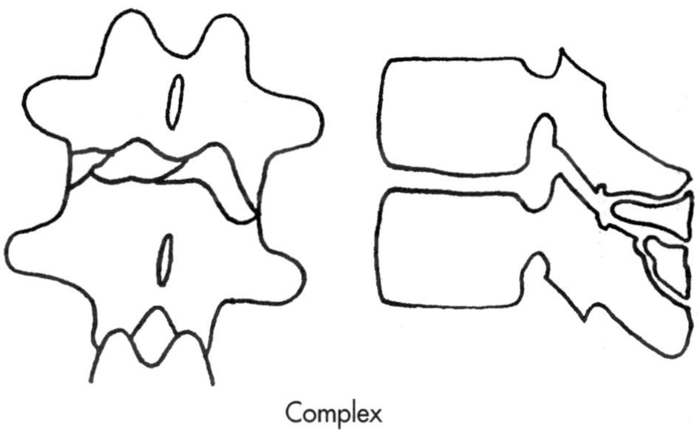


FIGURE 51-6

Schematic of complex pseudarthrosis.

When there is more than one adjacent defect in the fusion mass between adjacent vertebrae the pseudarthrosis is classified as complex (Fig. 51-6).

## AGE, SMOKING, METABOLIC, AND MEDICATION ISSUES

Whether or not a solid fusion is achieved after repair for pseudarthrosis, or even after primary arthrodesis, several factors play an important role for clinical success; the three more common factors that may predispose to pseudarthrosis are age, smoking habits, and medication.

Advanced age is frequently accompanied by degenerative changes at multiple levels. Multiple-level fusion increases the magnitude of surgery, and the lengthy postoperative recovery can exceed 6 months to 1 year. Esses and Huler state that the magnitude of multiple level arthrodesis, in the presence of osteoporotic bone and advancing age, invite significant perioperative morbidity.[8] Thus, in patients with advancing age requiring multiple fusion, nonoperative management may be the best solution. In the younger patient, moreover, the literature has suggested accelerated proximal and distal degenerative changes immediately adjacent to successful lumbar arthrodesis. Carpenter et al noted that there was no association between the age of the patient and the rate of pseudarthrosis.[4]

Carpenter et al and Silcox et al both reported the association between pseudarthrosis and smoking.[4,25] Of 72 patients who had primary attempts at repair of pseudarthrosis, 34 were smokers, and 38 were nonsmokers at the time of the operation. Patients who stopped smoking before the surgery faired better than those who had not stopped (less pain, less disability, more progress, and more patient satisfaction). Furthermore, Silcox et al reported that there is a direct correlation between the systemic presence of nicotine in an animal model and delayed bony healing.[25] In his experiment, 16 of 28 rabbits underwent single-level posterior lateral intertransverse process fusion and had a nicotine-filled mini osmotic pump and all had failed fusions. Furthermore, his results suggest the bone formed in the face of systemic nicotine has decreased biochemical properties.

Brown, et al also investigated the relationship of smoking with the rate of pseudarthrosis.[3] He compared

50 patients who had smoked and 50 patients who did not smoke; the patients selected were patients who had a two-level posterior lateral spine fusion from L4 to the sacrum. None of the patients had any type of internal fixation device, and it was the first fusion attempt for each. Brown reported that the oxygenation ($PO_2$) level in smokers averaged 78.5%, and that in the nonsmokers was within normal limits, between 95% to 97%. His results showed that smokers generally have lowered blood gas levels secondary to increased carbon monoxide (CO) absorption and arterial vasoconstriction. Therefore, it is postulated that pseudarthrosis is more likely to develop in smokers because of inadequate oxygenation to the healing graft.

Raney and Kolb have suggested that metabolic bone disease also contributes to the development of pseudarthrosis.[22] They reported that 47 of 66 patients with diagnoses of untreated postmenopausal estrogen deficiency with osteoporosis, malabsorption, phosphate depletion from excess antacid use, abnormalities of vitamin D, or excess use of alcohol and/or tobacco, healed after correction of the metabolic abnormality. Schofferman et al reported, however, that metabolic disorders may play a small role in the development of pseudarthroses, but that most pseudarthroses are not due to metabolic factors.[24]

It is clear that certain medications affect metabolism. Anticonvulsants, such as Dilantin, have been shown to inhibit bone formation. Patients on these medications may be prone to the development of a pseudarthrosis. It has also been thought that steroid use is a risk factor for pseudarthrosis formation.

New bisphosphonate medications have recently been developed. Although some of these may be useful in the treatment of metabolic disorders such as Paget's disease or osteoporosis they may have a deleterious effect on bone healing. Further studies are needed to document the effect of drugs such as Didronel and Fosomax on pseudarthrosis formation. For the moment, it is probably preferable to have patients so treated discontinue these drugs in the perioperative period.

## SUMMARY

It is clear that although the complication of thoracolumbar pseudarthrosis is frequent there has been little scientific investigation into its causes, identification, and histopathology. One should consider the diagnosis of a pseudarthrosis in any patient who has undergone a fusion and who continues to have symptoms. It needs to be reiterated, however, that the demonstration of a pseudarthrosis does not necessarily mean that the patient's symptoms are arising from it. Further work and research should be given to addressing this frequent cause for revision in spine surgery.

## REFERENCES


1. Albert TJ, Pinto M, Johnson E, Dennis F: Treatment of symptomatic lumbar pseudarthrosis with AP fusion: a functional and radiographic outcome study. Presented at the 28th Annual Meeting of Scoliosis Research Society, Dublin, Ireland, Sept. 19-23, 1993.
2. Brodsky AE, Kovalsky ES, Khalil MA: Correlation of radiologic assessment of lumbar spine fusions with surgical exploration, *Spine* 16:S261-S265, 1991.
3. Brown CW, Orme TJ, Richardson HD: The rate of pseudarthrosis (surgical nonunion) in patients who are nonsmokers: a comparison study. Presented at the Tenth Annual Meeting of the International Society for the Study of the Lumbar Spine, Cambridge, England, April 1983.
4. Carpenter CT, Dietz JW, Leung KYK, et al: Repair of pseudarthrosis of the lumbar spine, *J Bone Joint Surg* 78-A:712-720, 1996.
5. Cobb JR: Technique, after-treatment, and results of spine fusion for scoliosis. In Instructional Course Lectures, The American Academy of Orthopaedic Surgeons 9:65-70, 1952.
6. Dawson EG, Clader TJ, Bassett LW, et al: A comparison of different methods used to diagnose pseudarthrosis following posterior spinal fusion for scoliosis, *J Bone Joint Surg* 67A:1153-1159, 1985.
7. DePalma AF, Rothman RH: The nature of pseudarthrosis, *Clin Orthop* 59:113-118, 1968.
8. Esses SI, Huler RJ: Indications for lumbar spine fusion in the adult, *Clin Orthop* 279:87-100, 1992.
9. Grubb SA, Lipscomb HJ: Results of lumbosacral fusion for degenerative disk disease with and without instrumentation, *Spine* 17:349-355, 1992.
10. Hannon KM, Wetta WJ: Failure of technetium bone scanning to detect pseudarthrosis in spinal fusion for scoliosis, *Clin Orthop* 123:42-44, 1977.
11. Heggeness M, Esses SI: Classification of pseudarthroses of the lumbar spine, *Spine* 16:S449-S454, 1991.
12. Heggeness M, Esses S, Mody D: A histologic study of lumbar pseudarthrosis, *Spine* 18:1016-1020, 1993.
13. Heggeness M, Esses S, Mody D: Identification of pain sources in lumbar pseudarthrosis. Presented at North American Spine Society, Boston MA, USA, July 1992.
14. Lang P, Genant H, Chafetz N, et al: Three-dimensional computed tomography and multiplanar reforma-

tions in the assessment of pseudarthrosis in posterior lumbar fusion patients, *Spine* 13:69-75, 1988.

15. Larsen JM, Rimoldi RL, Capen DA, et al: Assessment of pseudarthrosis in pedicle screw fusion: a prospective study comparing plain radiographs, CT scanning, and bone scintigraphy with operative findings, *J Spinal Disord* 9:117-120, 1995.
16. Lauerman WC, Bradford DS, Ogilive JW, Transfeld EE: Results of lumbar pseudarthrosis repair, *J Spinal Disord* 5:149-157, 1992.
17. Lorenz M, Zindrick M, Schwaegler P, et al: A comparison of single-level fusions with and without hardware, *Spine* 16:S455-S458, 1991.
18. McMaster MJ, James JIP: Pseudarthrosis after spinal fusion for scoliosis, *J Bone Joint Surg* 58B:305-312, 1976.
19. McMaster MJ, Merrick MV: The scintigraphic assessment of the scoliotic spine after fusion, *J Bone Joint Surg* 62B(1):65-72, 1980.
20. Prothero SR, Parkes JC, Stinchfield FE: Complications after low-back fusion in 1000 patients, *J Bone Joint Surg* 48A:57-65. 1966.
21. Ralston EL, Thompson WA: The diagnosis and repair of pseudarthrosis of the spine, *Surg Gynecol Obstet* 37-44, 1949.
22. Raney FL, Kolb FO: *The effect of metabolic bone disease on spinal fusion.* In: White AM, Rothman R, Ray CD, editors: *Lumbar spine surgery, techniques and complications.* St. Louis, 1987, CV Mosby.
23. Rawlins BA, Michelsen CB: Failed lumbosacral fusions, *Spine: State of the Art Reviews* 8(3):563-571, 1994.
24. Schofferman J, Schofferman L, Zucherman J, et al: Metabolic bone disease in lumbar pseudarthrosis, *Spine* 15:687-689. 1990.
25. Silcox DH, Daftari T, Boden SD, et al: The effect of nicotine on spinal fusion: animal model, *Scoliosis Res Soc* 1996;601.
26. Slizofski WJ, Collier BD, Flatley TJ, et al: Painful pseudarthrosis following lumbar spinal fusion: detection by combined SPECT and planar bone scintigraphy, *Skeletal Radiol* 16:136-141, 1987.
27. Watkins MB: Posterolateral fusion in pseudarthrosis and posterior element defect of the lumbosacral spine, *Clin Orthop* 35:80-95, 1964.
28. Weber BG, Ceck O: *Pseudarthrosis.* Bern, 1976, Hans Huber Publishers.

# 52

# THORACOLUMBAR PSEUDARTHROSIS: TREATMENT CONSIDERATIONS

**Ramin Raiszadeh, B.S.**
**Michael H. Heggeness, M.D., Ph.D.**
**Stephen I. Esses, M.D.**



Degenerative disease continues to be the single greatest reason for performing a spine fusion in North America. Other indications for lumbar arthrodesis include deformity, unstable low lumbar fractures, painful spondylolisthesis, and pain after destabilizing decompression for spinal stenosis or disk disease. Moreover, pseudarthrosis remains the leading cause of failed spine fusion and is of paramount concern to surgeons attempting fusion procedures.[9] In all probability the published rates of pseudarthrosis underestimate the true frequency with which it occurs. This is because many pseudarthroses are not painful. It is of interest, however, that in patients who have documented asymptomatic pseudarthrosis symptoms will often develop at these areas when followed for long periods of time.[3,6,10] Clearly not all pseudarthroses need treatment. In those instances where treatment is considered there are both nonoperative and operative strategies. Operative alternatives include posterolateral, anterior, or anterior and posterior combined fusions.

## NONOPERATIVE MANAGEMENT

The presence of pseudarthrosis after attempted fusion can not automatically be assumed to be the primary cause of continuing symptoms; thus, operative repair is not always mandatory. A search for other causes of pain should be sought. Other causes for failure include biomechanical problems and chronic radiculopathy. Wetzel and LaRocca reviewed 12 cases of failed posterior lumbar interbody fusion.[39] Even after multiple operations, the accomplishment of a solid fusion did not correlate with satisfactory relief of pain. Adjacent unfused segments were noted to be symptomatic in 25% of patients. All patients had chronic radiculopathy and intraoperatively were noted to have extensive epidural fibrosis. The first problem of mechanical dysfunction can be addressed by stabilization of adjacent segments with rigid fixation, but the problem of chronic radiculopathy currently has no good solution and is usually managed nonoperatively. The problems of chronic radiculopathy and epidural fibrosis are more common with dural manipulation, such as posterolateral interbody fusion (PLIF).[6]

Lauerman et al showed that for management of pseudarthroses after arthrodesis of the spine for idiopathic scoliosis, it appears safe to observe an asymptomatic pseudarthrosis since the results of delayed repair did not differ from those of earlier repair.[19] Care must be taken, however, to observe for curve progression and evidence of hardware failure. If there is pain and if indeed pseudarthrosis is determined to be the cause of persistent pain, more time may be allotted in the hope that healing eventually ensues, given that the hardware is intact and that there is no increasing deformity. In failed lumbar fusions, usually 6 to 9 months are given to observe for evidence of fusion. An alternative for surgical exploration is the use of pulsing electromagnetic fields. Simmons showed that in patients with failed PLIFs, with an average of 40 months since the last surgical fusion attempt, pulsing electromagnetic fields (PEMFs) prompted significant increase in bone formation.[29] Eighty five percent (11 of 13) of patients showed increased bone formation and 77% (10 of 13) achieved body-to-body fusion throughout the intervertebral disk space. Tejano furthermore reported on the use of implantable direct stimulation in multilevel spine fusions without instrumentation. Fusion among 118 patients was 91.5%; two-level procedures had a fusion rate of 93%, and three-level procedures had a fusion rate of 91%.[34]

## OPERATIVE MANAGEMENT

With the persistence of pain and/or progression of the curve, the management of pseudarthrosis after arthrodesis for idiopathic scoliosis should be surgical. Lauerman et al showed that multiple pseudarthroses were commonly found at the time of repair and, therefore the entire fusion mass should always be explored.[19] They also report that use of a compression implant significantly improves the rate of healing. Erwin et al in a clinical review of patients with broken Harrington rods conclude that the clinical management of rod fractures must be individualized.[8] Reinstrumentation and fusion may be indicated in patients with early instrument failure or loss of correction but not in patients experiencing little or no loss of correction and no associated symptoms.

Repair of pseudarthroses requires meticulous surgical technique. Care must be taken during initial exposure of the fusion mass to avoid midline dissection into the spinal canal since many previously fused spines have had a wide midline decompression. Pseudomeningocele can exist posterior to the boundaries of the posterior canal and therefore, careful preoperative evaluation of the computed tomography (CT) scan or magnetic resonance imaging (MRI) is important.[27] Neural decompression is performed using blunt and sharp dissection, and the pedicle and associated nerve roots can be identified and freed from the encapsulating scar tissue. All fibrous tissue from the pseudarthrosis site is cleaned down to bleeding bone and autologous graft is packed at the site. Insertion of instrumentation is performed under direct vision or palpation of the pedicles, since landmarks have usually been obliterated by the previous fusion procedure. Autologous bone graft (either obtained locally or from the iliac crest) is placed at the pseudarthrosis site. Even though there are reports of use of allograft for lumbar fusion, there is currently no strong indication for bank bone in the repair of pseudarthroses.[16] If a bone stimulator is used, it is placed directly over the pseudarthrosis site, and electrocautery is not used so as not to disable the battery pack.

The repair of pseudarthroses of the lumbar spine may be accomplished by posterior fusion, anterior fusion, or combined anterior and posterior fusion.

### POSTERIOR

It is generally agreed that a posterolateral lumbar fusion for pseudarthrosis should be performed with instrumentation.[7,15,21,22,24,32,33,36] Lorenz noted a 58% rate of pseudarthrosis with uninstrumented single-level fusions and 0% with instrumented fusion.[23] Lauerman et al showed a 29% rate of fusion when no instrumentation was used for pseudarthrosis repair.[19] For pseudarthrosis repair, moreover, solid fusion was obtained at a rate of 50% when Luque sublaminar wires were used, 55% when Steffee screw-plate fixation was used, and 67% when Harrington compression instrumentation was used.[19] West et al had a similar (65%) fusion rate for repair of pseudarthrosis when instrumentation was used.[38] Clinically, Harmon, Sacks, Hoover, and Freebody reported that 65% to 96% of patients had complete relief of symptoms.[11,13,14,28] It thus follows that repair of pseudarthrosis should be supported by instrumentation.

Another surgical option is augmentation of the posterolateral fusion by PLIF.[15,21,22] PLIF may increase the rate of fusion because restoration of anterior column support helps unload the posterior instrumentation and increases the surface area for fusion. Disk space distraction, with the use of instrumentation, also permits decompression of the intraforaminal space and deformity correction. Fusion rates of up to 96% for pseudarthrosis repair were obtained by Enker et al.[7] Lin reported that out of 465 patients of PLIF over a 10-year period, 82% improved clinically and 88% showed satisfactory fusion rate.[21] Accomplishment of the PLIF may be made more difficult, however, if there is severe epidural fibrosis because scarring makes dural sac retraction and graft placement difficult.

### ANTERIOR

Excision of the disk by an anterior approach and spine fusion by interbody bone grafting is a method advocated by several surgeons dissatisfied with the more conventional methods of spine fusion. Stauffer and Coventry, however, reported that this technique should be used as a salvage procedure especially in patients with spondylolisthesis or one who has had a previous operation posteriorly with some compromise of the integrity of the joints between the articular processes and supporting ligamentous structures.[31]

There has been some disagreement amongst advocates of anterior spine fusion regarding the success rate;

Batchelor reported 26% success rate, Stauffer and Coventry reported 56%, Goldner reported 80%, Freebody reported 92%, and Harmon reported 95%.[31] Tiusanen et al reported on a series of 83 patients with 54% being reoperated for failed back surgery; 81% had solid fusion of levels.[35] Flynn and Hoques reported their series of anterior fusion of fifty patients with different diagnoses with the use of fibular and iliac autogenous bone grafts. The fusion rate was 56%.

Anterior fusion can also be performed with instrumentation. Different types of cages can also be used. The theoretic advantage of instrumentation use is maintenance of anterior disk height and avoidance of collapse of the graft. This has advantages in increase in the size of the neuroforaminal volume. Chen et al reported in a cadaver study using the BAK fusion system an increase in neuroforaminal volume by over 23%.[5] There are also recent reports of diskectomy and fusion and instrumentation being done laparoscopically.[25]

### Anterior and Posterior

It has been suggested that the most successful method of obtaining solid fusion, yet the most extensive, is anterior and posterior fusion. A pseudarthrosis rate of only 10% has been reported.[1] Seventy-two percent of patients demonstrated solid posterior and anterior fusion, 8% had solid posterior fusion with anterior pseudarthrosis, and 10% had solid anterior fusion with posterior pseudarthrosis.

At present, there are no major publications addressing the use of 360-degree fusion for the treatment of pseudarthrosis. Until more data is available, it is difficult to recommend this approach in most cases.

## POSTOPERATIVE IMMOBILIZATION

There is very marked controversy concerning postoperative immobilization following a spine fusion and following a repair of pseudarthrosis. Clearly, factors taken into consideration would include the presence of fixation, rigidity of the construct, and patient factors such as age and bone structure.

Lin has suggested that for satisfactory spine fusion in patients who have undergone PLIF, immobilization for 4 months after surgery with a Knight's brace is mandatory.[21] Half-knee bends (25 to 50 repetitions, twice daily) and brisk walking (10 min/km and 3 to 5 km per day) are helpful for general physical fitness and subsequent promotion of osteosynthesis. Swimming may also be helpful after the 4-month postoperative period. Jogging is not advocated during the 4-month postoperative period. Flexion of the lumbar spine should be avoided at all times during the 4-month postoperative period. If the osteosynthesis is not adequate as demonstrated on the tomogram 4 months after surgery, continuation of immobilization is suggested by Lin until satisfactory fusion is seen on roentgenogram. If fusion, however, has not occurred 9 months postoperatively, discontinuation of immobilization is suggested. At this stage, further treatment, such as an additional PLIF or lateral intertransverse process fusion, may be necessary if osteofibrous union is symptomatic. Later fusion performed for pseudarthrosis of PLIF often brings about a solid refusion of the PLIF.

Lauerman et al reported that the type of postoperative external immobilization showed no effect on the rate of pseudarthrosis[18,19]; 26 of the 44 procedures after which the patient wore a cast were successful, 11 of the 17 procedures after which the patient wore a brace were successful, and 1 of the 2 after which no immobilization was used was successful for arthrodesis.

## WORKERS' COMPENSATION ISSUES

Many observers have suggested that disability payments alter the response to treatment of injured patients. It is well known that therapy successful for noncompensated patients is not equally satisfactory for those receiving compensation, especially in patients who complain of low-back problems.[2] Krusen and Ford found that those receiving compensation had 33% less objective evidence of impairment, had twice as much physical therapy, and experienced 44% less long-term improvement compared to those not receiving compensation.[17] Mensor, who reported results from treatment for lumbar disk syndrome, reported an excellent result in 64% of private patients versus 45% in compensated patients.[26] Similarly, Slepian reported a 30% better result in private patients compared to compensated patients.[30] Furthermore, Esses and Huler reported that less than 60% of patients who had undergone one-level or two-level fusion to the sacrum ever return to their original heavy-labor occupation.[9] This figure is even lower if the patient is covered under compensable claim, has pending litigation, or has three or more degenerative levels that are included for fusion.

All explanations for the less favorable results among patients who are compensated is secondary to psychological factors.[2] Thus, the patient's psychosocial history, the patient's secondary financial gain through continued illness, and the patient's financial disincentives, all of which are provided through Workers' Compensation benefits, may increase the rate of failure after fusion.

## NUMBER OF PREVIOUS OPERATIONS

Following surgical procedures of the lumbar spine, some patients continue to suffer from back and/or leg pain. Conservative treatment (improved posture, trunk strength, spine mobility) may reduce the pain, but total relief is unlikely. Repeat surgery can significantly decrease the pain, however it can also exacerbate the pain. Patients who have undergone unsuccessful primary arthrodesis repair have had varying success rates on salvage procedures. The success rates reported by authors have ranged anywhere from Waddel et al (40%), Lehman and LaRocca (50%), Frymoyer et al (70%), to Finnegan (81%).[10,12,20,37] Furthermore, Carpenter reported that the likelihood of a successful salvage procedure after a failed primary arthrodesis decreases with increased number of levels fused.[4] Carpenter discussed 81 out of 86 patients who eventually obtained solid fusion; in patients who required subsequent salvage procedures, 10 of 15 obtained bony fusion after one, two, or three attempts. Of the five remaining patients, four refused additional attempts at repair, and one never had the pseudarthrosis repaired.

Satisfactory results can be expected when surgically correctable anomalies exist; if the etiology of continued pain is mechanical compression of nerve roots from any source but scarring, the prognosis is good with repeat surgery; if the problem is primarily neural scarring, the prognosis is poor.[20]

## SUMMARY

It is clear that pseudarthroses represents a very major cause of disability and pain following thoracolumbar surgery. It is as yet unclear as to why some patients with a pseudarthrosis are asymptomatic and others have significant symptoms. It is crucial in the management of a patient with back pain to have a pseudarthrosis to try and determine if there is any causal relationship. This may, in some patients, be extremely difficult. If the pseudarthrosis is not the cause of the pain, then surgical repair of the failed fusion is doomed to clinical failure. If, on the other hand, the patients pain can be shown to be coming from the nonunion then a technically successful operation yields clinically satisfying results.

## REFERENCES


1. Albert TJ, Pinto M, Johnson E, Dennis F: Treatment of symptomatic lumbar pseudarthrosis with AP fusion: a functional and radiographic outcome study. Presented at the 28th Annual Meeting of Scoliosis Research Society, Dublin, Ireland, Sept., 19-23, 1993.
2. Beals RK, Hickman NW: Industrial injuries of the back and extremities, *J Bone Joint Surg* 54A:1593-1611, 1972.
3. Bosworth DM: Technique of spinal fusion: pseudarthrosis and method of repair, *Instr Course Lect* 5: 295-313, 1948.
4. Carpenter CT, Dietz JW, Leung KYK, et al: Repair of pseudarthrosis of the lumbar spine, *J Bone Joint Surg* 78A:712-720, 1996.
5. Chen et al: Increasing neuroforaminal volume by anterior interbody distraction in degenerative lumbar spine, *Spine* 20:74-79, 1995.
6. Dawson EG, Clader TJ, Bassett LW, et al: A comparison of different methods used to diagnose pseudarthrosis following posterior spinal fusion for scoliosis, *J Bone Joint Surg* 67A:1153-1159, 1985.
7. Enker P, Steffee AD: Interbody fusion and instrumentation, *Clin Orthop* 300:90-101, 1994.
8. Erwin WD, Dickson JH, Harrington PR: Clinical review of patients with broken Harrington rods, *J Bone Joint Surg* 62A:1302-1307, 1980.
9. Esses SI, Huler RJ: Indications for lumbar spine fusion in the adult, *Clin Orthop* 279:87-100, 1992.
10. Finnegan WJ, Fenlin JM, Marvel JP, Nordini RJ, Rothman RH: Results of surgical intervention in the symptomatic multiply-operated back patient, *J Bone Joint Surg* 61A:1077-1082, 1979.
11. Freebody D, Bendall R, Taylor RD: Anterior transperitoneal lumbar fusion, *J Bone Joint Surg* 53B: 617-627, 1971.
12. Frymoyer JW, Hanley E, Howe J, et al: Disc excision and spine fusion in the management of lumbar disc disease, *Spine* 3:1-11, 1978.
13. Harmon PH: Anterior excision and vertebral body fusion operation for intervertebral isc syndromes of the lower lumbar spine, *Clin Orthop* 26:107-127, 1963.
14. Hoover NW: Methods of lumbar fusion, *J Bone Joint Surg* 50A:194-210, 1968.
15. Kiviluoto O, Santavirta S, Salenius P: Posterolateral spine fusion, *Acta Orthop Scand* 56:152-154, 1985.
16. Knapp DR, Jones ET: Use of cortical cancellous allograft for posterior spinal fusion, *Clin Orthop* 229:99-105, 1987.
17. Krusen EM, Ford DE: Compensation factor in low back injuries, *JAMA* 166:1128-1133, 1958.
18. Lauerman WC, Bradford DS, Ogilive JW, Transfeld EE: Results of lumbar pseudarthrosis repair, *J Spinal Disord* 5:149-157, 1992.
19. Lauerman WC, Bradford DS, Transfeldt EE, et al: Management of pseudarthrosis after arthrodesis of the spine for idiopathic scoliosis, *J Bone Joint Surg* 74A: 222-236, 1991.
20. Lehman TR, LaRocca HS: Repeat lumbar surgery: a review of patients with failure from previous lum-

bar surgery treated by spinal canal exploration and lumbar spinal fusion, *Spine* 6:615-619, 1981.
21. Lin PM: Posterior lumbar interbody fusion technique: complications and pitfalls, *Clin Orthop* 193:90-102, 1985.
22. Lin PM: Radiographic evidence of posterior lumbar interbody fusion with an emphasis on computed tomographic scanning, *Clin Orthop* 242:159-163, 1989.
23. Lorenz M, Zindrick M, Schwaegler P, et al: A comparison of single-level fusions with and without hardware, *Spine* 16:S455-S458, 1991.
24. Macnab I, Dall D: The blood supply of the lumbar spine and its application to the technique of intertransverse lumbar fusion, *J Bone Joint Surg* 53B:628-638, 1971.
25. Mathews NH, Evans MT, Molligan HJ, Long BH: Laparoscopic discectomy with interior lumbar interbody fusion: A preliminary review, *Spine* 20:1797-1802, 1995.
26. Mensor MC: Non-operative treatment, including manipulation for lumbar intervertebvral disc syndrome, *J Bone Joint Surg* 37A:925-936, 1955.
27. Rawlins BA, Michelsen CB: Failed lumbosacral fusions, *Spine: State of the Art Reviews* 8(3):563-571, 1994.
28. Sacks S: Anterior interbody fusion of the lumbar spine, *J Bone Joint Surg* 47B: 211-223, 1965.
29. Simmons JW: Treatment of failed posterior lumbar interbody fusion (PLIF) of the spine with pulsing electromagnetic fields, *Clin Orthop* 193:127-132, 1985.
30. Slepian A: Lumbar disc surgery. long follow-up results from three neurosurgeons, *N Y State J Med* 66: 1063-1068, 1966.
31. Stauffer RN, Coventry MB: Anterior interbody lumbar spine fusion, *J Bone Joint Surg* 54A:756-768, 1971.
32. Stauffer RN, Coventry MB: Posterolateral lumbar-spine fusion, *J Bone Joint Surg* 54A:1195-1204, 1972.
33. Stonecipher TK, Vanderby R, Sciammarella CA: The mechanical consequence of failure of ossified union in attempted posterior spinal fusion: a canine model, *Spine* 8:31-34, 1983.
34. Tejano NA, Puno R: The use of implantable direct current stimulation in multilevel spinal fusion without instrumentation. A prospective clinical and radiographic evaluation with long-term follow-up, *Spine* 21(16):1904-1908, 1996.
35. Tiusanen H, Hurri H: Functional and clinical results after anterior interbody lumbar fusion, *Eur Spine* J 5(5): 288-292, 1996.
36. Tunturi T, Kataja M, Keski-Nisula L, et al: Posterior fusion of the lumbosacral spine, *Acta Orthop Scand* 50:415-425, 1979.
37. Waddell G, Kummel EG, Lotto WN, et al: Failed lumbar disc surgery and repeat surgery following industrial injuries, *J Bone Joint Surg* 61A:201-207, 1979.
38. West JL, Bradford DS, Ogilvie JW: Results of spinal arthrodesis with pedicle screw-plate fixation, *J Bone Joint Surg* 73A:1179-1183, 1991.
39. Wetzel FT, LaRocca H: The failed posterior lumbar interbody fusion, *Spine* 16:839-845, 1991.

# 53

# FLAT BACK SYNDROME AND THE RELATED KYPHOTIC DECOMPENSATION SYNDROMES

Frank J. Schwab, M.D.
Jean-Pierre C. Farcy, M.D.



The first spinal fusion operations were performed at the beginning of this century to address spinal infection and progressive deformity from tuberculosis. Success of spinal fusion for this particular pathology led to application of the technique to other areas of spinal disease. The introduction of spinal instrumentation was a second tremendous catalyst in the development of spinal surgery. Today there is a wide range of indications for spinal fusion and placement of spinal instrumentation. While fusion and the use of instrumentation may have solved some of the original pathologic states of the spinal column, it is increasingly apparent that a new set of iatrogenic problems has been created. Aside from the perioperative surgical complications, spinal fusion has created a new set of disorders related to modifications of spinal biomechanics. Junctional degeneration and global decompensation are the two principal categories of late complications related to spinal fusion. Our discussion here will focus on the global decompensation syndromes of which flat back is one common example.

The flat back syndrome is a postural disorder of the spine described by affected patients as a feeling of leaning forwards or being "bent over" with difficulty or inability to stand erect without knees and hips flexed. The symptomatic loss of proper spinal alignment in this syndrome frequently leads to complaints of stumbling while walking, catching feet on carpets, and having particular difficulty walking on uneven ground. Due to the strain of trying to maintain erect posture, pain and fatigue develop in cervical, thoracic, and distal lumbar areas as well as in the thighs and buttocks, where muscles are under constant strain due to compensatory mechanisms. Although flat back syndrome can result from a variety of iatrogenic etiologies, it is most commonly attributed to instrumentation, such as Harrington rods, extending into the lumbar spine (L4, L5) or the sacrum for scoliosis correction.[2,4,5,6]

A related syndrome of pain and sensation of imbalance with spinal sagittal malalignment resulting from lumbosacral fusions in kyphosis can be termed kyphotic decompensation syndrome (KDS). KDS is differentiated from flat back not by clinical presentation or degree of sagittal malalignment but rather by the original surgery (and thus the levels of fusion). Flat back syndrome is a result of decompensation after scoliosis surgery and most frequently involves malaligned fusions from the thoracic spine extended into the lower lumbar spine (L4, L5). Kyphotic decompensation syndrome is a result of decompensation following spinal surgery mostly for degenerative pathology in adults and involves short fusions restricted to the lumbosacral region.

The sagittal malalignment of the flat back and KDS place high demands on the muscles, ligaments, and disks of the spine. Minimal disturbances in sagittal alignment can be compensated for by muscle action to maintain level gaze. Increasing loss of normal sagittal spinal alignment leads to a decrease in paraspinal muscle lever arm and thus greater forces are required to maintain erect posture.[8] The progressive decompensation in malalignment syndromes can be theorized as a gradual process of failure in the muscular mechanisms (dynamic stabilizers) to maintain posture followed by gradual failure of the ligamentous and capsular structures (rigid stabilizers). This creates a situation of progressive deformity with pain and limitation of function for the patient. A variety of compensatory mechanisms exist to accommodate sagittal plane malalignment. These include alteration of sagittal curvatures in nonfused segments (i.e., decreased lumbar or cervical lordosis), pelvic rotation, and hip and knee hyperextension or flexion.

Initial treatment for all patients with flat back and kyphotic decompensation syndromes is focused upon optimizing the compensatory mechanisms and paraspinal muscle function. When conservative management has failed, and pain and function are disabling, the spine surgeon must carefully plan surgical realignment addressing the three-dimensional deformity. The amount of correction attainable and overall prognosis for these patients are poorly defined in the current literature.

Doherty was the first to report on the malalignment complication seen with flat back as it is now called.[2] He reported in 1972 on treatment of the deformity with bilateral pelvic osteotomies in order to restore upright posture. In 1978, Grobler and Moe described the symptom complex of sagittal imbalance with forward thrust of the trunk accompanied by pain and fatigue.[4] Pain was seen as a result from hyperextension of the neck and constant flexion of the knees in order to maintain upright posture. Kostuik in 1988 reported on the treatment of 54 patients with sagittal malalignment.[5] Of these patients, 44 were fused to the sacrum originally, 8 were fused to L5, and 2 patients were fused to L4. LaGrone reported on treatment of 55 patients who had loss of lumbar lordosis after spinal fusion and were surgically corrected.[6] In 53 of the patients, Harrington distraction instrumentation had been employed at the initial surgery. Fusion had been performed to the sacrum in the majority of patients although 4 were fused to L5, 12 were fused to L4, and 2 were fused to L3. Inability to stand erect and back pain were the presenting chief complaints in approximately 90% of the patients. Sagittal plane imbalance averaged 8.2 cm anteriorly (range, −4.8 cm to 22.5 cm) preoperatively. Surgical correction was performed via osteotomies and Harrington compression instrumentation in the majority of cases. The amount of sagittal plane correction at follow up averaged 4.2 cm. Clinically at follow-up, 47% of patients still reported that they were leaning forward, 36% had moderate or severe pain, yet 95% felt they had benefitted from corrective surgery. The overall complication rate was 60% in the study. Although data was analyzed for a subgroup of patients with idiopathic scoliosis, no attempt was made to separate groups based upon level of initial fusion. Furthermore, no guidelines were proposed for systematically approaching sagittal plane imbalances based upon degree of deformity, levels of fusion, or status of intervertebral disks adjacent to previous fusions.

## PATIENT EVALUATION

The patient who presents for complications related to sagittal plane malalignment is most commonly in the late twenties to forties age range and has either had surgery as a teenager for scoliosis or had surgery as a young adult for disk- or instability-related pathology. Presenting complaints are usually back pain, progressive fatigue, and, in severe cases, the classic symptoms of falling forward and difficulty maintaining comfortable standing posture. Initial assessment should start with a careful history of not only the original diagnosis and surgical treatment but also an analysis of pain patterns and functional limitation. It is important to discern fatigue and alignment-related musculoskeletal complaints from radicular complaints or possible instrumentation-related local discomfort. Physical examination should include a detailed neurologic evaluation and may detect abnormal reflexes, associated radicular findings, weakness, and muscle contracture.

Radiographic studies should include a standing full-length standard scoliosis series. The patient must stand in a relaxed posture with hips and knees extended and upper extremities positioned on a bar at shoulder level. It is important that the upper extremities are not used to support upper body weight, this could lead to alterations in apparent spinal alignment. The full-length radiographs will permit calculation of frontal and sagittal plane offset of the plumb line. The latter is drawn from the center of the odontoid along the full length of the film perpendicular to the bottom of the radiograph (Fig. 53-1) In reference to this line, the offset of the midsacral line (on frontal radiograph) and anterior edge of the sacral promontory (on sagittal film) are measured. Should the radiographs reveal a possible nonunion, a series of regional anteroposterior, lateral, and oblique radiographs should be obtained. With suspected junctional instability, it is recommended to obtain dynamic radiographs to analyze the degree of intersegmental motion. Computed tomography, magnetic resonance imaging, and myelograms may be indicated to evaluate neurologic symptoms.

An additional radiographic measure that we have recently examined is the sagittal pelvic tilt index (SPTI). This index is a technique of quantifying the degree of pelvic sagittal plane rotation in the standing patient. In a healthy person the sagittal plane

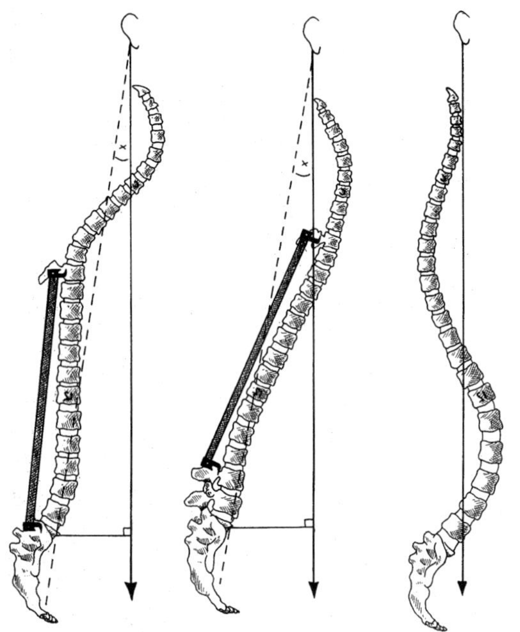

**FIGURE 53-1**

Illustration of plumb line measurement. Standing lateral radiographic analysis may reveal plumb line offset due to cephalad or caudal failure.

alignment of L5 in respect to S2 and the hip joints falls within a range of values (SPTI average 0.7). In patients with significant spinal malalignment, compensatory mechanisms come into play in order to maintain standing balance. Among these compensatory mechanisms are cervical extension, hip flexion, knee flexion, and pelvic rotation (retroversion). The degree of relative hip flexion and pelvic rotation quantified by radiographic measurement (SPTI) may be helpful in guiding treatment (Fig. 53-2)

## TREATMENT APPROACH

Flat back and the kyphotic decompensation syndromes present in a wide spectrum of radiographic malalignment and clinical symptoms and findings. Detailed evaluation will determine if there are associated pathologies (stenosis, disk herniation, instability, etc.), which must be considered in the overall treatment of the sagittal malalignment. We advocate an initial aggressive guided isometric back-strengthening program in all patients. In conjunction with weight loss for overweight patients, this may provide effective treatment for mild malalignment patients. Guided exercises will also

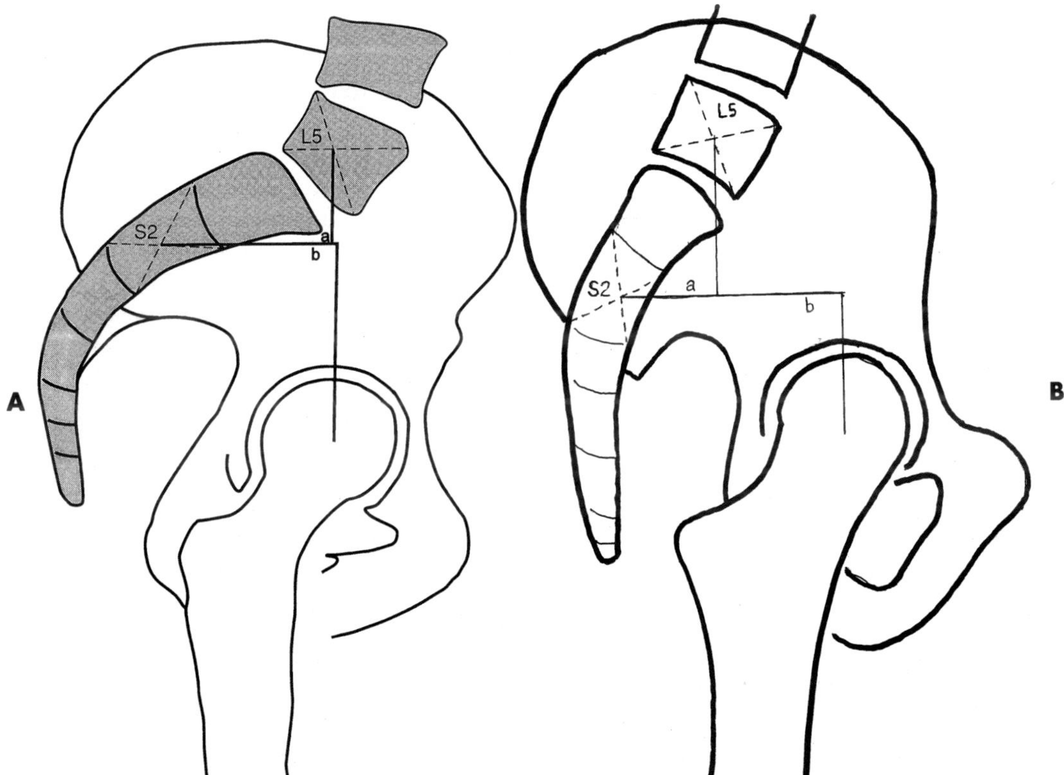


**FIGURE 53-2**

Illustration of sagittal pelvic tilt index measurement. **A,** Normal SPTI of around 1. **B,** Example of low SPTI due to pelvic rotation associated with sagittal spinal management. The centers of L5, S2, and the acetabulum are identified on the standing lateral radiograph. The relative offset of L5 in respect to the acetabulum is then quantified on the horizontal line.

optimize the overall condition for those patients who may require surgical treatment.

Removal of spinal instrumentation may be helpful in patients with prominent implants. This will also permit improved analysis of the spine by magnetic resonance imaging (MRI). In patients with flat back and fusion short of the sacrum, the evaluation of mobile segment disks is crucial. Well hydrated disks without evidence of advanced degeneration and annular tears may be preserved when considering realignment surgery. For patients with KDS, the status of disks cephalad to previous fusion must be carefully examined. Extension of fusion may be required in some cases. Once a decision has been made to realign a previous fusion, computed tomography (CT) and MRI will assist in determining the level of corrective osteotomy (level of conus, details of local morphology). The goal of the surgical intervention is global balance (plumb line), and treatment of any associated pathologies (stenosis, disk herniation, instability, pseudarthrosis).

## REVIEW OF TREATMENT OF FLAT BACK AND KYPHOTIC DECOMPENSATION SYNDROMES

Based upon the paucity of literature, our service designed a study to address questions regarding management of the aforementioned sagittal plane deformities based upon degree of deformity, previous level of fusion, and condition of disks adjacent to fused segments. Our series also sought to examine data on correction of sagittal plane deformities using newer instrumentation systems that were lacking in the literature. A group of patients treated by sagittal realignment and a group of nonrealigned patients were examined to determine the effectiveness of these treatment modalities and to increase our understanding on the prognosis for patients with these malalignment deformities.

## MATERIALS AND METHODS

A retrospective review of all patients treated for symptomatic sagittal malalignment syndromes of the spine by the senior author between 1985 and 1995 was performed. All patients had symptomatic complaints of falling forward and associated distal lumbar back pain. A total of 72 patients were identified. For a patient to be included in the study, preoperative, postoperative, and follow-up standing radiographs had to be available. The minimum follow-up after surgical intervention was 24 months. Charts were reviewed in order to determine the degree of pain (serial patient self-reported pain questionnaires included), medication taken for pain control, and the level of activity of the patient. The rating scale (completed by patient), applied to evaluate pain, was based upon a 10 point scale, in which 1 reflected no significant pain and 10 reflected maximal pain that is constant and requires morphine pump anesthesia (Table 53-1).

All spinal curvatures were measured applying the Cobb technique. Thus, frontal and sagittal plane alignment was measured on preoperative, postoperative, and follow-op standing, full-length radiographs. These radiographs were taken with the patient standing with knees and hips fully extended. When necessary to maintain balance, the patient was permitted to sustain the necessary position by using the arms to gently seek support against a horizontal bar at shoulder height. Overall sagittal alignment was determined by measuring the distance from the sacral promontory (anteriorly) on a horizontal to the intersection with a plumb line dropped from the center of the odontoid process. Positive values, in centimeters, reflected anterior displacement of the plumb line, negative values reflected posterior displacement of the plumb line.

In the study group of 72 patients, there were 17 males and 55 females. The average time elapsed from initial spinal fusion was 11.8 years. Diagnosis at time of the original surgery was idiopathic scoliosis in 60 patients. In this group the average age at revision was 26 years, and time elapsed from original surgery was 13 years (range 9 to 19 years). Diagnosis at time of original surgery was degenerative scoliosis in 12 patients. For this group the average age at original surgery was 45 years and average time elapsed since original surgery was 5.5 years. Original surgery involved Harrington distraction instrumentation in 51 patients, Wisconsin instrumentation in 6 patients,

**Table 53-1. Patient Pain Scale—Self-Evaluation**

| Score | Type of Pain |
|---|---|
| 1 | no significant pain |
| 2 | occasional pain |
| 3 | activity related, relief with rest |
| 4 | requiring occasional NSAIDs |
| 5 | interferes with work, constant NSAIDs |
| 6 | interferes with work, NSAIDs, pain modalities |
| 7 | requiring occasional opiates |
| 8 | constant, regular opiate use |
| 9 | constant, bed to chair activity only, opiates |
| 10 | morphine pump, high-dose constant opiates |

NSAIDs, nonsteroidal anti-inflammatory drugs.

Zielke anterior instrumentation in 8 patients, Cotrel-Dubousset instrumentation (CDI) in 5 patients, and Luque instrumentation in 2 patients. The diagnosis at time of presentation to our service was flat back syndrome in 60 patients and KDS in 12 patients.

## TREATMENT

Initial management of the patients in this study included intensive physical therapy in all instances. This served the dual purpose of deciding which patient required realignment surgery, and also optimized physical condition in the preoperative patient. Of the 72 patients, 28 (Group A), achieved significant improvement of pain such that patients did not wish major realignment surgery. Nonetheless, a limited surgical intervention of spinal instrumentation removal (no decompression) was performed in 22 patients in this group. In 5 cases of instrumentation removal, only the caudal portion of the Harrington rod was removed. The original fusion levels of patients in Group A ended at L4 in 24 patients, and L5 in 4 patients.

Decision to proceed with spinal instrumentation removal was based upon physical exam and character of the pain. Pain was attributed to the instrumentation when it was localized, reproduced by palpation over prominent components, and associated with motion in a direct correlation. This pain is different from what was felt to be pain secondary to malalignment: gluteal, quadriceps, and distal lumbar back stiffness and pain that is progressive over prolonged standing or motion. This pain is frequently tolerable at the beginning of the day yet clearly worsens with activity as the day proceeds.

Of the 72 patients in this study, surgical intervention with osteotomy and sagittal realignment was necessary in 44 patients (Group B) due to progressive pain and persistent sensation of imbalance. The surgical group (Group B) was divided into two subsets based upon the level of initial fusion. Group B1 was composed of 16 patients (9 females and 7 males) who had received initial fusion to the sacrum (Fig. 53-3). All patients in this group underwent anterior and posterior osteotomy with posterior instrumentation that involved caudal purchase with pedicle screws while proximal fixation was offered by either pedicle screws in the lumbar spine or segmental hooks and a claw configuration for fusions extending into the thoracic region. The anterior osteotomies were required due to dessication and contracture of the disks, thus not permitting adequate motion with a simple diskectomy. True bony osteotomy was necessary to obtain sufficient motion for a realignment of the fusion mass.

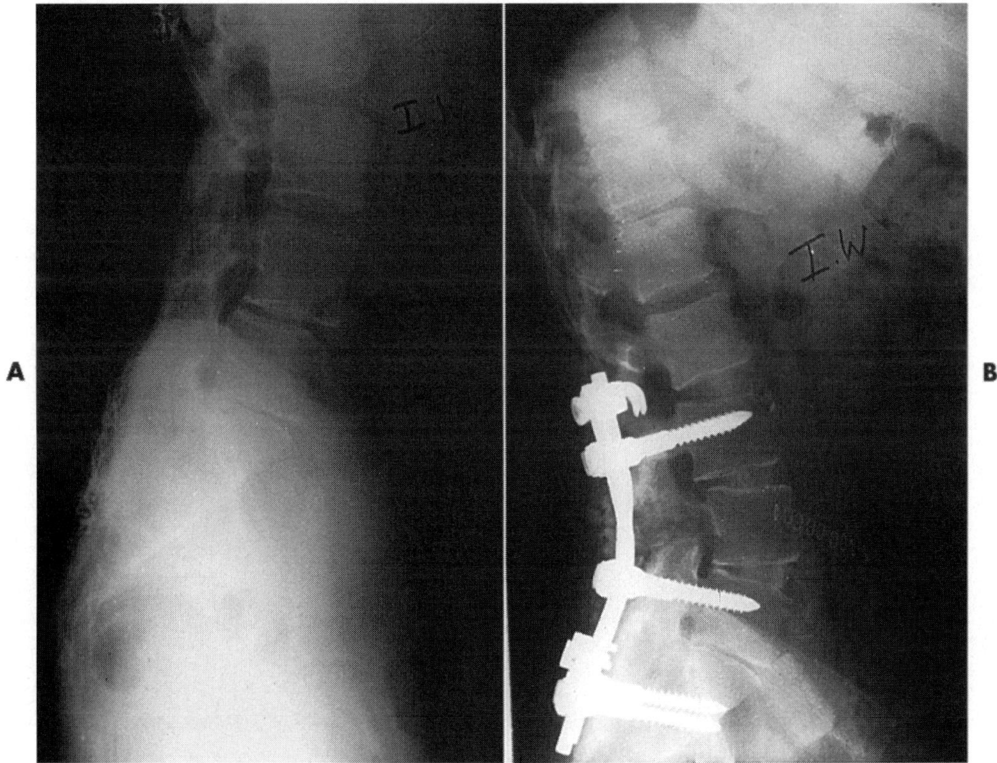


**FIGURE 53-3**

**A,** Lateral radiograph of patient with kyphotic decompensation syndrome (KDS) . A lumbosacral fusion in kyphosis led to progressive disabling pain and complaints of falling forward. **B,** Lateral postoperative radiograph. Anterior and posterior osteotomy permitted realignment of the fusion mass.

In Group B1 simultaneous anterior and posterior procedures were performed when feasible.[3] This approach, in the senior author's experience, appears to offer superior control of alignment due to visibility and access to both aspects of the spine simultaneously. The approach is technically challenging, but if two teams of experienced spine surgeons are familiar with the procedure, operating time, blood loss, and risks due to instability between stages may be decreased. An additional possible advantage of a simultaneous technique is control over the anterior graft that otherwise is vulnerable to displacement during sequential procedures that involve patient repositioning.

There are a few technical points that must be emphasized. Patients with an existing fusion to the sacrum can be corrected by a one- or two-level osteotomy, both anteriorly and posteriorly. The osteotomies must be located between L2 and L5, depending on the level of the conus. A simultaneous technique appears to offer the most advantageous approach to these cases. Posterior instrumentation in all of these cases was applied in compression and carried out high enough to obtain purchase on the cranial kyphosis above the fusion. When deemed necessary, two or three additional levels were fused cranially above a preexisting fusion, in order to avoid placing the end of the fixation at the apex of a kyphosis.

The second surgical realignment group, Group B2, consisted of 28 patients. There were 4 males and 24 females all of whom had been originally fused to L4 or L5. An MRI scan was performed in all cases to evaluate the disks below the original fusion. A viable disk was one that demonstrated no herniation, good hydration (high intensity) on T2 images, and lack of a high intensity zone within the annulus (Fig. 53-4).[1] In 8 patients, severe disk degeneration was found and revision surgery was thus extended to the sacrum after realignment osteotomies of the previous fusion mass. In these cases, circumferential fusions of levels below the old fusion were performed, involving anterior diskectomy and grafting. Posterior instrumentation involved a four-rod construct with screw fixation to the sacroilium (Fig. 53-5). One set of rods extended from the sacrum to L2 or L3. The second pair of rods, connected by dominos, extended to the proximal end of the old fusion mass. In some cases, in order to prevent ending on a kyphotic apex, fusion was extended proximally several levels. In four patients of Group B2, an MRI revealed acceptable viable disks caudal to the previous fusion. In that subgroup, realignment with anterior and posterior osteotomies of the previous fusion mass was performed without extension of the arthrodesis to the sacrum (Fig. 53-6).

## RESULTS

Complete records were available on all 72 of the patients treated in this series. Sixty patients were classified as having flat back syndrome while twelve patients had the related kyphotic decompensation syndrome. All patients were evaluated at a minimum 2-year follow-up with regard to alignment, success of arthrodesis, and distal lumbar back pain based upon serial pain score as filled in by the patient upon each visit. Patients in Group A had an average follow-up of 6 years. Of the 28 patients

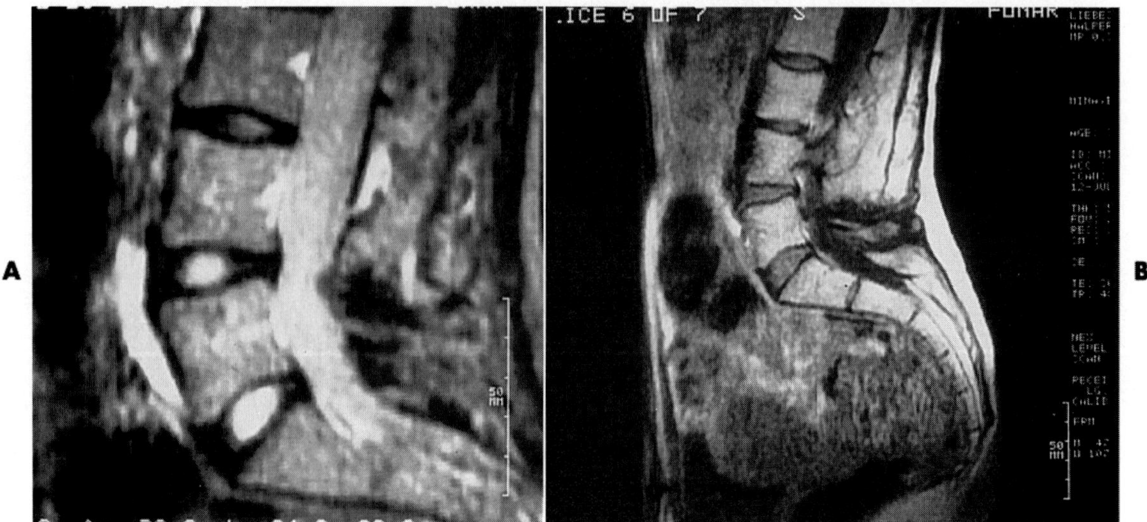


**FIGURE 53-4**

**A,** MRI of the lumbar spine in patient with long fusion ending above the sacrum. On this T2-weighted image, well-hydrated disks are noted without evidence of annular disruption or high intensity signal. **B,** MRI of lumbar spine on T1 image. Note the caudal extent of the fusion mass posteriorly. In this patient extension of fusion to the sacrum was not indicated due to the preservation of viable caudal disks.

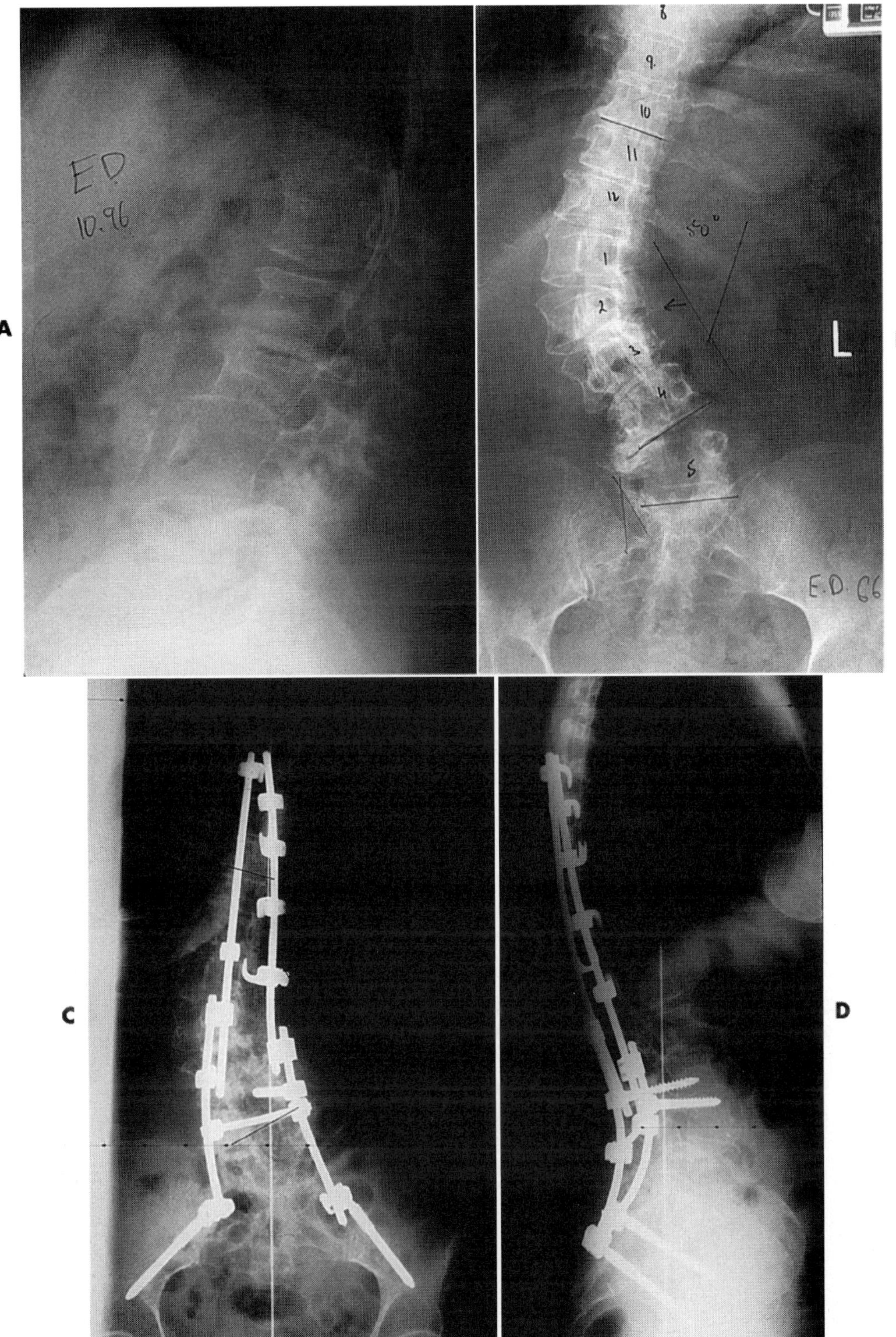


FIGURE 53-5

**A,** Lateral radiograph of a patient with flat back deformity. Progressive deformity has occurred below previous fusion. Posterior instrumentation had been removed at the time of a caudal decompression performed prior to presentation to our service. **B,** Anteroposterior radiograph demonstrating deformity below the original fusion. Note the area of decompression which was performed from L4 to the sacrum. **C,** Anteroposterior radiograph after surgical realignment. The four-rod technique was applied with use of iliac screws for caudal fixation. **D,** Lateral radiograph after realignment. Sagittal plane correction is evident with restoration of plumb line centering over the sacrum.

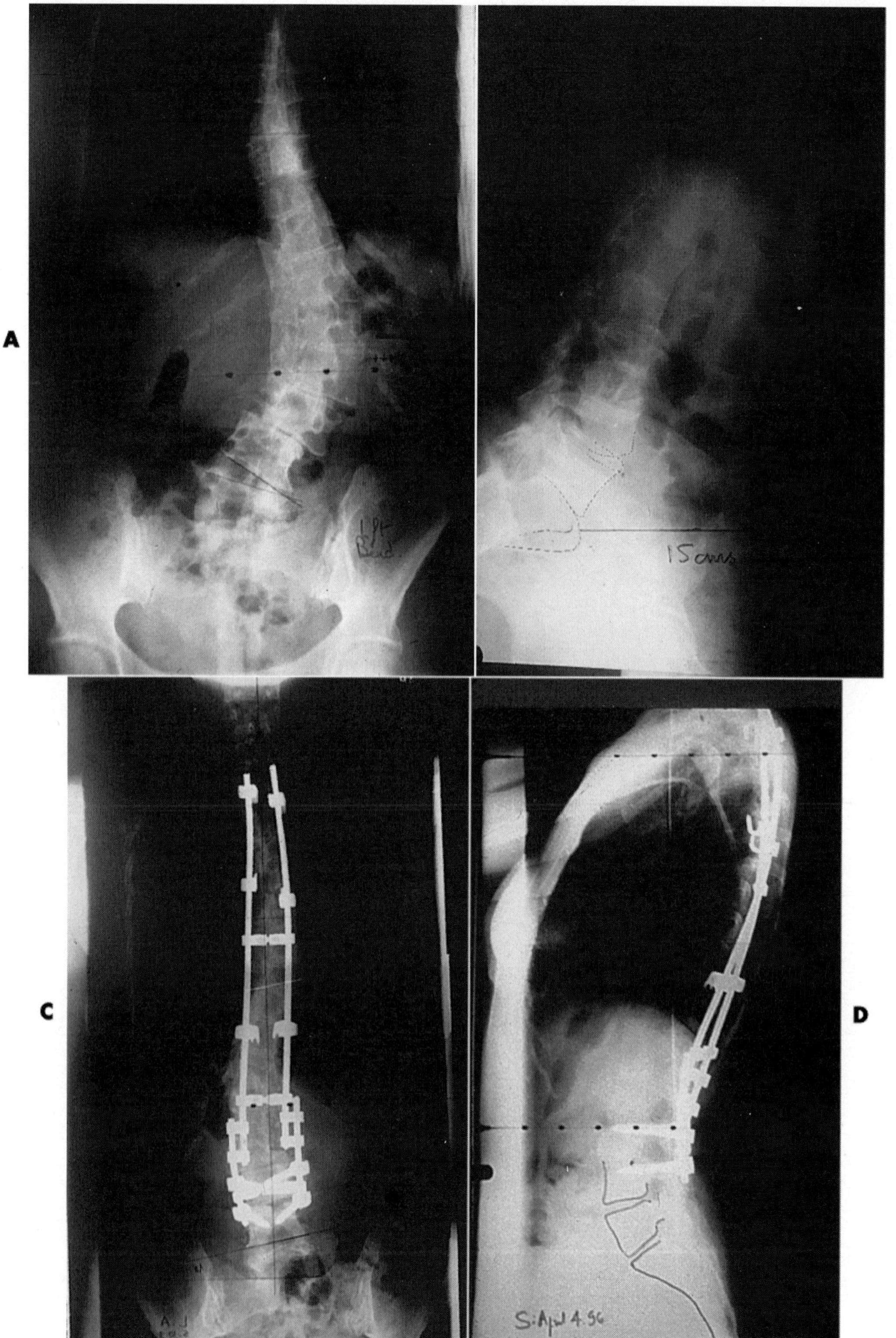


**FIGURE 53-6**

**A,** Anteroposterior radiograph of a flat back deformity with viable caudal disks by imaging studies. **B,** Lateral radiograph of this patient. Plumb line offset was measured at 15 cm. **C,** Postoperative standing radiograph, anteroposterior projection. Frontal plane alignment has been restored with fusion to L4. **D,** Postoperative lateral radiograph. Sagittal plane alignment has been restored with fusion ending at L4. Extension of fusion to the sacrum was spared with excellent clinical result.

in this group, 22 had spinal instrumentation removal performed due to suspected irritation from the latter. At time of surgery, loose or dislodged instrumentation was found in 50% of the cases, a notable bursa was found in 25% at the proximal extent of the instrumentation, no significant metallosis was noted in any case. The initial average sagittal malalignment upon presentation to our service for this group was 3.3 cm (range 2.3 to 6.5 cm). The median pain score at presentation was 4. This improved to a median value of 2 at 4 years and then increased to a median of 3 at last follow-up. Although all patients had improved by 4 years into the study, we are now beginning to notice some late deterioration in the conservative management group (i.e., Group A, no realignment surgery) and are aware of the possibility that realignment surgery and possibly extension of fusion may be necessary in 7 of the 28 original patients in Group A. This is based upon the gradually increasing distal lumbar back pain (to a median of 4), MRI signs of disk degeneration caudal to the original fusion, and gradual worsening of sagittal alignment noted in the 7 patients. The average initial plumb line in this group was 4.8 cm (range 4 to 6.5 cm), which increased to an average of 6.5 cm (range 4.7 to 7.5 cm) at latest follow-up. The progression does not correlate with the level at which the original fusion ended (L4, L5).

In Group B1 (those patients originally fused to the sacrum) realignment improved sagittal balance such that distance from the promontory to the plumb line decreased from an average of 13.6 cm (range 3.5 to 25 cm) to 1.5 cm average postoperatively (range 0 to 5.4 cm). Distal lumbar back pain was reduced from a preoperative median of 7 to 3 postoperatively (Table 53-2). Radiographic solid fusion occurred in 14 out of the 16 cases. In two patients, posterior exploration for suspected pseudarthrosis was performed. In both cases nonunion was noted and exposure of bone edges was performed to bleeding tissue followed by autologous grafting. Revision led to fusion of the 2 pseudarthroses by radiographic analysis.

In Group B2 (those patients originally fused to L4 or L5) sagittal malalignment was reduced from 8.7 cm (range 3.6 to 18 cm) to an average of 1.6 cm (range −3 to 4.5 cm). Within this group of 28 patients, the preoperative MRI revealed healthy, and thus salvageable, caudal disks in 10 patients. The preoperative plumb line in this subset averaged 5.5 cm (range 3.6 to 7 cm) and this was improved to an average plumb line offset of 0.9 cm (range 1.8 to −0.5 cm) with surgical realignment. At an average follow-up of 4.2 years, these patients have maintained their alignment and median pain score remains at 2. Distal lumbar back pain was reduced from a median in Group B2 of 6 preoperatively to 2 at follow-up. Successful fusion occurred in all but one case. The failed fusion occurred in a fusion which was extended to the sacrum for nonsalvageable disks at L4-l5 and L5-S1.

Overall complications in Groups B1 and B2 included four deep vein thrombosis, four wound infections (one requiring operative debridement), and two urinary tract infections. Six radiculopathies occurred that required instrumentation repositioning in 2 cases and decompression in 2 other cases. A traction phenomenon was suspected in 2 cases. In all instances no long-term sequelae resulted. Three cases of DIC developed, one of these was associated with adult respiratory distress syndrome. In all instances, significant perioperative blood loss occurred. The complication rate in the surgical realignment groups thus was 25%. There were a total of 5 pseudarthroses for a nonunion rate of 11%. In Group A (the patients who had spinal instrumentation removal) no complications were noted.

A unique problem occurred in one patient with flat back deformity from Group B2 who had a rigid hypokyphotic (nearly lordotic) thoracic spine in addition to her plumb line imbalance due to malaligned fusion. Upon realignment and lumbosacral extension of her original fusion, it was noted that an exaggerated posterior displacement of the fusion mass occurred. This posterior exaggeration of the spine beyond the anatomic limits obligated a kyphotic correction in the cervical region to maintain horizontal gaze. This patient is now developing progressive neck pain. The eventual result of

**Table 53-2. Results by Treatment Categories**

| | | Plumb Line Imbalance (Average cm) | | Pain Score (Median) | |
|---|---|---|---|---|---|
| Group | Treatment | Preop | Postop | Preop | Postop |
| A | no realignment | 3.4 | na | 4 | (3 at last f/u) |
| B1 | realignment | 13.5 | 1.5 | 7 | 3 |
| B2 | realignment | 8.6 | 1.6 | 6 | 2 |

na, not applicable; f/u, follow-up.

the cervical adaptation is poorly understood and therefore not easy to treat.

## DISCUSSION

The sagittal plane imbalance observed in flat back and kyphotic decompensation syndromes offers a spectrum of deformity and symptomatology. Appropriate diagnostic evaluation and initial physical therapy are essential. In our series, nearly 40% of the patients were initially effectively managed with spinal instrumentation removal and therapy. In Group A, average sagittal imbalance was however significantly less than in the patients requiring surgical realignment (Group B). For those patients originally treated with minimal surgery (instrumentation removal) and aggressive therapy, 7 out of 28 experienced significant initial clinical improvement yet demonstrated late deterioration. Failure to maintain sagittal alignment, increasing pain, and failure of disks below the original fusion in these 7 patients (25% of Group A) leads to the question of whether an earlier, and perhaps more aggressive sagittal realignment procedure could have averted the accelerated degeneration of the remaining caudal disks. We have noted that the 7 patients of the conservative treatment group who developed gradual increasing pain all had sagittal malalignment exceeding 4 cm of plumb line shift (average 4.8 cm). The average malalignment in patients effectively managed in Group A was 2.6 cm.

In Group B, surgical realignment with anterior and posterior approaches revealed good correction and significant pain reduction. Greater imbalance was noted in patients originally fused to the sacrum than those fused to L4 or L5 originally. The latter group (Group B2), in which patients still had mobile caudal segments, retained some ability to compensate for malalignment of the fusion mass. Once the flat back becomes symptomatic in patients fused to L4 or L5, therapy and spinal instrumentation removal can be effective assuming healthy disk spaces exist caudally. Those patients failing these "conservative" measures may require realignment osteotomies. In this study, greater than 4 cm of malalignment even in instances of viable disks was noted to lead to eventual increase in distal lumbar back pain and imbalance and may represent long term conservative treatment failure. In Group B2, an MRI helped identify those patients in whom fusion mass osteotomy and realignment without extension of fusion to the sacrum was considered a viable option due to disks that appeared well hydrated and without significant fissuring or herniation.

A clear limitation of our methods lies in the quantification of pain. Although a self-reporting pain scale was applied, the interpretation of pain and its intensity is certainly variable between individuals and thus comparison between groups based upon pain scores is open to bias.

## CONCLUSION

The flat back and kyphotic decompensation syndromes are iatrogenic pathologies related to spinal fusion. Although one can not reasonably recommend to never fuse the spine based upon possible long-term complications, it must be emphasized that fusion should be minimized, in terms of anatomic extent, and optimized in terms of rigorous patient selection and careful consideration of physiologic spinal alignment. As we are increasingly confronted with late sequelae of spinal fusion, an attempt to increase our understanding of ideal spinal contour is essential. The treatment of painful disability of global failure due to spinal malalignment must focus first on maximizing paraspinal muscular function and compensatory mechanisms. Removal of painful instrumentation can also be quite successful. When these less invasive approaches are unsuccessful, realignment surgery may be indicated.

In our series, treatment without realignment surgery was found to offer long-term success for cases of mild sagittal malalignment (less than 4 cm) when two intact disks were present below the fusion mass. In the operative groups, MRI evaluation guided surgical management. Viable levels below a previous fusion may obviate the need for extension of the preexisting fusion mass. Anterior and posterior osteotomies through the existing fusion mass with posterior instrumentation appear to yield good long-term results in respect to sagittal plane balance and pain. MRI evidence of significant disk degeneration was felt to necessitate an extension of a previous fusion in order to avoid later disk related problems despite realignment.

It is our hypothesis that the long-term clinical findings in treated flat back and kyphotic decompensation syndromes will be related to the amount of remaining sagittal imbalance as well as the rate and degree of degeneration of disks adjacent to the original fusion mass. Further follow up and addition of more patients to our series will hopefully more clearly define the essential issues and treatment approaches in the sagittal malalignment syndromes. At this time our preferred approach for patients failing conservative management is a surgical spine realignment performed as a simultaneous segmental anterior/posterior technique.

The pathology of the flat back and kyphotic decompensation syndrome is fairly new, and of an iatrogenic origin. Sagittal plane imbalance beyond physiologic limits anteriorly (and possibly posteriorly), in terms of plumb line displacement, can lead to the clinical symptom complex of a feeling of imbalance, increasing pain, fatigue and disability. The increasing awareness of long-term consequences of sagittal plane imbalance has already led to the development of techniques and instrumentation systems that avoid this complication from the outset. Perhaps there is also a role for more aggressive early intervention in cases of imbalance prior to the development of disabling deformity. Further investigation of this matter, including prospective studies involving MRI and cases of possibly salvageable levels below symptomatic spinal malalignment, is essential.

## REFERENCES


1. Aprill C, Bogduk N: High-intensity zone: a diagnostic sign of painful lumbar disc on magnetic resonance imaging, *Br J Radiol* 65:361-369, 1992.
2. Doherty JH: Complications of fusion in lumbar scoliosis, *J Bone Joint Surg* 55A:438, 1973.
3. Farcy J-P: Simultaneous anterior and posterior procedures for short segment spine pathology, Am Acad Orthop Surgeons, Video tape 23112, 1993.
4. Farcy J-PC, Schwab FJ: Management of flatback and the related kyphotic decompensation syndrome, *Spine* 22:2452-2457, 1997.
5. Grobler LJ, Moe JH, Winter RB: Loss of lumbar lordosis following surgical correction of thoracolumbar deformities, *Orthop Trans* 239:2, 1978.
6. Kostuik JP, Maurais GR, Richardson WJ, Okajima Y: Combined single stage anterior and posterior osteotomy for correction of iatrogenic lumbar kyphosis, *Spine* 13(10):257, 1988.
7. Lagrone MO, Bradford DS, Moe JH, Lonstein JE, Winter RB, Ogilvie JW: Treatment of symptomatic flat back after spinal fusion, *J Bone Joint Surg* 70A:569, 1988.
8. Tveit P, Daggfeldt K, Hetland S, Thorstensson A: Erector spinae lever arm length variations with changes in spinal curvature, *Spine* 19:199-204, 1994.

# 54

# FAILURES IN SPINE SURGERY DUE TO INFECTION

**Cameron Bruce Huckell, M.D.**



Infection rates have lessened with refinements in technique and prophylactic antibiotics, however, infection remains a complication that every surgeon must face occasionally. In the last 50 years, the developed world has seen great advancement in general medical care. Since World War II, great leaps forward in the field of antibiotic chemotherapy have been made. There has been a large decrease in spinal osteomyelitis mortality from over 50% in the preantibiotic era to approximately 2% in the 1960s.[49] Underlying conditions such as advanced age, alcoholism, diabetes, corticosteroid therapy, and chronic renal failure are associated with spinal infection and make treatment challenging.[6,13,43,48] Specific surgical factors such as revision surgery, the length and complexity of surgery, the addition of instrumentation, remote infections at the same surgical site, malnutrition, previous radiation, and perhaps obesity can increase infection rates.

## DEFINITIONS

The conditions of discitis, vertebral osteomyelitis, and epidural abscess tend to be regarded as separate entities in the medical literature and this is somewhat artificial since they represent a disease spectrum of pyogenic vertebral infection that many Europeans refer to as spondylodiscitis. Anatomically, the spine is unique since it encompasses both a bone, namely the vertebra, and joints, composed of the disk and facets. Furthermore, the structure is segmental and it lies adjacent to the dural sheath that creates the epidural space. In the spine, the separation of osteomyelitis from pyogenic discitis often fails since the bone and the disk or their border at the end plate are both involved.[33]

## PATHOPHYSIOLOGY AND PATHOLOGY

The etiology of postoperative pyogenic spinal infection is multifactorial. There are several possible sources for established pyogenic spinal infection. The first is hematogenous osteomyelitis that seeds itself in a recently operated vertebrae. Ratcliffe postulates that an arterial septic embolus seeds itself into the vertebral metaphysis and creeping septic thrombosis starts the infectious process in the endplate and that may spread to the adjacent avascular disk.[40] In my opinion, this theory has a sound basis and to the best of my understanding represents a clear picture of the pathogenesis.

The second mechanism for established pyogenic spinal infection is direct inoculation of the disk or vertebra that may follow surgery, trauma, or an invasive procedure. The source of the bacteria can be the patient's own skin, bacterial shedding from the staff to the wound itself or to hands and instruments that contact the wound.[44] Finally, pyogenic spinal infection may occur secondary to a contiguous focus of infection. Bacteremia may seed the wound hematoma causing wound infection in the early postoperative period.[3] The presence of foreign material, hematoma, and necrotic tissue increases the risk of infection.[39,52]

After infection has started it initiates acute suppurative inflammation.[52] In an experimental sheep model of discitis using inoculation with *Staphylococcus epidermidis,* the earliest change was endplate disorganization followed by breach in the endplate and herniation of nuclear material into adjacent bone that caused a cellular infiltrate with polymorphonuclear leukocytes around the nuclear material. Young granulation tissue replaced the marrow spaces of the adjacent bodies and vascular engorgement penetrated the hyaline lamina.[17] At 3 weeks there were extensive loss of the endplate, larger herniations of the nucleus pulposus into the adjacent bone, and hemorrhage into the center of the disk.[17] Adjacent bone resorption by granulation tissue infiltration was striking.[17] Fraser showed that by six weeks there was evidence of new bone forming at the periphery of the lesion.[17] In humans, if bone and disk destruction is extensive, then collapse and deformity may follow.[16,25] These factors together usually contribute to an increase in kyphosis because anterior structures are more often affected.[37] Finally, in chronic osteomyelitis bacteria may establish a microscopic colony on the necrotic bone (sequestrum) protected by a biofilm layer of polysaccharide that is resistant to elimination.[31]

Magnetic resonance imaging (MRI) correlated with intraoperative ultrasound and surgical confirmation has shown that epidural abscess is frequently associated with the adjacent infection of the bone and disk in greater than 90% of circumstances.[19] Epidural abscesses are usually associated with adjacent pyogenic spinal infection and this represents the failure of the immune response to contain the infection within the confines of the disk and bone and their surrounding ligaments. Occasionally, an epidural abscess in the absence of a contiguous paraspinal infection occurs that may stem from a hematogenous source or by iatrogenic or traumatic inoculation.[2]

## BACTERIOLOGY

The most common identified organism to cause pyogenic vertebral osteomyelitis, adult or childhood discitis, and epidural abscess is *Staphylococcus aureus.*[8,13,15,16,24,38,51] *S. aureus* is the leading cause of osteomyelitis in the postoperative setting. The virulence of gram-positive cocci in general depend on many genetic factors including antibiotic resistance genes,[45] its ability to bind to tissue proteins such as fibronectin,[28] the production of certain enzymes and exotoxins, and slime (abundant extracapsular polysaccharide) production.[10]

It is important to note that gram-negative organisms are usually opportunistic organisms that can be cultured from healthy individuals in the mouth skin and feces. Gram-negative organisms such as *Escherichia coli, Pseudomonas aeruginosa, Salmonella, Haemophilus, Klebsiella, Acinetobacter,* and *Proteus* organisms can cause serious and disabling infections.[18,21,38] Gram-negative infections may originate by direct inoculation through contamination or by hematogenous means such as after a postoperative urinary tract infection that follows catheterization and then results in bacteremia that establishes itself in the wound area. Gram-negative organism pathogenicity is partly related to endotoxin production,[34] exotoxin production,[41] bacterial transfer of resistant genes,[26] and ability to form pili that adhere to substrates.[23]

## PREVENTION OF INFECTION

Obviously, prevention is the best cure for postoperative infections. The spinal surgeon should consider this possible outcome carefully before undertaking any procedure. The literature suggests prophylactic antibiotics are probably indicated for simple laminectomy/diskectomy procedures and they reduce the risk of infection from 1% to 2% to 0.5%.[11] The risk of infection in posterior lumbar arthrodesis with instrumentation is between 2% and 5% and there is general agreement that prophylactic antibiotics are indicated.[39] Surgeons and operating room staff should limit the amount of traffic and follow strict sterile technique. Wound infections are prevented by gentle tissue handling since it decreases the amount of tissue necrosis. Reduction of the presence of foreign material, and avoidance of hematoma formation are also known to lessen the chance of infection. Long procedures that require vigorous retraction can be debrided and irrigated prior to closure; I release retractors intermittently to allow resumption of blood flow into tissues.

## DIAGNOSIS

Early recognition and treatment of discitis, osteomyelitis, and epidural abscess are almost always associated with a better outcome.[8,9] The early diagnosis of discitis allows simple administration of antibiotics for resolution of the condition.[51] If diagnosis of spinal infection is late then the infection may become life-threatening and vertebral osteomyelitis or epidural abscess may require urgent surgery and antibiotic therapy.

Delayed diagnosis of postoperative discitis is common. The key in early diagnosis of spinal infection is to keep a high index of suspicion for this diagnosis while evaluating the patient. Initially, the only complaint is back pain and it may not be easy to distinguish from incisional pain. The severity of pain from infection can cause a patient to have great emotional distress and in my opinion this is an important early indicator for the presence of a serious deep infection. Unfortunately, the surgeon can fail to recognize the magnitude of the problem, because the wound initially appears normal. On physical examination, there is usually paraspinal muscle spasm and local tenderness and for most patients, straight leg raising will only produce back pain. All of these findings overlap with a normal postoperative course. If there is significant neurological deficit, the diagnosis of epidural hematoma, epidural abscess, or recurrent disk herniation must be excluded by means of appropriate imaging studies followed by urgent surgery if indicated. Even with epidural abscess physical examination usually does not reveal any major findings in the initial stages of the disease.[9] Occasionally, local deep-seated back pain or tenderness with palpation and percussion can be noted. The patient may experience involuntary muscle spasm. Infection may lead to vertebral destruction that manifests itself on physical exam by obvious deformity or neurological deficit.[37] Late in the course of the disease spectrum focal neurological deficits and frank paralysis can occur. The patient should be examined for meningeal signs to help rule out meningitis.

Up to 68% of patients with epidural abscess have a white blood cell count (WBC) greater than $11,000/10^{-5}$ 1. However, a WBC that is less than $10,000/10^{-5}$ 1. bears no clear relationship to severity of disease.[24] The erythrocyte sedimentation rate (ESR) is elevated in greater than 90% of pyogenic spinal infections.[21,46] These tests are simple, inexpensive, and sensitive but not very specific because they are raised with any condition causing inflammation.[22] Approximately 30% of discitis, 50% of osteomyelitis,[50] and 69% of epidural abscess patients[8] present with positive blood cultures and this correlates to severity of infection and sepsis. Every effort should be made to identify the organism using blood cultures. Urine, sputum, and other indicated cultures should be performed to rule out remote sources.

All patients at this early postoperative stage have an elevated ESR. In normal postoperative patients, the peak ESR ranges from 65 to 100 four days after surgery. Most patients have a value under 40 by 2 weeks after surgery and by 6 weeks most have returned to approximately 20.[22] For this reason, a clinical index of suspicion has to remain high, factors such as persistent fever, incisional pain, and wound drainage are more important in diagnosing infections than any specific laboratory test although a persistently raised white count and ESR may aid in the diagnosis of infection.

## DIAGNOSTIC IMAGING

Initial plain films are normal, they take up to two weeks to show endplate erosion, and disk space narrowing helps make a presumptive diagnosis of pyogenic spinal infection. The earliest possible changes seen on the plain film are soft tissue widening in the retropharyngeal area, widening of the mediastinum in the thoracic spine, or distortion of the psoas contour in the lumbar spine. The indicator for vertebral osteomyelitis is a small lytic lesion of the vertebral body and endplate and it eventually is replaced by sclerotic bone.[1,49,53] At very early stages of infection it can be difficult to differentiate degenerative disease from pyogenic spinal infection using plain radiographs alone.

Modic showed plain films have sensitivity of 82%, specificity of 57%, and accuracy of 73% for the diagnosis of vertebral osteomyelitis. Bone scans (technetium-99m-DHP) have a sensitivity of 90%, a specificity of 78%, and an accuracy rate of 86% in the diagnosis of vertebral osteomyelitis.[33] When the bone scan is combined with a gallium-67 scan, sensitivity is 90%, specificity is 100%, and accuracy is 94%. Technetium-99m-DHP bone scan is very useful in ruling out multiple metastatic tumor sites. Indium-111 scans are not recommended because they are only 31% accurate for the diagnosis of osteomyelitis.[52]

Computerized tomography (CT) scans with myelographic enhancement show excellent bony detail and reasonable definition of soft tissue structures. Usually if there is infection then fibrovascular granulation tissue resorbs infected bone and disk in an attempt to clear the infection so high-resolution CT with axial and sagittal cuts is of great value in assessing the amount of bone destruction. These studies are also useful for postoperative patients who have stainless steel MRI artifact-producing hardware. Titanium causes less CT artifact than stainless steel but neither material negates the possibility of accurate interpretation. The presence of hardware should not deter the surgeon from obtaining a necessary study. Often, the plain myelogram including oblique studies provides critical information with regard to neural compression in the central canal and subarticular recess, but unfortunately the neural foramen is not outlined by the dye column so soft tissue changes in this area are difficult to evaluate. Fluid collections and epidural abscess often can be identified despite hardware artifact. It is important to send cerebrospinal fluid samples for culture cell count, chemistry, and glucose levels before performing the myelogram lumbar puncture.

The MRI diagnostic accuracy for vertebral osteomyelitis is high and is the best single diagnostic test that can be performed. It has a sensitivity of 96%, specificity of 92%, and accuracy of 94%,[33] but this applies to spontaneous vertebral osteomyelitis. After surgery, however, postoperative changes complicate interpretation because of edema, hematoma, granulation tissue, and scar that change their MRI appearance and vascularity in the bone and soft tissues over time.

In the postdiskectomy setting, an excellent prospective study has shown that the gadolinium-enhanced T1 image usually shows intermediate signal tissue mimicking the mass effect of the preoperative disk herniation and it is thought that it probably represents normal hematoma that is maturing into scar tissue; it is often seen in patients with little or no clinical symptoms.[5] There are other "normal" changes that occur after surgery, such as enhancement of nerve roots, endplates, facet joints, and paraspinal muscles. However, it is rare to have a T2-bright signal in the disk especially several months after surgery and often this a clue to the presence of postoperative discitis. MRI interpretation is clouded by artifact if there is hardware. However, in the late postoperative patient metal suppression MRI sequences with titanium hardware allow a reasonable interpretation of structures more than several millimeters away from the metal.

A diagnostic triad consisting of T2-weighted image hyperintensity of the disk and endplates with T1-weighted hypointensity and gadolinium T1-weighted hyperintensity of the adjacent marrow makes the diagnosis of pyogenic infection likely.[47] T2-weighted hyperintensity at the infection site usually exceeds the intensity of cerebrospinal fluid in pyogenic spinal infection and the infection often involves two adjacent vertebrae with an anterior bandlike swelling of the adjacent anterior soft tissue.[20] Gadolinium enhancement of the adjacent marrow is predictor of discitis in the postoperative setting and it helps to distinguish normal changes from inflammation due to surgery form changes due to infection.[4] Also the presence of a T2-bright disk space raises great suspicion about the possibility of discitis. MRI images provide the surgeon with precise anatomical information for a possible planned surgical procedure and they detect even small epidural abscesses. It is the best test to evaluate pyogenic spinal infection fully. However, MRI is not always useful in the immediate postoperative patient, since there may be edema, hematoma, and granulation tissue present that confound the interpretation of the tissues in the operative wound. The most important point for the clinician to remember about the use of diagnostic imaging is that the patient who presents with an uncertain diagnosis of pyogenic spinal infection can be evaluated using an early CT myelogram or MRI and the study may aid in the diagnosis but interpretation is difficult and it must be correlated to the clinical and pathological setting.

## TREATMENT GOALS

The first goal of treatment is to identify the exact organism that caused the disease. Then, the physician must make a plan to eradicate the organism and decrease the chance of chronic or recurrent infection. Consideration of spinal function must include the restoration or maintenance of spinal alignment and neurological function. Finally, appropriate treatment usually leads to a reduction in pain and resolution of infection.

## MEDICAL TREATMENT OF POSTOPERATIVE WOUND INFECTIONS

Patients with minor superficial infections, draining sterile hematomas, or a stitch abscess may benefit from medical treatment with antibiotics. The treating physician should resist the temptation of giving broad-spectrum antibiotics prior to organism identification unless the patient's life is threatened by sepsis, or neurological function is compromised by epidural abscess. In these circumstances urgent blood cultures and wound aspiration should precede antibiotic administration. Antibiotic sensitivities must be analyzed and their penetration into bone should be considered. In general, the best agents to use for the treatment of this disease are bacteriocidal agents and they should penetrate the infected tissues at sufficient concentrations. The importance of bone antibiotic concentrations is not clarified but the best single agent was clindamycin and it gave the best treatment results in experimental *Staphylococcus aureus* osteomyelitis.[30] Using this model it was also found that clindamycin had the greatest bone to serum ratio.[29] Clindamycin and tobramycin were found to have better penetration into the rabbit nucleus pulposus than cephalothin, which was poorly absorbed.[14] However, many factors play a role including changing antibiotic-resistant patterns and the development of new antibiotics so it is necessary to review and revise antibiotic regimens for specific organisms.

After identification of the organism there is general agreement that if osteomyelitis is identified the treatment should include a six-week course of appropriate intravenous antibiotics, possibly followed by a course of oral antibiotics for another six weeks. The length of treatment can probably be shortened in children and a three-week course of antibiotics is often sufficient, initially three to five days of intravenous therapy followed by oral antibiotic is sufficient.[51] These recommendations have been determined empirically. However, animal rabbit models show prolonged treatment of osteomyelitis resulted in a cure rate of 70% to 80% with less development of chronic osteomyelitis than short courses of treatment.[35,36] Animal studies seem to support the use of combination drug therapy of oxacillin or rifampin with an aminoglycoside but rabbits have higher renal excretion rates of most antibiotics and clinical observations have not clearly supported these laboratory findings.[50] Obviously, there are many variables in clinical practice including the presence of sequestrum, the local vascularity, and the addition of surgical debridement.

It is preferable to treat a known organism according to its known sensitivities but occasionally no organism can be identified but the diagnosis of spinal osteomyelitis is confirmed on histology. In my opinion either repeat biopsy or broad spectrum anti-staphylococcal antibiotic treatment can be considered. Great care to eliminate other possible pathogens such as mycobacteria species, gram-negative, rare bacterial, and fungal pathogens is required before instituting presumptive treatment for *Staphylococcus aureus*. The patient's response to treatment is measured by monitoring the patient's clinical response and ESR on a regular basis.

Intervention with intravenous antibiotics and medical treatment alone frequently completely cures spontaneous discitis or vertebral body osteomyelitis and this method can probably be used in some postoperative patients without instrumentation who are diagnosed early and who do not have established infections. If there was instrumentation used, this method is less likely to work because there is foreign material in the wound. The immune response and intravenous antibiotics alone can clear away the dead bone in the highly vascular anterior vertebral structures allowing the body to successfully resolve the infection. Depending on the virulence of the organism and the duration of the symptoms medical treatment may result in disk space narrowing or even spontaneous fusion at resolution. In trauma, significant spinal instability with neurological elements at risk necessitates some form of spinal immobilization to help preserve neurological function[12] and this is probably true in the case of infection. However, there are no direct data to support or refute the use of spinal bracing as an adjunct to the treatment of infection.

## SURGICAL TREATMENT OF PYOGENIC SPINAL INFECTION

The absolute indications for repeat surgery are the following: (1) failure of medical treatment, (2) deep (subfascial) postoperative infections with abundant drainage especially if foreign body materials were used, and (3) significant or increasing neurological deficit. A relative indication for surgery includes vertebral bony destruction and impending spinal deformity. The goals of surgery are resection of infected bone, decompression of neural structures, restoration of vertebral load-bearing capacity, and maintenance of normal spinal alignment.

## REPEAT SURGERY BY INCISION AND DRAINAGE OF THE SPINAL WOUND

In my opinion, if the surgeon suspects wound infection or a hematoma that is persistently draining, then the best course of treatment is to take the patient back to the operating room for definitive treatment. Occasionally, an early contaminated hematoma can be salvaged without removing bone graft and instrumentation by thorough irrigation and debridement followed by wound closure and antibiotic treatment, eliminating all dead space over large-diameter suction drains that exit from separate stab wounds. An aggressive surgical and medical approach to a contaminated hematoma is less likely to lead to a chronic spinal infection that becomes more difficult to treat especially in patients who have instrumentation for deformity correction.

At the time of irrigation and debridement, specimens should be sent to the laboratory for microbiological analysis. Necrotic material should be removed and it may be necessary to remove bone graft material.

If the wound is clearly infected then some wounds can be salvaged by thorough debridement and then placement of large bore inflow-outflow irrigation tubes incorporating appropriate antibiotic solution. This treatment is employed for three to five days, monitoring the patient clinically following fever and response to treatment.

The other alternative is to leave the wound open and allow healing by secondary intention. After the infection is eradicated then delayed secondary closure is possible. However, the metabolic load placed on the elderly patient is great, and for the aged, I prefer the inflow-outflow technique.

If the instrumentation is tight, another possible option is loose closure of the fascia to prevent bone desiccation and aid fusion; the skin is left open to facilitate drainage.

When there is loose instrumentation or infected bone graft material then it should be removed until resolution of infection. Resulting spinal deformity or pseudarthrosis can be treated surgically after the eradication of infection. Sometimes there is significant soft tissue loss and a local rotational flap or even a free flap from the latissimus dorsi may aid in bone healing.[42] Care to encourage increased nutritional intake orally, via enteral tube feeding or by total parenteral nutrition (TPN), should be started in patients with a high caloric requirement due to an open wound. At the same time, the patient should have intravenous antibiotics to cover a broad spectrum of organisms and when culture and sensitivity results are ready, antibiotics should be adjusted to focus on the infecting organisms. Intravenous antibiotic therapy should probably last six weeks, followed by six weeks of oral therapy. The ESR can be followed on a weekly basis to measure the success of treatment.

There is little doubt that deep wound infections increase the chance of a poor outcome by putting the patient at risk for chronic pain, an increased risk of pseudarthrosis, or the development of chronic pyogenic spinal infection. In my opinion it is probably better to have a very aggressive approach to a contaminated hematoma and perhaps even to over-diagnose the condition rather than to undertreat early wound healing problems that may go on to develop a chronic pyogenic spinal infection.

## BIOPSY

Sometimes it is necessary to diagnose the organism causing the infection in a patient in whom the infection was suppressed initially by oral antibiotic treatment but ultimately went on to develop an established infection. If the infection is indolent and the symptoms are not neurologically or life-threatening, then antibiotics may be stopped for several days in a closely observed setting. A Craig needle biopsy may identify the infecting organism and establish the diagnosis. If no antibiotics are given prior to biopsy then the organism identification yield increases from approximately 30% to 75% in the case of spinal osteomyelitis.[7] Accurate organism identification will improve long-term outcome by improving antibiotic selection.

## SURGICAL APPROACHES

If there is a large amount of bone destruction with paraspinal anterior abscess and osteomyelitis is established in the vertebral body and intervertebral disk, an anterior approach is most often used for definitive debridement. At the level of the odontoid, a lateral or transoral approach can be performed. Below C2, a standard anterior approach provides access, even down to the T1 level. At the T2-T3 level, I have found an anterior third rib thoracotomy provides adequate access. T4-T6 requires a fifth rib approach and T7-T11 should be entered from two ribs above. At T12 and L1, a transthoracic, transdiaphragmatic retroperitoneal approach through the tenth rib provides excellent access. From L2 to the sacrum, an oblique retroperitoneal incision provides excellent exposure but it is technically very difficult due to the significant scarring from infection and the proximity of the great vessels. If infected bone is posterior and there is a posterior epidural abscess without anterior osteomyelitis then the standard midline posterior approach is adequate. In the thoracic spine a costotransversectomy can provide access to the vertebral body.

## ESTABLISHED VERTEBRAL OSTEOMYELITIS/DISCITIS

If the predominant finding is bone destruction causing unacceptable deformity or neurological compromise then treatment with resection and debridement of the infected and necrotic bone with fusion of the involved motion segment will likely provide definitive treatment. In my experience, a significant amount of bone destruction would lead to surgical intervention and debridement because the dead bone may be sequestered from the bodies normal defense mechanisms. The surgeon must strive to remove all of the necrotic tissue to the level of healthy bleeding bone. In the vast majority of patients requiring surgery this means that anterior debridement with autogenous bone grafting is required.[6,13,16,27] One group of authors successfully treated lumbar infection in 13 out of 32 selected patients using bilateral lateral grafts and posterior debridement after nerve root mobilization and retraction.[32] Their recommendation at more proximal spinal cord levels was to debride anteriorly avoiding mobilization at the cord and fuse with structural autogenous graft from C1-L1 unless there was a psoas abscess, in which case anterior debridement and fusion were recommended even at the lumbar levels.[32] I feel that anterior debridement and structural autogenous graft via an anterior approach in the lumbar spine are preferable because they pose a smaller neurological risk to nerve roots than anterior debridement via a posterior approach. After anterior debridement and autogenous grafting, the surgeon has the option of augmenting the stability with a brace or with internal fixation into parts of the spine that are not affected by the infection. It is my opinion that this approach will probably reduce the chance of graft extrusion although if the patient cannot tolerate the second procedure either bed rest or bracing is valid. Treatment of vertebral osteomyelitis by laminectomy alone has been associated with a poor neurological outcome.[13]

One study of 10 elderly patients showed that bed rest can be well-tolerated after anterior debridement and bone grafting with good outcome.[6] In my experience thinner, healthier, younger people, can tolerate immobilization by a cast but these are poorly tolerated in older people. Well-selected patients may benefit from a posterior stabilization and fusion with instrumentation after anterior debridement but I recommend against having foreign material in contact with the source of infection. At the end of the surgical procedure, the surgeon will determine the inherent stability of the construct and may add bracing.

Autogenous iliac crest bone grafts are the best structural graft for corpectomy defects under 10 cm. The strength of the graft is not usually sufficient for anterior column support although the cancellous nature of the bone allows early revascularization and healing. The fate of autogenous bone graft is incorporation and fusion in over 95% of patients.[32] If the defect is longer than 10 cm, thought should be given to autogenous single or multiple fibular bone grafts but incorporation can be delayed. These grafts can be augmented with morselized bone of any autogenous source.

In my opinion the use of autogenous material is greatly superior to either allograft or metal cages, since they can incorporate and become healthy living tissue and they are less likely to provide a foreign body substrate to the infecting organisms. I feel it is often possible to use only autogenous material anteriorly and augment this with stable posterior fixation at a site that is not involved in the infection to obtain the benefit of immediate stable internal fixation in well-selected patients. Also there is a great advantage in spending time using a grafting technique that has inherent stability so there is no need to add instrumentation to achieve fusion across the infected region. In my opinion, allografts should not be used because this is a dead foreign material that can promote infection. However, anecdotal reports by some surgeons indicate success with cages, ceramics, and allograft with radical debridement prior to insertion, I feel this is a poor option and should be used only if no autogenous source of bone is available.

## SPECIAL CONSIDERATIONS REGARDING EPIDURAL ABSCESS

Modern MRI has shown us that an associated epidural extension of the infection is often found with vertebral osteomyelitis there are times that it is not the major component of the infection and the epidural component of the infection is contained by the inflammatory response. Treatment in these cases should be directed predominantly against the discitis or osteomyelitis at the source of the problem.

However, if there is a frank epidural abscess—especially if there are neurological symptoms—then treatment of this condition with surgical drainage and antibiotic intervention is an emergency. The chance of a good outcome is directly proportional to the severity of the neurological lesion at presentation; furthermore inaccurate initial diagnosis adversely affects neurological outcome.[9] The diagnosis of meningitis must be excluded clinically and cerebrospinal fluid examination and culture through an uncontaminated site may be indicated. Antibiotic treatment should immediately follow blood cultures. The surgical approach to the abscess should provide direct access to the infected material. I feel the anatomic site of the abscess should dictate whether an anterior or posterior approach is used and if there is an associated vertebral osteomyelitis there should also be debridement of infected bone and disk material with autogenous grafting.

## CONTROVERSIES IN TREATMENT

In my patients with established vertebral osteomyelitis I thoroughly debride the infected bone and fuse the involved motion segment and stabilize with a brace if the patient will tolerate it. I do not believe in implanting instrumentation into infected regions of the spine. However, sometimes I perform a posterior stabilization procedure after debridement of anterior osteomyelitis or discitis and I make every effort to keep the posterior instrumentation away from the infected area of the spine by inserting fixation at uninfected motion segments that span and bypass the infected area posteriorly. The advantages of this approach are that early mobilization and perhaps better control of spinal deformity are obtained. One drawback with the use of posterior instrumentation is that more segments must be included into the levels fused because the normal segments above and below the infected area must be included in the fusion to immobilize area where anterior debridement and bone grafting were performed. Also, I am always concerned that the instrumentation can act as a foreign body surface where resistant bacterial microcolonies can establish themselves so in many patients I make every effort to achieve inherent stability of the anterior grafting procedure using precise and careful carpentry techniques that resist graft extrusion and I often employ additional external immobilization with a cast, halo, or activity restriction.

There is controversy surrounding the use of anterior instrumentation after an anterior debridement, since the foreign body substrate can act as a nidus of infection for bacteria to attach and set up a resistant colony. If anterior instrumentation is used after debridement and bone grafting, usually fewer motion segments need to be included, but there is probably a higher risk of implant loosening. Without radical debridement there is a higher rate of unsuccessful infection eradication and there is an unacceptable remote risk of major organ erosion from a loose infected implant.

There have been recent unpublished preliminary reports of successful eradication of infection using anterior instrumentation after anterior debridement of infected tissue. This treatment may hold some promise in well-selected patients but its present role is unclear. The debridement must be extensive and there must be no remaining infected tissue for its theoretical success. Highly vascular areas such as the anterior lumbar and cervical spine may respond better to this approach. However, one of my concerns is that there is increased graft resorption in infection and this will lead to a load-bearing implant that will be at high risk for failure and loosening. I have had several patients referred to me by surgeons who used this plan of treatment and they had disturbing results. However, there may be a role for single-stage anterior debridement and instrumentation in the patient who has had infection eliminated by complete debridement of the infection in a highly vascular region especially if a very antibiotic-susceptible organism has been identified as the cause. I caution the use of this technique in the patient who has a high comorbidity due to diabetes, advanced age, renal failure, or reduced immunity.

In my opinion, the safest treatment of established osteomyelitis infections unlikely to respond to medical treatment is anterior debridement, autogenous grafting followed by casting, bracing, or posterior instrumentation and fusion if there is instability. Staging can be used if the patient cannot tolerate a lengthy procedure. The key to improving outcome in the infected patient is early recognition of the disease so that simple intervention provides excellent results. If the patient presents with more advanced stages of infection, the surgeon now has effective treatments that prevent or correct neurological disability, reduce spinal deformity, and eradicate infection.

## REFERENCES


1. Allen EH, Cosgrove D, Millard F: The radiological changes in infection of the spine and their diagnostic value, *Clin Radiol* 29:31-40, 1978.
2. Angtuaco EJC, McConnell JR, Chadduck WM, Flanigan S: MR imaging of spinal epidural sepsis, *Am J Neuroradiol* 8:879-883, 1987.
3. Blomgren G, Lindgren U: Post-operative infections resulting from bacteremia. An experimental study in rabbits, *Acta Orthop Scand* 51:761-765, 1980.
4. Boden SD, Davis DO, Dina TS, Sunner JL, Wiesel SW: Post-operative discitis: distinguishing early MR findings from normal post-operative disc space changes, *Radiology* 184:765-771, 1992.
5. Boden SD, Davis DO, Dina TS, Parker CP, O'Malley S, Sunner JL, Wiesel SW: Contrast-enhanced MR imaging performed after successful lumbar disc surgery: Prospective study, *Radiology* 182:59-64, 1992.
6. Cahill DW, Love LC, Rechtine GR: Pyogenic osteomyelitis of the spine in the elderly, *J Neurosurg* 74: 878-886, 1991.
7. Cotty P, Fouquet B, Pleskof L, Audurier A, Cotty F, Goupille P, Valat JP, Alison A, Lafont J: Vertebral osteomyelitis: value of percutaneous biopsy, *J Neuroradiol* 15:13-21, 1988.
8. Danner RL, Hartman BJ: Update on spinal epidural abscess: 35 cases and review of the literature, *Rev Infect Dis* 9:265-274, 1987.
9. Darouiche RO, Hamill RJ, Greenberg SB, Weathers SW, Musher DM: Bacterial spinal epidural abscess, *Medicine* 71(6):369-385, 1992.
10. Davenport DS, Massanari RM, Pfaller MA, Bale MJ, Streed SA, Hierholzer WJ: Usefulness of a test for slime production as a marker for clinically significant infections with coagulase-negative staphylococci, *J Infect Dis* 153:332-339, 1986.
11. Dempsey R, Rapp RP, Young B, Johnston S, Tibbs P: Prophylactic parenteral antibiotics in clean neurosurgical procedures: a review, *J Neurosurg* 69:52-57, 1988.
12. Ducker TB, Salcman M, Daniell HB: Experimental spinal cord trauma, III. Therapeutic effect of immobilization and pharmacologic agents, *Surg Neurol* 10: 71-76, 1978.
13. Eismont FJ, Bohlman HH, Prasanna LS, Goldberg VM, Freehafter AA: Pyogenic and fungal vertebral osteomyelitis with paralysis, *J Bone Joint Surg* 65A(1): 19-29, 1983.
14. Eismont FJ, Wiesel SW, Brighton CT, Rothman RH: Antibiotic penetration into rabbit nucleus pulposis, *Spine* 12:254-256, 1987.
15. Emery SE, Chan DP, Woodward HR: Treatment of hematogenous pyogenic vertebral osteomyelitis with anterior debridement and primary bone grafting, *Spine* 14:284-291, 1989.
16. Fang D, Chung KM, Dos Remedios ID, Lee YK, Leong JC: Pyogenic vertebral osteomyelitis: treatment by anterior spinal debridement and fusion, *J Spinal Disord* 7:173-80, 1994.
17. Fraser RD, Osti OL, Vernon-Roberts B: Discitis after discography, *J Bone Joint Surg* 69B(1):26-35, 1987.
18. Frederickson B, Yuan H, Olans R: Management and outcome of pyogenic vertebral osteomyelitis, *Clin Orthop* 131:160-167, 1977.
19. Friedmand DP, Hills JR: Cervical epidural spinal infection: MR imaging characteristics, *AJR Am J Roentgenol* 163:699-704, 1994.
20. Hovi I, Lamminen A, Salonen O, Raininko R: MR imaging of the lower spine, *Acta Radiol* 35:532-540, 1994.
21. Jones NS, Anderson DJ, Stiles PJ: Osteomyelitis in a general hospital, *J Bone Joint Surg* 69B(5):779-783, 1987.
22. Jönsson B, Söderholon R, Strömqvist B: Erythrocyte

sedimentation rate after lumbar spine surgery, *Spine* 16:1049-1050, 1991.

23. Keith BR, Harris SL, Russel PW, Orndorff PE: Effect of Type 1 piliation on in vitro killing of *Escherichia coli* by mouse peritoneal macrophages, *Infect Immunol* 58: 3448-3454, 1990.
24. Kemp HBS, Jackson JW, Jerimiah JD, Hall AJ: Pyogenic infection occuring primarily in the intervertebral discs, *J Bone Joint Surg* 55B(4):698-714, 1973.
25. Kulowski J: Pyogenic osteomyelitis of the spine, *J Bone Joint Surg* 18A(2):343-364, 1934.
26. Lampson BC, Parisi JT: Naturally occuring *Staphylococcal epidermidis* plasmid expressing constitutive macrolide-lincosamide-streptogranin B resistance contains a deleted attenuator, *J Bacteriol* 166:479-483, 1986.
27. Lifeso RM: Pyogenic spinal sepsis in adults, *Spine* 15: 1265-1271, 1990.
28. Lowrance JH, Baadour LM, Simpson WA: The role of fibronectin binding in the rat model of experimental endocarditis caused by *Streptococcus sanguis, J Clin Invest* 86:7-13, 1990.
29. Mader JT, Adams KR: *Experimental osteomyelitis.* In Schlossberg D, editor: *Orthopaedic infection,* New York, 1988, Springer/Verlag, pp 39-48.
30. Mader JT, Adams KR, Morrison L: Comparative evaluation of cefazolin and clindamycin in the treatment of experimental *Staphylococcal aureus* osteomyelitis in rabbits, *Antimicrob Agent Chemother* 33:1760-1764, 1989.
31. Marrie TJ, Costerton JW: Mode of growth of bacterial pathogens in chronic polymicrobial human osteomyelitis, *J Clin Microbiol* 22:924-933, 1985.
32. McGuire RA, Eismont FJ: The fate of autogenous bone graft in surgically treated pyogenic vertebral osteomyelitis, *J Spinal Disord* 7:206-215, 1994.
33. Modic MT, Feiglin DH, Piraino DW, Boumphrey F, Weinstein MA, Duchesneau PM, Rehm S: Vertebral osteomyelitis: assessment using MRI, *Radiology* 159: 157-166, 1985.
34. Morrison DC, Ryan JL: Endotoxins and disease mechanisms, *Annu Rev Med* 38:417-432, 1987.
35. Norden CW: Experimental osteomyelitis. II. Therapeutic trials and measurements of antibiotic levels in bone, *J Infect Dis* 124:565-567, 1971.
36. Norden CW: Experimental osteomyelitis. III. Treatment with cephaloridine, *J Infect Dis* 127:525-528, 1973.
37. O'Brien JP: Kyphosis secondary to infectious disease, *Clin Orthop* 128:56-64, 1977.
38. Perronne C, Saba J, Behloul Z, Salmon-Ceron D, Vilde JL, Kahn MF: Pyogenic and tuberculosis spondylodiscitis (vertebral osteomyelitis) in 80 adult patients, *Clin Infect Dis* 19:746-750, 1994.
39. Petty WP, Spanier S, Shuster JJ, Silverthorne C: The influence of skeletal implants on incidence of infection: experiments in a canine model, *J Bone Joint Surg* 67A(8):1236-1244, 1985.
40. Ratcliffe JF: Anatomic basis for the pathogenesis and radiological features of vertebral osteomyelitis and its differentiation from childhood discitis. A microarteriographic investigation, *Acta Radiol Diagn Stockh* 26:137-143, 1985.
41. Rice PA, Iglewski BH: The cell envelope of gram-negative bacteria. Structure and function. Summary of session, *Rev Infect Dis* 105:5277-5278, 1988.
42. Richards RR, McKee MD, Paitich CB, Anderson GI, Bertoia JT: A comparison of the effects of skin coverage and muscle flap coverage on the early strength of union at the site of osteotomy after devascularization of a segment of canine tibia, *J Bone Joint Surg Am* 73(9):1323-1330, 1991.
43. Rigamonti D, Liem L, Wolf AL, Fiandaca MS, Numaguchi Y, Hsu FP, Nussbaum ES: Epidural abscess in the cervical spine, *Mt Sinai J Med* 61(4): 357-362, 1994.
44. Ritter MA: Surgical wound environment, *Clin Orthop* 190:11-13, 1984.
45. Schaberg DR, Zervos M: Plasmid analysis in the study of the epidemiology of nosocomial gram positive cocci, *Rev Infect Dis* 8:705-712, 1986.
46. Silverthorn KG, Gillespie WJ: Pyogenic spinal osteomyelitis: a review of 61 cases. *N Z Med J* 99:62-65, 1986.
47. Smith AS, Blaser SI: Infections and inflammatory processes of the spine, *Radiol Clin North Am* 29:809-827, 1991.
48. Spencer JD: Bone and joint infection in a renal unit, *J Bone Joint Surg* 68B(3):489-493, 1986.
49. Waldvogel FA, Medhoff MD, Swartz MN: Osteomyelitis: a review of clinical features, therapeutic considerations and unusual aspects (first of three parts), *New Engl J Med* 282:198-206, 1970.
50. Waldvogel FA, Vasey H: Osteomyelitis: the past decade, *New Engl J Med* 303:360-370, 1980.
51. Wenger DR, Bobechko WP, Gilday DL: The spectrum of intervertebral disc-space infection in children, *J Bone Joint Surg* 60A(1):100-108, 1978.
52. Whalen JL, Brown ML, McLeod R, Fitzgerald RH: Limitations of leukocyte imaging for the diagnosis of spine infection, *Spine* 16:193-197, 1991.
53. Wiley AM, Truetta J: The vascular anatomy of the spine and its relationship to pyogenic vertebral osteomyelitis, *J Bone Joint Surg* 41B(4):796-809, 1959.

# 55

# SURGICAL TREATMENT OF THE COMPLICATIONS OF TUBERCULOSIS SPONDYLITIS

**Emre R. Acaroglu, M.D.**



Tuberculosis of the spinal column constitutes up to 50% of the cases with skeletal involvement. The most frequent location is the thoracic spine (50%), followed by the lumbar (40%) and the cervical spine (10%).[40] Sacral disease is usually associated with involvement of the lower lumbar spine.[33] Three forms of vertebral involvement have been described: peridiscal, central, and anterior.[6] Two-thirds of the classifiable cases present with peridiscal involvement, while in more than 50% of the cases the primary focus can not be determined because of the extension of the disease. Progression of vertebral disease is usually by direct subperiosteal or subligamentous spread. Prior to the era of antibiotics and improvements in general health, multisegmental involvement was thought to be the norm, usually diagnosed at autopsy, but today involvement of more than one noncontiguous region of the spine is very rare. The true incidence of primary posterior involvement is virtually unknown, however, the introduction of computed tomography (CT) and magnetic resonance imaging (MRI) have probably increased the rate of identifiable cases to up to 10% of the cases with extensive disease.[3,37]

Surgery in tuberculosis spondylitis is generally considered to be an adjuvant of effective chemotherapy. Indications for surgical treatment include: (1) neurologic involvement, (2) deformity and/or impending increase in deformity, and (3) the presence of large tuberculosis abscess and/or abundant necrotic tissue.

## NEUROLOGIC INVOLVEMENT

The prognosis associated with and the treatment of neurologic involvement in tuberculosis spondylitis are influenced by many factors such as the age and general medical condition of the patient, the location of the involved vertebrae, drug resistance, the severity of neurologic deficit, the cause and mechanism of the neurologic deficit, and the time of onset and duration of symptoms.[5,12,27] Paralysis occurring in children generally has a better prognosis compared with adults.[5] Deficits arising from cervical or high thoracic involvement are associated with a dismal prognosis.[17] Overall good response to chemotherapy carries a higher likelihood of improvement. Severe involvement (Fränkel grades A or B) has a bad prognosis and probably constitutes an indication for urgent decompression.[17] Several mechanisms for the occurrence of neurologic involvement have been described. During the early phases of the disease with active infection, possible reasons include direct compression of the neural structures by the abscess and/or sequestrated bone fragments, direct dural invasion, vascular compromise due to compression or thrombosis, acute instability, or severe deformity. Direct compression by abscess or necrotic tissue is the most frequent cause of early onset paralysis and generally has a good prognosis and a relatively high probability to resolve with effective treatment.[27] Deficits due to cord compression by sequestrated bone fragments or at the apex of the kyphotic deformity require surgical decompression and the prognosis depends on the duration and severity of the paralysis. Acute instability of the involved segments may rarely cause subluxation or dislocation and subsequent paralysis that is best addressed by immediate surgical stabilization.[5,19,37] Direct dural invasion and vascular thrombosis are very rare and probably carry the worst prognosis.[37] The mechanisms involved in late-onset paralysis are the development of anterior bony ridges, disease reactivation, chronic instability, increase in kyphotic deformity, and, rarely, degenerative changes adjacent to the segments healed with significant deformity.[18] Patients with active disease have been reported to respond well to surgical decompression; however, in cases with healed disease, decompressive surgery appears to be more prone to complications and is less reliable.[13]

Several approaches have been used for the treatment of paralysis due to tuberculosis spondylitis. These include chemotherapy alone, chemotherapy with immobilization (ambulatory or nonambulatory), chemotherapy with surgery, laminectomy, costotransversectomy, and anterior decompression.

Early Medical Research Council (MRC) studies focused on the treatment of tuberculosis spondylitis with nonsurgical measures regardless of the neurological status. In the first MRC report, 10 patients with neurologic involvement were included in the study.[20] During the course of treatment, five (50%) of these deteriorated to complete paraplegia, but returned to their original status within 5 months. Finally, eight of the original ten patients had complete resolution of their paralysis. In the fifth report, which also includes the group of patients studied in the first report, a total of 32 patients had paraparesis at some stage of the treatment, 20 of whom had complete resolution at the end of the 18-month treatment protocol, 8 required additional chemotherapy and/or surgery but at the end had complete resolution, 3 died, and 1 still had neurologic involvement on final evaluation at five years.[23] On the other hand, Tuli reported significant improvement in only 38.5% of patients treated by chemotherapy alone, compared to 69% full and 11% partial recovery in patients who had surgical treatment.[38]

Laminectomy probably has a very limited role in the decompression of the spinal canal. Patients with posterior element involvement should undergo laminectomy provided that surgical intervention is indicated, but apart from these, it should not be used in the majority of patients with anterior column involvement and collapse because of the additional instability caused by the procedure. Costotransversectomy was advocated as the treatment of choice for the evacuation of large paravertebral abscesses and decompression of the spinal canal before the anterior procedures were proven to be safe and effective.[45] The only advantage over anterior debridement is that the dissection plane is usually extrapleural obviating the need for the placement of a chest tube and underwater drainage in the postoperative period. Disadvantages on the other hand include often inadequate visualization of the pathology and less-than-ideal decompression, further destabilization of a kyphotic segment, inadequate (if any) correction of deformity, and the technical difficulties associated with the procedure. Based on a series of patients decompressed by costotransversectomies or anterolateral or posterolateral decompressions, Martin reported 60% recovery, while only a minority of the patients in this series had also received chemotherapy.[19]

The gold standard of decompressive surgery for Pott's paralysis appears to be the anterior procedures. Anterior procedures were first demonstrated to be safe and effective by Hodgson and coworkers and have been used for the treatment of a wide array of spinal disorders since then. Hodgson and coworkers treated 100 cases of Pott's paraplegia by either conservative inpatient immobilization or anterior decompression.[12] They reported a 74% complete recovery and an additional 10% incomplete recovery, but did not compare the two methods based on the rate of recovery. Lifeso and coworkers reported the results of 65 patients with neurologic deficits, 94% of whom had improvement with surgical decompression compared to a 79% recovery rate by chemotherapy alone and 55% after laminectomy.[17] Conversely, in a population of 63 adults and children with neurologic involvement, Moula et al divided the patients arbitrarily into conservative and surgery groups and demonstrated that the conservatively treated group had 68% complete and 19% partial recovery, compared to 38% complete and 31% partial recovery in patients treated by additional anterior decompression and grafting.[31] Mortality in the group that only had medical treatment was 5% in contrast with the 23% after surgery. My clinic's experience consists of 33 patients who were followed for an average period of 4 years, with paralysis that was Fränkel A in 1, Fränkel B in 2, and Fränkel C or D in 30, seen over a period of 15 years.[2,36] These patients were treated by either chemotherapy alone, posterior fusion, or anterior debridement and fusion; all were mobilized with external support. All patients received chemotherapy for at least two weeks prior to surgery, and all were immobilized with the use of Halter traction during this period. Seventy-five percent of the patients were found to have had complete resolution, and 19% had partial improvement in their neurologic status at final follow-up, regardless of the type of treatment used. The two patients who had no improvement were both treated surgically (1 in the posterior fusion [PF] group and the other in the anterior fusion [AF] group). The patient with Fränkel grade A involvement was found to have significant improvement (to grade D) with anterior surgery. Of the two grade B patients, one had a minor improvement to grade C, while the other deteriorated to grade A.

Results of anterior decompressive surgery in nonselected groups of patients with paralysis have been analyzed in several reports. Bailey and coworkers reported the results of 43 children with neurologic involvement who were treated with the procedure described by Hodgson.[5] Nineteen of the 23 (82.6%) patients with incomplete paralysis had total recovery within 12 months of the operation, and 3 others were independent walkers. For paraplegics, the total recovery rate was 85% (17 of 20) achieved at periods ranging from 2 to 36 months. In another study conducted on 200 patients with neurologic lesions, Vidyasagar and Murty reported 70% complete and 15% incomplete recovery using various decompressive procedures.[43] These authors strongly recommended surgical treatment for all patients with paralysis based on the relative uncertainty they have experienced in arriving at a definite diagnosis of tuberculosis spondylitis as the cause of neurologic involvement. The seventh report of the MRC, based on a study conducted in two centers in South Africa, includes the neurologic recovery rates of patients treated with anterior debridement or anterior debridement and fusion.[25] Mortality in patients with paralysis was 14%. Paraplegics were found to have responded less favorably in terms of recovery compared to paraparetics on analyses performed at 6 and 18 months, but results of both groups were similar at 21 months (72% and 69%, respectively).

The definition of late-onset neurologic involvement is not quite clear. In most of the reports dealing with paralysis associated with tuberculosis spondylitis, the duration of neurologic symptoms have been extremely variable, ranging from a few months to years. What I understand by late onset neurologic involvement is the paralysis that had developed after the active infection has subsided and bone and soft tissue pathology have healed. Possible causes can be listed as the development of anterior bony ridges, disease reactivation, chronic instability, increase in kyphotic deformity and rarely degenerative changes adjacent to the segments that healed with significant deformity.[18] Hsu and coworkers reported their experience with 22 patients with late-onset paraplegia presenting an average of 18 years after initial symptoms.[13] The cause of paralysis was disease reactivation in 14 and healed hard bony ridges in 8 patients. They have concluded that the results after anterior decompressive surgery were favorable in the disease reactivation group (9 complete and 3 partial recoveries), however, the operation was less effective (3 complete recoveries and 1 partial recovery) and more complicated if the paralysis was caused by hard bony ridges. My experience with late-onset Pott's paraplegia is similar and I can say that decompression of the spinal cord in the presence of rigid bony deformity may be prone to severe complications, and deterioration of neurologic status of the patients.[2,36]

As a conclusion for the treatment of neurologic involvement due to tuberculosis spondylitis, it can only be said that all patients with this disorder would not fit into one ideal treatment scheme, and the decision should be based upon the consideration of several factors, most important of which are probably the severity and duration of the paralysis and the exact cause of the neural compression.

## ABSCESS

The necessity of surgical treatment for the evacuation of paravertebral "cold" abscesses and/or debridement of necrotic tissue is as controversial as any other subject in the treatment of tuberculosis spondylitis. The first report of the MRC gives a detailed analysis of the course of mediastinal or psoas abscesses in a group of patients who did not receive any surgical treatment.[20] Seventy-six percent of inpatients and 72% of outpatients had clinically or radiologically evident abscesses or draining sinuses, or one developed during the course of medical treatment. On final evaluation at 3 years, 11% of inpatients and 5% outpatients still had residual abscesses or sinuses. On a further study, disappearance of the clinically or radiologically evident abscesses was reported in 100% of patients treated by chemotherapy alone, debridement, or anterior spinal fusion.[23] Moon et al have reported favorable results with conservative treatment in children and concluded that surgical drainage of a cold abscess is not required and should not be recommended.[28] In my experience, however, 89 out of 100 patients retrospectively evaluated had cold abscesses at presentation, and nine of these developed actively draining sinuses, five of which persisted longer than one year. Of interest, only one of these nine patients had been treated by anterior debridement and fusion (1 in 33), the rest by posterior fusion without evacuation of the abscess (8 in 56), but the difference was not statistically significant. The no-drainage patients were observed to require a longer period of chemotherapy.[36] Thus, I still think that the presence of a large paravertebral abscess constitutes a relative indication for surgery. Several other methods of abscess drainage including costotransversectomy, anterior extrapleural approach, and transpedicular drainage have been recommended in several reports, without any demonstrated advantages over anterior drainage or debridement.[8,15,45]

## DEFORMITY

The term deformity generally depicts kyphosis in tuberculous spondylitis. The anterior spinal column is most frequently involved, and the natural history of the disease is that of progressive bone loss, resulting in the collapse of the involved segments. The resulting deformity carries an intrinsic instability and tends to progress in a manner directly related to the amount of bony destruction, independent of the activity of the infection.[34] This concept of instability is different from the classical definitions based on spinal functional units, and is more like the instability involved in the development of late deformity following thoracolumbar fractures.[7,44] The natural end result in the surviving patient is expected to be the healing of the infection with bony and/or fibrous union of the involved segments regardless of the type of treatment used.

Kyphosis is generally classified into two types based on the flexibility.[30] The mobile type is usually that seen with active disease, or before the complete healing of the lesion, and becomes rigid after bony or fibrous union. Therefore, I prefer to classify deformity due to spinal tuberculosis into two types, early deformity and late deformity, based on the activity of the disease. Early deformity is associated with active disease and tends to be relatively flexible, and late deformity occurs after the active infection has healed by fibrous or bony union. Several procedures have been proposed for the management of either type of deformity. A list of the procedures and an overview of the advantages and disadvantages of each procedure is cited in Box 55-1.

**Box 55-1. Advantages and Disadvantages of Each Procedure for the Management of Deformities**

A. Early deformity
- Posterior fusion
- Anterior debridement
- Anterior debridement and fusion
- Posterior fusion and instrumentation
- Posterior fusion and instrumentation with anterior fusion

B. Late deformity
- Anterior osteotomy and fusion with strut grafting
- Eggshell procedure
- Posterior fusion and instrumentation with anterior fusion
- Anterior osteotomy, halo traction, posterior osteotomy and fusion followed by anterior fusion (three-stage procedure)
- Simultaneous anterior and posterior osteotomies and fusion

## POSTERIOR FUSION

Posterior fusion had been the standard surgical procedure for the limited correction and prevention of progression of deformity in many centers, before the safe and liberal use of anterior spinal surgery became feasible. The rationale behind this procedure are: (a) stabilization of the spinal column once the fusion is achieved, preventing the progression of the deformity; (b) enhancing the rate of healing of the infection by obtaining a stable spinal segment; and (c) obtaining a posterior epiphysiodesis so as to counter the deforming effect of the loss of anterior growth potential. My experience with this procedure has so far been disappointing. On a review of 56 patients who had undergone posterior fusion, 14 patients were found to have completed the treatment with severe deformity (local kyphosis exceeding 50 degrees) despite prolonged periods of immobilization with plaster of Paris jackets.[2,36] I saw that pseudarthrosis was very common especially in the group of patients who were already severely kyphotic, and even if fusion could be achieved, bending of the fusion mass resulted in progression of the deformity in several patients.[2] Furthermore, the overall healing of the infection was not more rapid compared to those who did not have any surgical treatment. Other reports in the literature support these findings.[42] Moreover, evidence confirming the role of unopposed posterior spinal growth in the progression of kyphosis appears not to be conclusive.

## ANTERIOR DEBRIDEMENT

Anterior debridement without fusion in the treatment of spinal tuberculosis has been evaluated in MRC studies performed in Hong Kong and Bulawayo.[21,22] The results of these studies demonstrated that the magnitude and the rate of progression of the kyphotic deformity were similar in patients who had no surgery and those who had anterior debridement without fusion, and were significantly inferior compared to anterior debridement and fusion. Longitudinal follow-up of the same group of patients revealed that bony fusion occurred later in those who had anterior grafting compared to only debridement, but the rates of fusion were similar at 5 years.[24] Over 10 years, debridement patients exhibited mean increases in kyphosis of 9.8 degrees for thoracic and thoracolumbar lesions and 7.6 degrees for lumbar lesions, compared to minor changes in the fusion group.[26] Upadhyay and coworkers reported the latest follow-up of the same group of patients, concluding that the debridement patients demonstrated increases in kyphotic deformity for up to six months. Adult patients then demonstrated an arrest in progression, while some spontaneous correction of the deformity occurred in the pediatric patients.[39-42]

## ANTERIOR DEBRIDEMENT AND FUSION

Anterior debridement and fusion for the treatment of tuberculosis spondylitis (Hong Kong operation) was popularized by Hodgson et al in 1960.[11] Since then it has been tested against other treatment modalities by several studies. The MRC trials demonstrated that an increase in kyphotic deformity occurred in only 17% of patients treated with this procedure compared to 39% of patients treated with chemotherapy, and compared to patients treated with anterior debridement alone, the progression of the kyphotic deformity was considerably less with the Hong Kong procedure, especially during the first six months of the treatment.[21,22,24,26] As mentioned above, kyphotic deformity did not significantly increase in these patients regardless of the treatment method after six months. Rajasekaran and Soundarapandian retrospectively analyzed 81 patients treated by anterior arthrodesis.[35] Fifty-nine percent of their patients had favorable results (excellent or good), 19% were rated as fair, and 22% as poor. Favorable results were obtained in patients (1) who had minimum destruction of vertebral bodies, (2) required limited surgical excision of bone resulting in a small postdebridement defect that needed only a short graft, (3) with marked intraoperative correction of the deformity, and (4) in those with lumbar spine disease. The amount of intraoperative correction of the deformity is usually not included in the analysis of other studies, and generally appears to be negligible.

Graft material has been pointed out as being one of the most important factors governing a favorable outcome in several other studies as well. Hodgson and Stock reported problems associated with graft failure in 12% of their cases.[11] Bailey et al reported the same incidence for graft fracture in a series of 100 children, and slippage of the graft in further 5 patients.[5] Seventy-four patients exhibited some increase in their kyphotic deformity in this series (average 22.2 degrees). Progression was associated with graft slippage in 5, protrusion of the grafts into adjacent vertebral bodies in 9, graft fracture in 10, resorption and shortening of the grafts in 40, and posterior overgrowth of the fusion mass in only 5 cases. Rajasekaran and Soundarapandian reported graft slippage in 24%, resorption in 20%, and fracture in 12% of their cases.[34,35] Rib grafts were used in the majority of these patients, and were demonstrated to be unable to prevent vertebral collapse in patients in whom the length of the graft exceeded two disk spaces. The use of tricortical iliac crest grafts appears to yield better results compared to rib grafts. Kemp and coworkers reported 32% graft fractures using rib grafts resulting in a significant increase in the deformity.[14] The overall fusion rates were 62% for rib grafts and 94.5% for iliac crest grafts in their series. On the other hand, Yazici and coworkers demonstrated a limited rate of graft incorporation and secondary remodeling using MRI in a series of patients who had undergone anterior fusion with tricortical iliac crest grafts at 2-years' follow-up, although the preservation of the correction of deformities in this series was very good.[48]

The use of anterior instrumentation supplementing the strut graft has been performed on a limited number of series. Oga et al evaluated the adherence properties of mycobacterium tuberculosis to stainless steel and demonstrated that adherence was negligible, and the use of implants in regions with active tuberculosis infection may be safe.[32] Kostuik reported his experience on cases with healed or inactive disease.[16] Anterior plate fixation, along with debridement and fusion of the active disease, has been used for a very limited number of patients with active disease.[4] Addition of the implant does not seem to increase the overall correction, and whether it is going to be effective in decreasing the graft related complications is yet to be seen. Nevertheless, a very limited number of cases in whom posterior instrumentation may not be advisable because of complications of previous posterior surgery appear to be suitable for anterior instrumentation along with a complete debridement and strut grafting (Fig. 55-1).

## POSTERIOR FUSION AND INSTRUMENTATION

The necessity of prolonged immobilization following anterior procedures, and the relatively high rates of progression of kyphosis frequently related to the problems with strut grafts prompted the idea that tuberculosis spondylitis may be stabilized by posterior instrumentation. Oga and coworkers reported their experience with this method in a series consisting of 11 patients, 4 of whom had only posterior surgery. Their indication for the use of posterior instrumentation alone was basically posterior element involvement. Good clinical results were reported but the instrumentation was extended to an alarming average of 8.5 levels, in spite of the fact that 3.5 levels on average were involved by the disease.[32] Güven et al reported their experience on the treatment of anterior column tuberculosis with posterior instrumentation and fusion on a series of 10 patients.[8] Pedicle screws were used in the majority of cases, and the paravertebral abscesses were drained transpedicularly in two cases. Some kyphosis correction could be obtained in only five cases, however the instrumentation appeared to be effective in preventing the progression of the deformity. Short-segment fixation was pointed out as a risk

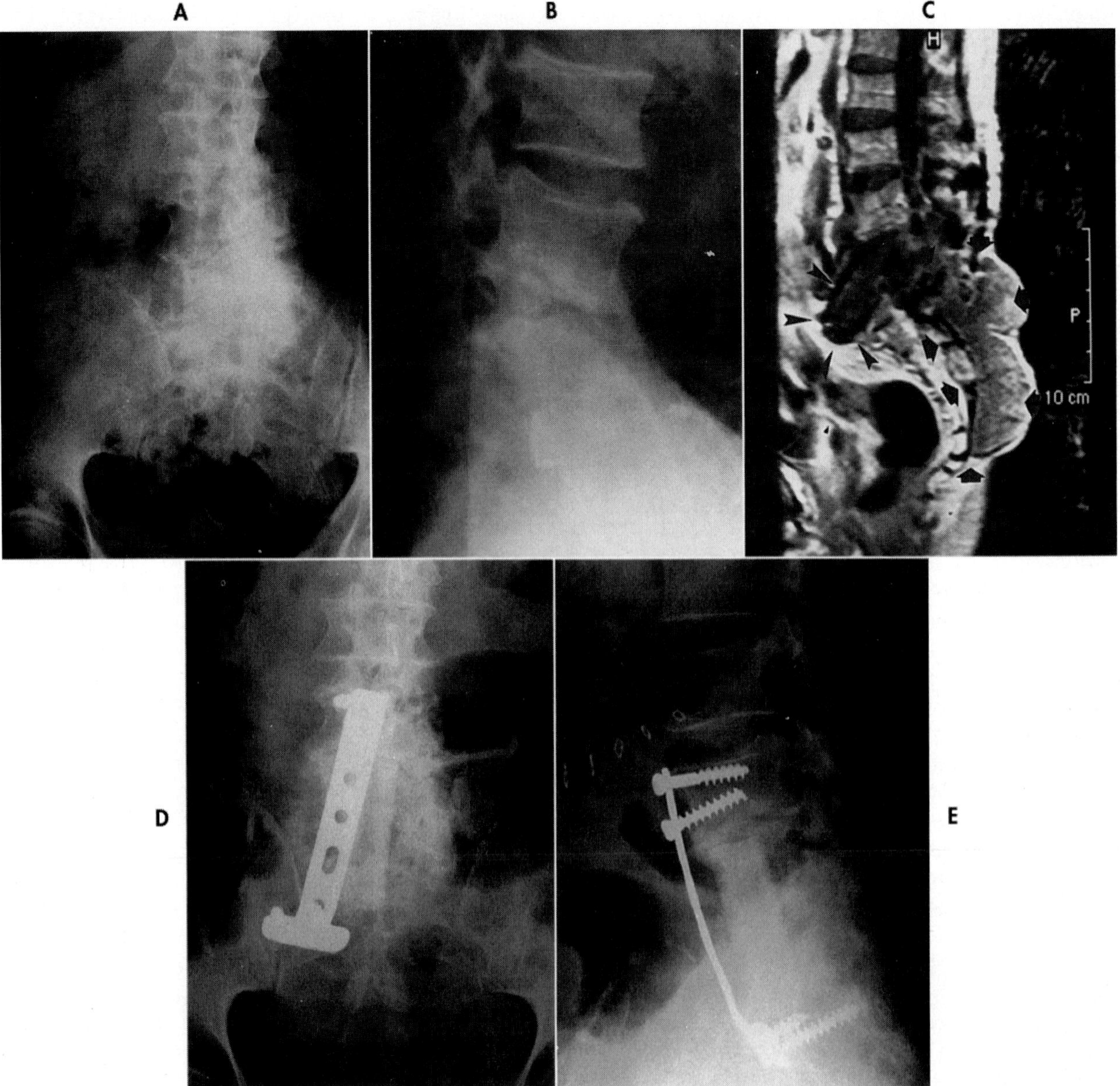


**FIGURE 55-1**

A 54-year-old man who had four previous operations (two posterior and two anterior transperitoneal) for tuberculosis spondylitis at the lumbosacral junction. At presentation he had not been sitting or standing for the last three months because of incapacitating low back pain and had complete bilateral L5 and S1 paralysis, along with a large pseudomeningocele located at the lower lumbar area. AP **(A)** and lateral **(B)** x-rays demonstrate complete destruction of the L5 body. Magnetic resonance imaging **(C)** further revealed a dislocated tricortical graft in place of the L5 body (*small arrows*) and the large pseudomeningocele extending to the laminectomy defect at L5 (*large arrows*). As further posterior surgery so as to stabilize this segment was deemed not possible, anterior debridement and decompression along with a L4 to S1 anterior fusion using a tibial allograft and spongious autograft chips with internal fixation was performed. Early postoperative AP **(D)** and lateral **(E)** x-rays illustrate a marked decrease of segmental kyphosis despite the slight misplacement of the internal fixation material.

factor for losses of correction. The long-term results of this approach have not been reported to date. It appears that posterior instrumentation prevents the increases in kyphosis that were usually encountered during the first six months of this treatment, but the problems frequently reported in series of posterior instrumentation and fusion in fractures devoid of any anterior column support may raise some concern.

## ANTERIOR AND POSTERIOR FUSION WITH POSTERIOR INSTRUMENTATION

Both Oga et al and Moon et al have reported satisfactory results using anterior and posterior fusion with posterior instrumentation.[29,32] Both advised performing the posterior surgery first, followed by the anterior debridement and fusion either sequentially, or after a period of a couple of weeks. Moon et al reported very good rates of correction and good maintenance of correction for both children and adults, fusion occurred in four months in single-level spondylodesis cases and in six months in two levels.[29] I have performed a similar procedure executing the anterior stage first, followed by posterior fusion and instrumentation, never sequentially, for patients in whom anterior column destruction exceeded two disk spaces. For this sequence, the amount of correction is limited to that obtained in the anterior fusion. I believe this method to be superior in safety especially in patients with incomplete paralysis due to active disease as spinal cord decompression is carried out directly as the primary stage.

## LATE DEFORMITY

Indications for surgical approaches aiming the correction of deformity after the active disease has completely healed are less clear and somewhat controversial. In my belief, this clinical entity is profoundly different compared to the deformity with active disease, and much more complex. In many instances it may be considered as being a similar problem with a kyphotic deformity following a fracture malunion, but the ligaments and soft tissues are far more contracted, the anatomic planes may be nonexistent because of fibrosis, and furthermore, several vertebral levels may be involved. Staged operations are usually required and the functional cosmetic end results have so far not been uniformly good.

Kostuik reported favorable results with anterior osteotomy, decompression and fusion with instrumentation in a large series of patients with various diagnoses.[16] In only two cases the deformity was related to healed tuberculous spondylitis, but, nevertheless he concluded that supplementary posterior fixation was not necessary except for those cases with more than single level involvement.

The eggshell procedure as devised by Heinig consists of the decancellation of the body of the deformed vertebra via a transpedicular route.[10] The posterior wall is then fractured and pushed anteriorly while the kyphotic deformity is corrected, under direct vision obtained by complete laminectomy of that level. Güven and coworkers reported their experience with this method in the treatment of kyphosis due to tuberculosis.[9] The average correction obtained in three patients was 53 degrees, and no major complications were encountered.

Three-stage operations have been advocated for the treatment of rigid severe kyphosis. Yau and coworkers reported the results of a combination of spinal osteotomy, halopelvic traction, and anterior and posterior fusion performed on 23 patients with severe kyphosis.[46] Deformity correction in this series averaged 28.3% in spite of the fact that all patients had undergone at least three major operations. Eleven of the 23 patients were reported to have severe restrictions in their vital capacities, leading to a mortality rate of 10%. Although several other studies that include some patients treated with three-stage operations reported more favorable results, the correction rates appear to be similar to those obtained with two-stage operations.

An alternative for the three-stage operation is the simultaneous anterior-posterior approach as defined by Farcy et al.[7,44] This operation consists of the simultaneous exposure of both the anterior and the posterior elements of the involved segments by two separate surgical teams. In this way, the anterior and posterior osteotomies can be performed at the same time, not only totally mobilizing the segment, but also allowing the surgeons to effectively shorten the posterior column prior to the application of any distractive force to the anterior column, thereby decreasing the risk of overall lengthening of the deformed segment. Very favorable results have been reported in the treatment of late kyphotic deformity following thoracolumbar fractures by the original authors.[1] My experience with this technique has been as favorable when performed for the same indication, although being slightly disappointing in cases of kyphosis due to tuberculosis spondylitis.[47] The average preoperative sagittal index was 45 degrees in this series, the cases of tuberculosis kyphosis being significantly more severe compared to those of fracture complications, average sagittal indexes being 79.5 and 27.75 degrees, respectively. The trauma group could be corrected to an average sagittal index of 2.5 degrees (91% correction), while in the tuberculosis group the average final sagittal index was 35 degrees (56% correction) due to the severe fibrosis and contracture of ligaments encountered. Average blood loss and the duration of surgery were similar for both groups (Fig. 55-2).

It therefore appears that an ideal treatment for late deformity following tuberculosis spondylitis does not exist. The approach to this difficult problem should be tailored according to the expectations of the patients as well as the experience and the ability of the involved medical center.

## AUTHOR'S PREFERRED TREATMENT

The indications for operative treatment in patients with active disease are:

1. Failure to establish a definitive diagnosis by nonsurgical methods
2. Fränkel grades A or B neurologic involvement
3. Failure of conservative measures (chemotherapy and strict bed rest for adults, halter traction is added to this regimen in children) to completely restore neurologic function in Fränkel grade C or D patients
4. Presence of a large paravertebral abscess

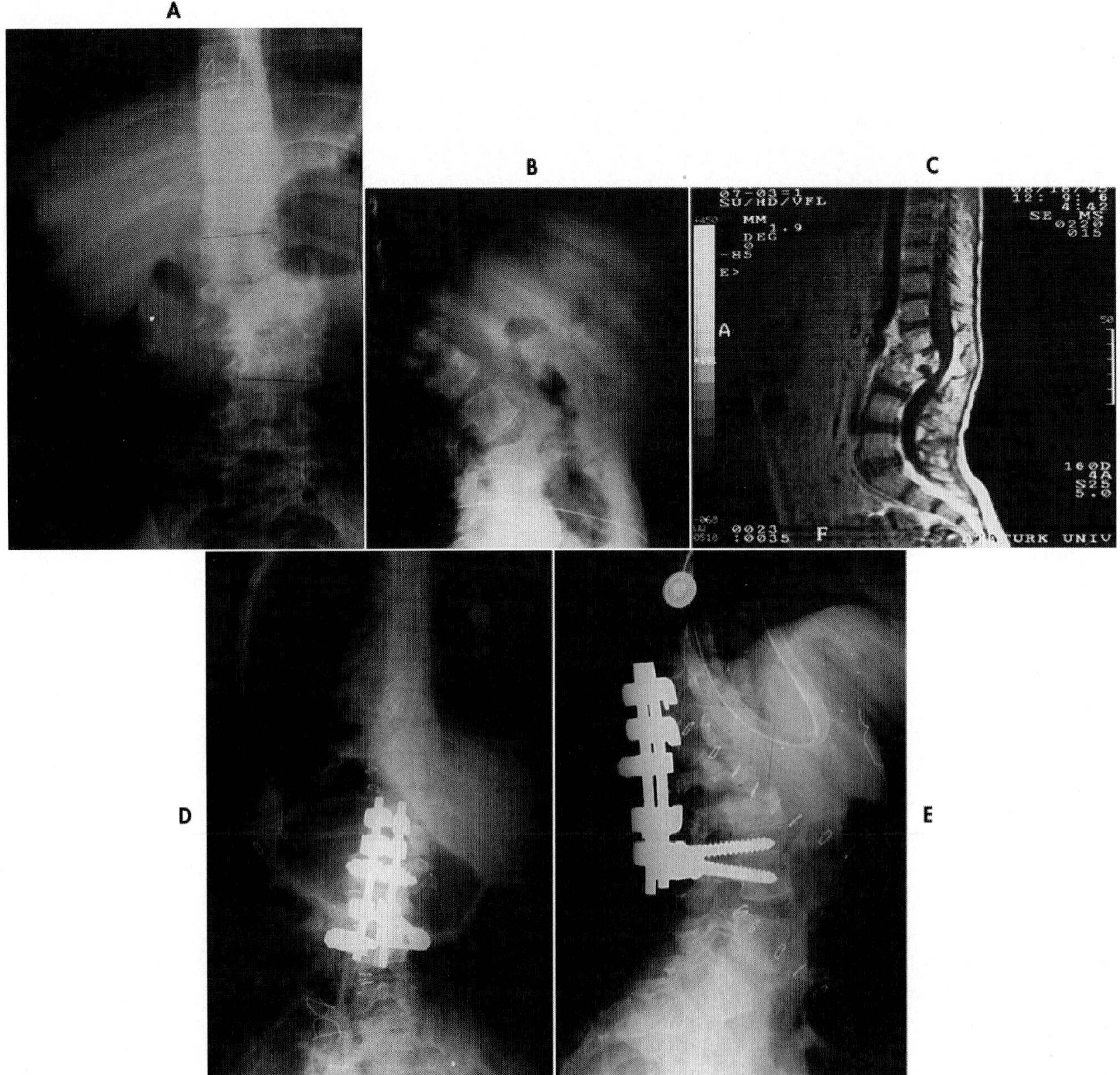

FIGURE 55-2

A 9-year-old girl referred because of severe kyphosis located at the thoracolumbar area that had developed during the previous year as the patient received chemotherapy for tuberculosis spondylitis. Pain and neurological symptoms were absent. AP **(A)** and lateral **(B)** x-rays demonstrate the presence of a significant translation in the frontal plane (L1 over L2) and a severe kyphosis. The problem is further delineated on MRI **(C)** as the almost complete destruction of L2 that causes encroachment of the spinal canal. This deformity could be corrected with reasonable safety using a simultaneous anterior-posterior approach, utilizing a tricortical iliac crest anteriorly and rigid posterior instrumentation. Early postoperative AP **(D)** and lateral **(E)** x-rays show good correction of the frontal translation as well as the kyphotic deformity. Some residual translation in the sagittal plane still remains and may be a matter of concern in the long term follow-up of this patient.

5. Kyphotic deformity with sagittal index exceeding 15 degrees, or destruction of more than 50% of one vertebral body impending an increase in deformity
6. Multilevel involvement

Surgery is always aimed at the site of involvement, anterior for the majority of cases. A complete decompression of the spinal cord can thus be achieved, followed by anterior fusion using strut grafts. Rib grafts have been associated with a high incidence of graft related complications, so tricortical iliac grafts are preferred. I have limited, but so far favorable, experience with the use of fibular or femoral allografts. A second-stage posterior fusion is then performed in cases in which the lesion extended more than two disk levels.

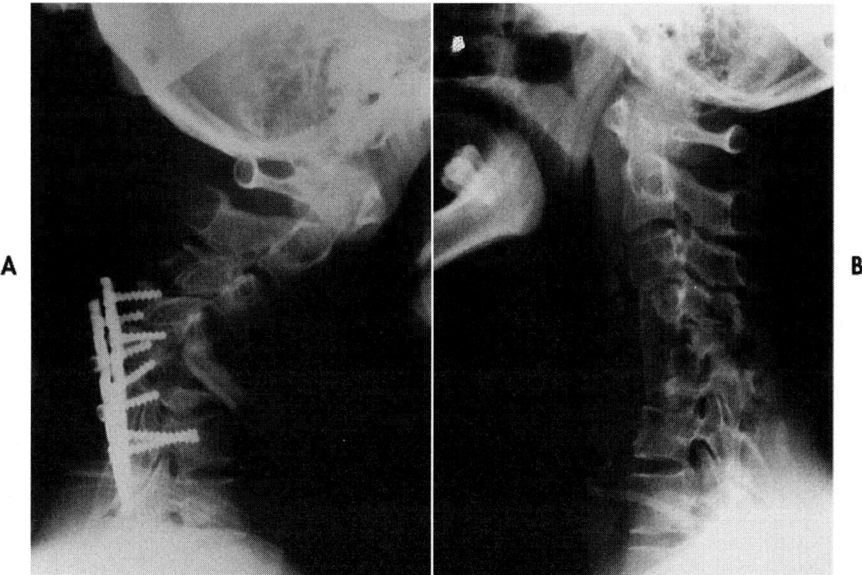


**FIGURE 55-3**

A 34-year-old woman referred for marked cervical kyphosis and spastic quadriparesis that had developed over a period of six months. She had undergone several anterior debridements for tuberculosis spondylitis at the cervical spine, and finally staged anterior and posterior surgical stabilization had been performed eleven months prior to the onset of her latest symptoms. Her lateral x-ray **(A)** at presentation reveals a dislodged anterior graft and failed posterior lateral mass fixation resulting in severe kyphosis. This deformity failed to exhibit any flexibility even under halo traction, so a two-stage operation, consisting of hardware removal and multilevel osteotomies from posterior followed by anterior decompression and fusion with a tricortical iliac crest graft was performed. Her follow-up lateral x-ray **(B)** shows good correction of kyphosis. Her neurological status was found to have improved from Fränkel grade C to grade E at 6-month follow-up.

I recommend the use of internal fixation in adults undergoing posterior fusion, but not so for the pediatric population because the results of uninstrumented anterior-posterior fusions have so far been very good. Finally, I do not recommend the use of posterior fusion and instrumentation alone for anterior column disease until the relatively late results in patients treated with this modality are known.

For the patients with predominantly posteriorly located diseases, the approach should be posterior. I do not have adequate experience with this group of patients so as to suggest indications for posterior fusion or instrumentation. In the limited number of cases I have operated my indications were based on the extent of the laminectomy defect produced by the disease or the surgeon.

For late deformities, one of the major problems confronting the surgeon is the decision of whether to operate. I have so far adopted my indications as being a kyphotic deformity with a sagittal index exceeding 30 degrees and/or severe patient dissatisfaction due to the unsightly deformity or impairment of respiratory functions because of the deformity. The only absolute indication is late-onset paralysis. The type of surgical approach depends on the location of the deformity as well as the respiratory status of the patient. For most of the thoracic and lumbar lesions I prefer to use the simultaneous anterior-posterior approach, unless the general status of the patient indicates that the performance of a thoracotomy may be dangerous. In such cases, the eggshell procedure or other posterior osteotomies of the vertebral column can be performed. For high thoracic and cervical lesions, a simultaneous approach is not feasible, and a multistaged operation should be tailored according to the severity and the rigidity of the deformity (Fig. 55-3). My experience with high thoracic kyphosis due to tuberculosis has been less than satisfactory so far and I would recommend extreme caution in patient selection and avoidance of causing an even minor elongation of the bony vertebral column.

## REFERENCES

1. Acaroglu E, Schwab F, Farcy JPC, Weidenbaum M: Simultaneous anterior and posterior approach for correction of late deformity due to thoracolumbar fractures, *Eur J Spine* 5:56-62, 1996.
2. Aksoy MC, Acaroglu RE, Tokgözoglu AM, Özdemir N, Surat A: Retrospective evaluation of treatment methods in tuberculosis spondylitis, *Hacettepe J Orthop Surg* 5:207-209, 1995.
3. Arthornthurasook A, Chongpieboonpatana A: Spinal tuberculosis with posterior element involvement, *Spine* 15:191-194, 1990.
4. Aydin E, Solak S, Kis M, Gider M, Benli T, Yücesoy C: Pott's disease: retrospective evaluation of treatment results, *J Tur Spinal Surg* 5:166-169, 1994.
5. Bailey HL, Gabriel SM, Hodgson AR, Shin JS: Tuberculosis of the spine in children, *J Bone Joint Surg* 54A:1633-1657, 1972.
6. Doub HP, Badgley CE: The roentgen signs of tuberculosis of the vertebral body, *AJR Am J Roentgenol* 27:827-837, 1932.
7. Glasman SD, Farcy JPC: *Late deformities.* In Floman Y, Farcy JPC, Argenson C, editors: *Thoracolumbar spine fractures,* New York, 1993, Raven Press, pp 449-462.
8. Güven O, Kumano K, Yalçin S, Karahan M, Tsuji S: A single stage posterior approach and rigid fixation for preventing kyphosis in the treatment of spinal tuberculosis, *Spine* 19:1039-1043, 1994.
9. Güven O, Yalçin S, Karahan M; Egg shell procedure in correction of neglected cases of Pott's kyphosis. Trans ESDS 5th Biannual Conference, 84, 1994.
10. Heinig CF: *Eggshell procedure.* In Luque E, editor: *Segmental spinal instrumentation,* New Jersey, 1984, Slack, pp 221-234.
11. Hodgson AR, Stock FE: Anterior spine fusion for the treatment of tuberculosis of the spine. The operative findings and results of treatment in the first one hundred cases, *J Bone Joint Surg* 42A:295-310, 1960.
12. Hodgson AR, Yau A, Kwon JS, Kim D: A clinical study of 100 consecutive cases of Pott's paraplegia, *Clin Orthop* 36:128-150, 1964.
13. Hsu LC, Cheng CL, Leong JC: Pott's paraplegia of late onset: the cause of compression and results after anterior decompression, *J Bone Joint Surg* 70B:534-538, 1988.
14. Kemp HBS, Jackson JW, Jeremiah JD, Cook J: Anterior fusion of the spine for infective lesions in adults, *J Bone Joint Surg* 55B:715-734, 1973.
15. Korkusuz Z, Binnet MS, Isiklar ZU: Pott's disease and extrapleural anterior decompression, *Arch Orthop Trauma Surg* 108:349-352, 1989.
16. Kostuik JP: Anterior spinal cord decompression for lesions of the thoracic and lumbar spine: techniques, new methods of internal fixation, *Spine* 8:512-531, 1983.
17. Lifeso RM, Weaver P, Harder EH: Tuberculous spondylitis in adults, *J Bone Joint Surg* 67A:1405-1413, 1985.
18. Luk KDK, Krishna M: Spinal stenosis above a healed tuberculous kyphosis: a case report, *Spine* 21:1098-1101, 1996.
19. Martin NS: Pott's paraplegia. A report on 120 cases, *J Bone Joint Surg* 53B:596-608, 1971.
20. Medical Research Council Working Party on Tuberculosis of the Spine: A controlled trial of ambulant outpatient treatment and in-patient rest in bed in the management of tuberculosis of the spine in young Korean patients on standard chemotherapy: A study in Masan, Korea, *J Bone Joint Surg* 55B:678-697, 1973.
21. Medical Research Council Working Party on Tuberculosis of the Spine: A controlled trial of debridement and ambulatory treatment in the management of tuberculosis of the spine in patients on standard chemotherapy: A study in Bulawayo, Rhodesia, *J Trop Med Hyg* 77:72-92, 1974.
22. Medical Research Council Working Party on Tuberculosis of the Spine: A controlled trial of anterior spinal fusion and debridement in the surgical management of tuberculosis of the spine in patients on standard chemotherapy. A study in Hong Kong, *Br J Surg* 61: 853-866, 1974.
23. Medical Research Council Working Party on Tuberculosis of the Spine: A five-year assessment of controlled trials of in-patient and out-patient treatment and of plaster-of-Paris jackets for tuberculosis of the spine in children on standard chemotherapy: Studies in Masan and Pusan, Korea, *J Bone Joint Surg* 58B:399-411, 1976.
24. Medical Research Council Working Party on Tuberculosis of the Spine: Five-year assessments of controlled trials of ambulatory treatment, debridement and anterior spinal fusion in the management of tuberculosis of the spine: Studies in Bulawayo (Rhodesia) and in Hong Kong, *J Bone Joint Surg* 60B:163-177, 1978.
25. Medical Research Council Working Party on Tuberculosis of the Spine: A controlled trial of anterior spinal fusion and debridement in the surgical management of tuberculosis of the spine in patients on standard chemotherapy: a study in two centers in South Africa, *Tubercle* 59:79-105, 1978.
26. Medical Research Council Working Party on Tuberculosis of the Spine: A ten-year assessment of a controlled trial comparing debridement and anterior spinal fusion in the management of tuberculosis of the spine in patients on standard chemotherapy in Hong Kong, *J Bone Joint Surg* 64B:393-398, 1982.
27. Moon MS, Ha KY, Sun DH, Moon JL, Moon YW, Chung JH: Pott's paraplegia: 67 cases, *Clin Orthop* 323: 122-128, 1996.
28. Moon MS, Kim I, Woo YK, Park YO: Conservative treatment of tuberculosis of the thoracic and lumbar spine in adults and children, *Int Orthop* 11:315-322, 1987.
29. Moon MS, Woo YK, Lee KS, Ha KY, Kim SS, Sun DH: Posterior instrumentation and anterior interbody

fusion for tuberculosis kyphosis of dorsal and lumbar spines, *Spine* 20:1910-1916, 1995.

30. Moon MS; Spine update: Tuberculosis of the spine, Controversies and a new challenge, *Spine* 22:1791-1797, 1997.
31. Moula T, Fowles JV, Kassab MT, Sliman N: Pott's paraplegia: A clinical review of operative and conservative treatment in 63 adults and children, *Int Orthop* 5:23-29, 1981.
32. Oga M, Arizono T, Takasita M, Sugioka Y; Evaluation of the risk of instrumentation as a foreign body in spinal tuberculosis: clinical and biologic study, *Spine* 18:1890-1894, 1993.
33. Pun WK, Chow SP, Luk KD, Cheng CL, Hsu LC, Leong JC: Tuberculosis of the lumbosacral junction. Long term follow-up of 26 cases, *J Bone Joint Surg* 72B:675-678, 1990.
34. Rajasekaran S, Shanmugasundaram TK: Prediction of the angle of gibbus deformity on tuberculosis of the spine, *J Bone Joint Surg* 69A:503-509, 1987.
35. Rajasekaran S, Soundarapandian S: Progression of kyphosis in tuberculosis of the spine treated by anterior arthrodesis, *J Bone Joint Surg* 71A:1314-1323, 1989.
36. Surat A, Acaroglu E, Özdemir N, Yazici M, Memikoglu S: Pott's disease, *Hacettepe J Orthop Surg* 2:73-76, 1992.
37. Tuli SM, Srivastava TP, Varma BP, Sinha GP: Tuberculosis of the spine, *Acta Orthop Scand* 38:445-458, 1967.
38. Tuli SM: Results of treatment of spinal tuberculosis by "Middle Path" regime, *J Bone Joint Surg* 57B:13-23, 1975.
39. Upadhyay SS, Saji MJ, Sell P, Sell B, Yau ACMC: Longitudinal changes in spinal deformity after anterior spinal surgery for tuberculosis of the spine in adults: a comparative analysis between radical and debridement surgery, *Spine* 19:542-549, 1994.
40. Upadhyay SS, Sell P, Saji MJ, Sell B, Hsu LC: Surgical management of spinal tuberculosis in adults: Hong Kong operation compared with debridement surgery for short and long term outcome of deformity, *Clin Orthop* 302:173-182, 1994.
41. Upadhyay SS, Saji MJ, Sell P, Sell B, Hsu LCS: Spinal deformity after childhood surgery for tuberculosis of the spine. A comparison of radical surgery and debridement, *J Bone Joint Surg* 76B:91-98, 1994.
42. Upadhyay SS, Saji MJ, Sell P, Yau ACMC: The effect of age on the change in deformity after radical resection and anterior arthrodesis for tuberculosis of the spine, *J Bone Joint Surg* 76A:701-708, 1994.
43. Vidyasagar C, Murthy HKRS: Management of tuberculosis of the spine with neurological complications, *Ann R Coll Surg Engl* 76:80-84, 1994.
44. Weidenbaum M, Farcy JPC: *Surgical management of thoracic and lumbar burst fractures.* In Bridwell KH, DeWald RL, editors: *The textbook of spinal surgery,* ed 2, Philadelphia, 1997, Lippincott-Raven, pp 1839-1880.
45. Wilkinson MC: Curettage of tuberculous vertebral disease in the treatment of spinal caries, *Proc R Soc Med* 43:114, 1950.
46. Yau ACMC, Hsu LCS, O'Brien JP, Hodgson AR: Tuberculous kyphosis: Correction with spinal osteotomy, halo-pelvic distraction, and anterior and posterior fusion, *J Bone Joint Surg* 56A:1419-1434, 1974.
47. Yazici M, Acaroglu RE, Alanay A, Surat A: Simultaneous anterior-posterior surgery in the treatment of acute thoracolumbar kyphosis, *Hacettepe J Orthop Surg* 6:194-197, 1996.
48. Yazici M, Atilla B, Gülman B: Anterior debridement and grafting in the treatment of Pott's disease, *Hacettepe J Orthop Surg* 6:190-193, 1996.

# 56

# PELVIC FRACTURES AFTER FUSION TO THE PELVIS

**Kirkham B. Wood, M.D.**



Long fusions of the lumbosacral spine are known to present with many potential adverse outcomes including adjacent level degeneration, pseudarthrosis, and failure to adequately relieve pain.[1,4,11,12,15,19] Additionally, fractures of the pelvic girdle have also been reported following such surgery.[2,6,23] Recently, Wood et al[23] reported a 5% clinical incidence of late fractures of the pelvis following long instrumented lumbosacral spine fusions in certain patient populations.

This chapter will examine the specific pathology of pelvic ring fractures following lumbosacral spine fusions, its incidence, predisposing factors, biomechanics, and treatment.

## PELVIC INSUFFICIENCY AND STRESS FRACTURES

As an introduction, pathologic fractures of the pelvis in bone rendered abnormally fragile by osteoporosis may be seen even without a prior history of spine fusion. Especially in elderly women with osteopenia, they may be an unsuspected cause of low back pain when a strong history of trauma is absent.

Weber et al[22] reported on twenty patients with sacral insufficiency fractures who were all women with dull low back pain, and all were between 58 and 94 years of age. Typically, the fractures are aligned vertically within the sacral ala, parallel with the sacroiliac joints.[13] Plain radiography establishes the diagnosis in less than 10% of cases, however; stress fractures through cancellous osteopenic bone are notoriously difficult to detect, especially in an anatomically complex area such as the sacrum. Most are confirmed on computed tomography (CT) images[13]; bone scintigraphy may also be useful.[3,5,13]

Vertically aligned insufficiency-type fractures may also be found more anteriorly in the pubis (Fig. 56-1), pubic symphysis, medial pubic rami, or more posteriorly in the ischium.[3,5,8,9,18]

## ILIAC FRACTURES AND SACROILIAC PATHOLOGY FOLLOWING LUMBOSACRAL FUSIONS

The harvesting of bone graft from the ilium for lumbar fusions has been complicated on occasion by instability through the sacroiliac joint[2,14] and/or fracture through the donor site.[6,7,10,20,21] Coventry and Tapper[2] reported six patients who developed instability at the sacroiliac joint following the removal of iliac bone for lumbosacral fusions. Symptoms consisted primarily of local pain and "clicking" with activity. Four of the six did require surgical stabilization to relieve symptoms. Grimm et al[6] described eight patients with late posterior iliac wing fractures though the donor site following lumbosacral fusions instrumented with pedicle screws. Their feeling was that the defect acts as a stress riser leading to fracture, its propagation and even potential displacement. One patient in their series required surgical stabilization.

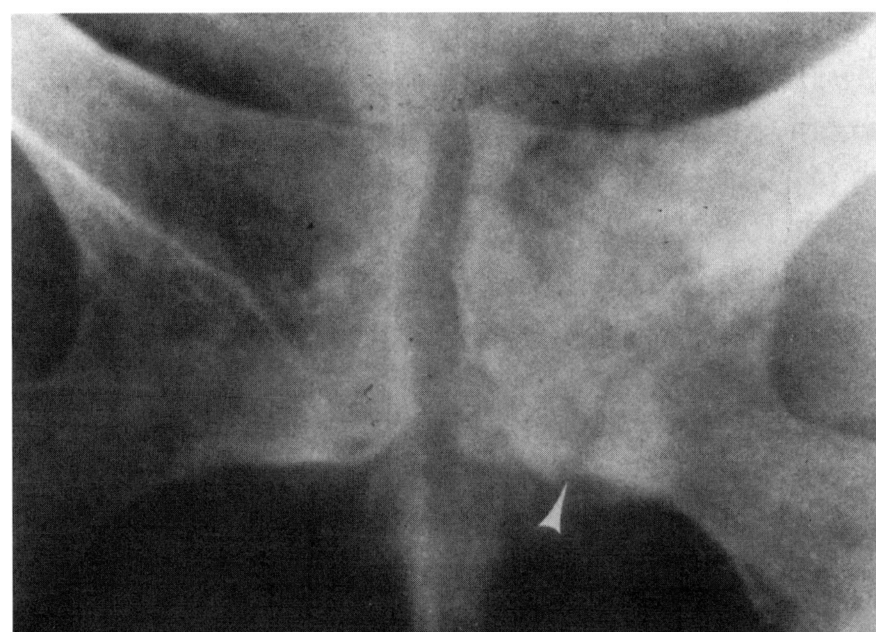

**FIGURE 56-1**

Vertical fracture of the pubis in a 69-year-old woman with steroid induced osteopenia (*arrow*).

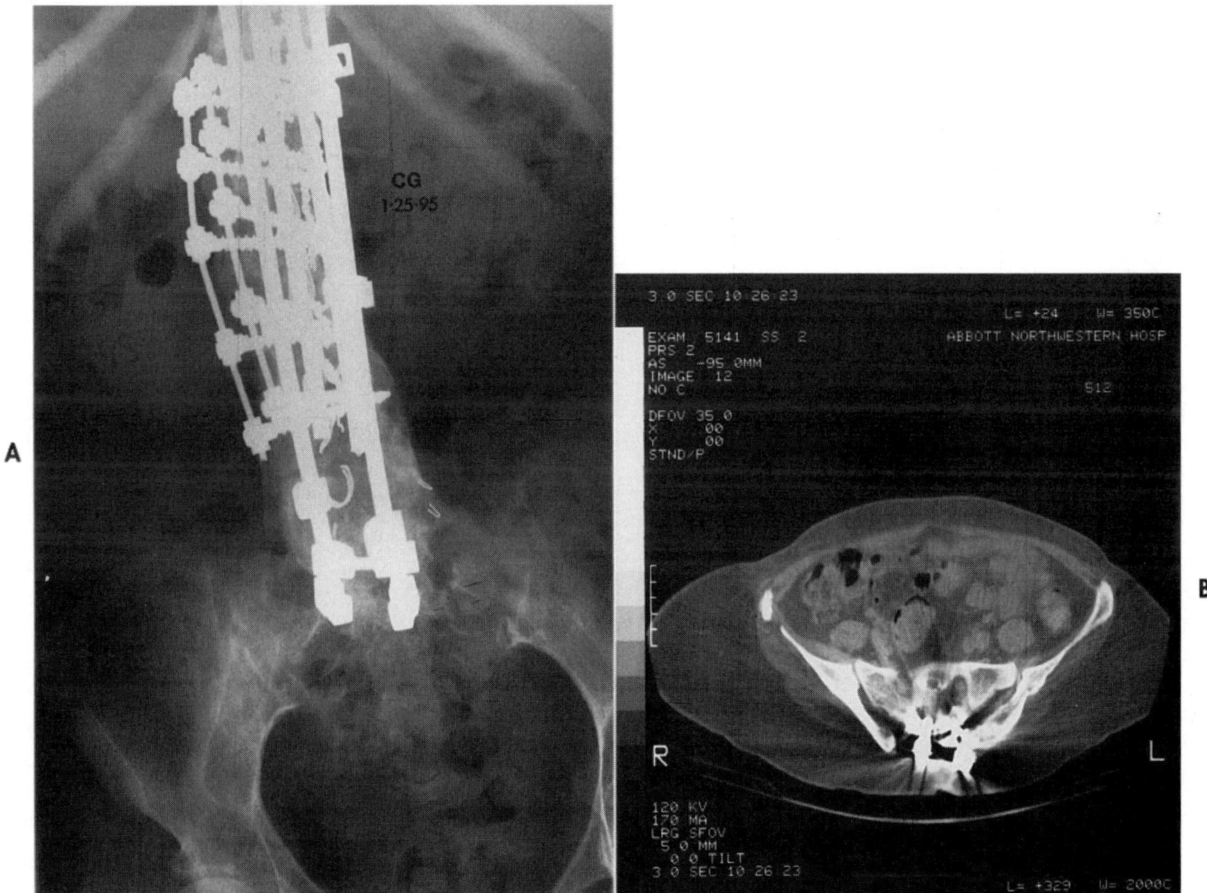


**FIGURE 56-2**

**A,** Oblique fracture of the right sacrum following long lumbosacral instrumentation. **B,** CT scan describes the fracture of the right sacrum (*arrow*).

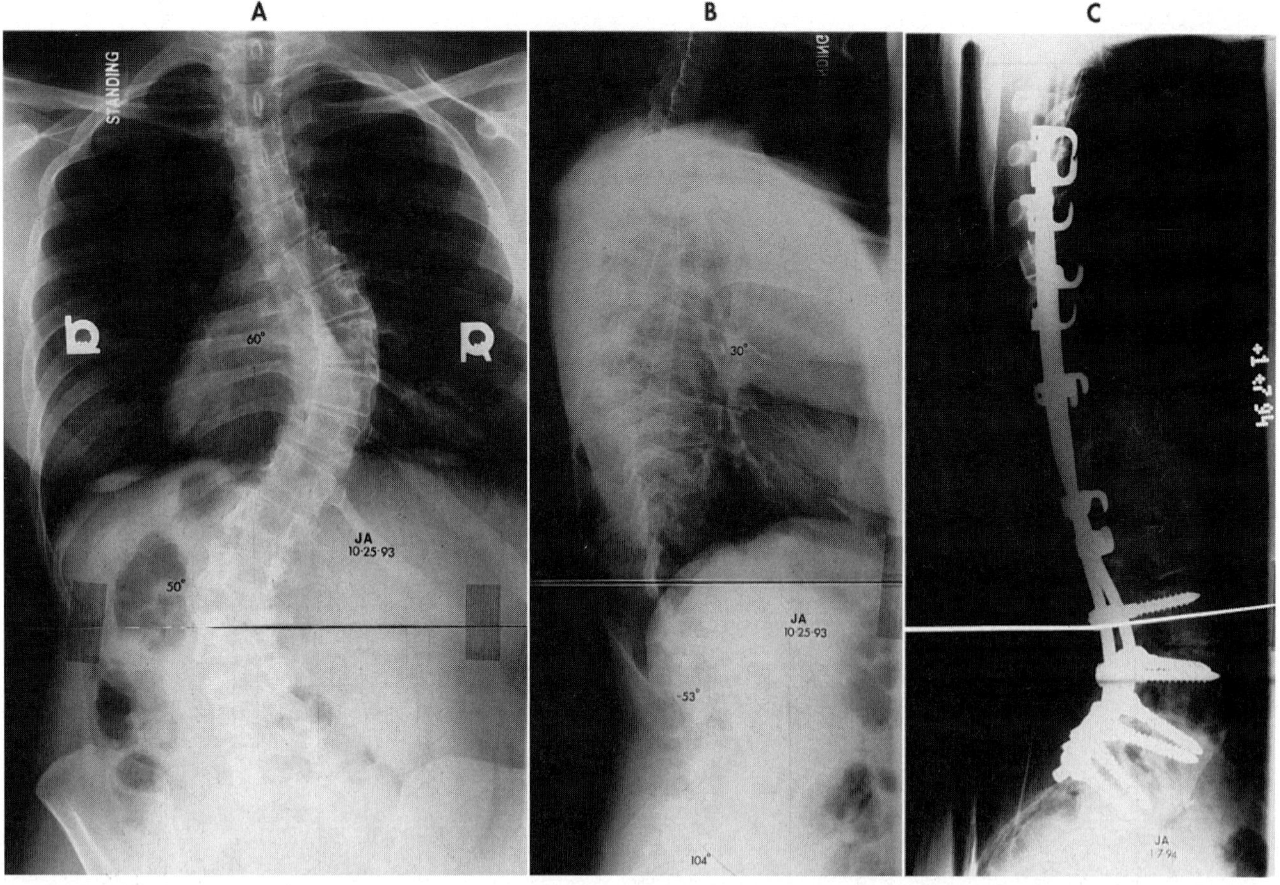


FIGURE 56-3

Standing AP **(A)** and lateral **(B)** radiograph of a 38-year-old woman with a double curve pattern idiopathic scoliosis. **C,** Anterior and posterior fusion from T5 to the sacrum demonstrates excellent postoperative sagittal balance.

*Continued*

## SACRAL FRACTURES

Isolated fractures of the sacrum following instrumentation and fusion to the lumbosacrum as an isolated event are rare, yet may be seen (Figs. 56-2 and 56-3). More typically, they are seen in combination with other fractures within the pelvic ring.

Radiographically they may be distinguished from typical insufficiency-type fractures in that the fracture line is not the characteristic vertical one parallel to the sacroiliac joint, but usually more oblique or even horizontal.

## ANTERIOR PELVIC FRACTURES FOLLOWING LONG FUSIONS TO THE PELVIS

Occasionally, patients will present at varying intervals following long lumbosacral fusions with the insidious onset of vague hip and/or groin pain, yet the exam and radiographs describe no new pathology within the instrumented and/or fused segment, nor in the iliac wings where bone may have been harvested.

At the Twin Cities Scoliosis Spine Center, my colleagues and I retrospectively reviewed records over a 10-year period for patients who had received long (from L1 or above) instrumented fusions down to the lumbosacral junction (L5, the sacrum, or the ilium, e.g., Galveston technique).[23] We identified six individuals who developed late fractures of the anterior pelvic ring in the absence of known trauma (Figs. 56-4 through 56-6) All six were women and at the time of the pelvic fracture all were aged 50 years or more. The group had had an average of 2.1 previous spine fusions (range 1-4). Noteworthy in the majority of cases was a history of pseudarthrosis requiring repeat surgeries. Autologous bone had been harvested from the posterior iliac crest at least once and in some cases bilaterally. Four fractures followed harvesting from the ipsilateral iliac crest yet two were after contralateral bone graft harvesting. All fractures were of the left pubic rami (one woman also fractured the right ramus) and

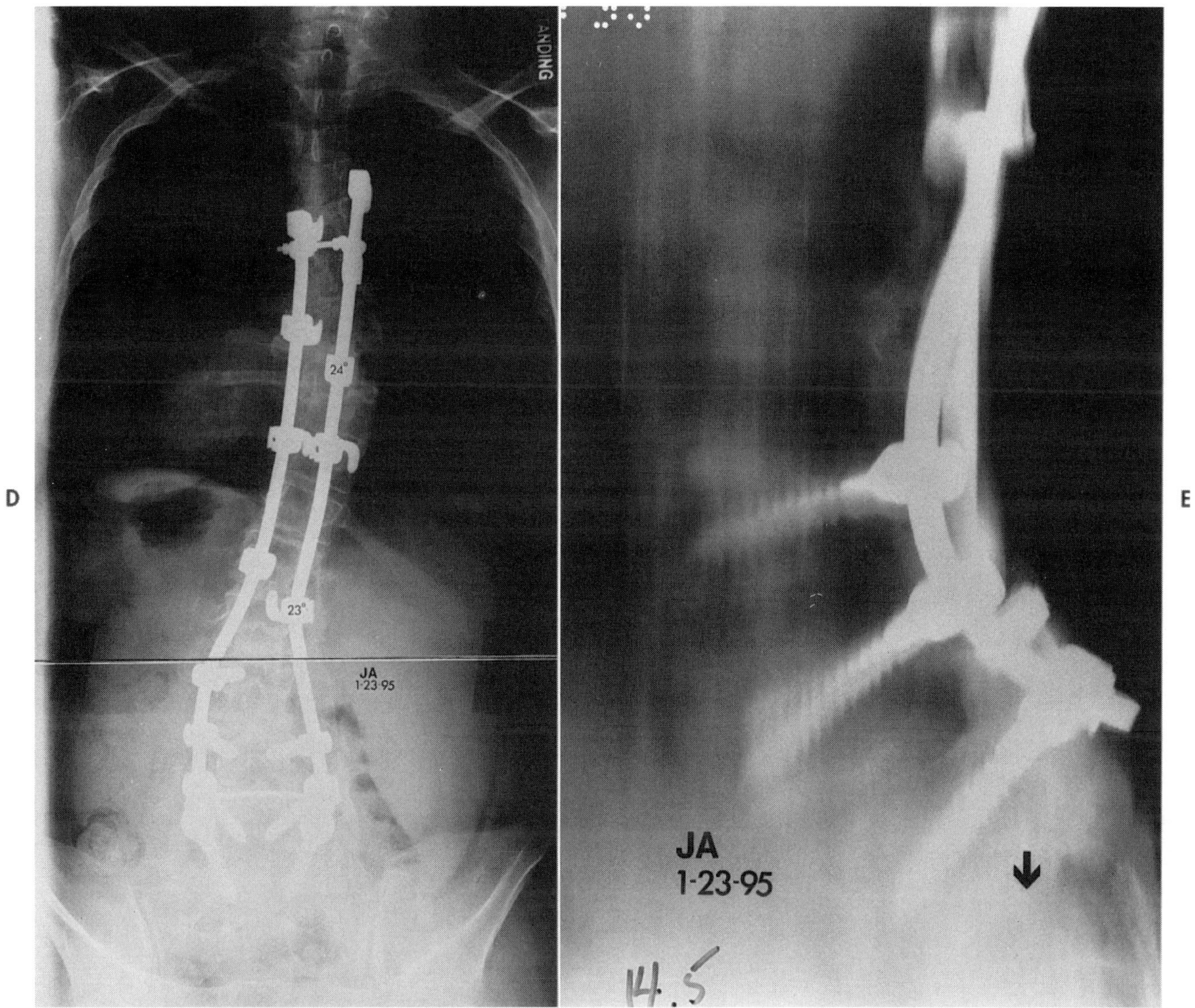


**FIGURE 56-3, CONT'D**

One year later, patient complained of sacral pain. AP radiographs **(D),** failed to disclose obvious pathology. Lateral tomographs of the sacrum **(E)** describe a horizontal fracture distal to the instrumentation (*arrow*).

*Continued*

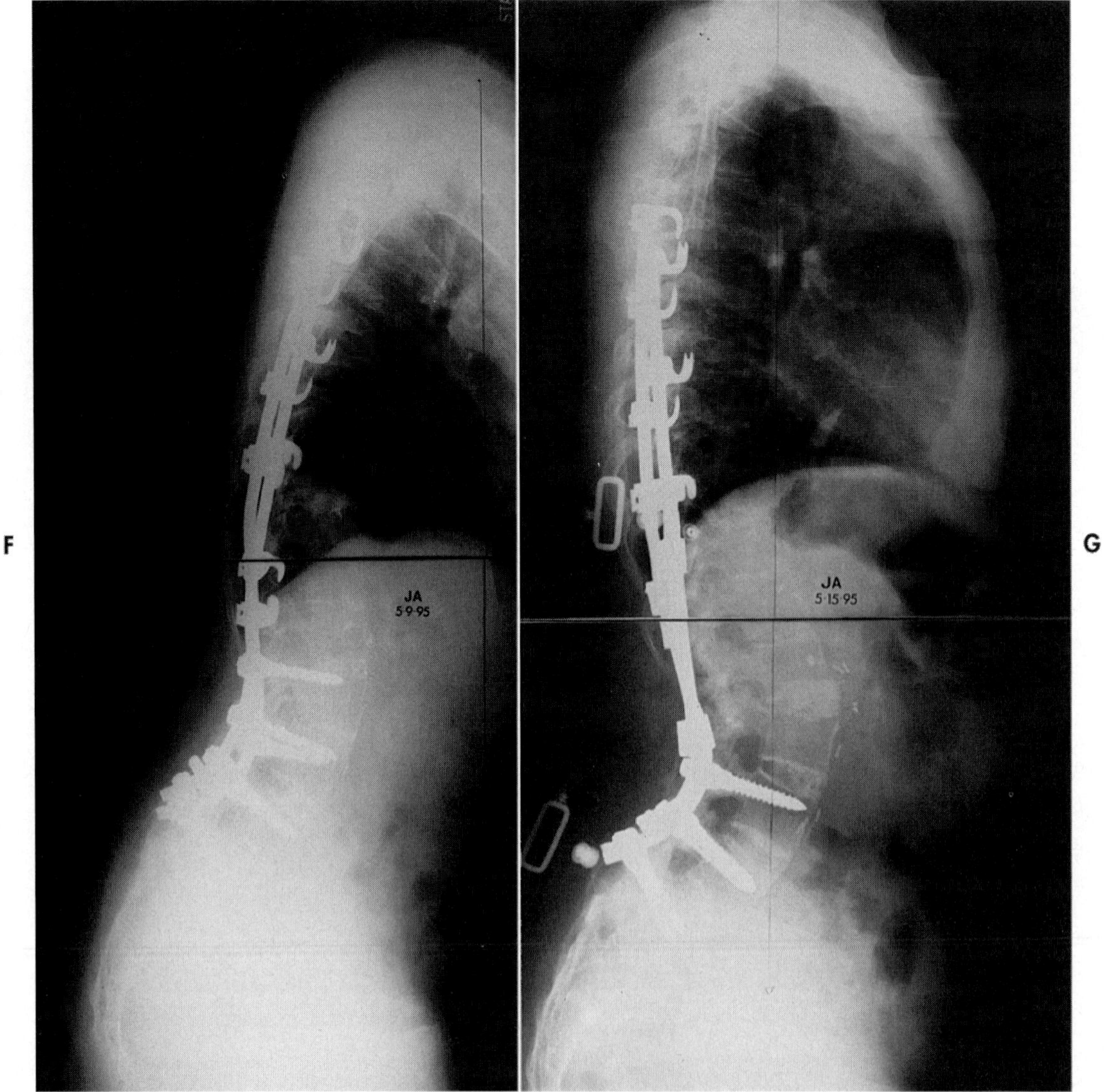


**FIGURE 56-3, CONT'D**

**F,** By 16 months postoperative, she had developed a painful flat back deformity and continued sacral pain. **G,** A revision anterior and posterior midlumbar osteotomy corrected the flat back deformity and allowed compression across the sacral fracture site, effecting successful healing. *(Courtesy of F. Denis, M.D.)*

were more laterally situated than insufficiency-type fractures. (Figs. 56-4 through 56-6) The length of time from last surgery to pelvic fracture ranged widely from 4 months to 7 years.

All individuals were treated with simple protected yet progressive weightbearing until comfortable. The time until pain free ranged from 6 to 31 months.

What this study cataloged was the experience many surgeons have anecdotally reported following long fusions to the lumbosacrum and pelvis, e.g., that late, seemingly insidious, pelvic fractures can occur. As with the earlier-described insufficiency-type fractures, the population at risk is the older, postmenopausal osteopenic female often with multiple medical problems.

In most cases, plain radiography will make the diagnosis. In early, or more subtle instances, bone scintigraphy, plain tomography, or computed tomography may be helpful (Fig. 56-5).

What distinguishes these fractures is the following: They tend to be found in a very characteristic location: at the caudad reflection of the inferior pubic ramus and the lateral aspect of the superior ramus in an almost periacetabular location (see Figs. 56-4 through 56-6). Insufficiency-type fractures of the anterior pelvic ring are more commonly seen within the pubic bone itself or within the peripubic rami and are typically more vertically aligned (see Fig. 56-1). The oblique fracture pattern of the post fusion fractures also suggests more rotational loading than insufficiency collapse (Fig. 56-6).

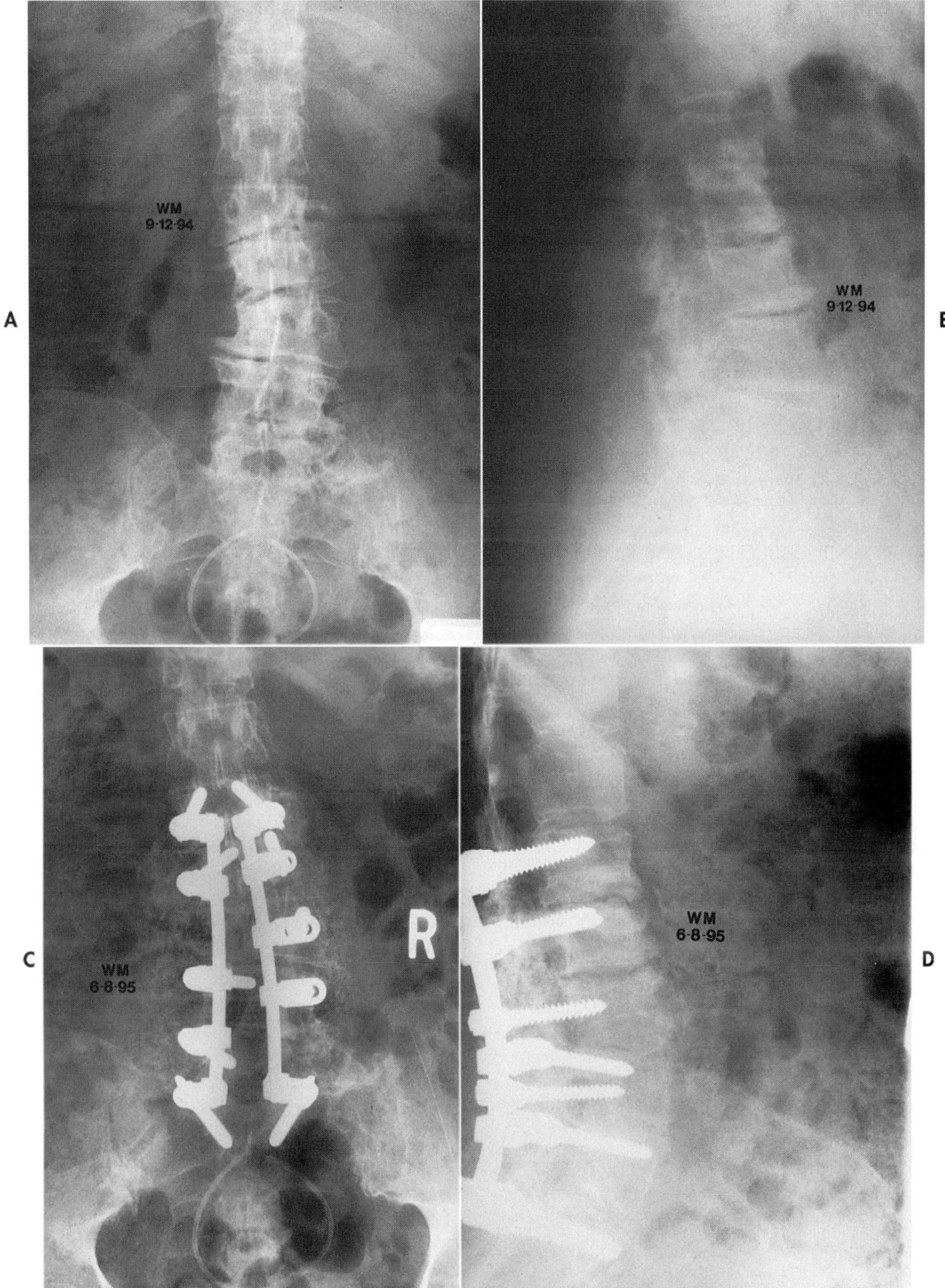


**FIGURE 56-4**

Preoperative AP **(A)** and lateral **(B)** radiographs of a 68-year-old woman with rheumatoid arthritis and degenerative lumbar scoliosis. Postoperative AP **(C)** and lateral **(D)** radiograph showing instrumented posterior spine fusion from L1 to the sacrum.

*Continued*

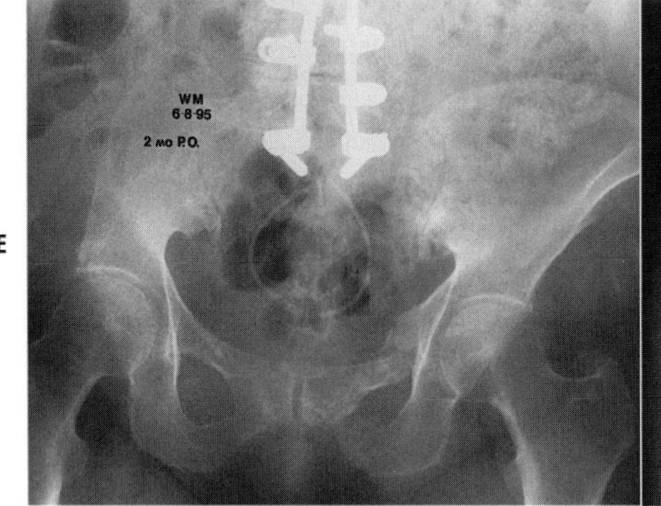


E

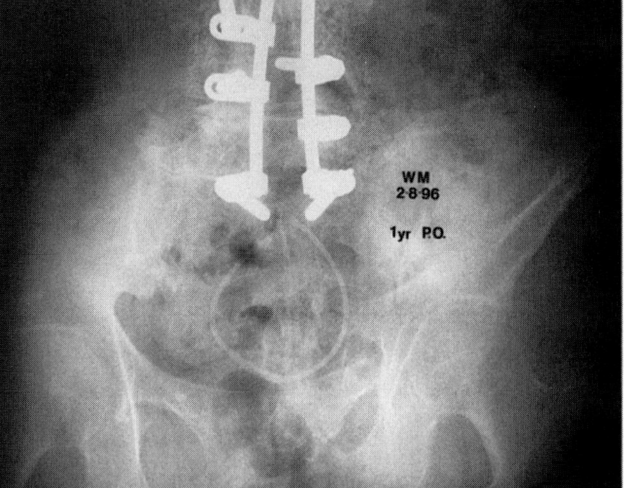


F

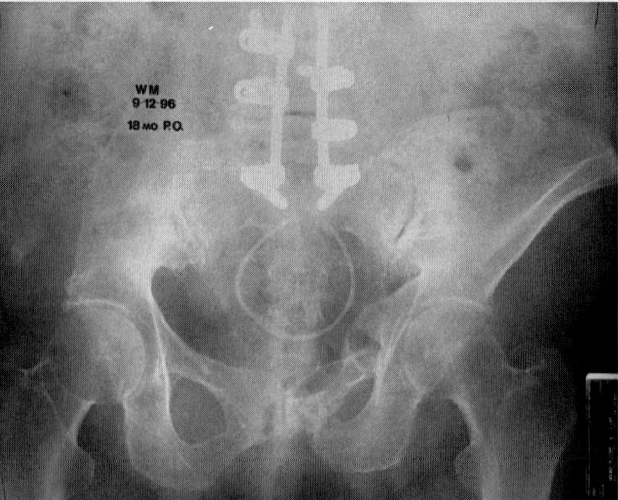


G

**FIGURE 56-4, CONT'D**

**E,** At 2 months postoperatively, the patient described the insidious onset of left groin discomfort. AP radiograph describes a fracture of the superior and inferior pubic ramus. Of note: 7 years previously the patient had had an anterior cervical spine fusion harvesting bone graft from the right anterior iliac crest. This had been complicated postoperatively by a complete avulsion fracture of the origin of the hip flexors. It had healed relatively unremarkably. **F,** At 1 year postoperatively, the patient continued to complain principally of groin discomfort and an antalgic gait, despite protective weightbearing. Very little callus is seen. **G,** Approximately 18 months postoperatively, however, a deposition of some callus formation is seen and the patient was by this time able to ambulate comfortably without assistance. Note, however, the increased subchondral sclerosis and joint degeneration taking place at the left sacroiliac joint when compared with earlier radiographs.

The relative frequency of postlumbosacral fusion pelvic ring fractures also bears noting. In the series reported above, of 99 women over the age of 50 treated with a long lumbosacral fusion, the risk of a late pelvic fracture was approximately 6%.[23] By contrast, in Weber's review of pelvic insufficiency fractures, the largest to date, their 20 patients represented only 1.8% of 1,015 females older than 55 seen in their department of rheumatology.[22]

One final point: the treating physician should be careful, because healing fractures, especially if early with relative osteolysis or less organized callus, may present a radiologic picture that may at times be confused with malignancy or infection. The clinical setting should be kept in mind so as to limit unnecessary biopsy.

## BIOMECHANICS OF POSTSURGICAL PELVIC FRACTURES

An understanding of how the strain distribution changes in the pelvic ring following lumbosacral and lumbosacroiliac instrumentation would be of some importance in understanding how and why these fractures take place, not only to surgeons but designers of instrumentation as well.

In our biomechanical labs, we studied human pelves (lumbar spines attached) with axis rosette strain gauges fixed to the previously described specific fracture sites (Fig. 56-7, *A*).[24] Each specimen was then axially loaded (445 N) in different pelvic positions according to that seen in the normal human gait cycle, e.g., stance phase, 15 degrees pelvic rotation, etc. (e.g., swing-through; Fig. 56-7, *B*). Five different instrumentation-fusion configurations were then studied: (1) normal or uninstrumented; (2) with a long fusion (instrumentation) to and including the sacrum via segmental interpedicular fixation and $\frac{1}{4}$-inch rods; (3) similar fixation but with additional iliac fixation as well via bolts (e.g., Galveston-type); and (4) and (5) each of the two previous configurations but also following standard posterior iliac bone graft harvesting (taking care to preserve the sacroiliac and sacropelvic ligaments).

As far as strain seen within the pelvic ring, our results showed that there was no real difference between

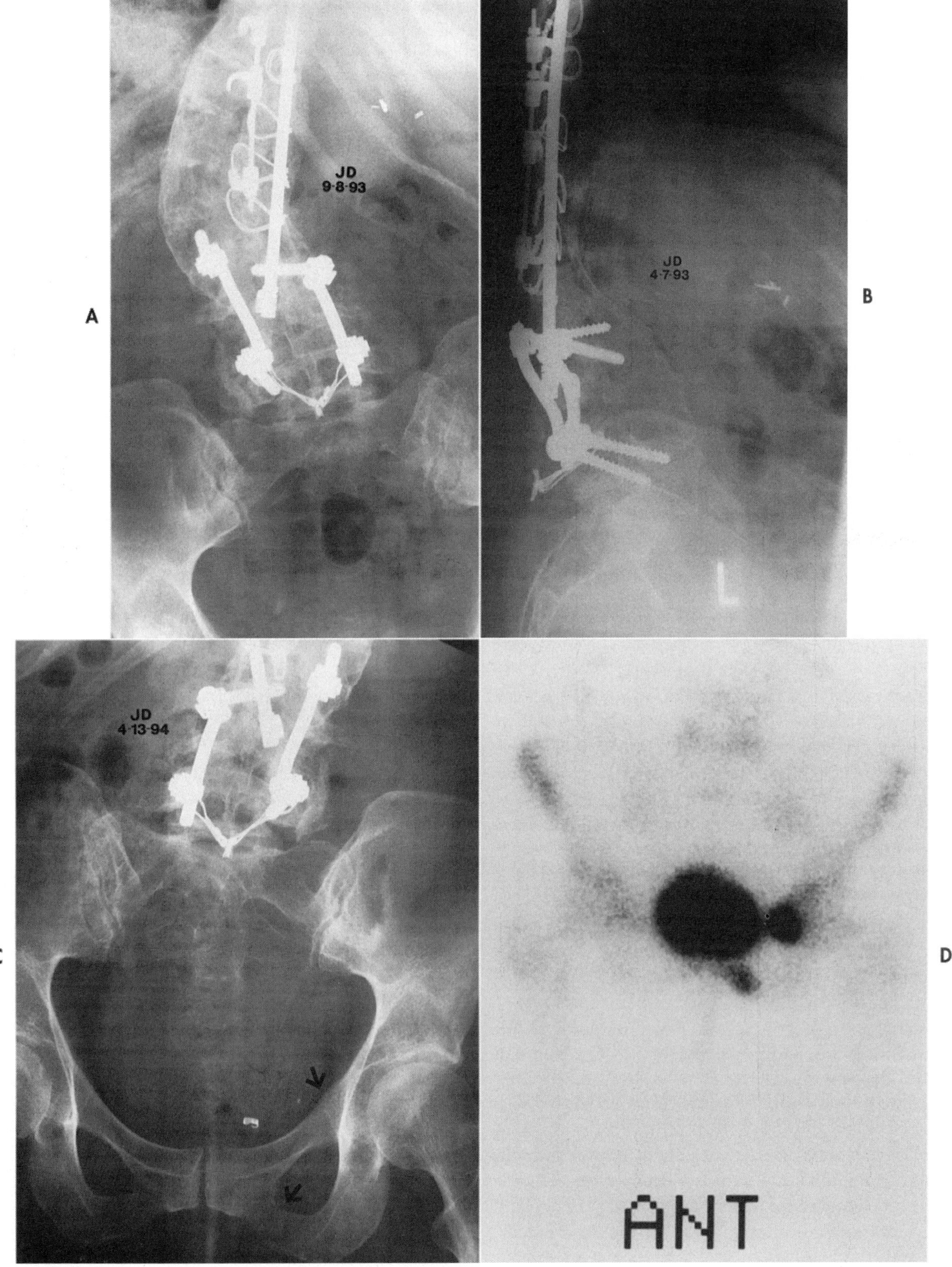


**FIGURE 56-5**

AP **(A)** and lateral **(B)** radiograph of the thoracolumbar spine in a 50-year-old woman. Eight years prior to these radiographs the woman had undergone instrumentation and fusion for scoliosis down to L4. Two years later, this was extended to L5. **C,** Six years after her last surgery, the patient began to complain of left-sided groin discomfort. An AP radiograph of the pelvis suggested possible fractures within the pubic rami (arrows). **D,** Bone scintigraphy taken at that time revealed increased uptake in the left inferior pubic ramus and the right superior ramus in a periacetabular position.

*Continued*

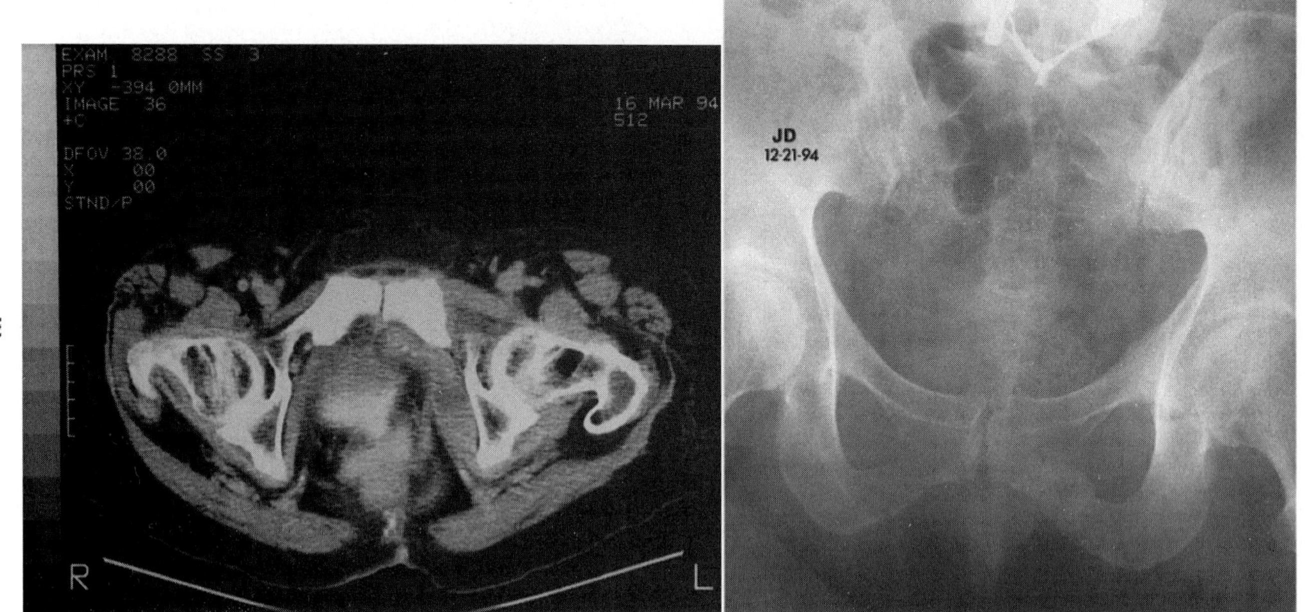


**FIGURE 56-5, CONT'D**

**E,** Subsequent CT examination of the pelvis confirmed disruption of the superior pubic ramus. **F,** Eight months after presentation and treatment with the protected weightbearing, radiographic callus formation can be seen and the patient was ambulating pain-free without assistance.

instrumentation that crossed the sacroiliac joint (Galveston) and that which ended in the sacrum. In addition, there was no change in strains seen, even within the iliac wing, following posterior iliac bone graft harvesting. What we did see was that after instrumentation to the pelvis, strain significantly decreased within the pubic rami when specimens were axially loaded, yet when the pelvis was dynamically rotated 15 degrees (e.g., keeping the limbs fixed); strain at the pubic rami significantly increased above that seen when the normal uninstrumented spine was similarly rotated.

What this study suggests is that under axial loading, significant stress shielding may be provided by the rigid lumbosacral and lumbosacroiliac instrumentation and may predispose to device-related osteopenia within the pelvic ring, the most distal aspect of long instrumentation and fusion.[16,17] Then, within this setting, dynamic activity, such as pelvic rotation during ambulation, significantly increases strain at certain sites and may lead to late fractures. Alternatively, rigid, multilevel instrumentation and fusion of the lumbosacral spine may immobilize so many previously available motion segments that stress is naturally transferred directly to the osteopenic pelvis, which then fails under the increased strains of torsional loading.

In a follow-up study, we segmentally instrumented from the thoracic spine into the upper lumbar spine, and then sequentially included more caudad levels, eventually extending all the way down to S1 (Wood et al, unpublished data). Similar load testing was then performed. As the instrumentation is extended down to L4 or lower, strain within the pubic rami significantly increased during rotational activities compared with instrumentation ending at higher levels, placing these structures at some risk for fracture.

Similarly, we sequentially built up constructs from the sacrum in a cephalad direction (i.e., L5-S1, L4-S1, etc.). Here again, there was a sudden, statistically significant, increase in strain seen at the pubic rami when the instrumentation reached L2 or above.

## TREATMENT

As a general rule, the treatment of most fractures of the anterior pelvis following long instrumented lumbosacral fusions is nonoperative. Pubic rami fractures can almost always be treated with protected weightbearing with progression from walker or crutches to cane ambulation until comfortable. Neither bed rest nor surgical stabilization appears necessary. Eventually most, if not all, become essentially pain-free. As well, most fractures of the ilium and sacrum can be managed without surgery, however, some iliac wing fractures may progress to a painful nonunion that benefits from stabilization.[2,6]

It is important to reemphasize, too, that some fractures, during healing, may take on an appearance similar to that of malignancy (osteolysis, bone disorganiza-

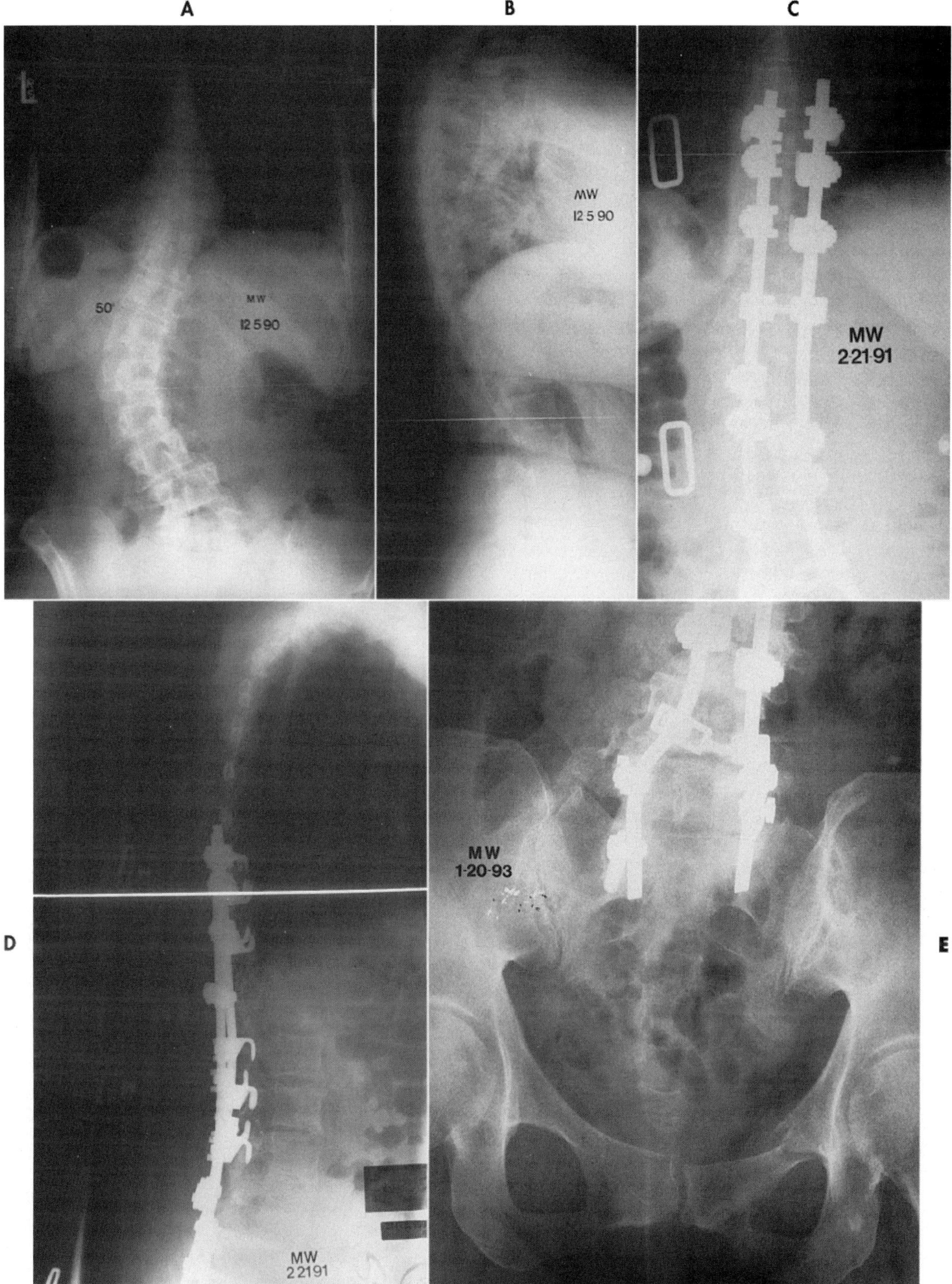


**FIGURE 56-6**

AP **(A)** and lateral **(B)** radiographs of a 49-year-old woman with long-standing thoracolumbar scoliosis. AP **(C)** and lateral **(D)** radiographs of the thoracolumbar spine following anterior and posterior spine fusion with instrumentation from T9 to the sacrum. **E,** Approximately 2 years postoperatively the patient noted the insidious onset of left groin pain. An AP radiograph of the pelvis describes an oblique fracture of the right superior periacetabular ramus and a fracture of the inferior pubic ramus.

*Continued*

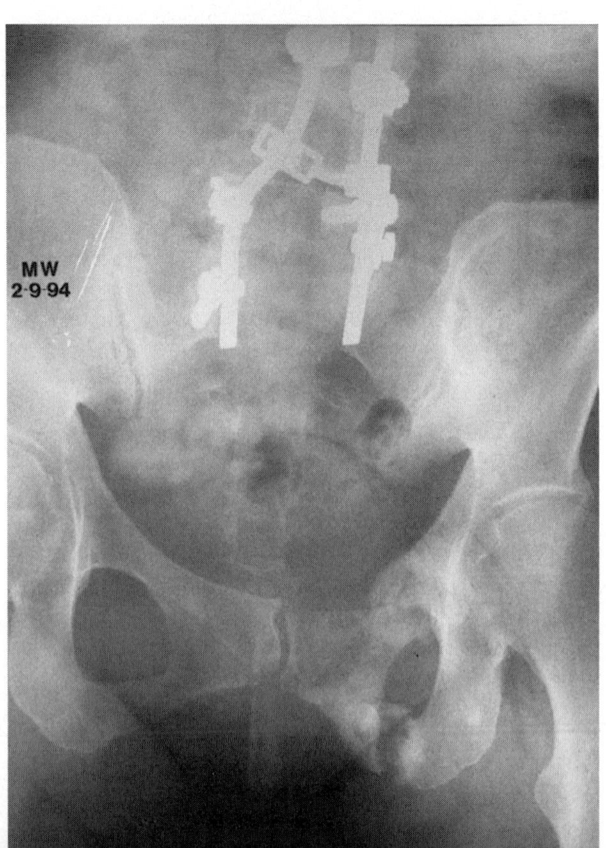


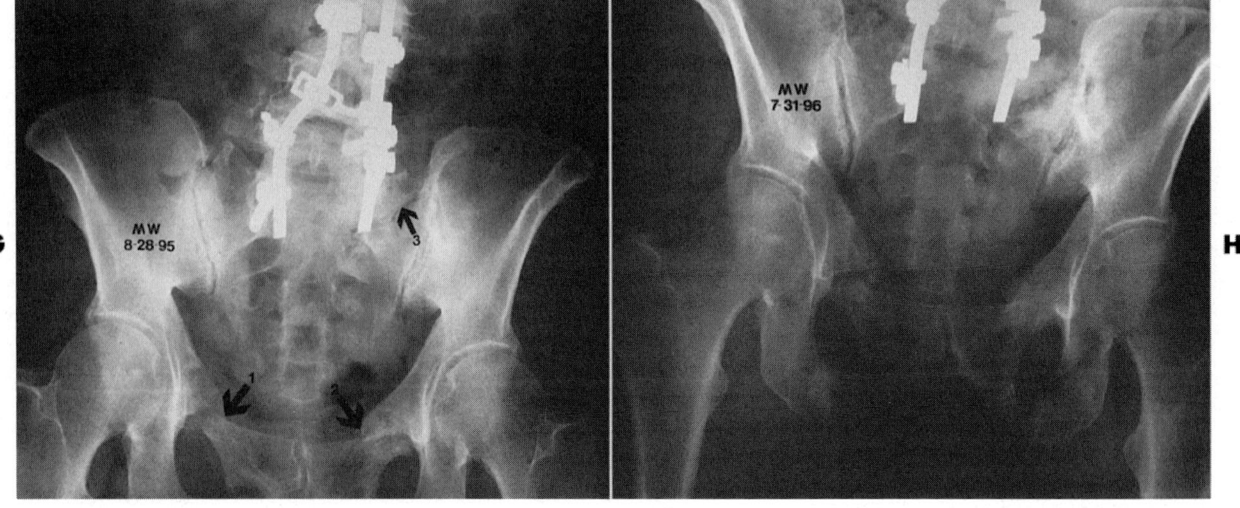


FIGURE 56-6, CONT'D

**F,** At 2 years postfracture, callus formation appears complete and the patient is ambulating without assistance or pain. **G,** Five months later, however, the patient noted the onset of new right-sided groin pain as well as left posterior buttock discomfort. An AP radiograph of the pelvis now shows a new fracture of the right superior and inferior pubic rami (*1*) in the presence of healed fractures on the left (*2*). In addition, there is an oblique fracture of the sacrum posteriorly on the left side (*3*). **H,** Eleven months later the patient is still complaining of mild, right-sided groin discomfort and incomplete callus bridging can be seen at the fracture sites, both at the right pubic rami and the left sacrum.

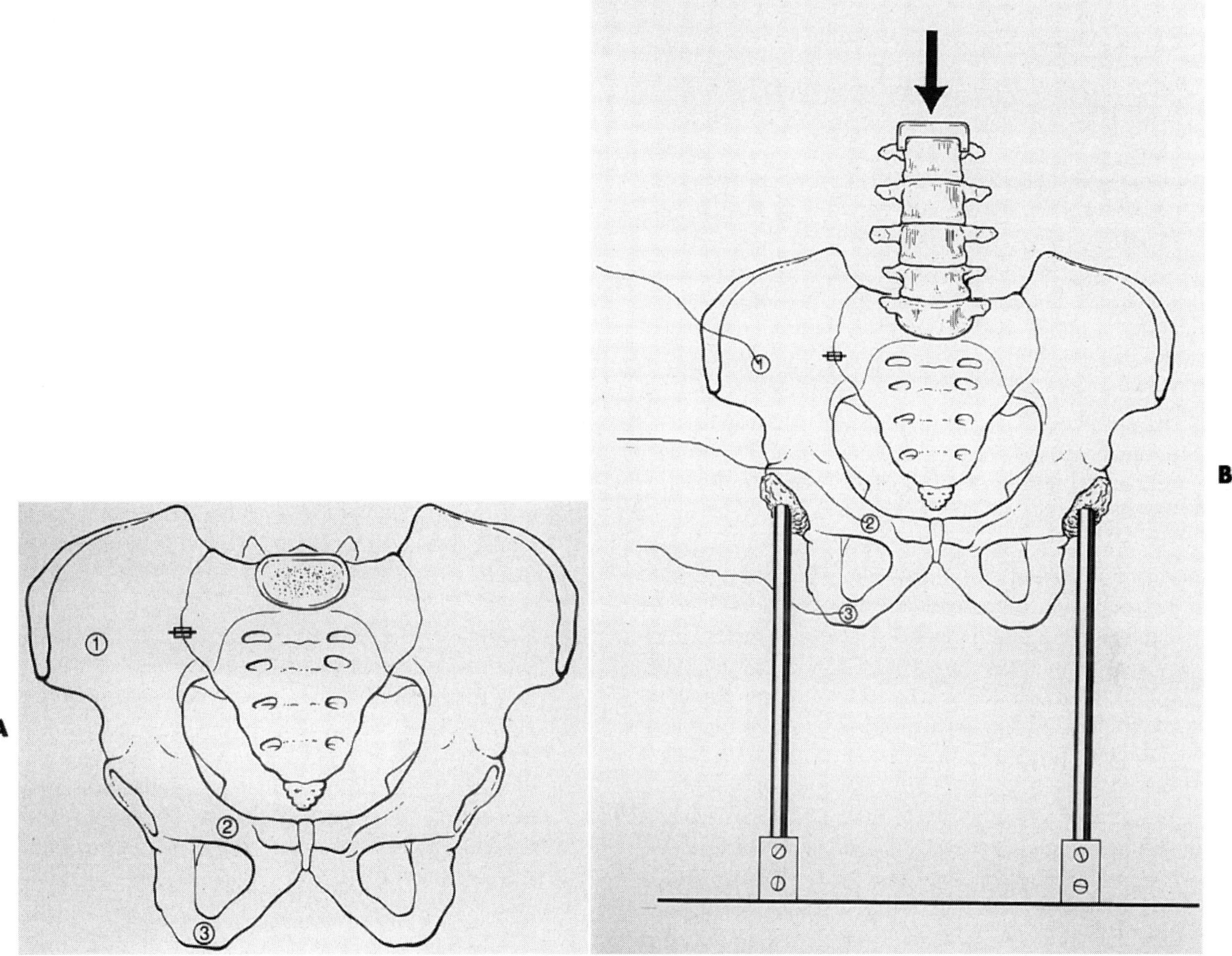


FIGURE 56-7

**A,** Placement sites of rosette strain gauges on the pelvic specimen. These sites were chosen because they represent typical sites of fractures following lumbosacral spine fusions. **B,** Diagram of the human pelvis subjected to axial loading with strain information recovered from rosette strain gauges placed at specific sites within the right hemipelvis.

tion, etc.). However, if one recognizes the characteristic fracture patterns and clinical setting, especially when present with multiple other fractures outside of the pelvis, biopsy is usually not necessary.

It is important to recognize that late fractures of the pelvis after long instrumented fusions can and do occur, especially in certain patient populations, so as to avoid unnecessary delays in diagnosis and increased morbidity. Awareness, thus, is probably the critical factor, yet there may be items that are under the surgeon's control, such as when harvesting bone graft from the posterior ilium care should be taken to preserve the sacroiliac ligaments as much as possible. Grimm and Jackson also suggest, whenever possible, avoiding the harvesting of the outer cortical ilium and removing only the cancellous bone from within the two cortical tables.[6]

It is important to educate the patient to be aware of the potential for late fracture (e.g., the warning signs to look for so as to avoid delays in treatment: new onset of groin pain, ambulation difficulty, etc.). Certainly if long fusions are extended to the lumbosacral area or extend up more than 3 levels from the sacrum, frequent evaluations, including radiography, should continue for years. Finally, the diligent medical management of osteoporosis plays an obvious and vital role.

## REFERENCES


1. Cochran T, Nachemson A: Long-term anatomic changes in patients with adolescent idiopathic scoliosis treated by Harrington rod fusion, *Spine* 9:576-584, 1983.
2. Conventry MB, Tapper EM: Pelvic instability: a consequence of removing iliac bone for grafting, *J Bone Joint Surg Am* 4(1):83-101, 1972.
3. De Smet AA, Neff JR: Pubic and sacral insufficiency fractures: clinical course and radiologic findings, American Roentgen Ray Society 145:601-606, 1985.
4. Edgar MA: Back pain assessment from a long-term follow-up of operated and unoperated patients with adolescent idiopathic scoliosis, *Spine* 4:519-20, 1979.
5. Gotis-Graham I, McGuigan L, Diamond T, Portek I, Quinn R, Sturgess A, Tulloch R: Sacral insufficiency fractures in the elderly, *J Bone Joint Surg Br* 76:822-826, 1994.
6. Grimm JO, Jackson RP, Hamilton AC: Stress fracture of the pelvis: a complication following instrumented lumbar fusion, 27th Annual Meeting of the Scoliosis Research Society, Kansas City, KS, Sept. 23-26, 1992.
7. Guha SC, Poole MD: Stress fracture of the iliac bone with subfascial femoral neuropathy: unusual complications at a bone graft donor site: a case report, *Br J Plastic Surg* 36:305-306, 1983.
8. Hall FM, Goldberg RP, Kasdon EJ, Glick H: Posttraumatic osteolysis of the pubic bone simulating a malignant lesion, *J Bone Joint Surg* 66A(1):121-126, 1984.
9. Hauge MD, Cooper KL, Litin SC: Subspecialty clinics: oncology. Insufficiency fractures of the pelvis that simulate metastatic disease, *Mayo Clin Proc* 63:807-812, 1988.
10. Hu RW, Bohlman HH: Fracture at the iliac bone graft harvest site after fusion of the spine, *Clin Orthop* 309:208-213, 1994.
11. Lee CK: Accelerated degeneration of the segment adjacent to a lumbar fusion, *Spine* 13(3):375-377, 1988.
12. Lehmann TR, Spratt KF, Tozzi JE, Weinstein JN, Reinarz SJ, El-Khoury GY, Colby H: Long-term follow-up of lower lumbar fusion patients, *Spine* 12(2):97-104, 1986.
13. Leroux JL, Denat B, Thomas E, Blotman F, Bonnel F: Sacral insufficiency fractures presenting as acute low-back pain: biomechanical aspects, *Spine* 18(16): 2502-2506, 1993.
14. Lichtblau S: Dislocation of the sacro-iliac joint: a complication of bone-grafting, *J Bone Joint Surg* 44A(1): 193-197, 1962.
15. Luk KDK, Lee, FB, Leong JCY, Hsu, LCS: The effect on the lumbosacral spine of long spinal fusion for idiopathic scoliosis: a minimum 10-year follow-up, *Spine* 12(10):996-1000, 1987.
16. McAfee PC, Farey ID, Sutterlin CE, Gurr KR, Warden KE, Cunningham BW: Device-related osteoporosis with spinal instrumentation, *Spine* 14(9): 919-926, 1989.
17. McAfee PC, Farey ID, Sutterlin CE, Gurr KR, Warden KE, Cunningham BW: The effect of spinal implant rigidity on vertebral bone density: a canine model, *Spine* 16(suppl):S190-S197, 1991.
18. McGuigan LE, Edmonds JP, Painter DM: Pubic osteolysis, *J Bone Joint Surg* 66A(1):127-129, 1984.
19. Nagata H, Schendel MJ, Transfeldt EE, Lewis JL: The effects of immobilization of long segments of the spine on the adjacent and distal facet force and lumbosacral motion, *Spine* 18:2471-2479, 1993.
20. Reale F, Gambacorta D, Mencattini G: Iliac crest fracture after removal of two bone plugs for anterior cervical fusion: case report, *J Neurosurg* 51:560-561, 1979.
21. Reynolds AF Jr, Turner PT, Loeser JD: Fracture of the anterior superior iliac spine following anterior cervical fusion using iliac crest: case report, *J Neurosurg* 48: 809-810, 1978.
22. Weber M, Hasler P, Gerber H: Insufficiency fractures of the sacrum: twenty cases and review of the literature, *Spine* 18(16):2507-2512, 1993.
23. Wood KB, Geissele AE, Ogilvie JW: Pelvic fractures after long lumbosacral spine fusions, *Spine* 21(11): 1357-1362, June 1, 1996.
24. Wood KB, Schendel MJ, Ogilvie JW, Braun J, Malcolm JR: Effect of sacral and iliac instrumentation on strains in the pelvis: a biomechanical study, *Spine* 21(10):1185-1191, May 15, 1996.

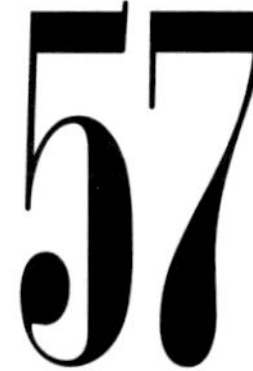

# POSTLAMINECTOMY SCAR FORMATION

**Michael Osipoff, P.A.**
**Jean-Jacques Abitbol M.D.**
**Laurence E. Mermelstein, M.D.**
**Steven R. Garfin, M.D.**
**Wayne H. Akeson, M.D.**



Postlaminectomy scar formation has been implicated as a possible source of persistent pain following spine surgery. Additionally, scar tissue increases the technical difficulty and risk during subsequent procedures. Early failure of spine surgery characterized by persistent or recurrent pain accounts for up to 20% of all patients after lumbar decompression and diskectomy, with long-term failure rates reportedly approaching 40%.[85] Recurrent disk herniation, postoperative degenerative changes, arachnoiditis, poor patient selection, inadequate surgery, and formation of extradural scar, have all been identified as possible causes of poor surgical outcome.[137]

Despite these and other studies, the association of postoperative perineural scar with pain remains controversial. This chapter will review the pertinent historical aspects, pathophysiology, and current recommendations for prevention of postlaminectomy adhesions.

## HISTORICAL ASPECTS

The genesis of scar following laminectomy remains debatable. Key and Ford first studied perineural scar following laminectomy and diskectomy reporting in 1948 that postoperative adhesions were derived from the surgically damaged annulus fibrosis.[98] Nachemson supported this early report implicating a proton leak from the disrupted intervertebral disk as a factor in perineural fibrosis.[132] Others claim that the primary source of scar after laminectomy originates from posterior tissues rather than anteriorly from the intervertebral disk. LaRocca described the layer of fibrosis that covers a laminectomy site and extends into the spinal canal as the "laminectomy membrane."[111] He suggested that migration of fibroblasts from the raw surface of the erector spiny musculature is a source of postoperative scar tissue. Foreign body reaction from surgical swab debris, as well as the systemic fibrinolytic defect, have also been reported as possible etiologies of post laminectomy scar formation.[45]

Numerous attempts have been made to prevent scar after laminectomy. LaRocca first studied the effects of Gelfoam and Silastic interpositional membranes after spine surgery in a dog model. He reported a decrease in perineural scar formation with use of such physical barriers. Autogenous fat grafts remain one of the most popular interpositional membranes used clinically. Several studies suggest long-term viability and clinical superiority of fat compared to interpositional membrane. However, this technique is not without reported complications. Most seriously, epidural migration of the free fat graft with resulting cauda equina syndrome has been reported. Donor site seroma, cosmesis, and lack of availability of fat in thin patients are also of concern.

A myriad of other substances, including Avitene (Alcon, Humacao, PR), Surgicel, heparinized collagen, bone wax, plastics, steroid topical and lamina bone graft have also been investigated. These studies have focused uniformly on the volume of scar formed, rather than the functional effect of scar on the surrounding neural tissues. In addition, a reliance on subjective criteria, such as grading of scar by dissection or histology, is common to all these reports.

The advent of magnetic resonance imaging (MRI) has allowed us to examine sequentially changes that occur following routine laminectomies. Kotilainen and coworkers performed MRI scans in 41 patients, both pre- and postoperatively at 3 and 6 months. The presence of an early postoperative hematoma was frequently associated with radiological presence of perineural fibrosis on subsequent scans.[104] These findings supported an earlier hypothesis that epidural scar tissue results from the organization of postoperative hematomas. Furthermore, Kotilainen noted that there was no correlation between the scar seen on MRI and the patient's clinical status, questioning the clinical significance of radiological epidural fibrosis.

Cooper et al reviewed the biochemical plasma fibrinolytic parameters in 70 patients who were suffering from chronic post surgical low back and radicular pain. These 70 patients exhibited significant impairment of plasma fibrinolytic activity when compared with 84 normal control subjects. An increased level of circulating plasminogen activator inhibitor-1 appears to have been related to the impairment of the fibrinolytic activity. It was further observed that patients with radiological abnormalities consistent with epidural fibrosis were more symptomatic. Additionally, the frequency of radiological abnormalities was higher for patients with fibrinolytic abnormalities. Although these results were suggestive, they did not demonstrate a significant association between clinical symptoms and biochemical and radiological abnormalities.[45]

Others have noted that iron derived from hemoglobin has been implicated in the production of cerebral vasospasm following subarachnoid hemorrhage.[115] This same subarachnoid blood has been felt to contribute to the production of basilar arachnoiditis and subsequent hydrocephalus. Additionally, Wan and Lewis studied the role of iron as a catalyst for the generation of hydroxyl radicals from hydrogen peroxide. They found free iron concentration to be significantly higher in hypertrophic scar when compared to normal skin. They have hypothesized that hypertrophic scar may result from free radical generation secondary to inflammatory processes in which free iron may be associated.[196]

## PATHOPHYSIOLOGY OF EPIDURAL FIBROSIS

Since Key and Ford,[98] in their classic article in 1948, proposed a likely central role for scar formation as a complicating factor following disk surgery, various authors have explored techniques to limit scar formation in the postlaminectomy wound. LaRocca and McNabb reported favorably on the use of Gelfoam as a barrier material following their canine studies in 1974,[111] but these findings were later refuted.[67,89,96,205] Subsequently, after favorable animal studies, fat graft application at the laminectomy site was proposed by other investigators for this purpose.[39,90,205] Corticosteroid use was found marginally useful in this application by Hinton et al,[82] but the high concentration required locally was found to carry significant risk due to increased wound infection postoperatively. Hyaluronan has been used locally to control scar in experimental laminectomy models in Akeson's laboratory, as well as by Songer and by Trotter et al.[1,176,189] Trotter et al also studied the effect of a carbohydrate polymer (GT1587) on postlaminectomy scar formation. A nonsteroidal anti-inflammatory drug, Keto-profen, was shown by He et al to decrease scar in the postoperative laminectomy wound in the rat.[76] These studies have each evaluated scar formation grossly and histologically. They generally suffer from the lack of functional neurological evaluation, and of course, cannot directly assess efficacy of reduction of pain, which may presumably result from perineural scar production.

Evidence points to epidural scarring, nerve root scarring and adhesions as important factors in postoperative complications after lumbar disk surgery.[22,32,67,98] Olmarker and colleagues have demonstrated reduction in cauda equina nerve conduction when autologous nucleus pulposus was applied to the cauda equina without creating any nerve root compression.[141] In this study, myelinated nerve fiber damage was also observed in the nucleus pulposus treated group, but not in a control fat graft treated group. The effects could be reduced dramatically by high dose methyl prednisone administration within 1 to 2 days following.[140] The nucleus pulposus in this model also produced marked leukotaxis.[127,139]

More definitive and directly effective candidates for postsurgical scar control have recently emerged following an explosion of progress in understanding and prevention of a variety of chronic fibrotic conditions of skin, lung, heart, liver, kidney, and vasculature. Extensive studies on the processes of leukocyte trafficking in wounds have broadened the understanding of the underlying processes at work in the early wound. These concepts have been clarified and phenomenologically synthesized by Butcher and others.[23,34,43,165]

Progress in this field now provides an exciting opportunity to approach the problem of control of fibrosis with a variety of new neutralizing agents.

Briefly, leukocyte-endothelial cell interactions are mediated by cell adhesion molecules (CAMs) and chemoattractants that are programmed in a sequential manner to form a leukocyte-endothelial cell adhesion cascade.[27,43,146,175,195] Platelets release TGF-β and TNF-α among other factors immediately after wounding. Cytokines and chemokines quickly up-regulate selectins on leukocytes and endothelial cells in the post capillary venules in the region of injury causing leukocyte slowing, margination, or "rolling," a phenomenon resulting in a reduced rate of passage of leukocytes through the venule and allowing the leukocytes to monitor the environment for chemoattractants.[29,160,161] Chemoattractants bind into serpentine receptors on the leukocytes, which then activate G proteins, which signal up-regulation of integrins on the leukocyte cell surface. The CD11 (beta 2) integrins leukocyte function-associated antigen-1 (LFA-1), and p150/95 integrins are thus up-regulated along with VLA-4 (beta 1, very late antigen) and LPAM-1 (beta 7, murine homing receptor). The leukocytes are arrested as their integrins lock onto immunoglobulins on the endothelial surface: ICAM-1, ICAM-2, VCAM-1 and MadCAM-1. The arrested cells subsequently undergo transmigration between the endothelial cells under the influence of the adhesion proteins described above plus platelet endothelial cell adhesion molecule-1 (PECAM-1), chemoattractant gradients aided by chemoattractant-proteoglycan binding,[126,198,201] and chemotaxins in the wound environment. After entry into the wound, these cells are free to react with matrix proteins, and to stimulate mitogenesis and additional chemotaxis through autocrine and paracrine functions.

The sequence of leukocyte classes recruited into the wound environment is observed to include neutrophils in the first few hours followed by monocytes at 18 hours and T cells at 36 to 48 hours. Sequential changes in the adhesion molecule system are presumably the mechanism of selection and control of specific leukocyte transendothelial migration. Of note is the observation that there are clear differences in adhesion requirements for particular types of inflammation.[6,103,123]

The production of scar through the stimulation of collagen synthesis by connective tissue growth factor (CTGF) in the injured tissue is believed to be coordinated by TGF-β. TGF-β has been called the "conductor of the symphony" of the healing response by Grotendorst.[40,71,86,87,88,95,99] TGF-β stimulates connective tissue cell growth, stimulates extracellular matrix synthesis and modulates the immune response. It acts on both fibroblasts and on smooth muscle cells. It increases messenger RNA (mRNA) for CTGF. CTGF is chemotactic and mitogenic for connective tissue cells and stimulates extracellular matrix production. TGF-β exists in tissue in a latent form, bound by latency-associated peptide (LAP) and latent TGF-β-binding protein (LTBP).[182] Recombinant LAP is a potent inhibitor of TGF-β in vivo and in vitro.[25,26,166] TGF-β exists in several isoforms including several models.[172] Different fibroblasts react differently to TGF-β, emphasizing the fact that all fibroblasts are not the same.[47,155] Work in our laboratory characterizing the differences between ligaments of the knee has clearly shown that ligaments that heal well (medial collateral ligaments) have quite different fibroblastic characteristics than ligaments that fail to heal (anterior cruciate ligaments).[7,65,118,133,168]

TGF-β is overproduced in fibrotic lesions and is a key factor in the pathogenesis of organ fibrogenesis.[4,5,6,94,172,199] Fibrosis resembles normal wound healing, but fails to terminate, leading to replacement of normal tissue with scar. Most fibrotic reactions (lung, heart, vascular system, kidney, liver, skin, brain, gastrointestinal tract, synovial joints) appear secondary to trauma, infection, or inflammation. Studies using immunohistochemical techniques have demonstrated that TGF-β is over produced in areas of chronic fibrosis. As mentioned above, CTGF is induced in fibroblasts by TGF-β and may drive the fibrotic reaction. The reason for the continued scar proliferation is not always clear, but it is possible that some fibroblasts become permanently altered and do not respond appropriately to the usual regulatory controls.[47] TGF-β 3 has been found to inhibit the actions of TGF-β 1 and 2 and may represent a local regulatory control element.[25,172,173] The exaggerated behavior of TGF-β in the fibrotic syndromes has been termed "The Dark Side of TGF-β" in a paper by Border and Roushlati,[24] and termed "The Good, the Bad and the Ugly" by Wahl.[196]

There has also been considerable progress in understanding the structure and function of the special class of mostly post inflammatory secreted peptides called chemokines. The recruitment of leukocytes into injured tissues has been called "the hallmark of inflammation." The nomenclature of the 22 presently known members of this class of peptides has been recently reviewed by Bacon and Schall and by Prieschl et al.[14,147] The term *chemokine* is derived from a combination of the two functional attributes of chemoattractant and cytokine. The group was originally characterized by structural similarity and conservation of four cysteinyl residues not shared with cytokines, but recent isolation of a novel subgroup of chemokines has shown that conservation of the four cysteinyl residues is not required for chemokine function.[97] The three phases of this process: rolling, firm adhesion, and transendothelial migration have been described earlier. Each of these phases are mediated by the interplay of endothelial and leukocyte surface molecule interactions that include the integrin, selectin, and chemokine families of molecules. Chemokines both activate the leukocytes to express adhesion molecules and lead to transendothelial migration via chemotaxis and haptotaxis. The early functional classification of the chemokine superfamily was based on the almost exclusive monocyte-activating effects of the C-C subgroup, which includes the MCP isomer as well as RANTES and a few other C-C chemokines. MCP-1 up-regulates the β2 integrin family important for leukocyte adhesion via CD18/CD11a, b, and c. Chemoattractants are distinguished by certain cell-target specificity.[164,167,174,179,185] Preischl et al speculate that this specificity may explain the predominance of mononuclear cells in hypersensitivity and autoimmune-associated events compared to the primarily neutrophilic infiltrates induced by classical chemoattractants such as C5a and the bacterial N-formyl peptides. The chemokine receptors are of the seven transmembrane serpentine type[15,84,167,174] and are found on most leukocytes. They couple G proteins.

Confusion in chemokine terminology has existed in recent years due to functional-based descriptions versus gene cloning. Present terminology is based on the first two conserved cysteines.[147] The subgroups are designated the CXC branch, the CC branch, the C branch and the fourth subgroup (which is a variant of the CXC branch differing in the three amino acids immediately upstream of the first cysteine residue) called the non-E-L-R-C-X-C subgroup. The CXC branch has also been called the "a" family, PF4 superfamily, or IL-8/NAP family. The CC family has also been called the "β" family or RANTES/sis family. The C branch currently has only one member called lymphotactin whose gene structure is not yet published. The non-E-L-R-C-X-C subfamily consists of IFN-γ-inducible protein-10 (IP-10), platelet factor-4 (PF-4), and mig (the monokine induced by IFN-γ). Space does not allow for detailed discussion of the individual aspects of the biology of each of these chemokines.

The exciting breadth of antifibrotic agents becoming available for research studies on fibrosis inhibition is illustrated by the following examples of neutralizing agents to consider.

Antagonists to TFG-β: mAbs to TFG-β 1,2 blocking peptides to TGF-β 1,2, LAP, TFG-β3 (which neutralizes isoforms 1 and 2), decorin, mannose-6-phosphate, TGF-β antisense nucleotides, nonviral gene therapy, soluble receptors to TGF-β-1,2, and peptidomimetics that react with and block the TGF-B receptors.[190]

Other classes of antifibrotics: these include the interferons, relaxin, certain peptidomimetics (such as RGD peptides or Fn fragments against integrins), certain glycomimetics, mAbs against selectins, lysyl oxidase inhibitors of collagen cross-linking, and collagen prolyl hydroxylase inhibitors, to name just some of the potential candidates. Recently anti-cd44 antibody has been shown to induce cultured fibroblast detachment from substratum and morphological change compatible with apoptosis.[80]

The significance of hyaluronan (hyaluronic acid, [HA]), lies in the need for a safe carrier of the antifibrotics to limit their rapid diffusion away from the local site of application. Further advantages of hyaluronan in this respect reside in its intrinsic anti-inflammatory and antifibrotic properties. High molecular weight (MW) (i.e., Healon MW $3.6 \times 10^6$, 10 mg/ml) and low molecular weight (i.e., ARTZ MW $8 \times 10^6$, 10 mg/ml) hyaluronan have been intensively studied in our laboratories over the past 10 years.[1,10,21,207]

Hyaluronan is a glycosaminoglycin that plays structural and regulatory roles in connective tissue and synovial fluid.[8,18,120] It is a linear single-chain molecule formed from disaccharide units containing N-acetylglucosamine and glucuronic acid. Its macromolecular structure of an inflexible expanded coil allows it to act as a space-occupying molecule in the matrix of connective tissues.[18] HA has been demonstrated to regulate a variety of leukocyte functions.[17,28,61,63,73,143,183] Migration and chemotaxis of inflammatory cells were inhibited in a concentration-dependent manner, but of note the low MW preparations were less effective than the high MW preparations.[28,62,143,181]

High MW HA also inhibited leukocyte, and mononuclear cell phagocytosis[61,73,145,183] adherence,[63] and mitogen-induced proliferation.[79,81] Although the above effects of HA on phagocytic cells was originally attributed to their physical exclusion or entrapment within the extended polymeric HA network,[16,19,197] the finding that oxygen-derived free radicals, generated by the exposure of leukocytes to serum-opsonized zymosan, were inhibited by high ($1.0 \times 10^6$ Da) or low ($0.8 \times 10^6$) MW HA suggested that other mechanisms were operative.[183] A specific membrane receptor for HA has now been identified.[62,73,124,145,183] This glycoprotein belongs to the CD44 adhesion glycoprotein family[46] and would appear to allow HA to modulate some cell functions directly. By modulating inflammatory cell activities, including their release of proinflammatory mediators, cytokines and free radicals, HA could indirectly influence the sensitization of pain receptors in post laminectomy wounds. Direct analgesic effects of HA have also been reported using experimental models of knee pain induced in rates by injection of bradykinin.[69,125]

Synovial cells from osteoarthritic patients were used to examine the in vitro effects of HA on the interleukin-1a (IL-1a)-induced prostaglandin E-2 (PGE-2) production by these cells. The levels of PGE-2 released in response to IL-1a activation was suppressed by HA in a concentration of MW-dependent fashion. HA of MW $2.0 \times 10^6$ was more effective in this regard than an H preparation of $0.3 \times 10^6$.[78,128,187,203,204]

## CLINICAL PRESENTATION

Symptomatic postoperative epidural fibrosis may produce recurrence of radicular symptoms and/or back pain at variable times following surgery. While sciatica in a postoperative patient may represent disk recurrence, perineural fibrosis should also be considered.

The postlaminectomy membrane has also been shown to tether the lumbar nerve roots in the neural foramen. Movements of the lumbar spine that are commonly associated with painless deformation of the lumbar thecal sac may also become tethered in the presence of scarring. Furthermore, the pathologic release of phospholipase A2 may ultimately lead to a chronic inflammatory condition at the surgical site. This inflammation may result in a greater perception of pain by the patient.[153,157] Abitbol et al, describing a new animal model for the study of postlaminectomy scar formation, suggested that fibrosis may increase the vulnerability of nerve roots to compression or tension.[1] Separately, Benoist and coauthors studied a series of patients presenting to their clinic ultimately requiring reoperation for removal of epidural scar and quantified the clinical symptomatology. Of the 38 patients in the series, all of them had sciatic-like pain (37 unilateral and 7 bilateral). Low back pain was a complaint in 28 of the 38 patients, while a positive straight leg raise occurred in 20 of the 38, and lumbar stiffness noted in 17 of the 38. Neurologic dysfunction occurred less frequently.[20]

Other studies have attempted to clinically differentiate patients with postoperative fibrosis, from those with recurrent disk disease. The data from both of these groups were compared with the same variables of patients with primary disk herniations. Pain at rest and night pain were equally common in all patients. Pain with coughing was more common in those with disk herniations, both primary and in addition to those with recurrent disk herniations in the presence of fibrosis. Separately, severe reduction of ambulation was found to be more common in patients with recurrent disks, while regular consumption of analgesics was reportedly more frequent in those with fibrosis.[91]

In addition to the clinical picture outlined above, patients with postoperative chronic back pain with associated epidural fibrosis, often exhibit varying forms of psychological dysfunction. This may vary from psychiatric disorder and maladaptive personalities to narcotic abuse and addiction.[114]

Epidural fibrosis is an inevitable consequence of spinal surgery. Any time spinal surgery is performed and the ligamentum flavum is opened, a variable amount of postoperative epidural scarring can occur. This scarring causes adherence of the dura of the thecal sac and lumbar nerve roots to the surrounding tissues. As a result of this fibrosis subsequent surgery becomes increasingly more technically difficult. The surgical anatomy becomes obscured making the dissection tedious and associated with increased intraoperative problems such as dural tears and nerve root injuries.

In addition to the increased difficulty encountered as a result of postoperative scarring there are numerous reports in the literature suggesting that fibrosis is a major cause of recurrent symptoms, or a failed back syndrome. Early failure of spine surgery characterized by persistent or recurrent pain occurs in up to 20% of patients undergoing laminotomy and diskectomy, long-term failure rates have been reported to approach almost 40%.[33] In 1991 North et al analyzed the 5-year follow-up for 102 patients who underwent repeat lumbosacral surgery at The Johns Hopkins Hospital as well as reviewed eighteen other series of patients who had undergone repeat surgeries (more than 1,000 patients). North concluded that the presence of significant epidural fibrosis was a negative prognostic indicator for patients who underwent repeat lumbosacral surgeries. He observed that those patients whose surgery involved a significant lysis of epidural scar tissue usually had poorer outcomes.[137] Many other observers have reached similar conclusions.[56,92] The association of epidural fibrosis and recurrent pain or failed back syndrome remains controversial.

There is ample clinical evidence that fibrosis may be a major cause of recurrent symptoms when no alternative bony or disk pathology can be found. Ross et al in a prospective, randomized, double blind study sought to correlate recurrent radicular pain and the MRI appearance of postoperative fibrosis. Patients were followed clinically and had MRI imaging at 6 months postoperatively. Patients having extensive peridural scar on MRI imaging were 3.2 times more likely to experience recurrent pain than those patients with less peridural scaring.[156]

A significant amount of literature is available to point out the lack of correlation between the amount of scaring as seen on MRI or CT scan and clinical symptomatology.[12,37] One hundred and fifty-six patients who were treated surgically for herniated lumbar disks were randomly assigned to one of three groups. Group 1 had Gelfoam placed in the postoperative epidural space, group 2 had a free fat graft placed into the postoperative epidural space, and group 3 had nothing placed in the postoperative epidural space and served as controls. These patients were followed prospectively. At 6 months, all patients underwent MRI and at a minimum of 1 year all had clinical follow-up. Thirty-six patients (19%) were unavailable for follow-up. The results indicated that 97% of the patients improved following surgery. They did not demonstrate a statistical difference between the three groups clinically and radiologically. MacKay et al concluded that clinical outcome after lumbar disk surgery does not correlate with the use or type of interpositional membrane used to prevent epidural fibrosis.[116] The study did not indicate if contrast enhanced MRI was utilized for the follow-up study. The addition of contrast may have demonstrated a more significant amount of fibrosis than was observed. The loss of 19% of the initial group may also skew the results as a large percentage of this group may have had poorer results and gone to seek medical attention elsewhere.

Over the years, numerous methods have been tried to reduce or eliminate postoperative epidural fibrosis. The placement of interpositional membranes, applications of topical agents and refinements in surgical techniques all attempted to reduce epidural scarring without any conclusive clinical evidence of success.

## RADIOLOGIC DIAGNOSIS

Increasingly, with the advent of newer radiological techniques, the causes and progress of postoperative epidural fibrosis may further be elucidated. In the immediate postsurgical period, epidural hematomas are commonly seen in asymptomatic patients, seen in either noncontrast CT scans or MRI. The short-term significance of these hematomas remains questionable, because no correlation has been demonstrated between the presence of an immediate postoperative hematoma or outcome in the short term period.[105] However, postoperative epidural fibrosis may result from organization of the extradural hematoma and subsequent possible toxic effects of iron derived from hemoglobin. Therefore, the size of the hematoma may prove to be an important factor in predicting the extent of the postoperative scarring, perhaps long-term outcome of the patient.[90,180,205]

Plain myelography has not been found to be as useful to differentiate scar from recurrent disk herniations.[103] Myelograms evaluate the epidural space indirectly and therefore cannot accurately distinguish between these two entities. The addition of a post-myelogram CT scan also does not appreciably increase its ability to differentiate between epidural fibrosis and recurrent/residual disk material.[37] The nonenhanced CT scan has less than a 60% accuracy rate in differentiating scar from disk. Heilbronner et al concluded that a positive nonenhanced CT scan in patients with failed back syndrome, has limited use.[37,74,77]

In contrast, plain MRI reportedly has an 85% accuracy rate in differentiating disk from scar.[37] The use of gadolinium-diethylenetriaminepentaacetic acid/dymalglumine (Gd-DTPA)-enhanced MRI, is currently felt to have greater than a 95% correlation with surgery, being able to differentiate postoperative scarring from recurrent disk.[57,83] Gd-DTPA rapidly diffuses the extravascular space of epidural scar through "leaky" cellular junctions in areas of endothelial discontinuity resulting in enhancement on MRI. Herniated disk material, being avascular, does not show this early enhancement pattern, but is also encased in an envelope of enhancing scar. However, enhancement of the disk may take place in a delayed fashion secondary to diffusion of contrast material from the adjacent scar tissue. Mass effect and continuity with the disk space, MRI characteristics are more compatible with recurrent disk herniations than scar. Gd-DTPA-enhanced T1-weighted spin echo MRI is the most useful imaging technique to differentiate scar from recurrent disk, as a scar shows heterogeneous enhancement. Potential interpreted difficulties arise from subtle contrast enhancement and distinction of enhancing tissue from epidural fat. Pre- and postcontrast T1 images are usually performed.[83]

The amount of time that has elapsed after surgery affects the Gd-DTPA-enhanced MRI ability to discern scars versus postoperative changes. Van De Kelft et al performed Gd-DTPA-enhanced MRI scans on 34 patients who had good clinical responses to lumbar diskectomy at 6 weeks and again at 6 months. Enhancing epidural scar was observed in all patients 6 weeks postoperatively, with significant anterior scar present in 87% and significant posterior scar present in 80%. At 6 months' time, only 15% of all patients still showed significant epidural enhancement. The conclusion therefore leads us to negate any areas of epidural enhancement for several weeks after surgery, as the majority of these will disappear in time.[194]

Nguyen et al looked at the ability to demonstrate epidural fibrosis using contrast-enhanced MRI techniques in an experimental design using beagle dogs. Their results indicated that epidural scar tissue enhanced more intensely between 2 and 15 minutes after Gd-DTPA administration than between 40 and 60 minutes after contrast administration. Consistently greater scar enhancement was observed when the dose of Gd-DTPA was increased from 0.1 mmol/kg to 0.3 mmol/kg.[129,134] Digitally subtracted contrast-enhanced MRI techniques[131] and fat-suppression techniques[122] did not appear to be useful adjuncts in being able to better differentiate scar from recurrent disk material.

Recently some interest in epidurography has emerged. The filling defects can be seen with a variety of pathologies such as epidural fibrosis, infection, tumor or compression from bony pathology. The addition of postcontrast CT epidurography may allow for more accurate diagnostic interpretation of epidural space pathology.[55,169,188] Devulder et al examined 34 patients using epidurography following three days of epidural treatment for fibrosis. The treatment consisted of hypertonic saline, local anesthetic, and a corticosteroid. Approximately 50% of patients with filling defects had an increase in spread of the epidurally placed contrast. There was however no clinically significant correlation with clinical improvement.[52] Epidural endoscopy allows one to look directly into the epidural space. Furthermore it can be a portal for surgical lysis of adhesions or instillation of therapeutic drugs.[158,159,174]

Positron emission tomography (PET) uses tissue metabolic activity to image internal structures. In the future it may be a useful tool to help determine whether a patient's pain is secondary to fibrosis, which would have a relatively higher metabolic rate, or recurrent disk in which we would expect the metabolic rate to be lower. PET scanning has been used extensively in trying to differentiate residual/recurrent tumor from postoperative or radiation induced changes.[13] The lack of universal availability and the very high cost of the examination at this time preclude its use in this area.

## SCAR PREVENTION: EXPERIMENTAL AND CLINICAL ALTERNATIVES

Since LaRocca and MacNabb's original experiment in 1974, numerous investigators have studied techniques of scar reduction or prevention.[111] The lack of uniformity in reporting the amount of scar formed in response to surgery and many treatment modalities proposed, imposes a significant handicap in being able to compare one study with another. Whereas some of the techniques that have been tried over the years may ultimately prove to be of some benefit, the lack of basic science research in addition to well-designed prospective randomized clinical studies further makes it difficult to advocate one method of scar reduction over another. Finally, the inability to correlate clinical outcome and the presence of substantial postoperative epidural fibrosis suggest that other variables may also be involved.

There are advantages as well as disadvantages of the various methods to reduce postoperative scarring that have been utilized over the years, bearing in mind the limitations outlined previously. The major categories of modalities are interpositional membranes, topical agents, refinements in surgical techniques, and miscellaneous treatment to improve symptoms of scarring.[184]

## INTERPOSITIONAL MEMBRANES

Gelfoam has been used extensively in the epidural space to reduce epidural fibrosis and enhance hemostasis since LaRocca's and MacNabb's 1974 article. These authors performed laminectomies in 18 dogs and placed Gelfoam in the epidural space at one level and Silastic material around the exposed nerve root at the other level. At 3 weeks, the Gelfoam had undergone considerable lysis. At 6 weeks, there was no evidence of any remaining Gelfoam. These investigators concluded that Gelfoam served as a effective barrier to scar invasion. They further observed that the nerve, which was covered by Gelfoam, remained free and mobile in the canal.[111]

In a 1980 publication Yong-Hing et al were unable to reproduce LaRocca's and MacNabb's results and found that Gelfoam was inferior to other materials as a method of reducing postoperative scarring in canine laminectomies.[156] These results were again confirmed by Pospiech et al in 1995 showing Gelfoam to be an inferior method to reduce postoperative fibrosis when compared to other materials.[13] Gelfoam was compared to microfibrillary bovine collagen when placed in the postoperative epidural space in canine laminectomy sites. Gelfoam demonstrated more granulation tissue earlier, which extended into the spinal canal. At 12 and 18 weeks there was a foreign body reaction associated with the Gelfoam, followed by the development of a mature scar, which in some cases contained new bone formation. Animals treated with Avitene showed minimal early granulation reaction, which progressed into a looser fibrous tissue formation than either the control or the Gelfoam-treated dog. Neither material appeared to decrease the formation of scar at the laminectomy site effectively, although the Avitene seemed to be superior to nothing, probably related to its hemostatic properties.[205] Krüger confirmed collagen's superior hemostatic properties compared to Gelfoam in neurosurgical operations.[106] In an experimental study in dogs, testing the efficacy of various types of interpositional membranes postoperative paralysis developed in one dog that had Gelfoam place in the epidural space.[67] Grillo et al reported compression of both the brain and spinal cord as a result of Gelfoam being placed in the postoperative epidural space.[70]

LaRocca and MacNabb also covered the exposed nerve root with a split Silastic tube 1.2 mm in thickness. The roots covered with Silastic remained free and mobile no matter how dense the surrounding scar was. There did not appear to be any adverse effects of the epidurally placed silastic to the nerve root. Electrical stimulation of the covered nerves showed the motor latency and root conduction times to be normal. Microangiographic studies and histological studies did not demonstrate toxic effects to the microvascular bed or myelin sheath. It appears the only reluctance to advocating the use of Silastic was the fact that it was not absorbable.[111] Epidurally placed silicone tubing was found to be superior to fat grafts in protecting against the development of postoperative epidural adhesions in rats.[72] In another investigation, Silastic sheeting was compared to free fat grafts and expanded polytetrafluoroethylene as an interpositional membrane to reduce postoperative epidural scarring in canine laminectomies. Twelve weeks after surgery, dense scarring was seen at all the sites; the scar density at the site treated with polytetrafluoroethylene was noted to be less than with the other materials. The significance of this is uncertain.[53]

In 1978, Field and McHenry described the preliminary results of an implantable silicone device, the lumbar shield, the purpose of which was to: (a) provide a radiopaque marker on the dorsal perimeter of the removed disk so that the presence or absence of a recurrent disk herniation could be seen on plain postoperative x-rays, (b) provide ready access to the operative site in the event of a recurrent disk herniation, (c) prevent postoperative perineural adhesions between the lumbar dural and the nerve root and the partially removed intervertebral disk, and (d) prevent postoperative adhesions between the lumbar dura and the nerve root and the paraspinal muscles. A follow-up report was made in 1980; 123 patients had the lumbar shield implanted. Statistical analysis indicated that at 3 months the recipients of the lumbar shield had less pain. Emphasized was the ease of secondary surgery. Although the preliminary results were encouraging, the lumbar shield never gained universal acceptance in lumbar disk surgery.[58,59]

Silastic implants have been used in neurosurgical procedures for many years as a dural substitute and to cover the edges of bone in craniosynostosis surgery. The material is tolerated by the nervous system without toxic effects. Like any foreign body, there is an increased incidence of infection associated with its use.[118] Epidural catheters are often composed of Silastic material and over the years have not demonstrated any neurotoxicity. In a comparison between silicone epidural catheters and a Hydrogel elastomer blend epidural catheters, the Silastic catheters elicited more of an epidural fibrotic reaction using both histopathology and quantitative imaging methods, indicating that Silastic is not a completely inert material in the epidural space.[44] Silastic gel sheeting has been used with success in the treatment of various types of hypertrophic scars, this type of silicone preparation has not been utilized in the post operative epidural space at this time.[54,66]

Avitene has been used as a hemostatic agent in spine surgery for many years. There has only been one study that has looked at the resulting changes in the epidural space after Avitene has been place in the postoperative epidural space. Jacobs et al felt that Avitene (and Gelfoam) did not appear to control scar tissue formation at the laminectomy site effectively, although its use was seemed superior to no treatment.[90] Avitene is a xenographic implant prepared from purified bovine corium collagen. It is by no means immunologically inert. In a comparative study with other collagen preparations of dermal origin, Avitene was found to be the most immunogenic.[51] There have been reports of severe systemic allergic reactions[100] and foreign body/granulomatous reactions to Avitene in abdominal and gynecological surgeries.[142]

As a preface to his own animal experiments using autogenous fat transplantation to prevent epidural scar formation, Kiviluoto did extensive historical research on the early use of fat transplantation. Experimental fat transplants have been done in animals since the mid-nineteenth century. Autogenous fat transplantation has been used with humans for over 100 years. Transplanted fat had been utilized for a variety of reasons and placed in a number of different locations, including: (a) repair of facial cosmetic deformity (1896), (b) postmastectomy breast augmentation (1895), (c) prevention of postoperative adhesions after peripheral nerve surgery (1913, 1914), (d) prevention of ankylosis after shoulder surgery (1914), (e) as a prosthesis after ocular enucleation (1901), (f) as a cranial dural substitute (1912, 1913), (g) as a method of decreasing surgical bleeding (biliary surgery,1913; renal, hepatic, and lung surgery, 1913). The early histological follow up on these fat transplants indicated that the fat grafts remained viable despite a modest decrease in size.[102]

In his own experimental work Kiviluoto placed epidural fat grafts at 92 sites in rabbits; controls consisted of nothing, surgical gelatin, and cortisone solution. Additionally combinations of fat and gelatin, or fat and cortisone, were used. The animals were sacrificed between 1 and 4 months after surgery at which time both gross and histological examination of the operated levels were performed. Kiviluoto found that all 92 fat grafts that had been placed had a practically normal appearance to them. Giant cells, fibrosis, fat cysts, and cellular infiltration were seen in the marginal parts of the grafts. The transplants had decreased in size, but he did not quantify this variable. The control sites all exhibited abundant scar formation and new bone growth. Cortisone did seem to have some effect on decreasing new bone growth. Kiviluoto went on to conclude that free fat grafts placed on the dura in disk surgery would facilitate a possible reoperation for recurrence.[102] In another experimental design comparing epidurally placed free fat grafts and Vicryl mesh to a control, Akdemir et al found the free fat graft produced the least amount of postoperative epidural fibrosis. They did point out that one of the ten sites to receive the fat graft showed evidence of neural compression from the fat graft.[3] Pospiech et al compared free fat grafts, cellulose mesh, Gelfoam, and triamcinolone suspension to a control consisting of nothing, in their abilities to decrease postoperative scarring. Again, the results of the study revealed that the free fat grafts reduced epidural fibrosis in a higher proportion of the cases, leading the group to conclude that free fat grafts are superior to other materials because of simple operative handling, good comparability, and effective prevention of the laminectomy membrane.[13]

Gill et al tested different materials for their ability to decrease postoperative epidural fibrosis in dogs. The material tested included: Gelfoam, Gelfilm, micropore tape, polyethylene, woven and smooth Silastic, Mylar, and free fat grafts. Like previous investigators, they found the free fat grafts to be superior to the other materials tested. Upon sacrifice of the animals at 12 weeks postoperatively (average) the investigators noted that the free fat grafts recruited a new local blood supply and that portions of the graft showed live fat cells with their nuclei intact. Hoping to improve the function of the graft, the team next used pedicle based fat grafts to cover the exposed nerve root and dura. Flaps averaging 2.5 cm in width by 7.6 cm in length were raised from the deep fascia, brought into the laminotomy site, wrapped around the nerve root, brought out to cover the dura, and than tacked down with a Dexon suture. When the results of the free fat graft were compared to those of the pedicle based graft with 25 animals, the number of excellent results increased from 2 to 9 and the number of failures decreased from 14 to 8. Additionally, with these 25 animals, the laminotomy site remained open (no bony closure) in 19 cases with the pedicle fat graft as compared to 7 with the free fat graft. The team also reported on the use of the pedicle based fat graft in 36 humans, without any operative difficulty. One of these patients needed to be reoperated on for recurrent disk. It was reported that the fat graft was easily stripped away from the dura and that histological examination of a section of the graft confirmed that it contained live fat cells.[67]

A follow-up report of the first 92 patients who had pedicle fat grafts placed by Gill et al was published in 1985. The grafts were placed in the following groups of patients: following primary disk surgery,[37] following reoperation of the multiply operated on low back for scar removal, with radiculopathy,[37] patients with spondylolisthesis who had prior decompression and developed L5 radiculopathy after lateral fusion,[6] spondylolisthesis with primary simple decompression,[3] and following decompression for lumbar spinal stenosis.[9] The results of follow-up 1 to 4 years after surgery were good to excellent in 66% of the reoperated spondylolisthesis group with L5 radiculopathy and the lumbar spinal stenosis group and 99% in the spondylolisthesis group with decompression only.[68] Sakamoto compared pedicle fat grafts to free fat grafts in rats and found that at 2 and 4 weeks after surgery the pedicle fat grafts contained more viable fat cells and were more effective in preventing dural scar formation.[162] Trevor et al came to the conclusion that there was no discernible difference between free fat grafts and pedicle based fat grafts in the healing characteristics after dorsal laminectomy and durotomy in dogs.[189]

Bryant et al reported on their experience using autogenic free fat transplants in 44 consecutive spine operations. There were no postoperative wound infections, one patient developed a sterile seroma at the fat donor site that required surgical intervention, no neurological deterioration was ascribed to the fat graft. The mean follow up in this series was 10.4 months. Grafts over 1 cm in size were able to be identified on follow up CT scans.[30]

The survival of fat grafts has been investigated in several manners. Saunders et al looked at both the survival of autologous fat grafts in mice and epidural fat grafts from humans that had been removed at reoperation up to 22 months after the original operation. In both cases the fat was found to be reduced in size, it underwent an initial breakdown of fat cells, which was followed by revascularization. In the humans, the fat had not been replace by scar tissue.[163] Free fat graft are able to be seen on postoperative CT scans. Several reports follow the fates of these epidurally placed free fat grafts over time and indicate their radiographic persistence on subsequent scans. Langenski and Valle were able to identify on CT scan epidurally placed free fat grafts that had been place on the dura between 15 and 18 years earlier.[49,110,193]

Epidural fat grafts are not without problems. In thin individuals, it is sometimes difficult to harvest local adipose tissue without increasing the size of the incision. We have observed objectionable cosmetic deformities from removing large pieces of fat to cover multilevel laminectomies. Occasionally a blood vessel is cut in the fat donor site, which may prove difficult to coagulate. Anecdotally there appeared to be an increased amount of postoperative seromas developing after fat grafts were harvested. Much more serious neurological complications resulting from migration of the epidurally place fat graft have been reported. Several reports of symptomatic nerve root compression from a surgically placed epidural fat graft have been reported.[35,41] The development of a Cauda equina syndrome following fat graft application has occurred multiple times as reported in the literature.[50,89,119,148,178,186,192] Such a devastating complication makes many spine surgeons very reluctant to utilize these grafts at all. Martin-Ferrer reported on a series of three patients who had had epidural fat grafts placed previously; reoperation in two and follow-up myelography in the third revealed dense fibrotic scar to be present where the fat graft was placed. Histopathological examination of the removed fat at the second operation demonstrated fibrotic infiltration of the fat graft.[117]

Over the years, a number of various membranes have been tried either in clinical studies or in animal research models to inhibit postoperative epidural scar formation. Some of these materials were tried as parts of larger experiments, with many materials being tested simultaneously and have included: bone wax;[90] Vicryl mesh;[3,138] polytetrafluorethylene;[53] ligamentum nuchae;[205] Heparinized Surgicel;[108] polylactic acid, elastase;[121] Gore-Tex;[184] Poloxamer 407;[150] Viscous Carboxymethylcellulose;[101] and various carbohydrate polymers.[152,202] Either for lack of further clinical applications or a result of initial unfavorable findings, none of these materials have made any substantial impact on reducing postoperative scarring.

## TOPICAL MEDICATIONS

In addition to the use of physical barriers to prevent postoperative epidural fibrosis, there have been many topical substances used clinically and experimentally. Unfortunately, the number of well-controlled, randomized clinical studies addressing the use of these topical medications is extremely small. In addition, in reviewing these studies, it is very difficult to correlate clinical outcomes with the degree of scarring seen. Nevertheless, some broad conclusions regarding the efficacy of these medications can be gleaned.

Perhaps the most common topical medication used in the epidural space has been corticosteroids. The first use of corticosteroids in the epidural space was reported in the 1960s and its use as a primary treatment for low back syndromes has undergone over thirty years of waxing and waning popularity. This treatment remains controversial. There have been several controlled studies that have evaluated the use of corticosteroids as an adjunct to open diskectomy procedures. Jacobs et al performed laminectomies in dogs and compared the use of corticosteroids in the laminectomy defects to the use of Gelfoam, fibrillar collagen, bone wax, or control (nothing).[90] Whereas the steroid-treated groups showed a decrease in fibrosis early (6 weeks), by 18 weeks, the findings were similar to the control groups. The authors were concerned about an increase in infection rate, but did not state how many abscesses were encountered as compared to controls. Hinton et al in an animal model for laminectomy (rat) demonstrated that the topical application of dexamethasone decreased the amount of scaring at 4 weeks postoperatively, but not when the steroid was placed in a low dosage, sustained-release polymer.[82] Again, high doses of steroids caused a high incidence of surgical infections. When compared to Jacobs' data, 4 weeks may be too early to correlate with late clinical outcomes.

Clinical data showing the efficacy of steroids is sparse. In a randomized, controlled trial of 84 consecutive patients, Lavyne and Bilsky failed to show any short-term benefit of the epidural instillation of methylprednisolone acetate after microdiskectomy as compared to saline.[112] No increase in morbidity was noted. Davis and Emmons used methylprednisolone acetate in a similar fashion in 43 patients and compared them to a matched cohort. These authors found a significant benefit to the use of steroids in the early postoperative period with decreased pain and need for pain medication. No increase in infection rate was noted. Unfortunately, there has been no randomized, prospective, controlled study evaluating the long-term follow-up of patients receiving epidural steroids intraoperatively either clonically or radiographically with respect to scar formation.[48]

The use of HA has been shown to decrease the degree of scarring in a variety of surgical models. Songer et al treated dogs that underwent a laminectomy and diskectomy with HA in the epidural space. He found that viscous hyaluronate significantly reduced the amount and tenacity of peridural fibrosis when compared to controls. This was shown to be true even anterior to the dura against the annulus fibrosis up to 26 weeks postoperatively.[176,177] Abitbol et al described a new, quantitative method for assessing epidural fibrosis and they too found a substantial decrease in scarring in dogs undergoing laminectomy/diskectomy treated with HA.[1] HA has yet to be evaluated clinically, but it has shown excellent promise in animal models.

As outlined above, many authors feel that the degree of postoperative scarring is directly proportional to the size of the postoperative epidural hematoma. Toward this end, the use of fibrinolytic agents such as urokinase and tissue plasminogen activator (TPA) has been tested in animals.[79,170] Unfortunately, neither of these agents has been able to demonstrate a significant decrease in peridural fibrosis when compared to the use of no medication in dog laminectomy models. In fact, they fared significantly worse than those animals treated with epidural fat grafts.

The use of new carbohydrate polymer gels is receiving attention as barriers to peridural scarring. Early clinical use of one of these products in Europe, ADCON-L, has been encouraging. A preliminary, randomized, controlled trial in laminotomy/diskectomy patients has reported significant decreases in pain scores and increases in activity scores for patients treated with ADCON-L up to six months postoperatively.[144] In eight patients requiring reoperation (4 controls, 4-study group), a significant reduction in epidural fibrosis was observed. Clinical trials in the

U.S. are ongoing and a repeat, randomized, controlled trial is pending.

## SURGICAL TECHNIQUES

Many authors have espoused the theory that surgical technique is the most important variable in the generation of epidural scarring. If one believes that LaRocca's and McNabb's theory of "postlaminectomy membrane" is important, limiting the amount of postoperative bleeding and muscle injury is of paramount importance. The development of microsurgical techniques has allowed surgeons to limit their dissections thereby decreasing postoperative muscle injury and bleeding. Clinical studies have shown that these techniques speed postoperative rehabilitation and lessen short-term postoperative morbidity, but studies of long-term outcomes have yet to show significant clinical differences when compared to traditional laminectomy/diskectomy techniques.[11,191] The microsurgical technique itself has been modified in an attempt to limit postoperative scarring. The preservation and reattachment of the ligamentum flavum ("flavum plasty") is described as a means to decrease invasion of epidural scar. Again, there have been no useful scientific evaluations of this approach when compared to established controls, and certainly no evidence that this technique has any effect on long-term clinical outcomes.

The decompression of neural elements without violating the spinal canal is perhaps the best way to avoid postoperative epidural fibrosis. Percutaneous diskectomy techniques were developed with this as a goal. The first percutaneous technique developed was the use of chymopapain for chemical nucleolysis. As this technique has fallen out of favor in North America, other percutaneous techniques have become popular. These techniques can be broken down into two separate approaches: (1) the removal of disk material from the center of the disk thereby achieving intradiscal decompression (automated percutaneous lumbar diskectomy [APLD]), or (2) the selective removal of nuclear material from the herniation using endoscopic control. The vast majority of the clinical literature regarding percutaneous techniques consists of retrospective, uncontrolled series of patients and case reports. One of the few randomized, controlled studies performed was by Chatterjee et al, who studied 71 patients randomized to receive APLD or microdiskectomy for contained disk herniations. Satisfactory outcomes were found in 29% of the APLD group and in 80% of the open microdiskectomy group.[38] These results are in stark contrast to the literally hundreds of uncontrolled series of APLD patients who uniformly have 80% to 90% satisfactory results. Several reports describe the postoperative MRI appearance of patients who underwent percutaneous diskectomies. Kotilainen, et al scanned 41 patients on the first postoperative day and then again 6 months later. Postoperative fibrosis presented in 53% of patients (64% of the microdiskectomy patients and 44% of the percutaneously treated patients). The amount of scarring at 6 months had a strong correlation to the amount of epidural hemorrhage initially. Most importantly, the degree of scarring had no correlation to the eventual clinical result. It is very interesting to point out that scarring presented anterior to the dura in the percutaneously treated patients, though the intraspinal space is not violated. We must point out that scarring is part of the "normal" reparative process seen in the healing of disk herniations that have not be violated surgically.[132,154]

Finally, the effects of chymopapain treatment of lumbar herniated disks should be mentioned. Over the past 40 years, extensive clinical experience with this approach has been gained, mostly in Europe. After the Food and Drug Administration released the drug for general use in 1982, use of this technique had all but vanished in this country, mainly because of the publicity surrounding anaphylactic reactions to the drug. Mortality associated with this procedure due to all causes was estimated at .022% and anaphylaxis incidence estimated at 0.5%.[2] Nordby and Wright reviewed the literature and found overall success rates with chymopapain to be 76% as compared to 88% for open surgery.[135] Concern over postoperative epidural scarring to the chymopapain itself has been unfounded, with experimental studies showing that direct epidural instillation of chymopapain does not induce scarring.[130,171] In addition, because it is a percutaneous technique, intraspinal trauma and bleeding are minimized, thereby decreasing epidural scarring when compared to open procedures.

## ADJUNCT METHODS TO TREAT EPIDURAL FIBROSIS

As evident by the previous discussions, there has not been any one method that has predictably been able to reduce postoperative epidural fibrosis. Over the years, various methods have been tried to treat the resulting symptoms of postoperative epidural fibrosis, the failed back syndrome. Reoperation primarily for the excision of epidural keloids or surgery where no other etiology for recurrent/residual pain can be found other than fibrosis, have a poor prognosis for improvement of pain.[20,64] Anecdotally, many surgeons apply topical steroid preparations at reoperation for its adhesiolysis properties, in an attempt to limit the development of additional scar and for postoperative comfort from operative nerve root manipulation. No studies to date have looked at the use of topical steroids specifically in reoperation.

In an experimental design, Colak et al pointed out that use of $CO_2$ laser on epidural fibrosis in the guinea pig resulted in a decreased amount of scaring three months after the laser treatment.[42] The use of the laser in the treatment of epidural keloids has not been addressed in humans.

The evolution of the interventional pain specialists has resulted in the development of different treatments for the pain syndromes that result from postoperative epidural fibrosis. Routine epidural steroid injections have been used for a considerable period of time, with marginal success in this clinical setting. More invasive catheter techniques of epidural lysis of adhesions using combinations of steroids, hypertonic saline, local anesthetics and/or hyaluronidase—sometimes incorporating "forceful" injections into the epidural space—have been advocated by the pain specialists. The caudal route is the preferred method for entering the epidural space. A catheter is inserted in the epidural space and the epidurography is performed to assess the amount of epidural scaring present. There are a variety of techniques that have been employed to try to treat epidural fibrosis once the catheter has been placed utilizing different combinations of the above mentioned drugs. Monitoring the success of treatment with sequential epidurograms has been suggested by some. Comparative and randomized studies have shown the benefits of differing combinations of medications in the hands of different examiners. These treatments are often multiple, sometimes with an indwelling epidural catheter, which would require hospitalization for the duration of treatment.[52,149,151] In Racz's series of 1,500 patients who underwent epidural adhesiolysis, depending upon the type of treatment given, 12% to 14% of patients received persistent relief of symptoms, 68% to 81% received partial improvement, and 6% to 18% had no relief.[52]

The symptoms that are a result of postoperative epidural fibrosis, both axial back pain and radicular pain can be treated indirectly utilizing implanted devices, both epidural spinal cord stimulators (SCS) and pumps to deliver intrathecal analgesics. For those patients who have continued complaints after surgery for which no structural reasons such as recurrent disk, stenosis, or instability are found, these procedures may afford considerable relief of symptoms. Trials of epidural stimulation or of intrathecal analgesics are done prior to the implantation of the device. Only those patients who have a positive trial with a reduction in pain of at least 50% should be considered for implantation.

Fiume et al looked at the results of 34 SCS that were implanted in patients with lumbosacral fibrosis over a 4-year period. The mean follow-up was 55 months. Patients who reported at least a 50% pain relief and satisfaction were regarded as successful, and 56% of the patients fell into that category. Ten patients (29%) returned to work. The data collected by Fiume et al led them to consider the SCS as a first choice treatment in failed back syndrome due to lumbosacral fibrosis.[60]

LeDoux and Langford found that in 26 patients with failed back syndrome secondary to fibrosis, 76% of patients at one year and 74% of patients at two years were receiving 50% or greater pain relief. (Nineteen of the original 26 patients still had the SCS implanted at 2 years.)[113] North and Kidd report success rates of 53%, 47%, and 52% at mean follow up of 2.2, 5 and 7.1 years, respectively.[136] Other investigators have found similar results using the SCS for the relief of pain in patients with epidural fibrosis.[31,109]

Intrathecal devices that deliver opiates are used extensively in the treatment of cancer pain. More recently, researchers have tried using morphine pumps in treating chronic pain from failed back syndrome. Carey et al followed 11 patients who had morphine pumps implanted for failed back syndrome type pain. At 3 years' follow-up, 8 (73%) of the patients were still getting excellent pain relief from the pump. There is considerable reluctance to use implantable morphine pumps in pain of nonmalignant origin, however Carey et al concluded that the device should be considered in the treatment options for these patients.[36]

Kanoff's results of the morphine pump in 15 patients being treated for intractable pain from reflex sympathetic dystrophy and postoperative arachnoiditis were that pain relief was reported as excellent in 8 patients, good in 3, and fair in 4. Six patients returned to work. Kanoff noted that few complications occurred, although he did point out that most patients required increasing doses of morphine over time to maintain pain relief.[93] Hassenbusch et al suggested that Clonidine may be an alternative to high-dose morphine.[75]

Yoshida et al, on the other hand, felt that intraspinal narcotic analgesia should not be used for the long-term management of chronic pain from nonmalignant causes. In their series of 18 patients who had morphine pumps implanted, only 4 patients (25%) at 2 years had objective evidence of benefit from the procedure. Patients with implanted morphine pumps had an average of 1.4 additional surgeries or hospitalizations after the initial pump insertion.[200]

## REFERENCES


1. Abitbol JJ, Lincoln TL, Lind BI, Amiel D, Akeson WH, Garfin SR: Preventing post-laminectomy adhesion: a new experimental model, NASS/AcroMed Manuscript Award, *Spine* 19(16):1809-1814, 1994.
2. Agre K, Wilson RR, Brim M, McDermott DJ: Chymodiactin post-marketing surveillance: demographic and adverse experience data in 29,075 patients, *Spine* 9:479, 1984.
3. Akdemir H, Pacsaoglu, Selçuklu A, Oztürk J, Kurstoy A: Prevention of adhesions after laminectomy: an experimental study in dogs, *Res Exp Med Berl* 193(1):39-46, 1993.
4. Akenson WH: Anti-adhesion therapy; regulation of adhesion molecule expression; peptidomimetic and glycomimetic rational design; anti-fibrotic therapy of reperfusion injury, Cambridge Health Institute Third Annual Conference on Cell Adhesion and Inflammation, San Diego, April 29-30, 1996.
5. Akenson WH: Biological mechanisms of fibrosis; new animal models of fibrosis; chronic fibrotic diseases; novel therapeutics intervention, IBC International Conference on Therapeutic Advances in Fibrosis, Washington, DC, April 18-19, 1996.
6. Albelda SM, Smith CW, Ward PA: Adhesion molecules and inflammatory injury, *FASEB J* 8:504-512, 1994.
7. Amiel D, Kuiper SD, Wallace CD, Harwood FL, VandeBerg JS: Age related properties of medial collateral ligament and anterior cruciate ligament: a morphologic and collagen maturation study in the rabbit, *J Gerontol* 46:B159-165, 1991.
8. Amiel D, Frey C, Wood SL-Y, Harwood F, Akeson WH: Value of hyaluronic acid in the prevention of contracture formation, *Clin Orthop* 196:15-25, 1985.
9. Amiel D, Harwood FL, Gelberman RH, Chu CR, Seller JG III, Abrahamsson S: Autogenous intrasynovial and extrasynovial tendon grafts: an experimental study of Pro l(l) collagen mRNA expression in dogs, *J Orthop Res* 13:459-463, 1995.
10. Amiel D, Ishizue K, Billings E Jr, Wiig M, Gelberman R, VandeBerg J, Akeson WH: Hyaluronan in flexor tendon repair, *J Hand Surg* 14A-837-844, 1989.
11. Andrews DW, Lavyne MH: Retrospective analysis of microsurgical and standard lumbar discectomy, *Spine* 15:329-335, 1990.
12. Annertz M, Jonsson B, Stromqvist B, Holtas S: No relationship between epidural fibrosis and sciatica in the lumbar postdiscectomy syndrome. A study with contrast-enhanced magnetic resonance imaging in symptomatic and asymptomatic patients, *Spine* 20(4): 449-453, 1995.
13. Austin JR, Wong FC, Kim EE: Positron emission tomography in the detection of residual laryngeal carcinoma, *Otolaryngol Head Neck Surg*: 113:404-7, 1995.
14. Bacon KB, Schall TJ: Chemokines as mediators of allergic inflammation, *Int Arch Allergy Immunol:* 109:97-109, 1996.
15. Baggiolini M, Dewald B, Moser B: Interleukin-8 and related chemotactic cytokines-CXC and CC chemokines, *Adv Immunol* 55:97-179, 1994.
16. Balazs EA, Denlinger JL: *Clinical uses of hyaluronan.* In Evered D, Whelan S, editors: *The biology of hyaluronan.* John Wiley (Ciba Found Symp No 143) 265-285, 1989.
17. Balazs EA, Jacobson B: In Balazs EA, Jeanio RW, editors: *The amino sugars: The chemistry and biology of compounds containing amino sugars,* vol. 11B, NY and London, 1966, Academic Press, p 386.
18. Balazs EA, Darzynkiewiz Z: *The effect of hyaluronic acid on fibroblasts, mononuclear phagocytes and lymphocytes.* In Kulonen E, Pikkaraihen J, editors: *Biology of the fibroblast.* London, NY, 1973, Academic Press, pp 237-262.
19. Balazs EA, Denlinger JL: Sodium hyaluronate and joint function, *Equine Vet Sci* 5:217-228, 1985.
20. Benoist M, Ficat C, Baraf P, Cauchoix J: Post operative lumbar epiduro-arachnoiditis (diagnostic and therapeutic aspects), *Spine:* 5(3) 432-436, 1980.
21. Berry S, Lee J, Green MH, Amiel D: Hyaluronan: a potential carrier for growth factors for the healing of ligamentous tissues. Wound Healing Soc Mtg, San Francisco, May 18-21, 1994. Abstract 4. *Wound Repair and Regeneration* 2(1):73, 1994.
22. Boot DA, Hughes SPF. The prevention of adhesion after laminectomy, *Clin Orthop* 215:296-302, 1987.
23. Border WA, Noble NA, Yamamoto T, Tomooka S, Kagami S: Antagonists to TGF-β: a novel approach to treatment of glomerulonephritis and prevention of glomerulosclerosis, *Kidney Int* 41:566-570, 1992.
24. Border WA, Ruoslahti E: Transforming growth factor —in disease: the dark side of tissue repair, *J Clin Invest* 90:1-7, 1992.
25. Bottinger EP, Factor VM, Tsang M L-S, Weatherbee JA, Kopp JB, Qian SW, Wakenfield LM, Roberts AB, Thorgeirsson SS, Spom MB: The recombinant proregion of transforming growth factor-β1 (latency-associated peptide) inhibits active transforming growth factor-β1 in transgenic mice, *Proc Natl Acad Sci USA* 93:5877-5882, 1996.
26. Bottinger E: *TGF-β: A therapeutic challenge in fibrosis.* In IBC International Conference on Therapeutic Advances in Fibrosis, April 18-19, 1996, Renaissance Washington DC Hotel, Washington DC.
27. Braide M, Bjursten LM: Optimized density gradient separation of leukocyte fractions from whole blood by adjustment of osmolarity, *J Immunol Methods* 93:183-191, 1986.
28. Brandt KD: The effect of synovial hyaluronate on the ingestion of monosodium urate crystals by leukocytes, *Clin Chim Acct* 55:307-315, 1974.
29. Brown Z, Gerristen ME, Carley WW, Strieter RM,

Kunkel SL, Westwick J: Chemokine gene expression and secretion by cytokine-activated human microvascular endothelial cells—differential regulation of monocyte chemoattractant protein-1 and interleukin-8 in response to interferon, *Am J Pathol* 45:913-921, 1994.

30. Bryant MS, Bremer AM, Nguyen TQ: Autogenic fat transplants in the epidural space in routine lumbar spine surgery, *Neurosurgery* 13(4):367-370, 1983.
31. Burchiel KJ, Anderson VC, Brown FD, Fessler RG, Friedman WA, Pelofsky S, Weiner RL, Oakley J, Shatin D: Prospective, multicenter study of spinal cord stimulation for relief of chronic back and extremity pain, *Spine* 21(23):2786-2794, 1997.
32. Burton CV, Kirkaldy-Willis WH, Yong-Hing K, Heithoff KB: Causes of failure of surgery on the lumbar spine, *Clin Orthop* 157:191-199, 1981.
33. Burton CV: Lumbosacral arachnoiditis, *Spine* 3:24-30, 1978.
34. Butcher EC: Leukocyte endothelial cell recognition: three (or more) steps to specificity and diversity, *Cell* 67:1033-1036, 1991.
35. Cabezudo JM, Lopez A, Bacci F: Symptomatic root compression by a free fat transplant after hemilaminectomy, *J Neurosurg* 63:633-635, 1985.
36. Carey M, Gould H, Angel I: Intrathecal morphine pump as a treatment option in chronic pain of nonmalignant origin. Paper presented at The Congress of Neurological Surgeons, September 1996.
37. Cervellini P, Curri D, Volpin L, Bernardi L, Pinna V, Benedetti A: Computed tomography of epidural fibrosis after discectomy: a comparison between symptomatic and asymptomatic patients, *Neurosurgery* 23(6): 710-713, 1988.
38. Chatterjee S, Foy PM, Findlay GF: Report of a controlled clinical trial comparing automated percutaneous lumbar discectomy and microdiscectomy in the treatment of contained lumbar disc herniations, *Spine* 20(6):734-738, 1995.
39. Chen PQ, Yang C-Y, Su C-J, Lee F: Prevention of post-laminectomy membrane: experimental and clinical observations, *J Formosan Med Assoc* 88:57-61, 1989.
40. Chomczynski P, Sachi N: Single step method of rna isolation by acid guanidinium thiocyanate-phenol-chloroform extraction, *Anal Biochem* 162:156-159, 1987.
41. Cobanoíglu S, Imer M, Ozylmaz F, Memis M, Complication of epidural fat graft in lumbar spine: case report, *Surg Neurol* 44(5) 479-481,1995.
42. Colak A, Bavbek M, Aydin NE, Renda N Acikgíoz B: Effect of $CO_2$ laser on spinal epidural fibrosis, *Acta Neurochir Wein* 138(2):162-166, 1996.
43. Collins T: Adhesion molecules in leukocyte emigration, *Sci Am Sci Med* Nov/Dec:28-37, 1995.
44. Coombs DW, Colburn RW, DeLeo JA, Hoopes PJ, Twitchell BB: Comparative histopathology of epidural hydrogel and silicone elastomer catheters following 30 and 180 implant in the ewe, *Acta Anaesthesiol Scand* 38(4), 388-395, 1994.
45. Cooper RG, Mitchell WS, Illingworth KJ, Forbes WS, Gillespie JE, Jayson MI: The role of epidural fibrosis and defective fibrinolysis in the persistence of postlaminectomy back pain, *Spine:* 16(9):1044-1048, 1991.
46. Culty M, Miyake K, Kincade PW, Silorski E, Butcher EC, Underhil C: The hyaluronate receptor is a member of the cd44 (hcam) family of cell surface glycoproteins, *J Cell Biol* 111:2765-2774, 1990.
47. Davidson JM: *Cell biology of tissue repair and fibrosis.* In IBC International Conference on Therapeutic Advances in Fibrosis.
48. Davis R, Emmons SE: Benefits of epidural methylprednisolone in a unilateral lumbar discectomy: a matched controlled study, *J Spinal Disord* 3(4):299-306, 1990.
49. Deburge A, Benoist M, Lassale B, Blamoutier A, [The Fate of Fat Grafts Used in Surgery of the Lumbar Spine], *Rev Chir Orthop* 74(3):238-242, 1988.
50. Deburge A, Bitan F, Lassale B, Vaquin G: [Cauda Equina Syndrome Caused by Migration of a Fat Graft after Laminoarthrectomy], *Rev Chir Orthop* 74(7): 677-678, 1988.
51. DeLustro F, Condell RA, Nguyen MA, McPherson JM: A comparative study of the biological and immunological response to medical devices derived from dermal collagen, *J Biomed Mater Res* 20(1):109-120, 1986.
52. Devulder J, Bogaert L, Castille F, Moerman A, Rolly G: Relevance of epidurography and epidural adhesiolysis in chronic failed back surgery patients, *Clin J Pain* 11(2):147-150, 1995.
53. Difazio FA, Nichols JB, Pope MH, Frymoyer JW: The expanded polytetrafluoroethylene as an interpositional membrane after lumbar laminectomy, *Spine* 20(9):986-991, 1995.
54. Dockery GL, Nilson RZ: Treatment of hypotrophic and keloid scars with silastic gel sheeting, *J Foot Ankle Surg* 33(2):110-119, 1994.
55. Du Pen SL, Williams AR, Feldman RK: Epidurograms in the management of patients with long-term catheters, *Reg Anesth* 21(1):61-67, 1996.
56. Ebeling U, Kalbracyk H, Reulen HJ: Microsurgical reoperation following lumbar disc surgery. Timing, surgical findings and outcomes in 92 patients, *J Neurosurg* 70(3):397-404,1989.
57. Fan YF, Chong VF: MRI findings in failed back surgery syndrome. *Med J Malaysia* 50(1):76-81, 1995.
58. Field JR, McHenry H: The lumbar shield: a preliminary report, *Neurosurgery* 3(1):26-36, 1978.
59. Field JR, McHenry H: The lumbar shield: a progress report, *Spine* 5(3):264-278, 1980.
60. Fiume D, Sherkat S, Callovini GM, Parzizle G, Gazzeri G: Treatment of the failed back surgery syn-

drome due to lumbo-sacral epidural fibrosis, *Acta Neurochir Wein* 64(suppl):116-118, 1995.

61. Forrester JV, Balazs EA: Inhibition of phagocytosis by high molecular weight hyaluronate, *Immunology* 40: 435-436, 1980.
62. Forrester JV, Lackie JM: Effect of hyaluronic acid on neutrophil adhesion, *J Cell Sci* 50:329-344, 1981.
63. Forrester JV, Wilkinson PC: Inhibition of leukocyte locomotion by hyaluronic acid, *J Cell Sci* 48:315-331, 1981.
64. Fritsch EW, Heisel J, Rupp S: The failed back surgery syndrome reasons, intraoperative findings and long-term results: a report of 182 operative treatments, *Spine* 21(5):626-633, 1996.
65. Geiger MH, Amiel D, Green MH, Most D, Berchuck M, Akeson WH: Rates of migration of ACL and MCL derived fibroblasts, *Orthop Trans* 16: 409, 1992.
66. Gibbons M, Zucker R, Brown, Candlish S, Snider L, Zimmer P: Experience with Silastic gel sheeting in pediatric scarring, *J Burn Care Rehab* 15(1):69-73, 1994.
67. Gill GG, Sakovitch L, Thompson E: Pedicle fat grafts for prevention of scar formation after laminectomy, *Spine* 4:176-186, 1979.
68. Gill GG, Scheck M, Kelley ET, Rodrigo JJ: Pedicle fat grafts for the prevention of scar in low-back surgery. a preliminary report on the first 92 cases, *Spine* 10(7):662-667, 1985.
69. Gotoh S, Miyazaki K, Onaya J, Sakamoto T, Toku-Yasu K, Namiki O: Experimental knee pain model in rats and analgesic effect of sodium hyaluronate (PH), *Folia Pharm Japanica* 92:17-27, 1988.
70. Grillo HC, Riseborough EJ, Rich JC Jr: Compression of the brain and spinal cord following the use of Gelfoam, *Arch Surg* 104(1):107, 1972.
71. Grotendorst GR: Connective tissue growth factor as a mediator of fibrosis. In IBC International Conference on Therapeutic Advances in Fibrosis, April 18-19, 1996, Renaissance Washington DC Hotel, Washington, DC.
72. Hadani M, Ram Z, Horowitz A, Shacked I: Silicon prevents post laminectomy epidural root adhesions. an experimental study in rats, *Acta Neurochir Wien* 123(3-4):153-156, 1993.
73. Hakansson L, Hallgren R, Venge P: Regulation of granulocyte function of hyaluronic acid in vitro and in vivo effects on phagocytosis, locomotion, and metabolism, *J Clin Invest* 66:298-305, 1980.
74. Hashizume H, Tamaki T, Kawakami M, Nish H, Senba E, Danjo S: Nitric oxide in herniated lumbar discs. In Final Programme and Abstracts SIROT 96, 7th World Congress Societe Internationale de Recherche Orthopedique et de Traumatologie, page 359.
75. Hassenbusch SJ, Stanton-Hicks M, Covington EC: Spinal cord stimulation versus spinal infusion for low back and leg pain, *Acta Neurochir Wein* 64(suppl):109-115, 1995.
76. He Y, Revel M, Lotoy B: A quantitative model of post laminectomy scar formation, *Spine* 20:557-563, 1995.
77. Heilbronner R, Fanlhauser H, Schnyder P, de Tribolet N: Computed tomography of the postoperative intervertebral disc and lumbar spinal canal: serial long-term investigation in 19 patients after successful operation for lumbar disc herniation, *Neurosurgery* 29: 1-7, 1991.
78. Heinrich JN, Bravo R: The orphan mouse receptor interleukin(il)-βrb binds N51, *J Biol Chem* 270:4987-4989, 1995.
79. Henderson R, Weir B, Davis L, Mielke B, Grace M: Attempted experimental modification of the post-laminectomy membrane by local instillation of recombinant tissue-plasminogen activator gel, *Spine* 18(10):1268-1272, 1993.
80. Henke C, Bitterman P, Roogta U, Ingbar D, Polunovky V: Induction of fibroblast apoptosis by anti-cd44 antibody: implications for the treatment of fibroproliferative lung disease, *Am J Pathol* 149: 16339-16350, 1996.
81. Hills BA, Butler BD: Surfactants identified in synovial fluid and their ability to act as boundary lubricants, *Ann Rheum Dis* 43:641-648, 1984.
82. Hinton JL, Warejcka DJ, Mei Y, McLendon RE, Laurencin C, Lucas PA, Robinson JS Jr: Inhibition of epidural scar formation after lumbar laminectomy in the rat, *Spine* 20:564-570, 1995.
83. Hueftle MG, Modic MT, Ross JS et al: Lumbar spine: postoperative MR imaging with gadolinium-DTPA, *Radiology* 167: 817-824,1988.
84. Hurwitz AA, LymanWD, Berman JW: Tumor-necrosis factor and transforming growth factor up-regulate astrocyte expression of monocyte chemoattractant protein-1, *J Neuroimmunol* 57:193-198, 1995.
85. Hutadilok N: Studies on the synthesis and degradation of hyaluronan. PhD Thesis. Univ of Sydney, Sydney, Australia, 1990.
86. Igarashi A, Nashiro K, Kikuchi K, Sato S, Inh H, Grotendorst GR, Takehara K: Significant correlation between connective tissue growth factor gene expression and skin sclerosis in tissue section from patients with systemic sclerosis, *J Invest Derm* 105:280-285, 1995.
87. Igarashi A, Okoch H, Bradham DM, Grotendorst GR: Regulation of connective tissue growth factor gene expression in human skin fibroblasts and during wound repair, *Mol Biol Cell* 4:637-645, 1993.
88. Igarashi A, Nashiro K, Kikuchi K, Sato S, Ihn H, Fujimoto MO, Grotendorst GR, Takehara K: Connective tissue growth factor gene expression in tissue sections from localized sclerodern, keloid, and other fibrotic skin disorders, *J Invest Derm* 106:729-733, 1996.

89. Israel Z, Constantini S: Compressive epidural autologous fat graft in a patient with failed back syndrome: case report, *J Spinal Disord* 8(3):240-242, 1995.
90. Jacobs RR, McClain O, Neff J: Control of post laminectomy scar formation. An experimental and clinical study, *Spine* 5:223-229, 1980.
91. Jonsson B, Stromqvist B: Clinical characteristic of recurrent sciatica after lumbar discectomy, *Spine* 21(4):500-505, 1996.
92. Jonsson B, Stromqvist B: Repeat decompression of lumbar nerve roots. A prospective two-year evaluation, *J Bone Joint Surg Br* 75(6):894-897, 1993.
93. Kanoff RB: Intraspinal delivery of opiates by an implantable, programmable pump in patients with chronic intractable pain of nonmalignant origin, *J Am Osteopath Assoc* 94(6):487-493, 1994.
94. Kavanaugh A, Heudebert G, Cush J, Jain R: Cost Evaluation of Novel Therapeutics in Rheumatoid Arthritis (CENTRA), *Semin Arth Rheum* 25:1-12, 1995.
95. Kawakami M, Tamari T, Hishizume H: *Pathomechanisms of radicular pain secondary to intervertebral disc herniation.* In Final Programme and Abstracts SIROT 96, 7th World Congress Societe Internationale de Recherche Orthopedique et de Traumatologie, page 56.
96. Keller JT, Dunsker SB, McWhorter JM, Ongkiko CM, Saunders MC, Mayfield FH: The fate of autogenous grafts to the spinal dura, *J Neurosurg* 49:412-418, 1978.
97. Kelner GS, Kennedy J, Bacon KB, Kleyensteuber S, Lagaespada DA, Jenkins A, Copeland NG, Bazan JF, Moore KW, Schall TJ, Zlotnik A: Lymphotactin: a cytokine that represents a new class of chemokine, *Science* 266:1395, 1994.
98. Key JT, Ford LT: Experimental intervertebral-disc lesions, *J Bone Joint Surg* 30A:621-630, 1948.
99. Kikuchi K, Kadono T, Inh H, Sato S, Igarashi A, Nakagawa H, Tamari K, Takehara K: Growth regulation in scleroderma fibroblasts: increased response to transforming growth factor-1, *J Invest Derm* 105:128-132, 1995.
100. Kitamura K, Yasuoka R, Ohara M, Shimotsuma M, Hagiwara A, Yamane T, Yamaguchi T, Takahashi T: How safe are the xenogenic hemostats?—report of a case of sever systemic allergic reaction, *Surg Today* 25(5):433-435, 1995.
101. Kitano T, Zerwekh JE, Edwards MS, Usui Y, Allen MD: Viscous carboxymethylcellulose in the prevention of epidural scar formation, *Spine* 16(7):820-823, 1991.
102. Kiviluoto O: Use of free fat transplants to prevent epidural scar formation, *Acta Orthop Scand* 164(suppl): 3-75, 1976.
103. Knutsson F: The myelogram following operation for herniated disc, *Acta Radiology* 32:60-65, 1949.
104. Kotilainen E, Alanen A, Erkinatalo M, Valtonen S, Kormano M: Magnetic resonance image changes and clinical outcome after microdiscectomy or nucleotomy for ruptured disc, *Spine* 41: 432-440, 1994.
105. Kotilainen E, Anu A, Erkiatalo M, Helenius H, Simo V: Postoperative hematomas after successful lumbar microdiscectomy or percutaneous nucleotomy: a magnetic resonance imaging study, *Surg Neurol* 41:98-105, 1994.
106. Krüger J: [Hemostasis in neurosurgical operations. a comparative study between collagen fleece (Lyostat) and gelatin sponge (Marbagelan)], *Zentralbl Neurochir* 53(1):33-36, 1992.
107. Kudo C, Araki A, Matsuchima K, Sendo F: Inhibition of IL-8-induced W3/25 + (CD4+) T lymphocyte recruitment into subcutaneous tissue of rats by selective depletion of in vivo neutrophils with a monoclonal antibody, *J Immunol* 147:2196-2201, 1991.
108. Kuivila T, Berry JL, Bell GR, Steffee AD: Heparinized materials for control of the formation of the laminectomy membrane in experimental laminectomies in dogs, *Clin Orthop* 236:166-174, 1988.
109. Kumar K, Nath R, Wyant GM: Treatment of chronic pain by epidural spinal cord stimulation: a 10 year experience, *J Neurosurg* 75(3):402-407, 1991.
110. Langenskiöld A, Valle M: Epidurally placed free fat grafts visualized by CT scanning 15-18 years after discectomy, *Spine* 10(1):7-8, 1985.
111. LaRocca H, McNabb I. The laminectomy membrane. Studies in its evolution, characteristics, affects, and prophylaxis in dogs, *J Bone Joint Surg Br* 56:545-550, 1974.
112. Lavyne MH, Bilsky MH: Epidural steroids, postoperative morbidity and recovery in patients undergoing microsurgical lumbar discectomy, *J Neurosurg* 77(1): 90-95, 1992.
113. LeDoux MS, Langford KH: Spinal cord stimulation for the failed back syndrome, *Spine* 18(2):191-194, 1993.
114. Long DM, Filtzer DL, BenDebba M, Hendler NH: Clinical features of the failed-back syndrome, *J Neurosurg* 69(1):61-71, 1988.
115. Lou Z, Harada T, London S, Gajdusek C, Mayberg MR: Antioxidant and iron-chelating agents in cerebral vasospasm, *Neurosurgery:* 37(6):1154-1158, 1995.
116. Mackay MA, Fischgrund JS, Herkowitz LY, Hecht B, Schwartz M: The effect of interposition membrane on the outcome of lumbar laminectomy and discectomy, *Spine* 20(16):1793-1796, 1995.
117. Martrin-Ferrer S: Failure of autologous fat grafts to prevent postoperative epidural fibrosis in surgery of the lumbar spine, *Neurosurgery* 24(5):718-721, 1989.
118. Matson DP: *Neurosurgery of infancy and childhood,* ed 2, 1969, Charles C. Thomas Publisher, pp 122-167.
119. Mayer PJ, Jacobsen FS: Cauda equina syndrome after surgical treatment of lumbar spinal stenosis with application of free autogenous fat graft: A report of two cases, *J Bone Joint Surg Am* 71(7):1090-1093, 1989.
120. McGregor DH, MacArthur RI, Carter T: Avitene

granulomas of colonic serosa, *Ann Clin Lab Sci* 16(4): 296-302, 1986.

121. Mikawa Y, Hamagami H, Shikata J, Higashi S, Yamamuro T, Suong-Hyu H, Ikada Y: An experimental study on prevention of postlaminectomy scar formation by the use of new materials, *Spine* 11(8): 843-846, 1986.
122. Mirowitz SA, Shady KL: Gadopentetate dimeglumine-enhanced MR imaging of the postoperative lumbar spine: comparison of fat-suppressed and conventional T1-weighted images, *AJR Am J Roentgenol* 159:385-389, 1992.
123. Miyahara K, Ishida T, Hukuda S, Tojo H: Group II phospholipase A2 in human intervertebal discs. In Final Programme and Abstracts SIROT 96, 7th World Congress Societe Internationale de Recherche Orthopedique et de Traumatologie, p 365.
124. Miyake K, Underhill CB, Lesley J, Kincade PW: Hyaluronate can function as a cell adhesion molecule and cd44 participates in hyaluronate recognition, *J Exp Med* 172:69-75, 1990.
125. Miyazaki K, Goto S, Okawara H, et al: Sodium hyaluronate (SPH): studies on analgesic and anti-inflammatory effects of sodium hyaluronate (SPH), *Pharmacometrics* 28:1123-1135, 1984.
126. Muller WA, Weigl SA, Deng X, Philips DM: PECAM-1 is required for transendothelial migration of leukocytes, *J Exp Med* 178:449-460, 1993.
127. Mulligan MS, Jones ML, Bolaanowski MA, Baganoff MP, Deppeler CL, Meyers DM, Ryan US, Ward PA: Inhibition of lung inflammatory reactions in rats by an anti-human IL-8, *J Immunol* 150(12):5585-5595, 1993.
128. Mulligan MS, Johnson KJ, Todd RF III, Issekutz TB, Miyasaka M, Tamatani T, Smith CW, Anderson DC, Ward PA: Requirements for leukocyte adhesion molecules in nephrotoxic nephritis, *J Clin Invest* 91:577-587, 1993.
129. Mulligan MS, Paulson JC, De Frees S, Zheng Z-L, Lowe JB, Ward PA: Protective effects of oligosaccharides in p-selectin-dependent lung injury, *Nature (London)* 364:149-151.
130. Mulligan MS, Watson SR, Fennie C, Ward PA: Protective effects of selectin chimeras in neutrophil-mediated lung injury, *J Immunol* 151:6410-6417, 1993.
131. Murray JG, Stack JP, Ennis JT, Behan M: Digital enhancement in contrast-enhanced MR imaging of the postoperative lumbar spine, *AJR Am J Roentgenol* 162 (4):893-894, 1994.
132. Nachemon A: Intradiscal measurements of pH in patients with lumbar rhizopathies, *Acta Orthop Scand* 40:23-42, 1969.
133. Nagineni CN, Amiel D, Green MH, Berchuck M, Akeson WH: Characterization of the intrinsic properties of ACL and MCL cells: an in vitro cell culture study, *J Orthop Res* 10:465-475, 1992.
134. Nguyen CM, Haughton VM, Khang-Cheng H, An HS: MR contrast enhancement: an experimental study in postlaminectomy epidural fibrosis, *Am J Neuroradiol* 14:997-1002, 1993.
135. Nordby EJ, Wright PHCM, Haughton VM, Ho KC: Efficacy of chymopapain in chemonucleolysis: a review. *Spine* 19(22): Effect of repeated injections of chymopapain in the epidural space, *Radiology* 174(2):417-419, 1990.
136. North RB, Kidd DA: A prospective, randomized clinical efficacy and cost analysis study of spinal cord stimulation versus reoperation, *AANS and CNS Joint Section on Pain Newsletter* 4(1):7, 1997.
137. North RB, Campbell JN, James CS, Conover-Walker MK, Wang H, Piantadosi S, Rybock JD, Long DM: Failed back surgery syndrome: 5-year follow-up in 102 patients undergoing repeated operation, *Neurosurgery* 28(5):685-691, 1991.
138. Nussbaum CE, McDonald JV, Baggs RB: Use of Vicryl (polyglactin 900) mesh to limit epidural scar formation after laminectomy, *Neurosurgery* 26(4):649-654, 1990.
139. Olmarker K, Blomquist J, Stromberg J, Nannmaark U, Thomsen P, Rydevik, B: Inflammatogenic properties of nucleus pulposus, *Spine* 20:665-669, 1995.
140. Olmarker K, Byrod G, Comefjord M, Nordborg C, Rydevik B: Effects of methylprednisolone on nucleus pulposus-induced nerve root injury, *Spine* 19:1803-1808, 1994.
141. Olmarker K, Rydevik B, Nordborg C: Autologous nucleus pulposus induces neurophysiologic and histologic changes in porcine cauda equina nerve roots, *Spine* 18:1425-1432, 1993.
142. Park SA, Giannattasio C, Tancer ML: Foreign body reaction to the intraperitoneal use of Avitene, *Obstet Gynecol* 58(5):664-667, 1981.
143. Partsch G, Schwarzer C, Neumuller J, Dunky A, Petera P, Broll H, Ittner G, Jantsch S: Modulation of the migration and chemotaxis of PMN cells by hyaluronic acid, *Z Rheumatol* 48:123-128, 1989.
144. Petrie JL, Ross JS: Use of ADCON-L to inhibit post-operative peridural fibrosis and related symptoms following lumbar disc surgery: a preliminary report, *Eur Spine J* 5(suppl):S10-S17, 1996.
145. Pisko E, Turner RA, Soderstrom LP, Panetti M: Inhibition of neutrophils, phagocytosis, and enzyme release by hyaluronic acid. *Clin Exp Rheumatol* 1:41-44, 1983.
146. Pober JS, Cotran RS: The role of endothelial cells in inflammation, *Transplantation* 50:537-544, 1990.
147. Prieschl EE, Klumburg PA, Baumruker T: The nomenclature of chemokines, *Int Arch Allergy Immunol* 107:475-483, 1995.
148. Prussick VR, Lint DS, Bruder WJ: Cauda equina syndrome as a complication of free fat-grafting. A report of two cases and a review of the literature, *J Bone Joint Surg Am* 70(8):1256-1258, 1988.
149. Racz GB, Heavner JE, Diede JH: *Lysis of epidural ad-*

*hesions utilizing the epidural approach.* In Waldman SD, Winnie AP, editors: *Interventional pain management,* Philadelphia, 1996, WB Saunders.

150. Reigel DH, Bazmi B, Shih S, Marquaardt MD: A pilot investigation of poloxamer 407 for the prevention of leptomeningeal adhesions in the rabbit, *Pediatr Neurosurg* 19:250-255, 1993.
151. Revel M, Auleley GR, Alaoui S, Nguyen M, Duruoz T: Forceful epidural injections for the treatment of lumbosciatic pain with post-operative lumbar spinal fibrosis, *Rev Rheum Engl Ed* 63 (4) 270-277, 1996.
152. Robertson JT, Meric AL, Dohan C, Schweitzer JB, Wujek JR, Ahmad S: The reduction of postlaminectomy peridural fibrosis in rabbits by a carbohydrate polymer, *J Neurosurg* 79:89-95, 1993.
153. Robertson JT: Role of peridural fibrosis in the failed back: a review, *Eur Spine J* 5(suppl 1):S2-S6, 1996.
154. Ross JS: Magnetic resonance assessment of the postoperative spine, *Radiol Clin North Am* 29:793-808, 1991.
155. Ross JS, Delamarter R, Hueftle MG et al: Gadolinium-DTPA enhanced MR imaging of the postoperative lumbar spine: time course and mechanisms of enhancement, *Am J Neuroradiol* 10:37-46, 1989.
156. Ross JS, Robertson JT, Frederickson RCA, Petrie JL, Obuchowski N, Modic MY, deTribolet N: Association between residual scar and recurrent pain after lumbar discectomy. magnetic resonance evaluation, *Neurosurgery* 38(4):855-861, 1996.
157. Saal JS, Franson RC, Dobrow R, Saal JA, Goldwaite N: High levels of inflammatory phospholipase A2 activity in lumbar spine disc herniations, *Spine* 15: 674-678, 1990.
158. Saberski LR, Brull SJ: Spinal and epidural endoscopy: a historical review, *Yale J Biol Med* 68:7-15, 1995.
159. Saberski LR, Kitahata LM: Review of the clinical basis and protocol for epidural endoscopy, *Conn Med* 60(2):71-73, 1996.
160. Saiki I, Murata J, Yoneda J, Kobayashi H, Azuma I: Influence of fibroblasts on the invasion and migration of highly or weakly metastatic B16 melanoma cells, *Int J Cancer* 56:867-873, 1994.
161. Saiki I, Murata J, Watnabe K, Fji H, Abe F, Azuma J: Inhibition of tumor cell invasion by Ubenimex (bestatin) in vitro, *Jap J Cancer Res* 80:873-878, 1990.
162. Sakamoto K: [Experimental study on pedicle fat grafts after laminectomy: comparison of pedicle and free fat grafts], *Nippon Seikeigeka Gakkai Zasshi* 61(6):743-753,1987.
163. Saunders MC, Keller JT, Dunsker SB, Mayfield FH: Survival of autologous fat grafts in humans and mice, *Connect Tissue Res* 8(2):85-91, 1981.
164. Schall TJ, Bacon K, Toy KJ, Goeddel DV: Selective attraction of monocytes and t lymphocytes of the memory phenotype by cytokine RANTES, *Nature* 347:669, 1990.
165. Schall TJ, Bacon KB: Chemokines, leukocyte trafficking and inflammation, *Curr Opin Immunol* 6:865-873, 1994.
166. Schall TJ: Biolog of the RANTES/SIS cytokine gene family, *Cytokine* 3:165-183, 1991.
167. Schall, TJ: *The chemokines.* In Thompson A, editor: *The cytokine handbook,* ed 2, New York, 1994, Academic Press, pp 419-460.
168. Schreck PJ, Kitabayashi LR, Amiel D, Akeson WH, Woods VL Jr: Integrin receptor display increases in the wounded rabbit medial collateral ligament but not in the anterior cruciate ligament, *J Orthop Res* 13:174-198, 1995.
169. Seeling W, Tomczak R, Merk J, Mrakovic N: [CT-epidurography. A comparison of conventional and CT-epidurography with contrast medium injection through a thoracic peridural catheter], *Anaesthesist* 44(1):24-26, 1995.
170. Selcklu A, Pasaoglu A, Akdemir H, Kurtsoy A, Patiroglu TE: Urokinase for control of scar formation after laminectomy, *Spine* 18(1):165-168, 1993.
171. Shah M, Foreman DM, Ferguson WJ. Control of scarring in adult wounds by neutralizing antibody to TGF-β, *Lancet* 339:213-214, 1992.
172. Shah M, Foreman DM, Ferguson MWJ: Neutralization of TGF-β1 and TGF-β2 or exogenous addition of TGF-β3 to cutaneous rat wounds reduces scarring, *J Cell Sci* 108:985-1002, 1995.
173. Shah M, Whitby DJ, Ferguson MWJ: *Fetal wound healing and scarless surgery.* In Jackson D, Sommerlad BC, editors: *Recent advances in plastic surgery,* ed 5, Edinburgh, 1996, Churchill Livingstone.
174. Shutse G, Kurtse G, Groll O, Enns E: [Endoscopic method for the diagnosis and treatment of spinal pain syndromes], *Anesteziol Reanimatol* 4:62-64, 1996.
175. Smith CW: Endothelial adhesion molecules and their role in inflammation, *Can J Physiol Pharmacol* 71:76-87, 1993.
176. Songer MN, Rauchning W, Carson EW, Suchaker MP. Analysis of peridural scar formation and its prevention after lumbar laminectomy and discectomy in dogs, *Spine* 20:571-580, 1995.
177. Songer MN, Ghosh L, Spencer DL: Effects of sodium hyaluronate on peridural fibrosis after lumbar laminotomy and discectomy, *Spine* 15(6):550-4, 1990.
178. Ströqvist B, Jönsson B, Annertz M, Holtas S: Cauda equina syndrome caused by migrating fat graft after lumbar spinal decompression. A case report demonstrated with magnetic resonance imaging, *Spine* 16(1):100-101, 1991.
179. Sung K-LP, Whittemore D, Shi Y, Jin G, Akeson WH, Sung LA: The differential adhesion of acl and mcl ligament fibroblasts: effects of tropomodulin, talin, vinculin and actin, *Proc Natl Acad Sci USA* 93(17):9182-9187, 1996.
180. Sung K-LP, Whittemore D, Yang L, Akeson WH: Signal pathway and ligament cell adhesiveness, *J Orthop Res* 14:729-735, 1996.

181. Sung K-LP, Steele LL, Whittemore D, Hagan J, Akeson WH: Adhesiveness of human ligament fibroblasts to laminin, *J Orthop Res* 13:166-173, 1995.
182. Tamaki K, Okuda S, Miyazono K, Nakayama M, Fujishima M: Matrix-associated latent TGF-beta with latent TGF-beta binding protein in the progressive process in adriamycin-induced nephropathy, *Lab Invest* 73:81-89, 1995.
183. Tamoto K, Tada M, Shimada S, Nochi H, Mori Y: Effects of high molecular weight hyaluronates on the function of guinea pig polymorphonuclear leukocytes, *Semin Arthritis Rheum* 22(suppl 1):4-8, 1993.
184. Tator CH, Park Y: Prevention of arachnoiditis and postoperative tethering of the spinal cord with GORE-TEX surgical membrane: an experimental study. Poster presentation, Congress of Neurological Surgeons Annual Meeting Sept. 1996.
185. Taub DD, Conlon K, Lloyd AR, Oppenheim JJ, Kelvin DJ: Preferential migration of activated CD4+ and CD8+ T cells in response to MIP-1 and MIP-1, *Science* 260:355, 1993.
186. Teplick JG, Haskin ME: Computed tomography of the post-operative lumbar spine, *Am J Radiol* 141: 865-884, 1983.
187. Tobetto K, Nakai K, Akatsuka M, Yasui T, Ando T, Hirano S: Inhibitory effects of hyaluronan on neutrophil-mediated cartilage degradation, *Connect Tissue Res* 29:181-190, 1993.
188. Tomczak R, Seeling W, Rieber A, Sokiranski R, Rilinger N, Brambs H: [Epidurography: comparison with CT, spiral CT and MR epidurography], *Rofo Fortschr Geb Rontgenstr Neun Bildgeb Vefahr* 165(2): 123-129, 1996.
189. Trevor PB, Martin RA, Saunders GK, Trotter EJ: Healing characteristics of free and pedicle fat grafts after dorsal laminectomy and durotomy in dogs, *Vet Surg* 20(5):282-290, 1991.
190. Trotter EJ, Crissman J, Robson D, Babish J: Influence of nonbiologic implants on laminectomy membrane formation in dogs, *Am J Vet Res* 49:634-643, 1988.
191. Tullegerg T, Isacson J, Weidenhielm L: Does microscopic removal of lumbar disc herniations lead to better results than the standard procedure? Results of a one year randomized study, *Spine* 18(1):24-27, 1993.
192. Urvoy P, Perlinski S, Berger M, Butin E, Mestdagh H: [Cauda equina syndrome due to early postoperative migration of an adipose tissue flap following laminectomy], *Acta Orthop Belg* 56(2):513-516, 1990.
193. Van Akkerveeken PF, Van De Kraan W, Muller JW: The fate of the free fat graft. a prospective study using CT scanning, *Spine* 11(5):501-504, 1986.
194. Van De Kleft EJZ, Van Goethem JWM, De Le Porte C, Verlooy JSA: Early postoperative gadolinium-DTPA-enhanced MR imaging after successful lumbar discectomy, *Br J Neurosurg* 10(1):41-49, 1996.
195. Von Andrian UH, Chambers JD, McEvoy LM, Bargatze RF, Arfors K, Butcher EC: Two-step model of leukocyte-endothelial cell interaction in inflammation: distinct roles for LECAM-1, and the leukocyte β2 integrins in vivo, *Proc Natl Acad Sci USA* 88:7538-7542, 1991.
196. Wahl SM: Transforming growth factor beta: the good, the bad and the ugly, *J Exp Med* 180:1587-1590, 1994.
197. Wan KC, Lewis WH: Study of free iron and pyridinoline in hypertrophic scars and normal skin, *Br J Biomed Sci* 53(3):196-302, 1996.
198. Webb LMC, Ehrengruber MU, Clark-Lewis I, Baggiolini M, Rot A: Binding to heparin sulfate or heparin enhances neutrophil responses to interleukin 8, *Proc Natl Acad Sci USA* 90:7158-7162, 1993.
199. Weyrich AS, Ma X, Lefer DJ, Albertine KH, Lefer AM: In vivo neutralization of P-selectin protects feline heart and endothelium in myocardial ischemia and reperfusion injury, *J Clin Invest,* 91:2620-2629, 1993.
200. Witkowski J, Yang L, Sung K-LP: Migration and healing of ligament cells under inflammatory conditions, *J Orthop Res* 15:269-277, 1997.
201. Witt DP, Lander AD: Differential binding of chemokines to glucosaminoglycan subpopulations, *Curr Biol* 4:394-400, 1994.
202. Wujek JR, Ahmad S, Harel A, Maier KH, Roufa D, Silver J: A carbohydrate polymer that effectively prevents epidural fibrosis at laminectomy sites in the rat, *Exp Neurol* 114:237-245, 1991.
203. Yasui T, Akatsuka M, Tobetto K, et al: Effects of hyaluronan on the production of stromelysin and tissue inhibitor of metalloproteinase-1 (TIMP-1) in bovine articular chondrocytes, *Biomed Res* 12:343-348, 1992.
204. Yasui T, Akatsuka M, Tobetto K, Hayaishi M, Ando T: The effect of hyaluronan on interleukin-1-induced prostaglandin-$e_2$ production in human osteoarthritic synovial cells, *Agents Actions* 37:155-156, 1992.
205. Yong-Hing K, Reilly J, de Korompay V, Kirkaldy-Willis WH: Prevention of nerve root adhesions after laminectomy, *Spine* 5:59-64, 1980.
206. Yoshida GM, Nelson RW, Capen DA, Nagelberg S, Thomas JC, Rimoldi RL, Haye W: Evaluation of continuous intraspinal narcotic analgesia for chronic pain from benign causes, *Am J Orthop* 25(10):693-694, 1996.
207. Yoshioka M, Cshimizu C, Harwood F, Coutts RD, Amiel D: The effect of hyaluronan during the development of osteoarthritic. *Osteoarth Cart* 5:251-260, 1997.

# IX
# BALANCING THE SPINE

# 58

# RATIONALE FOR REALIGNMENT SURGERY OF THE SPINE

**Frank J. Schwab, M.D.**
**Jean-Pierre C. Farcy, M.D.**



Prior to any discussion regarding alignment or realignment surgery of the spine one must at first examine the criteria defining alignment. In the evolution of mankind and the acquisition of bipedal posture the spinal column assumed a series of sagittal plane curvatures.[2] Various studies have attempted to define the normal alignment of the human spine. It is evident that quite some variability in the degree of spinal curvatures and global spinal balance exists. With aging, the spine also undergoes a characteristic change in sagittal curvatures.[13] A significant limitation of studies regarding alignment and curvatures of the spine is that these have examined the static alignment of osseous structures and only rarely the positional variations. It is evident that significant motion of spinal segments is physiologically performed. A coupling of motion patterns has also been identified. Most importantly, physiologic motion of the spine falls within the limits of anatomy and balance such that the body is not injured nor destabilized nor does it lose posture and fall.

Normal spinal alignment has principally been studied in the standing position by obtaining scoliosis series radiographs. It is evident that these studies give only an impression of normal ranges for that particular standing position. The most common techniques employed to measure alignment are based upon a radiographic plumb line. A line is drawn perpendicular to the base of a standing radiograph and the horizontal distance from various bony elements are tabulated. Stagnara in 1982 examined sagittal contour of healthy adults without spinal problems. He found significant variations in contour amongst a volunteer population.[10] Jackson more recently examined sagittal plane contour in volunteers and patients with back pain. Although significant variability in thoracic and lumbar contour were noted, the plumb line fell within a small distance from the sacral promontory in all subjects.[8] Our research service has examined sagittal balance in the context of flat back deformity and found that plumb line variations when drawn from the odontoid were well tolerated with up to 4 cm displacement from the anterior sacral promontory.[7] Deviation greater than that was associated with pain and poor response to conservative clinical management. Dubousset has proposed the concept of the cone of stability to illustrate the narrow range within which the center of gravity must fall for the standing patient in order to minimize energy consumption and maintain balance (Fig. 58-1). Mangione has closely examined the relationship between regional curvatures of the spine, pelvic rotation, and hip extension. Direct correlation between loss of lumbar lordosis and pelvic retroversion was noted in pathologic conditions as well as the aging spine.[9]

In order to accurately define spinal alignment on a segmental level, the position of each vertebrae should be defined in a three-dimensional coordinate system. The proposed system consisting of x, y, and z axes has been outlined by Stokes.[11] Displacement in the three

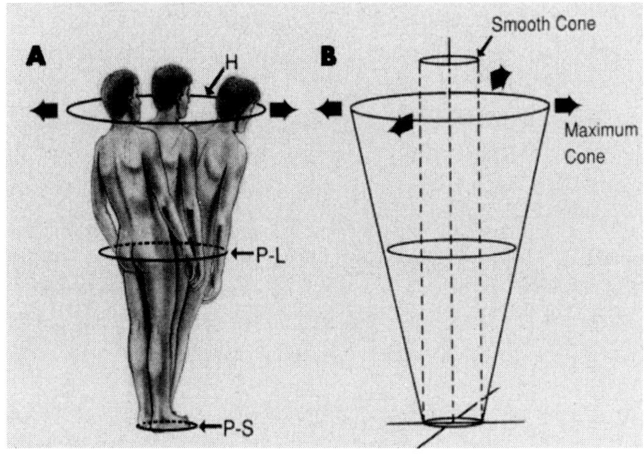


**Figure 58-1**

Illustration of conus of stability as proposed by Dubousset. For balance, the center of gravity must fall within a narrow circle at the feet. Limited amount of upper body displacement is possible, this range is the "maximum cone" described by Dubousset.[5]

planes can be linear or rotational. Accurate analysis of each spinal segment has thus been analyzed by plain radiographs and by computed tomography.[1,3]

It is now accepted that normal standing balance of the human spine should fall within a range of radiographic values. From a more functional perspective, it is evident that the center of gravity of the body as a whole during all activities of the standing person should fall within a narrow circle about the position of the feet.[6] As Dubousset has outlined, any displacement of the center of gravity near or beyond this circle requires increased energy use (muscles to stabilize) or the use of a support structure (cane, crutch, walker) in order to prevent loss of balance and fall (Fig. 58-1).

Effective and efficient function of the locomotor apparatus, standing, sitting, displacement of the extremities, and maintenance of level vision thus require physiologic function of the spinal column as an organ. Limited compromise of spinal physiology can be tolerated due to the recruitment of compensatory mechanisms which include cervical and lumbar spinal motion as well as pelvic rotation and hip and knee positioning.

## EFFECTIVENESS OF SAGITTAL SPINAL CURVATURES

From an anthropomorphic viewpoint, the sagittal curvatures of the human spine have several important roles. One of these is to minimize energy use in the maintenance of overall body balance during standing. Another important role involves the ability to absorb energy from daily compressive (and other) forces across the trunk in addition to accepting large loads (trauma) while protecting neurologic structures from injury. From a mechanical standpoint, the arrangement of the spine into a set of sagittal plane curvatures permits minimal muscular contraction to maintain upright balance.[4] Mechanical lever arms are optimized with several short curves as compared to one long straight spine. The curvatures of the healthy spine also offer a superb arrangement for effective displacement and orientation of the trunk and extremities in space.

## SPINAL FUSION AND COMPENSATORY MECHANISMS

The most evident effect of spinal fusion is the conversion of mobile spinal segments into a solid unit. Much less evident and more significant is consequent effect on not only adjacent structures but the overall function of the spine, pelvis, and extremities. Due to the dynamic nature of spinal function, the loss of one or more mobile levels will augment the demands for motion as well as absorption of energy by the remaining levels. The loss of motion at one or more levels can occur for a variety of reasons. With the normal aging process a certain loss of intersegmental motion may occur and spontaneous ankylosis can be observed in healthy aging individuals. In a variety of pathologic conditions, spinal alignment can also be significantly affected. The latter can affect not only static alignment in the standing posture but more significantly the overall functioning during the wide variety of postures involved in activities of daily living from lying to sitting, walking, and extremity displacement (upper and lower).

Fusion, or ankylosis of spinal segments, will evidently reduce not only normal motion but also eliminate any possibility of compensatory adjustments required by the affected segments during daily function. Consequently, remaining mobile segments will be recruited during all activities to function in an increased capacity (compensatory function). In the cervical spine this may involve loss of normal lordosis or exaggerated segmental kyphosis and hyperlordosis. The latter entity has been named the swan neck deformity by some. The thoracic spine is limited in its ability to increase motion or positional changes due to rigidity imposed by the rib cage. The lumbar spine can be recruited to compensate to changes in motion or alignment by an increase in segmental lordosis. The pelvis appears to have a remarkable ability to adapt to positional changes and pathologic alignment of the spine. Through pelvic retroversion the hip joints are displaced anteriorly, this hip extension permits balanced acetabuli over the feet; by hip extension, the feet are displaced anteriorly. This may enable an otherwise abnormally anterior displaced gravity line to remain within a narrow circle around the feet in stance. The lower extremities can also play a crucial role in compensation to spinal malalignment. With hip hyperextension or flexion significant variations in gravity line displacement can be accommodated. Overall balance of an individual can thus be maintained by a concerted interaction of these various mechanisms. All of these mechanisms will drive up the energy requirements for normal functioning in all activities of daily living. Aside from the energy consideration, painful syndromes may develop when muscles and ligaments are exerted beyond usual physiologic demands. With progressive or continuous significant spinal malalignment, the compensatory mechanisms may be recruited increasingly, leading to progressive pain and disability.[7]

## REGIONAL CONSIDERATIONS IN DEFORMITY

Iatrogenic deformity of the spinal column in conjunction with a fusion is almost invariably in kyphosis (relative or absolute when compared to normal regional contour). Aside from global considerations and the primary diagnosis prior to fusion, the altered regional contour can lead to problems itself based just upon the deformity. Most evident to the patient may be the aesthetic effect of a change in spinal contour. This can be quite striking particularly in the deformities involving rotation in the thoracic region. Rib cage asymmetry can be readily apparent. Deformity may also affect the comfort of standing and sitting postures as well as ambulation. As discussed above, additional muscle recruitment may be necessary in these activities making them more strenuous or painful. In significant deformity, upper extremity recruitment can be required for support with use of a cane, crutch, or walker.

Another significant effect of the deformity itself, particularly in the thoracic region, concerns pulmonary function. Fusions extending into the thoracic region with deformity can significantly impact vital capacity, tidal volume, forced expiratory volume, and thus lead to restrictive pulmonary disease. Long-standing pulmonary changes can induce vascular and cardiac disease that may have significant morbidity and affect life expectancy.

Extreme alterations of regional spinal contour during primary surgery can lead to neurologic compromise. Aside from instances of abrupt change in contour or direct injury to neurologic structures related to spinal pathology or trauma, iatrogenic malalignment of the spinal column can lead to neurologic pathology. In the acute setting, tenting of the cord over osseous structures or abrupt manipulation with stretching of roots or the cord can result in neurologic compromise. The latter can occur in overzealous correction of a deformity or fracture. Aside from a mechanism of direct mechanical neuronal injury, regional vascular compromise has been postulated to play a role in some cases of neurologic deterioration.

Aside from acute neurologic injury, long-term or late neurologic compromise can occur with iatrogenic spinal deformity. Malalignment of an attempted fusion may lead to non-union and progressive regional deformity with consequent compression, stretching or microvascular insult to cord and nerve roots. Even solid fusion has the potential for remodeling over time. The concave side of a deformity loaded in compression will thicken over time (Wolff's law) while the tension side of a fusion will tend to be absorbed and thus be remodeled.

## DEFORMITY AND ITS EFFECTS ON ENERGY CONSUMPTION AND MUSCLE EFFECTIVENESS

Optimal functioning of the spinal column from a biomechanical perspective requires minimal energy consumption in maintaining posture and effecting displacement in space. Pathologic as well as aging changes in contour of the spine will lead to increases of energy consumption in activities of daily living. As Dubousset has outlined, energy use to maintain balance is significantly increased by muscle recruitment when the center of gravity falls near or outside the "cone of economy." Aside from the use of paraspinal musculature, deformity can lead to the recruitment of muscles involved in compensatory mechanisms. These mechanisms were discussed above and range from regional curvature changes to pelvic rotation and hip and knee hyperextension or flexion.

Deformity of the spine will affect the mechanical axis, lever arms, and acting lengths (from origin to insertion) of the paraspinal musculature. Investigations into skeletal muscle physiology have revealed ideal ranges of muscle length for maximal force generation. Thus, it appears evident that spinal deformity may not only reduce the effectiveness of muscle groups by changing lever arms and axis but also by shifting a muscle into a less functional range of length by either shortening or lengthening the distance between origin and insertion. It has been shown in volunteers that changes in lumbar lordosis significantly affect muscle effectiveness.[12] In a pathologic state such as a malunion of the lumbar spine in kyphosis, a significant shortening of the lever arm of the paraspinal musculature (distance from sagittal plane center of rotation) as well as shortening in the distance between origin and insertion of the muscle groups may occur. Both of these factors can lead to a clear reduction in effectiveness of the muscle groups to maintain an extension force across the lumbar spine. Significantly greater recruitment of muscle units may thus be necessary to maintain balance and displacement of the trunk than in the well aligned spine.

## LONG-TERM EFFECTS OF SPINAL FUSION

Contour of the spine must permit standing balance, level vision, and effective displacement of the trunk and extremities. Ideally, these conditions are met with minimal energy consumption and absence of pain. Spinal deformity or fusion can lead to not only increased energy consumption but with increasing severity of the deformity, to limitation of the above functions. A host of dynamic mechanisms (compensatory positions, muscular contractions) can accommodate deformity and fusion of spinal segments. Over time, a spinal fusion or deformity may lead to a new equilibrium state with well adapted compensatory mechanisms and muscular adaptation (hypertrophy). When these mechanisms fail though, a global decompensation can occur. Aside from decompensation by failure of dynamic mechanisms, gradual degenerative changes in osteo-ligamentous structures may occur. The latter can also lead to painful syndromes, which are categorized as junctional phenomena.

### GLOBAL DECOMPENSATION

The most common syndrome of late global failure of spinal alignment due to fusion and malalignment is the flat back. In this disorder, an imposed poor alignment of a spinal segment leads to painful and progressive muscle failure with an inability to accommodate kyphotic collapse by compensatory mechanisms (Fig. 58-2) Thus, a combined failure of static and dynamic stabilizers has occurred. The static stabilizers consist of osseoligamentous structures such as the anterior disks and ligaments as well as posterior facets (with capsules) and inter- as well as supraspinous ligaments. The dynamic stabilizers consist of the paraspinal musculature providing support essentially by contraction.

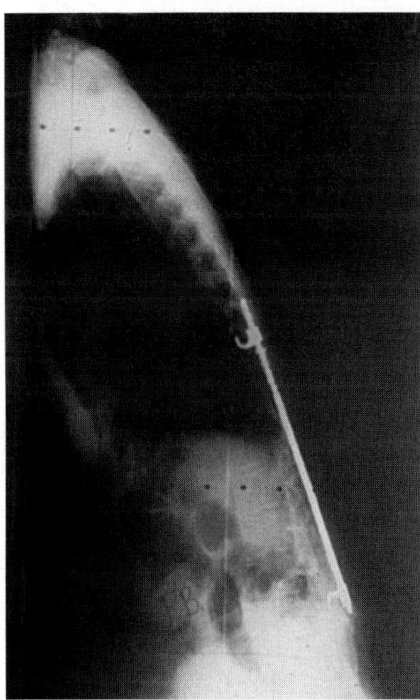

**FIGURE 58-2**

Lateral radiograph of patient with flat back deformity. Harrington distraction instrumentation was originally placed to correct scoliotic deformity.

### JUNCTIONAL PROBLEMS

Regional pathology with painful degeneration adjacent to fusion and malalignment of the spine is grouped into a set of disorders entitled junctional failure. As outlined earlier, the increased mechanical demands on the first mobile segment adjacent to the fusion are particularly prone to accelerated degeneration. It appears that the classic cascade of degeneration is merely accelerated from the normal aging process (Fig. 58-3). Disk dehydration with loss of height and biomechanical performance is followed by facet arthrosis and ligamentous hypertrophy (and laxity).

Junctional problems can develop at the cephalad (Fig. 58-4) (often thoracic) or caudal (usually lumbar) end of a fusion. It appears that the caudal mobile level is more prone to this process possibly due to increasing forces more distally along the spine, coupled with more inherent mobility in the lumbar than the thoracic spine due to rib cage support in the thoracic levels. The length of a fusion as well as the degree of malalignment are important risk factors to junctional pathology since they are independent yet cumulative in their impact on pathomechanics.

## CONCLUSIONS

The problems associated with spinal fusions are become increasingly clear as the follow-up and sheer number of fusion procedures has drawn attention to the iatrogenic complications. To outright avoid spinal fusions based upon the complications and long-term sequelae is unreasonable. It can be stressed, however, that fusion should be minimized and careful patient selection optimized. Great efforts have been undertaken to limit the extent of fusions in scoliosis and trauma surgery, much of it made possible by the application of pedicle screw instrumentation techniques. Newer instrumentation systems and surgical techniques will certainly lead to more optimally aligned, and shorter fusions in all aspects of spinal surgery in which fusion is indicated.

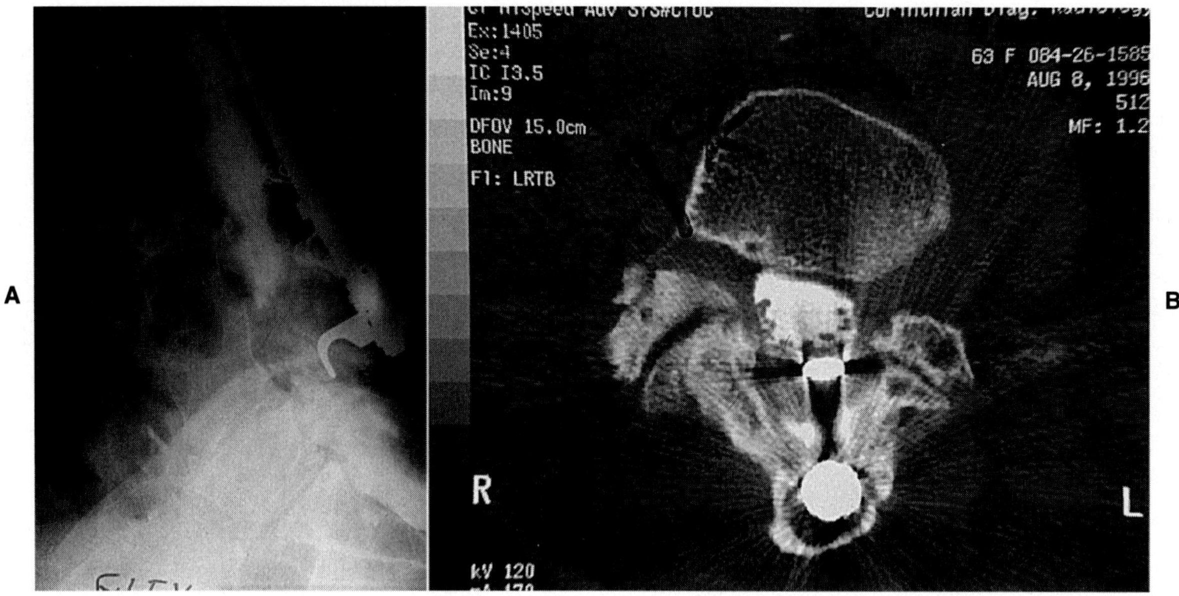


**Figure 58-3**

**A,** Lateral myelogram demonstrating significant stenosis at inferior junction of previous fusion, which was instrumented in distraction creating malalignment. **B,** CT scan at the junctional level of a longstanding fusion. Although this level was not fused, significant arthrosis is evident. The tip of the Harrington rod is noted posteriorly.

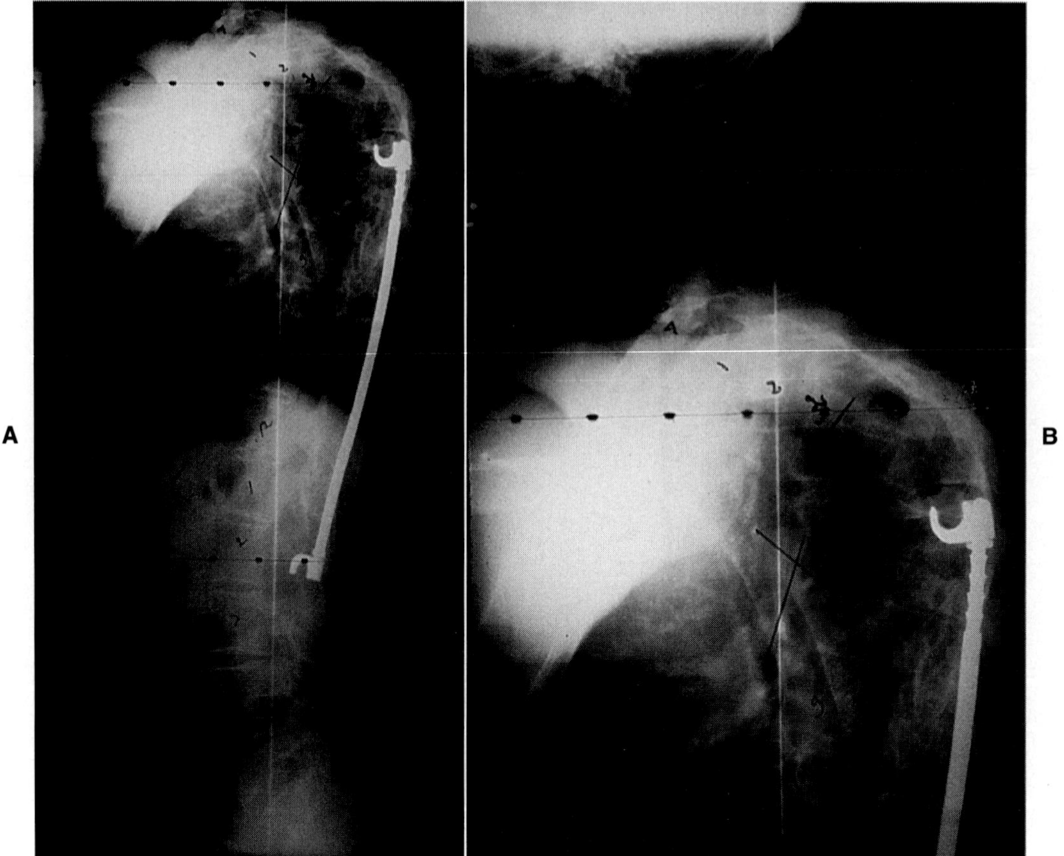


**Figure 58-4**

**A,** Lateral standing radiograph of patient who was treated with Harrington distraction instrumentation for scoliosis. A cephalad junctional collapse in kyphosis has occurred with obligatory cervical hyperlordosis to maintain level vision. This deformity (swan neck) has been progressive and painful. **B,** Lateral radiographic close-up of the junctional upper thoracic kyphosis with compensatory cervical hyperlordosis.

In revision surgery, the rationale for realignment becomes evident in view of the considerations discussed above. Correction of frontal and sagittal plane contour can lead to significant reduction of muscle forces required to maintain balance. The function of the spine as supportive structure can be optimized with surgical realignment. Painful and energy consuming compensatory mechanisms can be unloaded with restoration of proper spinal contour. The global and regional failure of the spine as biomechanical structure and organ can also be addressed surgically. As our understanding of ideal spinal contour expands, the timing for realignment surgery will become more precisely defined. With increased understanding of the natural history of malalignment syndromes, strong arguments can be made for early surgical intervention prior to the failure of mobile segments adjacent to a fusion. Such an approach may be able to save motion segments from inevitable accelerated degeneration. A question that remains unanswered to date is whether realignment surgery can alter the natural history of junctional disk failure.

## REFERENCES


1. Aaro S, Dahlborn M: Estimation of vertebral rotation and the spinal and rib cage deformity in scoliosis by computer tomography, *Spine* 6:461-467, 1981.
2. Abitbol M: Evolution of the lumbosacral angle, *Am J Physiol Anthropol* 72:361-372, 1987.
3. Bernhardt M, Bridwell KH: Segmental analysis of the sagittal plane alignment of the normal thoracic and lumbar spines and thoracolumbar junction, *Spine* 14:717, 1989.
4. Delmas A: L'homme devant l'hominisation, *Quaderni di Anatomica Practica* S XXVIII N1-4:22-56, 1972.
5. Dubousset J: *Pelvic obliquity correction in lumbosacral and spinopelvic fixation.* In: Margulies JY, Floman Y, Farcy J-P, Newell, editors: *Lumbosacral and spinopelvic fixation.* Philadelphia, 1996, Lippincott-Raven, p 40.
6. Duval-Beaupere G, Schmidt C, Cosson PH: A barycentremetric study of the sagittal shape of spina and pelvis, *Annals Biomed Eng* 20:451-462, 1992.
7. Farcy J-P, Schwab F: Management of flatback and related kyphotic decompensation syndromes, *Spine,* 22(20):2452-2457, 1997.
8. Jackson R, McManus A: Radiographic analysis of sagittal plane alignment and balance in standing volunteers and patients with low back pain matched for age, sex, and size, *Spine* 19:1611-1618, 1994.
9. Mangione P, Senegas J: L'equilibre rachidien dans le plan sagittal, *Rev Chir Orthop* 83:22-32, 1997.
10. Stagnara P, Mauroy JC, Dran G, Bonon B, Costanzo G, Dimnet J, Pasquet A: Reciprocal angulation of vertebral bodies in a sagittal plane: approach to references for the evaluation of kyphosis and lordosis, *Spine* 7:335-342, 1982.
11. Stokes I, Bigalow L, Moreland M: Measurement of axial rotation of vertebrae in scoliosis, *Spine* 11:213-218, 1986.
12. Tveit P, Daggfeldt K, Hetland S, Thorstensson A: Erector spinae lever arm length variations with changes in spinal curvature, *Spine* 19:199-204, 1994.
13. Vital JM, Senegas J, Pointillart V: *Cyphoses degeratives lombaires. Le rachis vieillissant.* Paris, 1992, L Simon, Masson, p 146-154.

# 59

# SAGITTAL BALANCE CONSIDERATIONS IN ADULTS

**Lawrence G. Lenke, M.D.**
**Douglas A. Linville, M.D.**
**Keith H. Bridwell, M.D.**



With the introduction of segmental spinal instrumentation and three-dimensional assessment of the spinal column, analysis of sagittal plane alignment has come into the forefront of spinal surgeons pre- and postoperative considerations. Inherent to the importance of the sagittal plane is global assessment of overall sagittal balance and various factors that may affect it. This chapter will first describe ideal sagittal alignment from the segmental, regional, as well as global perspective. Next, specific types of sagittal malalignments that are commonly seen will be reviewed. Lastly, various types of revision surgery to correct sagittal imbalance in the adult will be described.

## NORMAL SAGITTAL ANATOMY: PRINCIPLES OF ALIGNMENT AND BALANCE

Normal sagittal alignment has become increasingly recognized as an important aspect in the management of the spinal deformity patient. Prior to the early 1980s, no study existed that described the acceptable norms for sagittal balance and alignment. Treatment of spinal deformities centered either upon the coronal plane only, as in scoliosis where long cassette lateral films often were not obtained, or assumed a general range of acceptable thoracic kyphosis and lumbar lordosis based upon anecdotal information. Historically, this generalization for all patients was that a thoracic kyphosis in the range of 20 to 40 degrees seemed appropriate for the majority.[16] In response to these assumptions, Fon, Pitt, and Thies reported on thoracic kyphosis in a group of 316 normal patients referred for chest radiographs without any previous history of spinal pathology.[6] Their conclusion was that kyphosis increased with age and was of a greater degree in females than males. Also established by their data was the fact that there was a very wide distribution of normals, making mean values almost useless for application to the population as a whole.

These initial studies, however, did not address the spine as an entire functional unit. Thus, analysis was performed segmentally and regionally, but not globally. Segmental analysis refers to the relationships between two vertebral bodies and their intervening disk. Regional areas considered are the cervical, thoracic, and lumbar spines and the thoracolumbar junction. In order to evaluate the complex balance and interrelationships between these regions, a global approach must be taken. The global spinal alignment is what is referred to when speaking in terms of sagittal balance. These definitions are useful when discussing sagittal anatomy and should be used in a standardized fashion to avoid confusion.

Features that have been examined for their contribution to sagittal spinal alignment include: patient age, gender, height, race, weight, smoking, and scoliosis.[7,15,26] None, however, has consistently shown significant correlation with sagittal balance and/or alignment. Therefore, it seems that numerous factors including genetic predisposition may dictate a person's sagittal spinal alignment and balance. Several publications have addressed some of these issues in both the lumbar and thoracic spine and are discussed.

## CERVICAL SAGITTAL PLANE

There is little mention of normal cervical spinal alignment. It is known clinically that the cervical spine is normally lordotic, with this development occurring as a person begins upright posture. This lordosis is a secondary curvature forming in order to balance the initial kyphosis of the entire spine that is present in the infant. What degree this cervical curvature contributes to the overall sagittal balance, however, has not been reported until recently. It appears that much of this lordosis is at the atlantoaxial junction. Hardacker et al noted that approximately 75% of cervical lordosis was formed by the junction of these two segments.[8] Comparing the absolute measurements, −40 degrees of lordosis occurred occiput to C7, −30 degrees from occiput to C2, and the subaxial segment contributes collectively only −10 degrees.[9] The occurrence of vertebral wedging combined with disk morphology also contributes to the overall balance of the cervical spine.

Sagittal balance has also been evaluated with attention to the correlation with the thoracic and lumbar regional curves, global alignment, and balance. Confirmed by Hardacker et al was the fact that a plumb line dropped from C7 falls posterior to the posterior superior corner of the lumbosacral disk, and the odontoid plumb fell slightly anterior to this position.[8] Global sagittal balance was noted to be correlative as increased cervical lordosis resulted from increased thoracic kyphosis. A similar relationship between thoracic kyphosis and lumbar lordosis was also noted, with the lumbar spine compensating with lordosis for any increased thoracic kyphosis. What can be taken from this information is that, like other regions of the spine, the sagittal alignment and balance of the cervical spine are important in the consideration of global spinal balance, and appear to compensate for thoracic kyphosis when present, keeping the global balance intact. It is important, therefore, that the surgeon be cautious in maintaining this anatomic and physiologic relationship during operative interventions so as not to create a sagittal imbalance in which the "cure" is worse than the initial pathology.

## THORACIC SAGITTAL PLANE

The primary sagittal curvature of the human spine is that of a long kyphosis that evolves in the infant as upright posture ensues. The initial spinal alignment of the neonate is a global kyphosis from occiput to sacrum that subsequently evolves its final form over time. This primary curvature changes shape with the aging of the child to reach adult normative range by the adolescent years. Initial formation of thoracic kyphosis is most rapid in the first 5 years of life. Thereafter, it slows and progresses only a few degrees from age 5 to 20 years. Males and females show no significant variations in the degree of physiologic thoracic kyphosis once final alignment is reached.[26] Several studies have documented normal ranges in both pediatric and adult patients (Table 59-1). Kyphosis begins at the first thoracic vertebra and

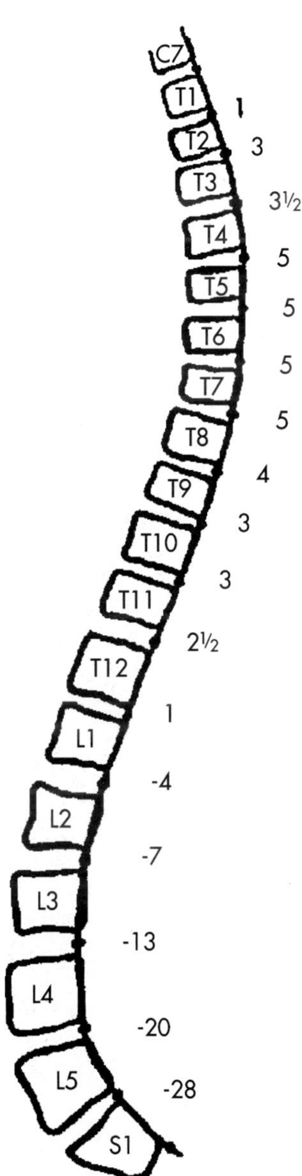


**FIGURE 59-1**

Segmental contributions throughout the thoracic and lumbar spine. *(From Bernhardt M, Bridwell KH: Segmental analysis of the sagittal plane alignment of the normal thoracic and lumbar spines and thoracolumbar junction,* Spine *14(7):717-721, 1989.)*

continues incrementally to reach its segmental maximum at the apex of the thoracic spine, which is most commonly T6, T7, or the intervening disk. Thereafter, segmental kyphosis slowly decreases and ends at the T12-L1 disk.[1,7] (Fig. 59-1, Table 59-2).

Ranges of thoracic kyphosis in normal patients, adult and pediatric, have been reported from 9 to 63 degrees. Mean kyphosis is fairly consistent in the 27- to 39-degree range.[1,6,7,15,19,26] Care must be maintained when interpreting these values since studies reported are not consistent in the end vertebrae measured when describing kyphosis. Ideally, the end vertebrae are the superior endplate of T1 to the inferior endplate of T12. Unfortunately, due to varying radiographic technique, especially when obtaining long cassette lateral films, the endplates of T1 are not often well visualized due to the overlying shadows of the shoulder girdle. The T4 or T5 vertebrae seem to be best visualized and thus are the most frequently reported upper end vertebrae in these sagittal analyses. Gelb et al reported that upper thoracic kyphosis, that is from T1-T5, measured 14 ± 8 degrees (range −4 to +35 degrees).[7] The segmental contribution of these levels is approximately 1 to 3 degrees per level, which was determined by Bernhardt and Bridwell,[1] allowing the observer to make an educated inference of the contribution of the upper thoracic segment to global kyphosis when radiographs do not allow proper measurements.

What one can ascertain from these studies is that no one normal value exists for thoracic kyphosis, when

**Table 59-1. Mean Global Measures for Thoracic Kyphosis and Lumbar Lordosis in Normal Patients**

| Study | Patient Age | Thoracic End Vertebrae | Mean Thoracic Kyphosis | Lumbar End Vertebrae | Mean Lumbar Lordosis | SVA |
|---|---|---|---|---|---|---|
| Bernhardt & Bridwell[1] | 12.8 yrs (5–30 yrs) | T3-T12 apex T6-T7 disk | 36 ± 10° (9–53° ) | T12-L5 apex L3-L4 disk | −44 ± 12° (−14–69°) | |
| Fon et al[6] | (2–77 yrs) | T2-T12 | 21–45° (5–66°)† | | | |
| Gelf et al[7] | 57 ± 11 yrs (40–82 yrs) | T5-12 apex T7 | 34 ± 11° (9–66°) | T12-S1 apex L4 | −64 ± 10° (−38–84°) | −3.2 ± 3.2 cm |
| Jackson & McManus[11] | 38.9 ± 9.4 yrs (20–63 yrs) | T1-T12 apex T7-T8 | 42.1 ± 8.9° (22–68°) | L1-S1 | −60.9 ± 12° (−31–88°) | −0.05 ± 2.5 cm (−6–6.5 cm) |
| Propst-Proctor & Bleck[15] | Children 2–>19 yrs | T5-T12 | 27° (21–33°) | L1-L5 | −40° (−31–49.5°) | |
| Stagnara et al[19] | 20–29 yrs | T4-IVB# | 37° (7–63°) | IVB-S1# | −50° (−32–84°) | |
| Voutsinas & MacEwen*[26] | 5–20 yrs | T2-T12 | 36.7–38.5° | L1-S1 | 52.2–56.6° | |
| Wambolt & Spencer[27] | 18 yrs | | | T12-S1 | −59° (−31–79°) | |
| Vedantam et al[25] | 14.3 (10–18 yrs) | T3-T12 apex T6 | 38 ± 9.8° | T12-S1 apex L4 | −64° ± 12° | −5.7 ± 3.5 cm |

*Values reported were means for three groups of patients grouped by age, ranges reported are upper and lower means for these groups.
#IVB-intermediate vertebral body that is transitional vertebra at thoracolumbar junction (L1 1/3, T12 1/5, L2 1/5).
†Range is that of means for all ages male and female, range in parentheses is that of minimum and maximum values for all ages, male and female.

**Table 59-2. Segmental Measurements of Thoracic Spine**

| Study | T1-2 | T2-3 | T3-4 | T4-5 | T5-6 | T6-7 | T7-8 | T8-9 | T9-10 | T10-11 | T11-12 | T12-L1 |
|---|---|---|---|---|---|---|---|---|---|---|---|---|
| Bernhardt & Bridwell[1] | +1° | +3° | ±3.5° | +5° | +5° | +5° | +5° | +4° | +3° | +3° | +2.5° | +1° |
| Stagnara et al[19] | | | | +5 | +5 | +6 | +5 | +4 | +3 | +2 | +2 | +1 |

comparing similar end vertebrae. A range of between 30 to 50 degrees of global thoracic kyphosis seems appropriate for most of the population, though clinical factors must be considered carefully before judging a patient's alignment as pathologic. Therefore, a 65-degree thoracic kyphosis may be perfectly acceptable as long as sagittal balance is maintained. The point to be made is that consideration of the patient globally is much more important than generalizations regarding norms for thoracic kyphosis.

## THORACOLUMBAR SAGITTAL PLANE

Joining the kyphotic thoracic spine and the lordotic lumbar spine is a transition zone—the thoracolumbar junction. This portion of the spine is an area of transition both of alignment and force transmission. The relatively rigid thoracic segment with its smaller vertebral bodies and disks transforms into the lumbar spine, which has much more flexibility due to larger disks, sagittal facet orientation, and the lack of intrinsic support by both ribs and sternum. No published data exists regarding the development of this specific region of the spine in the pediatric population. It seems safe to extrapolate that the adult alignment occurs simultaneously with the compensatory development of the lumbar lordosis once upright posture and later ambulation occurs.

Much is happening to the patient's overall alignment in the sagittal plane in this area. The thoracic spine is increasingly kyphotic segmentally up to its apex and then begins to be less kyphotic until reaching the lumbar spine. The disk at L1-L2 is the first lordotic segment as reported by Gelb et al.[7] Normal thoracolumbar contour, therefore, is either neutral or slightly lordotic when the segment from T12-L2 is examined. Bernhardt and Bridwell also confirmed that this region was usually lordotic and segmentally measured: 3 ± 7 degrees with a range of −23 to +13 degrees. The T10-T12 segment just above, however, remains kyphotic. This region segmentally measured +5.5 ± 4 degrees with a range of −3 to 20 degrees.[1] It is evident from this study in adults that the transition from kyphosis to lordosis appears in the T12-L2 region, which is the functional transition zone between the thoracic kyphosis and lumbar lordosis. Attention must be directed towards maintenance of this relationship during reconstructive procedures in order to prevent junctional kyphosis which can be cosmetically undesirable, though long-term functional effects are presently unknown.

## LUMBAR SAGITTAL PLANE

Normal lumbar sagittal alignment is lordosis which begins at L1 and arches smoothly to S1. This compensatory curve forms and progresses from age 5 years to 15 years in females and age 20 years in males.[26] The rate of progression of the lordosis is greater in females, however, after the male spine completes its compensation and attains adult alignment at age 20 years, the degree of lordosis has equalized. The normal apex of the lumbar spine is at L3-L4, and can be either of these vertebrae or the disk space itself.[1,7,25] Segmentally, L1-L2 begins this lordosis which increases segmentally throughout the lumbar spine. The segments at L4-L5 and L5-S1 show similar contributions to the overall lumbar lordosis and together account for 60% of the overall lumbar lordosis.[1,7,11] Segmental contributions of the respective lumbar vertebral levels are listed in Table 59-3. It is important to note in published data that lordosis values reported include the L5-S1 segment, as earlier studies only evaluated lordosis from T12-L5. Due to the significant contribution of the L5-S1 segment, it is recommended that all measures of sagittal alignment in the lumbar spine include this level in calculations. This will ensure that global measures can be better evaluated and that there is consistency in comparison of data among other examiners.

The question that has been posed recently is, what contribution of this lordosis is from the disk, and what is from the wedging of the vertebral bodies? This would have application in anterior compression instrumentation in which diskectomy is performed, or even in degenerative disk disease in which disk desiccation and collapse occur causing segmental imbalance. Wambolt et al addressed this subject by measuring the

**Table 59-3. Segmental Measurements of Lumbar Spine**

| Study | T12-L1 | L1-2 | L2-3 | L3-4 | L4-5 | L5-1 |
|---|---|---|---|---|---|---|
| Gelb et al[7] | +2 ± 5° | −4 ± 5° | −10 ± 5° | −14 ± 17° | −24 ± 7° | −24 ± 7° |
| Jackson & McManus[11] | | −2 ± 4° | −7 ± 4° | −11 ± 4° | −16 ± 5° | −25 ± 6° |
| Bernhardt & Bridwell[1] | +1° | −4° | −7° | −13° | −20° | −28° |
| Stagnara et al[19] | +1 | −2° | −7° | −11° | −15° | −21° |

Cobb angle of each of the disks and then each of the vertebrae from T12 to the sacrum. It was noted that the disks combined for −47 degrees of the lordosis while the vertebrae accounted for only −12 degrees of lumbar lordosis.[27] This research emphasizes the necessity of restoring or preserving disk height when using anterior instrumentation for the treatment of spinal deformity. Also, collapse of the lower most segments due to degenerative disease will result in more significant decompensation than in the upper lumbar spine due to the relative contribution of the lower two disks to sagittal balance. These disk contributions should be understood when dealing with distal lumbar disk disease and degenerative conditions in the adult patient so that global balance is maintained.

## SAGITTAL BALANCE

Another important consideration in the sagittal plane of the thoracic spine is the sagittal vertical axis or SVA (Fig. 59-2). This is a parameter that quantifies the global sagittal balance of the spine as a unit. The SVA is constructed by dropping a plumb from the center of C7, which is almost always identified on a long cassette lateral radiograph. The center of the dens is also an acceptable point of reference, however, it is not consistently present on long cassette radiographs limiting usefulness. Therefore, further reference to the SVA will assume the C7 plumb is used. The SVA normally falls anterior to the thoracic spine, through or slightly anterior to the apical lumbar vertebral bodies and finally through the first sacral body. Positive SVA is considered present when this line is anterior to the anterior most aspect of S1. Negative SVA, on the contrary, is present when this axis passes posterior to the anterior body of S1. Studies in the adult and pediatric population have elucidated that normal SVA is usually negative. Vedantam et al showed in the pediatric population that a normal SVA was −5.7 ± 3.5 cm.[25] Adults seem to be slightly less negative in their balance according to Gelb et al with SVA measuring −3.2 ± 3.2 cm.[7] Thus, this index provides information that is additive to the individual segmental analysis of curvatures in the sagittal plane. Age would seem to affect SVA as disks desiccate and lose height, though this has not been statistically proven. The small difference in values in these two studies can only provide stimulus for further research into this issue and comparison of patients longitudinally (Fig. 59-3).

Understanding SVA is important in global assessment of the spine. Also important is comprehension of the dynamic relationships of the spine in the maintenance of sagittal balance. It appears that the body attempts to maintain the sagittal vertical axis in as physiologic a position as is possible by compensating with sagittal curvature. There is a direct correlation between increasing thoracic kyphosis and lumbar lordosis which act in concert to maintain balance. Similar to the lumbar spine, the cervical spine reacts with a compensatory lordosis in cases of accentuated thoracic kyphosis.[9,19] This was suggested by Stagnara et al. in their early study and has been substantiated by the aforementioned study. This dynamic relationship may call for more of a "dependent estimation" of lumbar lordosis. That is, for a patient with a "normal" kyphosis for their spine, a normal lumbar lordosis appears to be a dependent variable. The apparent normal relationship between these curves is that lumbar lordosis should be in the range of 20 to 30 degrees greater in magnitude than the kyphosis. For example, a patient with a normal thoracic kyphosis of +36 degrees should have a lumbar lordosis in the range of −56 to 66 degrees. This allows adequate global balance with maintenance of a negative sagittal vertical axis.

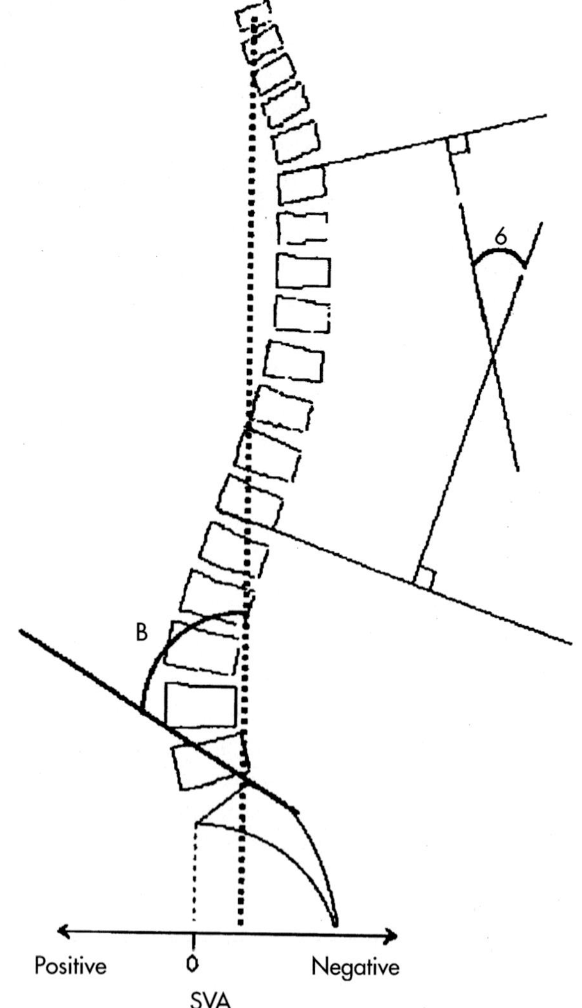


**FIGURE 59-2**

Construction of sagittal plumb line in evaluation of sagittal vertical axis. *(From Gelb DE, Lenke LG, Bridwell KH, Blanke K, McEnery KW: An analysis of sagittal spinal alignment in 100 asymptomatic middle and older aged volunteers,* Spine *20(12):1351-1358, 1995.)*

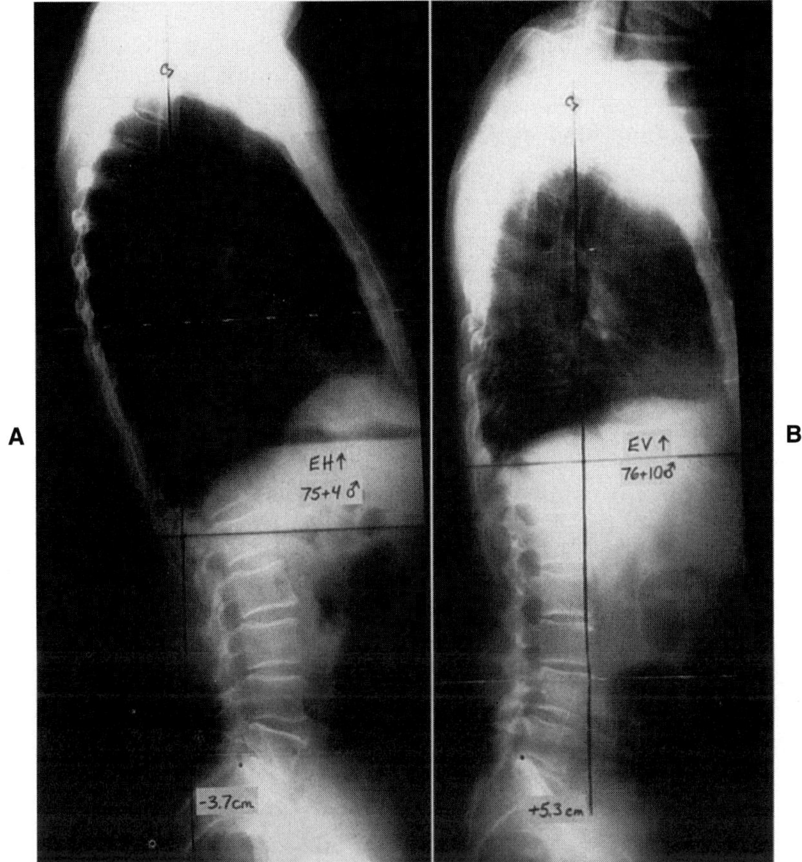


**FIGURE 59-3**

**A,** A 75-year-old asymptomatic man who participated in a standing sagittal alignment study of asymptomatic adult volunteers. The sagittal vertical axis (C7 sagittal plumb line) is situated 3.7 cm behind the lumbosacral disk. Note the normal lumbar lordosis with relatively well maintained disk spaces anteriorly in the lumbar spine. **B,** This is a 76-year-old volunteer who also is completely asymptomatic in regards to his spine, but has a sagittal vertical axis that lies in front of the lumbosacral disk by 5.3 cm. Note the flattened thoracic, thoracolumbar, and lumbar regional alignments.

Radiographic comparisons of these values are useful for assessment of alignment and balance done serially. What is important, though, is to be aware of positional variations that can influence angular and plumb measurements. Stagnara et al stated that when measurements were performed of lumbar lordosis and thoracic kyphosis at intervals of five to ten years that these were reproducible to "within a few degrees, provided the position is clearly stipulated."[19] Unpublished data from our institution differs from this slightly in both adult and pediatric patients either with or without previous fusion surgery. Our results show that sacral inclination and segmental measurements are not significantly affected by arm position either in a 30- or 90-degree arm position from the vertical. The SVA additionally is affected unpredictably in either a positive or negative direction and no correlation in this regard could be made. We are in agreement with Stagnara et al that for the most reproducible sagittal measurements over time, a standard position and radiographic technique should be enforced.

## SUMMARY

Many factors are important in understanding normal sagittal alignment and balance. Cervical lordosis, thoracic kyphosis, thoracolumbar and lumbar lordosis all contribute to global balance which is evident by measuring sagittal vertical axis. There is a constantly changing, complex relationship between these spinal regions and their vertebral segments. It is, thus, the surgeon's undertaking to maintain these relationships in a state that is most near the physiology for that particular patient. Using reported "normals" will not be appropriate for all patients, therefore, guidelines have been presented in order to help understand the principles of sagittal anatomy, so that appropriate application to deformity patients in practice is possible.

## TYPES OF SAGITTAL MALALIGNMENT

Having defined normative sagittal alignment from a segmental, regional, as well as global perspective, various types of postoperative sagittal malalignments become apparent. We will concentrate our discussion on those that tend to produce global sagittal imbalance that almost invariably occurs in an anterior or forward position with the cervical thoracic junction lying anterior to the sacrum. Sagittal imbalance may occur following a "successful" spinal fusion such as a lumbar flat back syndrome following Harrington distraction instrumentation into the lumbar spine; or it may also occur following an unsuccessful fusion as in lumbar pseudarthrosis with settling of the lumbar spine via loose instrumentation, loss of anterior disk height, and poor lumbar spinal extensor musculature, all of which lead to a more forward sagittal balance. In addition, the spine may "autofuse" in a forward posture in disease states such as ankylosing spondylitis and diffuse idiopathic skeletal hyperostosis (DISH). Finally, a frequently encountered mechanism for sagittal imbalance in the elderly is multilevel thoracic, thoracolumbar, and/or lumbar compression fractures that may produce a fixed anterior sagittal imbalance with incapacitating pain. All of these sagittal malalignments become increasingly more complex when associated with coronal imbalance.

Probably the most common type of postoperative global sagittal imbalance that is encountered by a spinal surgeon currently is still the detrimental effect of distraction type instrumentation such as Harrington rods when placed into the lumbar spine (Fig. 59-4).[3,4] The posterior distraction forces decrease the segmental as

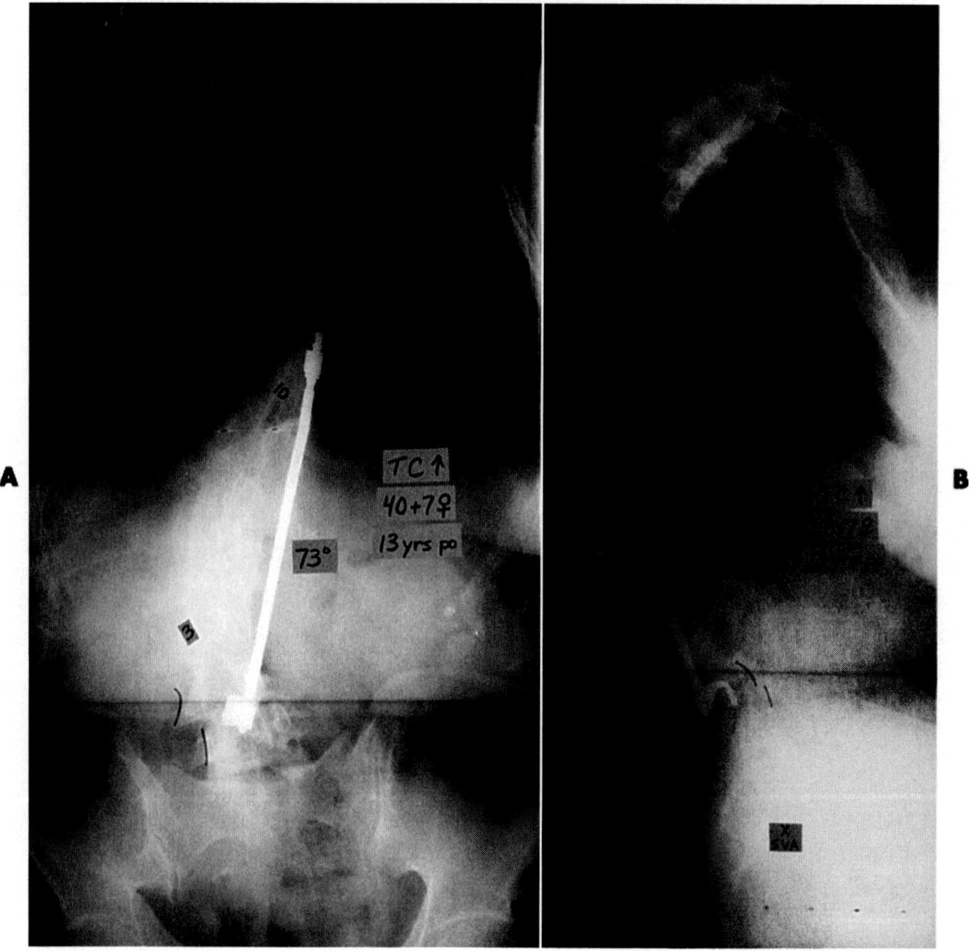


**Figure 59-4**

A 40-year-old woman who is 13 years status post Harrington rod placement from T9-L4 for correction of a thoracolumbar idiopathic scoliosis. **A,** Her long cassette coronal x-ray shows a residual 73-degree lumbar curve, with a rotatory subluxation of L3 on L4. **B,** The lateral view shows segmental kyphosis of the thoracolumbar and lumbar spine with a retrolisthesis of L4 on L5. The sagittal vertical axis falls through the midpoint of the sacrum.

well as regional thoracolumbar and lumbar lordosis, with possible anterior sagittal imbalance. The degree of sagittal imbalance depends on several factors including: alignment of the thoracic kyphosis and thoracolumbar junction; the hyperextensibility of any unfused distal lumbar disks, and the flexibility of the hip joints. However, hyperextension of the L4-L5 and/or L5-S1 disk is only a temporary solution to the loss of lumbar lordosis. A hyperextended disk produces accelerated degeneration in these disks with a tendency towards retrolisthesis, and further loss of disk height in these segments.[4,13] This commonly produces low lumbar pain and is often the primary reason for presentation to a spine specialist. These patients may present in either a neutral global sagittal alignment, or in an anterior or forward sagittal alignment primarily based on the degree of regional alignments of the thoracic, thoracolumbar, and lumbar spine. In a patient with a flat thoracic spine, often the sagittal plumb line will fall at or near the lumbosacral disk when the lumbar spine is flat as well (Fig. 59-5). However, in patients with more normal degrees of thoracic kyphosis, along with a flat or kyphotic thoracolumbar and lumbar regional alignment, then an anterior global sagittal imbalance is inevitable. Thus, it is imperative to document regional sagittal alignments (thoracic kyphosis, T1-T12; thoracolumbar junction, T10-L2; and lumbar alignment, T12-sac) in patients presenting with global sagittal imbalance to determine the specific regional etiologies for the imbalance. In those patients instrumented and fused flat all the way to the pelvis, one must carefully assess any hip flexion contractures to determine their role in the overall sagittal balance. In patients fixed flat to their pelvis, forward sagittal imbalance normally ensues with resultant flexion contractures of the hips that propagates the clinical and radiographic malalignment. These patients tend to stand with varying degrees of knee flexion as a compensatory mechanism to try and maintain an upright posture (Fig. 59-6).[13]

Spinal surgeons also may encounter patients with "autofusions" of their spine such as those with

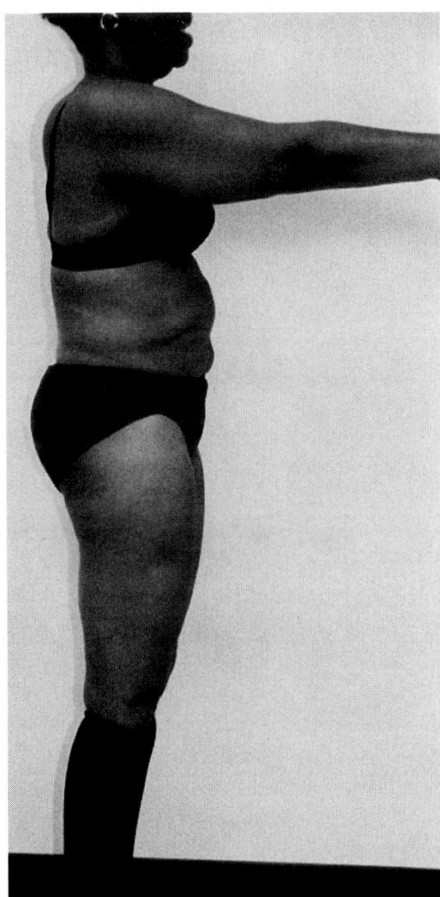

**FIGURE 59-5**

This 45-year-old woman had a Harrington rod placed down to L4 for adult idiopathic scoliosis 15 years ago. Her sagittal posture shows a flat thoracic, thoracolumbar, and lumbar spine, with her overall global balance being clinically acceptable.

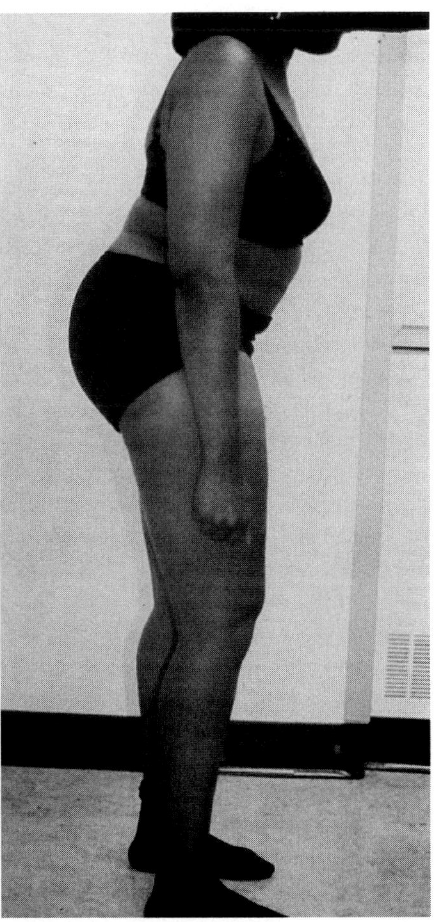

**FIGURE 59-6**

This 34-year-old woman had a Harrington distraction rod placed from T10 to the sacrum 20 years ago. She presents with clinical global sagittal forward imbalance, with a flat lumbar spine, prominent buttocks, flexion between the spinal pelvic and femoral axes, and slight flexion of the knees as an attempt to obtain a more upright posture.

ankylosing spondylitis and DISH in which the patient falls into a forward global sagittal imbalance (Fig. 59-7). A similar analysis of their regional thoracic, thoracolumbar and lumbar alignments is required, as well as an assessment of the cervical region because of associated fixed cervical kyphotic malalignments.[2,17]

Another cause of sagittal imbalance are transition syndromes, defined as the breakdown of a spinal segment either above and/or below a solid spinal fusion. These can occur when the fused spine is in a normative sagittal alignment, but appear to occur much more commonly when the spine is fused in a regional malalignment, specifically with loss of lumbar lordosis. In a review from our institution, Chapman et al found both radiographic and clinical factors that placed patients at higher risk of developing transition syndromes above or below their solid spine fusions. The most common radiographic abnormality was fusing the lumbar spine in a flat position of either hypolordosis or frank kyphosis. As expected, distal transition syndromes were more commonly seen below a long fusion that ended at L4-L5 making the L4-L5 and/or L5-S1 segments susceptible to radiographic degeneration and clinical symptomatology. In contrast, proximal transition syndromes were more common in lumbar degenerative fusions producing a junctional kyphosis with fall-off of the thoracic spine anteriorly. Proximal transition syndromes occur at an increasingly higher incidence the closer a fusion ends near the apex of the thoracic kyphosis. Thus, in adults undergoing fusion to the lower thoracic spine and thoracolumbar junction, it is imperative to determine the preoperative apex of thoracic kyphosis. If the planned proximal fusion level is within 2 to 3 spinal segments of the thoracic apex, then it is probably advantageous to consider extending the fusion above the apex to the

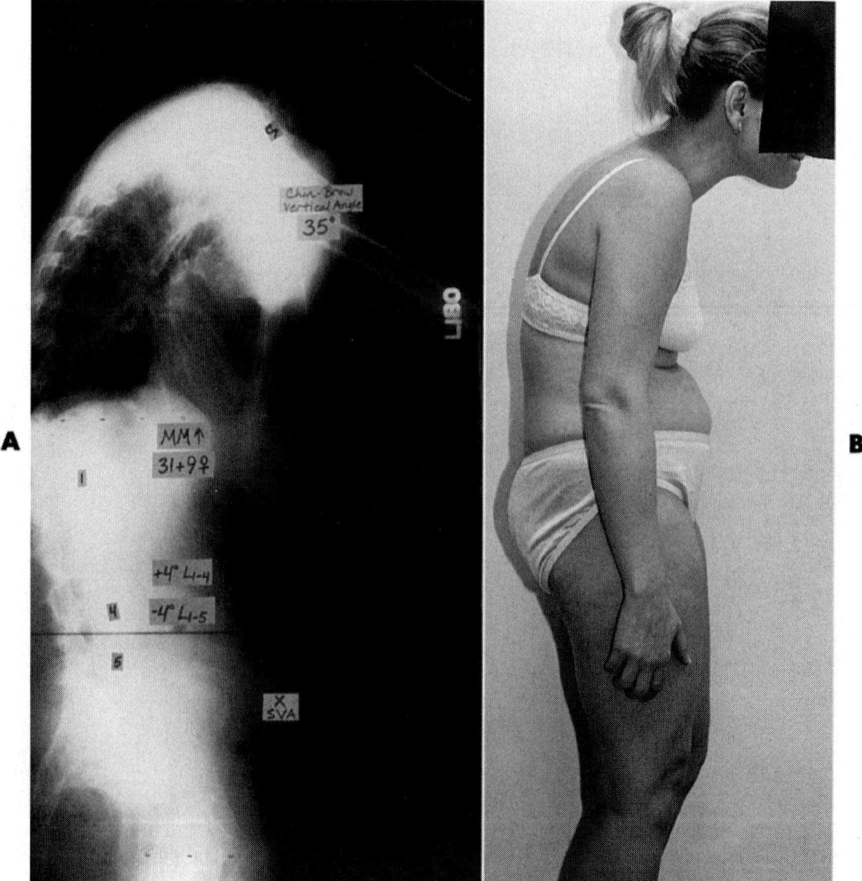


**Figure 59-7**

This 31-year-old woman with ankylosing spondylitis presented with complaints of poor posture, and increasing difficulty with forward gaze. **A,** Her lateral long cassette x-ray shows an ankylosed spine, a completely flat thoracolumbar and lumbar spine, and a marked anterior sagittal vertical axis. **B,** Her clinical appearance correlates with the radiographic alignment seen with a flat lumbar spine, protruding thoracic and cervicothoracic alignment, and forward position of her head and neck on her pelvis. She also demonstrated mild knee flexion as a compensatory mechanism to maintain a more upright posture and thus a more forward gaze.

upper thoracic spine. The same principle also holds true when fusing patients beyond the sixth decade (especially females) as these patients appear to have an increased risk of a proximal transition syndrome when fused proximally to the lower thoracic spine or even their thoracolumbar junction.

Surgical technique also plays an important role in preventing proximal and distal transition syndromes.[5] Specifically, maintenance of the ligamentous structures (intraspinous ligament, ligamentum flavum, and facet capsules) of adjacent nonfused segments must be stressed. In addition, injury to the facet joints themselves should be completely avoided. Proximally, avoidance of bilateral supralaminar hooks will limit the soft tissue damage that may occur during placement of these hooks and subsequent proximal breakdown. When using pedicle screws proximally at the thoracolumbar junction, it is important to elevate the connection of the screw and rod above the adjacent facet joint so as not to disturb the joint during implantation of the instrumentation.

When analyzing distal transition syndromes, the degree of disk degeneration present in the lower lumbar spine must be assessed. Disk degeneration may be manifested by the loss of disk height with traction spurs, retrolisthesis of the cephalad segment on the caudad segment, or via hyperextension of a low lumbar disk that produces a triangulated pattern.[3] This occurs as the body attempts to improve global sagittal balance by hyperextending the unfused distal lumbar motion segments. Although the hyperextended disks may improve sagittal balance temporarily, this invariably leads to accelerated degeneration of these disks and subsequent pain, with eventual loss of anterior disk height, and forward migration of the sagittal plumb line.

When assessing a suspected transition syndrome, several points are exceedingly important. The first is to document a solid spinal fusion throughout the entire arthrodesis. Next, the segmental and regional alignments of the sagittal spine throughout the fused area must be analyzed critically, especially since it appears that segmental hypolordosis is a significant etiology of proximal and distal transition syndromes. Next, regional and segmental alignments of the unfused spine above and below the solid spine fusion must be critically assessed to note the contributions of these to the overall global sagittal imbalance as noted on a long cassette lateral radiograph of the entire spine. Last, flexibility of the unfused spine above and below must be determined for proper positioning of the patient during subsequent revision surgery and the ability to produce a more normal global balance. In general, patients with more flexible regions of their unfused spine may be rebalanced without an osteotomy, while those patients with inflexible spines and a forward sagittal imbalance will almost always require an osteotomy procedure to rebalance (Fig. 59-8).

The third type of sagittal malalignment commonly seen postoperatively occurs with pseudarthrosis of the thoracolumbar and/or lumbar spine. Often these patients present as a "multi-operated spine" with several surgeries that commonly include diskectomies, laminectomies, and either uninstrumented and/or instrumented fusion attempts. Usually, they are posterior-only procedures and have not had any previous anterior surgery. They usually have loose instrumentation that may or may not be painful with motion. They invariably have poorly conditioned spinal extensor muscles from the surgical insult(s), as well as the poor muscle physiology occurring with constant irritation by any instrumentation that may be in place. They may present with slight or marked global sagittal imbalance because of a combination of all these factors that must be sorted out individually (Fig. 59-9). Documentation of a lumbar pseudarthrosis may or may not be obvious. Besides upright anteroposterior (AP) and lateral radiographs of the spine, oblique ra-diographs, flexion-extension lateral radiographs, fine-cut CT scans with sagittal reformations, and tomography (if available) may be of assistance. The number and type of previous surgeries must be delineated as well as any early and/or late complications occurring from previous surgeries. The two important surgical goals in these patients include both correction of any global sagittal imbalance and production of a solid spinal arthrodesis.[5]

## SPECIFIC SURGICAL PROCEDURES

There are a variety of surgical procedures that may be indicated to revise and correct global sagittal imbalance. These include a posterior-only revision; an anterior procedure as well as a revision posterior procedure; the addition of a spinal osteotomy performed posteriorly,[14,18,22-24] both anteriorly and posteriorly,[12] or all posteriorly but spanning all three columns of the spine via a pedicle subtraction three-column osteotomy[21]; and lastly, an anterior and posterior vertebrectomy procedure for correction of massive sagittal as well as coronal imbalance.[3]

Revision posterior surgery only is indicated when the overall standing sagittal balance is only slightly altered preoperatively and can be readily corrected with the patient positioned in a suitable operative frame under general anesthesia.[20] This would include situations of proximal and/or distal transition syndromes where the spine is readily correctable through the pathologic levels. This is assessed preoperatively on a supine hyperextension radiograph of the involved level(s). The previously fused level(s) must be documented to have a successful arthrodesis, and no large gaps should be present in the disk spaces anteriorly following the repositioning of the spine. A typical

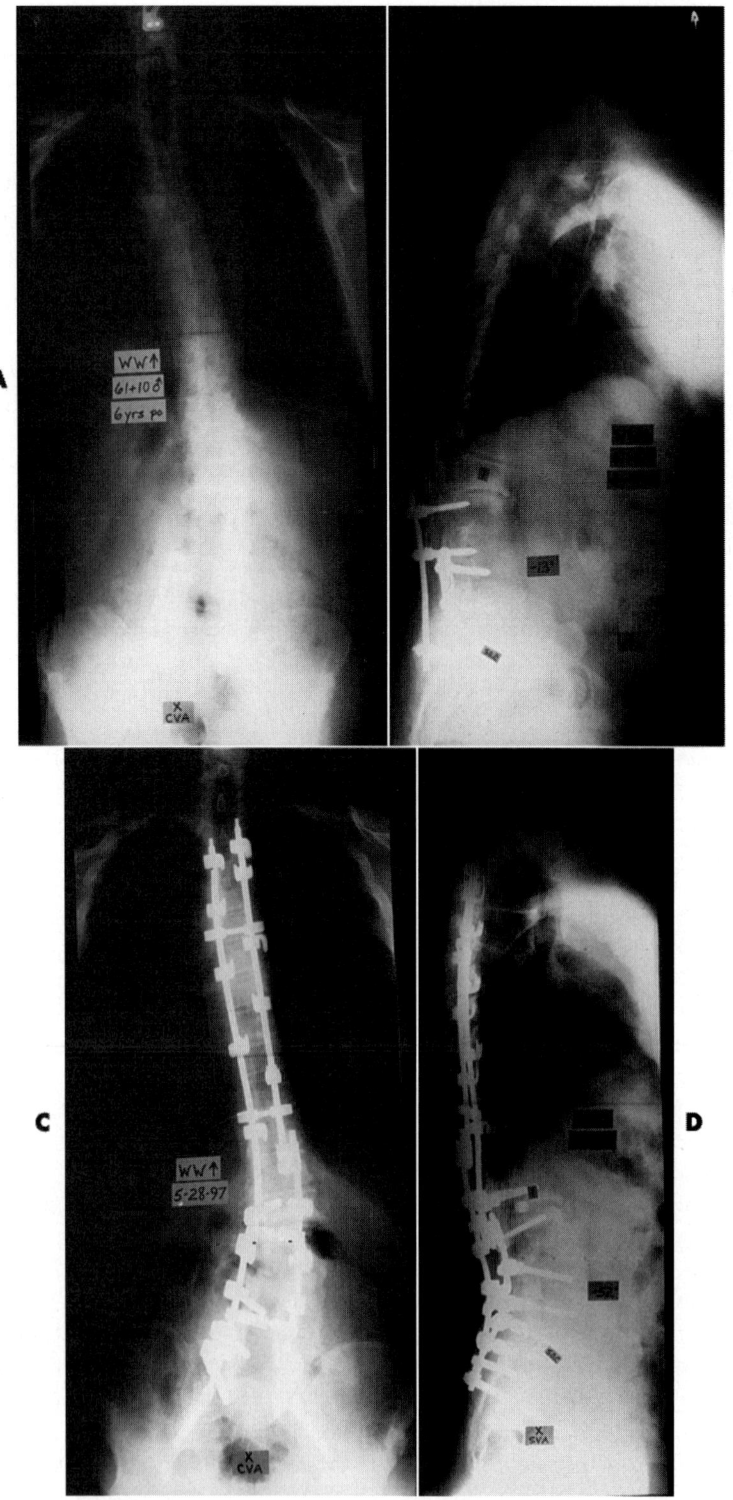


**FIGURE 59-8**

A 61-year-old man presented 6 years following three lumbar spine surgeries including laminectomies and instrumented fusions. At the time of his presentation, he was noted to have a solid spine fusion from L2-L5 with his **(A)** coronal alignment being slightly off to the left, but more impressively, **(B)** his sagittal vertical alignment being 12 cm anterior to his sacrum due to a lumbar spine fused in a flattened position, as well as a transitional segment at L1-L2 in segmental kyphosis. He underwent a revision posterior instrumentation removal, fusion documentation, and a posterior three-column transpedicular osteotomy at L3 with revision instrumentation extending from T3 to the pelvis. His postoperative coronal x-ray **(C)** showed a balanced spine, and his lateral x-ray **(D)** showed rebalancing in the sagittal plane with his sagittal vertical axis falling at the posterior aspect of the lumbosacral disk, with reduction and secure fixation spanning his L1-L2 transition segment.

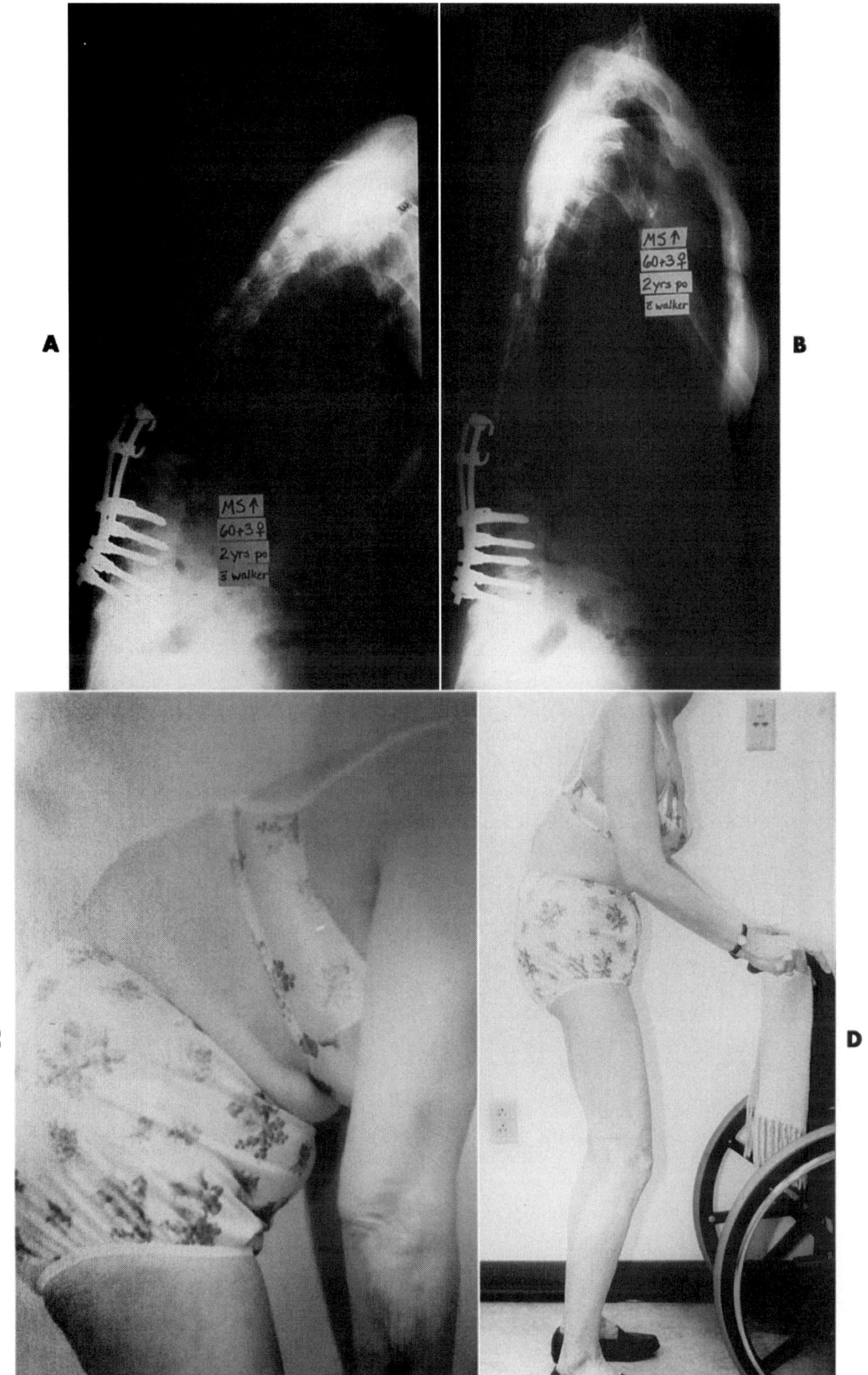


**FIGURE 59-9**

This 60-year-old woman presented 2 years following a series of three lumbar spinal surgeries including decompressions, uninstrumented, and lastly an attempted instrumented lumbar fusion. She complained of severe lumbar spinal pain and the inability to stand upright. **A,** Her long cassette lateral spine x-ray taken without her supporting herself on a walker shows marked forward sagittal imbalance, loose instrumentation, and a kyphotic lumbar spine. **B,** Her anterior sagittal balance was somewhat improved by the use of a walker clinically which is what she was relying upon constantly for support. **C,** Her clinical appearance unsupported with a marked falling forward of her entire trunk and torso on her pelvis, as well as the prominent lumbar instrumentation noted on her dorsal lumbar skin. **D,** Her clinical appearance holding onto a wheelchair as was her routine showing continued sagittal imbalance, prominent instrumentation, and knee flexion in an attempt to maintain a more upright posture.

situation where revision posterior only surgery is required is a fall-off junctional kyphosis at the thoracolumbar junction following instrumentation and fusion for a primary lumbar spinal pathology. In this example, the posterior instrumentation and fusion should be extended up into the upper thoracic spine above the apex of thoracic kyphosis if required to achieve and maintain global sagittal balance. This should produce acceptable sagittal balance in and of itself, otherwise consideration for osteotomy surgery of the lumbar spine should be performed if marked sagittal imbalance will still be present following the proximal extension of the instrumentation and fusion.

Combined anterior surgery and posterior revision surgery is often required to rebalance a patient in the sagittal plane. The anterior surgery provides increased mobility of the disk spaces whether performed in the thoracic, thoracolumbar, or lumbar spine assuming there is no posterior resistance over the released levels to limit flexibility (i.e., previously placed posterior instrumentation and fusion). Normally, these types of procedures are indicated for those patients with only mild global imbalance (approximately 5 cm) and can be somewhat corrected on a preoperative supine hyperextension film. A typical situation where this type of procedure is indicated is extension of a previous fusion to L3 or L4 down to the sacrum secondary to degenerative disk disease changes with loss of disk height of the lower disks (Fig. 59-10). Anterior surgery to restore disk height with structural grafts or cages, followed by posterior extension of the previously placed instrumentation and fusion is performed to achieve and maintain a global sagittal balance.[3]

In those patients with greater sagittal imbalance

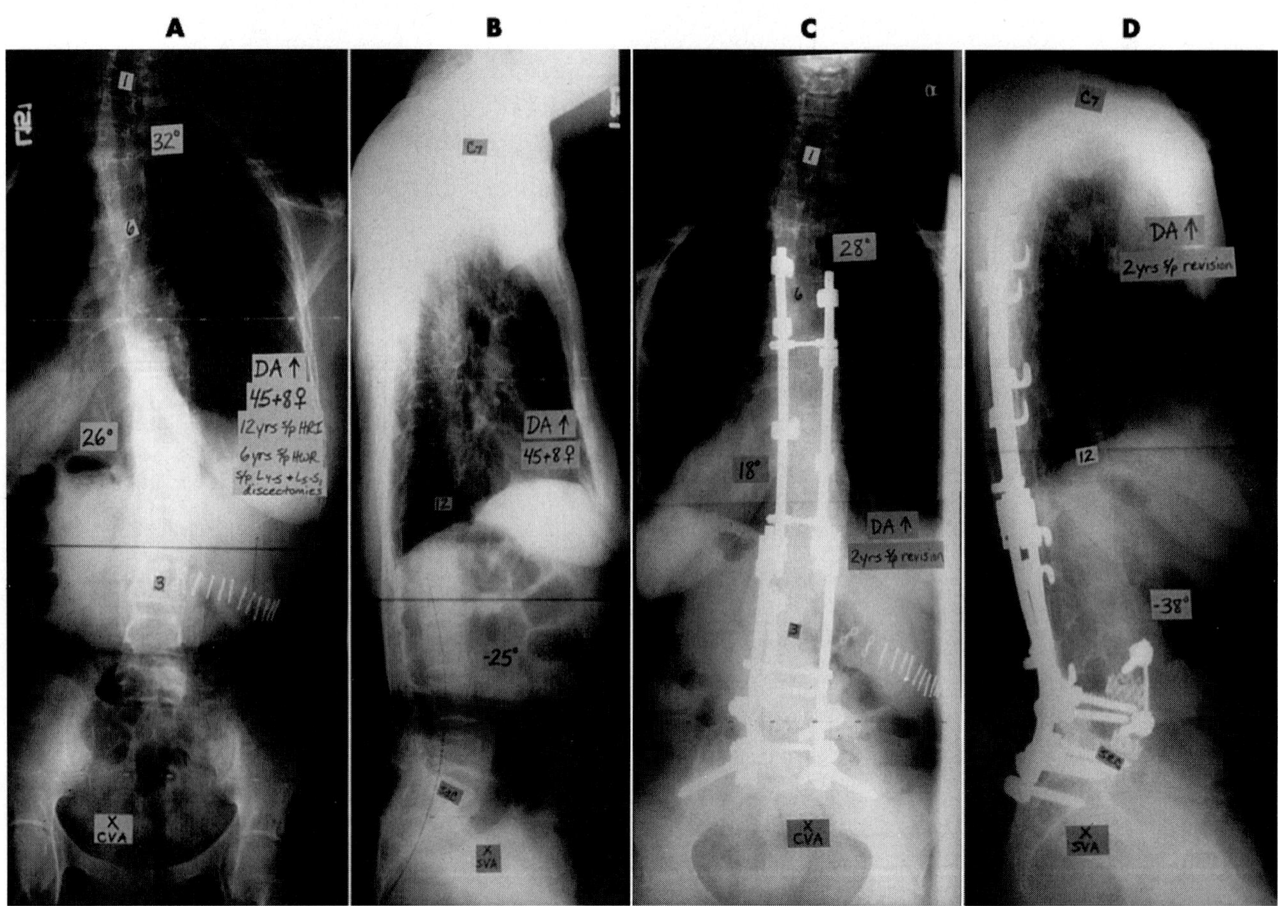


**Figure 59-10**

A 45-year-old woman treated with a Harrington rod to L4 twelve years previously for idiopathic scoliosis. She presented with discogenic pain in her lower two unfused disks at L4-L5 and L5-S1. **A,** Her long cassette coronal x-ray shows a solid spine fusion to L4. **B,** Her presenting long cassette lateral x-ray showed a flattened thoracic, thoracolumbar, and lumbar spine, with hyperextension of the L4-L5 and L5-S1 disks in order to maintain an upright posture. Her overall sagittal vertical axis was 4 cm anterior to her posterior lumbosacral disk. She underwent an anterior and posterior surgery whereby her L4-L5 and L5-S1 disks were fused with structural bone grafting utilizing cages, and posteriorly she had a single Smith-Petersen osteotomy performed at L2-L3 in an attempt to move her sagittal vertical axis slightly more posterior. Her postoperative coronal x-ray **(C)** showed the extension of her instrumentation and fusion to her pelvis, and her postoperative lateral x-ray **(D)** showed mild improvement in her overall sagittal vertical axis now located at the posterior superior corner of the lumbosacral disk.

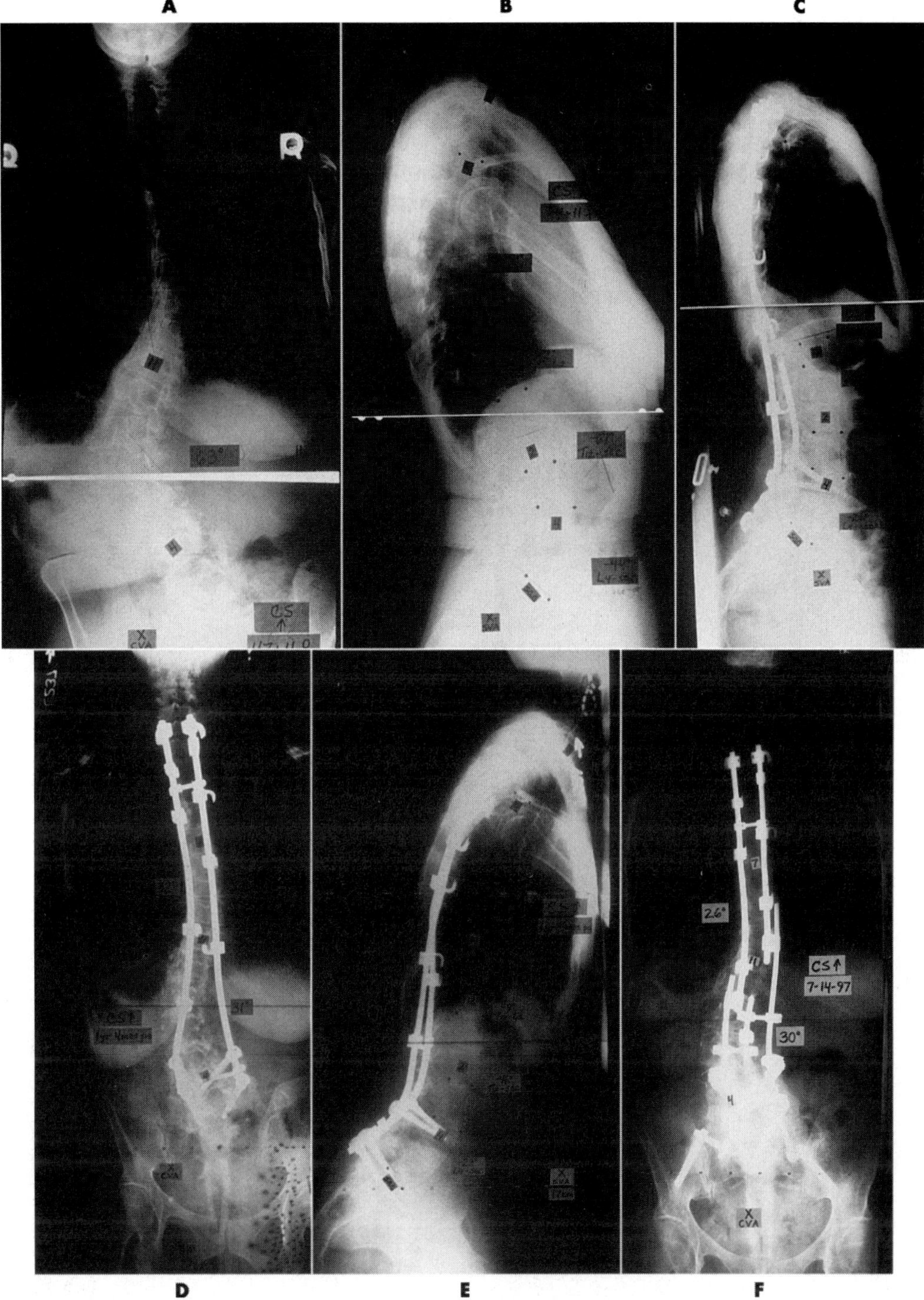


**FIGURE 59-11**

**A,** A 47-year-old woman who underwent operative treatment for a 63-degree adult lumbar idiopathic scoliosis with coronal imbalance. **B,** Her preoperative sagittal plane showed excellent sagittal alignment with her sagittal vertical axis 4 cm behind the lumbosacral disk. She was treated with an anterior spinal fusion from T12 to the sacrum using morselized rib (nonstructural) bone graft, and a posterior instrumentation and fusion from T2 to the sacrum with autogenous iliac crest graft. **C,** Her 1-week postoperative long cassette lateral x-ray showed slight forward migration of her sagittal vertical axis falling just anterior to her lumbosacral disk, but still quite acceptable. Her 18-month postoperative coronal x-ray **(D)** showed continued mild coronal imbalance to the left, while the lateral long cassette x-ray **(E)** demonstrated migration of the sagittal vertical axis now 17 cm in front of the sacrum. Her anterior sagittal imbalance gradually occurred via a combination of non-structural anterior bone graft in her lower lumbar disks, and inadequate sacral pelvic fixation for such a long instrumented scoliosis fusion. She underwent a revision posterior operation with complete instrumentation removal, documentation of a solid arthrodesis, posterior transpedicular 3-column osteotomy of L3 with re-instrumentation including improved sacral pelvic fixation points. Her postoperative revision coronal x-ray **(F)** shows near complete rebalancing in the coronal plane.

*Continued*

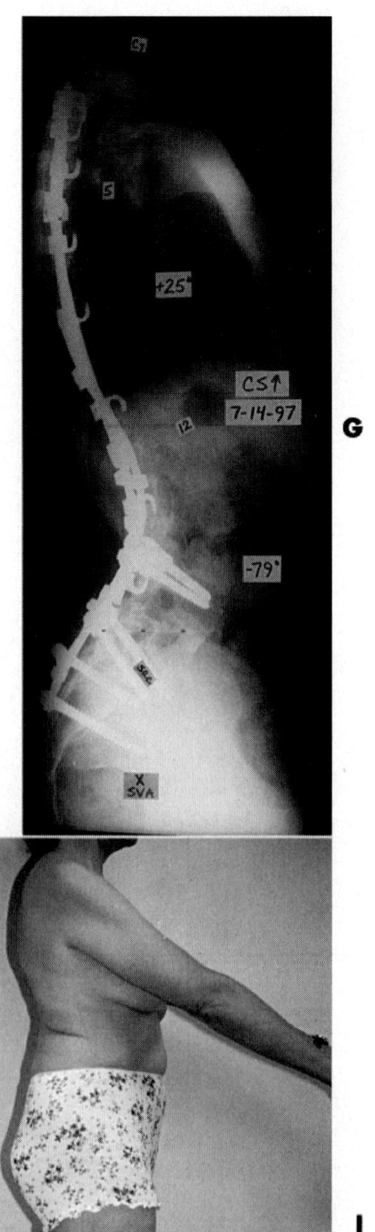


**FIGURE 59-11, CONT'D**

Her postoperative revision lateral spinal x-ray **(G)** shows complete correction of her anterior sagittal imbalance with a sagittal vertical axis that is positioned at the posterior edge of the lumbosacral disk. **H,** Here is her pre-revision clinical appearance demonstrating her marked anterior sagittal imbalance. **I,** Her postrevision clinical appearance shows restoration of a more appropriate upright posture.

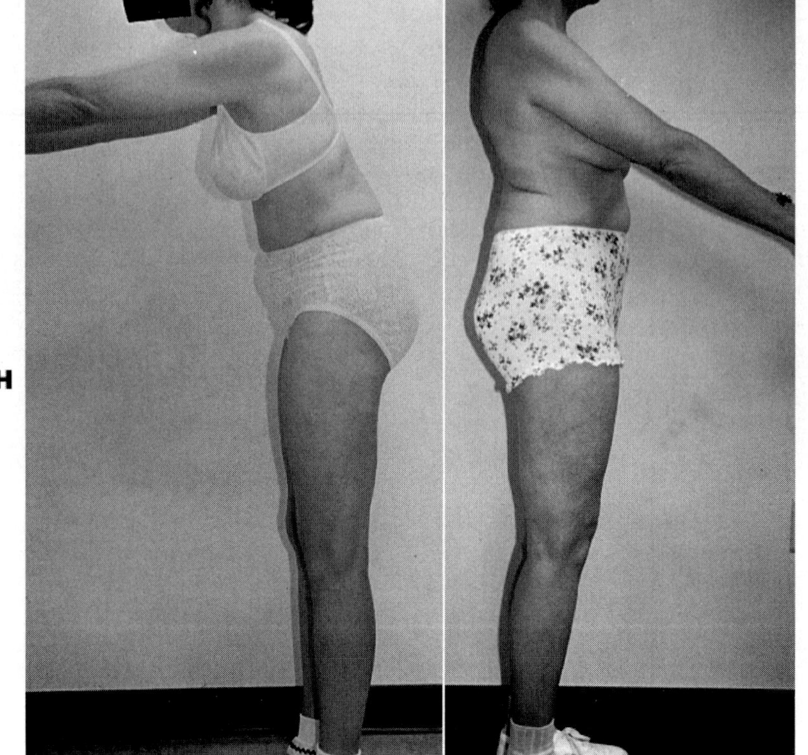


that is fixed, then some type of osteotomy procedure will be necessary to rebalance the spine. Osteotomies can be performed in several manners: as a single or multilevel Smith-Peterson type of posterior osteotomy centered between the pedicles with or without previous release of the anterior disk spaces[18]; both anterior through a previous intradiscal fusion, followed by posterior Smith-Peterson osteotomies at the corresponding levels osteotomized anteriorly; or posteriorly via a three-column pedicle subtraction osteotomy that shortens the posterior column, and to a lesser extent the middle column, and hinges on the anterior column.[21] Although there is certainly some overlap as to when these specific osteotomies are

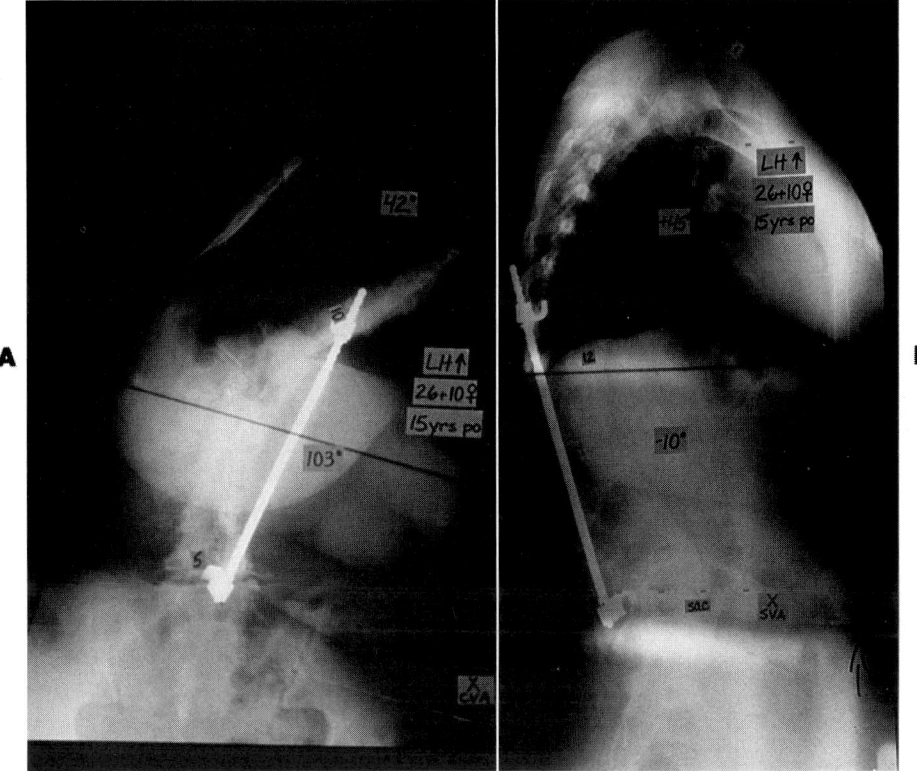


**FIGURE 59-12**

A 26-year-old woman who is 15 years status post-Harrington instrumentation and fusion from T10-L5 for an adolescent idiopathic lumbar scoliosis. She presented with complaints of increasing forward and right-sided postural imbalance, as well as debilitating lumbosacral back pain. **A,** Her upright coronal radiograph showed a residual 103-degree lumbar scoliosis (her immediate postoperative curve was only 40 degrees) with the coronal plumb line deviated 18 cm to the right of her mid sacrum. Also noted were degenerative changes of the unfused L5-S1 joint. **B,** Her lateral radiograph demonstrated a segmentally kyphotic thoracolumbar and lumbar spine and a sagittal vertical axis 5 cm in front of the sacrum. Goals in this type of spinal reconstruction are three fold: (1) to relieve her lumbosacral discogenic pain by fusing her L5-S1 joint; (2) to improve her marked coronal imbalance; and (3) to improve her moderate sagittal imbalance. Because of the marked coronal imbalance noted, it would be impossible to completely correct her malalignment with multiple Smith-Petersen osteotomies, or a posterior transpedicular osteotomy. The only way to obtain the amount of correction required to try and rebalance her is through a spinal vertebrectomy procedure. She underwent a three-stage spinal reconstruction. The first stage involved a two-level anterior corpectomy of L1 and L2, as well as an anterior spinal fusion of L5-S1 with a structural cage and autogenous bone graft. In the same setting, she underwent posterior Harrington rod removal, and placement of pedicle screw fixation points in her lumbar spine. Her second stage procedure performed five days later consisted of a large convex based closing wedge osteotomy centered at L1 and L2 (previous sites of the anterior corpectomies) to complete the spinal vertebrectomy procedure. This dissociated her proximal and lower spinal columns, which were then re-instrumented with convex compression forces to correct her coronal and sagittal imbalance simultaneously. Her instrumentation and fusion was extended up to T3 and down to the sacrum. Her third stage procedure done one month later, was a revision anterior thoracolumbar approach to place a structural cage that was locked in with anterior instrumentation, into the large residual anterior and middle column defect present between T12 and L3. This was performed because of her large body habitus, and the concern of leaving such a large anterior and middle column gap in her spine with subsequent risk of losing correction on her. *Continued*

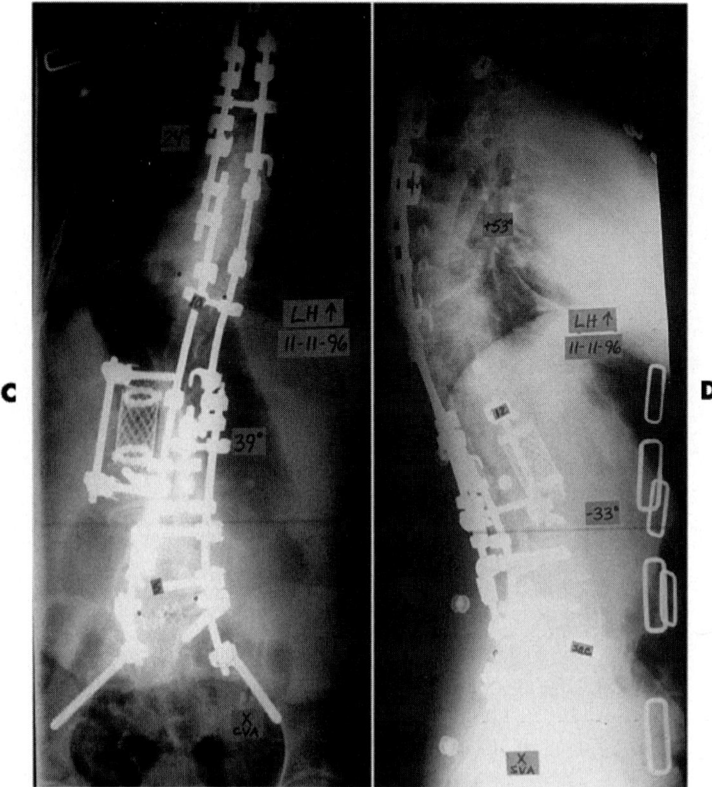


**Figure 59-12, cont'd**

Her postoperative upright coronal x-ray **(C)** demonstrated 13 cm of improvement in her coronal balance, with her long cassette lateral x-ray **(D)** showing obtainment of physiologic sagittal alignment including a sagittal vertical axis falling posterior to the sacrum.

indicated, there are some general guidelines that can be discussed regarding each of these.

Single or multilevel posterior Smith-Peterson osteotomies are probably the most common osteotomies performed in attempt to improve thoracolumbar and lumbar lordosis and correspondingly improve global sagittal balance.[18] These can be performed either through a previous posterior fusion mass or through an unfused spine by removing posterior element and facet bone to be able to compress posteriorly and thus shorten the posterior column. One should never lengthen the spinal column when trying to correct sagittal imbalance; it is always much safer to shorten the posterior column of the lumbar spine to improve sagittal balance. The osteotomy is centered between the pedicles, performed in a mild "V" fashion with the tip of the "V" pointing distal, so as to limit any tendency towards medial-lateral translation of the spine to occur. Approximately 10 to 12 degrees of lordosis can be obtained per osteotomy, assuming the anterior structures of the spine (anterior longitudinal ligament, anterior annulus) are flexible enough to allow the osteotomy to completely close posteriorly. A classic indication for occurrence of multiple posterior Smith-Peterson osteotomies is in patients with ankylosing spondylitis, and an autofused flat lumbar spine with forward sagittal imbalance and the inability to look forward. In these patients, the autofused anterior column will crack open with the posterior osteotomy closure.[2,10,17]

Simultaneous anterior and posterior osteotomies are indicated in patients with previous anterior and posterior fusion as well as marked sagittal imbalance.[12] These patients can either be managed with several corresponding anterior and posterior osteotomies, or a single posterior three-column pedicle subtraction osteotomy. The only absolute indication to perform anterior and posterior surgery on these patients is if both anterior and posterior instrumentation are present in the lumbar spine, and thus removal will be required prior to any osteotomy procedure being performed. If the anterior and posterior osteotomies are to be performed, the remnants of the anterior disks can usually be identified, and osteotomy is performed back to the spinal canal, and deep to the anterior and middle vertebral columns as well. Corresponding posterior Smith-Peterson osteotomies are then performed between the pedicles at each level where an anterior osteotomy has been previously performed.[18] Depending on the amount of the opening of the anterior and middle columns, subsequent structural grafting of any large "gaps" present may also be required as a third-stage procedure in these complex reconstructive patients.[3] For those patients with sagittal imbalance and a solid posterior instrumentation and fusion to the lower lumbar spine or sacrum, with or without a previous anterior fusion, an alternative procedure to rebalance these patients is the posterior three-column pedicle subtraction osteotomy.[21] Ideally, these are performed at L3, the normal apex of lumbar lordosis. Following removal of any posterior instrumentation, and the attainment of appropriate fixation points above and below the osteotomy, a 2- to 3-cm posterior column of bone is removed followed by decancellation of the pedicles, middle column including the floor of the spinal canal, and the side walls of the vertebral body down to but not through the anterior column. By tightly closing the posterior column defect, between 20 and 30 degrees of lordosis can be obtained through this one level. Adequate fixation points (at least 6) are required both above and below the osteotomy to maintain its closure and restore sagittal balance (Fig. 59-11, p. 765). This is a demanding procedure and should only be performed by those with adequate intraoperative assistants and training. However when properly performed, the osteotomies can provide significant improvement in global sagittal imbalance through a single posterior approach.

Occasionally, a patient presents with marked coronal and sagittal imbalance in whom osteotomy procedures will not be able to fully correct the deformity. In these rare patients, a spinal vertebrectomy may be required to realign the marked coronal and/or sagittal imbalance present. Ideally, the vertebrectomy should be performed if possible in the upper or midlumbar spine, preferably below the level of the conus. It is imperative that the spinal column is always shortened and never lengthened during these procedures. Anteriorly, the disks above and below the body to be resected are removed, including the entire body and ipsilateral pedicle back to the spinal canal, leaving the distal and anterior shell of the vertebral body intact. Posteriorly, the corresponding posterior elements and pedicles are removed thereby effectively separating the proximal and distal limbs of the spinal column, which are re-approximated and held with strong fixation following realignment of the spinal column (Fig. 59-12, p. 767). These again are challenging procedures that should be performed by those who are properly trained and have adequate intraoperative assistants.

## CONCLUSION

Sagittal plane analysis has become increasingly important for spinal reconstructive surgeons, especially when performing long fusions to the lower lumbar spine and/or sacrum. It is imperative to achieve a global sagittal balance whereby the C7 plumb line falls at or behind the lumbosacral disk following these reconstructive surgeries. When confronted with a postoperative patient with anterior global sagittal imbalance, careful analysis of the regional alignments of the thoracic, thoracolumbar, and lumbar spine is essential, as well as assessment of any hip flexion contractures that may be present. The specific surgical solution to these patients depends on many factors, but often requires osteotomy procedures to shorten the posterior column of the lumbar spine in order to move the sagittal plumb line posterior to the lumbosacral disk. Hopefully, the increased awareness placed upon the sagittal plane will lessen the need for revision surgery for sagittal imbalance and prove beneficial to the patients whom we treat.

## REFERENCES


1. Bernhardt M, Bridwell KH: Segmental analysis of the sagittal plane alignment of the normal thoracic and lumbar spines and thoracolumbar junction, *Spine* 14(7): 717-21, 1989.
2. Bradford DS et al: Ankylosing spondylitis: experience and surgical management of 21 patients, *Spine* 12:238-243, 1987.
3. Bridwell KH: *Osteotomies for fixed deformities in the thoracic and lumbar spine.* In Bridwell KH, DeWald RL, editors: *The textbook of spinal surgery,* ed 2, vol 1, Philadelphia, 1997, Lippincott-Raven, p 821.
4. Denis F: *The iatrogenic loss of lumbar lordosis: the flat back and flat buttock syndromes.* In Farcy JP, editor: *Complex spinal deformities, Spine: State Art Rev* 8(3):659, Philadelphia, 1994, Hanley & Belfus.
5. De Wald RL: Revision surgery for spinal deformity: adult spinal deformity, *Instr Course Lect* 41:235-250, 1992.
6. Fon GT et al: Thoracic kyphosis: range in normal subjects, *AJR Am J Roentgenol* 134:979-983, 1980.
7. Gelb DE et al: An analysis of sagittal spinal alignment in 100 asymptomatic middle and older aged volunteers, *Spine* 20(12):1351-1358, 1995.
8. Hammerberg KW: *Ankylosing spondylitis.* In Bridwell KH, DeWald RL, editors: *The textbook of spinal surgery,* vol 1, Philadelphia, 1991, JB Lippincott, p 525.
9. Hardacker JW et al: Radiographic standing cervical segmental alignment in adult volunteers without neck symptoms, *Spine* 22(13):1472-1479, 1997.

10. Hehne H-J, Zielke K: *Correction of long, curved deformities in ankylosing spondylitis.* In Bridwell KH, DeWald RL, editors: *The textbook of spinal surgery,* vol 1, Philadelphia, 1991, JB Lippincott, p 547.
11. Jackson RP, McManus AC: Radiographic analysis of sagittal plane alignment and balance in standing volunteers and patients with low back pain matched for age, sex, and size: a prospective controlled clinical study, *Spine* 19(14):1611-1618, 1994.
12. Kostuik JP et al: Combined single stage anterior and posterior osteotomy for correction of iatrogenic lumbar kyphosis, *Spine* 13(3):257-266, 1988.
13. LaGrone MO et al: Treatment of symptomatic flatback after spinal fusion, *J Bone Joint Surg* 70A(4):569-580, 1988.
14. Law WA: Osteotomy of the spine, *Clin Orthop* 66: 70-76, 1969.
15. Propst-Proctor SL, Bleck EE: Radiographic determination of lordosis and kyphosis in normal and scoliotic children, *J Ped Orthop* 3:344-346, 1983.
16. Roaf R: Vertebral growth and its mechanical control, *J Bone Joint Surg* 42B(1):40-59, 1960.
17. Simmons EH: The surgical correction of flexion deformity of the cervical spine in ankylosing spondylitis, *Clin Orthop* 86:132-143, 1972.
18. Smith-Petersen MN et al: Osteotomy of the spine for correction of flexion deformity in rheumatoid arthritis, *J Bone Joint Surg* 27:1-11, 1945.
19. Stagnara P et al: Reciprocal angulation of vertebral bodies in a sagittal plane: approach to references for the evaluation of kyphosis and lordosis, *Spine* 7(4):335-342, 1982.
20. Tan SB et al: Effect of operative position of sagittal alignment of the lumbar spine, *Spine* 19(3):314-318, 1994.
21. Thiranont N, Netrawinchien P: Transpedicular decancellation closed wedge vertebral osteotomy for treatment of fixed flexion deformity of the spine in ankylosing spondylitis, *Spine* 18(16):2517-2522, 1993.
22. Thomasen E: Vertebral osteotomy for correction of kyphosis in ankylosing spondylitis, *Clin Orthop* 194: 142-152, 1985.
23. Twomey LT, Taylor JR: Age changes in lumbar vertebral and intervertebral discs, *Clin Orthop* 224:97-104, 1987.
24. Urist MR: Osteotomy of the spine: report of a case of ankylosing rheumatoid spondylitis, *J Bone Joint Surg* 40A:833-843, 1958.
25. Vedantam R et al: Comparison of standing sagittal alignment in asymptomatic adolescents versus adults, *Spine* 23(2):211-215, 1998.
26. Voutsinas SA, MacEwen GD: Sagittal profiles of the spine, *Clin Orthop* 210:235-242, 1986.
27. Wambolt A, Spencer DL: A segmental analysis of the distribution of lumbar lordosis in the normal spine, *Orthop Trans* 11:92-93, 1987.

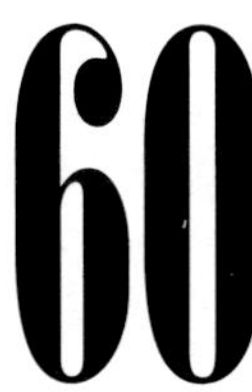

# SAGITTAL SPINOPELVIC ALIGNMENTS AND POSITIONING FOR SURGERY

**Roger P. Jackson, M.D.**



Successful surgery on the lumbar spine requires careful patient positioning with primary concerns for controlling ventilation and the sagittal spinopelvic alignments as well as reducing pressure points and blood loss. Adjusting the lumbopelvic contour for less lordosis can facilitate some neurodecompressive procedures. Appropriate positioning can also provide more lordosis for fusion procedures, specifically lower lumbar lordosis which is important in correcting the standing spinopelvic compensations that occur around the hip axis.[30,31,33,35-38,50-52] Table and pad designs for supporting the patient that allow for unrestricted intraoperative imaging of the entire spine and pelvis and that minimize skin pressure point problems, including those on the face, as well as positioning techniques to decompress the abdomen and diminish intraoperative bleeding are also critically important considerations.[5,50,55] In addition, positioning the patient to decrease the overall nerve root length and relieve any sciatic nerve stretch can be beneficial in certain cases.[53] During the past 5 decades many frames, tables, and techniques have been developed and promoted to position and support the patient during lumbar spinal surgery.[5,6,8,12,13,17,46,49,50,54,55,59,60,67,70] The described devices and techniques are quite different in their philosophy and approach. Furthermore recent studies have shown considerable differences in how these frames and tables affect sagittal lumbar and pelvic alignments, particularly segmental lordosis at the L4-L5 and L5-S1 levels.[3,48,50,62,63,65,66] As many of these frames, tables, and positioning techniques have unique advantages and disadvantages, the surgeon is obligated to select a position that, again, facilitates the planned procedure as best possible and does not contribute to intraoperative or postoperative morbidity. This is especially true for revision spine surgery.

Placing the patient in a certain position may not accomplish all that is needed or desired with respect to both the planned surgical procedure and the spinopelvic alignments.[49] For example, entrance into the spinal canal during lumbar laminectomy can, again, be simplified somewhat by operative positions that reduce lordosis and increase the interlaminar space.[5,8,50,54,59,60] Since physiologic lordosis is felt to be a very important factor affecting long-term results of spinal fusions,[11,15,18,32,36,37,40-44,56] intraoperative positions should be used that preserve or increase the lordosis and that help correct or improve the lumbopelvic alignment when using instrumentation or other spinal implants, particularly in revision spine surgery. Therefore, for patients who are undergoing both laminectomy and fusion with implants in the lumbosacral region at the same surgery, each of these procedures and their importance needs to be considered and, perhaps, prioritized.

Although the importance of sagittal lumbopelvic alignment and its relationship to intraoperative positioning seem intuitively evident, the literature provides few detailed reports and some conflicting and confusing information. It has been reported that 90-90 knee-chest positioning on various spinal frames, such as the Hastings or Andrews, produces lumbar hyperextension.[54,57] More recent studies looking specifically at the segmental distributions of lordosis have shown that the 90-90 positions significantly decrease lumbar lordosis, particularly at the L4-L5 and L5-S1 levels.[48-50,62,63,66] The Wilson frame has been advocated and frequently used to apparently reduce lumbosacral lordosis by positioning the patient over the arches of the device, thereby opening up the L5-S1 interlaminar space for diskectomy or other neurodecompressive procedures in the spinal canal at this level. However, more current reports have shown that when awake adult volunteers are positioned over a Wilson frame, which is fully domed, and even with the subjects' hips flexed a mean 28 degrees, L5-S1 lordosis is not decreased but actually increased over that measured when standing upright in these same subjects.[3,65] Therefore, in certain situations these studies may not support some of our beliefs and/or actual practices, as well as what has been published in some textbooks.[54,57]

Standing balance and, in particular, spinopelvic alignments and compensatory relationships around the hip axis[36] are very important considerations in lumbar arthrodesis procedures, especially with the increasing use of instrumentation and other spinal implants designed for the lumbosacral region. Segmental fixation systems have the capacity to significantly alter these alignments and relationships and improve or aggravate compensations of the spinopelvic axis that occur with and for standing balance. This is true whether or not the insertion of these spinal systems is performed to the sacropelvis. Studies of spinopelvic balance and of standing compensatory lumbopelvic relationships are, therefore, potentially helpful.[14,16,30,31,36-38,51,52,61,64,69] While values for vertebral angular alignments in the sagittal plane have been reported,[4,14,61,72] standing physiologic relationships of the spinopelvic axis, specifically with respect to lumbopelvic compensations and balance around the hip axis, have only been recently established and defined.[27,30,31,33,35-38,51,52] It is often advantageous to first measure "normal" asymptomatic subjects for such alignments and relationships (Table 60-1). The data from this research can then be used in the analysis of other studies, such as those involving patients with specific spinal disorders.[30,31,34-38,52,72] By so doing, different treatments of these disorders can be more completely compared, particularly with respect to patient outcome, as recommended by Swank et al.[64]

## SAGITTAL SPINOPELVIC ALIGNMENTS

### STANDING LUMBOPELVIC ANGULATIONS, COMPENSATIONS, AND MEASUREMENTS FOR SAGITTAL BALANCE IN NORMAL SUBJECTS

Using various techniques to measure segmental angulations of the lumbar vertebrae, studies have shown that half to three-fourths of the total lordosis between L1 and S1 is normally located at the two most distal motion segments (Table 60-1).[4,30,51,60] These studies and measurements in normal standing subjects should be given careful consideration when reconstructive lumbar spine surgery is performed in patients, with or without the use of instrumentation or other spinal implants (Figs. 60-1, 60-2, 60-3, and 60-4). Although the ultimate goal is to get a solid fusion it is also very important to have a well aligned, balanced spine segmentally, regionally and globally with corrections, or at least improvements, in the spinopelvic compensations and decompensations that occur in these patients.[23,26,30,36-38,52] In the sagittal plane, for many patients this can be largely achieved by obtaining or preserving, as well as increasing and maintaining on a long-term basis, lordosis in the lower lumbar spine.

Studies of "normal" volunteers, as well as of patients with spinal disorders, have shown a close association between standing sagittal sacropelvic angulation (sacral base slope or sacral inclination) and total lumbar lordosis (Figs. 60-4 and 60-5).[14,30,31,38,51,52,61,69] In addition to total lumbar lordosis, Jackson and McManus also found significant correlations between the sacral inclination and segmental lordosis measurements in their standing subjects.[30] In this study, the sacral inclination was an indication not only of the sacropelvic angulation, but also of standing hip extension through the acetabula, or pelvic "hip axis," for the authors (Figs. 60-1 and 60-4). In their studies the pelvic hip axis was located midway along a line drawn between the centers of the femoral heads on the lateral radiographs (Figs. 60-1, 60-3, and 60-4). The significant Pearson correlation coefficients reported by Jackson and McManus for standing sacral inclination or sacropelvic angulation around the "hip axis," as defined, with segmental and total lordosis in the volunteers were as follows: L1-L2, $r = -0.30$ ($p = 0.0020$); L2-L3, $r = -0.40$ ($p = 0.0001$); L3-L4, $r = -0.35$ ($p = 0.0040$); L4-L5, $r = -0.49$ ($p = 0.0001$); L5-S1, $r = -0.28$ ($p = 0.0043$); and L1-S1, $r = -0.70$ ($p = 0.0001$).[30] The authors found similar correlations in the patients with low back pain and degenerative lumbar disk disease that they also studied.[30] In these static studies, done with the subjects' knees fully extended or as straight as possible, the correlations indicated that as both segmental and total lordosis decreased the sacropelvis rotated posteriorly around the hip axis

**Table 60-1. Sagittal Plane Normative Data — Mean Measurements (SEM, Range)**

| | Stagnara et al<br>n = 100; 43F, 57M<br>(ages 20 to 29 yrs) | Bernhardt and Bridwell<br>n = 102; 55F, 47M<br>(ages 4.6 to 29.8 yrs) | Jackson and McManus<br>n = 100; 50F, 50M<br>(ages 20 to 63 yrs) | Peterson et al<br>n = 50; 25F, 25M<br>(ages 22 to 63 yrs) |
|---|---|---|---|---|
| (T1-12) | | +41 | +42.1 (8.9, +22 to +68) | +47.1 (9.7, +26 to +75) |
| T1-T2 | | +1 | | |
| T2-T3 | | +3 | | |
| T3-T4 | | +3.5 | | |
| T4-T5 | +5 (4, −2 to +17) | +5 | | |
| T5-T6 | +5 (4, −2 to +23) | +5 | | |
| T6-T7 | +6 (4, +1 to +22) | +5 | | |
| T7-T8 | +5 (4, 0 to +22) | +5 | | |
| T8-T9 | +4 (5, −5 to +36) | +4 | | |
| T9-T10 | +3 (5, −6 to +24) | +3 | | |
| T10-T11 | +2 (5, −5 to +17) | +3 | | |
| T11-T12 | +2 (5, −7 to +17) | +2.5 | | |
| T12-L1 | +1 (5, −7 to +17) | +1 | | |
| L1-L2 | −2 (5, −13 to +13) | −4 | −1.7 (4.2, −12 to +11) | −1.9 (3.5, −8 to +7) |
| L2-L3 | −7 (5, −17 to +7) | −7 | −7.0 (4.3, −18 to +5) | −7.2 (4.0, −15 to +1) |
| L3-L4 | −11 (5, −26 to 0) | −13 | −11.3 (3.8, −19 to 0) | −12.0 (3.4, −20 to −6) |
| L4-L5 | −15 (6, −2 to −10) | −20 | −16.5 (5.0, −28 to +3) | −17.0 (4.4, −29 to −10) |
| L5-S1 | −21 (6, −35 to −10) | −28 | −24.6 (6.2, −39 to −11) | −24.0 (5.4, −37 to −12) |
| L1-S1 | −56 (10, −79 to −33) | −72 | −60.9 (12.0, −88 to −31) | −62.1 (10.8, −86 to −41) |
| Sacral Base Slope (from horizontal) | 41 (35, 35 to 71) | | | |
| Sacral Inclination (from vertical) | | | 50.4 (7.7, 28 to 68) | 47.9 (6.7, 35 to 61) |
| Lumbar Apex | | L3-L4 disk | | L3-L4 disk |
| Thoracic Apex | | T6-T7 disk | T7-T8 disk | T7 body |
| S1 to C7 Vertical Lines | | | −0.05 cm (2.5, −6 to +6.5) | +0.38 cm (2.1, −5.7 to +5.2) |
| Hip Axis to C7 Vertical Lines | | | | −3.9 cm (2.1, −8.8 to +0.5) |
| Hip Axis to S1 Vertical Lines | | | | −4.2 cm (1.4, −1.2 to −7.2) |
| Pelvic Angle | | | | 17.4 (5.5, 5.0 to 29.0) |
| Pelvic Radius | | | | 13.5 cm (0.86, 11.4 to 15.0) |

SEM = standard error of the mean; all data given in degrees unless otherwise indicated. (+, kyphotic; −, lordotic); +, anterior to reference point; −, posterior to reference point

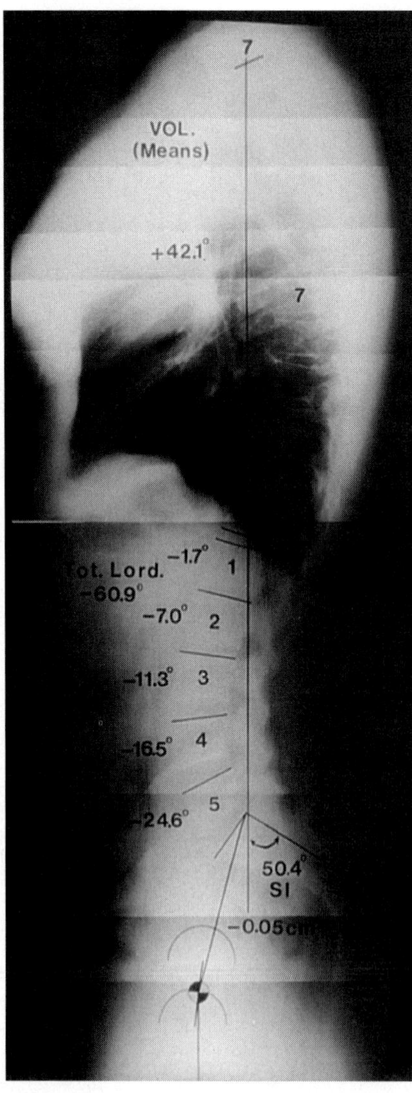


**FIGURE 60-1**

Standing 36-inch lateral radiograph of the spine and pelvis showing the methodology used and mean measurements obtained for 100 adult volunteers. Segmental lordosis is measured using a modified Cobb method from adjacent superior vertebral lumbar endplates, as marked and shown, and total lordosis (*Tot Lord*) is measured from the superior endplates of L1 to S1 (S1 endplate technique).[30] Total thoracic kyphosis is measured using the Cobb method from the top of T1 to the bottom of T12. The apex of lordosis and kyphosis are recorded. A sagittal vertical axis line or plumb line extending down from the center of the C7 body is drawn and measured. The sacral inclination (SI) angle is measured. The pelvic hip axis is determined by locating the mid-point along a line drawn between the centers of the femoral heads. A line is then drawn from the center of the hip axis to the sacral reference point (posterior superior corner of S1). This line is the pelvic radius. *(From Jackson RP: Spinal balance, lumbopelvic alignments around hip axis and positioning for surgery. In Margulies JY, ed: Adult L5-S1 surgery issue of SPINE, State of the art reviews 11(1):33-58, 1997.)*

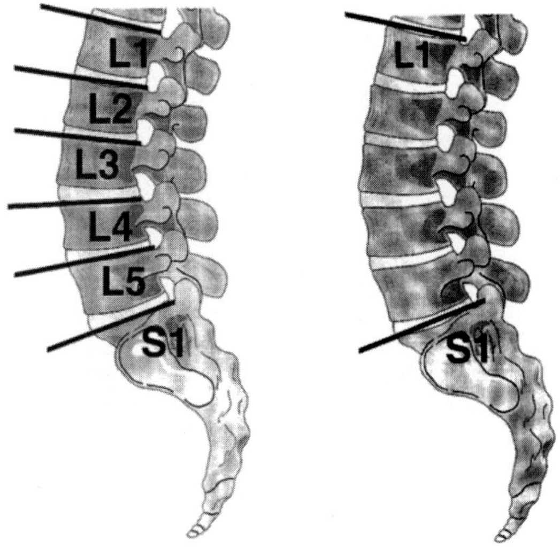


**FIGURE 60-2**

Modified Cobb methodology used to measure segmental (*left*) and total (*right*) lumbar lordosis from L1 to S1 on the lateral radiographs (S1 endplate technique).

resulting in a more vertical sacral inclination or slope with an associated increase in standing hip extension, if possible, to compensate for sagittal balance (Fig. 60-4).[16,30] Jackson and McManus felt this to be an important lumbopelvic relationship for balance that deserved further study.[30] Since spinopelvic balance and lifting are closely related it is not surprising that similar changes in the lumbopelvic angulation, i.e., decreased lordosis and corresponding pelvic rotation (which occurs posteriorly around the hips) have also been reported with static and dynamic loading of the spine.[7,68]

A sagittal vertical axis (SVA) line, such as the C7 plumb line, for standing spinal balance has been evaluated and measured in different ways.[9,14,30,31,36,38,43,44,51,52,58,64] Jackson and McManus were the first to publish normative sagittal C7 plumb line measurements for standing spinal balance in asymptomatic adult volunteers with well defined methodology (Table 60-1).[30] The authors found that the C7 plumb line measurements had wide variation (range, −6.0 to +6.5 cm) and no association with sacral inclination as a measurement for sacropelvic angulation around the hip axis.[30,36] In addition, they found that segmental as well as total lordosis had strong correlation with the standing sacral inclination and that these lumbopelvic relationships were also tied to the pelvic hip axis. The authors of this study pointed out that the sagittal C7 plumb line was not the center of gravity line for spinal balance that they felt to be globally over the hip axis when standing upright in the balanced subject. In their discussion they stated that measurements on standing lateral radiographs for the sagittal C7 plumb line and the sacropelvic angulation (sacral inclination and pelvic rotation around the axis through the hips) were important, but independent determinates of spinopelvic balance and that both should be carefully considered in the assessment of patients with disorders of the spine. However, the wide range of "normal" values reported by the authors for these spinopelvic

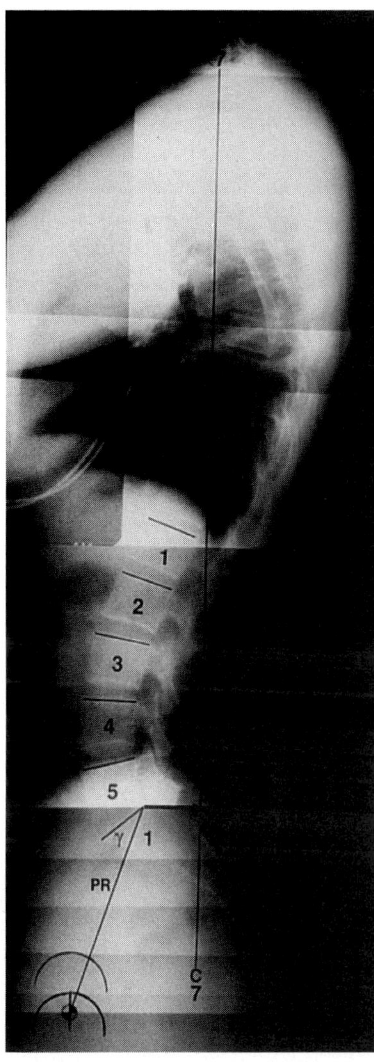


**FIGURE 60-3**

Methodology used to measure the standing sagittal C7 plumb line from the S1 reference point and lumbopelvic angles by the pelvic radius technique on the lateral radiographs. The plumb line extends down from the center of the C7 body. The perpendicular distance and direction from the posterior superior corner of the S1 vertebra to the C7 plumb line was recorded as the measurement for this line (horizontal arrow directed posteriorly). The hip axis is located in the pelvis midway along a line drawn between the centers of the femoral heads. The hip axis is also important because it is the center or axis of the pelvis for tilting and rotating in the frontal and transverse planes, respectively. The line from the center of the hip axis to the reference point is the PR. The angle (γ) is measured from the PR to the S1 superior endplate and is constant for each patient or subject. Lumbopelvic angles for segmental and total lordosis can be more reliably measured from the PR line to the lines along the superior endplates of the L5, L4, L3, L2 and L1 vertebrae (pelvic radius technique).[38]

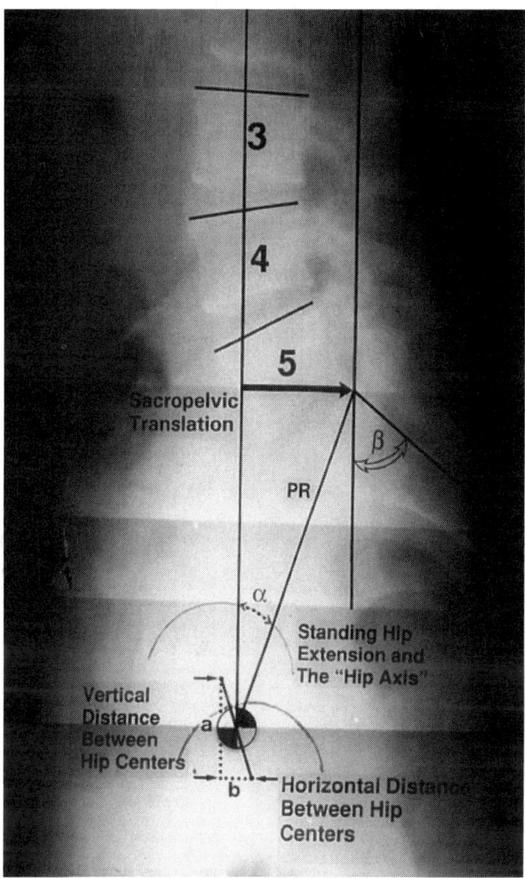


**FIGURE 60-4**

Methodology used to measure pelvic rotation and balance (alignment of the sacropelvis over the hips) on the standing lateral radiographs taken with the cassette positioned 72 inches from the x-ray source. The angle "β" between a vertical line through the posterior superior corner of the S1 vertebral body and the line drawn parallel along the back of S1 and S2 is determined (*hollow curved arrow*). This angle is the sacral inclination and is considered to be a determinant for standing hip extension with compensatory sacropelvic translation and angulation (α) around the hip axis. The hip axis is located in the pelvis midway along a line drawn between the centers of the femoral heads. Sacropelvic translation is measured as the horizontal perpendicular distance from the vertical line through the hip axis to the S1 vertical line (*horizontal arrow* directed posteriorly to the posterior superior corner of S1). Pelvic rotation in the transverse plane occurs with positioning of the patient from one radiograph to the next thereby affecting the compensatory sacropelvic translation measurements and the other measurements. As long as the perpendicular distance "*b*" between the centers of the femoral heads is 40-mm or less on standardized radiographs (source to cassette distance of 72 inches), the pelvic rotation in the transverse plane is less than 15 degrees and the true sacropelvic translation is no greater than 3.5% of the actual measured length.[38] The divergence of the x-ray beams also causes one hip (closest to the film) to appear higher than the other hip giving the impression of pelvic tilting in the frontal plane (vertical distance "*a*" between the hip centers). Whereas this finding on the films does not affect the linear measurements for compensatory sacropelvic translation measurements it does affect angular measurements, including the sacropelvic angle α, the sacral inclination β, and the lumbopelvic angles from the PR line to the lines along the superior vertebral endplates. The PR line is drawn from the center of the hip axis to the posterior superior corner of S1.[38]

parameters needs to be recognized (Table 60-1).[30] Consequently, in the actual care of patients the relationships and congruencies between these parameters would appear to be more meaningful and useful than any absolute values.

The lumbopelvic relationships described by

Jackson and McManus[30] have been found to be true not only for standing, but also with lifting,[68] and with sitting,[2] as well as with positioning on different devices, including the Andrews table and frame (Andrews Table and Andrews Frame, Orthopedic Systems, Inc., Union City, Calif.), the Children's Hospital of Philadelphia four-poster frame (CHOP Spine Frame, U.S. Medical, Inc., Colwyn, Pa.), the Relton-Hall four-poster frame and the Hastings frame.[17,55] As the hips are passively flexed during standard positioning on these devices, the top of the pelvis rotates posteriorly around the hip axis[36] with respect to the lumbar spine. As a result there are associated and significant decreases in both total and segmental lordosis, the latter occurring mostly at the L4-L5 and L5-S1 levels.[48-50,62,66] However, on the Wilson frame (even fully domed for lumbar flexion) and on the Jackson table (Jackson Modular Table System, Orthopedic Systems, Inc., Union City, Calif.), with the hips flexed a mean 28 degrees to 33 degrees on both devices, L5-S1 segmental lordosis has been documented to be increased compared with standing measurements.[3,50,65] Positioning on these two devices then would appear to be favorable for most fusion procedures across the lumbosacral level with spinal implants.

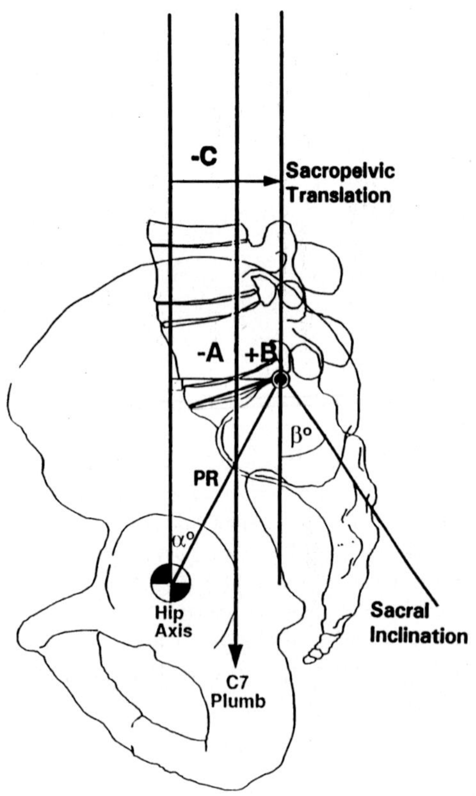


**FIGURE 60-5**

Methodology used for measuring standing sagittal lumbopelvic angular alignments and the A, B, C measurements for spinopelvic balance (alignment of the spinal vertebrae over the sacropelvis and hips). The three vertical lines extend through the S1 reference point, the center of the C7 body, and the hip axis. The hip axis is centered between the acetabula. *A* and *B* are the perpendicular distances for balance from the hip axis and S1 vertical lines to the vertical C7 plumb line, respectively. *C* is the perpendicular distance between the hip axis and S1 vertical lines and represents the compensatory sacropelvic translation around the hip axis for balance. The PR line is measured as the distance between the center of the hip axis and the S1 reference point. The angle α is the sacropelvic angle measured between the hip axis vertical line and the PR. The angle β is the sacral inclination.

## DEFINITIONS AND DETERMINATES OF STANDING SPINOPELVIC BALANCE

Standing physiologic relationships and apparent compensations for spinopelvic balance have been further studied by Peterson et al.[51] The authors evaluated 50 asymptomatic "normal" adult volunteers without history of hip or spinal pathology (males = 25, females = 25, mean age 39.4 years, height = 67 inches, weight = 168 pounds). Each person had a standing 36-inch lateral radiograph of the pelvis and entire spine measured by two observers for segmental and total lumbar lordosis (Cobb method from adjacent superior endplates and from superior endplates of L1 to S1, Figs. 60-1 and 60-2), apex of lumbar lordosis and apex and degree of thoracic kyphosis (Cobb method from T1 to T12, Fig. 60-1). The pelvic hip axis was located midway along a line drawn between the centers of the femoral heads on the lateral radiographs (Figs. 60-3, 60-4, and 60-5). Radiographic studies have shown the center of rotation for the hips, or the center of rotation for the sacropelvis in the sagittal plane with respect to the hip joints, to be along the axis through the center of the femoral heads.[39] The length of the line from the center of the pelvic hip axis between the femoral heads to the sacral reference point (posterior superior corner of S1 body) was recorded in centimeters as the "pelvic radius" (indicated as "PR" in Figs. 60-3, 60-4, and 60-5). Measurements for the standing sagittal sacropelvic angulation involved the pelvic angle and the sacral inclination (angles "α" and "β," recorded in degrees, formed by a vertical line through the hip axis with the pelvic radius line and a line drawn parallel along the back of the proximal sacrum with a vertical line through the posterior superior corner of the S1 body, respectively; Figs. 60-4 and 60-5). Additional assessments for spinopelvic balance were made by perpendicular distance measurements between the sagittal C7 plumb line and vertical lines drawn through the posterior superior corner of the S1 vertebral body and the pelvic hip axis. Distance "A" was measured from the hip axis to the C7 plumb line, distance "B" from S1 to the C7 plumb line and distance "C" from the hip axis to the S1 vertical line (Figs. 60-5 and 60-6). Because the sacrum rotates and translates around the hip axis along the "pelvic radius," as defined, the linear perpendicular distance measurement "C" was referred to as the "compensatory sacropelvic translation" (Figs. 60-4, 60-5, and 60-6). This measurement was also an assessment of the standing sagittal sacropelvic angulation due to the fact that these measurements were expected to be closely correlated. Twenty percent of the study group was randomly selected and remeasured by each observer. The data were statistically analyzed for interobserver and intraobserver reliability, normative values and significant relationships. The interobserver and intraobserver measurements were highly correlated and not significantly different.

Peterson et al found the following mean values for the standing sagittal spinopelvic parameters measured (Table 60-1): T1-12 total kyphosis, +47 degrees; segmental lordosis at L1-L2, −1.9 degrees; L2-L3, −7.2 degrees; L3-L4, −12.0 degrees; L4-L5, −17.0 degrees; L5-S1, −24.0 degrees; and L1-S1 total lordosis, −62.1 degrees; measurement "A" (hip axis to C7 plumb line), −3.9 cm; measurement "B" (S1 to C7 plumb line), +0.38 cm; measurement "C" (hip axis to S1 vertical line for compensatory sacropelvic translation), −4.2 cm; pelvic angle, 17.4 degrees; sacral inclination, 47.9 degrees; and pelvic radius, 13.5 cm.[51] Many of the mean values are, again, similar to those previously reported in other studies (Table 60-1).[4,30,61] Of the different A, B, C measurements for spinal balance, compensatory sacropelvic translation (C) for pelvic balance had the smallest range and standard deviation (−1.2 to −7.2 cm and 1.36 cm, respectively).

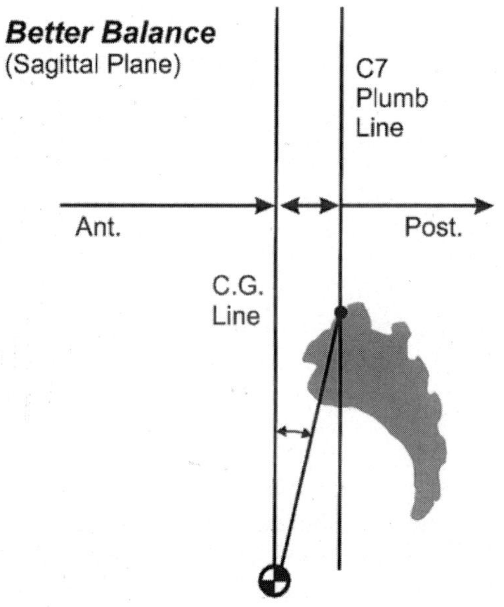


**FIGURE 60-6**

The vertical C7 plumb line extends through the center of the C7 vertebral body (not shown) and is superimposed on a vertical line through the posterior superior corner of the S1 body. The center of gravity (*CG*) line is over the hip axis and anterior (*Ant*) to the superimposed S1 vertical line and C7 plumb line. As the sacrum rotates and translates anteriorly around the hip axis the distance (↔), or compensatory sacropelvic translation, between the vertical line through S1 and the CG line over the hip axis gets shorter and the spinal balance appears to be better in the sagittal plane. In this situation, the C7 plumb line and S1 vertical line may not and usually are not exactly superimposed.

This Peterson et al study of 50 standing adult volunteers found thoracic kyphosis to have positive correlation with lower lumbar segmental lordosis at L4-L5 and L5-S1, and with total lordosis ($r = 0.50$, $p = 0.0005$), i.e., as kyphosis increased or decreased so did lordosis.[51] Others have also reported similar correlations for total kyphosis and lordosis.[31,36,38,61,69] In the study by Peterson et al, significant correlations ($p < 0.05$) also existed between measurement "B" for balance and lower lumbar segmental lordosis at L4-L5 and L5-S1, total lordosis, pelvic angle (α), and between the other 2 vertical line measurements "A" and "C" from the pelvic hip axis vertical line to both the C7 plumb line and the S1 vertical line, respectively (Fig. 60-5).[51] In their study the measurement "B" for sagittal balance was not correlated with the lumbar and thoracic apex; degree of kyphosis; upper or middle lumbar segmental lordosis at L1-L2, L2-L3, L3-L4; nor with sacral inclination (β). Again, Jackson and McManus had also found no association between the S1 to C7 plumb line measurement "B" and sacral inclination for assessment of sacropelvic angulation around the hip axis.[30] In addition, Gelb et al found no correlation between their S1 to C7 plumb line and sacral inclination measurements.[14]

Other significant lumbopelvic relationships or apparent compensations reported in the study by Peterson et al, again, included correlations for sacral inclination (β) with segmental lordosis (L1-L2, L3-L4, L4-L5) and with total lordosis (L1-S1).[51] These findings were also similar to those published previously in the Jackson and McManus study.[30] In addition, strong correlations existed for the pelvic angle (α), sacral inclination (β), and compensatory sacropelvic translation (C, measured as the perpendicular distance between the hip axis and S1 vertical lines), which would all be expected since these are assessments of standing sacropelvic angulation (Figs. 60-4 and 60-5). Of all the spinopelvic parameters measured pelvic angle (α) and compensatory sacropelvic translation (C) had the strongest correlation ($r = 0.97$, $p = 0.0001$). Again, the vertical line measurements for compensatory sacropelvic translation (C) had some association with the other 2 vertical line measurements "A" and "B" ($r = 0.31$, $p = 0.0300$ and $r = 0.31$, $p = 0.029$; respectively). While sacral inclination (β) had correlation with compensatory sacral translation (C), it had no such association with the other 2 vertical line measurements "A" and "B". Also, sacral inclination (β) had no association with lumbar and thoracic apex or degree of kyphosis. The mean PR length was not significantly different between the sexes and showed no correlation to height or weight. Correlation analyses of ratios using measured values as numerators, and the PR as the denominator produced the same relationships previously noted.

The correlations in this Peterson et al study of 50 standing volunteers showed that as the lumbopelvic angulation increased (or as the lordotic angles increased between the pelvic radius line and the lines along the superior endplates of the lumbar vertebrae, see Fig. 60-3) the lumbar spine translated anteriorly with respect to the C7 plumb line measurement "B" for sagittal balance.[51] Perhaps more importantly the correlations showed that as the segmental lordosis at L5-S1 increased the top of the sacrum translated superiorly and anteriorly toward the hip axis vertical line along an arc defined by the "pelvic radius" centered through the hip joints themselves ($r = 0.34$, $p = 0.016$). As a result, the sacropelvis appeared to be better balanced over the hips in the sagittal plane (Figs. 60-3, 60-4, 60-5, and 60-6). When lordosis decreased the sacral inclination became more vertical as the sacropelvis rotated posteriorly along this same arc around the hip axis with an associated increase in standing hip extension ($r = 0.56$, $p = 0.0001$), the perpendicular distance "B" increased as the S1 body and its vertical line moved posteriorly away from the C7 plumb line ($r = 0.37$, $p = 0.01$), and the perpendicular distance "C" increased as S1 and its vertical line, again, translated posteriorly away from the vertical line through the pelvic hip axis ($r = 0.34$, $p = 0.015$; Figs. 60-4, 60-5, and 60-6). In "normal" adult volunteers with a full complement of compensatory mechanisms for spinopelvic balance, the authors of this study found that the measurement "A" between the hip axis and C7 plumb line was fairly constant and not correlated with lordosis (segmental, total) or sacral inclination suggesting that the other spinopelvic parameters adjusted around this relationship to keep the center of gravity over the hips in the sagittal plane. These findings supported the previous Jackson and McManus study.[30] The findings also supported the concept that the sacrum and, therefore, the pelvis act like a sixth lumbar vertebra or "pelvic vertebra," as suggested by Dubousset,[10] but with an added restraint of having to translate along an arc defined by the "pelvic radius" centered through the hips (i.e., compensatory sacropelvic translation around the hip axis [Figs. 60-1, 60-3, 60-4, 60-5, and 60-6]). It should, therefore, be pointed out that disorders of the hips, such as flexion contractures, might compromise this compensatory mechanism for spinal balance by sacropelvic translation and in so doing cause other, perhaps less desirable, compensations to occur. These compensations could include knee flexion and muscle contraction in the back to decrease thoracic kyphosis and shift segmental lordosis proximally into the upper lumbar spine and even into the thoracic spine in an attempt to get or keep the C7 plumb line around or behind the hip axis and S1 under C7.[16,30,43] In some patients, the pelvic hip axis would then appear to be under S1 and the C7 plumb line and the vertical lines for compensatory sacropelvic translation would all be closely approximated. Movement of the lines away from each other would be an indication of spinopelvic decompensation over time in certain patients. This would be particularly so if the C7 plumb line moved closer or even more anterior to the hip axis and the compensatory sacropelvic translation increased in a negative direction (Fig. 60-6).

This Peterson et al study is important because data for physiologic standing sagittal spinopelvic angulations and balance are established and significant compensatory relationships identified.[51] The authors stated that many of the spinopelvic correlations that they found may represent compensatory mechanisms for maintaining the center of gravity over the hips in the sagittal plane. Specifically the authors of this study described spinopelvic balance in terms of the lumbopelvic angulation and the compensatory sacropelvic translation (C) around the hip axis, as defined, in conjunction with the C7 plumb line measurements (A and B). While the C7 plumb line "B" measurement for balance was dependent on the lumbar lordosis (total, lower segmental) and compensatory sacropelvic translation, it was independent of the sacral inclination, as well as the upper and middle segmental lordosis, the lumbar and thoracic apex and the degree of kyphosis. However, other authors have reported correlations for S1 to C7 plumb line measurements with the lumbar and thoracic apices.[14] In the Peterson et al study,[51] the lumbar and thoracic apices, sacral inclination and the C7 plumb line (B) measurements were all independent of each other. The authors, therefore, felt that the hip axis to C7 plumb line measurement (A) and the pelvic angle measurement ($\alpha$) from the "pelvic radius" were more clinically useful and reliable in evaluating sagittal balance. This would be particularly so when compared with measuring a spinal vertical axis line alone from some lower lumbar or sacral reference point. In fact, it is these authors' strong opinion that the lumbopelvic angulations (from the pelvic radius to the superior endplates of the lumbar vertebrae; Fig. 60-3), the pelvic angle, and the compensatory sacropelvic translation be carefully evaluated (Figs. 60-4, 60-5, and 60-6), and that their relationships with the C7 plumb line around the hip axis be closely assessed. Unfortunately, the authors pointed out that C7 plumb line measurements required standing lateral radiographs of the entire spine and can involve localization of vertebrae in the often difficult to visualize cervicothoracic region. The lumbopelvic angle, pelvic angle, and compensatory sacropelvic translation measurements, on the other hand, can be made on routine standing lateral lumbar radiographs that simply show the sacrum and hips (Figs. 60-3, 60-4, and 60-5). Of the different vertical line measurements (A, B, C) for spinopelvic balance, compensatory sacropelvic translation (C) had the narrowest range and smallest standard deviation in this study (Table 60-1) and high reliability. The authors concluded that by studying such ra-diographic parameters, but more so their relationships, it may be possible to further define congruent sagit-tal alignment, as well as recognize and better treat the spinopelvic compensations that occur for compensated or uncompensated balance in patients with different spinal disorders.[51,52]

I feel that the spinopelvic angulations and compensations for congruent sagittal alignment and balance on standing lateral radiographs should be considered in the assessment of all patients with spinal disorders. This is particularly so in their preoperative and postoperative radiographic evaluations. The following are felt to be important spinopelvic parameters for measurement on available standing radiographs: thoracic kyphosis (total, segmental and the distribution); thoracic apex (vertebra or disk); lumbar lordosis (total, segmental, and the lower, middle, and upper distribution); lumbar apex (vertebra or disk); total kyphosis/total lordosis ratio; vertical line measurements for spinopelvic balance (where, if at all, the lines cross the spine, their relationship to the thoracic apex, the lumbar apex and to a reference point on the sacrum, as well as more importantly the defined axis through the hips); pelvic angle, sacral inclination, and compensatory sacropelvic translation measurements as indicators for standing hip extension (since the sacropelvis angulates and translates around the axis through the hips); lumbopelvic angles (pelvic radius to superior endplates of the lumbar vertebrae) and a careful consideration for the center of gravity in the sagittal plane, which is generally located globally above the axis through the hips while standing upright in the balanced static subject. In addition, any disorders of the hips should be recognized. To reiterate, the relationships of these spinopelvic parameters, especially those involving measurements for the pelvic hip axis to the sagittal C7 plumb line and for the pelvic rotation, are much more clinically useful than any absolute values. Also, the kyphosis/lordosis ratio would appear to be important for congruent sagittal spinopelvic alignment.

Each person has a unique posture and spinopelvic balance with a particular set of alignments that can be influenced or altered by such variables as age, sex, weight, and pelvic anatomy, including degree of acetabular anteversion.[1,14,30,68,72] In addition, subjects may stand and/or be positioned differently from one exam to the next. No good longitudinal studies have been completed concerning normal variations for repeated measurements of these spinopelvic parameters within the same subject or patient. For example, varying degrees of pelvic rotation in the transverse plane can occur with positioning of the subject against the x-ray cassette, which would make the compensatory sacropelvic translation appear shorter in the sagittal plane than it really is from one measurement to the next on the lateral radiographs (Fig. 60-4). In comparative studies this would affect reproducibility and reliability. However, careful positioning of the subject by keeping the pelvic rotation to the right or left less than 15° in the transverse plane can greatly minimize errors due to this variable (Fig. 60-4).[38] Nevertheless, basic sagittal spinopelvic angulations and compensations for balance should be assessed and, in patients, corrected, improved or, at least, not aggravated by the treatment. This also applies to the care of patients with degenerative spinal disorders who undergo short one- and two-level lumbar or lumbosacral fusion procedures.[15,32]

## POSITIONING FOR SURGERY

### Positioning Studies and Sagittal Lumbopelvic Angulations

How patients are positioned at surgery is extremely important as this largely determines the sagittal alignment, especially in the lumbopelvic spine, but also in the cervical and thoracic spines. Studies looking at the effect of operative position on spinopelvic alignment are, therefore, not only of interest, but clinically very relevant. Peterson et al evaluated the effect of operative position on lumbar lordosis in a group of patients under general anesthesia.[50] To determine how the 90-90 knee-chest and the prone positions affect lordosis, two patient groups were analyzed by these authors. All patients were selected from the practice of the same surgeon. Inclusion criteria for this study required adequate preoperative (standing 36-inch lateral spine) and intraoperative radiographs (lateral lumbar spine L1 to the sacrum) in either the knee-chest position on a Hastings frame with the hips flexed approximately 90 degrees (Group I, n = 20), or the prone position on a Jackson table with the hips flexed approximately 30 degrees (Group II, n = 20). Radiographs were measured twice by two observers using Cobb methodology for total and segmental lordosis between L1 and S1 (Fig. 60-2). The data were analyzed for intraobserver and interobserver error, and significant changes in total and segmental lordosis between preoperative and intraoperative radiographs. Repeat measurements of total and segmental lordosis by the same intraobserver were highly correlated (mean, $r = 0.87$, $p \le 0.01$) and not significantly different. Between interobservers, measurements were also highly correlated (mean, r = 0.84, p ≤0.05); however, mean standing segmental lordosis at L5-S1 was different between the observers (p <0.01). Standing segmental lordosis at all other levels, standing total lordosis, and intraoperative measurements were not significantly different between these two groups in this study.

Group I (Fig. 60-7) radiographic mean segmental and total lordosis measurements in the standing position for the Peterson et al study were: L1-L2, −2.7 degrees; L2-L3, −6.4 degrees; L3-L4, −9.6 degrees; L4-L5, −13.5 degrees; L5-S1, −20.5degrees; and L1-S1, −52.7 degrees.[50] Mean segmental and total lordosis measurements in the 90-90 position on the Hastings frame for this group of patients were: L1-L2, −2.4 degrees; L2-L3, −3.2 degrees; L3-L4, −4.0 degrees; L4-L5, −5.6 degreees; L5-S1, −18.4 degrees; and L1-S1, −33.6 degrees. Compared with standing, segmental lordosis was significantly reduced (p <0.01) at all levels except L1-L2, which showed no significant change. Total lordosis (L1-S1) also was significantly reduced (p <0.01).

Group II (Fig. 60-8) radiographic mean segmental and total lordosis measurements in the standing position for the Peterson et al study were: L1-L2, −4.2 degrees; L2-L3, −6.5 degrees; L3-L4, −10.4 degrees; L4-L5, −14.8 degrees; L5-S1, −25.7 degrees; and L1-S1, −61.7 degrees.[50] Mean segmental and total lordosis measurements in the standard prone position on the Jackson table for this group of patients were: L1-L2, −4.4 degrees; L2-L3, −5.7 degrees; L3-L4, −9.2 degrees; L4-L5, −13.9 degrees; L5-S1, −29.2 degrees; and L1-S1, −62.8 degrees. Compared with standing, segmental lordosis at L5-S1 was significantly increased (p <0.01). Segmental lordosis at all of the other levels and total lordosis (L1-S1) showed no significant change.

Peterson et al in this anesthetized patient positioning study concluded that preservation of normal segmental angulation during reconstructive lumbar spine surgery is important, and largely determined by the intraoperative positioning.[50] Although the 90-90 position often gave the impression of preserving lordosis, this was not necessarily so. It was presented by the authors that hip flexion with sitting (Fig. 60-9) or with prone positioning (Fig. 60-10) produced muscle and ligament tethering across or between the back of the hip joints and the pelvic ischii. The positioning and tethering caused posterior pelvic rotation around the hip axis, as defined in this chapter, with respect to the lumbar spine that resulted in a significant reduction of total and segmental lumbar lordosis.[49] These changes were most prominent at the L4-L5 and L5-S1 levels. Also such positioning of the patient made anterior pelvic rotation during surgery very difficult. Patients positioned on the Jackson table with the hips flexed approximately 30 degrees, however, showed no change in segmental lordosis above the lumbosacral level. Segmental lordosis at L5-S1 actually increased, and, again, total lordosis was preserved (Fig. 60-8).[50] The authors further presented that this may be due to

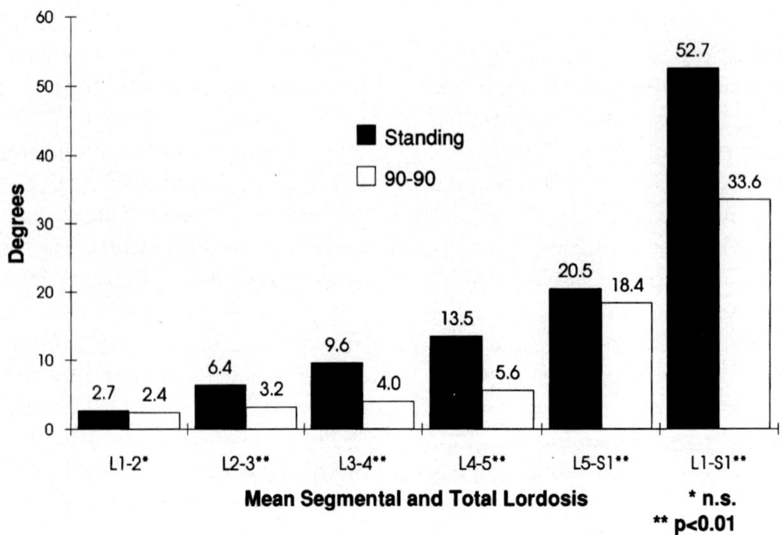


FIGURE 60-7

Mean segmental and total lordosis in degrees (Cobb method) measured on lateral radiographs in 20 patients standing preoperatively and at surgery in a 90-90 position on a Hastings frame under general anesthesia. Lordosis was significantly decreased at all levels except at L1-L2. *(From Peterson MD, Nelson LM, McManus AC, Jackson RP: The effect of operative position on lumbar lordosis—a radiographic study of patients under anesthesia in the prone and 90-90 positions,* Spine *20(12):1419-1424, 1995.)*

anterior pelvic rotation around the hip axis caused by less hip flexion and muscle and ligament tethering on the anterior iliac crests across the front of the hips with the associated knee flexion (Fig. 60-11).[49] Also, it was felt by the authors that such anterior pelvic rotation was promoted and facilitated by the location, orientation and function of the anterior pelvic and proximal thigh pads designed for the Jackson table, which distributed the weight fairly equally between the pelvis and the proximal femora (Jackson Modular Table System, Orthopedic Systems, Inc., Union City, Calif.). The authors noted that interobserver differences in segmental lordosis at L5-S1 were likely due to difficulty in identifying and using the same line for the S1 endplate. Given no significant intraobserver differences existed, the authors concluded that the significant changes in lordosis measured were valid in their study.[50]

This Peterson et al study was the first to show that in surgical patients with low back pain under general anesthesia the 90-90 knee-chest position resulted in significant reduction of both total and segmental lordosis, especially at the L4-L5 and L5-S1 levels, and that prone positioning on a Jackson table maintained the standing sagittal segmental angulations of the lumbar spine and actually increased lumbosacral lordosis.[50] This study also supported previously reported findings for 90-90 and prone positioning that had been carried out in a smaller group of 10 awake volunteers with no apparent spinal disorders.[66]

Nelson et al studied the effects of positioning on lumbar lordosis in a group of 17 awake asymptomatic volunteers (Table 60-2).[48] The authors' objectives were to measure total and segmental lordosis on standing lateral radiographs and on lateral lumbar radiographs taken with the subjects in four different operative positions. The positions studied were on the Hastings frame, the Relton-Hall frame, the Jackson table, and chest rolls. Standard positioning was carried out on each device and on the chest rolls according to the description of Tan et al[66] The hips were flexed 90 degrees on the Hastings frame, 60 degrees on the Relton-Hall frame, 30 degrees on the Jackson table, and neutral on the chest rolls. Total and segmental lordosis between L1 and S1 were measured twice by two observers using Cobb methodology with the S1 endplate technique (Fig. 60-2). Data were analyzed for intraobserver and interobserver reliability and for changes in total and segmental lordosis between the radiographs of the subjects in the five different positions. The authors' data in this study showed that the intraobserver and interobserver reliability measurements were very reproducible and not significantly different. Although lordosis was decreased in all four positions, compared with standing in these awake volunteers, it was much better maintained on the Jackson table (Table 60-2).[48] In addition, the Jackson table appeared to allow for more unrestricted pelvic rotation around the hip axis because of the different

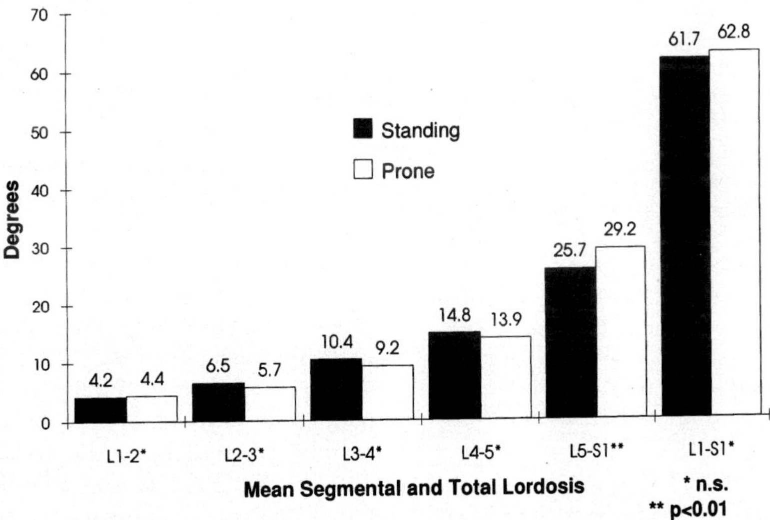


**FIGURE 60-8**

Mean segmental and total lordosis in degrees (Cobb method) measured on lateral radiographs in 20 patients standing preoperatively and positioned prone at surgery on a Jackson table under general anesthesia. Segmental lordosis was not different at L1-L2, L2-L3, L3-L4, and L4-L5. L5-S1 segmental lordosis was significantly increased on the Jackson table and total lordosis was slightly increased. *(From Peterson MD, Nelson LM, McManus AC, Jackson RP: The effect of operative position on lumbar lordosis—a radiographic study of patients under anesthesia in the prone and 90-90 positions,* Spine *20(12):1419-1424, 1995.)*

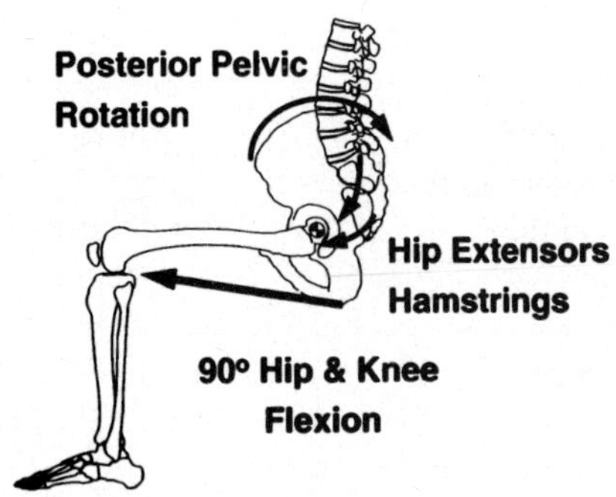


**FIGURE 60-9**

The sitting position with 90 degrees of hip and knee flexion produces muscle and ligament tethering of the hip extensors and hamstrings attaching on the ischii behind the hip joints. This results in posterior pelvic rotation around the Hip axis, as shown and defined in this chapter, with reduction in lordosis, especially in the lower lumbar spine. *(From Jackson RP: Spinal balance, lumbopelvic alignments around hip axis and positioning for surgery. In Margulies JY, ed: Adult L5-S1 surgery issue of SPINE, State of the art reviews 11(1):33-58, 1997.)*

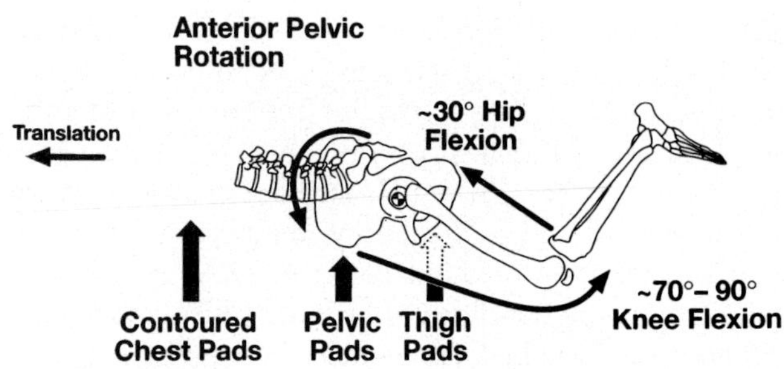


**FIGURE 60-11**

Prone positioning on the Jackson table, with approximately 30 degrees of hip flexion and 70 to 90 degrees of knee flexion, causes anterior pelvic rotation around the hip axis due to muscle and ligament tethering by the hip flexors on the anterior iliac crests across the front of the hip joints. Anterior pelvic rotation is also promoted by the location, orientation, and function of the pelvic and proximal thigh pads designed for the Jackson table. Positioning on the Jackson table is shown to approximate the standing lumbar lordosis and generally to increase the lumbosacral segmental lordosis with the patient relaxed under general anesthesia.

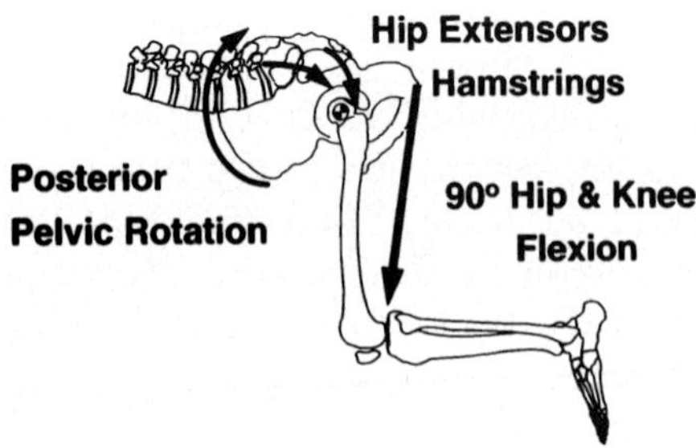


**FIGURE 60-10**

Prone knee-chest positioning with 90 degrees of hip and knee flexion produces muscle and ligament tethering by the hip extensors and hamstrings on the ischii behind the hip joints. This results in posterior pelvic rotation around the hip axis, as shown and defined in this chapter, with reduction in lordosis, especially in the lower lumbar spine and particularly at the L4-L5 level. With posterior pelvic rotation and loss of lordosis the erector spinae and other extensor muscles of the back are lengthened. Fusing the lumbar spine in this position with the muscles more elongated can interfere in their function and rehabilitation following surgery. *(From Jackson RP: Spinal balance, lumbopelvic alignments around hip axis and positioning for surgery. In Margulies JY, ed: Adult L5-S1 surgery issue of SPINE, State of the art reviews 11(1):33-58, 1997.)*

designs and functions for the pads, including their geometric orientations and locations for positioning on the participants.

Stephens et al carried out similar comparative studies for the sagittal segmental lumbar angulation produced by different operative positions.[62,63] This study also involved normal healthy awake subjects. Ten volunteers under the age of 30 with no prior history of lumbar disease had lateral lumbar radiographs taken in four different positions. The positions were: (1) standing; (2) prone on a Jackson table with the hips neutral; (3) prone on an Andrews table (Andrews Table, Orthopedic Systems, Inc., Union City, Calif.) with the hips flexed 60 degrees; and 4) prone on the Andrews table with the hips flexed 90 degrees. Lumbar lordosis was measured at all motion segments (intervertebral disk space angle) from L1-S1 for all subjects in each position.

Stephens et al found an average total lumbar lordosis from L1-S1 in the standing position of 51.7 degrees.[63] Mean contribution from the upper and middle lumbar spine (L1-L4) was 24.2 degrees and from the lower lumbar spine (L4-S1), 27.5 degrees. Average total lumbar lordosis on the Jackson table was 52.7 degrees, with 26.1 degrees contributed from L1-L4 and 26.6 degrees from L4-S1. There was no statistically significant difference between standing and standard positioning on the Jackson table. In fact, total lordosis was somewhat slightly increased on the Jackson table in this group of awake volunteers. Again, Peterson et al found the same thing in a group of anesthetized patients positioned on the Jackson table.[50] Average total lumbar lordosis on the Andrews table with 90 degrees of hip flexion was only 17 degrees, with the upper and middle lumbar spine (L1-L4) contributing 8.3 degrees and the lower lumbar spine (L4-S1) contributing 8.7 degrees. On the Andrews table with 60 degrees of hip flexion, average total lordosis was 27.3 degrees, with 16.2 degrees measured between L1-L4 and 11.1 degrees between L4-S1.

In the Stephens et al study, the difference between lordosis on the Jackson table compared with both positions on the Andrews table was statistically signifi-

**Table 60-2. Segmental and Total Lumbar Lordosis Mean Measurements (SEM*) In Volunteers (n = 17, Cobb method)**

| | Lateral Lumbar Radiographs — Standing Neutral vs. Four Prone Positions | | | | |
|---|---|---|---|---|---|
| | Standing | Jackson | Chest Rolls | Relton-Hall | Hastings |
| L1-L2 | 3.4 (4.1) | 4.6 (3.0) | 2.6 (3.9) | 2.0 (2.5) | 1.2 (3.0)[4] |
| L2-L3 | 7.0 (3.7) | 7.6 (2.0) | 5.2 (2.5) | 4.2 (2.5)[1,3] | 1.9 (2.5)[1,3] |
| L3-L4 | 10.9 (2.7) | 9.9 (2.5) | 7.2 (2.0)[1] | 6.9 (3.0)[1,4] | 3.7 (1.9)[1,3] |
| L4-L5 | 16.3 (3.7) | 13.2 (3.2)[1] | 12.1 (3.3)[1] | 9.2 (3.3)[1,3] | 3.7 (2.0)[1,3] |
| L5-S1 | 27.6 (4.7) | 25.4 (5.2)[2] | 24.6 (4.5)[1] | 21.4 (5.5)[1,3] | 16.9 (7.7)[1,3] |
| L1-S1 | 65.9 (7.9) | 60.8 (7.7)[2] | 51.7 (10.2)[1,3] | 43.7 (10.7)[1,3] | 27.5 (10.9)[1,3] |

All lordotic degrees
[1]Significantly different ($p < 0.01$) compared to standing.
[2]Significantly different ($p < 0.05$) compared to standing.
[3]Significantly different ($p < 0.01$) compared to Jackson table.
[4]Significantly different ($p < 0.05$) compared to Jackson table.
Lumbar lordosis in 17 adult volunteers with no history of spinal problems (9 women and 8 men, mean age 36 years, range 20 to 47 years old): standing vs positioned prone on Jackson table with hips flexed 30°, chest rolls with hips extended, Relton-Hall frame with hips flexed 60° and in the "90-90" position on Hastings frame with hips flexed 90°.
*SEM = standard error of the mean.
From Jackson RP: *Spinal balance, lumbopelvic alignments around hip axis and positioning for surgery*. In: Margulies JY, editor: *Adult L5-S1 surgery issue of SPINE, State of the art reviews* 11(1):33-58, 1997.

cant.[62,63] There was also a significant difference between lordosis measured for both positions on the Andrews table as compared with standing. Decreasing the amount of hip flexion on the Andrews table produced a significant increase in lumbar lordosis, but again it was still substantially less than standing. The authors in this study concluded from their data that for lumbar or lumbosacral fusions utilizing spinal instrumentation, physiologic standing sagittal lumbosacral angulations can best be maintained by: (1) intraoperative positioning on the Jackson table; and (2) avoidance of positions producing very much hip flexion.[62]

Like Peterson et al[50] and Nelson et al,[48] Stephens et al[63] confirmed and supported the findings previously reported by Tan et al.[66] Tan had also studied ten awake volunteers with no prior history of back pain.[66] The volunteers in the study by Tan et al had lateral lumbar radiographs taken standing and after standard positioning on chest rolls, the Andrews frame, the Hastings frame, and a four-poster CHOP spinal frame.[66] Total lordosis from L1-S1 was measured, as well as segmental lordosis (intervertebral disk space angle) at each level on all films. Mean total lumbar lordosis measurements for the various positions evaluated were as follows: standing, −55.6 degrees; chest rolls, −45.8 degrees; Hastings frame, −29.6 degrees; four-poster CHOP frame, −28.3 degrees; and Andrews frame, −23.8 degrees. While positioning on chest rolls caused about a mean 10-degree reduction of total lordosis, the difference was not statistically significant in this small study group and L5-S1 segmental lordosis was actually increased somewhat. All of the other positions showed a statistically significant reduction of lordosis, primarily at the L4-L5 and L5-S1 levels and the Andrews frame realized the largest reduction.[66]

In summary, preservation of segmental lumbar lordosis is important for some surgical procedures on the spine and positioning of the patient should be carefully assessed, particularly when using instrumentation or other spinal implants. From these studies it would appear that sagittal lumbopelvic angulation is largely dependent upon how the person is positioned, and this would seem to be especially so for patients relaxed or paralyzed under general anesthesia.

## SPINAL CORRECTION TECHNIQUES FOR IMPROVED SAGITTAL ALIGNMENTS

### SPINOPELVIC CORRECTIONS WITH JACKSON BENDERS AND BIOMECHANICS OF THE INSTRUMENTED SPINE

Although positioning of the patient is very important, specifically with respect to vertebral alignment and spinopelvic angulation in the sagittal plane, force application after fixation with instrumentation can also significantly change the spinopelvic alignments. Various strategies and techniques with spinal implants have been used to segmentally realign the spine and improve compensations and balance in different spinal disorders. I have defined and developed IntraSacral Fixation (ISF) (Liberty and CD IntraSacral Fixation

Systems, Sofamor Danek, Memphis, Tenn.) and in situ rod contouring principles and techniques with the Jackson Benders (Figs. 60-12 through 60-17, Sofamor Danek, Memphis, Tenn.) to correct scoliosis, other deformities and malalignments, and the associated spino-pelvic compensations that occur with these spinal disorders.[20-23,25,27,30,33,35-38] ISF and in situ contoured spinal correction (CSC) are concepts and techniques largely based on: (1) an analysis of the spinopelvic studies for sagittal alignments done by this author and his colleagues, as well as (2) an evolving understanding by this author of the biomechanics governing the instrumented spine.[15,19-38] It was found that posterior spinal instrumentation with rigid implant to implant fixation shifted the actual or potential axes for segmental angular motion (flexion, extension), normally in the middle column for the intact spinal motion segments, posteriorly and away from the center of gravity in the sagittal plane (Figs. 60-18 and 60-19). More specifically it was observed that the potential axes and loads were shifted to the necks of the screws, if used, and to the posterior rods or plates. With the use of stiffer and stronger implants, the axes became less active with loading. Also more unloading of the anterior and middle spinal column occurred. This was true for both static and cyclic loading within the flexibility or elastic limits of the implants. However, with stiffer and stronger implants the stresses on the implants and their bone interfaces were increased.

The center of gravity for sagittal spinopelvic balance can vary, but in its stable state is more commonly anterior to the sacrum and generally located globally over the axis through the hips when standing upright, as described by Jackson and McManus (Figs. 60-5, 60-6, 60-18, and 60-19).[30] The more posteriorly the rods or plates are positioned on the spine, and away from the center of gravity and the intervertebral disk spaces in the sagittal plane, the longer and stronger can be the moment arms acting on them, especially at the lumbosacral level (Fig. 60-18). It occurred to this author that a biomechanical advantage could be created by the insertion of spinal rods, and therefore the axes or potential axes, closer to the intervertebral disk space from a posterior approach. This was a fundamental principle in the further development of the ISF technique with the Liberty Spinal System (Fig. 60-19).[33,35]

With the insertion of less rigid and more ductile rods, which still have sufficient stiffness and strength to resist the high physiologic levels of loading to which they are subjected, and with the ISF technique providing increased purchase in the pelvis and leverage across the lumbosacral level, then application of in situ contouring principles with Jackson Benders for spinal and lumopelvic manipulation in the patient can be performed (Figs. 60-12 through 60-17). The use of these techniques has now become the preferred approach by this author for the correction of most all spinal disorders.[23,26,27,28,29,33,34,35,36,37] In 1992, I learned that with the use of stiff, strong and ductile rods or plates on the spine posteriorly it was easy to realize and clinically control "translating axes" for segmental corrections with the Jackson Benders. Specifically it was found that contouring with the benders created a "contoured translating axis" in the rod for realignment of the lumbopelvis and other regions of the spine. The axis could be "adjusted" along the rod, especially over the apex of any deformity, and an Adjustable Contoured Translating Axis (ACTA) could be developed and used for preservation or correction of alignments (including vertebral angulations as well as translations, such as retrolisthesis and spondylolisthesis) with improvement in the spinopelvic balance. The surgical techniques and biome-

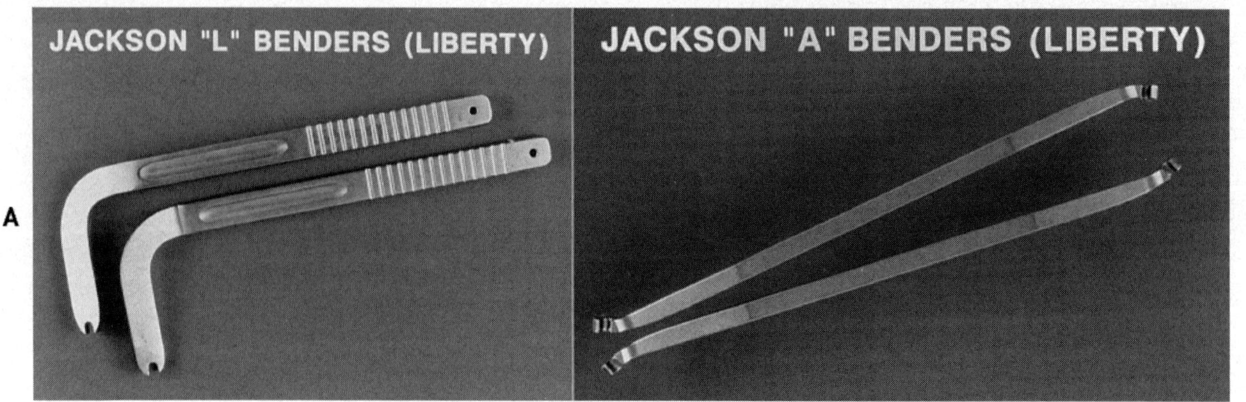


**Figure 60-12**

**A,** Jackson L-Benders for in situ rod contouring primarily in the frontal plane. **B,** Jackson A-Benders for in situ rod contouring primarily in the sagittal plane. Contouring with the instruments is carried out to facilitate implant-to-implant connections and in situ contoured spinal connection (CSC) at surgery. With the Jackson Benders, the axis for correction is over the apex of the deformity, or malalignment, and it is translated with the spine as the correction occurs. *(Liberty Spinal System, Sofamor Danek, Memphis, TN.)*

chanical principles for the creation of translational corrections with the Jackson Benders as well as the clinical results were first published in 1994.[27]

Lordotic contouring of the rod in the lower lumbar spine and at the lumbopelvic level in conjunction with ISF causes superior and anterior sacral translation around and over the pelvic hip axis, as previously defined; this axis through the hips being relatively fixed after patient positioning at surgery.[36] In addition, and as a consequence, ventral and vertical translation of the lumbar spine occurs with the increased lordosis. This is true provided the patient is positioned to allow for pelvic angulation with sacral translation around the hips and the associated lumbar translations in the sagittal plane that need to occur (Fig. 60-11). Therefore, when standing upright after surgery, a ventral shift or translation (i.e., "contoured translation") for the rods with respect to the spinopelvic center of gravity and the back of the intervertebral disk spaces in the sagittal plane can be realized. This can further reduce the length of the moment arms acting on the rods since the rods can now be even closer to the center of gravity while standing upright in a static position (Fig. 60-19). At the same time better segmental, regional, and global spinopelvic alignments and balance can be obtained, especially with respect to the hip axis and associated lumbopelvic relationships described previously by this author along with his coauthors (Figs. 60-1, 60-3, 60-4, 60-5, 60-6, and 60-17). In most cases, these techniques try to maintain or realign the vertical line through the S1 vertebral body as closely as possible to the pelvic hip axis vertical line, as discussed in this chapter (Figs. 60-4 to 60-6 and 60-17 to 60-19). The author has found these two techniques, ISF and in situ contoured spinal correction (CSC), with Jackson Benders, to provide greater control of the lumbopelvic alignments around the hip axis, especially lumbopelvic angulations in the sagittal plane. With these techniques, and with the patient carefully and properly positioned at surgery (Fig. 60-11), more complete corrections of spinopelvic compensations, particularly posterior pelvic rotation, due

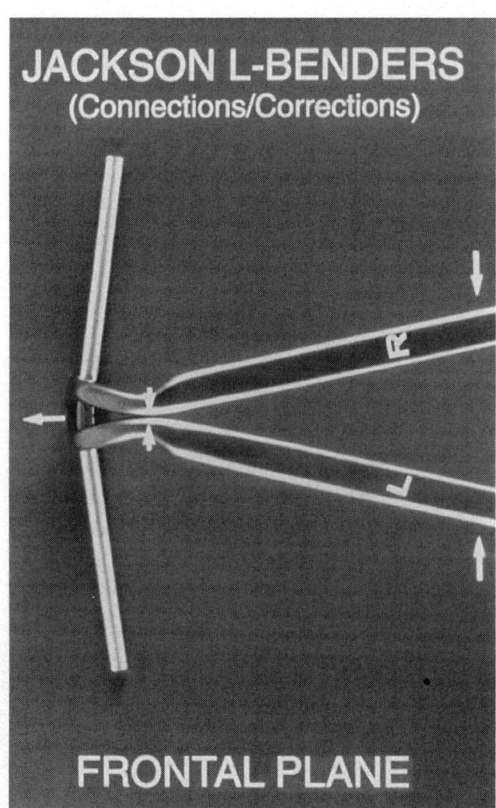


**FIGURE 60-13**

The rod is contoured in situ laterally or medially in the frontal plane with the Jackson L-Benders until its over the open implants. The rod is then rotated down or further contoured down into the open implants with the Jackson A-Benders to facilitate connections of the implants with insertion of less metal in the patient at surgery. After the rod is connected to the other implants in situ contoured spinal correction (CSC) in all planes can also be performed with the Jackson Benders. *(Liberty Spinal System, Sofamor Danek, Memphis, TN.)*

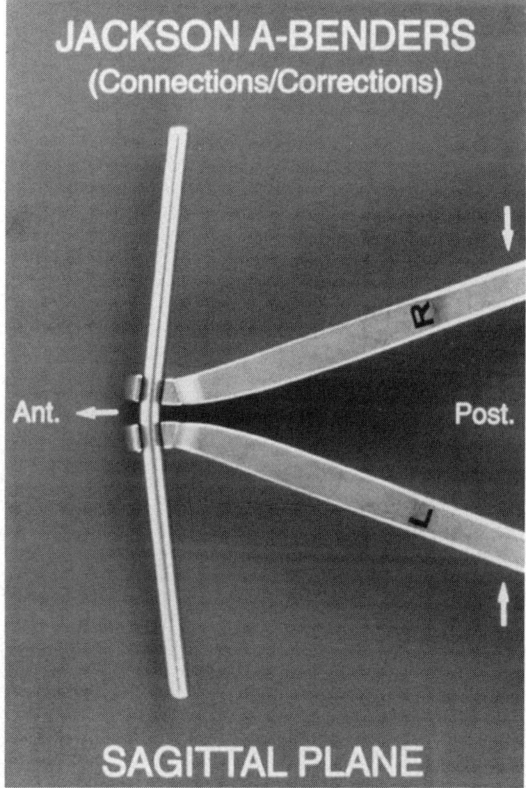


**FIGURE 60-14**

The rod can be contoured in situ anteriorly or posteriorly in the sagittal plane with the Jackson A-Benders to facilitate not only connection of the rod to the other implants, but also correction of the spine. These connection and correction techniques can significantly improve lordosis. *(Liberty Spinal System, Sofamor Danek, Memphis, TN.)*

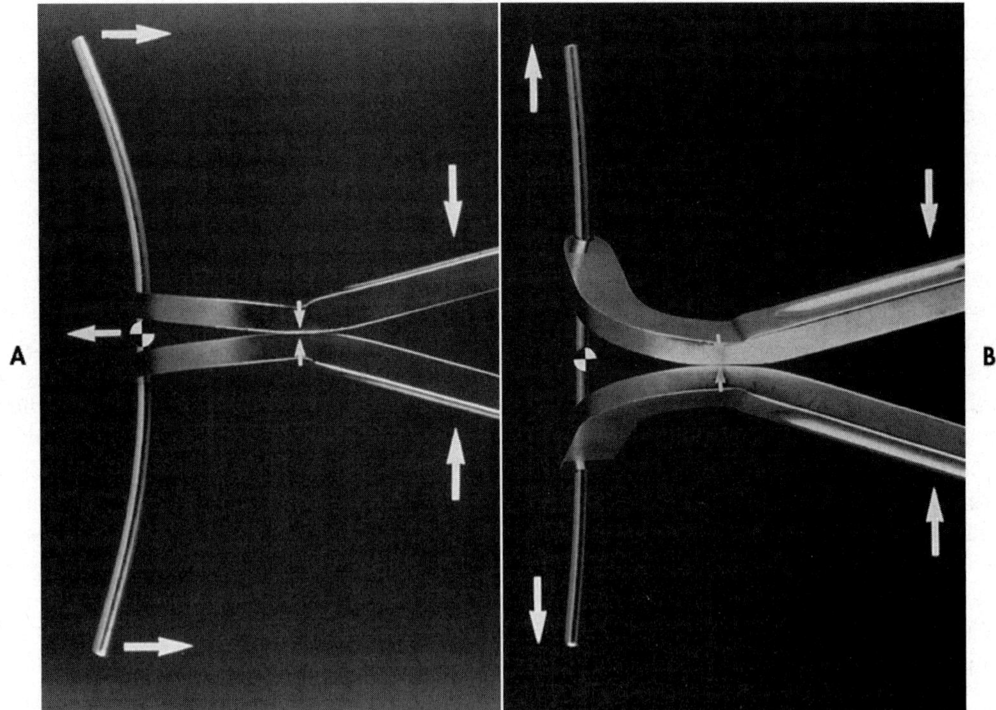


FIGURE 60-15

**A, B,** With the Jackson L-Benders in situ contoured spinal correction (CSC) of scoliosis and other angular deformities in the frontal plane can be carried out using the technique of an adjustable contoured translating axis (ACTA) in the rod, as shown. Direct contoured translation and distraction (*arrows*) occur simultaneously and this is more efficient than distraction alone. In situ contouring in the sagittal plane with the Jackson A-Benders can also be performed to develop kyphosis or lordosis, again, using the same principles and techniques. With the Jackson Benders the translating axis is over the apex of deformity, which is biomechanically very efficient. *(Liberty Spinal System, Sofamor Danek, Memphis, TN.)*

FIGURE 60-16

Lateral view of a lumbar burst fracture stabilized with pedicle instrumentation and partially reduced with in situ contoured spinal correction (CSC) techniques using the Jackson A-Benders. As in situ contouring progresses, with the Jackson Benders now somewhat more separated on the rod, continued angular correction occurs. The rod can be contoured down onto the back of the spine. Corrections with ACTA in the rod, as shown, provide good realignment. Also, three or more points of fixation are possible when the rod is contoured down onto the back of the spine. In addition, the spine does not translate away from the rod as correction occurs due to the use of a translating axis, as opposed to a fixed axis technique used in other spinal instrumentation systems. The axis for correction can be directly over the apex of injury or deformity and this is biomechanically more efficient because of the location for the axis and the fact that it can be translated. *(Jackson Benders, Sofamor Danek, Memphis, TN.)*

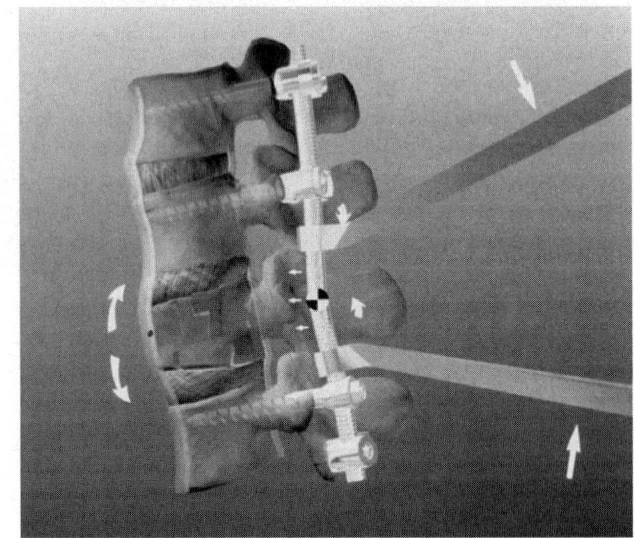

to deformities, degenerative changes, and malalignments with loss of lordosis have been possible. With physiologic lordosis appropriately distributed and improved spinopelvic balance after surgery, the erector spinae and other extensor muscles of the back can have a more optimal working length which can facilitate their function and rehabilitation postoperatively. This is true even with short lumbosacral fusions.

## CHANGES IN SEGMENTAL LORDOSIS FOLLOWING SHORT LUMBOSACRAL FUSIONS

Hardacker et al studied pre- and postoperative segmental lumbar lordosis in patients with uninstrumented and instrumented solid posterior lumbosacral fusions between L3 and S1.[15] The authors of this study stated that a primary goal in reconstructive lumbar surgery was to obtain solid fusion preferably with anatomically correct, or at least improved, alignments in all three planes. They commented that much attention had been paid to loss of lordosis with long fusions into the lumbar spine, and the development of the iatrogenic "flat back syndrome" with its sequelae.[16,40-45,58,71] However, in their work the authors pointed out that little attention had been paid to the sagittal spinopelvic alignments of shorter lumbar and lumbosacral fusions and any postoperative compensations in the spine that may contribute to complications such as junctional degeneration and segmental stenosis over time.[56]

The Hardacker et al study reviewed bilateral posterolateral one-, two-, and three-level solid lumbar fusions to the sacrum (Table 60-3).[15] To be included in this study the patient required two separate observers concluding solid fusion on recumbent Ferguson and lateral flexion-extension lumbar radiographs taken a minimum of 2 years postoperatively. A total of 119 patients were involved for the review. The authors stated that while sagittal alignments and compensations for spinopelvic balance are best assessed on standing lateral radiographs, many of their patients did not have such a study. However, all of their patients had recumbent extension lateral lumbar films taken pre- and postoperatively. A retrospective review by Nelson et al of neutral standing versus recumbent extension lateral lumbar radiographs in 2 groups of patients with different spinal disorders showed that segmental lordosis was not significantly different at L3-L4 and L4-L5 levels, and only about 4 degrees different at the L5-S1 level (Table 60-4).[47] It was, therefore, concluded that a valid comparison could be made by using recumbent extension lateral lumbar films pre- and postoperatively in the Hardacker et al study.[15]

The 119 patients in this study by Hardacker et al (Table 60-3) were divided into three fusion groups: group 1 uninstrumented (n = 37); group 2 instrumented using standard constructs (n = 42, 22 with CD rods and pedicle screws and 20 with bilateral translaminar facet screws); and group 3 instrumented using ISF with pedicle screws followed by in situ rod contouring with the Jackson Benders (n = 40).[15] Indications for fusion included failure of conservative care and continued disabling low back pain with a diagnosis of lumbar segmental instability, spondylolisthesis, and/or symptomatic degenerative lumbar disk disease with and without disk herniation and/or stenosis. All of the patients were operated on by me. All patients in groups 2 and 3 who had insertion of screws in the lumbar and sacral pedicles were positioned prone at surgery on the Jackson table for lordosis and promotion of anterior pelvic rotation (Fig. 60-11). This also allowed for unrestricted intraoperative radiographic imaging of the lumbopelvic region. All other procedures were performed with the patients positioned on the Hasting frame. All uninstrumented and standard instrumented patients were braced to solid fusion. Group 3 patients, who had ISF, required no bracing. Demographics reviewed included age, sex, levels fused, and the number of prior surgeries. Pre- and postoperative pain and functional outcome scores on self-assessment analog scales were compared. Segmental lordosis at all levels fused was measured pre- and postoperatively using the Cobb angle method on the extension lumbar radiographs (Fig. 60-2). Average follow-up for all patients was 54.8 months (range, 24 to 148 months). The pre- and postoperative mean total segmental lordosis measurements of all levels fused for the three groups are shown in Table 60-3 for this study.

The total segmental lordosis change (minus = loss) and average number of levels fused for each group in the Hardacker et al study were as follows: group 1 (n = 37) −385 degrees, average levels fused 1.7; group 2 (n = 42) −545 degrees, average levels fused 2.0; and group 3 (n +40) −67 degrees, average levels fused 2.0.[15] Group 3 was significantly different from group 1 and group 2 (p = 0.01). Demographics found the three groups to be different with regard to age, number of prior surgeries, and levels fused. Therefore, a comparison of pain and functional capacity assessment analog scores between the three groups is not very appropriate. However, group 1 patients had the most favorable factors for outcome (younger age and fewest number of three level fusions) and group 3 the least. In spite of these differences, group 3 patients did as well or better than the other two groups on all of the self-assessment analog scales and, again, they also had significantly more lordosis over the levels operated.

Hardacker et al in this spinal fusion study found that: group 1 and group 2 patients (uninstrumented and instrumented fusions) lost statistically significant segmental lordosis at the levels operated (p = 0.01)

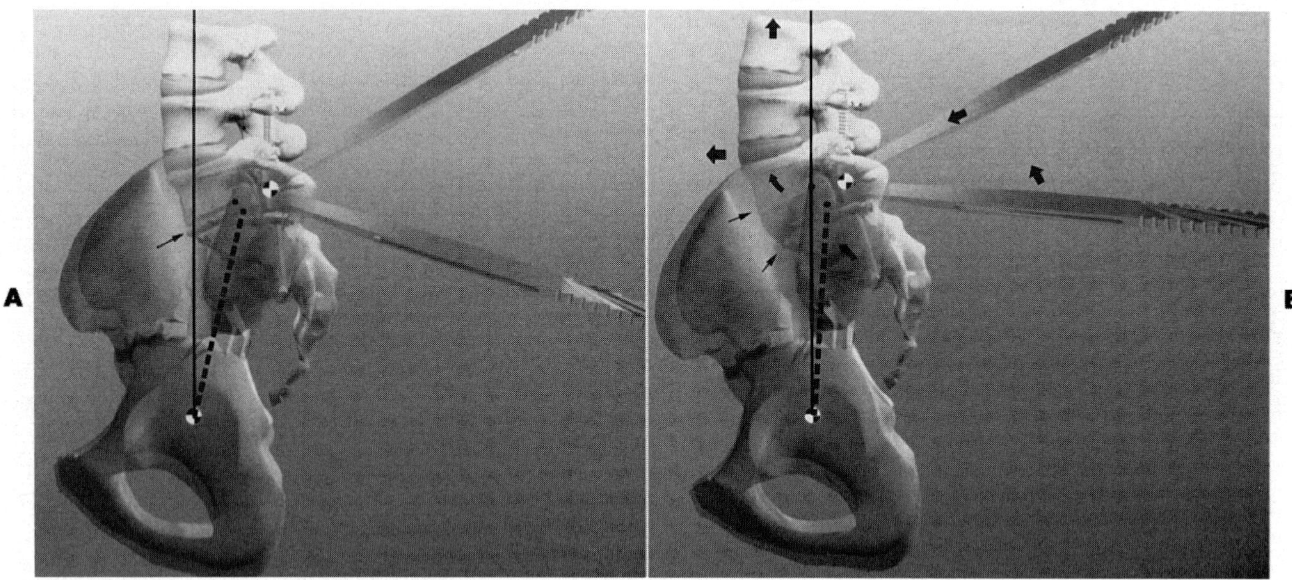


**FIGURE 60-17**

L4 to the sacrum instrumentation using screw fixation and Jackson intrasacral rod insertion before **(A)** and after **(B)** in situ contouring with Jackson Angled A-Benders. Contouring with the screws locked on the rod puts the hinge or axis for segmental angular motion through the rod and between the heads of the benders. By contouring, the axis of angulation is translated with the rod, (i.e., contoured translating axis.) Segmental angulation at L5-S1 is developed with associated angulation of the pelvis around the lower axis located through the hips, which are relatively fixed. In addition, anterior disk space distraction (*narrow straight arrows*) and opening of the neuroforamina at this level is created (*small dots posteriorly at L5 and S1*) because of where the axis in the rod is located. Ventral and vertical translation of the lumbar spine (*larger straight arrows*) and posterior column shortening, which is favorable for fusion, also occur. As a result the S1 vertebral body is translated closer to a vertical center of gravity line through the hip axis when standing upright and the sacrum appears to be better balanced over the pelvic hip axis. *(Jackson Benders, Sofamor Danek, Memphis, TN.)*

and group 3 patients (fusions with ISF and in situ CSC techniques using Jackson Benders) maintained preoperative segmental lumbar lordosis at the levels operated without significant change.[15] The authors concluded that in lumbar spine fusions care should be taken to preserve preoperative levels of segmental lordosis. In their study this was only consistently achieved and maintained, with a relatively short follow-up of 2 to 5 years, in the group 3 patients.

Jackson et al studied a group of patients operated between August 1979 and August 1987 who underwent bilateral posterolateral one-, two-, and three-level lumbar fusions to the sacrum without instrumentation.[32] To be included in this study, a minimum 2-year clinical and radiographic follow-up was required, as well as two observers concluding solid fusion on postoperative recumbent anteroposterior Ferguson and lateral flexion-extension lumbar radiographs. A preoperative recumbent lateral extension lumbar radiograph was also required for comparison, as well as pre- and postoperative self-assessment analog pain and functional capacity scores and pain drawings for outcomes analysis. In this study patients with anterior and posterior lumbar interbody fusions were excluded. During this period a total of 192 patients underwent one-, two-, and three-level uninstrumented lumbosacral fusions and were possible candidates for the study. One hundred sixty were excluded for the following reasons: no preoperative extension film available or taken (76); not solidly fused (32); follow-up less than 2 years, lost, deceased, (28); chymopapain injection within 1 year before surgery (15); and free-floating lumbar fusion (2). Seven patients with internal bone growth stimulators were also excluded. A total of 32 patients met the criteria. All of the patients had the same surgeon and all of the operations were performed with the patients positioned on the Hastings frame. All of the patients were ambulated soon after surgery in a brace.

Jackson et al also stated that sagittal spinal alignments and compensations for spinopelvic balance are best assessed on standing lateral radiographs.[32] However, many of their patients did not have such a study, but all had pre- and postoperative recumbent extension lateral lumbar films for comparison. The authors, again, used the study of Nelson et al to extrapolate from standing neutral to recumbent extension measurements and to support their methodology and comparisons in this study (Table 60-4).[47]

This fusion study by Jackson et al involved 18 men and 14 women.[32] At index surgery, the patients had a mean age of 41.5 years (range, 21 to 66 years). Average follow-up was 83 months (range, 36 to 148 months). The primary preoperative diagnoses were as follows: degenerative lumbar disk disease, with stenosis (7 patients), with herniated nucleus pulposus (11 patients),

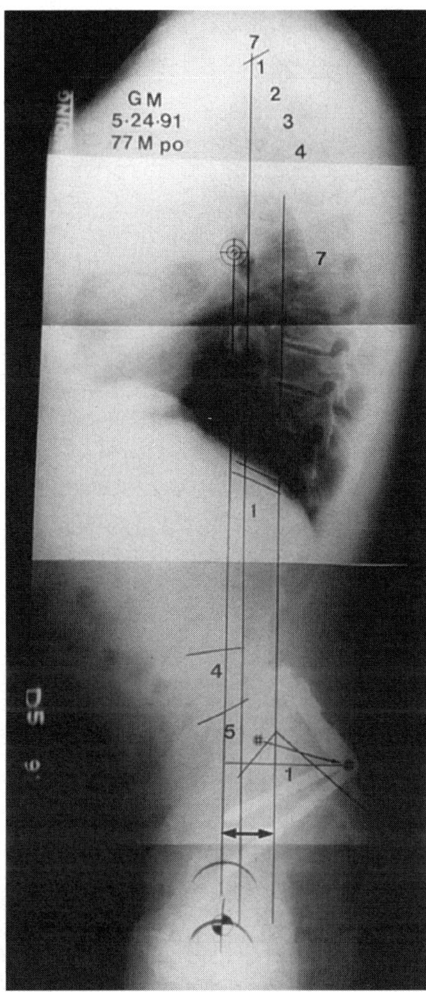


**FIGURE 60-18**

Standing lateral radiograph of a well-balanced spine in patient following L4 to the sacrum fusion with a Galveston construct for lumbopelvic fixation. Constrained posterior spinal instrumentation shifts the segmental axis or potential axis for angulation at L5-S1 posteriorly to the rod and away from the center of gravity, (*more proximal smaller straight arrow directed posteriorly*). With the implants in this position longer moment arms can act on them because they are so far behind the L5-S1 disk space. The three vertical lines extend through the hip axis, center of the C7 vertebral body (sagittal C7 plumb line) and, posterior superior corner of S1 body.

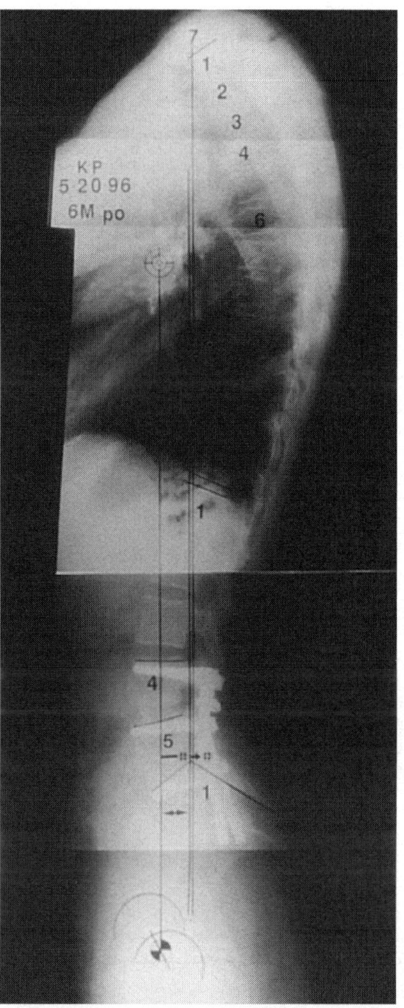


**FIGURE 60-19**

Standing lateral radiograph of a well-balanced spine in patient following L4 to the sacrum fusion with the Jackson ISF technique for lumbosacral fixation. With constrained posterior spinal instrumentation the segmental axis or potential axis for angulation at L5-S1 moves posteriorly to the rod and away from the center of gravity (*more proximal smaller straight arrow directed posteriorly*). Positioning the Liberty screws and rods more anteriorly in the lateral sacral mass and closer to the back of the L5-S1 disk space results in shorter moment arms acting on the implants in the upright static standing state. This can create a biomechanical advantage when compared with other techniques and spinal instrumentation systems. The three vertical lines extend through the hip axis, posterior superior corner of the S1 vertebral body, and center of the C7 body (sagittal C7 plumb line).

and without herniated nucleus pulposus or stenosis (2 patients); grade I isthmic spondylolisthesis (4 patients); degenerative spondylolisthesis with stenosis (1 patient); pseudarthrosis with stenosis (4 patients), and without stenosis (3 patients). The diagnosis of stenosis and/or herniated nucleus pulposus involved the performance of laminectomy and/or diskectomy surgery at the involved level(s), unilaterally or bilaterally. All of the isthmic (lytic) spondylolisthesis patients had L5 laminectomy for resection of the loose neural arch. Nineteen patients (59%) had a total of 31 lumbar spine surgeries (1.6 per patient) prior to their index surgery (resulting in solid fusion). A total of 54 levels were fused. Eleven patients had a one-level fusion; 20 a two-level fusion; and 1 a three-level fusion. The pre- versus postoperative total segmental lordosis mean measurements for the one-, two-, and three-level fusions were as follows: L5-S1, 26.4 degrees versus 16.9 degrees ($n = 11$, $p < 0.01$); L4-S1, 30.7 degrees versus 22.6 degrees ($n = 20$, $p < 0.01$); L3-S1, 52 degrees versus 58 degrees ($n = 1$). Across all the levels fused, a total of 263 degrees of lordosis was lost, a finding similar to that of the Hardacker et al study (Table 60-3).[15]

**Table 60-3. Preoperative versus Postoperative Additive Segmental Lordosis Mean Measurements (Cobb Method)**

| | 1, 2, and 3 Level Solid Posterior Lumbosacral Fusions in 119 Patients | | | | |
|---|---|---|---|---|---|
| | **Levels** | **Pre-op** | **vs.** | **Post-op** | **p-values** |
| Group 1 (fusion in situ without implants, n = 37): | | | | | |
| | L5-S1: | 25.8 | | 14.6 (n = 12) | p = 0.01 |
| | L4-S1: | 28.0 | | 17.8 (n = 24) | p = 0.01 |
| | L3-S1: | 48.0 | | 43.0 (n = 1) | — |
| Group 2 (standard constructs/sacral fixations, n = 42): | | | | | |
| | L5-S1: | 13.4 | | 9.4 (n = 7) | n.s. |
| | L4-S1: | 35.2 | | 21.1 (n = 29) | p = 0.01 |
| | L3-S1: | 47.0 | | 30.3 (n = 6) | p = 0.05 |
| Group 3 (ISF/Jackson benders, n = 40): | | | | | |
| | L5-S1: | 23.8 | | 25.1 (n = 9) | n.s. |
| | L4-S1: | 38.1 | | 35.1 (n = 22) | n.s. |
| | L3-S1: | 43.3 | | 41.9 (n = 9) | n.s. |

All lordotic degrees.
Standard constructs involve 1 pair of bilateral screws for sacral fixations.
The additive segmental lordosis change (minus = loss) and average number of levels fused for each group were as follows: Group1 (n = 37) −385°, average levels fused 1.7; Group 2 (n = 42) −545°, average levels fused 2.0; Group 3 (n = 40) −67°, average levels fused 2.0. Group 3 was significantly different from Group 1 and Group 2 (p = 0.01) and consisted of patients treated with ISF and in situ CSC techniques using Jackson Benders.
From Jackson RP: *Spinal balance, lumbopelvic alignments around hip axis and positioning for surgery*. In Margulies JY, editor: *Adult L5-S1 surgery issue of SPINE, State of the Art Reviews* 11(1):33-58, 1997.

**Table 60-4. Segmental and Total Lumbar Lordosis Mean Measurements (SEM) Standing Neutral Versus Recumbent Extension Lateral Lumbar Radiographs in Patients with Spondylolisthesis and Degenerative Lumbar Disk Disease**

| | Spondylolisthesis (30) | | Degenerative (30) | | Totals (60) | |
|---|---|---|---|---|---|---|
| | **Standing vs.** | **Extension** | **Standing vs.** | **Extension** | **Standing vs.** | **Extension** |
| Observer 1 | | | | | | |
| L1-L2 | 3.7 (4.5) | 4.8 (3.3) | 2.6 (3.4)* | 4.2 (3.4) | 3.1 (4.0)* | 4.5 (3.3) |
| L2-L3 | 7.5 (3.2)* | 9.7 (3.4) | 7.9 (3.7) | 8.8 (3.7) | 7.7 (3.4)* | 9.2 (3.6) |
| L3-L4 | 11.3 (3.5) | 11.2 (3.2) | 10.3 (3.6) | 11.7 (2.7) | 10.8 (3.6) | 11.5 (2.9) |
| L4-L5 | 19.5 (5.4) | 18.2 (4.0) | 15.9 (4.0) | 15.8 (5.0) | 17.7 (5.1) | 17.0 (4.7) |
| L5-S1 | 26.7 (10.2)† | 30.7 (9.6) | 23.9 (6.9)† | 26.2 (7.0) | 25.3 (8.8)† | 28.5 (8.6) |
| L1-S1 | 68.5 (11.8)† | 4.7 (13.0) | 60.9 (11.8)† | 67.0 (10.1) | 64.7 (12.3)† | 70.9 (12.2) |
| Observer 2 | | | | | | |
| L1-L2 | 3.3 (4.9) | 5.2 (4.3) | 3.4 (4.7)† | 5.8 (5.8) | 3.3 (4.7)† | 5.5 (5.1) |
| L2-L3 | 7.5 (3.4)† | 10.3 (3.9) | 7.9 (3.5)† | 10.3 (3.7) | 7.7 (3.4)† | 10.3 (3.8) |
| L3-L4 | 12.2 (4.2) | 12.5 (4.1) | 10.8 (3.8) | 12.1 (3.1) | 11.5 (4.0) | 12.3 (3.6) |
| L4-L5 | 20.8 (5.8) | 19.3 (4.7) | 15.2 (4.6) | 15.8 (4.9) | 18.0 (5.9) | 17.6 (5.1) |
| L5-S1 | 23.6 (9.7)† | 28.7 (9.3) | 21.1 (7.7)† | 24.6 (7.2) | 22.4 (8.8)† | 26.7 (8.5) |
| L1-S1 | 67.5 (11.4)† | 76.1 (13.8) | 58.7 (11.0)† | 68.6 (11.4) | 63.1 (12.0)† | 72.4 (13.1) |

SEM = standard error of the mean. All lordotic degrees (Cobb method).
*$p < 0.05$, †$p < 0.01$.
Segmental lordosis was not different at the L3-L4 and L4-L5 levels on standing neutral versus recumbent extension lateral lumbar radiographs.
From Jackson RP: *Spinal balance, lumbopelvic alignments around hip axis and positioning for surgery*. In Margulies JY, editor: *Adult L5-S1 surgery issue of SPINE, State of the Art Reviews* 11(1):33-58, 1997.

In this Jackson et al spinal fusion study without implants a change in segmental lordosis at a given level following fusion was not related to laminectomy with or without diskectomy.[32] Again, 54 levels in 32 patients were fused. Eighteen levels had fusion only: 5 levels gained an average of 2.8 degrees of lordosis, 1 stayed the same, and 12 lost an average of 7.7 degrees of lordosis. Nineteen levels had fusion with laminectomy only: 6 levels gained an average of 5.3 degrees of lordosis, 1 stayed the same, and 12 lost an average of 7.9 degrees of lordosis. Seventeen levels had fusion with laminectomy and diskectomy: 3 levels gained an average of 5.0 degrees of lordosis, and 14 levels lost an average of 7.4 degrees of lordosis. Overall the total loss of lordosis was: fusion only (18 levels) = 97 degrees, fusion with laminectomy only (19 levels) = 72 degrees, fusion with laminectomy and diskectomy (17 levels) = 94 degrees.

Outcomes analysis in the Jackson et al study found 25 patients to be a little to a lot "better," 2 to be the same, and 5 to be worse.[32] One-level did better than two-level fusions; however, the outcomes may have been influenced by the fact that only 36% of one-level fusion patients had prior surgeries (one or more), as compared with 70% of the two-level fusion patients. Pain frequency was improved 14%, pain severity 23%, work capacity 35%, and limitations in social and recreational activities 32%, with a mean overall improvement of only 26% on the self-assessment analog scales used.

The authors of the last two studies commented that their work was the first they could find comparing lumbar segmental lordosis before and after short one-, two-, and three-level lumbosacral fusions for degenerative disk disorders and instabilities involving low-grade isthmic and degenerative spondylolisthesis, spinal stenosis, herniated nucleus pulposus and pseudoarthrosis with disabling low back pain.[15,32] Jackson et al stated in their study that the loss of lordosis was not related to the performance of a laminectomy or diskectomy at a given level.[32] Possible explanations offered were postoperative bracing, iatrogenic muscle injury, and other causes such as further deterioration and desiccation of the disk(s) due to immobilization from posterior fusion of the spinal motion segment(s) with the possibility of decreasing anterior column support over time. However, disk space heights and any anterior or posterior translational malalignments (spondylolisthesis, retrolisthesis) were not measured in these studies. The authors stated that approximately two-thirds of total lordosis is normally distributed between the bottom two lumbar disks. They found that in situ posterior intertransverse fusion procedures did not maintain the lordosis between L4 and S1 in most of their patients. The long-term clinical consequences for such loss of segmental lordosis at the levels operated and for the levels above were not part of their present studies. The authors stated that the loss of lordosis was both undesirable and worrisome, that with longer follow-ups further loss of lordosis might be expected and that additional studies were needed. In fact, the authors felt that future longitudinal studies may show that it is easier to obtain lordosis than it is to maintain it over time. Also the authors of these last two studies commented that the overall clinical results were not as good as expected in the solidly fused groups of patients who have loss of segmental lordosis.[15,32]

Jackson et al in their study concluded that one- and two-level uninstrumented solid lumbosacral fusions lost significant segmental lordosis at the levels operated ($p < 0.01$) and showed that the changes in lordosis were not due to the other procedures performed at a given level (i.e., laminectomy and/or diskectomy).[32] The authors stated that a more careful assessment of pre- and postoperative segmental lordosis was indicated, especially when reporting outcome studies. Again, Hardacker et al found better clinical outcomes in the patients with more segmental lordosis at the lumbar levels fused.[15]

## CONCLUSIONS AND RECOMMENDATIONS

In the upright standing position most of the segmental lordosis is located in the lower lumbar spine (L4-S1). Lower lumbar lordosis is very important for compensated spinopelvic balance and the lumbopelvic alignments are closely related to the hip axis, as defined in this chapter. Sacral slope or inclination around the hip axis has no association with the standard sagittal C7 plumb line measurement for spinal balance, however, this measurement is highly correlated with lumbar lordosis. The key to understanding spinopelvic balance in the sagittal plane involves the hip axis and the associated lumbopelvic angulations and compensations that occur around this axis, especially pelvic rotation. Active or passive extension and flexion of the femoral heads in their acetabula cause pelvic rotation around the hip axis, which increases and decreases the lordosis, respectively, and this is particularly so in the lower lumbar spine. In terms of positioning, the increase or decrease in lordosis appears to be influenced somewhat by the subject or patient being awake or asleep under anesthesia. Therefore, the pelvic hip axis is important not only in standing spinopelvic balance, but also in positioning of the patient for surgery and manipulation of the spine and pelvis at the lumbosacral level during surgery. These lumbopelvic angulations and relationships around the hip axis deserve further consideration and study.

In awake volunteers, lumbosacral lordosis has been shown to be (1) significantly decreased compared to standing with standard positioning on the Andrews table (hips flexed 90 degrees and 60 degrees),[62] CHOP, Hastings and Andrews frames,[66] and on the Hastings and Relton-Hall frames, the Jackson table, and on chest rolls;[48] and (2) not significantly different on chest rolls,[66] the Wilson frame,[3,65] and the Jackson table.[62] In anesthetized patients lordosis at L5-S1 has also been shown to be significantly decreased after 90-90 knee-chest positioning on the Hastings frame,[50] essentially unchanged after standard positioning on the Wilson frame[3] and significantly increased after standard positioning on the Jackson table,[50] compared with preoperative standing measurements in these same patients. Therefore, if segmental lordosis in the lumbosacral region is to be decreased, especially at the L4-L5 and L5-S1 levels, then standard positioning on the Andrews table or on the Andrews, Hastings, CHOP, or Relton-Hall frames would appear to be appropriate. If segmental lordosis in this region is to be maintained or increased, then positioning on chest rolls, the Wilson frame or the Jackson table, as discussed in this chapter (Fig. 60-11), would be better. In addition, abdominal decompression would appear to be less complete on chest rolls and on the Wilson frame and intraoperative spinal imaging also may be more restricted, compared to the Jackson table.

Findings from my studies, those reported in the literature, and more recently at national meetings, support the following recommendations for patient positioning. If the primary objective is reduction of lordosis for posterior surgical decompression of the spinal canal in the lumbosacral region without spinal fusion, this can be accomplished by flexing the hips and knees approximately 90 degrees and positioning the patient on knee-chest devices such as the Hastings and Andrews frames or the Andrews table. Other options include standard positioning on the four-poster CHOP and Relton-Hall frames where the hips are flexed beyond 45 degrees. If the primary objectives are both abdominal decompression for laminectomy and posterior lumbosacral fusion using instrumentation, without lumbopelvic manipulation, the most optimal patient positions for segmental spinal alignments, at least in the lower lumbar spine, would appear to be either on the Jackson table, or on the Wilson frame which provide less abdominal decompression; and, with lumbopelvic manipulation, on the Jackson table. Other options would include patient positioning on 4-poster frames with the hips fully extended or on chest rolls, again with the hips out straight. If intraoperative imaging is required, this is best performed on a fully radiolucent frame or table such as that provided by the Jackson table. If canal decompression and posterior spinal fusion using instrumentation is planned, then initial lumbopelvic flexion followed later by adjustments of the hips for lumbopelvic lordosis, preferably with the knees flexed to further rotate the pelvis and reduce sciatic nerve tension, can be considered. Such hip repositioning is possible on most of the frames and tables currently in use today, but few studies exist to show how effectively these devices accomplish this. Close attention and careful assessment with lateral lumbar radiographic imaging intraoperatively are recommended.

## REFERENCES


1. Anda S, Svenningsen S, Grontvedt T, Benum P: Pelvic inclination and spatial orientation of the acetabulum. A radiographic, computed tomographic and clinical investigation, *Acta Radiologica* 31:389-394, 1990.
2. Andersson GBJ, Murphy RW, Ortengren R, Nachemson AL: The influence of backrest inclination and lumbar support on lumbar lordosis, *Spine* 4(1):52-58, 1979.
3. Benfanti PL, Geissele AE: The effect of intraoperative hip position on maintenance of lumbar lordosis. Presented at the Scoliosis Research Society 30th Annual Meeting, Asheville, NC, September 13, 1995.
4. Bernhardt M, Bridwell KH: Segmental analysis of the sagittal plane alignment of the normal thoracic and lumbar spines and thoracolumbar junction, *Spine* 14(7): 717-721, 1989.
5. Bostman O, Hyrkas J, Hirvensalo E, Kallio E: Blood loss, operating time, and positioning of the patient in lumbar disc surgery, *Spine* 15:360-363, 1990.
6. Callahan RA, Brown MD: Positioning techniques in spinal surgery, *Clin Orthop* 154:22-26, 1981.
7. Cholewicki J, McGill SM: Lumbar posterior ligament involvement during extremely heavy lifts estimated from fluoroscopic measurements, *J Biomechanics* 25 (1):17-28, 1992.
8. DiStefano VJ, Klein KS, Nixon JE, Andrews ET: Intraoperative analysis of the effects of position and body habitus on surgery of the low back: a preliminary report, *Clin Orthop* 99:51-56, 1974.
9. DeWald RL: Revision surgery for spinal deformity, *Am Acad Orthop Surg Instr Course Lect* 41:235-250, 1992.
10. Dubousset J: *Pelvic obliquity correction*. In Margulies JY, Floman Y, Farcy J-PC, Neuwirth MG, editors: *Lumbosacral and spinopelvic fixation*, Philadelphia, 1996, JB Lippincott-Raven, pp 39-49.
11. Edwards CC, Levine AM: *Complications associated with posterior instrumentation in the treatment of thoracic and lumbar injuries*. In Garfin SR, editor: *Complications of spine*

*surgery,* Baltimore, 1989, Williams and Wilkins, pp 164-199.

12. Eie N, Solgaard T, Kleppe H: The knee-elbow position in lumbar disc surgery: A review of complications, *Spine* 8:897-900, 1983.
13. Eker A: Kneeling position for operations on the lumbar spine. Especially for protruded intervertebral disc, *Surgery* 25:51-56, 1949.
14. Gelb DE, Lenke LG, Bridwell KH, Blanke K, McEnery KW: An analysis of sagittal spinal alignment in 100 asymptomatic middle and older aged volunteers, *Spine* 20(12):1351-1358, 1995.
15. Hardacker JW, Jackson RP, Nelson LM, Ebelke DK, McManus AC: Loss of segmental lordosis in instrumented and uninstrumented solid posterior lumbosacral fusions. Poster exhibit at the International Society for the Study of the Lumbar Spine 20th Annual Meeting, Marseille, France, June 15-19, 1993.
16. Hasday CA, Passoff TL, Perry J: Gait abnormalities arising from iatrogenic loss of lumbar lordosis secondary to Harrington instrumentation in lumbar fractures, *Spine* 8(5):501-511, 1983.
17. Hastings DE: A simple frame for operations on the lumbar spine, *Can J Surg* 12:251-253, 1969.
18. Herkowitz HN: Lumbar spinal stenosis: indications for arthrodesis and spinal instrumentation, *Am Acad Orthop Surg Instr Course Lect* 43:425-433, 1994.
19. Jackson RP, Cain JE: Correction and stabilization of kyphotic deformity in spondylolisthesis. 5th Proceeding of the International Congress on Cotrel-Dubousset Instrumentation-1988, GICD Textbook, Sauramps Medical, 1989, pp 131-134.
20. Jackson RP, Hamilton AC: CD screws with oblique canals for improved sacral fixation: a prospective clinical study of the first fifty patients. 7th Proceeding of the International Congress on Cotrel Dubousset Instrumentation-1990, GICD Textbook, Sauramps Medical, 1991, pp 75-86.
21. Jackson RP: IntraSacral Fixation—principles and techniques. Presented at the GICD-USA course on intrasacral fixation and other new methods with spinal instrumentation, Kansas City, MO, October 24, 1992.
22. Jackson RP, Ebelke DK, McManus AC: The "sacroiliac buttress" and new methods for correction with CD pedicle instrumentation. 8th Proceeding of the International Congress on Cotrel-Dubousset Instrumentation-1991, GICD Textbook, Sauramps Medical, 1992, pp 135-139.
23. Jackson RP, Ebelke DK, McManus AC: Clinical results and standing radiographic sagittal spinal analysis in spondylolisthesis instrumented to the sacrum with new techniques. Presented at the International Society for the Study of the Lumbar Spine 19th Annual Meeting, Chicago, IL, May 20-24, 1992.
24. Jackson RP, The Midwest Spine Foundation: Translating axes of segmental spinal motion in 3 planes. Presented at the GICD-USA course on intrasacral fixation and other new methods with spinal instrumentation, Kansas City, Missouri, October 24, 1992.
25. Jackson RP, McManus AC: The "iliac buttress"—a computed tomographic study of sacral anatomy, *Spine* 18(10):1318-1328, 1993.
26. Jackson RP, McManus AC: Radiographic sagittal spinal analysis in lumbar and thoracolumbar adult scoliosis instrumented to the sacrum with new techniques. Presented at the North America Spine Society 8th Annual Meeting, San Diego, California, October 14-16, 1993.
27. Jackson RP: *Jackson intrasacral fixation and segmental corrections with adjustable contoured translating axes.* In Errico TJ, editor: *Spinal Instrumentation issue of SPINE: State of the Art Reviews,* Philadelphia, 1994, Hanley & Belfus, 8(2):307-341.
28. Jackson RP: Biomechanics of lumbar burst fracture reductions with short segment screw fixation systems. Presented at the 6th Annual Rae Jacobs Memorial Lecture, Kansas City, MO, June 10-11, 1994.
29. Jackson RP, McManus AC: Evaluation of junctional kyphosis following surgical correction for developmental thoracic hyperkyphosis. Presented at the 6th Annual Rae Jacobs Memorial Lecture, Kansas City, MO, June 10-11, 1994.
30. Jackson RP, McManus AC: Radiographic analysis of sagittal plane alignment and balance in standing volunteers and patients with low back pain matched for age, sex, and size: a prospective controlled clinical study, *Spine* 19(14):1611-1618, 1994.
31. Jackson RP, Peterson MD, McManus AC: Standing sagittal balance and lumbopelvic relationships in adult volunteers and patients with degenerative lumbar disc disease, scoliosis and spondylolisthesis. Presented at the Scoliosis Research Society 29th Annual Meeting, Portland, OR, September 21-24, 1994.
32. Jackson RP, Nelson LM, Hardacker JW, Ebelke DK, McManus AC: Loss of segmental lordosis in uninstrumented solid posterior lumbosacral fusions. Presented at the Scoliosis Research Society 30th Annual Meeting, Asheville, NC, September 13-17, 1995.
33. Jackson RP: *Jackson sacral fixation and contoured spinal correction techniques.* In Margulies JY, Floman Y, Farcy J-PC, Neuwirth MG, editors: *Lumbosacral and spinopelvic fixation,* Philadelphia, 1996, JB Lippincott-Raven, pp 357-379.
34. Jackson RP: *Lumbar burst fractures: fixation with pedicle instrumentation and reduction by adjustable contoured translating axes using in situ Jackson benders.* In Bridwell K, DeWald R, editors: *The textbook of spinal surgery,* ed 2, Philadelphia, 1997, JB Lippincott-Raven, pp 1881-1898.
35. Jackson RP: *Insertion of intrasacral rods for sacral fixation and spinal correction with in situ rod contouring techniques.* In Bridwell K, DeWald R, editors: *The textbook of spinal surgery,* ed 2, Philadelphia, 1997, JB Lippincott-Raven, pp 2187-2209.

36. Jackson RP: *Spinal balance, lumbopelvic alignments around the hip axis and positioning for surgery.* In Margulies JY, editor: *Adult L5-S1 surgery issue of SPINE: State of the Art Reviews,* Philadelphia, 1997, Hanley & Belfus, 11(1):33-58.
37. Jackson RP: *Sagittal plane abnormalities in disorders of the adult spine.* In An H, editor: *Principles and techniques of spine surgery,* Baltimore, 1998, Williams and Wilkins, pp 489-516.
38. Jackson RP, Peterson, MD, McManus AC, Hales C: Compensatory spinopelvic balance over the hip axis and better reliability in measuring lordosis to the pelvic radius on standing lateral radiographs of adult volunteers and patients, *Spine* 23(16):1750-1767, 1998.
39. John JF, Fisher PE: Radiographic determination of the anatomic hip joint center. A cadaver study, *Acta Orthop Scand* 65(5):509-510, 1994.
40. Kostuik JP, Hall BB: Spinal fusions to the sacrum in adults with scoliosis, *Spine* 8:489-500, 1983.
41. Kostuik JP, Maurais GR, Richardson WJ, Okajima Y: Combined single stage anterior and posterior osteotomy for correction of iatrogenic lumbar kyphosis, *Spine* 13:257-266, 1988.
42. Kostuik JP: Treatment of scoliosis in the adult thoracolumbar spine with special reference to fusion to the sacrum, *Orthop Clin North Am* 19:371-381, 1993.
43. La Grone MO: Loss of lumbar lordosis: a complication of spinal fusion for scoliosis, *Orthop Clin North Am* 19:383-393, 1988.
44. LaGrone MO, Bradford DS, Moe JH, Lonstein JE, Winter RB, Ogilvie JW: Treatment of symptomatic flatback after spinal fusion, *J Bone Joint Surg Am* 70: 569-580, 1988.
45. Luk KD, Lee FB, Leong JC, Hsu LC: The effect on the lumbosacral spine of long spinal fusion for idiopathic scoliosis. A minimum 10-year follow-up, *Spine* 12:996-1000, 1987.
46. Mouradian WH, Simmons EH. A frame for spinal surgery to reduce intra-abdominal pressure while continuous traction is applied, *J Bone Joint Surg Am* 59: 1098-1099, 1977.
47. Nelson LM, McManus AC, Jackson RP: Standing neutral versus recumbent extension lordosis in patients with spondylolisthesis and degenerative lumbar disc disease. (Unpublished Abstract).
48. Nelson LM, Peterson MD, McManus AC, Jackson RP: Effect of positioning on lumbar lordosis—a radiographic study of awake adult volunteers. Presented at the International Society for the Study of the Lumbar Spine 23rd Annual Meeting, Burlington, VT, June 25-29, 1996.
49. Peterson MD, Nelson LM, McManus AC, Jackson RP: The effect of operative position on lumbar lordosis—a radiographic study of patients under anesthesia in the prone and 90-90 positions, Presented at the Scoliosis Research Society 29th Annual Meeting, Portland, OR, September 21, 24, 1994.
50. Peterson MD, Nelson LM, McManus AC, Jackson RP: The effect of operative position on lumbar lordosis—a radiographic study of patients under anesthesia in the prone and 90-90 positions, *Spine* 20(12):1419-1424, 1995.
51. Peterson MD, Jackson RP, McManus AC: Standing sagittal spinal balance, alignments and lumbopelvic relationships: part I—a study of adult volunteers, Presented at the Scoliosis Research Society 30th Annual Meeting, Asheville, NC, September 13-17, 1995 and at the North American Spine Society 10th Annual Meeting, Washington, DC, October 18-21, 1995.
52. Peterson MD, Jackson RP, McManus AC: Standing sagittal spinal balance, alignments and lumbopelvic relationships: Part II—a study of patients with spinal disorders, Presented at the Scoliosis Research Society 30th Annual Meeting, Asheville, NC, September 13-17, 1995 and the North American Spine Society 10th Annual Meeting, Washington, DC, October 18-21, 1995.
53. Petraco DM, Spivak JM, Cappadona JG, Kummer FJ, Neuwirth MG: An anatomic evaluation of L5 nerve stretch in spondylolisthesis reduction, *Spine* 12(10): 1133-1139, 1996.
54. Ray CD. *Positioning the patient for lumbar decompressions or fusions.* In White AH, Rothman RH, Ray CD, editors: *Lumbar spine surgery: techniques and complications,* St. Louis, 1987, CV Mosby, pp 95-102.
55. Relton JES, Hall JE: An operation frame for spinal fusion: a new apparatus designed to reduce hemorrhage during operation, *J Bone Joint Surg Br* 49:327-332, 1967.
56. Schlegel JD, Smith JA, Schleusener RL. Lumbar motion segment pathology adjacent to thoracolumbar, lumbar and lumbosacral fusions, *Spine* 21(8):970-981, 1996.
57. Selby DK: *Posterior spinal fusion.* In Weinstein JN, Wiesel SW, editors: *The lumbar spine,* Philadelphia, 1990, WB Saunders, p 459.
58. Shufflebarger HL, Clark CD: Thoracolumbar osteotomy for postsurgical sagittal imbalance, *Spine* 17(suppl):S287-S290, 1992.
59. Smith RH, Gramling ZW, Volpitto PP: Problems related to the prone position for surgical operations, *Anesthesiology* 22:189-193, 1961.
60. Smith RH: One solution to the problem of the prone position for surgical procedures, *Anesth Analg* 53: 221-224, 1974.
61. Stagnara P, De Mauroy JC, Dran G, Gonon GP, Costanzo G, Dimnet J, Pasquet A: Reciprocal angulation of vertebral bodies in a sagittal plane: approach to references for the evaluation of kyphosis and lordosis, *Spine* 7(4):335-342, 1982.
62. Stephens GC, Wilber RG, Yoo JU: Comparison of lumbar sagittal alignment produced by different operative positions. Presented at the Scoliosis Research

Society 29th Annual Meeting, Portland, OR, September 21-24, 1994.

63. Stephens GC, Yoo JU, Wilber G: Comparison of lumbar sagittal alignment produced by different operative positions, *Spine* 21(15):1802-1807, 1996.
64. Swank SM, Mauri TM, Brown JC: The lumbar lordosis below Harrington instrumentation for scoliosis, *Spine* 15(3):181-186, 1990.
65. Taddonio RF, L'Heureux EA, Doyle SM: Radiographic analysis of lumbar spine sagittal alignment and the effect of operative position during posterior lumbar spine surgery. Presented at the North American Spine Society 10th Annual Meeting, Washington, DC, October 18-21, 1995.
66. Tan SB, Kozak JA, Dickson JH, Nalty TJ: Effect of operative position on sagittal alignment of the lumbar spine, *Spine* 19(3):314-318, 1994.
67. Tarlov IM. The knee-chest position for lower spinal operations, *J Bone Joint Surg Am* 49:1193-1194, 1967.
68. Vanneuville G, Garcier JM, Poumarat G, Guillot M, Chazal J: Mechanisms of orientation of the pelvifemoral base during static loading of the lumbar spine in weight lifters, *Surg Radiol Anat* 14:29-33, 1992.
69. Voutsinas SA, MacEwen GD: Sagittal profiles of the spine, *Clin Orthop* 210:235-242, 1986.
70. Wayne SJ. The tuck position for lumbar disc surgery, *J Bone Joint Surg Am* 49:1195-1197, 1967.
71. Willers U, Hedlund R, Aaro S, Normelli H, Westman L: Long-term results of Harrington instrumentation in idiopathic scoliosis, *Spine* 18:713-717, 1993.
72. Wood KB, Kos P, Schendel M, Persson K: Effect of patient position on the sagittal plane profile of the thoracolumbar spine, *J Spinal Disord* 9(2):165-169, 1996.

# X
# REHABILITATION

# 61

# REHABILITATION AFTER REVISION SPINE SURGERY

**Gerard P. Varlotta, D.O.**
**Thomas J. Errico, M.D.**



The need for revision spinal surgery and postoperative rehabilitation exists despite technical progress in the surgical treatment of spinal disorders. Ever since the first internal spinal instrumentation by Wilkins in 1887 physicians and engineers have improved the technical aspects of spinal instrumentation maximizing stability and hastening restoration of maximum function. Despite this progress a number of patients require revision spine surgery for disorders ranging from adjacent degenerative changes to deformities. Progression from cumbersome orthotics and casts after gross spinal implantation, to limited fusion segments with pedicle screws and intradiscal cages have accelerated the need for early rehabilitation programs. Patients undergoing revision spine surgery instrumentation range from those with localized segmental disorders requiring limited surgical stabilization and minimal postoperative rehabilitation to those with catastrophic spinal fractures with neurologic deficit requiring intensive inpatient rehabilitation programs with permanent changes in functional and recreational activities. This chapter addresses those patients requiring revision spine surgery without spinal cord injury.

Instability requiring instrumentation of the cervical, thoracic, and lumbar spine may result from a variety of degenerative, infectious, carcinogenic, and traumatic etiologies. The purpose of spinal instrumentation procedures is to maximize function by diminishing abnormal painful motion, preventing progression of deformity, and maintaining correction after realignment procedures. The postoperative rehabilitation of patients undergoing spinal instrumentation is dependent upon numerous factors including age of the patient, the extent of the spinal disease, the association and degree of neurologic involvement, the duration of symptoms, the overall debilitation of the patient, associated medical ailments, and the social background and psychological constitution of the patient. A comprehensive rehabilitation program should be primarily focused on maximizing function and ultimately improving the quality of life rather than the treatment of pain. Postoperative scar, inflammation of the myofascial elements, and progression of adjacent intervertebral degeneration may be provocative and interpreted by the patient as a recurrence of the original disorder and a failure of the original surgical procedure. Thus, the integrity of the instrumentation and fusion should be radiographically established and reassurance should be given to the patient by the surgeon and the rehabilitation team. Once it has been determined that there is a need for revision spine surgery, the patient's functional deficits, level of function, reasons for failure to progress, and tasks that produce pain should be communicated by the rehabilitation team to the surgeon.

The primary goal of a postoperative spine revision rehabilitation program is to efficiently maximize function, limit the progression of adjacent intervertebral degeneration, recondition the adjacent soft tissues, reverse negative effects of the pre- and perioperative convalescent period (aerobic deconditioning and pain management), develop a preventative maintenance program, and reintroduce recreational and sports activities. Reestablishing "control" over their lives now that their spinal disorder is "under control" should be taught and reinforced throughout the rehabilitation program. Small obtainable goals should be individually established and reinforced to progress toward complete functional restoration of the patient.

The major postoperative factors that influence a revision rehabilitation program are the type and inherent degree of stiffness of the instrumentation, the surgical approach, the type and duration of immobilization, the extent and degree of preoperative disability, the associated medical illnesses, postoperative medical and surgical complications, the extent and degree of adjacent axial and appendicular pathology, the diagnostic accuracy and definitive implementation of the surgical procedure, and the motivation of the patient to achieve functional restoration.[53] The majority of patients undergoing spine revision surgery for degenerative conditions (not traumatic, infectious, or carcinogenic etiologies) would have been involved in a preoperative and postoperative rehabilitation program. The preoperative program should have included conceptual teaching of pathology, factors related to pain perception and modulation, and functional and exercise formats including aerobic conditioning. The postoperative program should have consisted of a bracing or fusion period followed by a progressive rehabilitation program to improve flexibility, strength, aerobic conditioning, and function. The spine revision procedure should be viewed as an adjunct to the overall functional restoration process and should not be perceived by the patient as a failure. A preoperative program should be titrated

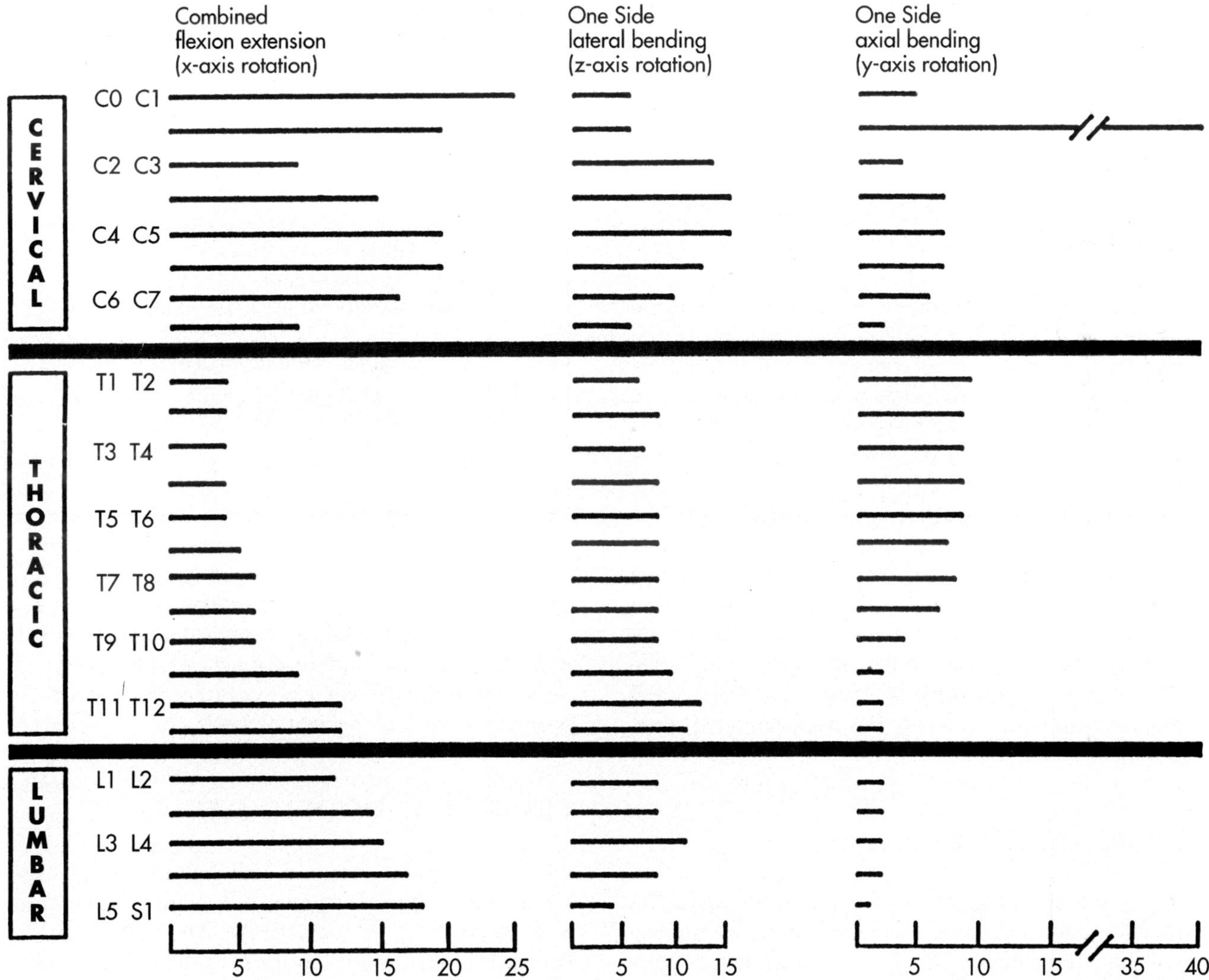


FIGURE 61-1

Segmental range of motion.[122]

to the patient's tolerance to specific exercise formats (stretching, strengthening, and aerobics). Despite the lack of supportive research stronger and more flexible and aerobically conditioned patients require a shorter postoperative recovery and rehabilitation period.

## ORTHOTIC DEVICES

Selection of a comfortable yet supportive orthosis is important in the rehabilitation of the patient undergoing revision spine surgery. A comprehensive discussion of spinal orthoses can be found elsewhere.[119]

The choice of external immobilization is dependent upon the length of fusion, type of fixation used and the location of the neutral axis and instantaneous axis of rotation of the spine.[98] Internal fixation provides stability and alignment until bony fusion occurs. Instrumentation that provides minimal internal rigidity requires maximal external support to ensure spine fusion. The final decision for the type and extent of postoperative bracing should be made by the surgeon with attention given to the quality of bone stock, nutritional status of the patient, amount and type of bone graft, the patient's body habitus, strength, and compliance, in addition to the type and security of instrumentation.

## SPINAL MOTION AND POSTOPERATIVE REHABILITATION

An in-depth discussion of normal spinal motion can be found elsewhere.[122] An understanding of the potential loss of a motion segment(s) and its implications on adjacent levels needs to be emphasized in a patient undergoing spine revision surgery with instrumentation. Elimination of one or more motion segments results in greater forces in both intersegmental and coupled-motion patterns at levels adjacent to the fusion. The increased forces may accelerate a preexisting degenerative process at adjacent levels if abnormal motion is not controlled.[127] Normal segmental range of motion (Fig. 61-1) is significantly reduced in postoperative patients. In those patients undergoing revision surgery the majority of motion is in abnormal coupled patterns and to date has not been adequately studied.

## SPINAL ORTHOSES

The efficacy of spinal orthoses depends upon the direction and magnitude of applied forces by the patient and the forces resisted by the orthosis. A tight comfortable fit allows for a more secure application of forces. A classification of spinal orthoses is most commonly ordered by the section of the spine immobilized (Box 61-1).[119] White and Panjabi[122] have grouped orthotic devices according to the extent of control over segmental and coupled motions (minimal, intermediate, and maximum) (Table 61-1). An understanding of both classifications is necessary in proper selection of a spinal orthosis.

### BOX 61-1. ORTHOTIC CLASSIFICATION

I. Cervical
   - Soft-Foam Collar

II. Occipitomandibular—Cervical
   - Collar and Chin Piece
   - Queen Anne Collar

III. Cervicothoracic
   - A. Occipitomandibular—High Thoracic
     - Philadelphia
     - Thomas (Four-Poster)
   - B. Occipitomandibular—Low Thoracic
     - Extended Philadelphia
     - SOMI (Sternooccipitomandibular Immobilizer)
     - Guilford (Two-Poster)
     - Yale

IV. Craniothoracic
   - Minerva
   - Halo Vest

V. Lumbosacral
   - Chairback
   - Knight
   - Cowhorn
   - Williams Flexion
   - McAusland Brace
   - Corsets

VI. Thoracolumbosacral
   - Taylor
   - Taylor-Knight
   - CASH (Cruciform Anterior Spinal Immobilizer)
   - Jewett Hyperextension
   - Korsair (Jewett with Anterior Abdominal Pad)
   - TLSO with and without thigh extension

VII. Cervicothoracolumbosacral
   - Cervical Extensions added to Custom TLSO
   - Jewett
   - Knight-Taylor

## CERVICAL SPINE ORTHOSES

The appropriate cervical orthosis needs to be chosen according to the degree of limitation in range of motion required postoperatively (Table 61-2). In the cervical spine, minimal control is achieved with various cervical orthoses (collars). Advantages of these collars include minimal expense, convenience, and easy fabrication and fitting. Soft collars (Fig. 61-2) provide essentially no immobilization but do provide warmth

**Table 61-1. Functional Control of Spinal Orthoses**

| | | | Controlled Motion | | |
|---|---|---|---|---|---|
| | | | F/E | LB | AR |
| Cervical: | Minimal: | Soft Collar (5–10%) | + | + | − |
| | Intermediate: | Hard Plastic Collar (75–90%) | + | + | ± |
| | | Philadelphia | + | + | ± |
| | | Four-Poster (Thomas) | + | + | + |
| | | *Long Two-Poster (Guilford, Duke) | + | + | + |
| | Maximum: | Minerva Cast | + | + | + |
| | | (>90%) *Halo | + | + | + |
| Thoracic: | Minimal: | Long Thoracic Corset | + | + | − |
| | Intermediate: | Jewett, *Griswold | + | − | − |
| | | Taylor | + | − | − |
| | | Taylor & Lateral Supports | + | + | − |
| | | *Taylor & Clavicle Pads | + | + | + |
| | Maximum: | Milwaukee | + | + | ± |
| | | Risser Plaster Cast/Jacket | + | + | + |
| | | *Halo Pelvic Device | + | + | + |
| Upper Lumbar: | Minimum: | NONE | | | |
| (T12-L4) | Intermediate: | Williams | + | + | − |
| | | Knight | + | ± | − |
| | | Taylor | + | + | + |
| | | *Norton & Brown | + | + | + |
| | Maximum: | Molded Plastic Jacket | + | + | + |
| Lower Lumbar: | Minimum: | Corsets | + | + | − |
| (L4-S1) | Intermediate: | NONE | | | |
| | Maximum: | Taylor & Thigh Attachment | + | + | + |
| | | Molded Plaster/Plastic Jacket & Thigh Attachment | + | + | + |
| | | *Halo Pelvic Device | + | + | + |

*Highest control within group.
Adapted from references 45, 57, 115.

**Table 61-2. Overall Range of Motion Occiput-T1 (Percent) with Various Cervical Orthoses**

| | F/E | Lateral Bending | Rotation |
|---|---|---|---|
| Normal (57) | 100% | 100% | 100% |
| Soft Collar (57) | 74% | 92% | 83% |
| Philadelphia Collar (57) | 29% | 66% | 44% |
| SOMI Brace (57) | 28% | 66% | 34% |
| Four-Poster Brace (57) | 21% | 46% | 27% |
| Yale Brace (57) | 13% | 51% | 18% |
| Halo (57) | 4% | 4% | 1% |
| Halo Cast/ Plastic (117) | 12% | 8% | 2% |
| Minerva Body Jacket (71) | 14% | 16% | 0% |

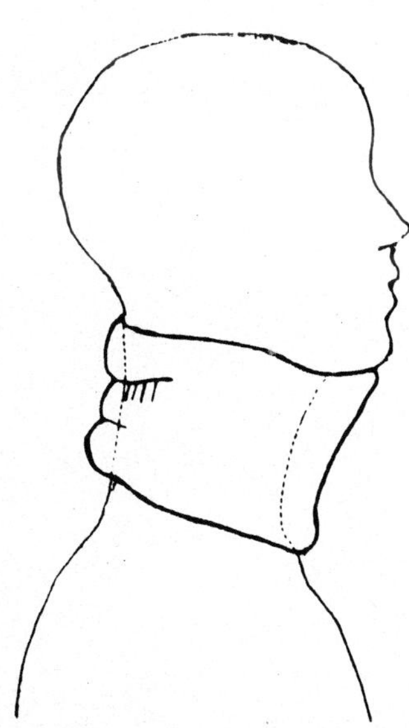

**FIGURE 61-2**

Soft cervical collar (cervical orthosis). Lateral view. *(From Berger N, Edelstein J, Fishman S, et al: Spinal Orthotics. NYU Medical Center Post-Graduate Prosthetics and Orthotics, New York, 1987.)*

and psychologic comfort. Intermediate control with a Philadelphia collar (Fig. 61-3) provides rigidity in flexion and extension and less restriction in axial rotation. Greater limitation in all planes can be obtained with a four-poster, Duke, or Guiliford brace.[121]

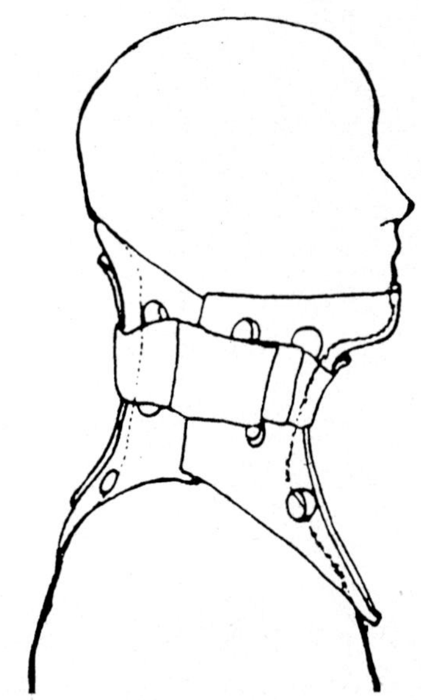

**FIGURE 61-3**

Philadelphia cervical collar. *(From Berger N, Edelstein J, Fishman S, et al. Spinal Orthotics. NYU Medical Center Post-Graduate Prosthetics and Orthotics, New York, 1987.)*

Cervicothoracic orthoses (CTO) also provide intermediate control of cervical motion. The sternooccipitomandibular immobilizer (SOMI) (Fig. 61-4) is effective in minimizing upper cervical motion (C1-5) in flexion.[27] It is less effective than the four-poster and rigid CTOs in controlling rotation and lateral bending. The advantage of the SOMI is its low cost and ease of application. The major disadvantage is allowing more extension than other CTOs. Molded cervicothoracic braces (Yale) orthoses are the most restricting of the nonhalo orthoses. They primarily control flexion, extension, and axial rotation, but only limit lateral bending by 50%.[57]

Maximum control of the cervical spine motion is obtained with the Minerva jacket (Fig. 61-5) and ultimately with a halo apparatus (Fig. 61-6) with limitation of greater than 95% of motion in all planes.[122]

Posterior plating of the cervical spine has been shown to be superior to posterior wiring techniques by providing stability in all planes. Wiring sustains only tensile loads, allows greater rotation and translation, and requires additional external immobilization.[32,89,105]

In the cervical spine longer and stiffer devices provide greater support and restriction in motion,[29] especially below C3-4. The Minerva orthosis and halo device maximally restrict motion in the upper cervical spine but skull-thoracic "paradoxical snaking" motion can occur.[58] Despite the reports of significant limitation in motion with a halo device[61] loss of reduction[121] and increased motion up to 70% with activities of daily living have been reported.[70]

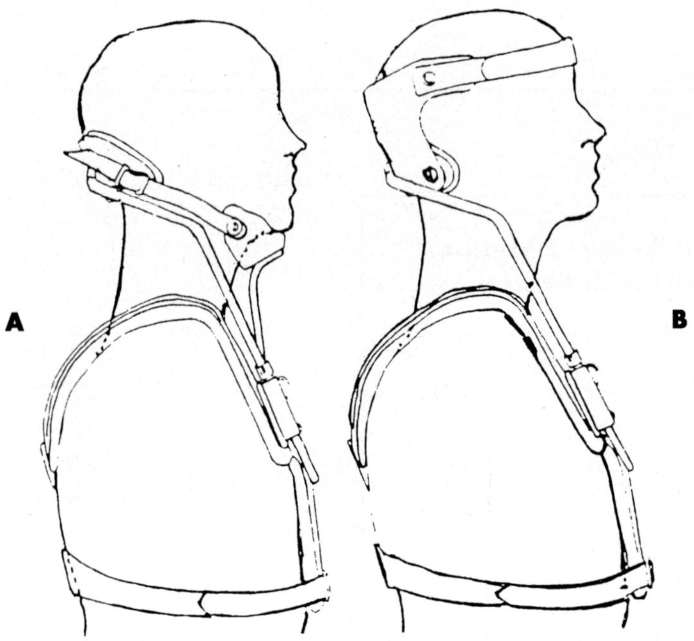


**FIGURE 61-4**

**A,** SOMI brace. Lateral view. **B,** Modified SOMI brace. Lateral view. *(From Berger N, Edelstein J, Fishman S, et al. Spinal Orthotics. NYU Medical Center Post-Graduate Prosthetics and Orthotics, New York, 1987.)*

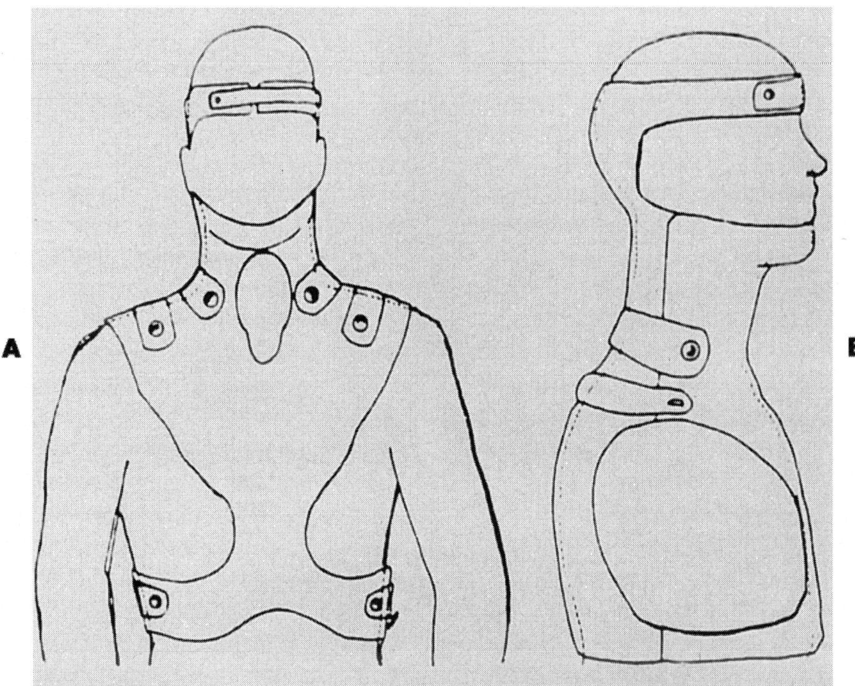


**FIGURE 61-5**

Minerva orthosis. **A,** Anterior view. **B,** Lateral view. *(From Fishman S, Berger N, Edelstein JE, Springer WP. Spinal Orthoses. In Bunch WH, Keagy R, Kritter AE et al. Atlas of Orthotics: Biomechanical principles and application, ed 2. American Academy of Orthopaedic Surgeons. St. Louis: CV Mosby, 1985: 238-256.)*

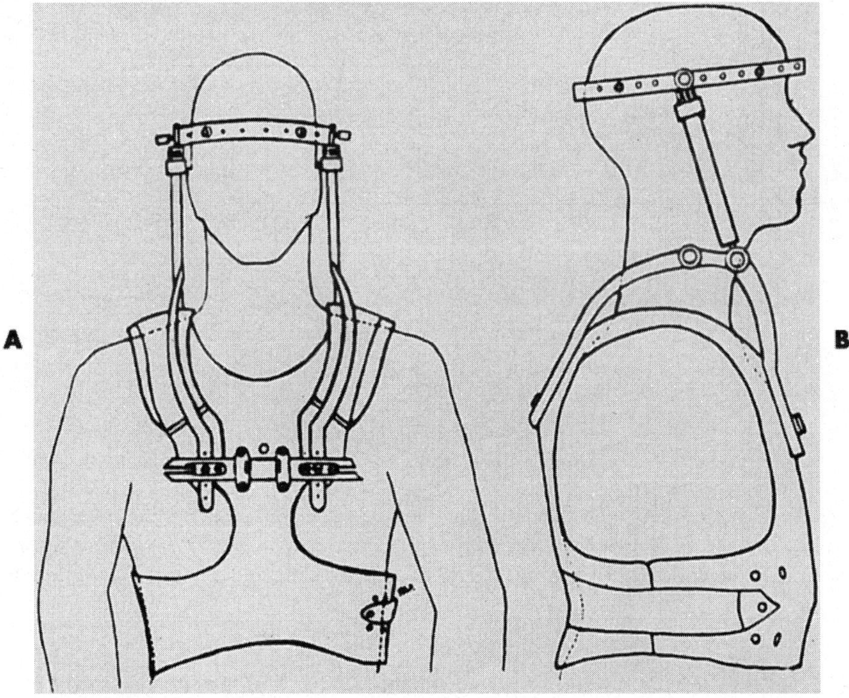


**FIGURE 61-6**

Halo vest. **A,** Anterior view. **B,** Lateral view. *(From Berger N, Edelstein J, Fishman S, et al. Spinal Orthotics. NYU Medical Center Post-Graduate Prosthetics and Orthotics, New York, 1987.)*

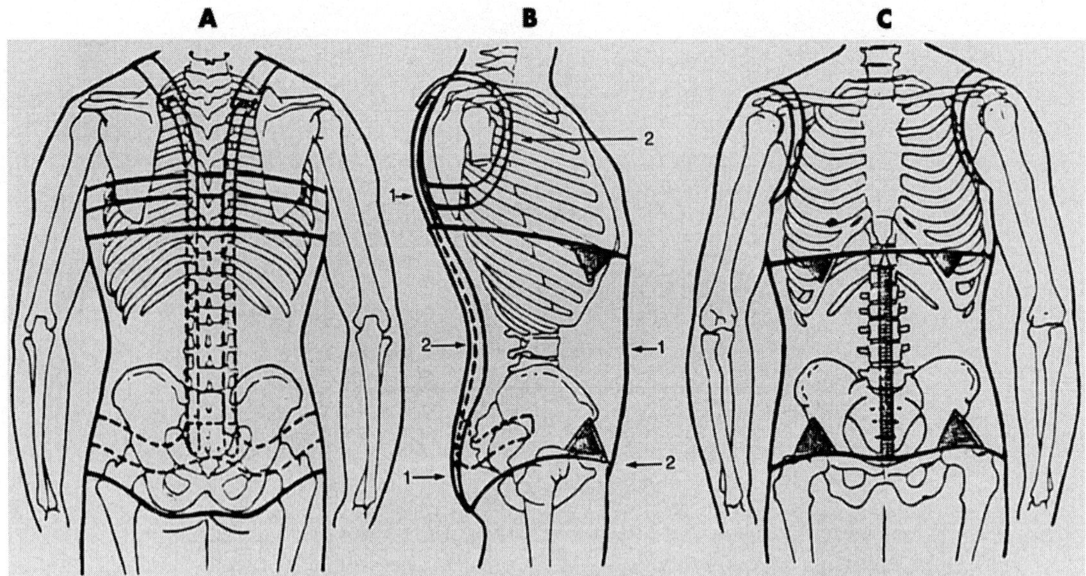


**FIGURE 61-7**

Taylor orthosis. **A,** Posterior view. **B,** Lateral view. *Arrows* represent two independent three-point applications of force. **C,** Anterior view. *(From Fishman S, Berger N, Edelstein JE, Springer WP. Spinal Orthoses. In: Bunch WH, Keagy R, Kritter AE et al. Atlas of Orthotics: Biomechanical principles and application, ed 2. American Academy of Orthopaedic Surgeons. St. Louis: CV Mosby, 1985:238-256.)*

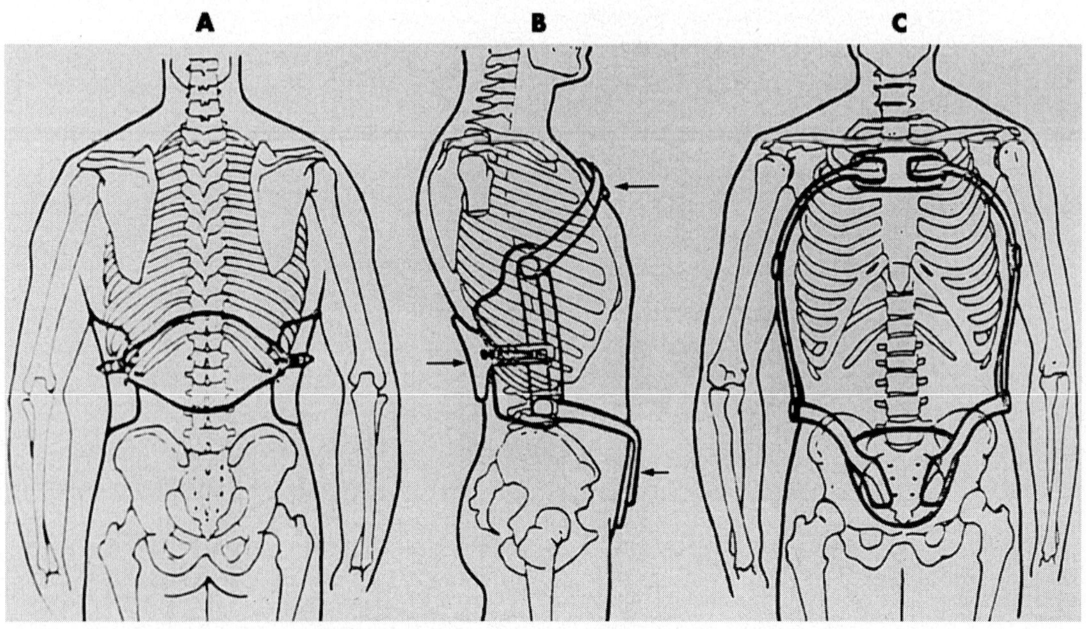


**FIGURE 61-8**

Jewett hyperextension orthosis. **A,** Posterior view. **B,** Lateral view. *Arrows* represent three-point application of forces. *(From Fishman S, Berger N, Edelstein JE, Springer WP. Spinal Orthoses. In Bunch WH, Keagy R, Kritter AE et al: Atlas of Orthotics: Biomechanical principles and application, ed 2. American Academy of Orthopaedic Surgeons. St. Louis: CV Mosby, 1985:238-256.)*

## THORACIC SPINE ORTHOSES

Thoracic spine instrumentation with Harrington rods allows for less inherent stability than Cottrell-Dubousset Instrumentation and thus requires immobilization postoperatively with thoracolumbosacral orthosis (TLSO) or body cast.[15,26]

Minimum control in the thoracic spine can be obtained with the use of a long corset. Taylor (Fig. 61-7), Jewett (Fig. 61-8), and CASH (Fig. 61-9) orthoses

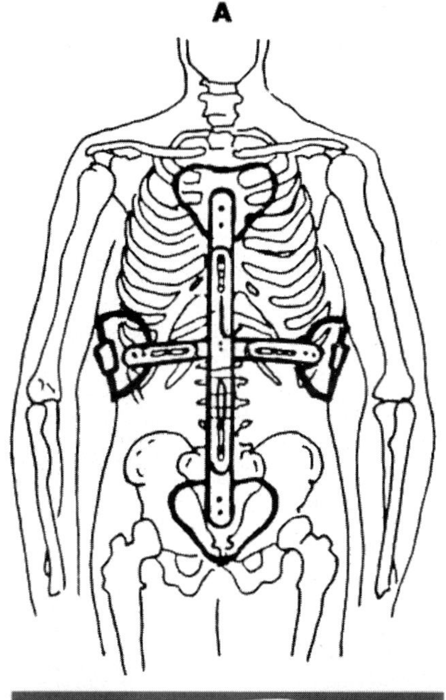


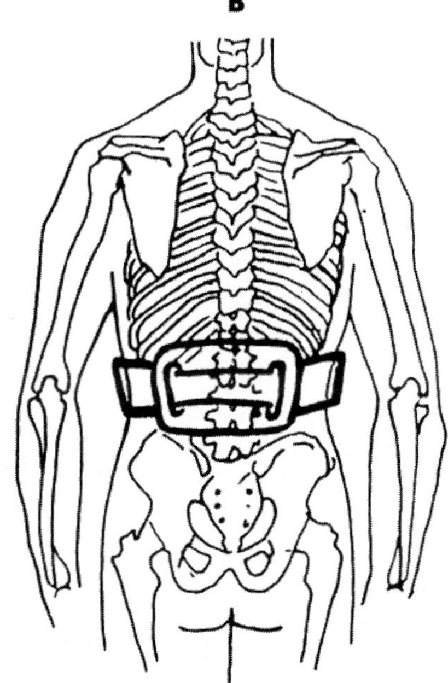


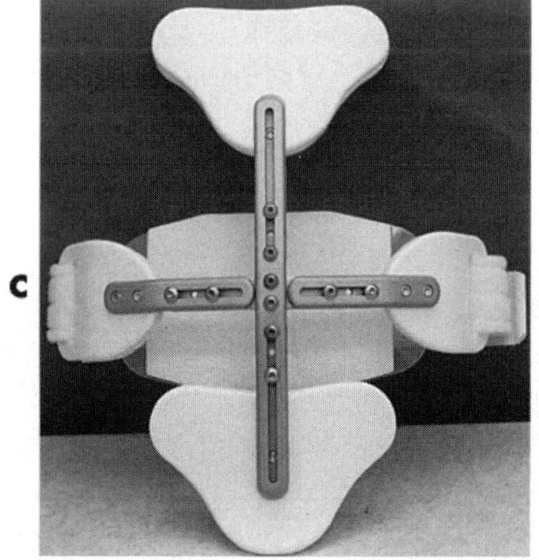


**FIGURE 61-9**

Cruciform anterior spinal hyperextension (CASH) orthosis. **A** and **C,** Anterior view. **B,** Posterior view. *(From Berger N, Edelstein J, Fishman S, et al. Spinal Orthotics. NYU Medical Center Post-Graduate Prosthetics and Orthotics, New York, 1987.)*

provide intermediate control with a three-point fixation system. These afford limitations in flexion and extension. Lateral control uprights can be added to limit lateral bending and clavicular pads and straps can be added to control rotation. Maximum control is obtained with a Milwaukee brace or a Risser cast. These control motion in all planes by pelvic molding, pads, and straps.

## LUMBAR SPINE ORTHOSES

Lumbar pedicle fixation provides maximum stability in all planes including axial rotation and requires minimal external support.[98] Anterior lumbar instrumentation with transverse fixators doubles the stiffness of the system and requires less external support.[1]

In the lumbar spine corsets with various metallic or molded structures ("warm and form" or metal stays) provide minimal control of motion in all planes. Intermediate control can be obtained with a Knight (Fig. 61-10) or chair-back (Fig. 61-11) orthosis with limitation of all motions except rotation. Maximal control can be obtained with a molded lumbosacral orthosis (LSO), with a thigh extension and a drop lock, and with a halopelvic apparatus. Limitation in axial motion is obtained with stabilization of the hip. TLSOs have been found to restrict upper lumbar flexion and rotation by 80% and extension and lateral bending by 50%.[63] Lumbar spine orthoses have been shown by Norton and Brown[95] and Lumsdens and Morris[72] to increase intersegmental motion while limiting only gross motions. Lumbosacral motion was reduced by only 30% but the addition of a thigh extension decreased flexion and extension by over 90% at the L4-5 and L5-S1 levels.[25]

Fidler and Plasmans[25] and Green and Dean[41] concluded that the rigid custom braces restrict motion better than the "off the shelf" orthoses. Corsets have been shown to result in a decrease in intradiscal pres-

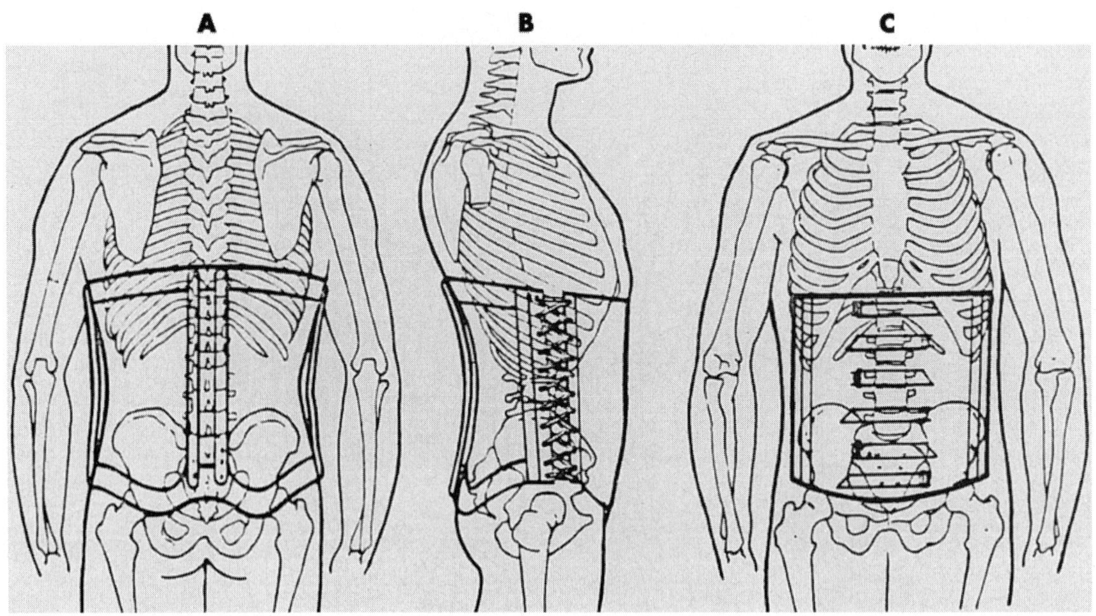


**FIGURE 61-10**

Knight orthosis. **A,** Posterior view. **B,** Lateral view. **C,** Anterior view. *(From Fishman S, Berger N, Edelstein JE, Springer WP. Spinal Orthoses. In: Bunch WH, Keagy R, Kritter AE et al. Atlas of Orthotics: Biomechanical principles and application. 2nd ed. American Academy of Orthopaedic Surgeons. St. Louis: CV Mosby, 1985:238-256.)*

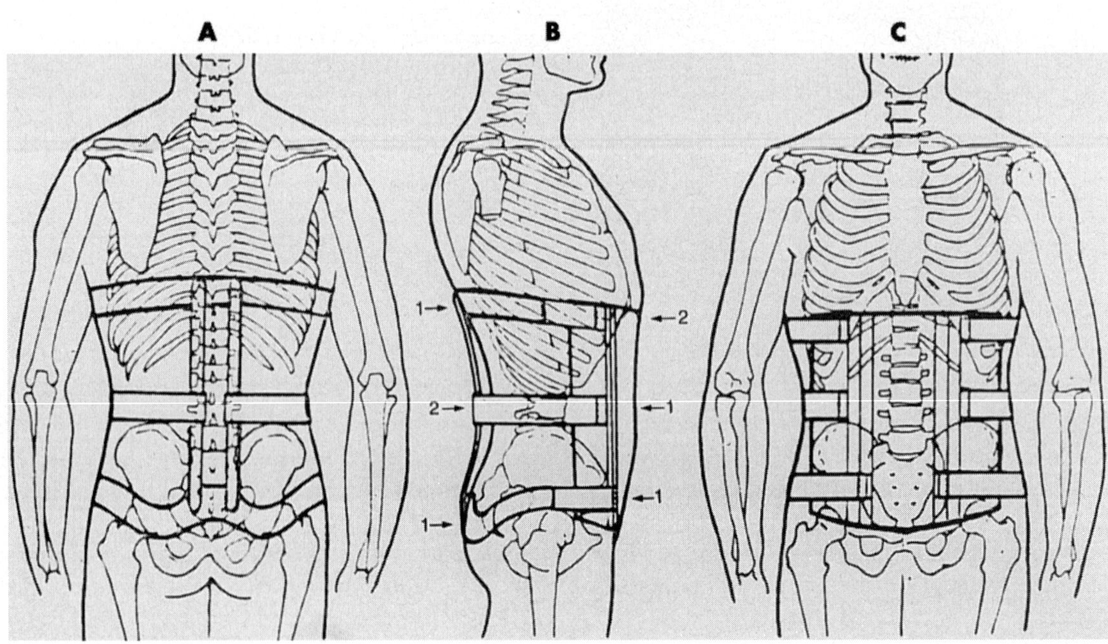


**FIGURE 61-11**

Chair back orthosis. **A,** Posterior view. **B,** Lateral view. **C,** Anterior view. *(From Fishman S, Berger N, Edelstein JE, Springer WP. Spinal Orthoses. In: Bunch WH, Keagy R, Kritter AE et al. Atlas of Orthotics: Biomechanical principles and application, ed 2. American Academy of Orthopaedic Surgeons. St. Louis: CV Mosby, 1985:238-256.)*

sure[92] and an increase in intradiscal pressure and paraspinal muscle activity.[60] Quantification of EMG activity with orthotic usage has yielded equally conflicting results.[13,56] Contrary to conventional wisdom lumbar orthoses do not decrease or substitute for muscle activity. An actual increase in myoelectric activity by 33% has been reported.[64,93] Specifically designed biofeedback orthoses may be able to limit intersegmental forces and postural stresses.[116]

The most common orthosis used in postoperative patients is the custom-molded TLSO (Fig. 61-12). Addition of a chest piece (Fig. 61-13) has been used

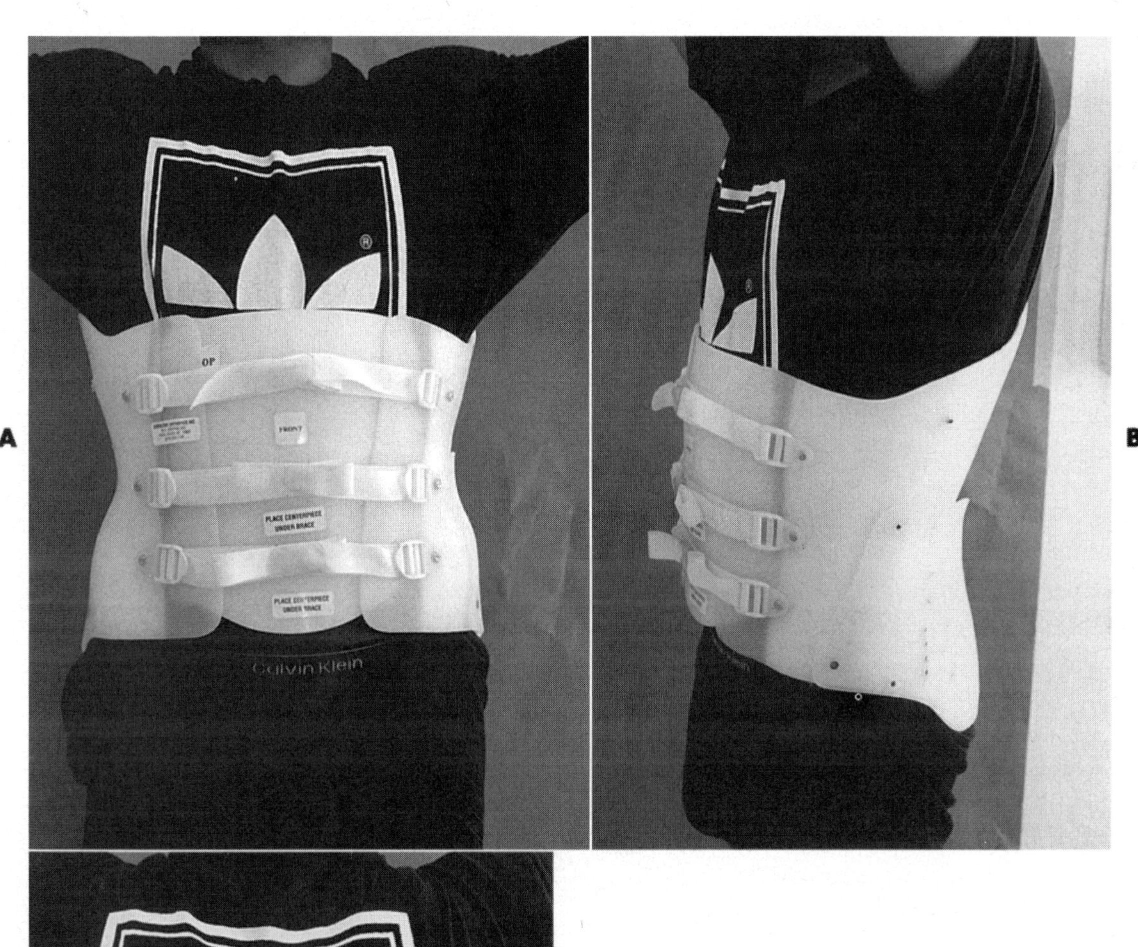

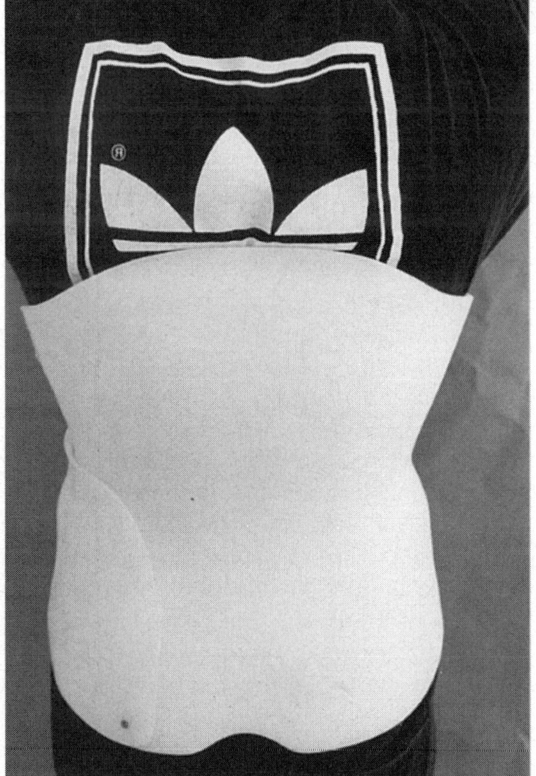

**FIGURE 61-12**

Custom-molded TLSO. **A,** Anterior view. **B,** Lateral view. **C,** Posterior view. *(Courtesy of Daniel Sciscente from Gibralter Orthotics, Pear River, NY.)*

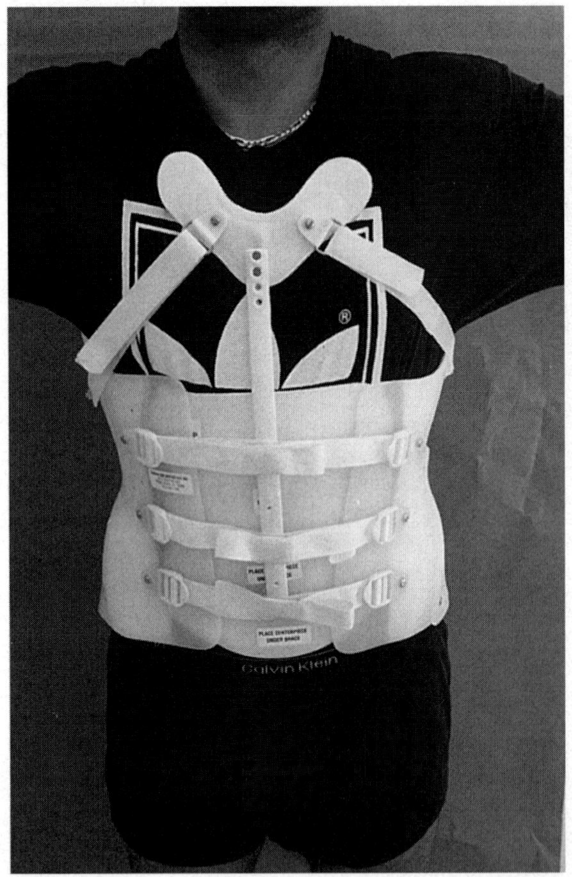


**FIGURE 61-13**

Custom-molded TLSO with chest piece. *(Courtesy of Daniel Sciscente from Gibralter Orthotics, Pear River, NY.)*

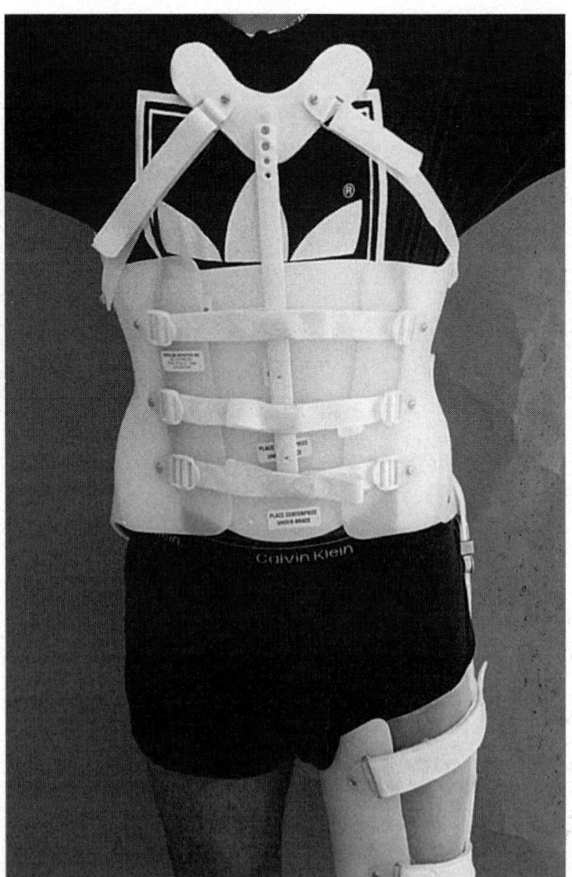


**FIGURE 61-14**

Custom-molded TLSO with leg piece.

routinely to control upper trunk flexion and subsequent spinal motion from above. A unilateral leg extension (Fig. 61-14) creates less motion at the lumbosacral junction but the patient must use a circumduction gait pattern. If the patient is not properly trained or performs ambulation more vigorously there may be an increase in rotational motion at the lumbosacral junction during the stance phase of the unbraced leg.

## ORTHOTIC WEANING

Orthotic weaning is usually begun 2 to 3 weeks prior to its discontinuation. Weaning is more efficacious when the orthotic is removed early in the day, when the soft tissues are less extensible, and prior to the onset of muscular fatigue. Isometric exercises are started when soft tissue healing has occurred. Specific neck, trunk, and lower back strengthening exercises after spinal instrumentation is rarely indicated beyond isometrics for patients. A further discussion of the postoperative rehabilitation program is found later in this chapter.

## PAIN

To adequately design and modulate a comprehensive rehabilitation program an understanding of the potential sources and management of pain must be reviewed. Weinstein's clinical review provides a more in-depth discussion of the mechanism of pain production.[121]

Two types of receptors are found in the spine, local nociceptors (free nerve endings and specialized encapsulated nerve endings) and local neuronal structures (spinal nerves, dorsal root ganglia, motor and sensory roots).[101,106] Sensory innervation from the posterior longitudinal ligament and posterior annulus is derived from the sinuvertebral nerve. The sensory stimulation of the posterior elements including the facet joint capsules, supraspinous and interspinous ligaments, periosteum of the lamina and pedicle, paraspinal muscles, and skin are transmitted by the posterior primary ramus of the spinal nerve. The anterior longitudinal ligament, vertebral bodies and lateral aspect of the disk are innervated by the anterior primary ramus and communicating rami from the sympathetic trunk.[12]

The nociceptors in the capsules of the facet joints respond to excessive mechanical strain, which results in heavy local pressure or movements beyond the physiological barriers of joint motion.[108] Brief nociceptive input from the joint capsule and peripheral tissues reflexively increases the excitability of the antagonist muscles of a joint, resulting in a reactive neurogenic immobilization of that joint.[125] Fatigue of these muscles would cause greater stresses on the capsular and ligamentous structures and ultimately lead to ligamentous and capsular laxity. Cerebral modulation of the motoneuron increases the reflex excitability of postural muscles and may initiate or amplify mechanical pain. Any therapeutic intervention that decreases the motoneuron excitability results in a decrease in muscle tension (spasm) and pain. Blocking of the afferent nociceptive drive can be achieved with the use of nonsteroidal antiinflammatory drugs (NSAIDs), transcutaneous electrical nerve stimulation (TENS), acupuncture, and trigger point, facet joint, or epidural injections. Good long-term results are obtained by combining a reduction in afferent stimulation with voluntary postural motion adjustments including EMG biofeedback.[4,5]

Numerous anatomical locations of the intersegmental motion units can perceive pain. It is well known that not all degenerated segments are painful. More than 37% of asymptomatic patients were found to have lumbar disk herniations and disk degeneration on myelogram[51] and 20% and 60%, respectively, on MRI.[8] Injections into the disk of neurotoxic contrast only produced pain in 37% of asymptomatic subjects.[52] Hypertonic saline injections into the facet joints, interspinous and supraspinous ligaments, intervertebral disks, and dorsal fascia reproduced pain in symptomatic patients.[50,75] Sclerotomal referral patterns can be seen with irritation of the paraspinal muscles and lumbodorsal fascia.[48] The most severe pain was seen with injection of the posterior longitudinal ligament and peripheral annular fibers of the intervertebral disk. Convergence facilitation, projection patterns, and reflex pathways of the spinal segments need to be understood to best localize the source of pain.[29,84]

There are numerous neurogenic and nonneurogenic pain mediators in the spine that play a role in pain provocation in inflammatory and degenerative spinal disorders (Box 61-2).[44,121]

The release of serotonin and histamine by mast cells located near the free and specialized nerve endings in the posterior longitudinal ligament and peripheral annulus may be responsible for the intense pain perception in this region.[97] Substance P released by afferent nerve endings initiates the release of serotonin and histamine.[69] Substance P has been found in high concentrations in the posterior longitudinal ligament.[60] High levels of phospholipase A2 have been found in herniated nucleus pulposus and may contribute to inflammation and pain. The inhibition of the production of prostaglandin synthetase with NSAIDs would decrease the diskogenic component of the patient's discomfort and allow the patient to exercise to restore strength and flexibility without discomfort.[31,109]

Physiologic mechanisms of sleep play a role in the modulation of musculoskeletal pain perception in degenerative joint diseases. Fragmented sleep and associated alpha-EEG non-REM sleep anomaly have been shown to be present in patients with "secondary fibrositis" and contribute to the severity and chronic nature of symptoms.[86,111] The recognition of sleep disturbance in postoperative patients with diffuse pain and fatigue improves a patient's response to a physical reactivation program. The use of analgesics at bedtime with neck or trunk support is beneficial in addition to the use of tricyclic antidepressants (amitriptyline) and antispasmodics (cyclobenzaprine).[7,12] Selected benzodiazepines can also reduce restlessness and improve sleep quality.[87]

Despite reports of limited therapeutic utility selective corticosteroid injections including facet joint, epidural, and nerve root injections may have a role in select patients.[16,54,73,118] Diagnostic localization of the pain generator and a temporary decrease in inflammation may be effective in helping complex patients to facilitate an active exercise program.

In patients having undergone spine revision surgery a systematic approach to identifying the source of the pain having an impact on function needs to be applied using an armamentarium of manual stretching, modalities, medications, bracing, pain provocation, and alleviating-injection techniques.

### Box 61-2. Spinal Pain Mediators

Angiotensin
Bombesin gastric-related peptide
Calcitonin gene-related peptide
Cholecystokinin
Enkephalin
Neurotensin
Somatostatin
Substance P
Vasoactive intestinal polypeptide (VIP)

## MODALITIES

Heating modalities can be effective in the post-spinal revision surgical patient by increasing the extensibility of collagen tissue, decreasing joint stiffness, providing pain relief, relieving muscle spasm, and increasing blood flow to assist in the removal of noxious substances.[67] The choice of heating modalities used is dependent on the localization of the discomfort and

**Table 61-3. Choice of Heating Modality According to Desired Anatomic Level**

| Level of Heating | Modality |
|---|---|
| Skin and subcutaneous tissue | Infrared light<br>Hot packs & heated air<br>Hydrotherapy |
| Subcutaneous tissue and superficial muscle | Shortwave diathermy |
| Muscle | Microwave |
| Joints, myofascial interface, tendon, and nerve sheaths | Ultrasound |

the desired anatomic level of heating (Table 61-3). Mental confusion and application over areas of grossly impaired sensation, ischemia, and malignancy are contraindications to the application of heating modalities.

All superficial heating devices can be used safely in the instrumented patient. Deep-heating modalities should be used with greater care. Ultrasound (US) may be used with caution in patients who have undergone a laminectomy and spinal instrumentation. Direction of the US beam away from the uncovered dura and towards the facet joints and paraspinal musculature would eliminate the likelihood of dural heating.[20] Increased temperature does not occur in areas of metallic implants and thus can be used in areas of spinal instrumentation.[33,67,68] Reflex heating of the deeper tissues can be accomplished with the use of superficial heating modalities.

Cooling modalities (cryotherapy) may be used clinically to reduce muscle spasm and spasticity, decrease bleeding and edema, and reduce pain and inflammation. Blood flow is decreased and joint stiffness is increased with cooling modalities. Additionally resistance to stretching may help to provide initial stability and pain relief by minimizing myofascial extensibility and irritability caused by overstretching of the soft tissues.[67]

Phonophoresis, the introduction of hydrocortisone into the deep tissues using US, has been reported to have beneficial effects in reducing inflammation.[42] More recent clinical trials found no statistical difference between US with and without hydrocortisone.[88] Specific anatomical delivery and dosage can not be controlled and may not provide the intended desirable effect over US alone.

Electrical muscular stimulation can result in a significant decrease in pain by increasing blood flow and interfering with the creation of spasm. It also initiates contraction of the stimulated muscle and can increase muscular strength. Studies in normal patients yielded variable results[80,114] but studies in patients with muscular atrophy revealed an increase in strength,[30] a decrease in succinic dehydrogenase activity,[21] and a decreased rate of protein degradation.[35] All of these are important in maintaining normal healthy muscle.

TENS has been widely used in postoperative pain management. The mechanism of pain reduction may occur via the spinal gate theory of Melzac and Wall[83] or via an increase in endorphin and enkephalin.[34] Low-frequency TENS application is thought to have central and peripheral effects by the actions of endogenous endorphins whereas high-frequency TENS application affects the gating mechanism in the substantia gelatinosa.

The use of modalities as an adjunct to a well-designed restoration program can greatly enhance recovery. Sole use of modalities in the postoperative phase of spine revision surgery is not advisable. The combination of modalities used should be individualized depending on the source of pain and intended result.

## ACUPUNCTURE

Acupuncture can be used as a means of achieving nonmedicinal pain relief. It has been shown by Pasternack[99] that there are endogenous pain suppression systems mediated by specific neuropeptides and neurohormones within the brain and spinal cord. It has been demonstrated that appropriate central and peripheral stimulation can activate these endogenous systems to produce analgesia. Its major effect is through activation of somatosensory pathways, including central neurohormonal and endorphinergic systems, which play a role in modulation of nociceptive impulses in the central nervous system.[71] Usually, a trial of 6 to 8 treatments is necessary to adequately determine if pain relief can be obtained.

## BIOFEEDBACK

The principle action of biofeedback is to influence motor activity and thus retrain muscles to modulate pain either through visual or auditory electromyographic feedback. Lee, et al have reported significant benefit with the use of biofeedback in patients with lower back pain.[66] Thermal and electrodermal techniques have been used but the most consistent and reliable results are with the use of surface EMG biofeedback.[102]

## PSYCHOTHERAPY

Behavioral inhibition, repression, and the effects of disclosure have been found to effect chronic pain and other psychosomatic processes. Treatment sessions with a psychologist trained in pain modulation techniques have been demonstrated to statistically reduce perception of pain and are a good adjunct to an active rehabilitation program.[24]

## THERAPEUTIC EXERCISE

The beneficial effect of exercise in spine disorders has been established. Aggressive exercise programs incorporating spinal stabilization techniques are the recommended treatment of choice in the spine revision patient. No studies have evaluated the effects of exercise on the spinal instrumented or revision patients but the principles from various reports can be extrapolated to this population.

Authors have emphasized exercise in the maintenance of nutritional health of the spinal structures.[78,94] Nutter believes that endorphin and improved circulation are beneficial effects of exercise in all patients with spinal disorders.[96] Aerobic exercise in rheumatoid and osteoarthritic patients resulted in improved aerobic capacity and a reduction in morning stiffness, pain, and swelling.[45,86] Bone mineral density has been found to be greater in patients involved in a variety of sports activities compared with more sedentary subjects.[40,55,62] One can speculate as to the beneficial effect on the spine-fusion mass in patients who perform regular exercise with trunk muscular contractions. Additionally, endurance exercises increase tensile strength of tendons and ligament-bone interface and reduce the stresses placed on adjacent structures.[117] Extreme overuse (destructive loading) or underuse (stress deprivation) of the synovial joints has a deleterious effect on the articular cartilage and the surrounding connective tissue.[3] Therefore, an exercise program must be started at an appropriate level individualized to the patient and titrated according to clinical response.

The efficacy of a comprehensive exercise program has been established in patients with chronic low back pain with a significant improvement in strength, flexibility, pain perception, and disability.[5,17,19,75,83] Functional restoration exercises incorporating specific strengthening and endurance exercises with functional and work simulation tasks have yielded an 85% return-to-work rate in patients with chronic low back pain.[47,79] In this population of patients a comprehensive, controlled, and supervised program has been found to be superior to independent exercise programs in achieving the goals of pain reduction and return to work through strength training, aerobic conditioning, and flexibility.[103]

## STRETCHING

The use of a systematic stretching program can reduce pain in patients after spinal instrumentation and revision surgery. The stretching of joints and associated paraspinal muscles adjacent to the fusion should have a desirable effect of reducing contracture and restoring motion, cartilaginous lubrication, and nutrition by increasing synovial fluid production.[77] Resolution of lumbar spine pain has been reported with a well-designed stretching program.[58,101]

Stretching can be achieved in a variety of methods including active and passive positioning, mobilization, manipulation, proprioceptive neuromuscular facilitation (contract-relax methods), and muscle-energy techniques. The last two techniques physiologically stretch contracted muscles and soft tissues while using the patient's musculature to maintain the stretched position.

Maintaining adequate muscle length allows for greater strength development and dynamic muscular stabilization in the cervical and lumbar spine.[108] A stretching program for the neck and trunk including the paraspinals, trapezius, and quadratus lumborum reduces muscular spasm, increases soft tissue extensibility, and restores functional muscular length and thus the capacity for normal movement patterns. Flexibility of the upper and lower extremities allows for arm and leg motion without compensatory spinal motion. Increasing pelvic tilt has been shown to decrease the compressive stress in the spine with trunk exercises.[38] Flexibility of the lower extremity provides greater absorption of forces directed toward the spine. Limitation in compensatory adjustments increases and abnormally directs the loads.[82]

Manipulation of the spine after instrumentation is not advisable but limited, well-directed soft tissue and facet joint mobilization and muscle energy techniques can be used to free and stabilize restricted motion segments above and below the levels of instrumentation. Restoration of normal balanced muscle function would reduce abnormal joint forces and delay progression of articular degradation.[127] Muscle energy techniques are employed to reduce localized tissue edema and to stretch intramuscular and fascial fibrosis. These techniques provide a concentric or eccentric isotonic or isometric contraction applied in a controlled counterforce. Reciprocal innervation (agonist reflexively inhibiting antagonist) and autogenic inhibition (activation of a lengthened muscle) reduce imbalances and normalize segmental motion patterns. Functional patterns of motion can be established within the physiologic pain-free range and slowly extended into more restricted and previously painful arcs of motion. Because the magnitude of force is low and specifically directed with mobilization and muscle energy techniques they can be safely used in the instrumented patient after the fusion has matured. They should be performed by those physicians and therapists qualified in their application and experienced in their use. Both should be used as an adjunct to, not a replacement of, an active restoration and stabilization program. High-velocity manipulation should be avoided after cervical spinal instrumentation and should be used with caution, if at all, in the lumbar instrumented patient.

## MUSCULAR STABILIZATION PROGRAM

Dynamic internal muscular stabilization is the goal of a spinal instrumentation rehabilitation program. Synergistic activity between all trunk musculature creates a corset-like effect with stabilization and control of spinal motion. Dynamic muscular "fusion" can be obtained in the cervical and lumbar spine to protect the instrumentation and adjacent segments from single overload and repetitive microtrauma. The elimination of shear forces in the intervertebral segments is achieved through coactivation of anterior and posterior musculature. Inability to control segmental stability results in an increase in repetitive flexion and torsional stresses leading to abnormal intervertebral disk and facet (and cervical uncovertebral) joint loading. Nuclear degradation and narrowing of the intervertebral disk also creates greater joint loading. An increase in load and shear forces accelerates mechanical wear in the articular cartilage and increases the inflammatory process.[2,22,23]

Cervical and lumbar muscular stabilization in a neutral spine position reduces abnormal shear and absorb greater forces. In the spinal instrumented patient this would protect the instrumented segment from abnormal stresses and minimize the force at adjacent uninstrumented motion segments. Muscular stabilization also minimizes motion at the fusion level and can allow protected healing to occur. Potentially, an increased fusion mass may occur secondary to repetitive loading and unloading from muscular contractions and a myogenic piezoelectric effect. Additionally, increased muscular activity has the capacity to absorb excessive external forces and vibration creating a stress-shielding effect. An exact quantification of loading necessary to promote fusion and protect the instrumentation has yet to be established.

In the cervical spine shortening of the suboccipital, the splenius, longissimus, spinalis and semispinalis capitis, the upper trapezius, the levator scapulae, and the sternocleidomastoid musculature straightens the lower cervical spine and provides a neutral orientation of the coronal occipitoatlantoacromion line. Lengthening of the posterior musculature by contraction of the anterior flexors physiologically achieves a balanced neutral spine position. Shortening of the anterior shoulder girdle musculature (pectoralis major and minor, anterior deltoid) protracts the scapula and increases the stress in the posterior scapular stabilizers. Retraining of the posterior scapular stabilizers (middle and lower trapezius, rhomboids, and serratus anterior) in a retracted position creates a more balanced cervical spine position. Flexibility and strength of the posterior muscles are needed to maintain a neutral spine/scapular retracted position. Obtaining a balanced neutral cervical spine position provides an appropriate starting point for segmental mobility and stabilization retraining. A neutral cervical spine position results in a reduction in facet-compression force, posterior soft tissue strain, and intervertebral disk loads.[115]

In the lumbar spine an increase in intraabdominal pressure has been reported to have a stabilizing effect.[91] In electromyographic studies an increase in intraabdominal pressure lessened the load on the spine by balancing the forward bending moments with erector spinae activity.[6,49,90] Synergistic muscular coactivation of the erector spinae muscles, hip extensors, latissimus dorsi, and abdominal muscles onto the lumbodorsal fascia are needed to assist in maintaining a neutral spine alignment, axial stability, and reduction (possibly elimination) of segmental shear forces.[9,10,36,37,39,107] Dynamic stabilization of muscular forces in a slightly reduced lumbar lordotic position minimizes shear forces in the lower lumbar motion segments. The lumbar lordosis can be controlled with adjustments in the lumbosacral angle.[38] Additionally, extension decreases the compressive forces on the nerve roots within the intervertebral foramen.[111] Thus, lower extremity and spinal flexibility and coordinated muscle-trunk strengthening are essential in assuming and maintaining neutral and balanced spine forces while minimizing neural and fascial irritation. Once dynamic stabilization is achieved carryover to functional activities is necessary to establish cortical engrams (preprogrammed, automatic multimuscular patterns of motion without conscious control) in an attempt to prevent future spinal impairment and disability.

## POSTOPERATIVE REHABILITATION PROGRAM

The postoperative rehabilitation program can be divided into the postoperative hospital phase (Phase I), the posthospital perfusion phase (Phase II), the posthospital postfusion phase (Phase III), and the maintenance and reactivation phase (Phase IV) (Table 61-4).

The program should begin at an appropriate level and progress according to gains in range of motion, flexibility, strength, and pain reduction within each phase. Progression into the next phase should include the introduction of new stretching and exercise techniques. Complex and stressful techniques including eccentric formats and plyometrics should be reserved for the end of the rehabilitation program (Tables 61-5 and 61-6). Return to recreational sports activities should be considered after achieving pain-free axial range of motion, upper extremity, lower extremity, and trunk strength, and flexibility and an increased aerobic capacity.

**Table 61-4. Phases of Rehabilitation After Spinal Instrumentation and Revision Surgery**

|  | | | | |
|---|---|---|---|---|
| PHASE I: | Brace fitting and modification<br>Bed mobility and transfer training<br>Balance and gait training<br>Abdominal/cervical dynamic bracing exercises | | | |
| PHASE II: | **Modalities**<br>All except ultrasound | **Massage**<br>Longitudinal | **Stretching**<br>Passive and contract/relax | **Extremity Exercise**<br>Light resistive lunges<br>Wall slides |
| | **Trunk Exercise**<br>Isometrics | **Aerobics**<br>Nonpercussive (Bicycle, UBE, Stairmaster) | | |
| PHASE III: | **Modalities**<br>All | **Massage**<br>Horizontal frictional | **Stretching**<br>Active and PNF | **Extremity Exercise**<br>Full resistive PRE program, eccentrics and plyometrics |
| | **Trunk Exercises**<br>Isotonic and Isokinetic<br>Stabilization | **Aerobics**<br>Percussive (treadmill, jogging)<br>Complex nonpercussive (Nordic Track, Versa climber) | | |
| PHASE IV: | Maintenance program (progression of speed and complexity of trunk and extremity resistive training and aerobics with enforcement of stabilization principles)<br>Reintroduction of sports activities | | | |

**Table 61-5. Stretching Program**

| | Cervical | Lumbar |
|---|---|---|
| PHASE II: | Cross arm (triceps/rhomboid)<br>Corner (pectoral) | Hamstring — Passive and seated with quadriceps co-contraction<br>Quadriceps — Active lunge/lean<br>ITB — Standing cross-leg |
| PHASE III: | Same as above plus lateral, diagonal and rotation cervical spine | Same as above plus knee to chest<br>prone press-up<br>trunk rotation |

## SPORTS PARTICIPATION

There are no scientific studies documenting the successful return to sports after spinal instrumentation and revision surgery. Empirically some physicians allow return to competitive athletics as early as 6 months postoperatively.[85] Wright,[126] through a questionnaire to the members of the North American Spine Society, found no agreements as to the postoperative rehabilitation program for return to active sports participation. Seventeen percent of respondents stated they never had an athlete return to the same level of participation after spine fusion. There are reports of isolated return to professional baseball, ice hockey, tennis, cycling, and skiing. Up to 36% discouraged return to football, gymnastics, wrestling, and ice hockey. Chance of participation appeared to decrease with increasing levels of competition, with 80% having a patient return at the high school level, 62% at the college level, and 18% at the professional level. All respondents would permit patients undergoing spine fusion to return to sports after 18 months, 91% after 12 months, 49% after 9 months, and 29% after 6 months.

Return to sports activity needs to be individualized in patients who have undergone spinal instrumentation. Factors leading to successful return to sports par-

**Table 61-6. Strengthening Program**

| Cervical | | Lumbar |
|---|---|---|
| PHASE II: | 1. Cervical isometrics (in collar)<br>2. Positional: supported to unsupported dying bug (supine)<br>3. Shoulder girdle (no weight to light weight PREs)<br>– Arm raises (ant. deltoid)<br>– Rowing (rhomboid)<br>– Pulldowns (latissimus dorsi)<br>– Lateral raises (middle deltoid) (with above elbow weight)<br>– IR/ER at neutral shoulder abduction<br>4. Aerobics: Upper body ergometer<br>Stationary bicycle<br>Stairmaster | 1. Lumbar/abdominal/gluteal isometrics (in brace)<br>2. Controlled lunges<br>3. Wall slides<br>4. Knee extensions<br>5. Hamstring curls<br>6. Toe raises<br>7. Aerobics: as per cervical program |
| PHASE III: | As above plus<br>1. Gravity-resisted cervical<br>2. Supraspinatus raises<br>3. Complex rows in variable trunk positions<br>4. IR/ER at progressive angles to 90-degree shoulder abduction<br>5. Shoulder shrugs<br>6. Arm raises & flys with progressive hip flexed position from 0 to 90 degrees<br>7. Upper extremity exercises on PNF ball | As above plus<br>1. Leg-press machine<br>2. Lumbar stabilization program<br>3. Abdominal crunches<br>4. Trunk extension (prone)<br>5. Single/unilateral then diagonal prone to quadruped raises<br>6. Complex lunges with weights |

ticipation are numerous and depend on the etiology of the spinal pathology, duration and severity of symptoms, level of competition, type and intensity of the sports participation, the location, levels, and extent of instrumentation and fusion, integrity of the adjacent spinal segments and reconstitution of normal range of motion, flexibility, strength, and endurance.

A patient undergoing cervical spine instrumentation at one level may be allowed to participate safely in contact sports. Instrumentation at more than one level would create too great of a lever arm and the risk of serious injury would be too great to allow participation. Instrumentation at the atlantooccipital and atlantoaxial levels would preclude participation in contact sports. Instrumentation after unstable fractures, healed fractures with persistent pain, incongruously healed facet fractures, or comminuted fractures with a retropulsed fragment would also preclude participation in contact sports.

The major question in determining return to contact sports after cervical spine instrumentation and fusion is: "Do the risks of potential catastrophic neurologic compromise outweigh the benefits of participation?" The patient (together with his/her family and coach) should be counseled: if the risk outweighs the benefits, the patient should be encouraged to participate in less high-risk sports activities. The risk in the lumbar spine is significantly reduced, and participation in contact sports is permitted after solid fusion is obtained (usually after 6 to 12 months).

For noncontact sports, a patient undergoing posterior cervical and lumbar spine instrumentation may return to participation at 4 months whereas patients undergoing anterior instrumentation may return after 6 months.

Percussive and running activities cause over 2000 N of force (2.5 to 3 times body weight) at heel strike and should be introduced with caution.[15,66] Significant loads are transmitted to the spine[18] in correlation to changes in intraabdominal pressure.[43] Disk height decreases by an average of 3.2 mm after a 6-km run and 8 mm after a 19-km run.[102] Selection of running shoes, surface, distance, duration, and speed all impact on loading in the spine. Postural pelvic control during running may have an influence on transmission of forces to the spine.[112] A progressive running program should be started controlling running distance, speed, and surface with increases no greater than 10% in speed or distance in a given week.[28]

Swimming is usually recommended for patients after spinal instrumentation and with other spinal disorders. Adequate upper and lower extremity, neck and trunk strength, and flexibility are necessary for formal swimming. The advantages to noncompetitive swimming are in providing buoyancy to minimize compressive axial forces, increasing hydrostatic pressure to enhance the corset-like effect, and providing resistance to muscular forces. Pool walking and floating may be needed prior to actual swimming in very deconditioned patients. The majority of swimming strokes promote truncal extension with the side stroke minimizing extension and rotation and the breast stroke minimizing rotation while creating greater extension forces in the cervical and lumbar spine.[75,80]

Prior to the return to outdoor cycling retraining with a stationary bicycle is usually necessary. For aerobic exercise an initial warmup phase of 2 to 5 minutes at 50 to 80 rpm, a 10 to 20 minute cadence at 80 to 90 rpm (with a maximum predicted heart rate of 65% to 85%), and a cool down phase with light pedaling for 2 to 5 minutes is necessary. The program should be increased by 5 minutes weekly until a maximum level is achieved. If the patient is deconditioned a lower rate should be started with a slower rate of progression. Anaerobic conditioning with increasing resistance and higher rpm sprints should be titrated to the patient's tolerance and goals for return to competitive cycling. Proper frame size and adjustments in seat and handle bar height need to be individualized to reduce cervical and lumbar spine forces and stress through a neutral spine position.

## REFERENCES


1. Abuni K, Panjabi MM, Durancean J: Biomechanical evaluation of spinal fixation devices: Part III: stability provided by six spinal fixation devices and interbody bone graft, *Spine* 14:1249-1255, 1989.
2. Adams MA, Hutton WC: The mechanical function of the lumbar apophysial joints, *Spine* 8:327-330, 1983.
3. Akison WH, Gartin S, Hansel D, Woo SL-Y: Para-articular connective tissue in osteoarthritis, *Sem Arthritis Rheum* 18(suppl 2):41-50, 1989.
4. Andrews DR: Procedures used in the diagnosis of pain, *Hosp Pract 21*:108-121, 1986.
5. Asfour SS, Khalil TM, Waly SM, et al: Biofeedback in back muscle strengthening, *Spine* 15:510-513, 1990.
6. Bartelink DL: The role of abdominal pressure in relieving the pressure on the lumbar intervertebral discs, *J Bone Joint Surg* 39B:718-723, 1957.
7. Bennett RM, Gatter RA, Campbell SM, et al.: A comparison of cyclobenzaprine and placebo in the management of fibrositis, *Arthritis Rheum* 31:1535-1542, 1988.
8. Boden SD, Davis DO, Dina TS, et al: Abnormal magnetic resonance scans of the lumbar spine in asymptomatic subjects, *J Bone Joint Surg* 3:403-408, 1990.
9. Bogduk N: A reappraisal of the anatomy of the human lumbar rector spinae, *J Anat* 131:525-540, 1980.
10. Bogduk N, Macintosh JE: The applied anatomy of the thoracolumbar fascia, *Spine* 9:164-170, 1984.
11. Bogduk N, Tynan W, Wilson AS: The nerve supply to the human lumbar intervertebral discs, *J Anat* 132:39-56, 1981.
12. Cavette S, McCain GA, Bell DA: Evaluation of amitriptyline in primary fibrositis, *Arthritis Rheum* 29:655-659, 1986.
13. Collins GA, Cohen MJ, Naiboff BD, Schandler SL. Comparative analysis of paraspinal and frontalis emg, heart rate and skin conductance in chronic low back pain patients and normals to various postures and stress, *Scand J Rehab Med* 14:39-46, 1982.
14. Cotrel Y, Dubusset J, Guillaunat M: New universal instrumentation in spinal surgery, *Clin Orthop* 227:10-23, 1988.
15. Cavaugh PR, Lafortune MA. Ground reaction forces in distance running, *J Biomech* 13:397-406. 1980.
16. Deyo RA: Fads in the treatment of low back pain, *N Engl J Med* 325(14):1039-1340, 1991.
17. Deyo RA, Walsh NE, Martin DC, et al: A controlled trial of transcutaneous electrical nerve stimulation (TENS) and exercise for chronic low back pain, *N Engl J Med* 322:1627-1634, 1990.
18. Dickenson JA, Cook SD, Leinhardt TM: The measurement of shock waves following heel strike while running, *J Biomech* 18:415-420, 1985.
19. Donchin M, Wodfo O, Kaplan L, Floman Y: Secondary prevention of low back pain, *Spine* 15:1317-1320, 1990.
20. Dussick CT, Fritch DJ, Kyraizidan M, Gear RS: Measurement of articular tissues with ultrasound, *Am J Phys Med* 37:160-165, 1958.
21. Eriksson E, Haggmark T: Comparison of isometric muscle training and electrical stimulation supplementing isometric muscle training in the recovery after major knee ligament surgery, *Am J Sports Med* 7:169-171, 1979.
22. Farfan HF: Effects of torsion on the intervertebral joints, *Can J Surg* 12:336-341, 1969.
23. Farfan HF: Muscular mechanism of the lumbar spine and the position of power and efficiency, *Orthop Clin North Am* 6:135-144, 1975.
24. Feinblatt A, Sarno JE, Flom MA, Diller L: Group psychotherapy for chronic pain disorders. American Psychosomatic Society Meeting. April 3, 1992.
25. Fidler MW, Plasmans CM: The effect of four types of support on the segmental mobility of the lumbosacral spine, *J Bone Joint Surg* 65A(7):943-947, 1983.
26. Fiore SM: Posterior spinal instrumentation, *Spine: State Art Rev* 6(2):347-357, 1992.

27. Fischer SV, Bowar JF, Awad EA, Gullickson G: Cervical orthosis effect on cervical spine motion: roentgenographic and goniometric method of study, *Arch Phys Med Rehab* 58:109-115, 1977.
28. Fixx J: *The complete book of running*. New York, 1977, Random House.
29. Foreman RD: Convergence of muscle and cutaneous input into primate spinothalamic tract neurons, *Brain Res* 124:555-560, 1977.
30. Fournier A, Goldberg M: A medical evaluation of the effects of computer assisted muscle stimulation in paraplegic patients, *Orthopedics* 7:1129-1133, 1984.
31. Franston RC: Human disc phospholipase A2 is inflammatory, *Spine* 17:129-132, 1992.
32. Garfin SR, Moore MR, Marshall LF: A modified technique for cervical facet fusions, *Clin Orthop* 230: 149-153, 1988.
33. Gensten JW: Effects of metallic objects on temperature rises produced in tissues by ultrasound, *Am J Phys Med* 37:75-82, 1958.
34. Gersh MR, Wolf SL: Applications of transcutaneous electrical nerve stimulation in the management of patients with pain, *Phys Ther* 65:314-323, 1985.
35. Goldberg AL, Etlinger JD, Goldspink DF, Jablecki C: Mechanism of work-induced hypertrophy of skeletal muscle, *Med Sci Sports* 7:185-198, 1975.
36. Gracovetsky S, Farfan H: The optimum spine, *Spine* 11:543-73, 1986.
37. Gracovetsky S, Farfan H, Helleur C: The abdominal mechanism, *Spine* 10:317-24, 1985.
38. Gracovetsky S, Kary M, Pitchen I et al: The importance of pelvic tilt in reducing compressive stress in the spine during flexion-extension exercises, *Spine* 14:412-416, 1989.
39. Gracovetsky S, Kary M, Levy S et al: Analysis of spinal and muscular activity during flexion extension and free lifts, *Spine* 15:1333-1339, 1990.
40. Granhed H, Jenson R, Hansson T: The loads on the lumbar spine during extreme weight lifting, *Spine* 12:146-149, 1987.
41. Green ND, Deane G: The physical effect of lumbar spinal supports, *Prosthet Orthot Int* 6:79-87, 1982.
42. Griffin JE, Echternach JL, Price RE, Touchstone JC: Patients treated with ultrasonic driven hydrocortisone and with ultrasound alone, *Phys Ther* 47:594-601, 1967.
43. Grillner S, Nilsson J, Thorstensson A: Intraabdominal pressure changes during natural movements in man, *Acta Physiol Scand* 103:275-283, 1978.
44. Gronblad M, Weinstein JN, Santavirta S: Immunohistochemical observations on spinal tissue innervation, *Acta Orthop Scand* 62:614-622, 1991.
45. Harkcom TM, Lampn RM, Bauwell BF et al: Therapeutic value of graded aerobic exercise training in rheumatoid arthritis, *Arthritis Rheum* 28:32-39, 1985.
46. Hartman JT, Palumbo F, Hill BJ: Cineradiography of the braced normal cervical spine, *Clin Orthop* 109: 97-102, 1975.
47. Hayard R, Fenwick JW, Kalisch SN et al: Functional restoration with behavior support, *Spine* 14:157-161, 1989.
48. Hellgren JH: Observations on referred pain arising from muscle, *Clin Sci* 3:175-190, 1938.
49. Hemborg B, Moritz U: Intraabdominal pressure, Part II: chronic low back pain patients, *Scand J Rehab Med* 17:5-13, 1985.
50. Hirsch C, Ingelmark B, Miller M: The anatomical basis for low back pain, *Acta Orthop* 33:1-17, 1963.
51. Hitselberger WE, Witten RM: Abnormal myelograms in asymptomatic patients, *J Neurosurg* 28:204-206, 1968.
52. Holt EP: The question of lumbar discography, *J Bone Joint Surg* 50A:720-726, 1968.
53. Hurme M, et al: Factors predicting the results of surgery for lumbar intervertebral disc herniation, *Spine* 12:933-938, 1987.
54. Jackson RP, Broom MJ: Facet injection in low back pain: a controlled study. Quebec, 1989, North Am Spine Society, pp 24-25.
55. Jacobson PC, Beaver W, Grubb SA et al: Bone density in women: college athletics and older athletic women, *J Orthop Res* 2:328-332, 1984.
56. Janda U: *Muscle, central nervous motor regulation and a back problem*. In Korr JM, editor: *The neurobiological mechanisms in manipulative therapy*, New York, 1977, Plenum Press.
57. Johnson RM, Hart DL, Owen JR, Lerner E, Chapin W, Zeleznick R: The Yale orthosis: an evaluation of its effectiveness in restricting cervical motion in normal subjects and a comparison with other cervical orthoses, *Phys Ther* 58:865-871, 1978.
58. Johnson RM, Hart DL, Simmons EF, Ramsby GR, Southwich WO: Cervical orthoses. A study comparing their effectiveness in restricting cervical motion in normal subjects, *J Bone Joint Surg* 59A:332-339, 1977.
59. Khalil TM, Asfour SS, Martinez MS et al: Stretching in the rehabilitation of low back pain patients, *Spine* 17:311-317, 1992.
60. Krag MH, Gilbertson L, Pope MH: Intra-abdominal and intrathoracic pressure effects upon load bearing at the spine, *Orthop Trans* 9:358, 1985.
61. Krag MH, Beynnon BD: A new halo-vest: rationale, design and biomechanical comparison to standard halo-vest designs, *Spine* 13:228-235, 1988.
62. Lane NE, Bloch DA, Jones HH et al: Long distance running, bone density, osteoarthritis, *JAMA* 255:1147-1151, 1986.
63. Lantz SA, Schultz AB: Lumbar spine orthosis gearing. I: Restriction of gross body motion, *Spine* 11:834-837, 1986.
64. Lantz SA, Schultz AB: Lumbar spine orthosis wearing, II. Effects on trunk myoelectric activity, *Spine* 11:838-842, 1986.
65. Lee PWH, Chow FL, Cham KC, Wong S: Psychosocial factors influencing outcome in patients with lower back pain, *Spine* 14:838-843, 1989.

66. Lees A, McCullagh PJ: A preliminary investigation into the shock absorbency of running shoes and shoe inserts, *J Human Mov Studies* 10:95-106, 1984.
67. Lehmann JF, deLateur BJ: *Diathermy, superficial heat, laser and cold therapy*. In Kothe FJ, Lehmann JF, editors: *Krusen's handbook of physical medicine and rehabilitation,* Philadelphia, 1990, WB Sanders, pp 283-367.
68. Lehmann JF, Brunner GD, McMillian JA: The influence of surgical implants on the temperature distribution in thigh specimens exposed to ultrasound, *Arch Phys Med Rehab* 39:692-695, 1958.
69. Levine JD, Dardick SJ, Roizen MF, et al: Contribution of sensory afferents and sympathetic efferents to joint injury in experimental arthritis, *J Neurosci* 6: 3423-3429, 1986.
70. Lind B, Sihlbom H, Nordwall A: Forces and motions across the neck in patients treated with a halo vest, *Spine* 13:162-167, 1988.
71. Lorenz KY, Katims JJ, Lee MHM: *Acupuncture: a neuromodulation technique for pain control.* In Aronoff GM, editor: *Evaluation and treatment of chronic pain,* ed 2, Baltimore, 1992, Williams & Wilkins, pp 291-298.
72. Lumsden RM, Morris JM: An in vivo study of axial rotation and immobilization at the lumbosacral joint, *J Bone Joint Surg* 50(A):1591-1602, 1968.
73. Lynch MC, Taylor JF: Facet joint injection for low back pain: a clinical study, *J Bone Joint Surg* 68B: 138-141, 1986.
74. Maiman D, Millington P, Novak S, et al: The effects of the thermoplastic Minerva body jacket on cervical spine motion, *Neurosurg* 25:363-367, 1989.
75. Marks R: Distribution of pain provoked from lumbar facets and related structures during diagnostic infiltration, *Pain* 39:37-40, 1989.
76. Martin RB: *Swimming: forces on aquatic animals and humans.* In Vaugh, CL, editor: *Biomechanics of sport,* Boca Raton, FL, 1989, CRC Press, pp 35-51.
77. Mayer TG, Gatchel RJ: *Functional restoration of spinal disorders: the sports medicine approach,* Philadelphia, 1988, Lea & Febiger.
78. Mayer TG: Discussion: *Exercise, fitness and back pain.* In Bouchard C, Shepard RJ, Stephens T, et al, editors: *Exercise, fitness & health,* Champaign, Illinois, 1990, Human Genetics Books, p 541.
79. McAfee PC, Cassidy JR, Davis RF, Norris RB, Ducker TB. Fusion of the occiput to the upper cervical spine: a review of thirty-seven cases, *Spine* 16:S490-S496, 1991.
80. McDonagh MJN, Davies CTM: Adaptive response of mammalian skeletal muscle to exercise with high loads, *Eur J Appl Physical* 52:139-155, 1984.
81. McNeal RL: Aquatic therapy for patients with rheumatic diseases, *Rheum Dis Clin No Am* 1:919-929, 1990.
82. Mellin G: Correlations of hip mobility with degree of back pain and lumbar spine mobility in chronic low back pain patients, *Spine* 13:668-670, 1988.
83. Melzac R, Wall PD: Pain mechanisms: a new theory, *Science* 150:971-979, 1965.
84. Mense S: Considerations concerning the neurobiological basis of muscle pain, *Can J Phys Pharm* 69: 610-616, 1991.
85. Micheli LJ: *Spinal deformities and the athlete.* In Torg JS et al, editors: *Current therapy in sports medicine.* St. Louis, 1985, Mosby/BC Decker, pp 158-164.
86. Minor MA, Hewett JE, Webel RR, et al: Exercise tolerance and disease related measures in patients with rheumatic arthritis and osteoarthritis, *J Rheumatol* 15: 905-911, 1988.
87. Moldofsky H: Sleep and fibrositis syndrome, *Rheum Dis Clin North Am* 15:91-103, 1989.
88. Moll MJ: A new approach to pain: lidocaine and decadron with ultrasound, *USAF Med Serv Dig* 30(3): 8-11, 1979.
89. Montegano PX, Juach EC, Anderson PA, et al: Biomechanics of cervical spine internal fixation, *Spine* 16(suppl):510-516, 1991.
90. Morris JM, Lucas DB, Bresler B: The role of trunk muscles in stability of the spine, *J Bone Joint Surg* 43A:317-330, 1961.
91. Nachemson AL, Andersson BJ, Schultz AB: Valsalva maneuver biomechanics: effects on lumbar trunk loads of elevated intraabdominal pressures, *Spine* 11: 476-479, 1986.
92. Nachemson A, Morris JM: In vivo measurements of intradiscal pressure, *J Bone Joint Surg* 46A:1077-1092, 1964.
93. Nachemson A, Schultz AB, Anderson G: Mechanical effectiveness studies of lumbar spine orthosis, *Scand J Rehab Med* 9(suppl):139-140, 1983.
94. Nachemson AL: *Exercise, fitness and back pain.* In Bouchard C, Shepard RJ, Stephens T, et al, editors: *Exercise, fitness & health.* Champaign, IL, 1990, Human Genetics Books, p 533.
95. Norton PL, Brown T: The immobility efficiency of back braces; their effect on the posture and motion of the lumbosacral spine, *J Bone Joint Surg* 39A: 111-139, 1957.
96. Nutter P: Aerobic exercise in the treatment and prevention of low back pain, *Occup Med: State Art Rev* 3:137-145, 1988.
97. Olsson Y: Mast cells in human peripheral nerve, *Acta Neurol Scand* 47:357-368, 1971.
98. Panjabi MM, Vasarada A, White AA: Biomechanical principles of spinal fusion, *Spine: State Art Rev* 6(3): 435-443, 1992.
99. Pasternack GW: Multiple morphine and enkephalin receptors and the relief of pain, *JAMA* 259(9):1362-1367, 1988.
100. Peck CL, Kraft SM: Electromyographic biofeedback for pain related to muscle tension: a study of tension headache, back and jaw pain, *Arch Surg* 112:889-895, 1977.
101. Ralston HJ: Nerve endings in human fasciae, ten-

dons, ligaments, periosteum and joint synovial membrane, *Anat Rec* 136:137-148, 1960.

102. Reilly T, Leatt D, Troup JGD: Spinal loading during circuit weight training and running, *Br J Sports Med* 20(3):119-124, 1986.
103. Reilly K, Lovejoy B, William R, Roth H: Differences between a supervised and independent strength and conditioning program with chronic low back syndromes, *J Occup Med* 31:547-550, 1989.
104. Rider RA, Daly J: Effects of flexibility training on enhancing spinal mobility in older women, *J Sports Med Phys Fitness* 31:213-217, 1991.
105. Robinson RA, Southwick WO: *Surgical Approaches to the cervical spine.* In AOSS: *Instructional Course Lectures,* vol 17, St. Louis, 1960, CV Mosby.
106. Rydevik B, Brown MD, Lundberg G: Pathoanatomy and pathophysiology of nerve root compression, *Spine* 9:7-15, 1984.
107. Saal JA: *Biomechanics of lumbar dynamic muscular stabilization.* In *Aggressive Non-Surgical Rehabilitation of Lumbar Spine and Sports Injuries.* Daly City, CA, 1989, San Francisco Spine Institute.
108. Saal JA: Dynamic muscular stabilization in the nonoperative treatment of lumbar pain syndromes, *Orthop Rev* 19:691-700, 1990.
109. Saal JS, Franson FC, Dobrow R, et al: High levels of inflammatory phospholipase a2 activity in lumbar disc herniations, *Spine* 15:674-678, 1990.
110. Schaibel HG, Schmidt RF: Effects of an experimental arthritis on the sensory properties of the articular afferent units, *J Neurophysiol* 54:1109-1122, 1985.
111. Schnebel BE, Watkins RG, Dillin W: The role of spinal flexion and extension in changing nerve root compression in disc herniations, *Spine* 14:835-837, 1989.
112. Slocum DB, Bowerman W: Biomechanics of running, *Clin Orthop* 23:39-45, 1962.
113. Smythe H. The "repetitive strain injury syndrome" B referred pain from the neck, *J Rheumatol* 15:1604-1604, 1988.
114. Stetanovska A, Vodovnik L: Change in muscle force following electrical stimulation, *Scand J Rehab Med* 17:141-146, 1985.
115. Sweeney T: Neck school: cervical thoracic stabilization training. *Occup Med: State Art Rev* 7:43-54, 1992.
116. Szeto AY, Saunders FA: Electrocutaneous stimulation for sensory communication in rehabilitation engineering, *IEEE Trans Biomed Eng* 29:300-308, 1982.
117. Tipton CM, Schild RJ, Tomanck RJ: Influence of physical activity on the strength of knee ligaments in rats, *Am J Physiol* 212:783-787, 1967.
118. Trindle MR, McKay WR: Dorsal primary ramus nerve block for treatment of low back pain after epidural analgenisia, *Anaesth Analgesia* 75:1038-1040, 1992.
119. Varlotta GP: *Spinal orthoses.* In Tindall GT, Cooper PR, Barrow DL, editors: *The practice of neurosurgery,* Baltimore, 1996, Williams & Wilkins, pp 2609-2622.
120. Varlotta GP, Errico TJ: *Rehabilitation after spinal instrumentation.* In *Spine: State of the Art Reviews.* Philadelphia, 1994, Hanley & Belfus, Inc., pp. 501-521.
121. Weinstein JN: The role of neurogenic and nonneurogenic medication as they relate to pain and the development of osteoarthritis: a clinical review, *Spine* 17:5356-5361, 1992.
122. White AA, Panjabi MM: *Clinical biomechanics of the spine,* ed 2. Philadelphia, 1990, JB Lippincott.
123. Whitehill R, Richman JA, Glaser JS: Failure of immobilization of the cervical spine by the halo-vest. A report of five cases, *J Bone Joint Surg* 68A:326-332, 1986.
124. Wolf JW, Jones HC: Comparison of cervical immobilization in halo-casts and halo-plastic jackets, *Orthrop Trans* 5(1):118-121, 1981.
125. Woolf CJ: Long term alterations in the excitability of the flexion reflex produced by peripheral tissue injury in the chronic decerebrate rat, *Pain* 18:325-343, 1984.
126. Wright A, Ferree B, Tromanhauser S: Spinal fusion in the athlete, *Clin Sports Med* 12:599-602, 1993.
127. Yong-Hing K, Kirkaldy-Willis WH: The pathophysiology of degenerative disease of the lumbar spine, *Orthop Clin North Am* 14:491-504, 1983.

# XI
# EMERGING TECHNIQUES

# 62

# EARLY EXPERIENCE: COMPUTER-ASSISTED NAVIGATION AND PEDICLE SCREW PLACEMENT

**Allen L. Carl, M.D.**
**Harpal S. Khanuja, M.D.**
**Charles A. Gatto, M.D.**
**John C. vom Lehn, M.S.**
**Kirby Vosburgh, Ph.D.**
**John Schenck, M.D., Ph.D.**
**William Lorensen, M.S.**
**Kenneth Rohling**

Navigational System
Imaging
Integration
In Vitro Method
In Vivo Method

Today more than ever technological innovations find increasing application in the medical field. This relationship has always existed, and much of successful everyday medicine is based on this interface. In 1869, Dr. Roentgen's discovery of "a form of radiant energy, which was invisible, could cause fluorescence, and passed through objects opaque to light" revolutionized medicine. There was the subsequent development of tomography and computer tomography. Ultrasound technology, a routine procedure in many aspects of medicine, evolved from Defense Department research from the 1930s and 1940s. As research with light emission and laser technology has evolved we have seen many applications in surgery.

Medicine, along with the rest of society, is now experiencing the information age. The developments and exponential surge in computer technology are changing the everyday practice of medicine. Radiographic images are now stored digitally. Thousands of medical charts are being replaced by single disks. The ability to communicate electronically has opened up vast new opportunities for consultation and collaboration around the world.

Enhanced computer imaging and simulation has lead to virtual reality technology. There are many novel ideas for its application to medicine. Much of the work is exploring its use in education, and surgical simulation. Computer generated images not only allow for accurate depiction of anatomy, but also provide models to view dynamic changes. In most instances these computer images and models are based on reconstruction of data acquired with computed tomography (CT) and magnetic resonance imaging (MRI) scans. There are numerous centers and universities in the United States dedicated to the use of new computer technology in surgical education.

Beyond surgical simulation, the role of this technology in the operating room is being explored. The principle is based on these more accurate and detailed images to aid in and enhance surgical procedures, the greatest benefit being in those areas or procedures in which direct visualization of pertinent anatomy is not possible.

Numerous applications are being sought. It has been shown to be effective in both framed and frameless stereotactic localization of brain tumors.[2,5,11,19] In this instance, preoperative data from MRI reconstructions are used to enhance delineation and resection of brain tumors. Other areas of investigation include craniofacial, reconstructive, and orthopedic surgery.

Our application and experiences of this fledgling technology to spine pedicle screw placement is presented. There are many efforts, similar to the one presented here directed at computer-assisted placement of pedicle screws.

There has been much controversy in both the medical and layman's literature over the safety of pedicle screws. This is a result of incurred problems with malpositioned screws including neurologic and major vascular injury as well as suboptimal biomechanical fixation, loss of fixation, and possible late neurovascular complications.[4,6,7,15,16] There is also a steep learning curve for pedicle screw placement in the lumbar spine.[6,17] In the thoracic spine and in cases of severe deformity or rotation, poor results are reported.[14] The variability of anatomy and low pedicle diameter to screw diameter ratio leave little room for error.

In order to improve screw placement, anatomic studies have been done to delineate the pedicle anatomy and better correlate the pedicle to posterior surface anatomy of the lumbar spine.[13,15,16,18] Current guidelines for positioning are based on this anatomy and preoperative imaging. Various aids including probes, scopes, guide palpation, and electrical impulse instruments are available to help confirm proper screw track position. Additional methods to assist in pedicle screw placement include radiography and fluoroscopy. Both of these methods are two-dimensional, time-consuming, and limited by radiation exposure. Fluoroscopy has limited ability for real-time guidance only in two dimensions with a delay to check the third dimension.

The problems associated with the placement of pedicle screws have prompted many groups to pursue methods to enhance the precision and accuracy of screw placement. Among the efforts are systems relaying on computer based imaging, similar to the one presented here. In formulating such a system, our specific goals included the ability for trajectory planning and visualization, real-time feedback of information, three-dimensional anatomy viewing from any position, as well as transverse section viewing at any level. Relying on depiction of unseen anatomy, the intention was to provide a map to plan and track pedicle screw drilling and placement in near real time. The goal was to be accomplished with a frameless system available for use in the operating room with only slight modifications of current technique.

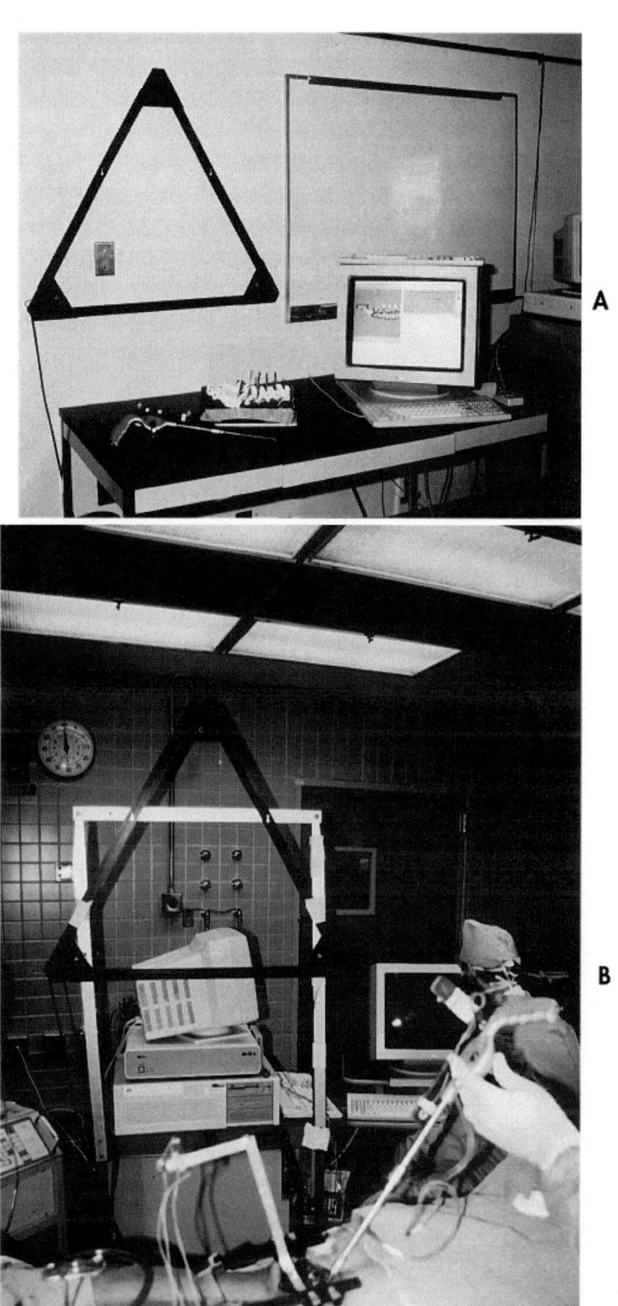


FIGURE 62-1

**A, B,** Laboratory set-up showing locator tool, computer with computed tomography reconstructed image and off-field receiver. Intraoperative set-up showing off-field receiver computer with reconstructed CT images and sterile locator tool in the surgical field.

## NAVIGATIONAL SYSTEM

A frameless stereotactic navigational system was devised allowing the surgeon to keep track of the tip of a probe in three dimensional space in near real time (Fig. 62-1). This was accomplished with a Science Accessories Acoustic Digitizer, model GP-12XL, as a sound locator. Three receivers for the acoustic digitizer were mounted on a three-dimensional triangular frame

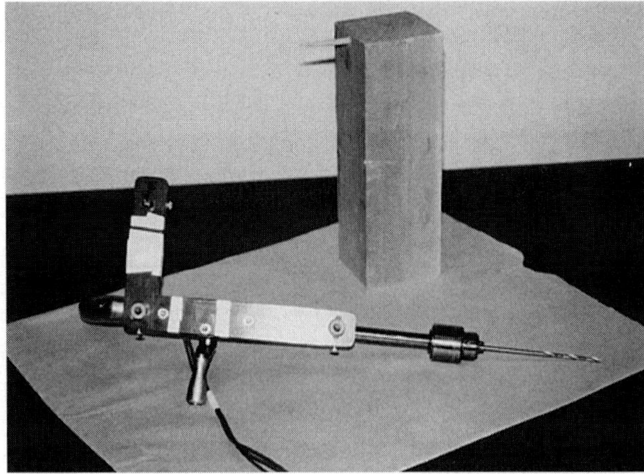

**Figure 62-2**

Locator tool with three fixed point triangular array of sound emitters.

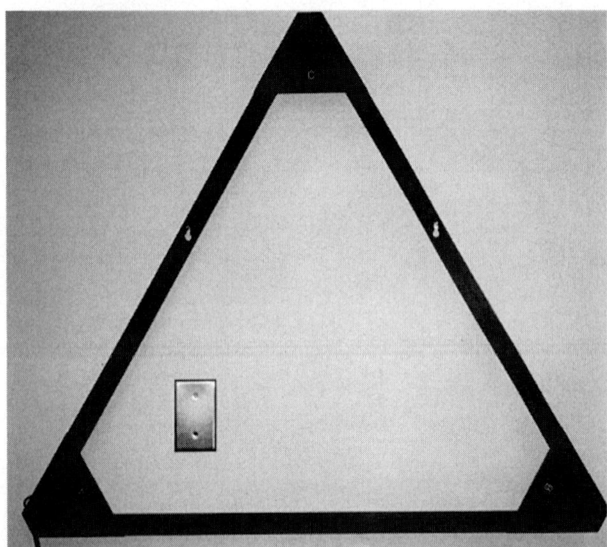

**Figure 62-3**

Off-field receiver to track sound emitters.

at a known fixed distance from one another. Three fixed point sound emitters were mounted in a three-dimensional triangular array on a hand operated surgical drill (locator tool) (Fig. 62-2). Emitter tracking is accomplished using an acoustic time-of-flight system off-field receiver (Fig. 62-3). Clicking pulses from the emitters mounted on the drill sound at regular intervals (six times per second) and are picked up at the stationary receiver at slightly different time intervals. This allows for calculation of the three-dimensional position of the emitters (and therefore the drill) in space within the set field. Calculation of the position of the emitters renders a new picture every second, thereby essentially giving immediate positional feedback and near real-time capability. Also, if the position of the tip of a probe, bit, or screw with respect to the hand drill emitters is known, then this tip can be tracked in space. This calculation is done dynamically by registering the tip to a fixed point in the field and then relating an emitter to the fixed point and thereby calculates the position of the registered tip with respect to the hand drill emitters (Fig. 62-4). The accuracy of this calculation was found to be ±0.25 mm.

## IMAGING

Model and cadaveric lumbosacral spines and then the lumbosacral spines of living patients were imaged in a GE helical CT scanner for the in vitro and in vivo portions of the study respectively. One millimeter spaced volumetric computed tomography slices were obtained for each spine. This data was then custom formatted into a three-dimensional (3D) computer reconstruction in both surface and volume on a Sun 4/670 workstation using GE research workstation software and a GE hardware rotate board as a rendering accelerator (GE, Milwaukee, WI).

## INTEGRATION

Once the preoperative data was acquired and formatted, the essential step of linking it with the navigational system was accomplished using novel GE software. This allowed for coordination of the real spine in space with the 3D reconstructed image on the computer screen (Fig. 62-5). Registration of the real anatomic structure to the 3D reconstruction image was done via the navigational system. This was accomplished in a similar manner to the registering of the probe tip to the hand drill: For in vitro anatomy, three asymmetric points on the fixed real vertebral structure were linked to their corresponding areas pictured on the 3D reconstruction image via the probe tip and the navigational system. For in vivo anatomy, this needed to be repeated at every level just prior to drilling in order to eliminate error secondary to changes in the relative position of the vertebral bodies since CT scanning was done supine and operative intervention prone. Additionally for in vivo application a second dynamic reference emitter positioned each time on the operative vertebral level was added to compensate and continually update the changes in position of the anatomy during surgical manipulation (Fig. 62-6).

## IN VITRO METHOD

Two lumbosacral plastic spine models and two fresh frozen human cadaver lumbosacral spines were used in this portion of the study. To mimic operative exposure

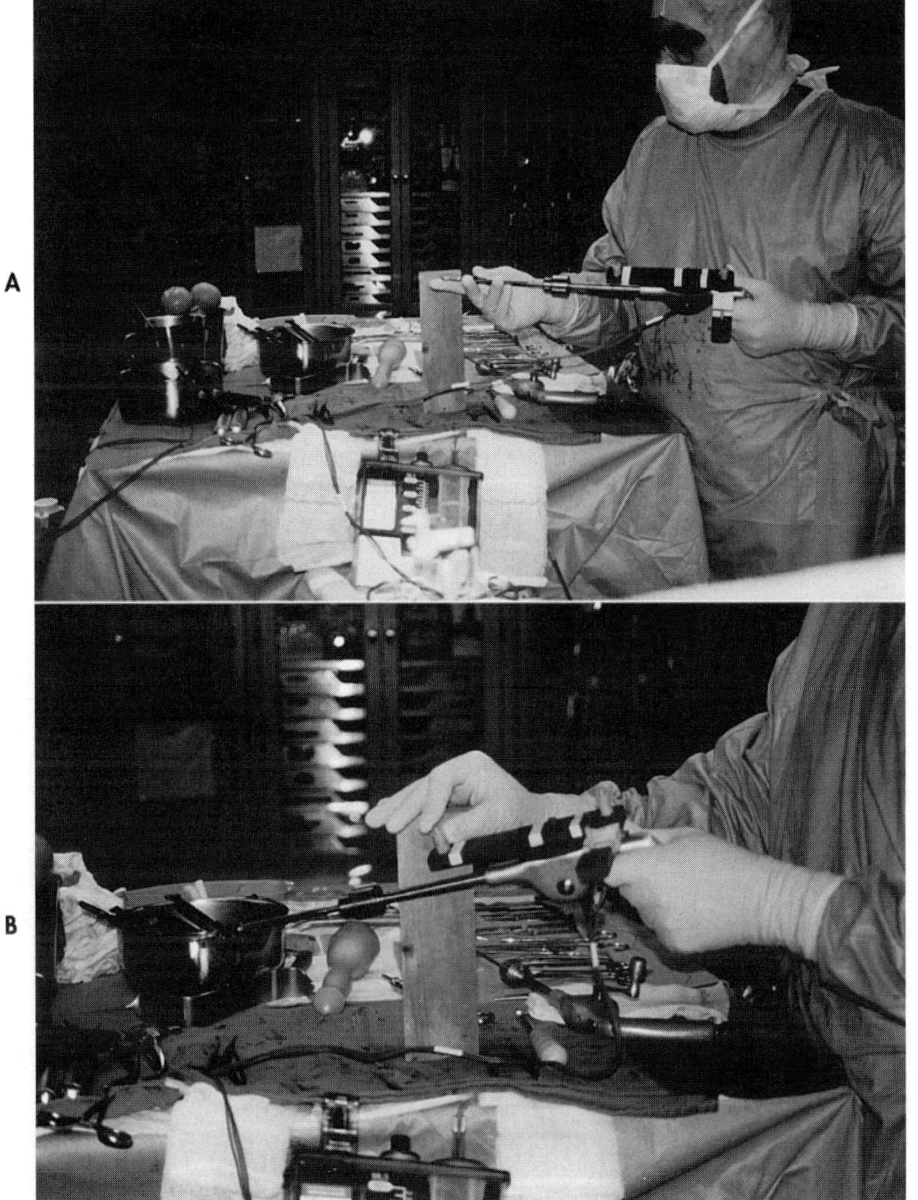

FIGURE 62-4

Registration of tool tip **(A)** and first emitter **(B)** to zero the tool to allow for tracking in space.

A

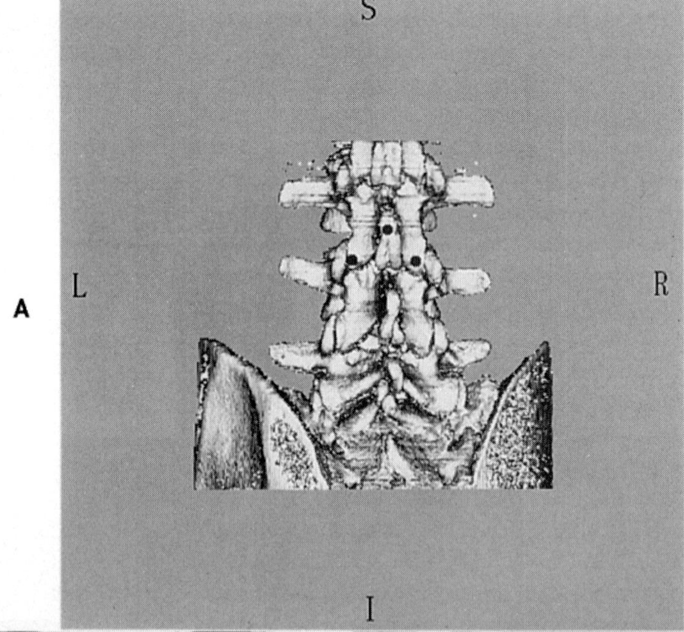


B

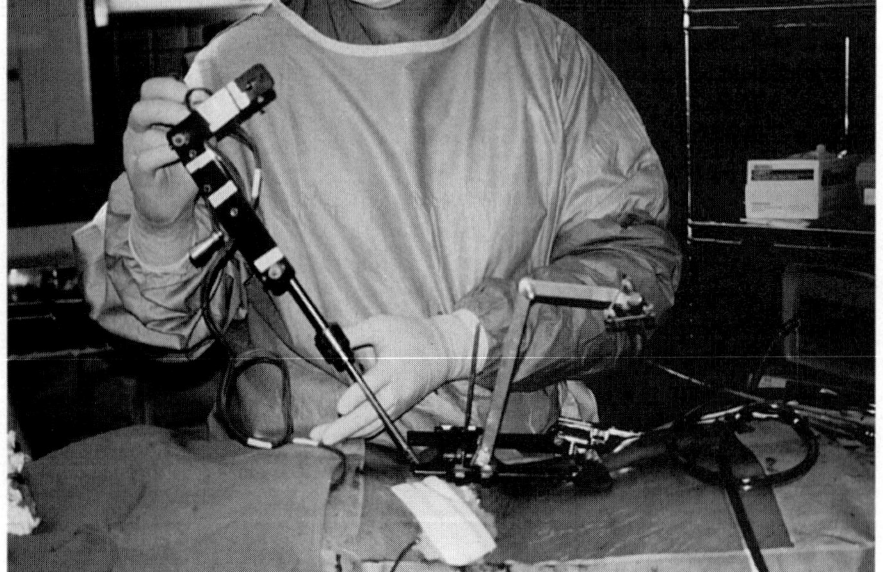

**FIGURE 62-5**

**A, B,** Once tool is zeroed (a) corresponding points are identified on the computer screen and meshed with the real spine anatomy.

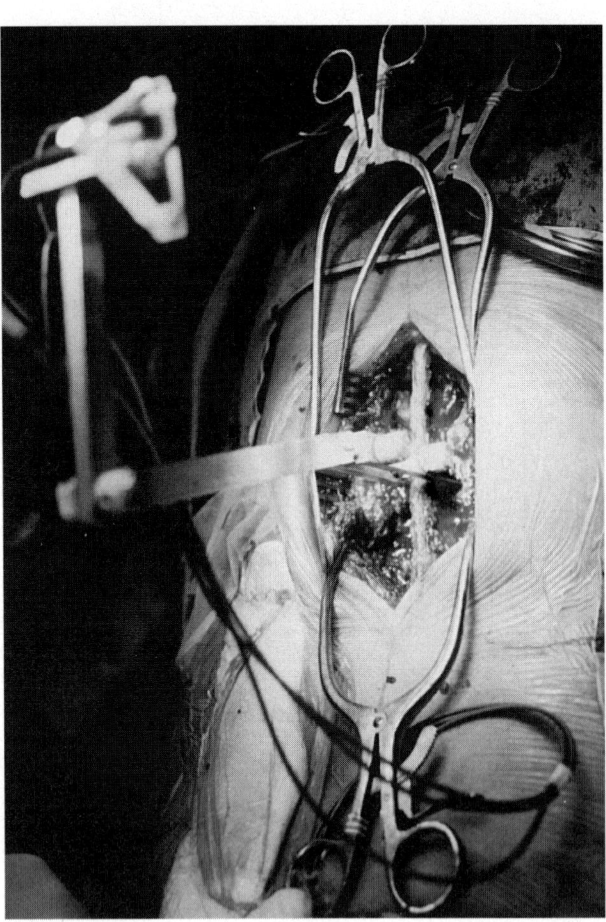

**FIGURE 62-6**

Second emitter positioned on each operative vertebral segment to account for its change in space.

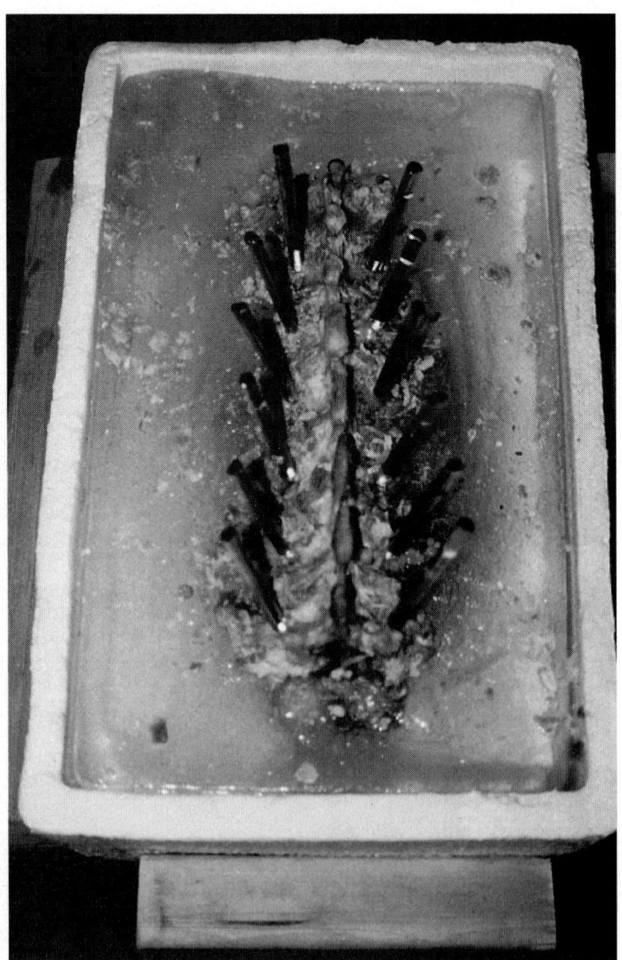

**FIGURE 62-7**

Opaque ice-embedded spine specimen with Schanz screws placed using stereotaxy tool.

and remove visual cues of pedicle position, these test models were imbedded in ice or black epoxy so that only the posterior elements were visualized (Fig. 62-7). This also held the spine and its vertebral bodies securely in position in the field and relative to each other. CT scans of the spines were obtained as above and 3D reconstructions were formatted for use on the screen of the navigation system. The cadaveric spines were registered to the 3D reconstruction using three reference points at each vertebral level as described above. First the drill bit and then the screw tip were registered to the navigational system as described above for each level of pedicle screws placed. Drilling was performed with a 3.2-mm diameter bit using the navigational system for guidance. Six-millimeter Schanz screws were used as pedicle screw implants and were also placed using the navigational system. In total, 44 pedicles were drilled and 44 pedicle screws were placed in this manner. For each screw placed an attempt was made to center the screw in the pedicle and to anchor it in the anterior vertebral cortex. Multiple views in the coronal, sagittal, and transverse planes were used at the discretion of the surgeon to plan and correct the trajectories of the drill tip and screws in real-time (Fig. 62-8). Trajectory pathway and final screw tip positions were recorded on the computer model. Postprocedure CT scans were performed on each specimen and then each vertebral body was sectioned to evaluate screw placement (Fig. 62-9). Correlation of perceived position using the navigational system compared to the actual position found by CT scan and sectioning was performed.

Postprocedural CT scans were calculated to have ±1.0 mm error secondary to implant beam scatter. These post procedure scans confirmed all 44 screws were embedded within the cortical margins of the pedicle. Sectioning of the plastic models showed accuracy of anterior cortical depth placement (closeness to the anterior vertebral cortex) to be within 1.4 mm ±0.6 mm. In the cadaver spines the accuracy of the depth placement was on average within 1.6 mm with standard deviation of 0.8 and range of 2.5 mm.

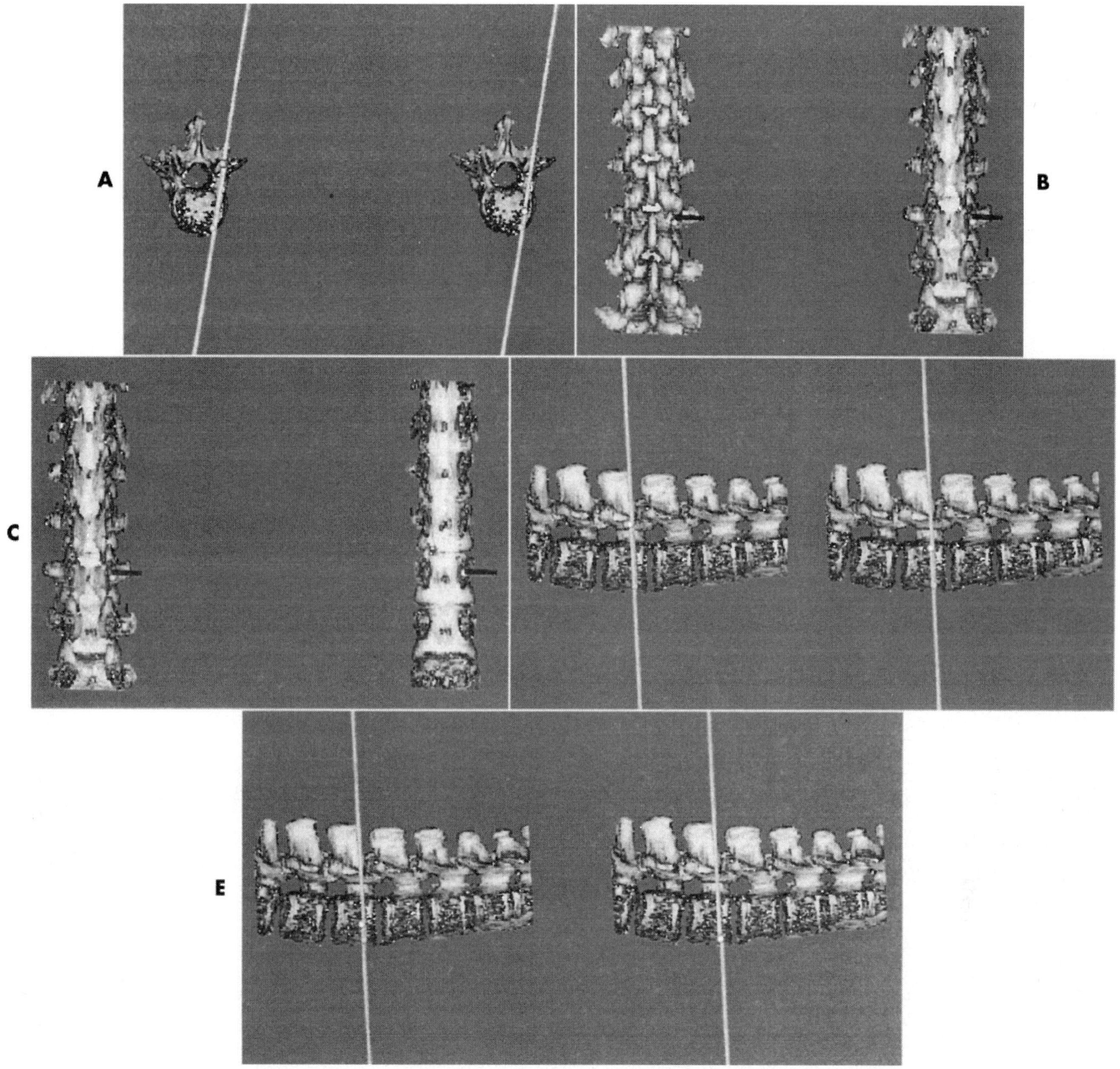

**FIGURE 62-8**

Sequential transverse **(A),** coronal **(B, C),** and sagittal **(D, E)** CT images of drill tip progression (*white ball*) identified during the actual procedure, which allows for tracking and immediate alignment to accomplish optimal accuracy.

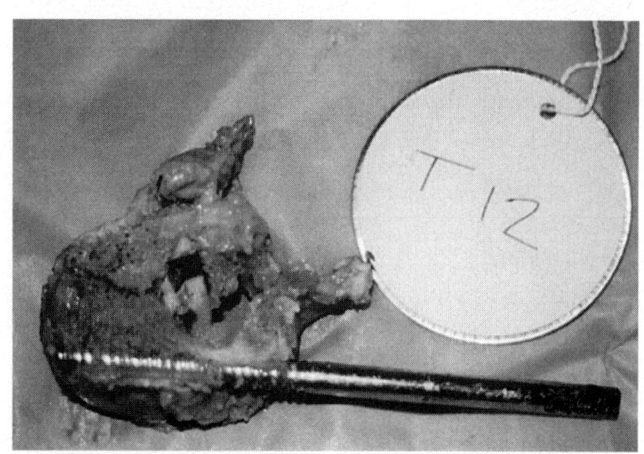


**FIGURE 62-9**

Sectioned vertebral body confirming visual results with post procedural CT scan findings.

## IN VIVO METHOD

After attaining Investigational Board approval and informed consent, eleven patients were scheduled for lumbosacral pedicle screw fixation. Consent and approval was for the passive tracking and positional confirmation of the drill tips and pedicle screws. One-millimeter cut computer tomography scans of the lumbosacral spines of the eleven patients were obtained and 3D reconstructions formatted for use on the video screen of the navigation system. The navigation system was set up in the standard operating room. After typical exposure of the lumbosacral spine segments selected for fusion, the registration of the navigational system was done at each level of screw placement. Three points for each vertebral level were registered to the corresponding points on the 3D computer model. The dynamic reference emitter was attached at each level prior to registration and drilling to track the operative vertebral body in order to compensate for intraoperative positional changes in the vertebral body secondary to operative manipulation (Fig. 62-10). All drilling and screw placement was done by a spine surgeon already experienced in the placement of pedicle screws. In total the drill trajectories and final screw tip positions for 32 pedicle screws placed in vivo were passively monitored and recorded in near real-time via the navigational system. Postprocedure CT scans were performed on each patient to evaluate the accuracy of screw position (Fig. 62-11). Correlation of the perceived screw positions via the navigational system versus the actual position as determined by postoperative CT scan was performed.

Postoperative CT scans were calculated to have a 1.0- to 2.0-mm error secondary to implant beam scatter. All screws were found to be within the pedicles but it was not possible to ascertain whether or not any screw threads were intracortical. Data was assessed in

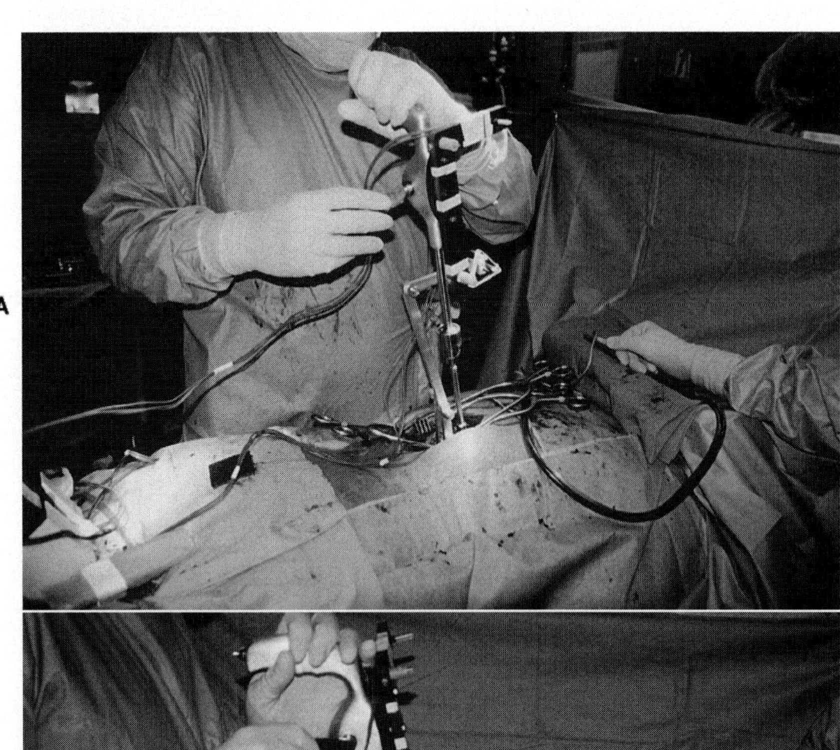

**FIGURE 62-10**

**A, B,** Intraoperative drilling with confirmation of position and trajectory by off-field computer monitor.

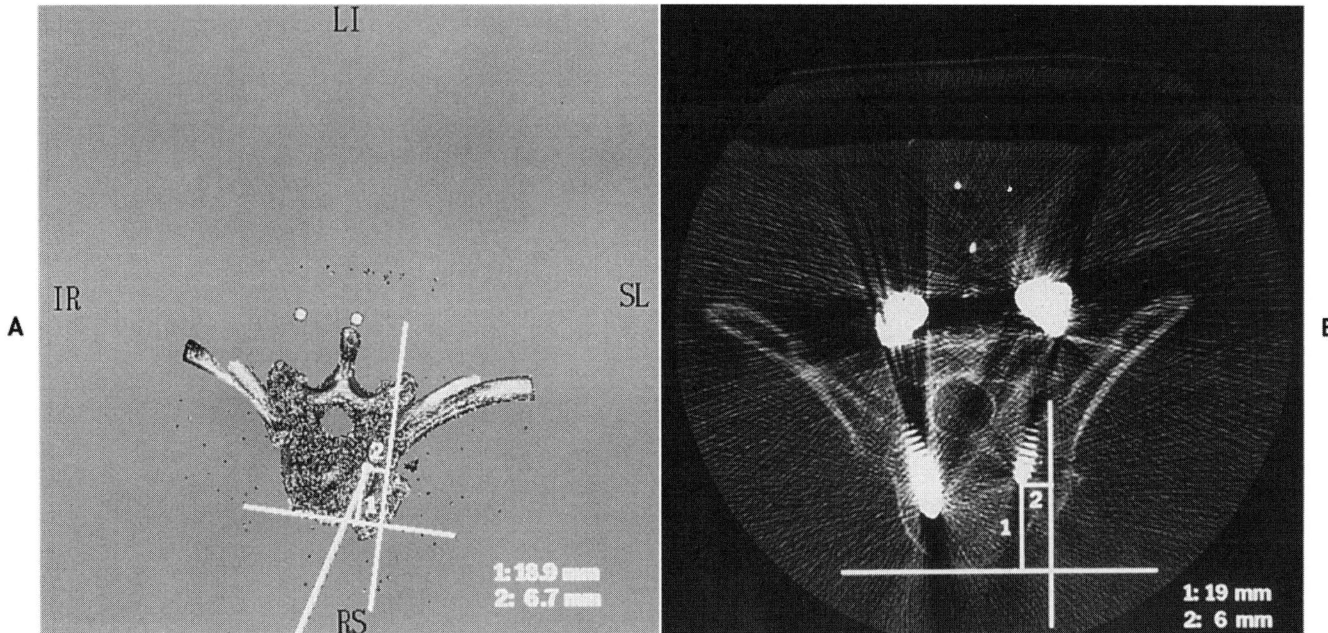


**Figure 62-11**

**A, B,** Comparison of intraoperative computer data with postoperative CT scan to compare the accuracy of navigational tool in placing the pedicle screw.

three planes. The greatest error occurred in the sagittal plane. In an attempt to control for scatter all measurements were made as a worst-case scenario measuring the largest distance differential between the perceived placement via the navigational system and the CT scan image position. The mean difference in the coronal plane was 1.1 mm, in the transverse plane 1.5 mm, and in the sagittal plane 5.5 mm. Overall accuracy for tip position with all planes combined was 2.0 mm.

This system for frameless stereotactic navigation based on reconstructed computer images has been shown to have reasonable accuracy and reproducibility in vitro as well as in the coronal and transverse planes in the in vivo model. The sagittal plane accuracy in the in vivo trials is less acceptable. This could be due to exaggerated lumbar lordosis in the prone operating position not matching the supine position of the preoperative CT scans. The majority of intraoperative motion is in flexion and extension (sagittal plane) and the second emitter that is placed on the operative vertebral body may not be tracking the vertebral body satisfactorily. This could be due to an unstable attachment to the vertebral body or to poor tracking of the emitter by the sensor array in the sagittal plane. Increasing the number of registration points prior to drilling is proving to be helpful in decreasing this error.

Some practical problems were encountered in the operating room. Regarding the use of a sonic localization system, minimal interference from noise and electronics were easily compensated for by positioning. The main problem was an occasional signal delay secondary to loss of line of sight of the emitters to the off field receiver. This can be corrected by mounting the sensor triangular array directly above the field instead of next to the field as in our study. There would be much less chance of someone or something interrupting the line of site with this arrangement.

In vivo registration with this prototype and the relative surgeon experience with it, combine to cause a lengthy average 15-minute time course for placement of pedicle screws at one level. This would improve considerably with surgeon familiarity with the system. Streamlining the hardware, improving the user friendliness of the software, and eliminating line of sight delays will help to decrease time. Also the need for intraoperative radiographs may be supplanted once accuracy is confirmed. This study was a preliminary one using a prototypical navigation system. It is based on computer-reproduced images, and a localization and coordinate reference system. Although not optimal in the sagittal place, and only limited to confirmation at this point, this system succeeds in the conceptual goal. It enables enhanced perception of anatomy to improve accuracy by providing a virtual map of areas not visible to the surgeon. The adjustments or enhancements to come to refine this procedure will be dependent upon development of the current technology.

There are numerous other trials based on the same concept. A similar setup using sonic localization, again based on preoperative CT scans as a confirmation tool has been described.[10] The clinical trials are promising: of 150 screws, 137 were felt to be optimum position,

12 satisfactory, and 1 unsatisfactory.[9] In this series, the operative time for screw placement was reduced when compared to standard technique as they did not use confirmatory intraoperative radiographs. The authors also stressed the advantage of this system in preoperative planning.

Other systems described rely on optic tracking instead of acoustic to establish a coordinate system.[12] Light-emitting diodes are detected by an off-field camera. In vitro results demonstrated ideal placement of 70 out of 77 screws placed with an optic tracking system. One feasibility study, based on tests with sheep vertebrae, concluded that their system would be useful for pedicle detection and "assessing the intervertebral location of a drilled hole."[1] In this latter system, localization was accomplished with a 3D position sensor operating on a magnetic field.

Another variation explored the use of an articulated arm as a locating device.[8] A pointer and cannulated probe attached to an arm that detected position in space provided for localization and registration. Using this instrumentation, the proper trajectory for pedicle screw placement was identified. Small guide wires were then placed into the cannulated probe and directed into a pedicle based on preoperative images and the spatial orientation of the probe. Again results were promising.

Technological advances have allowed for a modification of standard surgical equipment and procedure to enhance accuracy and decrease risk of pedicle screw placement. The above study shows that it is possible to enhance accuracy and decrease risk of pedicle screw placement. The above study also shows that it is possible to use this in the standard operating room, with standard surgical equipment.

It is important to note that in this and other studies referenced the use of the navigational system has been in the hands of experienced spine surgeons. Tactile feedback and anatomical familiarity are likely to enhance the apparent effectiveness of this system. We are currently investigating adding a component to the system that would also enhance tactile feedback, in order to provide the less experienced surgeon with another check to proper screw placement.

This developing technology may not aid the experienced spine surgeon in the placement of screws in the typical lumbar spine. Instead, it will prove beneficial in the severely deformed, distorted, or rotated spine, whether due to congenital anomalies or previous surgery and scarring. With further developments its use may allow for safe placement of pedicle screws into the thoracic area. The benefit of firm fixation in the thoracic spine is seen both in traumatic cases and in scoliosis treatment. With the latter, if pedicle screws could be safely placed in the thoracic and lumbar areas in scoliosis patients, this may then allow for such strong segment posterior fixation as to improve correction and obtain rotational control from the dorsum of the column. The precise placement of pedicle screws just into but not through the anterior cortex has already been shown to increase fixation strength and may be possible with computer aided placement, provided there is enough accuracy to dock into the anterior cortex.

The above application of current technology provides an example of the potential benefit of combining the enhanced accuracy of computer technology, imaging, and localization with complicated and higher risk procedures. This same technology used here may lend itself to surgery in other areas. There are numerous applications with the same principles where this may be applied. Any surgical device that can be applied to the drill, or have the emitters mounted on it, can be tracked in space within the sensor field. This ability also opens avenues for minimally invasive and percutaneous procedures with further advances.

From the onset of our work there have been many changes and enhancements in computer-guided surgery. Certainly technology exists for enhanced accuracy and precision by modifying the above systems. Robotics, ultrasonography, and laser technology are being explored. The limiting factor will be cost. As technology continues to improve, cost will diminish. So, although now based on theory and concept with proven feasibility, in the future these technological innovations certainly will be placed into practice.

Work is presently underway to use stereolithography and percutaneous ultrasound techniques to help with navigation in distorted structures such as revision spinal surgeries. Portable CT scanners are also being developed to be used as an intraoperative guidance tool for revision cases.

## REFERENCES


1. Amiot LP, Labelle H, Deguise JA, Sati M, Brodeur P, Rivard CH: Computer assisted pedicle screw fixation: a feasibility study, *Spine* 10:1208-1212, 1995.
2. Barnett GW, Kormos DW, Steiner CP, Weisenberger JP: Use of a frameless, armless stereotactic wand for brain tumor localization with two dimensional three dimensional neuro imaging, *Neurosurgery* 33:674-678, 1993.
3. Carl AL, Khanuja HS, Sachs BS et al: In vitro simulation. Early results of stereotaxy for pedicle screw placement, *Spine* 22(10);1160-1164.
4. Esses SI, Sachs BL, Dreyzin V: Complications associated with the technique of pedicle screw fixation-A selected survey of ABS members, *Spine* 18:2231-2239, 1993.
5. Galloway RL, Macinus RJ: Stereotactic neurosurgery, *Crit Rev Biomed Eng* 18:181-205, 1990.
6. George DC, Krag MH, Johnson CC, et al: Hole preparation techniques for transpedicular screws. Effect on pullout strength from human cadaveric vertebrae, *Spine* 16:181-184, 1991.
7. Gertzbein SD, Robbins SE: Accuracy of pedicular screw placement in vivo, *Spine* 15:11-14, 1990.
8. Glossop ND, Hu RW, Randle A: Computer-aided pedicle screw placement using frameless stereotaxis, *Spine* 21:2026-2034, 1996.
9. Kalfas IH, Kormos DW, Murphy MA et al: Application of frameless stereotaxy to pedicle screw fixation of the spine, *J Neurosurg* 83:641-647, 1995.
10. Lavallee S, Sautot P, Troccaz J, Cinquin P, Merloz P: Computer assisted spine surgery: a technique for accurate transpedicular screw fixation using CT data and a 3-D optical localizer, *J Image Guided Surg* 1:65-73, 1995.
11. Macinus RJ, Galloway RL, Fitzpatrick MJ, Mandave V, Edwards CA, Allen GS: A universal system for interactive image directed neurosurgery, *Stereotact Funct Neurosurg* 58:108-113, 1992.
12. Nolte LP, Zamoranoa LJ, Jiang Z, Wang Q, Langlotz F, Berlemann U: Image-guided insertion of transpedicular screws: a laboratory set-up, *Spine* 4:497-500, 1995.
13. Olsewski JM, Simmons EH, Kallen FC, Mendel FC, Severin CM, Beres DL: Morphometry of the lumbar spine, anatomical perspective related to transpedicular fixation, *J Bone Joint Surg* 72(A):541-549, 1990.
14. Vaccaro AR, Rizzoo SJ, Balderston RA, Allardyce TJ, Garfin SR, Dolinskas C: Placement of pedicle screws in the thoracic spine. Part II: An anatomic and radiographic assessment, *J Bone Joint Surg* 77(A);1200-1206, 1995.
15. Weinstein JN, Rydevik BL, Rauschning W: Anatomic and technical considerations of pedicle screw fixation, *Clin Orthop* 284:34-46, 1992.
16. Weinstein JN, Spratt KF, Spengler D, Brick C, Reid S: Spinal pedicle fixation: reliability and validity of roentgenogram based assessment and surgical factors on successful screw placement, *Spine* 13:1012-1018, 1988.
17. West JL, Ogilvie JW, Bradford DS: Complications of variable screw plate pedicle screw fixation, *Spine* 16:576-579, 1991.
18. Zindrick MR, Wiltse LL, Doornik A, Widell EH, Knight GW, Patwardhan AG, Thomas JC, Rothman SL, Fields BT: Analysis of the morphometric characteristics of the thoracic and lumbar pedicles, *Spine* 12:160-166, 1987.
19. Zinreich SJ, Tebo SA, Long DM, et al: Frameless stereotactic integration of CT imaging data: accuracy and initial applications, *Radiology* 188:735-742, 1993.

# INDEX

## A

**B**

**D**

**E**

## F

**G**



**H**

## I

## M

## N

## Q



## R

## S